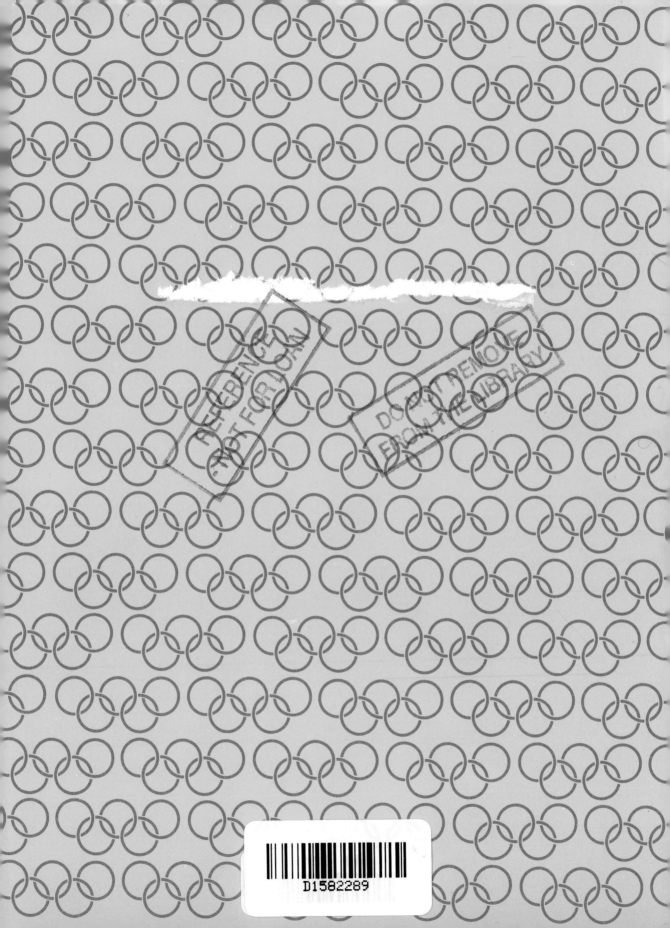

BIOMECHANICS IN SPORT

IOC MEDICAL COMMISSION

SUB-COMMISSION ON PUBLICATIONS IN THE SPORT SCIENCES

Howard G. Knuttgen PhD (Co-ordinator)
Boston, Massachusetts, USA

Francesco Conconi MD
Ferrara, Italy

Harm Kuipers MD, PhD
Maastricht, The Netherlands

Per A.F.H. Renström MD, PhD
Stockholm, Sweden

Richard H. Strauss MD
Los Angeles, California, USA

BIOMECHANICS IN SPORT

PERFORMANCE ENHANCEMENT AND INJURY PREVENTION

VOLUME IX OF THE ENCYCLOPAEDIA OF SPORTS MEDICINE
AN IOC MEDICAL COMMISSION PUBLICATION

IN COLLABORATION WITH THE
INTERNATIONAL FEDERATION OF SPORTS MEDICINE

EDITED BY

VLADIMIR M. ZATSIORSKY

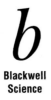

**Blackwell
Science**

© 2000 International Olympic Committee

Published by
Blackwell Science Ltd
Editorial Offices:
Osney Mead, Oxford OX2 0EL
25 John Street, London WC1N 2BL
23 Ainslie Place, Edinburgh EH3 6AJ
350 Main Street, Malden
  MA 02148-5018, USA
54 University Street, Carlton
  Victoria 3053, Australia
10, rue Casimir Delavigne
  75006 Paris, France

Other Editorial Offices:
Blackwell Wissenschafts-Verlag GmbH
Kurfürstendamm 57
10707 Berlin, Germany

Blackwell Science KK
MG Kodenmacho Building
7–10 Kodenmacho Nihombashi
Chuo-ku, Tokyo 104, Japan

First published 2000

Set by Graphicraft Limited, Hong Kong
Printed and bound in Great Britain
at the University Press, Cambridge

The Blackwell Science logo is a
trade mark of Blackwell Science Ltd,
registered at the United Kingdom
Trade Marks Registry

Part title illustration
by Grahame Baker

A catalogue record for this title
is available from the British Library

ISBN 0-632-05392-5

Library of Congress
Cataloging-in-publication Data

Biomechanics in sport: performance
improvement and injury prevention /
edited by Vladimir M. Zatsiorsky.
      p.   cm.—(Volume IX of
  the Encyclopaedia of sports medicine)
  "An IOC Medical Commission
  publication in collaboration with the
  International Federation of Sports
  Medicine."
  ISBN 0-632-05392-5
    1. Sports—Physiological aspects.
  2. Human mechanics.   3. Sports
  injuries. I. Zatsiorsky, Vladimir M.,
  1932– II. IOC Medical Commission.
  III. International Federation of Sports
  Medicine.   IV. Encyclopaedia of sports
  medicine; v. 10

RC1235 .B476   2000
617.1'027—dc21
                              99-054566

DISTRIBUTORS

Marston Book Services Ltd
PO Box 269
Abingdon, Oxon OX14 4YN
(Orders: Tel: 01235 465500
          Fax: 01235 465555)

USA
Blackwell Science, Inc.
Commerce Place
350 Main Street
Malden, MA 02148-5018
(Orders: Tel: 800 759 6102
              781 388 8250
          Fax: 781 388 8255)

Canada
Login Brothers Book Company
324 Saulteaux Crescent
Winnipeg, Manitoba R3J 3T2
(Orders: Tel: 204 837 2987)

Australia
Blackwell Science Pty Ltd
54 University Street
Carlton, Victoria 3053
(Orders: Tel: 3 9347 0300
          Fax: 3 9347 5001)

For further information on
Blackwell Science, visit our website:
www. blackwell-science.com

Contents

v

List of Contributors

A.S. ARUIN PhD, *Motion Analysis Laboratory, Rehabilitation Foundation Inc., 26 W171 Roosevelt Road, Wheaton, IL 60189, USA*

R.M. BARTLETT PhD, *Sport Science Research Institute, Sheffield Hallam University, Collegiate Hall, Sheffield S10 2BP, UK*

K. BARTONIETZ PhD, *Olympic Training Center Rhineland-Palatinate/Saarland, Am Sportzentrum 6, 67105 Schifferstadt, Germany*

G.-P. BRÜGGEMANN PhD, *Deutsche Sporthochschule Köln, Carl-Diem-Weg 6, 50933 Köln, Germany*

J.H. CHALLIS PhD, *Biomechanics Laboratory, Department of Kinesiology, 39 Rec. Hall, The Pennsylvania State University, University Park, PA 16802-3408, USA*

A.J. DALLMEIJER PhD, *Institute for Fundamental and Clinical Human Movement Sciences, Faculty of Human Movement Sciences, Vrije Universiteit Amsterdam, The Netherlands*

J. DAPENA PhD, *Biomechanics Laboratory, Department of Kinesiology, Indiana University, Bloomington, IN 47405, USA*

B. ELLIOTT PhD, *The Department of Human Movement and Exercise Science, The University of Western Australia, Nedlands, Western Australia 6907, Australia*

R.M. ENOKA PhD, *Department of Kinesiology and Applied Physiology, University of Colorado, Boulder, CO 80309-0354, USA*

M.D. GRABINER PhD, *Department of Biomedical Engineering, The Cleveland Clinic Foundation, 9500 Euclid Avenue, Cleveland, Ohio 44195, USA*

W. HERZOG PhD, *Faculty of Kinesiology, The University of Calgary, 2500 University Drive NW, Calgary, Alberta T2N 1N4, Canada*

M. HUBBARD PhD, *Department of Mechanical and Aeronautical Engineering, University of California, Davis, CA 95616, USA*

G.J. VAN INGEN SCHENAU PhD, *Institute for Fundamental and Clinical Human Movement Sciences, Faculty of Human Movement Sciences, Vrije Universiteit Amsterdam, The Netherlands (Professor G.J. van Ingen Schenau unfortunately passed away during the production of this volume.)*

D.L. KING PhD, *Department of Health and Human Development, Montana State University, Bozeman, MT 59717, USA*

P.V. KOMI PhD, *Neuromuscular Research Centre, Department of Biology of Physical Activity, University of Jyväskylä, 40351 Jyväskylä, Finland*

J.J. DE KONING PhD, *Institute for Fundamental and Clinical Human Movement Sciences, Faculty of Human Movement Sciences, Vrije Universiteit Amsterdam, The Netherlands*

J. LANKA PhD, *Department of Biomechanics, Latvian Academy of Sport Education, Brivibas 333, Riga LV-1006, Latvia*

P.E. MARTIN PhD, *Exercise and Sport Research Institute, Arizona State University, Tempe, Arizona 85287, USA*

J.L. McNITT-GRAY PhD, *Biomechanics Research Laboratory, Department of Exercise Sciences, University of Southern California, Los Angeles, CA 90089-0652, USA*

D.I. MILLER PhD, *School of Kinesiology, Faculty of Health Sciences, University of Western Ontario, London, Ontario, N6A 3K7, Canada*

C. NICOL PhD, *UMR 6559 Mouvement & Perception, CNRS-Université de la Méditerranée, Faculté des Sciences du Sport, 163, avenue de Luminy CP 910, F-13288 Marseille Cedex 9, France*

B.I. PRILUTSKY PhD, *Center for Human Movement Studies, Department of Health and Performance Sciences, Georgia Institute of Technology, Atlanta, GA 30332, USA*

V.A. RUMYANTSEV PhD, *Department of Swimming, Russian State Academy of Physical Culture, 4 Sirenevy Boulevard, Moscow 105122, Russian Federation*

D.J. SANDERSON PhD, *School of Human Kinetics, University of British Columbia, Vancouver, British Columbia, V6T 1Z1, Canada*

J.G. SEMMLER PhD, *Department of Kinesiology and Applied Physiology, University of Colorado, Boulder, CO 80309-0354, USA*

M.C. SIFF PhD, *School of Mechanical Engineering, University of the Witwatersrand, South Africa*

G.A. SMITH PhD, *Biomechanics Laboratory, Department of Exercise and Sport Science, Oregon State University, Corvallis, OR 97331, USA*

B.R. UMBERGER MS, *Exercise and Sport Research Institute, Arizona State University, Tempe, Arizona 85287, USA*

H.E.J. VEEGER PhD, *Institute for Fundamental and Clinical Human Movement Sciences, Faculty of Human Movement Sciences, Vrije Universiteit Amsterdam, The Netherlands*

M. VIRMAVIRTA PhLic, *Neuromuscular Research Centre, Department of Biology of Physical Activity, University of Jyväskylä, 40351 Jyväskylä, Finland*

A.S. VOLOSHIN PhD, *Department of Mechanical Engineering and Mechanics, Institute for Mathematical Biology and Biomedical Engineering, Lehigh University, Bethlehem, PA 18015, USA*

A.R. VORONTSOV PhD, *Department of Swimming, Russian State Academy of Physical Culture, 4 Sirenevy Boulevard, Moscow 105122, Russian Federation*

W.C. WHITING PhD, *Department of Kinesiology, California State University, Northridge, 18111 Nordhoff Street, Northridge, CA 91330-8287 USA*

K.R. WILLIAMS PhD, *Department of Exercise Science, University of California, Davis, CA 95616, USA*

L.H.V. van der WOUDE PhD, *Institute for Fundamental and Clinical Human Movement Sciences, Faculty of Human Movement Sciences, Vrije Universiteit Amsterdam, The Netherlands*

M.R. YEADON PhD, *Department of Sports Science, Loughborough University, Ashby Road, Loughborough, LE11 3TU, UK*

V.M. ZATSIORSKY PhD, *Department of Kinesiology, The Pennsylvania State University, University Park, PA 16802, USA*

R.F. ZERNICKE PhD, *Faculty of Kinesiology, University of Calgary, 2500 University Drive NW, Calgary, AB, T2N 1N4, Canada*

Forewords

On behalf of the International Olympic Committee, I welcome the publication of Volume IX in the IOC Medical Commission's series, *The Encyclopaedia of Sports Medicine.*

Citius, Altius, Fortius is our motto, which suggests the successful outcome to which all athletes aspire.

The role of the Olypmic movement is to provide these athletes with everything they require to attain this goal.

Biomechanics contributes to this end, through research into correct movement and the subsequent improvement in training equipment and techniques, by always keeping in view ways of improving performance while maintaining absolute respect for the health of the athletes.

Juan Antonio Samaranch
Président du CIO
Marqués de Samaranch

In the area of sports science, the last 20 years have witnessed the development of a remarkable number of advances in our knowledge of skill performance, equipment design, venue construction, and injury prevention based on the application of biomechanical principles to sport.

The accumulation of this wealth of biomechanical knowledge demanded that a major publication be produced to gather, summarize, and interpret this important work. It therefore became a logical decision to add 'biomechanics' to the list of topic areas to be addressed in the IOC Medical Commission's series, *The Encyclopaedia of Sports Medicine.*

Basic information is provided regarding skeletal muscle activity in the performance of exercise and sport; specific sections are devoted to locomotion, jumping and aerial movement, and throwing; and particular attention is given to injury prevention, rehabilitation, and the sports of the Special Olympics. An effort was made to present the information in a format and style that would facilitate its practical application by physicians, coaches, and other professional personnel who work with the science of sports performance and injury prevention.

This publication will most certainly serve as a reference and resource for many years to come.

Prince Alexandre de Merode
Chairman, IOC Medical Commission

Preface

The essence of all sports is competition in movement skills and mastership. Sport biomechanics is the science of sport (athletic) movements. Because of that, if nothing else, it is vital for sport practice. For decades, athletic movements have been performed and perfected by the intuition of coaches and athletes. We do have evidence in the literature that some practitioners understood the laws of movement even before Sir Isaac Newton described them. It was reported that Sancho Panza, when he saw his famous master attacking the windmills, told something about Newton's Third Law: he knew that the windmills hit his master as brutally as he hit them. Although it is still possible to find people who believe that intuitive knowledge in biomechanics is sufficient to succeed, it is not the prevailing attitude anymore. More fundamental lore is necessary. I hope this book proves that.

It was a great honour for me to serve as an editor of the volume on *Biomechanics in Sport: Performance Enhancement and Injury Prevention*. The book is intended to be a sequel to other volumes of the series of publications entitled *Encyclopaedia of Sports Medicine* that are published under the auspices of the Medical Commission of the International Olympic Committee. The main objective of this volume is to serve coaches, team physicians, and serious athletes, as well as students concerned with the problems of sport biomechanics.

Editing the volume was a challenging task: The first challenge was to decide on the content of the book. The problems of sport biomechanics can be clustered in several ways:

- General problems of sport biomechanics (e.g. muscle biomechanics, eccentric muscle action).
- Given sport movements (high jump) and sports (biomechanics of diving).
- Parts of the human body (biomechanics of spine).
- Blocks (constitutional parts) of natural athletic activities (athlete in the air, biomechanics of landing).

Each approach has its own pros and cons; it also has limitations. For instance, the number of events in the programme of Summer Olympic Games exceeds 200. Evidently, it is prohibitive to have 200 chapters covering individual events. After consideration, the plan of the book was selected and approved by the IOC Publications Advisory Committee (it is my pleasure to thank the Committee members for their support and useful advice).

The book is divided into the following six parts.
1 Muscle action in sport and exercise: This section is devoted to general problems of biomechanics of athletic movements.
2 Locomotion: After the introductory chapter, which covers material pertinent to all cyclic locomotions, the following sports are described: running, cycling, swimming, cross-country skiing, and skating.
3 Jumping and aerial movement: The opening chapter in this section highlights the biomechanics of aerial motion, while other chapters address high jumping, ski jumping, jumping in figure skating and diving.
4 Throwing and hitting: The section starts with two chapters that explain the basic principles of throwing and the aerodynamic aspects of the flight

of projectiles, respectively. Individual sports are shot putting, javelin throwing and hammer throwing.

5 Injury prevention and rehabilitation: Each chapter in this section addresses the problems that are pertinent to many sports.

6 Special Olympics sports: Biomechanics of wheelchair sports and sport for amputees are discussed.

Many recognized scholars participated in this project. The authors of the volume, 37 in total, have unique areas of expertise and represent 11 countries, including Austria, Canada, Finland, Germany, Holland, Latvia, Russia, Singapore, South Africa, United Kingdom and USA. Geography, however, did not play a substantial role in determining the authors. Their expertise did. The book contains chapters contributed by scholars who have established themselves as prominent world experts in their particular research or applied fields. To the extent that certain areas of sport biomechanics and eminent biomechanists have been omitted, apologies are offered. Evidently, a line had to be drawn somewhere. Outstanding experts are, as a rule, overworked people. Appreciation is acknowledged to the authors of this book who gave of their precious time to contribute to this endeavour. I am grateful to all of them.

Vladimir M. Zatsiorsky
Professor
Department of Kinesiology,
The Pennsylvania State University
2000

DEDICATION

A distinguished colleague and friend of the international biomechanics community, Dr. Gerrit Jan van Ingen Schenau, passed away during the production of this volume. During his academic career, Professor van Ingen Schenau conducted numerous studies of human performance and contributed dozens of publications to the literature of human biomechanics and sport. One of his last projects can be found in this volume, where he was a co-author of Chapter 11, Performance-Determining Factors in Speed Skating.

Participation of Professor van Ingen Schenau in international scientific activities will be sorely missed. The contributing authors and I wish to dedicate this volume to his memory.

VMZ

PART 1

MUSCLE ACTION IN SPORT AND EXERCISE

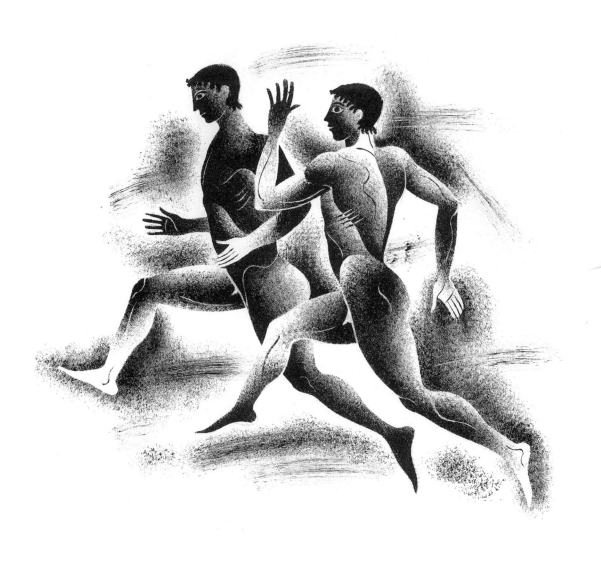

Chapter 1

Neural Contributions to Changes in Muscle Strength

J.G. SEMMLER AND R.M. ENOKA

Introduction

To vary the force that a muscle exerts, the nervous system either changes the number of active motor units or varies the activation level of those motor units that have been activated. For much of the operating range of a muscle, both processes are activated concurrently (Seyffarth 1940; Person & Kudina 1972). Motor units are recruited sequentially and the rate at which each discharges action potentials increases monotonically to some maximal level. Although most human muscles comprise a few hundred motor units, the order in which motor units are activated appears to be reasonably stereotyped (Denny-Brown & Pennybacker 1938; Henneman 1977; Binder & Mendell 1990). For most tasks that have been examined, motor units are recruited in a relatively fixed order that proceeds from small to large based on differences in motor neurone size, which is the basis of the Size Principle (Henneman 1957). Although variation in motor neurone size *per se* is not the primary determinant of differences in recruitment threshold, a number of properties covary with motor neurone size and thereby dictate recruitment order (Heckman & Binder 1993).

Despite current acceptance of the Size Principle as a rubric for the control of motor unit activity (Cope & Pinter 1995), our understanding of the distribution of motor unit activity among a group of synergist muscles is more rudimentary. One prominent example of this deficit in our knowledge is the lack of understanding of the role performed by the nervous system in the strength gains that are achieved with physical training. When an individual participates in a strength-training programme, much of the increase in strength, especially in the first few weeks of training, is generally attributed to adaptations that occur in the nervous system (Enoka 1988; Sale 1988). Because the assessment of strength in humans involves the activation of multiple muscles, the neural mechanisms that contribute to strength gains undoubtedly involve the coordination of motor unit activity within and across muscles. Nonetheless, the evidence that identifies specific neural mechanisms is rather weak. The purpose of this chapter is to emphasize our lack of understanding of the neural mechanisms that mediate strength gains and to motivate more systematic and critical studies on this topic.

To accomplish this purpose, we describe the relationship between muscle size and strength, discuss the significance of specific tension, present the case for a role of the nervous system in strength gains, and evaluate the potential neural mechanisms that contribute to increases in strength. Despite a substantial literature on training strategies for increasing muscle strength, less is known about the biomechanical and physiological mechanisms responsible for the changes in performance capacity.

Muscle size and strength

Each muscle fibre contains millions of sarcomeres (the force-generating units of muscle), which are arranged in series (end-to-end in a myofibril) and in parallel (side-by-side myofibrils) to one another. Theoretically, the maximum force that a muscle

3

fibre can exert depends on the number of sarco-meres that are arranged in parallel (Gans & Bock 1965). By extension, the maximum force that a mus-cle can exert is proportional to the number of muscle fibres that lie in parallel to one another. Because of this association, the strength of a muscle can be estimated anatomically by measuring its cross-sectional area (Roy & Edgerton 1991). This measure-ment should be made perpendicular to the direction of the muscle fibres and is known as the *physiological cross-sectional area*.

Despite the theoretical basis for measuring the physiological cross-sectional area of muscle to estimate its force capacity, it is typically more convenient to measure the *anatomical cross-sectional area*, which is a measurement that is made per-pendicular to the long axis of the muscle. This can be accomplished by using one of several imaging techniques (e.g. computed tomography (CT) scan, magnetic resonance imaging, ultrasound) to deter-mine the area of a muscle at its maximum dia-meter. Examples of the relationship between muscle strength and anatomical cross-sectional area are shown in Fig. 1.1 (Kanehisa *et al.* 1994). In these

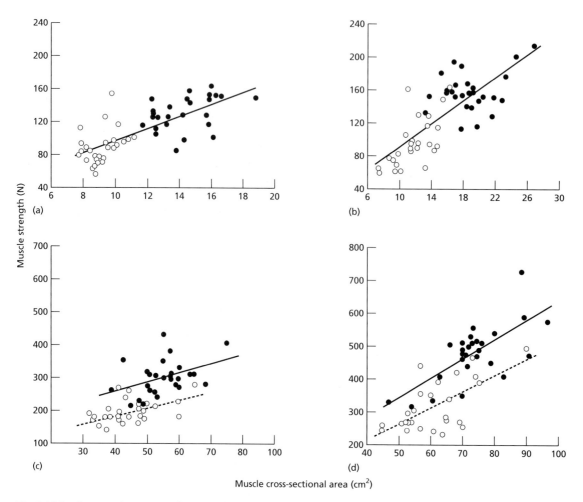

Fig. 1.1 Muscle strength varies as a function of the cross-sectional area of a muscle (adapted from Kanehisa *et al.* 1994). (a) Elbow flexors ($r^2 = 0.56$). (b) Elbow extensors ($r^2 = 0.61$). (c) Knee flexors ($r^2 = 0.17$ for men [solid line] and 0.35 for women [dashed line]). (d) Knee extensors ($r^2 = 0.54$ for men and 0.40 for women). Men are indicated with filled symbols and women with open symbols.

experiments, muscle strength was measured as the peak force exerted on an isokinetic device at an angular velocity of about 1.0 rad · s^{-1}, and the maximum anatomical cross-sectional area for each muscle group was measured with an ultrasound machine. Measurements were made on the elbow flexor and extensor muscles and on the knee flexor and extensor muscles of 27 men and 26 women.

For the elbow flexor and extensor muscles, the men were, on average, stronger than the women, but this was due to a greater cross-sectional area (Fig. 1.1a,b). The average strength (mean ± SE) of the elbow flexors, for example, was 130 ± 4 N for the men compared with 89 ± 4 N for the women; and the average cross-sectional area was 141 ± 0.4 cm^2 for the men and 91 ± 0.2 cm^2 for the women. Thus, the normalized force (force/cross-sectional area) was 9.2 N · cm^{-2} for men and 9.8 N · cm^{-2} for women. In contrast, the differences in strength between men and women for the knee muscles (Fig. 1.1c,d) were due to differences in both the cross-sectional area and the normalized force (force per unit area). For example, the average strength for the knee extensor muscles was 477 ± 17 N for the men and 317 ± 15 N for the women, and the average cross-sectional area was 74 ± 2 cm^2 for the men and 62 ± 2 cm^2 for the women. The normalized forces were 6.5 N · cm^{-2} and 5.1 N · cm^{-2}, respectively. The difference in normalized force is apparent by the y-axis displacement of the regression lines for the men and women (Fig. 1.1c,d). These regression lines indicate that for a cross-sectional area of 70 cm^2 for the knee extensor muscles, a man could exert a force of 461 N compared with 361 N for a woman.

These data demonstrate, as many others have shown (Jones *et al.* 1989; Keen *et al.* 1994; Kawakami *et al.* 1995; Narici *et al.* 1996), that the strength of a muscle depends at least partly on its size, as characterized by its cross-sectional area. This conclusion provides the foundation for the strength-training strategy of designing exercise programmes that maximize muscle hypertrophy, i.e. an increase in the number of force-generating units that are arranged in parallel. Nonetheless, there is substantial variability in the relationship between strength and cross-sectional area, which is indicated by the scatter of the data points about the lines of best fit in Fig. 1.1.

Some of this variability may be due to the use of anatomical rather than physiological cross-sectional area as the index of muscle size. However, variation in cross-sectional area accounts for only about 50% of the difference in strength between individuals (Jones *et al.* 1989; Narici *et al.* 1996).

Specific tension

The other muscular factor that influences strength is the intrinsic force-generating capacity of the muscle fibres. This property is known as *specific tension* and is expressed as the force that a muscle fibre can exert per unit of cross-sectional area (N · cm^{-2}). To make this measurement in human subjects, segments of muscle fibres are obtained by muscle biopsy and attached to a sensitive force transducer that is mounted on a microscope (Larsson & Salviati 1992). Based on such measurements, specific tension has been found to vary with muscle fibre types, to decrease after 6 weeks of bed rest for all fibre types, to decline selectively with ageing, and to increase for some fibre types with sprint training (Harridge *et al.* 1996, 1998; Larsson *et al.* 1996, 1997). For example, the specific tension of an average type II muscle fibre in vastus lateralis was greater than that for a type I muscle fibre for the young and active old adults but not for the sedentary old adults (Table 1.1). This finding indicates that the maximum force capacity of a type II muscle fibre

Table 1.1 Cross-sectional area (μm^2) and specific tension (N · cm^{-2}) of chemically skinned fibre segments from the human vastus lateralis muscle (Larsson *et al.* 1997).

Subject group	Cross-sectional area		Specific tension	
	Type I	Type II	Type I	Type II
Young control	2820 ± 620	3840 ± 740	19 ± 3	24* ± 3
Old control	3090 ± 870	2770† ± 740	18 ± 6	19 ± 1
Old active	2870 ± 680	3710 ± 1570	16 ± 5	20* ± 6

Values are mean ± SD. * $P < 0.001$ for type I vs. type II.
† $P < 0.001$ for old control vs. young control and old active.

in an old adult who is sedentary is less than that for young and active old adults because it is smaller (cross-sectional area) and it has a lower specific tension. Although such variations in specific tension probably contribute to the variability in the relationship between strength and cross-sectional area (Fig. 1.1), the relative role of differences in specific tension is unknown but is probably significant.

There are at least two mechanisms that can account for variations in specific tension. These are the density of the myofilaments in the muscle fibre and the efficacy of force transmission from the sarcomeres to the skeleton. The density of myofilaments can be measured from electron microscopy images of muscle fibres obtained from a biopsy sample. One of the few studies on this issue found that although 6 weeks of training increased the strength (18%) and cross-sectional area (11%) of the knee extensor muscles, there was no increase in myofilament density (Claasen et al. 1989). This was expressed as no change after training in the distance between myosin filaments (~38 nm) or in the ratio of actin to myosin filaments (~3.9). However, some caution is necessary in the interpretation of these data because the fixation procedures may have influenced the outcome variables. Nonetheless, even if these data are accurate, it is unknown if myofilament density changes with longer duration training programmes or with different types of exercise protocols (e.g. eccentric contractions, electrical stimulation, plyometric training).

Besides myofilament density, specific tension can also be influenced by variation in the structural elements that transmit force from the sarcomeres to the skeleton. This process involves the cytoskeletal proteins, which provide connections between myofilaments, between sarcomeres within a myofibril, between myofibrils and the sarcolemma, and between muscle fibres and associated connective tissues (Patel & Lieber 1997). Within the sarcomere, for example, the protein titin keeps the myofilaments aligned, which produces the banding structure of skeletal muscle and probably contributes significantly to the passive tension of muscle (Wang et al. 1993). Furthermore, there are several different isoforms of titin (Granzier et al. 1996), which may have different mechanical properties. Similarly, the intermediate fibres, which include the proteins desmin, vimentin and skelemin, are arranged longitudinally along and transversely across sarcomeres, between the myofibrils within a muscle fibre, and between muscle fibres (Patel & Lieber 1997). The intermediate fibres are probably responsible for the alignment of adjacent sarcomeres and undoubtedly provide a pathway for the longitudinal and lateral transmission of force between sarcomeres, myofibrils and muscle fibres. Because much of the force generated by the contractile proteins is transmitted laterally (Street 1983), variation in the intermediate fibres could contribute to differences in specific tension.

In contrast to changes in specific tension at the muscle-fibre level, some investigators determine 'specific tension' at the whole-muscle level by normalizing muscle force relative to the cross-sectional area of the muscle. This is misleading because the normalized force depends critically on the efficacy of the mechanisms that mediate excitation-contraction coupling. For example, Kandarian and colleagues found that the decline in normalized force exhibited by a hypertrophied soleus muscle was largely due to an impairment of calcium delivery to the contractile apparatus and not due to changes in the intrinsic force-generating capacity of muscle (Kandarian & White 1989; Kandarian & Williams 1993). For this reason, it is necessary to distinguish between the normalized force of a whole muscle and the specific tension of a single muscle fibre.

Although there is some uncertainty over the mechanisms that underlie the variation in specific tension of muscle fibres, it is clear that this factor can contribute significantly to differences in strength among individuals. Nonetheless, the magnitude of this effect is probably specific to each muscle (namely fibre-type proportions) and to the physical activity levels of the individual.

Evidence for a role of the nervous system in strength gains

Two sets of observations can be used to argue for a role by the nervous system in training-induced changes in muscle strength. These are the dissociation between changes in muscle size and strength and the specificity of the improvements in performance.

Dissociated changes in muscle size and strength

When an individual participates in a strength-training programme or experiences a decline in physical activity, the accompanying change in muscle strength precedes and exceeds the change in muscle size (Häkkinen *et al.* 1985; Narici *et al.* 1989). For example, although the loads that subjects could lift increased over an 8-week training period by 100–200%, there were no changes in the cross-sectional areas of muscle fibres in the vastus lateralis muscle (Staron *et al.* 1994). The maximum load that the men and women could lift in the squat exercise increased by about 200% (Fig. 1.2a), yet the size of the type I, IIa and IIb fibres did not increase significantly (Fig. 1.2b). However, there was a decrease in the proportion of the type IIb muscle fibres after 2 weeks of training for women and after 4 weeks of training for men (Fig. 1.2c), which may have influenced the average specific tension of the fibres in the muscle. Nonetheless, there was an increase in strength in the first few weeks of training that was not accompanied by an increase in muscle size or a change in the fibre-type proportions. By default, many investigators interpret this dissociation as evidence of a contribution to strength gains by so-called 'neural factors'.

Similarly, when muscle is subjected to a period of reduced use (e.g. bed rest, limb immobilization, tenotomy), the decline in strength is greater than the loss of muscle mass (Duchateau 1995; Berg *et al.* 1997; Yue *et al.* 1997). For example, a patient who sustained a closed bimalleolar fracture experienced a 25% decrease in the cross-sectional area of the triceps surae muscles after 8 weeks of immobilization but a 50% decline in muscle strength (Vandenborne *et al.* 1998). Furthermore, the force exerted by the triceps surae muscle was increased by an electric shock that was superimposed on a maximum voluntary contraction. Such dissociations between muscle size and strength are also evident in healthy subjects who experience a period of reduced use (Duchateau & Hainaut 1987).

Perhaps the most convincing case for a dissociation between muscle size and strength is made by findings that it is possible to increase muscle strength without even subjecting the muscle to

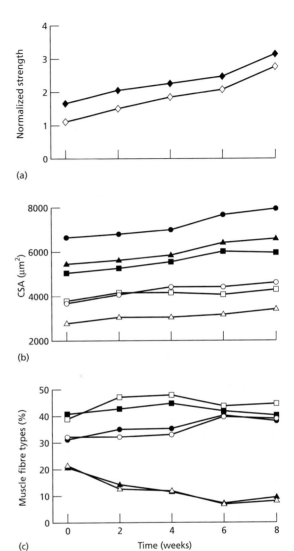

Fig. 1.2 Changes in strength, muscle fibre size, and fibre-type proportions over the course of an 8-week training programme (adapted from Staron *et al.* 1994). (a) Normalized strength (1RM load relative to fat-free mass) for the squat lift. (b) Cross-sectional areas (CSA) of muscle fibres from vastus lateralis. (c) The proportion (%) of the different muscle fibre types. Men are indicated with filled symbols and women with open symbols. In (b) and (c), type I fibres are shown with squares, type IIa fibres with circles, and type IIb fibres with triangles.

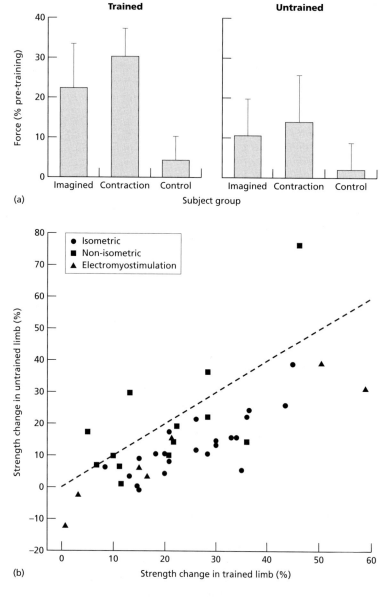

Fig. 1.3 The strength of a muscle can increase in the absence of physical training. (a) Increases (mean ± SD) in the maximum abduction force of the fifth finger after training with real or imagined maximal contractions (adapted from Yue & Cole 1992). Training was performed with the left hand but strength was measured in both hands. (b) Changes in muscle strength in homologous muscles of both limbs after training with a single limb. The data are derived from 29 studies reported in the literature.

physical training. Two protocols underscore this type of adaptation: imagined contractions and cross-education. When compared with subjects who either did no training or performed a 4-week strength-training programme, subjects who practised sets of imagined maximum voluntary contractions experienced a significant increase in the strength of a hand muscle (Yue & Cole 1992; however, cf. Herbert *et al.* 1998). Although electromyo-

gram (EMG) measurements indicated that the hand muscle was not activated during the training with imagined contractions, strength increased after 20 training sessions. The maximum abduction force exerted by the fifth finger increased by 30 ± 7% for the subjects who actually performed contractions, by 22 ± 11% for the subjects who did the imagined contractions, and by 4 ± 6% for the subjects who did no training (Fig. 1.3a). Furthermore, the abduction strength of the contralateral (untrained) fifth finger increased by $14 \pm 12\%$, $11 \pm 9\%$, and $2 \pm 7\%$, respectively.

The training effect that occurred in the untrained hand represents a phenomenon known as *cross-education*. Most studies that have examined this effect report that when the muscles in one limb participate in a strength-training programme, the homologous muscles also experience a significant increase in muscle strength despite the absence of activation during the training programme and no change in muscle fibre characteristics. For the data shown in Fig. 1.3b, the average increase in muscle strength for the trained limb was $24 \pm 13\%$ compared with an average of $16 \pm 15\%$ for the untrained limb. The magnitude of the cross-education effect was more variable for non-isometric contractions ($21 \pm 20\%$) compared with isometric contractions ($14 \pm 9\%$). Cross-education has also been demonstrated as a reduction in the quantity of muscle mass that is activated to lift submaximal loads after 9 weeks of unilateral strength training (Ploutz *et al.* 1994).

Specificity of strength gains

If the strength of a muscle is primarily dependent on its size, then whenever the muscle is activated maximally the peak force should be about the same. The fact that this is not the case underscores the dissociation between muscle size and strength and provides evidence for a significant contribution to strength gains from neural mechanisms. Whenever a muscle participates in a strength-training programme, the improvement in performance depends on the similarity between the training and testing procedures (Almåsbakk & Hoff 1996; Wilson *et al.* 1996). This effect, known as the specificity of training, is often demonstrated by comparing training-induced increases in the peak force exerted during a maximum isometric contraction with the maximum load that can be lifted once (1 repetition maximum [1RM] load). For example, when 11 men and 9 women trained the knee extensor muscles for 12 weeks by raising and lowering a load, the 1RM load increased by 200% for the men and 240% for the women compared with increases in the max-

imum isometric force of 20% for the men and 4% for the women (Rutherford & Jones 1986). Similarly, when Jones and Rutherford (1987) trained another group of subjects (11 men, 1 woman) with isometric, concentric, or eccentric contractions, the subjects who trained with eccentric contractions increased their 1RM load by 261% and maximum isometric force by 11%. Furthermore, the subjects who trained with isometric contractions experienced the greatest increase (35% vs. 11% and 15%) in the maximum isometric force.

The specificity of training is also evident with other training modalities. For example, O'Hagan *et al.* (1995) found that subjects who trained the elbow flexor muscles for 20 weeks on a device that provided a hydraulic resistance experienced significant increases in muscle cross-sectional area but task-dependent increases in muscle strength (Fig. 1.4). As determined by CT scan, the increase in cross-sectional area was greater for the brachialis muscle than the biceps brachii muscle, for both the men and women. The increases in peak force on the hydraulic device at the speed used in training and the increases in the maximum load that could be lifted once (1RM load) were about 50% for the men and 120% for the women. In contrast, the peak torque exerted on an isokinetic dynamometer at four angular velocities was largely unaffected (< 25% increase) by the training programme.

The specificity effects appear to be most pronounced for tasks that require more learning, such as less constrained movements (Rutherford & Jones 1986; Wilson *et al.* 1996; Chilibeck *et al.* 1998), those involving voluntary activation compared with electrical stimulation (McDonagh *et al.* 1983; Young *et al.* 1985), and those involving eccentric contractions (Higbie *et al.* 1996). For example, Hortobágyi *et al.* (1996) examined the adaptations in the force-velocity domain after subjects performed 36 training sessions on an isokinetic dynamometer over a 12-week period with the knee extensor muscles of the left leg. Some subjects trained with concentric contractions while others trained with eccentric contractions. For the subjects who trained with concentric contractions, the increase in peak force at a knee angle of 2.36 rad was similar for eccentric (46%), isometric (34%), and concentric (53%)

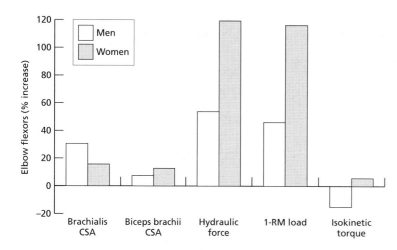

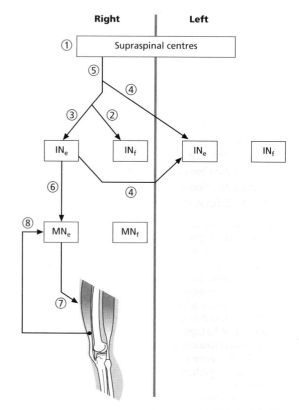

Fig. 1.4 Changes in the size and strength of the elbow flexor muscles in men and women after 20 weeks of training (adapted from O'Hagan *et al.* 1995). Muscle size was characterized by the measurement of cross-sectional area (CSA) for the brachialis and biceps brachii muscles. Muscle strength was represented by the peak force exerted on a hydraulic device, the 1RM load, and the peak torque on an isokinetic dynamometer (240 degrees · s^{-1}).

contractions. In contrast, the subjects who trained with eccentric contractions experienced a much greater increase in the peak force during eccentric contractions (116%) compared with isometric (48%) and concentric (29%) contractions. Furthermore, the cross-education effect was greatest for the subjects in the eccentric group when performing eccentric contractions (Hortobágyi *et al.* 1997).

These studies on the specificity of training demonstrate that improvements in strength-based performance are often unrelated to changes in muscle size. This dissociation is usually attributed to adaptations that occur in the nervous system, such as those associated with learning and improvements in coordination (Rutherford & Jones 1986; Laidlaw *et al.* 1999).

Neural activation of muscle

Despite the evidence that suggests a significant role for neural mechanisms in strength-training adaptations, it has proven difficult to identify specific mechanisms that underlie these changes. Figure 1.5 proposes sites within the nervous system where adaptations may occur, as suggested by current research findings. The proposed mechanisms range from a simple increase in the quantity of the neural drive to more subtle variations in the timing of motor unit activation. There is no consensus in the literature, however, on a significant role for any single mechanism.

Fig. 1.5 Scheme of the distribution of neural adaptations after strength training of the knee extensors of the right leg for 8 weeks. The numbers indicate the potential sites within the nervous system at which adaptations might occur, as suggested by various experimental findings: (1) enhanced output from supraspinal centres as suggested

Table 1.2 Percentage increases in performance and EMG for isometric contractions, 1RM contractions, and vertical jumps after 6 months of strength training by middle-aged (~40 years) and old (~70 years) men and women. (Adapted from Häkkinen *et al.* 1998.)

Subject group	Isometric contraction		1RM contraction		Vertical jump	
	Force	EMG	Load	EMG	Height	EMG
Men						
Middle-aged	36 ± 4	28 ± 13	22 ± 2	26 ± 13	11 ± 8	19 ± 12
Old	36 ± 3	33 ± 8	21 ± 3	15 ± 8	24 ± 8	14 ± 6
Women						
Middle-aged	66 ± 9	48 ± 13	34 ± 4	32 ± 14	14 ± 4	21 ± 7
Old	57 ± 10	33 ± 12	30 ± 3	24 ± 12	18 ± 6	34 ± 7

Values are mean ± SE. The EMG is based on the sum of the rectified and smoothed value for the vastus medialis and vastus lateralis of the right leg. All increases were statistically significant. Data provided by Dr. Keijo Häkkinen.

Activation maximality

Perhaps the most obvious neural adaptation that might contribute to strength gains is an increase in the quantity of the neural drive to muscle during a maximum contraction (sites 1, 6 and 7 in Fig. 1.5). This possibility has been examined by measuring changes in the absolute magnitude of the EMG and by testing activation maximality with the twitch interpolation technique. Although numerous investigators

by findings on imagined contractions; (2) altered drive that reduces coactivation of the antagonist muscles; (3) modified drive that causes greater activation of the muscles that assist the prime movers; (4) more effective coupling in spinal interneuronal pathways between limbs that produces cross-education; (5) changes in the descending drive that influence the bilateral deficit; (6) coupling of the input to motor neurones that raises the degree of synchronization in the discharge of action potentials; (7) greater muscle activation as indicated by an increased EMG, perhaps due to greater neural drive or a more effective excitation-contraction coupling for the same level of activation; and (8) heightened excitability of motor neurones as indicated by reflex potentiation and motor neurone plasticity. Abbreviations: IN_e, interneurones that project to the motor neurones innervating extensor muscles; IN_f, interneurones that project to the motor neurones innervating flexor muscles; MN_e, motor neurones innervating the extensor muscles; and MN_f, motor neurones innervating the flexor muscles.

have compared the EMG before and after strength training as an index of changes in the neural drive, the results are equivocal. Some studies have found significant increases in EMG amplitude after several weeks of training (Narici *et al.* 1989; Häkkinen *et al.* 1998), some have found task-specific increases in EMG (Thépaut-Mathieu *et al.* 1988; Higbie *et al.* 1996; Hortobágyi *et al.* 1996), and some have found no change in the EMG (Carolan & Cafarelli 1992).

One of the reasons for such diverse results is the variability associated with EMG measurements across subjects and sessions. The absolute amplitude of an EMG signal, for example, can vary across sessions due to such factors as differences in the placement of the electrodes and changes in the impedance of the skin and subcutaneous tissue. This variability can be reduced by averaging the EMG from several recording sites over a single muscle (Clancy & Hogan 1995) or by normalizing the recorded signal relative to the M wave (Keen *et al.* 1994). For example, when Häkkinen *et al.* (1998) summed the rectified and integrated EMG across the vastus lateralis and vastus medialis muscles, they detected significant training-related increases in the EMG for isometric contractions, for lifts with 1RM loads, and for maximum vertical jumps in various groups of subjects (Table 1.2). Similarly, Higbie *et al.* (1996) found significant increases in the summed EMG of vastus medialis and vastus lateralis after 10 weeks of strength training on an isokinetic device. The increase in EMG, however, was specific to the training task. For example, subjects who trained with eccentric contractions experienced a 36% increase in the peak torque and a 17% increase in the EMG during eccentric contractions but increases of only 7% for the peak torque and EMG during concentric contractions.

Others, however, have found that the increase in EMG peaked after a few weeks of training whereas strength continued to increase for the duration of the training programme. For example, Keen *et al.* (1994) found that linear improvements in the strength of a hand muscle were associated with a non-monotonic increase in the average EMG. In both young and old adults, the maximum voluntary contraction (MVC) force increased by about 40% after 12 weeks of strength training but the average EMG, when normalized to the peak-to-peak M wave, peaked at week 8 and was not different from initial values at week 12 for both groups of subjects. The normalized EMG increased by 10% at week 8 compared with an increase of 15–20% for MVC force. Because muscle volume only increased by 7% in this study, the increase in MVC force over the final 4 weeks of training must have been due to other factors.

Alternatively, the adaptation might involve a greater activation of the available muscle mass for the same EMG input (site 7 in Fig. 1.5). This possibility requires that individuals be unable to maximally activate muscle in an untrained state; the evidence on this issue is mixed. When the maximality of a contraction is tested by superimposing an electric shock (interpolated twitch) on an MVC, most investigators (Merton 1954; Bélanger & McComas 1981; Rutherford *et al.* 1986; Herbert & Gandevia 1996; De Serres & Enoka 1998), but not all (Dowling *et al.* 1994; Kent-Braun and Le Blanc 1996), find that subjects can maximally activate a muscle with a voluntary command. For example, subjects appear able to exert, on average, about 95% of the maximum force, and in 25% of the trials the force was indeed maximal (Allen *et al.* 1995). In contrast, when whole-muscle activation was assessed by measuring the

transverse relaxation time (*T*2) of muscle water with magnetic resonance imaging (Fisher *et al.* 1990; Tesch 1993; Yue *et al.* 1994; Ray & Dudley 1998), the MVC torque of the knee extensors seemed to be achievable by activating only ~71% of the cross-sectional area of the quadriceps femoris muscles (Adams *et al.* 1993). Similarly, the discharge rates of motor units during high-force contractions appear to place the motor units on the upper part of the force–frequency relationship but not on the plateau (Enoka 1995). These observations suggest that the force exerted during an MVC is less than the maximum tetanic force, but the magnitude of the difference is unclear.

Coactivation of antagonist muscles

In contrast to the apparent lack of an association between changes in strength and whole-muscle EMG, strength training does seem to affect the function of the relevant motor neurone pools. These changes can involve both the relative activation of different motor neurone pools and the connectivity within and between pools (Fig. 1.5). For example, strength training, at least with isometric contractions, appears to involve a reduction in the coactivation of the antagonist muscle (site 2 in Fig. 1.5) within the first week or so of training (Carolan & Cafarelli 1992). Similarly, elite athletes exhibit reduced coactivation of the semitendinosus muscle compared with sedentary subjects when performing isokinetic contractions with the knee extensor muscles (Amiridis *et al.* 1996). As a consequence, the net torque about a joint will increase due to removal of the negative torque contributed by the antagonist muscle. In short-term training studies, however, the reduction in coactivation is minimal. Häkkinen *et al.* (1998) found that substantial increases in knee extensor strength after 6 months of training were accompanied by mixed declines in coactivation of the antagonist muscle (biceps femoris). Coactivation of biceps femoris during an isometric MVC did not change in middle-aged men and women, whereas it declined by an average of 3% and 7% in older men and women, respectively. Furthermore, there was no change in coactivation during the

1RM task for all groups except the older women. Although these changes in antagonist activation may occur at the level of the descending drive from the supraspinal centres (site 3 in Fig. 1.5), they do not appear to be significant contributors to short-term increases in muscle strength.

Spinal cord plasticity

Of all the purported neural mechanisms, the most convincing case can be made for changes in neuronal connectivity with strength training. Two examples underscore this adaptation. The first example is related to the phenomenon of cross-education (site 4 in Fig. 1.5). In normally active individuals, the maximum force that a muscle can exert decreases when the homologous muscle in the contralateral limb is activated concurrently (Ohtsuki 1983; Secher *et al.* 1988; Schantz *et al.* 1989; however, cf. Jakobi & Cafarelli 1998). This effect is known as the *bilateral deficit* and appears to be caused by neural interactions between the limbs (site 5 in Fig. 1.5; Howard & Enoka 1991). The magnitude of this effect is usually small (5–10%), but can be quite substantial (25–45%), especially for rapid contractions (Koh *et al.* 1993). Because the size of the deficit can be altered by training (Taniguchi 1998), it is considered to depend on the neural connections between limbs. For example, individuals who train both limbs concurrently (e.g. rowers, weightlifters) exhibit a bilateral facilitation rather than a deficit (Secher 1975; Howard & Enoka 1991). In these subjects, muscle force is maximal during bilateral rather than unilateral contractions. This adaptation is presumably mediated by the long-term patterns of muscle activation that affect the descending drive to the interneuronal pools (Fig. 1.5).

The second example of neuronal plasticity concerns the connections between motor neurones in the same pool (site 6 in Fig. 1.5). Despite initial reports to the contrary, the discharge of action potentials by a motor neurone is temporally related to the discharge by other motor neurones. The degree of association can be quantified as the measurement of motor unit synchronization (Sears & Stagg 1976; Datta & Stephens 1990; Nordstrom *et al.*

1992), which indicates the patterns of shared synaptic input onto motor neurones either directly or through last-order interneurones (Kirkwood *et al.* 1982). The magnitude of this synchronized discharge among motor units is variable and is influenced by such factors as the task that is examined, the motor units and muscles involved in the task, and the type of habitual physical activity performed by the individual (Bremner *et al.* 1991; Schmied *et al.* 1994; Semmler & Nordstrom 1995, 1998; Huesler *et al.* 1998). The level of synchronization appears to be reduced between motor units in the individuals who require greater independent control of the fingers. This includes musicians and the dominant hand of control subjects (Semmler & Nordstrom 1998). In contrast, motor unit synchronization is greater among motor units in the hand muscles of individuals who consistently perform strength-training activities (Milner-Brown *et al.* 1975; Semmler & Nordstrom 1998). Nonetheless, computer simulations by Yao *et al.* (2000) indicate that motor unit synchronization does not increase the maximum force exerted by a muscle during steady-state isometric contractions (Fig. 1.6).

The altered connectivity among neurones as a consequence of training is also evident through the testing of reflexes (site 8 in Fig. 1.5). When an electric shock sufficient to elicit a maximal M wave (compound muscle action potential) is applied to a muscle nerve during an MVC, two reflex responses (V1 and V2) can also be elicited. Initial studies of these responses normalized them to the maximal M wave and used the ratio as an index of reflex potentiation (Sale 1988). Reflex potentiation (enhancement of V1 and V2) was found to occur in all muscles, to be more pronounced in weightlifters than sprinters, to increase with strength training, and to decrease with limb immobilization (Sale *et al.* 1982; Sale 1988). Subsequent work by Wolpaw and colleagues on operant conditioning of the spinal stretch reflex and the H reflex suggests that much of this plasticity appears to be located in the spinal cord, to involve the motor neurones, and also to be expressed in the contralateral, untrained limb (Wolpaw & Lee 1989; Carp & Wolpaw 1994; Wolpaw 1994).

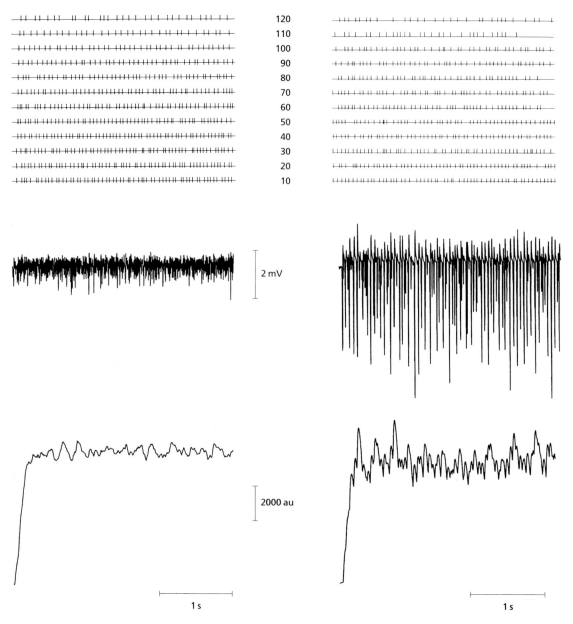

Fig. 1.6 Comparison of the EMG and force from computer simulations of maximal isometric contractions in the presence (right column) and absence (left column) of motor unit synchronization. In each column, the top set of traces indicate the timing of the action potentials discharged by some of the motor neurones in the pool ($n = 120$), the middle trace shows the interference EMG, and the bottom trace represents the net force. Adjusting the timing (synchronization), but not the number, of action potentials had a marked effect on the amplitude of the simulated EMG, no effect on the average simulated force, and a significant effect on the smoothness of the force profile.

These studies demonstrate that participation in a strength-training programme can induce changes in the connections between motor neurones located in the spinal cord. These adaptations are manifested as cross-education, the bilateral deficit (or facilitation), motor unit synchronization, and reflex potentiation. Nonetheless, the contributions of such changes to increases in muscle strength remain unknown.

Coordination

One of the most oft-cited reasons for an increase in strength is an improved coordination among the muscles involved in the task. A role for coordination is often invoked when strength gains are found to be specific to the training task (Rutherford & Jones 1986; Chilibeck *et al.* 1998). For example, subjects who performed strength-training exercises with a hand muscle (first dorsal interosseus) for 8 weeks experienced a 33% increase in the MVC force but only an 11% increase in the tetanic force evoked by electrical stimulation of the muscle (Davies *et al.* 1985). Furthermore, when another group of subjects trained the muscle with electrical stimulation for 8 weeks, there was no change in the evoked tetanic force whereas the MVC force declined by 11% (Davies *et al.* 1985). Because electrical stimulation evokes a muscle contraction by generating action potentials in intramuscular axonal branches, such findings suggest that activation by the nervous system is important in the expression of muscle strength.

A significant role of training-induced changes in neural activation can also be made based on post-training improvements in submaximal performance. One such example involves the steadiness of submaximal isometric contractions. When subjects exert an abduction force with the index finger, the normalized force fluctuations (co-efficient of variation) are usually greater for older adults compared with younger adults, especially at low forces (Galganski *et al.* 1993). After participation in a strength-training programme, however, the steadiness exhibited by the older adults improved and was similar to that of younger adults

(Keen *et al.* 1994). Because this improvement in performance was not associated with a change in the distribution of motor unit forces, the adaptations may have involved an enhancement of the muscle activation by the nervous system. Another example of the training-induced improvement in submaximal performance is the reduced volume of muscle that was activated to lift a submaximal load after participation in a strength-training programme (Ploutz *et al.* 1994). This effect appears to be largely mediated by neural mechanisms because there was no hypertrophy of the different muscle fibre types and the improvement was also evident in the untrained contralateral knee extensor muscles.

These findings suggest that the coordination of activity within and across muscles has a significant influence on the expression of muscle strength. In general, such adaptations influence two features of a strength manoeuvre: the postural foundation for the task and the goal-directed movement itself. Because the human body can be characterized as a linked mechanical system, it is necessary to orientate the body segments and to set the base of support on which the movement is performed (Horak & Macpherson 1996). For example, the elbow flexor muscles could lift a hand-held load with the body in a variety of postures, including standing, sitting, prone or supine positions. Such variations in posture appear to influence the outcome of a training programme, as indicated in several studies on the specificity of training. In one of the most comprehensive studies on this issue, Wilson *et al.* (1996) had subjects train for 8 weeks and then examined the improvement in performance of several tasks. They found, for example, increases of 21% for the squat lift and the vertical-jump height, but only a 10% increase in a 6-second-test on a cycle ergometer and no change in the performance by the knee extensor muscles on an isokinetic test. The improvements in performance were greatest in the tests involving postures that were used during training. Despite this recognized role for the specificity of posture, no studies have explicitly demonstrated a significant role for adaptations in postural support as contributing to strength gain.

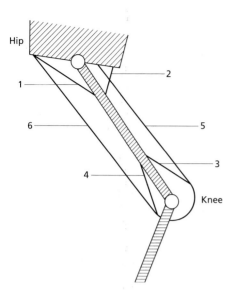

Fig. 1.7 Model of the human leg with six muscles arranged around the hip and knee joints. Muscles 1 to 4 cross one joint while muscles 5 and 6 cross both joints. (From van Ingen Schenau *et al.* 1990; Fig. 41.6.)

Similarly, muscles that act across other joints can influence the mechanical action about a joint. The classic example of this effect is the use of two-joint muscles to distribute net moments and to transfer power between joints (van Ingen Schenau *et al.* 1992). This scheme is represented in Fig. 1.7, where the human leg is modelled as a pelvis, thigh and shank with several one- and two-joint muscles crossing the hip and knee joints. In this model, muscles 1 and 3 are one-joint hip and knee extensors, muscles 2 and 4 are one-joint hip and knee flexors, and muscles 5 and 6 are two-joint muscles. Concurrent hip and knee extension can be performed by activation of the two one-joint extensors (muscles 1 and 3). Because muscle 5 exerts a flexor torque about the hip joint and an extensor torque about the knee, concurrent activation of muscle 5 with muscles 1 and 3 will result in a reduction in the net torque at the hip but an increase in the net torque at the knee. Based on this interaction, the two-joint muscle is described as redistributing some of the muscle torque and joint power from the hip to the knee.

Conversely, activation of muscle 6 will result in redistribution from the knee to the hip. Although rarely considered, such interactions are undoubtedly significant in the measurement of muscle strength.

In addition to the postural support and the transfer of actions between joints, an improvement in coordination can involve an enhancement of the timing of motor unit and muscle activity. At the motor-unit level, for example, van Cutsem *et al.* (1998) found that the gains obtained by training with rapid, low-load contractions involved reductions in the recruitment threshold, increases in motor unit force, and an increased rate of action-potential discharge. Twelve weeks of training the dorsiflexor muscles resulted in a pronounced increase in the initial discharge rate of motor units and an improvement in the maximal rate of force development. Similarly, although the timing of action potentials between motor units (motor unit synchronization) does not increase steady-state force, it may influence the rate of increase in force. Because of technical limitations, the magnitude of motor unit synchronization during anisometric contractions is unknown. However, there must be some functional benefit from short-term synchronization because it is greater in a hand muscle of weightlifters (Milner-Brown *et al.* 1975; Semmler & Nordstrom 1998) and it increases during the performance of attention-demanding tasks (Schmied *et al.* 1998).

At the whole-muscle level, the timing issues related to coordination involve task-specific variation in the activation of muscle. For example, the relative EMG amplitude in biceps brachii, brachialis and brachioradialis varied for constant-force (isometric) and constant-load (isoinertial) conditions despite a similar net elbow-flexor torque (Buchanan & Lloyd 1995). Similarly, the relative EMG activity of brachioradialis and biceps brachii varied for shortening and lengthening contractions (Nakazawa *et al.* 1993) and the relative contributions of motor unit recruitment and modulation of discharge rate varied for shortening and lengthening contractions (Kossev & Christova 1998). Presumably, early gains in a strength-training programme are related to learning the appropriate activation pattern for the task, especially if it is a novel task.

Conclusion

Although a compelling case can be made for a significant role of adaptations in the nervous system for training-induced increases in muscle strength, the specific mechanisms remain elusive. There is neither a consensus on individual mechanisms nor evidence that suggests the relative significance of the various mechanisms. These deficits in our knowledge exist partly because of technical limitations but mainly because of the narrow view taken in the search for neural mechanisms.

Acknowledgements

This work was partially supported by a grant from the National Institutes of Health (AG 13929) that was awarded to RME.

References

Adams, G.R., Harris, R.T., Woodard, D. & Dudley, G. (1993) Mapping of electrical muscle stimulation using MRI. *Journal of Applied Physiology* **74**, 532–537.

Allen, G.M., Gandevia, S.C. & McKenzie, D.K. (1995) Reliability of measurements of muscle strength and voluntary activation using twitch interpolation. *Muscle and Nerve* **18**, 593–600.

Almåsbakk, B. & Hoff, J. (1996) Coordination, the determinant of velocity specificity? *Journal of Applied Physiology* **80**, 2046–2052.

Amiridis, I.G., Martin, A., Morlon, B. *et al.* (1996) Co-activation and tension-regulating phenomena during isokinetic knee extension in sedentary and highly skilled humans. *European Journal of Applied Physiology* **73**, 149–156.

Bélanger, A.Y. & McComas, A.J. (1981) Extent of motor unit activation during effort. *Journal of Applied Physiology* **51**, 1131–1135.

Berg, H.E., Larsson, L. & Tesch, P.A. (1997) Lower limb skeletal muscle function after 6 wk of bed rest. *Journal of Applied Physiology* **82**, 182–188.

Binder, M.D. & Mendell, L.M. (eds) (1990) *The Segmental Motor System*. Oxford University Press, New York.

Bremner, F.D., Baker, J.R. & Stephens, J.A. (1991) Effect of task on the degree of synchronization of intrinsic hand muscle motor units in man. *Journal of Neurophysiology* **66**, 2072–2083.

Buchanan, T.S. & Lloyd, D.G. (1995) Muscle activity is different for humans performing static tasks which require force control and position control. *Neuroscience Letters* **194**, 61–64.

Carolan, B. & Cafarelli, E. (1992) Adaptations in coactivation after isometric resistance training. *Journal of Applied Physiology* **73**, 911–917.

Carp, J.S. & Wolpaw, J.R. (1994) Motoneuron plasticity underlying operant conditioned increase in primate H-reflex. *Journal of Neurophysiology* **72**, 431–442.

Chilibeck, P.D., Calder, A.W., Sale, D.G. & Webber, C.E. (1998) A comparison of strength and muscle mass increases during resistance training in young women. *European Journal of Applied Physiology* **77**, 170–175.

Claasen, H., Gerber, C., Hoppeler, H., Lüthi, J.-M. & Vock, P. (1989) Muscle filament spacing and short-term heavy-resistance exercise in humans. *Journal of Physiology* **409**, 491–495.

Clancy, E.A. & Hogan, N. (1995) Multiple site electromyograph amplitude estimation. *IEEE Transactions on Biomedical Engineering* **42**, 203–211.

Cope, T.C. & Pinter, M.J. (1995) The Size Principle: still working after all these years. *News in Physiological Sciences* **10**, 280–286.

van Cutsem, M., Duchateau, J. & Hainaut, K. (1998) Neural adaptations mediate increase in muscle contraction speed and change in motor unit behaviour after dynamic training. *Journal of Physiology* **513**, 295–305.

Datta, A.K. & Stephens, J.A. (1990) Synchronization of motor unit activity during voluntary contraction in man. *Journal of Physiology* **422**, 397–419.

Davies, C.T.M., Dooley, P., McDonagh, M.J.N. & White, M.J. (1985) Adaptation of mechanical properties of muscle to high force training in man. *Journal of Physiology* **365**, 277–284.

De Serres, S.J. & Enoka, R.M. (1998) Older adults can maximally activate the biceps brachii muscle by voluntary command. *Journal of Applied Physiology* **84**, 284–291.

Denny-Brown, D. & Pennybacker, J.B. (1938) Fibrillation and fasciculation in voluntary muscle. *Brain* **61**, 311–334.

Dowling, J.J., Konert, E., Ljucovic, P. & Andrews, D.M. (1994) Are humans able to voluntarily elicit maximum muscle force? *Neuroscience Letters* **179**, 25–28.

Duchateau, J. (1995) Bed rest induces neural and contractile adaptations in triceps surae. *Medicine and Science in Sports and Exercise* **27**, 1581–1589.

Duchateau, J. & Hainaut, K. (1987) Electrical and mechanical changes in immobilized human muscle. *Journal of Applied Physiology* **62**, 2168–2173.

Enoka, R.M. (1988) Muscle strength and its development: new perspectives. *Sports Medicine* **6**, 146–168.

Enoka, R.M. (1995) Morphological features and activation patterns of motor units. *Journal of Clinical Neurophysiology* **12**, 538–559.

Fisher, M.J., Meyer, R.A., Adams, G.R., Foley, J.M. & Potchen, E.J. (1990) Direct relationship between proton T2 and exercise intensity in skeletal muscle MR images. *Investigative Radiology* **25**, 480–485.

Galganski, M.E., Fuglevand, A.J. & Enoka, R.M. (1993) Reduced control of motor output in a human hand muscle of elderly subjects during submaximal contractions. *Journal of Neurophysiology* **69**, 2108–2115.

Gans, C. & Bock, W.J. (1965) The functional significance of muscle architecture: a theoretical analysis. *Advances in Anatomy, Embryology, and Cell Biology* **38**, 115–142.

Granzier, H., Helmes, M. & Trombitas, K. (1996) Nonuniform elasticity of titin in cardiac myocytes: a study using immunoelectron microscopy and cellular mechanics. *Biophysics Journal* **70**, 430–442.

Häkkinen, K., Komi, P.V. & Alén, M. (1985) Effect of explosive type strength training on isometric force- and relaxation-time, electromyographic and muscle fibre characteristics of leg extensor muscles.

Acta Physiologica Scandinavica **125**, 587–600.

Häkkinen, K., Kallinen, M., Izquierdo, M. *et al.* (1998) Changes in agonist-antagonist EMG, muscle CSA, and force during strength training in middle-aged and older people. *Journal of Applied Physiology* **84**, 1341–1349.

Harridge, S.D.R., Bottinelli, R., Canepari, M. *et al.* (1996) Whole-muscle and single-fibre contractile properties and myosin heavy chain isoforms in humans. *Pflügers Archives* **432**, 913–920.

Harridge, S.D.R., Bottinelli, R., Canepari, M. *et al.* (1998) Sprint training, in vitro and in vivo muscle function, and myosin heavy chain expression. *Journal of Applied Physiology* **84**, 442–449.

Heckman, C.J. & Binder, M.D. (1993) Computer simulations of the effects of different synaptic input systems on motor unit recruitment. *Journal of Neurophysiology* **70**, 1827–1840.

Henneman, E. (1957) Relation between size of neurons and their susceptibility to discharge. *Science* **126**, 1345–1347.

Henneman, E. (1977) Functional organization of motoneuron pools: the size-principle. In: *Integration in the Nervous System* (eds H. Asanuma & V.J. Wilson), pp. 13–25. Igaku-Shoin, Tokyo.

Herbert, R.D. & Gandevia, S.C. (1996) Muscle activation in unilateral and bilateral efforts assessed by motor nerve and cortical stimulation. *Journal of Applied Physiology* **80**, 1351–1356.

Herbert, R.D., Dean, C. & Gandevia, S.C. (1998) Effects of real and imagined training on voluntary muscle activation during maximal isometric contractions. *Acta Physiologica Scandinavica* **163**, 361–368.

Higbie, E.J., Cureton, K.J., Warren, G.L. III & Prior, B.M. (1996) Effects of concentric and eccentric training on muscle strength, cross-sectional area, and neural activation. *Journal of Applied Physiology* **81**, 2173–2181.

Horak, F.B. & Macpherson, J.M. (1996) Postural orientation and equilibrium. In: *Handbook of Physiology*. Section 12. *Exercise: Regulation and Integration of Multiple Systems* (eds L.B. Rowell & J.T. Shepherd), pp. 255–292. Oxford University Press, New York.

Hortobágyi, T., Hill, J.P., Houmard, J.A., Fraser, D.D., Lambert, N.J. & Israel, R.G. (1996) Adaptive responses to muscles lengthening and shortening in humans. *Journal of Applied Physiology* **80**, 765–772.

Hortobágyi, T., Lambert, N.J. & Hill, J.P. (1997) Greater cross education following strength training with muscle lengthening than shortening. *Medicine and Science in Sports and Exercise* **29**, 107–112.

Howard, J.D. & Enoka, R.M. (1991) Maximum bilateral contractions are modified by neurally mediated interlimb effects. *Journal of Applied Physiology* **70**, 306–316.

Huesler, E.J., Hepp-Raymond, M.C. & Dietz, V. (1998) Task dependence of muscle synchronization in human hand muscles. *Neuroreport* **9**, 2167–2179.

van Ingen Schenau, G.J., Bobbert, M.F. & van Soest, A.J. (1990) The unique action of bi-articular muscles in leg extensions. In: *Multiple Muscle Systems* (eds J.M. Winters & S.L.-Y. Woo), pp. 639–652. Springer-Verlag, New York.

van Ingen Schenau, G.J., Boots, P.J.M., de Groot, G., Snackers, R.J. & Woenzel, W.W.L.M. (1992) The constrained control of force and position in multi-joint movements. *Neuroscience* **46**, 197–207.

Jakobi, J.M. & Cafarelli, E. (1998) Neuro-muscular drive and force production are not altered during bilateral contractions. *Journal of Applied Physiology* **84**, 200–206.

Jones, D.A. & Rutherford, O.M. (1987) Human muscle strength training: the effects of three different regimes and the nature of the resultant changes. *Journal of Physiology* **391**, 1–11.

Jones, D.A., Rutherford, O.M. & Parker, D.F. (1989) Physiological changes in skeletal muscle as a result of strength training. *Quarterly Journal of Experimental Physiology* **74**, 233–256.

Kandarian, S.C. & White, T.P. (1989) Force deficit during the onset of muscle hypertrophy. *Journal of Applied Physiology* **67**, 2600–2607.

Kandarian, S.C. & Williams, J.H. (1993) Contractile properties of skinned fibers from hypertrophied skeletal muscle. *Medicine and Science in Sports and Exercise* **25**, 999–1004.

Kanehisa, H., Ikegawa, S. & Fukunaga, T. (1994) Comparison of muscle cross-sectional area and strength between untrained women and men. *European Journal of Applied Physiology* **68**, 148–154.

Kawakami, Y., Abe, T., Kuno, S.Y. & Fukunaga, T. (1995) Training-induced changes in muscle architecture and specific tension. *European Journal of Applied Physiology* **72**, 37–43.

Keen, D.A., Yue, G.H. & Enoka, R.M. (1994) Training-related enhancement in the control of motor output in elderly humans. *Journal of Applied Physiology* **77**, 2648–2658.

Kent-Braun, J.A. & Le Blanc, R. (1996) Quantification of central activation failure during maximal voluntary contractions in humans. *Muscle and Nerve* **19**, 861–869.

Kirkwood, P.A., Sears, T.A., Tuck, D.L. & Westgaard, R.H. (1982) Variations in the time course of the synchronization of intercostal motoneurones in cat. *Journal of Physiology* **327**, 105–135.

Koh, T.J., Grabiner, M.D. & Clough, C.A. (1993) Bilateral deficit is larger for step than for ramp isometric contractions. *Journal of Applied Physiology* **74**, 1200–1205.

Kossev, A. & Christova, P. (1998) Discharge pattern of human motor units during dynamic concentric and eccentric contractions. *Electroencephalography and Clinical Neurophysiology* **109**, 245–255.

Laidlaw, D.H., Kornatz, K.W., Keen, D.A., Suzuki, S. & Enoka, R.M. (1999) Strength training improves the steadiness of slow lengthening contractions performed by old adults. *Journal of Applied Physiology* **87**, 1786–1795.

Larsson, L. & Salviati, G. (1992) A technique for studies of the contractile apparatus in single human muscle fibre segments obtained by percutaneous biopsy. *Acta Physiologica Scandinavica* **146**, 485–495.

Larsson, L., Li, X., Berg, H.E. & Frontera, W.R. (1996) Effects of removal of weight-bearing function on contractility and myosin isoform composition in single human skeletal muscle cells. *Pflügers Archives* **432**, 320–328.

Larsson, L., Li, X. & Frontera, W.R. (1997) Effects of aging on shortening velocity and myosin isoform composition in single human skeletal muscle cells. *American Journal of Physiology* **272**, C638–C649.

McDonagh, M.J.N., Hayward, C.M. & Davies, C.T.M. (1983) Isometric training in human elbow flexor muscles. The effects on voluntary and electrically evoked forces. *Journal of Bone and Joint Surgery* **65**, 355–358.

Merton. P.A. (1954) Voluntary strength and fatigue. *Journal of Physiology* **123**, 553–564.

Milner-Brown, H.S., Stein, R.B. & Lee, R.G. (1975) Synchronization of human motor units: possible roles of exercise and supraspinal reflexes. *Electroencephalography and Clinical Neurophysiology* **38**, 245–254.

Nakazawa, K., Kawakami, Y., Fukunaga, T., Yano, H. & Miyashita, M. (1993) Differences in activation patterns in elbow flexor muscles during isometric, concentric and eccentric contractions. *European Journal of Applied Physiology* **59**, 310–319.

Narici, M.V., Hoppeler, H., Kayser, B. *et al.* (1996) Human quadriceps cross-sectional area, torque and neural activation during 6 months of strength training. *Acta Physiologica Scandinavica* **157**, 175–186.

Narici, M., Roi, G., Landoni, L., Minetti, A.E. & Cerretelli, P. (1989) Changes in force, cross-sectional area and neural activation during strength training and detraining of the human quadriceps. *European Journal of Applied Physiology* **59**, 310–319.

Nordstrom, M.A., Fuglevand, A.J. & Enoka, R.M. (1992) Estimating the strength of common input to human motoneurons from the cross-correlogram. *Journal of Physiology* **453**, 547–574.

O'Hagan, F.T., Sale, D.G., MacDougall, J.D. & Garner, S.H. (1995) Response to resistance training in young women and men. *International Journal of Sports Medicine* **16**, 314–321.

Ohtsuki, T. (1983) Decrease in human voluntary isometric arm strength induced by simultaneous bilateral exertion. *Behavioral Brain Research* **7**, 165–178.

Patel, T.J. & Lieber, R.L. (1997) Force transmission in skeletal muscle: from actomyosin to external tendons. In: *Exercise and Sport Sciences Reviews*, Vol. 25 (ed. J.O. Holloszy), pp. 321–363. Williams & Wilkins, Baltimore.

Person, R.S. & Kudina, L.P. (1972) Discharge frequency and discharge pattern of human motor units during voluntary contraction of muscle. *Electroencephalography and Clinical Neurophysiology* **32**, 471–483.

Ploutz, L.L., Tesch, P.A., Biro, R.L. & Dudley, G.A. (1994) Effect of resistance training on muscle use during exercise. *Journal of Applied Physiology* **76**, 1675–1681.

Ray, C.A. & Dudley, G.A. (1998) Muscle use during dynamic knee extension: implication for perfusion and metabolism. *Journal of Applied Physiology* **85**, 1194–1197.

Roy, R.R. & Edgerton, V.R. (1991) Skeletal muscle architecture and performance. In: *Strength and Power in Sport* (ed. P.V. Komi), pp. 115–129. Blackwell Scientific Publications, Oxford.

Rutherford, O.M. & Jones, D.A. (1986) The role of learning and coordination in strength training. *European Journal of Applied Physiology* **55**, 100–105.

Rutherford, O.M., Jones, D.A. & Newham, D.J. (1986) Clinical and experimental application of percutaneous twitch superimposition technique for the study of human muscle activation. *Journal of Neurology, Neurosurgery, and Psychiatry* **49**, 1288–1291.

Sale, D.G. (1988) Neural adaptation to resistance training. *Medicine and Science in Sports and Exercise* **20**, S135–S145.

Sale, D.G., McComas, A.J., MacDougall, J.D. & Upton, A.R.M. (1982) Neuromuscular adaptation in human thenar muscles following strength training and immobilization. *Journal of Applied Physiology* **53**, 419–424.

Schantz, P.G., Moritani, T., Karlson, E., Johansson, E. & Lundh, A. (1989) Maximal voluntary force of bilateral and unilateral leg extension. *Acta Physiologica Scandinavica* **136**, 185–192.

Schmied, A., Pagni, S., Sturm, H. & Vedel, J.P. (1998) Selective enhancement of motoneuron short-term synchronization in an attention-demanding motor task. *Society for Neuroscience Abstracts* **24**, 424.

Schmied, A., Vedel, J.-P. & Pagni, S. (1994) Human spinal lateralization assessed from motoneurone synchronization: dependence on handedness and motor unit type. *Journal of Physiology* **480**, 369–387.

Sears, T.A. & Stagg, D. (1976) Short-term synchronization of inter-costal motoneurone activity. *Journal of Physiology* **263**, 357–381.

Secher, N.H. (1975) Isometric rowing strength of experienced and inexperienced oarsmen. *Medicine and Science in Sports* **7**, 280–283.

Secher, N.H., Rube, N. & Ellers, J. (1988) Strength of one- and two-leg extension in man. *Acta Physiologica Scandinavica* **134**, 333–339.

Semmler, J.G. & Nordstrom, M.A. (1995) Influence of handedness on motor unit discharge properties and force tremor. *Experimental Brain Research* **104**, 115–125.

Semmler, J.G. & Nordstrom, M.A. (1998) Motor unit discharge and force tremor in skill- and strength-trained individuals. *Experimental Brain Research* **119**, 27–38.

Seyffarth, H. (1940) The behaviour of motor-units in voluntary contractions. *Avhandlinger Utgitt Norske Videnskap-Akad Oslo. I. Matematisk-Naturvidenskapelig Klasse* **4**, 1–63.

Staron, R.S., Karapondo, D.L., Kraemer, W.J. *et al.* (1994) Skeletal muscle

adaptations during early phase of heavy-resistance training in men and women. *Journal of Applied Physiology* **76**, 1247–1255.

Street, S.F. (1983) Lateral transmission of tension in frog myofibers: a myofibrillar network and transverse cytoskeletal connections are possible transmitters. *Journal of Cell Physiology* **114**, 346–364.

Taniguchi, Y. (1998) Relationship between the modifications of bilateral deficit in upper and lower limbs by resistance training in humans. *European Journal of Applied Physiology* **78**, 226–230.

Tesch, P.A. (1999) *Target Bodybuilding*. Human Kinetics, Champaign, IL.

Thépaut-Mathieu, C., van Hoecke, J. & Maton, B. (1988) Myoelectric and mechanical changes linked to length specificity during isometric training. *Journal of Applied Physiology* **64**, 1500–1505.

Vandenborne, K., Elliott, M.A., Walter, G.A. *et al.* (1998) Longitudinal study of skeletal muscle adaptations during immobilization and rehabilitation. *Muscle and Nerve* **21**, 1006–1012.

Wang, K., McCarter, R., Wright, J., Beverly, J. & Ramirez-Mitchell, R. (1993) Viscoelasticity of the sarcomere matrix of skeletal muscles: the titin-myosin composite filament is a dual-stage molecular spring. *Biophysics Journal* **64**, 1161–1177.

Wilson, G.J., Murphy, A.J. & Walshe, A. (1996) The specificity of strength training: the effect of posture. *European Journal of Applied Physiology* **73**, 346–352.

Wolpaw, J.R. (1994) Acquisition and maintenance of the simplest motor skill: investigation of CNS mechanisms. *Medicine and Science in Sports and Exercise* **26**, 1475–1479.

Wolpaw, J.R. & Lee, C.L. (1989) Memory traces in primate spinal cord produced by operant conditioning of H-reflex. *Journal of Neurophysiology* **61**, 563–572.

Yao, W.X., Fuglevand, A.J. & Enoka, R.M. (2000) Motor unit synchronization increases EMG amplitude and decreases force steadiness of simulated contractions. *Journal of Neurophysiology* **83**, 441–452.

Young, K., McDonagh, M.J.N. & Davies, C.T.M. (1985) The effects of two forms of isometric training on the mechanical properties of the triceps surae in man. *Pflügers Archives* **405**, 384–388.

Yue, G. & Cole, K.J. (1992) Strength increases from the motor program: comparison of training with maximal voluntary and imagined muscle contractions. *Journal of Neurophysiology* **67**, 1114–1123.

Yue, G., Alexander, A.L., Laidlaw, D., Gmitro, A.F., Unger, E.C. & Enoka, R.M.

(1994) Sensitivity of muscle proton spin-spin relaxation time as an index of muscle activation. *Journal of Applied Physiology* **76**, 84–92.

Yue, G.H., Bilodeau, M., Hardy, P.A. &

Enoka, R.M. (1997) Task-dependent effect of limb immobilization on the fatigability of the elbow flexor muscles in humans. *Experimental Physiology* **82**, 567–592.

Chapter 2

Mechanical Properties and Performance in Skeletal Muscles

W. HERZOG

Introduction

The mechanical properties of skeletal muscle determine its performance. Mechanical properties are defined here as those properties of skeletal muscle that can be measured by parameters derived from mechanics: force, length, velocity, work and power. The performance achieved in many sports depends to a large degree on these parameters, for example, on the power an athlete can produce or the velocity (speed) he or she can achieve or impart on an implement. Human joints are typically crossed by many muscles; therefore, athletic performance depends typically on the properties of many muscles, as well as their exact coordination. Coordination is defined here as the interaction of the force–time histories of muscles that contribute to a movement, and thus, because of the geometry of the musculoskeletal system, the moment–time histories of these muscles about joints. The coordination of muscles is tremendously important for achieving precise movements or movements that maximize the work performed or the power produced, features that are of primary significance for optimal performance in many sports. However, coordination of muscles is an issue of motor control rather than mechanics; it will only be included in this chapter when required for clarity.

Despite the well-accepted relationship between the mechanical properties of skeletal muscle and performance in many sports, there is a sparsity of muscle mechanics research in sports. Also, in the practical application of physical training aimed at improving sport performance, athletes and coaches rarely consider the mechanical properties of skeletal muscles with the exception of force (strength); strength training is a well-accepted mode for improving muscular strength. The reasons for this rather sad state of affairs is not clear; however, the following factors might be partly responsible for the lack of muscle mechanics research in sport.

• Most mechanical properties of skeletal muscle are non-linear, therefore their mathematical description is not always trivial.

• It is virtually impossible to determine even the most basic properties of individual skeletal muscles *in vivo* and non-invasively.

• The time dependence of the mechanical properties (e.g. with increasing fatigue) are virtually unknown.

Because muscle mechanics research in sports is rare, it is not appropriate to write a literature review here. Such a review would reveal a sketchy, incomplete picture that might confuse rather than enlighten, or worse yet, might lead to inappropriate interpretations and generalizations. Therefore, the goals of this chapter are:

• to present some basic considerations regarding the mechanical properties of skeletal muscle; and

• to give examples of how principles of muscle mechanics might be applied to evaluate or improve sports performance

Basic considerations

In this section, five considerations regarding muscle mechanics will be presented. First, the proposed mechanism of muscular force production is introduced. From this mechanism, many mechanical properties of muscle can be derived directly. Second, selected mechanical properties of skeletal muscle are introduced. Third, the *in vitro* or *in situ* mechanical properties of skeletal muscle derived from laboratory experiment cannot be directly used for *in vivo* human skeletal muscles. Selected examples will be shown to illustrate this point. Fourth, athletes are injured frequently or have musculoskeletal pain. It is discussed how pain and injury might influence muscular performance. Fifth, skeletal muscle is a biological tissue with a tremendous ability to adapt. Issues of muscular adaptation and the possible influence of such adaptations are discussed. Increases in mass and strength of muscles, arguably the most important factor for muscular performance, will be deliberately omitted from this discussion because this topic is covered elsewhere in this book and would require too much space for proper coverage. Here, we discuss muscular adaptations that are typically ignored in sports sciences.

Mechanism of muscular force production

The accepted mechanism of muscular contraction and force production is the sliding filament theory (Huxley & Hanson 1954; Huxley & Niedergerke 1954) combined with the cross-bridge theory (Huxley 1957; Huxley & Simmons 1971). According to the sliding filament theory, shortening and lengthening of muscle is brought about by the sliding of actin relative to myosin filaments. Force transmission from the myosin to the actin filament is thought to occur by a series of periodically arranged myosin-sidepieces (the cross-bridges) that can attach to periodically arranged, specialized sites on the actin filament. Some of the basic assumptions underlying the cross-bridge theory that are directly relevant for deriving the mechanical properties of skeletal muscle are:

• cross-bridges are periodically arranged on the myosin filament;
• cross-bridges attach to specialized sites that are periodically arranged on the actin filament;
• each cross-bridge produces the same average force and has the same capacity to perform mechanical work;

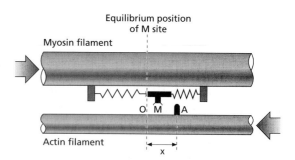

Fig. 2.1 Schematic illustration of a cross-bridge link between myosin and actin filaments as proposed by Huxley (1957). The so-called 'x-distance' is defined as the distance from the cross-bridge equilibrium position (O) to the nearest cross-bridge attachment site on the actin filament (A). (Reprinted from Huxley (1957), pp. 255–318, with permission from Elsevier Science.)

• actin and myosin filaments are essentially rigid;
• cross-bridges attach and detach according to rate functions that are dependent exclusively on the so-called 'x-distance', the distance from the cross-bridge head in its equilibrium position (Fig. 2.1) to the nearest attachment site (A in Fig. 2.1) on the actin filament;
• the instantaneous force of a cross-bridge depends on the x-distance exclusively; and
• each cross-bridge cycle is associated with the hydrolysation of one adenosine triphosphate (ATP).

For a thorough review of the cross-bridge theory and its mathematical formulation, the reader is referred to Huxley (1957), Huxley and Simmons (1971), Pollack (1990) and Epstein and Herzog (1998).

When expressing the cross-bridge theory mathematically, mechanical parameters such as the force, work or the energy required for a given contractile process can be calculated. Also, many of the mechanical properties can be derived directly from the cross-bridge theory. For example, the shape and extent of the so-called plateau and descending limb of the sarcomere force–length relationship (Gordon *et al.* 1966), and the concentric part of the force–velocity relationship observed experimentally (Hill 1938) can be approximated and explained by the theory. However, it must be pointed out that many experimental observations cannot be explained or are not part of the original formulation of the cross-bridge theory; such observations include the long-lasting effects of contraction history on force, or the heat production and force during eccentric contraction. Nevertheless, the cross-bridge theory provides, at present, the best basis for understanding and explaining the mechanical properties of skeletal muscle.

Although it may be argued that there is no need for athletes and coaches to understand the cross-bridge theory in its details, it should be recognized that muscular properties and performance in a given situation can be predicted reasonably well when equipped with some basic knowledge of the mechanisms underlying muscular contraction. The mechanical properties arising from the cross-bridge model should be known by every coach as they might influence sport performance dramatically.

Mechanical properties of skeletal muscle

Five mechanical properties of skeletal muscle will be discussed here. Only the basic characteristics of these properties are emphasized. Details that are not directly relevant for muscular or sport performance are ignored, therefore the following must be viewed as a 'simplified' or 'textbook' version of reality,

and other references should be consulted if more detailed information is sought. The five properties introduced here include:
- the force–length relationship;
- the force–velocity relationship;
- the power–velocity relationship;
- the endurance time–stress relationship; and
- selected history-dependent force properties.

THE FORCE–LENGTH RELATIONSHIP

The force–length relationship of skeletal muscle relates the maximal, isometric force to length. The term 'isometric' may relate to any specified level. For example, when talking about the muscle or sarcomere force–length relationship, the whole muscle or the sarcomeres are kept at a constant length, respectively. The force–length relationship is a static property of skeletal muscle; that means, a point on the force–length relationship is obtained by setting the muscle length, activating the muscle maximally, and then measuring the corresponding steady-state force (Fig. 2.2a). In order to obtain a second point, the muscle is relaxed (deactivated), set at the new length of interest and then reactivated maximally. It is not possible to go from point 1 (F_1) to point 2 (F_2) along the force–length relationship (Fig. 2.2b),

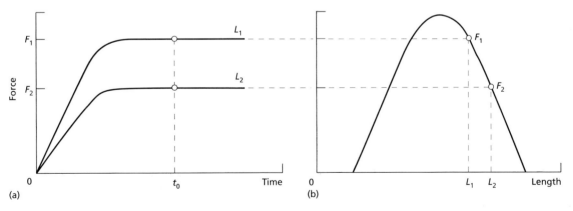

Fig. 2.2 Schematic illustration of how force–length relationships of muscles are determined, thereby emphasizing the static, non-continuous nature of the force–length relationship. (a) Force–time curves for two separate, fully activated contractions, one at a length L_1, the other at a length L_2. In both contractions, a steady-state force is measured, F_1 and F_2, respectively. (b) Force–length curve illustrating how the results of the experiment shown in (a) are used to determine the force–length relationship. Note that it is not possible to take a fully activated muscle and stretch it from L_1 to L_2 (or shorten it from L_2 to L_1) such that the force trace follows that shown in (b), because of the static, discontinuous nature of the force–length relationship.

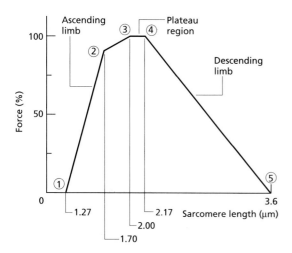

Fig. 2.3 Sarcomere force–length relationship as first described by Gordon *et al.* (1966) for frog skeletal muscle.

except, possibly, if the length change was carefully controlled by a complex and varying activation of the muscle during the experiment.

The sarcomere force–length relationship may be derived accurately based on the cross-bridge theory (Gordon *et al.* 1966). Specifically, the plateau region and the descending limb of the force–length relationship can be determined directly from the amount of myofilament overlap and the assumptions of the cross-bridge theory that: (i) the actin and myosin filaments are essentially rigid; (ii) they have periodically aligned attachment sites and cross-bridges, respectively; and (iii) each cross-bridge exerts the same amount of force and work independently of other cross-bridges and its own time history (Fig. 2.3).

In principle, the muscle force–length relationship states that the maximal force of a muscle depends on its length. In the human musculoskeletal system, the length of a muscle can be related to the angle(s) of the joint(s) the muscle is crossing. Therefore, there is an optimal length or joint angle at which muscular force is maximal. Knowing this length may be important for optimal sport performances. For example, during bicycling, the geometry of the bike dictates directly over which range of the force–length relationship the leg muscles work. Choosing the appropriate bike geometry for each individual

athlete therefore is of utmost importance for success in bicycling (Yoshihuku & Herzog 1990).

THE FORCE–VELOCITY RELATIONSHIP

The force–velocity relationship describes the relation between the maximal force at optimal length (the length at which the muscle can exert its maximal isometric force) and the corresponding speed of muscle shortening. For shortening (concentric) contractions, the force–velocity relationship has been described in mathematical form for over 60 years (Fenn & Marsh 1935; Hill 1938). In fact, Hill's (1938) force–velocity equation is still used today more often than any other equation to describe the force–velocity relationship of shortening muscle. It states:

$$F = \frac{F_0 b - av}{b + v} \qquad (2.1)$$

where F is the maximal force of a muscle at optimal length, F_0 is the maximal isometric force at optimal length, v is the speed of shortening, and a and b are constants with units of force (N) and speed (m · s^{-1}), respectively. A corresponding well-accepted equation for the force–velocity relationship of lengthening (eccentric) contractions does not exist.

For concentric contractions, the maximal force a muscle can produce at optimal length decreases with increasing speeds of shortening (Fig. 2.4) until it reaches a critical speed, v_0, at which the external

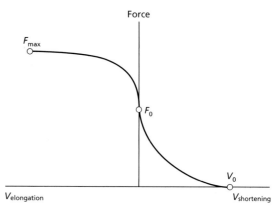

Fig. 2.4 Schematic force–velocity relationship for shortening and lengthening muscle.

force of the muscle becomes zero. The speed, v_0, can be calculated from Eqn 2.1 by setting F to zero, therefore:

$$v_0 = \frac{F_0 b}{a} \quad (2.2)$$

For eccentric contractions, the force a muscle can exert increases with increasing speeds of lengthening until a critical speed is reached at which the force becomes constant independent of the speed and equals about 1.5–2.0 times the maximal isometric force at optimal length, F_0 (Fig. 2.4). Since the force of a muscle depends on its contractile speed, force also depends on movement speed. For example, it has been well described that the force that can be exerted on the pedals during bicycling decreases with increasing speed of pedalling (Hull & Jorge 1985; Patterson & Moreno 1990; Sanderson 1991).

The shape of the force–velocity relationship depends strongly on the fibre type distribution within a muscle. Although the force per cross-sectional area (stress) of a slow-twitch and fast-twitch muscle fibre is about the same, the maximal speed of shortening differs by a factor of about 2 (Fig. 2.5). Therefore, for a given speed of shortening a predominantly fast-twitch fibred muscle can exert more force than a predominantly slow-twitch fibred muscle, although their isometric force (per cross-sectional area) is about equal. This observation explains why athletes with a high percentage of fast-twitch fibres typically perform better than athletes with a high percentage of slow-twitch fibres in events where a high speed of movement execution is combined with high force requirements—for example, in all sprinting, throwing and jumping events of track and field.

THE POWER–VELOCITY RELATIONSHIP

The power–velocity relationship can be derived directly from the force–velocity relationship since power, P, is the vector dot product of force ($\mathbf{F}$, vector) and velocity ($\mathbf{v}$, vector):

$$P = \mathbf{F} \cdot \mathbf{v} \quad (2.3)$$

which might be reduced to the scalar multiplication of the force magnitude, F, and the speed, v, for the special case of power in a skeletal muscle; i.e.

$$P = Fv \quad (2.4)$$

For concentric contractions, the power a muscle can exert is zero for isometric contractions (because $v = 0$) and for contractions at the maximal speed of shortening, v_0 (because $F = 0$). Power output of a muscle reaches a peak at a speed of about 30% of the maximal speed of shortening (Fig. 2.6). Therefore, in an athletic event in which power output should be maximized, it is of advantage to perform the movement at such a speed (if possible) that the major muscles contributing to the task contract at about 30% of their maximal speed of shortening. It has been suggested that animals take advantage of the

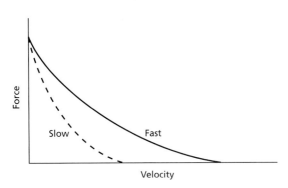

Fig. 2.5 Schematic force–velocity relationship for shortening contractions of a slow-twitch and a fast-twitch muscle fibre.

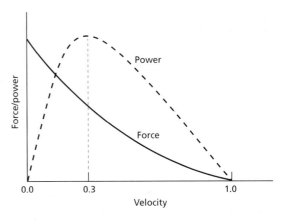

Fig. 2.6 Force–velocity and corresponding power–velocity relationship for shortening muscle.

power–velocity relationship of their muscles when escaping from predators. For example, it has been proposed that the frog leg muscles that contribute to jumping all contract close to 30% of their maximal shortening velocity, and so are able to produce near maximal power output of the legs (Lutz & Rome 1993). Quick, large jumps are taken by frogs to avoid being eaten by predators.

In some sports, movement speed can be selected by the athletes. Again, I would like to use the example of bicycling. When cycling at 40 km · h^{-1}, the athlete has a variety of gear ratios available to produce a given power output. Therefore, the athlete can directly manipulate movement speed (pedalling rate) for a given performance (cycling at 40 km · h^{-1}). The choice of proper gearing (pedalling rate) may be a decisive factor in the success of a cyclist.

THE ENDURANCE TIME–STRESS RELATIONSHIP

The three properties of skeletal muscle discussed so far do not take fatigue into account. Fatigue of skeletal muscle is defined here as the inability of a muscle to maintain a required force. Fatigue occurs fast when a muscle exerts large forces (or stresses). Maximal forces may only be sustained for a few seconds. However, a muscle that exerts a very small force relative to its maximal force may do so for an almost infinite amount of time (Fig. 2.7).

A predominantly slow-twitch fibred muscle

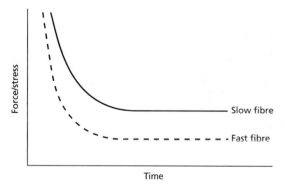

Fig. 2.7 Schematic force/stress–time relationship for a fast-twitch and a slow-twitch fibre.

can maintain a given amount of stress for a longer period of time than a predominantly fast-twitch fibred muscle (Fig. 2.7). Therefore, athletes with predominantly slow-twitch fibred muscles typically perform better than athletes with predominantly fast-twitched fibred muscles in sports that require long periods of muscular involvement at relatively low force levels—for example, long-distance running.

SELECTED HISTORY-DEPENDENT PROPERTIES

History-dependent properties of skeletal muscles have largely been ignored in muscle mechanics despite the fact that they have been observed experimentally and well described for at least half a century (e.g. Abbott & Aubert 1952; Maréchal & Plaghki 1979; Edman & Tsuchiya 1996; Herzog & Leonard 1997). History-dependent properties refer to properties of skeletal muscle (e.g. its ability to produce force) that depend on the contractile history. These properties are dynamic in nature and therefore are different from the static properties described so far.

The two history-dependent properties selected for this chapter are the force depression following muscle shortening and the force enhancement following muscle stretching. Force depression following muscle shortening refers to the observed phenomenon that the isometric force following muscle shortening is reduced compared with the corresponding purely isometric force (Fig. 2.8). Although this phenomenon has been well accepted for a long time (Abbott & Aubert 1952; Maréchal & Plaghki 1979) the mechanism causing force depression is not understood (Maréchal & Plaghki 1979; Herzog 1998). Also, force depression following muscle shortening has only recently been observed in human skeletal muscle (De Ruiter et al. 1998) and has been demonstrated to occur during voluntary human contractions in only a single study to date (Lee et al. 1999).

Force enhancement following muscle elongation refers to the experimentally observed result that the isometric force following muscle stretch is higher and remains higher than the corresponding purely

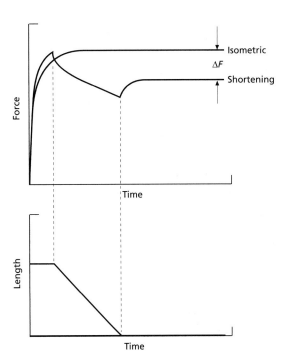

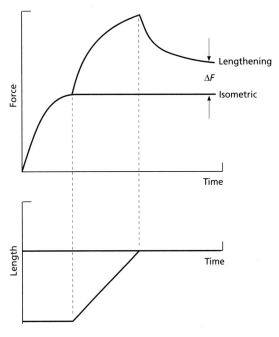

Fig. 2.8 Schematic illustration of force depression following muscle shortening. When comparing the maximal force of a purely isometric contraction to that of an isometric contraction that is preceded by a shortening of the muscle, it is observed that the isometric force following shortening is decreased (ΔF) compared with the purely isometric force at the corresponding muscle length.

Fig. 2.9 Schematic illustration of force enhancement following muscle lengthening. When comparing the maximal force of a purely isometric contraction to that of an isometric contraction that is preceded by a lengthening of the muscle, it is observed that the isometric force following lengthening is increased (ΔF) compared with the purely isometric force at the corresponding muscle length.

isometric force (Fig. 2.9). Force enhancement following muscle stretch has only been observed in artificially stimulated non-human muscle preparations (Abbott & Aubert 1952; Edman & Tsuchiya 1996); therefore, the possible significance of this property in human skeletal muscle during voluntary contractions must still be established. Nevertheless, the idea that stretching a muscle before concentric use might be beneficial for performance enhancement appears attractive and is used by many athletes. For example, movements such as a golf swing, jumping or throwing of any object are typically (if the rules of the game allow and if time permits) preceded by a counter-movement in which the major muscles required for the task are actively prestretched.

Muscle properties in humans (special considerations)

With few exceptions, the mechanical properties of skeletal muscles described in the previous section were obtained from isolated preparations of animal muscles. Human muscles may differ from animal muscles, and furthermore human muscles are voluntarily activated in sports and exercise rather than artificially stimulated. Therefore, some of the properties described above might only apply to a limited degree to *in vivo* human skeletal muscles. I would like to give two conceptual examples why *in vivo* human skeletal muscle properties may differ substantially from those of isolated *in situ* (or *in vitro*) animal muscles.

These two conceptual examples may be broadly grouped into activation- and adaptation-dependent phenomena.

When determining force–length, force–velocity, power–velocity, stress-endurance time, or history-dependent phenomena of isolated skeletal muscles, activation of the muscle is controlled, constant and artificial. Muscular contractions during human movement, and sport, are voluntary, and even maximal contractions are not performed at constant levels of activation. It has been proposed that during human voluntary contractions, activation may be increased when a muscle or muscle group contracts at full effort but the contractile conditions are not well-suited for large force production. For example, Hasler *et al.* (1994) argued that maximal voluntary activation of the knee extensor muscles (as recorded by surface electromyography, EMG) was increased towards full knee extension compared with levels of EMG at intermediate knee angles. The increase in EMG activity towards full knee extension was interpreted as an attempt of the neural control system to partly offset the unfavourable contractile conditions of the knee extensors at or near the fully extended knee.

Also, during maximal effort eccentric knee extensor contractions, the knee extensors should be 1.5–2.0 times as strong as during maximal effort isometric contractions, but they are not. Knee extensor activation is inhibited in this situation (presumably for reasons of safety) such that the eccentric force is about the same as that produced isometrically at the corresponding lengths (Westing *et al.* 1990).

Finally, pain or injury may not allow athletes to fully activate their muscles. For example, anterior knee pain, knee ligament injury, and knee effusion have all been shown to reduce the activation of the knee extensors achieved during maximal voluntary contractions in normal people and athletes (Suter *et al.* 1996; Huber *et al.* 1998). All these factors must be considered when assessing the potential for force, work and power output of muscles during athletic activities.

Although the mechanical properties of skeletal muscle, such as the force–length and force–velocity relationships, are typically treated as constant, invariant properties, it is well recognized that muscular properties may adapt to the requirements of everyday exercise and athletic training. For example, the force–length properties of high-performance cyclists and runners were found to differ significantly between the two groups of athletes, and appeared to have adapted to maximize cycling and running performance, respectively (Herzog *et al.* 1991a). Adaptations of strength following strength training and of endurance following aerobic training of skeletal muscles are other well-documented and well-accepted adaptations in athletes. These examples should serve to illustrate the possible danger of transferring muscle properties determined on *in situ* or *in vitro* preparations to the *in vivo* musculature of human athletes during competition.

Selected examples

Few examples exist in which muscle properties or muscle mechanics were used thoroughly and systematically to gain insight into the performance of an athlete or to maximize performance in a given sport. The possible exception to this rule is bicycling. Bicycling is an attractive sport to study from a muscle mechanics point of view because it is an essentially two-dimensional motion with few degrees of freedom. It can easily and realistically be studied in the laboratory, and output measures of mechanical performance (power, force, speed) can be determined in a straightforward way. Corresponding physiological measures, particularly those relating to the energetics of bicycling, have been determined for years using well-established testing procedures. Therefore, bicycling appears in many of the examples cited in the following pages.

When seated, the excursions of a cyclist's lower limb joints are basically given by the geometry of the bicycle, particularly the seat height, the handle bar length and the crank length. Therefore, the excursions of the lower limb muscles, as well as the area of the force–length relationship over which the lower limb muscles are working during a full pedal revolution is, to a large extent, given by the bicycle geometry and the anatomy of the athlete. In the ideal case, bicycle geometry should be chosen such that all major cycling muscles operate at or near the plateau region of the force–length relationship. It has been determined theoretically that such a geometry is achieved when the seat height is about 510 mm and the crank length is about 170 mm for a subject with thigh and shank length of 430 and 440 mm, respectively (Andrews 1987; Yoshihuku & Herzog 1996).

Once the bicycle geometry is set, the speed of muscular contraction depends exclusively on the pedalling rate. For minimal oxygen consumption, pedalling rates of 50–65 revolutions per minute (r.p.m.) have been shown to be optimal (Seabury *et al.* 1977; Coast & Welch 1985; Marsh & Martin 1993). Power output on a street bicycle (free gear selection) is maximized at about 120 r.p.m. (Sargeant *et al.* 1981; McCartney *et al.* 1983; Beelen & Sargeant 1991; MacIntosh & MacEachern 1997) and on a track bicycle (no gear selection, 200 m sprint) at about 150 r.p.m. (Yoshihuku & Herzog 1990). Finally, during long-distance racing, top athletes prefer to pedal at rates of about 90 r.p.m. (Hagberg *et al.* 1981; Patterson & Moreno 1990; Marsh & Martin 1993). According to the power–velocity relationship, a pedalling rate of about 120 r.p.m. would be optimal. However, the constraints of track cycling (one gear,

maintenance of maximal power for about 15–20 s in a 200 m sprint with the corresponding preparation phase), or the goals in long-distance cycling require different pedalling rates for success. Although pedalling at 60 r.p.m. uses less oxygen than pedalling at higher rates, the power that can be produced at 60 r.p.m. is relatively low because for a given (high) power output, the pedal forces need to be high causing local muscular fatigue to occur quickly.

Sprinting at 150 r.p.m. on the track or 120 r.p.m. during road racing allows for a high power output with relatively small muscular forces. However, at these high pedalling rates oxygen consumption for a given power output becomes prohibitive, and so this cannot be the strategy of choice for long-distance riding. Riding at 90 r.p.m. is a good compromise between the force–velocity, power–velocity and endurance time–stress relationships, although why most top cyclists prefer to ride at or near 90 r.p.m. still awaits complete and satisfactory explanation.

For maximal power output, athletes should use the primary muscles required for the task at optimal muscle length, at the optimal speed of shortening, and preferably after a stretch of the muscle (Fig. 2.10). Obviously, the musculoskeletal system is not built exclusively to maximize performance in a given sport, such as bicycling. However, muscles probably adapt to everyday exercise and training. The force–length properties of the human rectus femoris (RF) in cyclists are negative, those

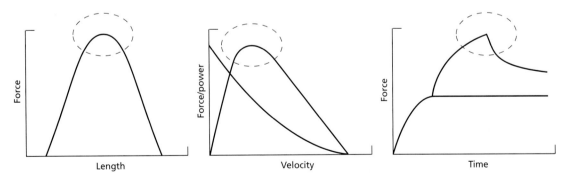

Fig. 2.10 Schematic force–length, force/power–velocity, and force–time curves illustrating that for maximal muscle power output, a muscle should be at a length close to optimal, should shorten at a speed close to optimal (i.e. at about 30% of the maximal speed of shortening), and should be used following a muscle stretch.

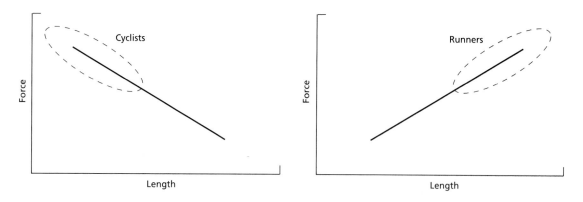

Fig. 2.11 Schematic illustration of the experimentally observed force–length relationships of human rectus femoris muscles in elite cyclists and elite runners.

of runners are positive (Herzog *et al*. 1991a), indicating that bicyclists are relatively stronger at short RF lengths and runners are relatively stronger at long RF lengths, as required for cycling and running, respectively (Fig. 2.11). This observation suggests that RF properties adapted in these athletes to accommodate the everyday demands of training and exercise. It has been speculated that such an adaptation could have occurred because of a change in the sarcomeres that are arranged in series in the RF fibres of these athletes (Herzog *et al*. 1991a), an attractive but as yet unproven speculation.

Independent of the mechanism of the muscular adaptation, it is safe to suggest that the RF force–length properties of the cyclists are not optimal for running and vice versa. This result has two interesting implications. First, cycling is not a good cross-training for running and vice versa, or in more general terms, cross-training could limit performance in the target sport. Second, in multievent sports, such as triathlon, even the most talented athlete will likely never be able to compete with the specialists in a particular discipline. For example, a highly talented runner who turns to triathlon cannot run with world-class runners even if the running training in terms of time, mileage and attempted intensity is the same for the triathlete as for the runners. The reason is not the amount or intensity of running but the fact that the properties

of the leg musculature will likely never be optimal for running because the triathlete also swims and cycles.

Final comments

Strength, power and endurance are attributes of skeletal muscles that often determine athletic success. The physiological adaptations of muscle to strength- and endurance-training are well known and documented. It was not the intent of this chapter to review the corresponding literature here. However, strength, power and endurance of a muscle are dramatically influenced by the length, speed and contractile history. This influence might be evaluated by knowing some of the mechanical properties of *in vivo* human skeletal muscles. Here, I have attempted to introduce some of these properties and demonstrate with selected examples how they might influence sport performance.

Two main difficulties arise when attempting to relate the properties of skeletal muscle to athletic performance:
• very little is known about the properties of individual, *in vivo* human skeletal muscles; and
• very little is known about the contractile conditions of the major task-specific muscles in sports.

Therefore, the current chapter cannot be viewed as a textbook chapter with all the answers. Rather, it represents considerations that might turn out to be useful in the analysis of the biomechanics of sports. It is hoped that this chapter might motivate sports biomechanists to systematically and thoroughly investigate sports activities and performances in the light of muscle mechanics. This approach is sorely lacking and offers new opportunities to gain exciting insights into the biomechanics of sports.

References

Abbott, B.C. & Aubert, X.M. (1952) The force exerted by active striated muscle during and after change of length. *Journal of Physiology* **117**, 77–86.

Andrews, J.G. (1987) The functional roles of the hamstrings and quadriceps during cycling: Lombard's paradox revisited. *Journal of Biomechanics* **20**, 565–575.

Beelen, A. & Sargeant, A.J. (1991) Effect of fatigue on maximal power output at different contraction velocities in humans. *Journal of Applied Physiology* **71**, 2332–2337.

Coast, J.R. & Welch, H.G. (1985) Linear increase in optimal pedal rate with increased power output in cycle ergometry. *European Journal of Applied Physiology* **53**, 339–342.

De Ruiter, C.J., de Haan, A., Jones, D.A. & Sargeant, A.J. (1998) Shortening-induced force depression in human adductor pollicis muscle. *Journal of Physiology* **507** (2), 583–591.

Edman, K.A.P. & Tsuchiya, T. (1996) Strain of passive elements during force enhancement by stretch in frog muscle fibres. *Journal of Physiology* **490** (1), 191–205.

Epstein, M. & Herzog, W. (1998) *Theoretical Models of Skeletal Muscle: Biological and Mathematical Considerations.* John Wiley, New York.

Fenn, W.O. & Marsh, B.O. (1935) Muscular force at different speeds of shortening. *Journal of Physiology* **85**, 277–297.

Gordon, A.M., Huxley, A.F. & Julian, F.J. (1966) The variation in isometric tension with sarcomere length in vertebrate muscle fibres. *Journal of Physiology* **184**, 170–192.

Hagberg, J.M., Mullin, J.P., Giese, M.D. & Spitznagel, E. (1981) Effect of pedaling rate on submaximal exercise responses of competitive cyclists. *Journal of Applied Physiology* **51**, 447–451.

Hasler, E.M., Denoth, J., Stacoff, A. & Herzog, W. (1994) Influence of hip and knee joint angles on excitation of knee extensor muscles. *Electromyography and Clinical Neurophysiology* **34**, 355–361.

Herzog, W. (1998) History dependence of force production in skeletal muscle: a proposal for mechanisms. *Journal of Electromyography and Kinesiology* **8**, 111–117.

Herzog, W. & Leonard, T.R. (1997) Depression of cat soleus forces following isokinetic shortening. *Journal of Biomechanics* **30** (9), 865–872.

Herzog, W., Guimaraes, A.C., Anton, M.G. & Carter-Erdman, K.A. (1991a) Moment-length relations of rectus femoris muscles of speed skaters/cyclists and runners. *Medicine and Science in Sports and Exercise* **23**, 1289–1296.

Herzog, W., Hasler, E.M. & Abrahamse, S.K. (1991b) A comparison of knee extensor strength curves obtained theoretically and experimentally. *Medicine and Science in Sports and Exercise* **23**, 108–114.

Hill, A.V. (1938) The heat of shortening and the dynamic constants of muscle. *Proceedings of the Royal Society of London* **126**, 136–195.

Huber, A., Suter, E. & Herzog, W. (1998) Inhibition of the quadriceps muscles in elite male volleyball players. *Journal of Sports Sciences* **16**, 281–289.

Hull, M.L. & Jorge, M. (1985) A method for biomechanical analysis of bicycle pedalling. *Journal of Biomechanics* **18**, 631–644.

Huxley, A.F. (1957) Muscle structure and theories of contraction. *Progress in Biophysics and Biophysical Chemistry* **7**, 255–318.

Huxley, A.F. & Niedergerke, R. (1954) Structural changes in muscle during contraction. Interference microscopy of living muscle fibres. *Nature* **173**, 971–973.

Huxley, A.F. & Simmons, R.M. (1971) Proposed mechanism of force generation in striated muscle. *Nature* **233**, 533–538.

Huxley, H. & Hanson, J. (1954) Changes in cross-striations of muscle during contraction and stretch and their structural interpretation. *Nature* **173**, 973–976.

Lee, H.D., Suter, E. & Herzog, W. (1999) Force depression in human quadriceps femoris following voluntary shortening contractions. *Journal of Applied Physiology* **87**, 1651–1655.

Lutz, G.J. & Rome, L.C. (1993) Built for jumping: The design of the frog muscular system. *Science* **263**, 370–372.

MacIntosh, B.R. & MacEachern, P. (1997) Paced effort and all-out 30-second power tests. *International Journal of Sports Medicine* **18**, 594–599.

Maréchal, G. & Plaghki, L. (1979) The deficit of the isometric tetanic tension redeveloped after a release of frog muscle at a constant velocity. *Journal of General Physiology* **73**, 453–467.

Marsh, A.P. & Martin, P.E. (1993) The association between cycling experience and preferred and most economical cadences. *Medicine and Science in Sports and Exercise* **25**, 1269–1274.

McCartney, N., Heigenhauser, G.J. & Jones, N.L. (1983) Power output and fatigue of human muscle in maximal cycling exercise. *Journal of Applied Physiology* **55** (1), 218–224.

Patterson, R.P. & Moreno, M.I. (1990) Bicycle pedalling forces as a function of pedalling rate and power output. *Medicine and Science in Sports and Exercise* **22**, 512–516.

Pollack, G.H. (1990) *Muscles and Molecules: Uncovering the Principles of Biological Motion.* Ebner & Sons, Seattle.

Sanderson, D.J. (1991) The influence of cadence and power output on the biomechanics of force application during steady-rate cycling in competitive and recreational cyclists. *Journal of Sports Sciences* **9**, 191–203.

Sargeant, A.J., Hoinville, E. & Young, A. (1981) Maximum leg force and power output during short-term dynamic exercise. *Journal of Applied Physiology* **51**, 1175–1182.

Seabury, J.J., Adams, W.C. & Ramey, M.R. (1977) Influence of pedalling rate and power output on energy expenditure during bicycle ergometry. *Ergonomics* **20**, 491–498.

Suter, E., Herzog, W. & Huber, A. (1996) Extent of motor unit activation in the quadriceps muscles of healthy subjects. *Muscle and Nerve* **19**, 1046–1048.

Westing, S.H., Seger, J.Y. & Thorstensson, A. (1990) Effects of electrical stimulation on eccentric and concentric torque-velocity relationships during knee extension in man. *Acta Physiologica Scandinavica* **140**, 17–22.

Yoshihuku, Y. & Herzog, W. (1990) Optimal design parameters of the bicycle-rider system for maximal muscle power output. *Journal of Biomechanics* **23**, 1069–1079.

Yoshihuku, Y. & Herzog, W. (1996) Maximal muscle power output in bicycling as a function of rider position, rate of pedalling and definition of muscle length. *Journal of Sports Sciences* **14**, 139–157.

Chapter 3

Muscle-Tendon Architecture and Athletic Performance

J.H. CHALLIS

Introduction

Athletic activities place a wide range of demands on the human muscular system. Some activities require small amounts of muscle force adjusted in fine increments, some require the rapid production of high forces, while yet others demand the slow production of very high forces. The purpose of this chapter is to identify the key properties of muscle and explain how they influence muscle function during athletic activities. The focus will be on skeletal muscle as opposed to the other two forms of muscle, smooth and cardiac, as skeletal muscle can be controlled voluntarily. As the skeletal muscle system has to perform a variety of functions its design is generally a compromise; it is specialized only in the sense that it can perform a variety of tasks.

Newton's First Law basically states that we need forces to stop, start or alter motion, therefore as the muscle fibres are the sources of force production in the human body they are responsible for our voluntary movement or lack of it. The muscle fibres produce forces which are transmitted via tendons to the skeleton, and transformation of these forces to moments at the joints either causes motion or restrains motion caused by other forces (e.g. maintaining upright posture when standing in a strong breeze). Therefore, it is useful not only to consider the forces the muscles produce but also to analyse how these muscles operate across joints. When referring to muscle-tendon architecture we are referring to the structure and arrangement of the components of the muscle-tendon system. This chapter will examine how the muscle-tendon system is arranged to produce movement, and the structures that permit this.

The contractile machinery

Reference is often made to 'muscle' when we are really referring to a muscle-tendon complex. The muscle-tendon complex is composed of muscle fibres, which are the actively controlled force generators that are attached to the skeleton via lengths of tendon at either end of the muscle belly. There are a variety of ways in which the muscle fibres can orientate themselves to the tendon. This aspect of their organization can be very important, as can the relative amounts of tendon and muscle fibre composing the muscle-tendon unit; these will be reviewed later. It is the building blocks of the muscle fibres, the myofilaments, which reveal the properties of the muscle fibres and these will be reviewed in this section.

We are all familiar with skeletal muscles as our own musculoskeletal system contains nearly 700 of them, and we come across it everyday in the form of meat. The whole muscle is surrounded by a layer of connective tissue, the fascia, beneath which is a further sheath of connective tissue, the epimysium. Whole muscle is composed of a large number of fascicles, which consist of bundles of 10–100 muscle fibres surrounded by the perimysium, another connective tissue sheath. The muscle fibres are surrounded by a further layer of connective tissue, the endomysium. The number of fibres comprising a whole muscle varies; for example, the medial head of the gastrocnemius comprises over one million fibres, whilst the finger muscle, the first dorsal interosseous, comprises around 40 000 (Feinstein *et al.* 1955). Typically a muscle fibre is approximately 50 µm in diameter, but will be smaller during infancy, and larger if adaptations have been made, for example due to strength training. Closer inspection of the muscle fibres reveals that they are in turn composed of myofibrils all organized side by side. The myofibrils are strings of sarcomeres arranged in series, with the sarcomere being the functional unit where the generation of muscle force takes place. A typical muscle fibre will be composed of as many as 8000 myofibrils. Figure 3.1 illustrates the hierarchical structure of muscle. The figure shows that muscle is composed of a large number of sarcomeres bundled together to form a whole muscle. In bundling together these sarcomeres there are significant amounts of connective tissue.

The sarcomere contains two major sets of contractile proteins, the thick myosin filaments and the thin actin filaments. It is the active interdigitation of these thick and thin filaments which is responsible for the generation of force. In experiments performed in the 1960s it was shown how the degree of overlap between these thick and thin filaments corresponded with the amount of force the sarcomere could produce under isometric conditions (Gordon *et al.* 1966). In these experiments small sections of muscle were held at a fixed length and stimulated, the degree of overlap between the filaments was measured as was the amount of force produced, then the length was changed and the process repeated. Figure 3.2 shows the isometric force–length properties of the sarcomere of frog skeletal muscle. More sophisticated experimental work by Edman and Reggiani (1987) has shown that the curve is much smoother than at first thought, with a much less defined plateau. Despite these deficiencies the original curve helps to explain the phenomena associated with the generation of muscle forces.

The production of force by muscle can be explained by the cross-bridge theory. Whilst this is only a theory it is the one most commonly accepted by muscle physiologists. The theory is that the force is due to the formation of myosin cross-bridges connecting with the binding sites on the actin filaments. The amount of force produced is proportional to the number of cross-bridges formed (Huxley 1957). As can be seen in Fig. 3.2 the maximum isometric force occurs when sarcomere lengths are in their mid-range. This length is called the optimum length and corresponds with the length at which the maximum number of cross-bridges can be formed. For frog muscle the optimum sarcomere length is between 2.00 and 2.25 µm (Gordon *et al.* 1966), whilst for human muscle it is slightly longer, between 2.60 and 2.80 µm (Walker & Schrodt 1973). At the shorter lengths the actin filaments from one side overlap with those from the other side, thus interfering with the formation of cross-bridges. As the amount of overlap is increased, from these short lengths, more cross-bridges can form so force is increased until the plateau region is reached where the maximum force is produced. Beyond the plateau region the force produced by the sarcomere decreases with increasing length because fewer cross-bridges can be formed. At the upper extreme of sarcomere lengths there is no overlap between the actin and myosin filaments and no force can be produced.

Although it is a tedious process, a number of researchers have taken whole human muscle and measured the number of sarcomeres comprising the length of the muscle. From these data it is possible to infer the properties of whole muscle. From the analysis of eight human cadavers, Huijing (1985) estimated that on average nearly 18 000 sarcomeres are arranged in series in the myofibrils of the medial head of the gastrocnemius. Meijer *et al.* (1998), taking measures from two cadavers, estimated that on average over 41 000 sarcomeres make up the myofibrils of the vastus medialis. Many myofibrils make up a whole muscle and they will not all contain precisely the same number of sarcomeres; there will be a range, which will affect the properties of whole muscle. Based on the data in Meijer *et al.* (1998) it is possible to examine the force–length profile of a whole muscle made up of 1000 myofibrils with a mean of 41 800 sarcomeres making up each myofibril and a standard deviation of 5300 sarcomeres. Figure 3.3 shows the shape of the

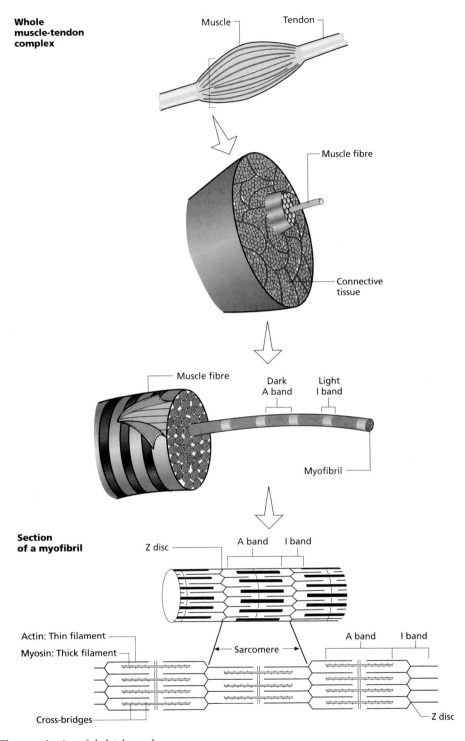

Fig. 3.1 The organization of skeletal muscle.

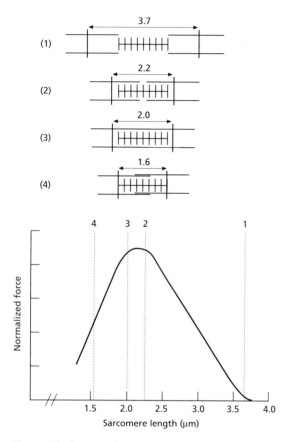

Fig. 3.2 The isometric force–length properties of the sarcomere of frog skeletal muscle, with examples of sarcomere overlap. (Based on data in Gordon *et al.* 1966.)

force–length curve for this theoretical muscle. The first thing to note is that variation in the number of sarcomeres in series gives a muscle with an active range from 6.5 cm to 21 cm, which is typical of the lengths we expect from the vastus medialis. The active range is much broader than it would be for the uniform number of sarcomeres; this is because some myofibrils will have their peak at shorter lengths and others at longer lengths. The optimum length of this muscle is around 12 cm.

The preceding analysis has assumed that muscles are arranged in bundles which transmit force along their length to the end regions, where they attach to tendon. Muscles often taper at the ends, which would mean that certain fibres would have to be longer than others; this constraint would accentuate the effects shown in Fig. 3.3. Loeb *et al.* (1987) examined the cat sartorius and showed that not all muscle fibres ran from one tendon plate to another. This arrangement has implications for the force–length properties of whole muscle, also it makes more complex the mechanism for force transmission to the external tendon. Such an arrangement has not been demonstrated in human muscle but may exist.

If, for a given activity, the production of maximum force from a muscle is desired then it makes sense that when performing the activity the muscle's range of motion should occur around the

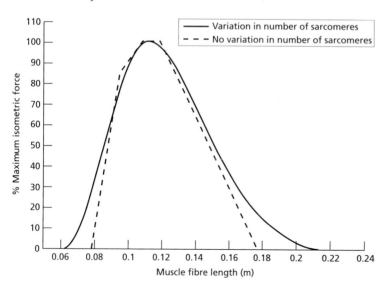

Fig. 3.3 The isometric force–length properties of a muscle composed of 1000 myofibrils with a mean of 41 800 sarcomeres making up each myofibril and a standard deviation of 5300. (Values based on data in Meijer *et al.* 1998.)

muscle's optimum length. Invasive studies on the semimembranosus of *Rana pipiens* (a species of frog), have shown that during the leaping motion this muscle operates near its optimum length throughout the movement (Lutz & Rome 1994). This example from the frog is not a general functional adaptation of muscle. *In vivo* measures have been made on the degree of sarcomere overlap of the human extensor carpi radialis longus, a wrist extensor muscle, and show that this muscle works on the descending limb of the force–length curve (Lieber *et al.* 1994). In a study of elite runners and cyclists it was found that the rectus femoris, over its active range *in vivo*, was operating on the descending limb for the runners and the ascending limb for the cyclists (Herzog *et al.* 1991). It is possible that these are self-selected groups, for example that success comes for the cyclist with a rectus femoris which works predominantly on the ascending limb of the force–length curve. It is more likely, though, that these are functional adaptations caused by changing the number of sarcomeres in series. There is evidence in animal studies that such adaptations can occur; for example, rats made to run downhill showed increased numbers of sarcomeres in their vastus intermedius (Lynn & Morgan 1994).

As the velocity of a muscle changes so does the force that muscle can produce, as illustrated in Fig. 3.4. This relationship was experimentally first quantified by Fenn and Marsh (1935), and the classic study was performed a few years later by A.V. Hill (Hill 1938). Hill's study was performed using whole frog sartorius muscle and investigated the variation in force production at different shortening velocities. More recent work has shown that single muscle fibres do not produce the same curve as Hill obtained, with a deviation for the high force/low speed part of the relationship (Edman *et al.* 1976). To understand the force–velocity properties of muscle fibres it is necessary to define a few terms. A stimulated muscle which shortens is performing a *concentric contraction*. If the ends of the muscle are constrained in some way so that the distance between the ends is fixed, then a stimulated muscle is performing an *isometric contraction*. If a force is applied to a stimulated muscle which exceeds its

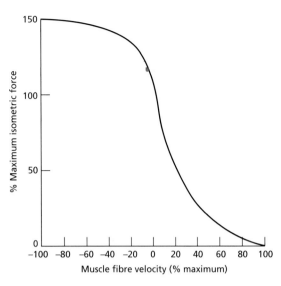

Fig. 3.4 The force–velocity curve for muscle (positive velocities—concentric phase, negative velocities—eccentric phase).

capacity for generating an isometric force then that muscle will lengthen, and this is called an *eccentric contraction*. By convention, concentric contractions are given positive velocities, whilst eccentric contractions have negative velocities. As the velocity of a concentric contraction increases, the force the fibres can produce decreases. As the magnitude of the velocity increases during eccentric contractions the force the fibres can produce increases. Some authors object to the use of the term contraction, when discussing eccentric activity. This is because there is no evidence of anything contracting, the muscle actually lengthens, and muscle volume remains constant (Baskin & Paolini 1967).

The maximum velocity of shortening is obtained during the concentric phase; this happens under the no-load or zero-force condition. Such a velocity of shortening is not likely to occur *in vivo* because a no-load condition is difficult to achieve as the muscle has to contend with the inertia of the limbs to which it is connected. The force that can be produced falls rapidly as velocity increases—a phenomenon familiar to athletes, who generally cannot move heavier objects with as high a velocity as lighter ones.

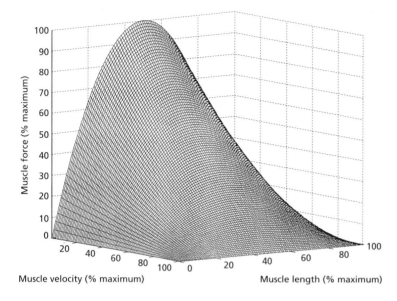

Fig. 3.5 The force–length–velocity curve for an idealized muscle; only the concentric phase of the force–velocity curve is represented.

Katz (1939) performed some of the earliest studies of eccentrically contracting muscle, and noted that the forces are higher during the eccentric phase compared with the concentric phase. Eccentric contractions only occur when muscle is yielding to a force. For example, our muscles often work eccentrically when controlling the landing from a drop. During many weight training exercises the major muscle groups work concentrically to raise the weight and eccentrically to lower it. The basic force–velocity properties of muscles immediately inform us that lowering the weight should be, and feel, easier than raising it. Weight trainers often find they can continue to lower weights which they can no longer raise. Such lowering of a weight after failing to raise the weight emphasizes the muscles working eccentrically and is often referred to as 'negatives', which is correct since if the muscles are lengthening the muscle fibre velocity will be negative. The eccentric phase of the force–velocity curve produces the highest muscle forces, unfortunately few experiments have been performed precisely to quantify this force, but estimates range from 110 to 180% of the maximum isometric force (e.g. Katz 1939; Joyce & Rack 1969; Mashima 1984).

The force–velocity properties of muscle can be explained using cross-bridge theory (Huxley 1957). The maximum velocity of shortening appears to be related to the maximum rate at which the cross-bridges can cycle (Barany 1967; Edman *et al.* 1988). If this is the case then maximum rate of shortening would not be affected by the degree of overlap of the sarcomeres, and therefore the force–length properties. Edman (1979) has shown this to be the case.

It would be incorrect to consider the force–length and force–velocity properties of muscles in isolation because during many movements the length and velocity of the muscle change simultaneously. Figure 3.5 illustrates the force–length–velocity properties of an idealized muscle. It should also be pointed out that this is the curve for a maximally activated muscle, and there are many other values obtainable for the muscle forces by varying the degree of muscle activation.

Muscle fibre organization

The next question to ask is how are the properties of a muscle affected by their muscle fibre organization or architecture. The main variations in muscle fibre architecture relate to the number of sarcomeres in parallel and the number in series. Rather than discuss this aspect of architecture in terms of sarcomeres we will focus on muscle fibres. If we arrange more muscle fibres in parallel then they can produce more force, with muscle force being directly proportional to muscle cross-sectional area. Intuitively we expect such a relationship as individuals with larger muscles are assumed to be stronger, i.e. capable of producing more muscular force than others, but we can also have muscle fibres of different lengths. Longer muscle fibres have more sarcomeres in series and so have a larger range of motion. They can produce force for a greater range of muscle lengths. They will not be able to produce muscle forces at as short a length as a short muscle, but will have a much greater operating range. This is not the only property which is enhanced for longer muscles —they can also shorten at higher velocities. Each sarcomere can shorten at a given rate and the shortening rate of a fibre will be a direct function of the number of these in series.

To illustrate the effects of muscle fibre organization, Fig. 3.6 shows the properties of two hypothetical muscles. Both muscles have the same volume, so they have the same amount of contractile machinery, but in one the muscle is relatively long and thin whilst the other is short and thick. Note that for both muscles the contraction time will be the same as this does not vary with muscle size. The peak isometric force is greater for muscle B, but it has half the working range of muscle A. Muscle A is able to shorten at twice the maximum velocity of muscle B due to its greater length, but muscle B can generate greater amounts of force for the lower contraction velocities. Power production, particularly peak power, is strongly correlated with performance in dynamic athletic activities. The power produced by a muscle is the product of the force it is producing and the velocity of contraction, and Fig. 3.6 shows that both muscles produce the same peak power. Muscle A due to its greater peak velocity produces peak power at a higher velocity than muscle B.

Human muscle fibres differ in their precise properties. Basically there are two types, fast (type II) and slow (type I), although these can be divided up into more detailed subcategories. Fast fibres can contract quickly and have the enzymes which make them specialized for anaerobic glycolysis. Slow fibres contract more slowly and are specialized for prolonged or sustained activities obtaining energy via aerobic glycolysis. Human muscle is not homogeneous in terms of fibre type content, so the relative distribution of the fibre types in a muscle helps determine its properties. In the preceding example it was assumed that both muscles had the same muscle fibre types. There is conflicting evidence as to whether the different fibre types can produce different maximum forces per unit of cross-sectional area, but the current balance of evidence suggests that there is no difference. The curvature of the force–velocity curve does depend on fibre type (Faulkner et al. 1986), with greater concavity for the slow fibres (see Fig. 3.7). This greater concavity will result in reduced force production particularly in the mid-range of the muscle's range of shortening velocities. The maximum shortening velocity of human muscle has been measured to be $6 \, \text{fl} \cdot \text{s}^{-1}$ (fibre lengths per second) for type II fibres, and $2 \, \text{fl} \cdot \text{s}^{-1}$ for type I fibres (Faulkner et al. 1986). The ratio of these velocities corresponds well with studies on the properties of different fibre types in other animals (e.g. Close 1964). Figure 3.7 illustrates the force–velocity curve for three hypothetical muscles, all of the same length and cross-sectional area: one muscle is composed of 100% slow fibres and the other two are 100% fast fibres. Peak force is the same for all three muscles, but the maximum velocity of shortening is three times greater for the 'fast' muscles compared with the slow muscle. This reflects the normal case where fast fibres can shorten at much higher velocities than slow fibres. The difference in concavity of the force–velocity curve also has a significant effect on the force-producing capabilities of the muscle. To illustrate this in Fig. 3.7 fast muscle II has been given the same concavity in its force–velocity properties as slow fibres. Fast muscle II produces less force for a given velocity of shortening than fast muscle I, even if it has the same maximum shortening velocity.

	Hypothetical muscle A	Hypothetical muscle B
Length	2 units	1 unit
Cross-sectional area	1 unit^2	2 units^2

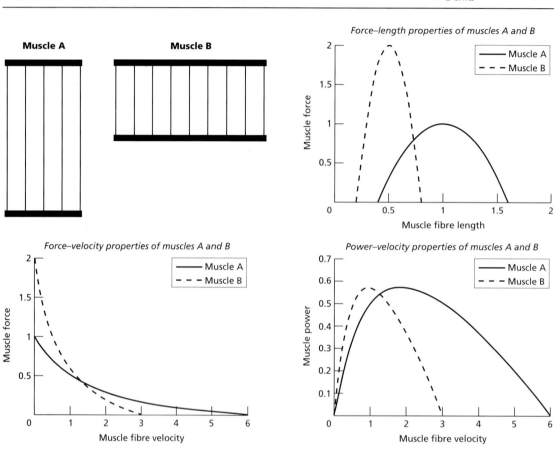

Key functional properties summary

	Hypothetical muscle A	Hypothetical muscle B
Contraction time	1	1
Maximum force	1	2
Range of motion	2	1
Maximum velocity	2	1
Peak power	2	2

Fig. 3.6 The influence of the arrangement of muscle fibres on the force–length, force–velocity, and velocity–power properties of two hypothetical muscles.

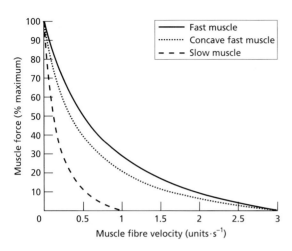

Fig. 3.7 The concentric phase of the force–velocity curve for three muscles. These muscles are equivalent in their properties, except in their fibre type distributions.

Connective tissue

In examining the structure of whole muscle (see above), it was seen that there are significant amounts of connective tissue in muscle (fascia, epimysium, perimysium, endomysium). The component of this connective material which dictates its properties is collagen, although there is also some elastin. Both materials have important elastic properties. As well as holding everything together, the connective tissue also provides the framework within which

muscle fibres form, and acts as the ducting through which blood vessels and nerves run. Forces produced by the muscle fibres are, in part, conveyed through this connective tissue (Street & Ramey 1965), and it has important properties which influence the force output of muscle. If this connective tissue is thought of as an elastic band acting in parallel to the contractile machinery, at certain lengths the contractile machinery will produce force and the band will be slack, but as the length of the contractile machinery increases the band will eventually become taut and also exert a force. At extreme lengths, the forces caused by the connective tissue will stop overextension of the muscle fibres (Purslow 1989). The properties of the connective tissue are not purely elastic; the force they produce also depends on the velocity at which they change length. However, the elastic band analogy stresses an important feature, namely that at a certain point in the force–length curve of muscle the connective tissue is stretched to longer than its resting length and produces a force.

In Fig. 3.8 the force–length curve is demonstrated for two different muscles. Each of the muscles starts to produce force from the parallel elastic component at a different point in the force–length curve, indicating different relative resting lengths of the parallel elastic component in each of the muscles. The amount of force produced as the parallel elastic component is extended beyond its resting length is

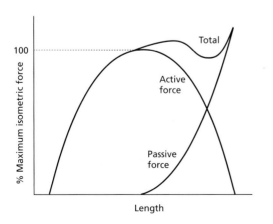

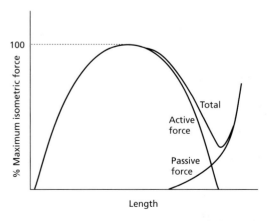

Fig. 3.8 The force–length curve of two muscles with different parallel elastic component contributions to the force output of the muscle. (Adapted from Wilkie 1968.)

different for each muscle depending on the parallel elastic component's resting length. In whole muscles the contributions to force from the parallel elastic component will vary and will be a function of the amount of connective tissue in each muscle—the greater the amount of tissue the larger the forces.

If a limb is forced to rotate about a joint but with no muscular activity of the muscles crossing the joint, there will still be a resistance to that motion caused by the passive structures crossing that joint. This passive resistance to motion has been assessed for most human joints (e.g. Hayes & Hatze 1977; Siegler *et al.* 1984; Engin & Chen 1986; Vrahas *et al.* 1990) and is largest towards either extreme of the joint's range of motion. Johns and Wright (1962) examined the sources of this resistance to passive motion in the wrist of the cat. Their analysis showed that in the mid-range of movement 51% of the resistance was caused by the muscle-tendon complexes crossing the joint, while the joint capsule was responsible for the majority of the remainder of the resistance (47%). Assuming similar ratios in humans, the passive properties of muscle contribute significantly to the passive moment profile at joints. This passive moment can provide an important contribution to human movement. To activate muscle takes time as the appropriate signals are sent to the muscles to produce force, and even when the signal reaches the muscle the generation of force is not instantaneous. During an unexpected perturbation there is a delay before the muscles respond appropriately to resist the externally caused motion. The parallel elastic components do not require nervous activation to produce force, and are present before the muscles can respond. These passive forces can help to halt unwanted joint extension in contact sports when the body experiences an unexpected impact, especially in view of the fact that these forces are largest at the extremes of a joint's range of motion.

The forces muscle fibres generate are applied to the skeletal system via tendon. Tendon consists predominantly of the protein collagen. Harkness (1961) examined the Achilles tendon of man, and found it to be composed of 86% collagen. When viewed under a light microscope tendons have a crimped wavelike appearance. Dale and Baer (1974) showed

that this crimping (actually in the collagen) unfolds during the initial loading of the tendon. Tendon is not uniform along its whole length; for example, the insertion onto the bone is a gradual transition from tendon to fibrocartilage. The tendon is anchored onto the bone by fibres from the periosteum of the bone (Cooper & Misol 1970).

The properties of tendon are normally examined by applying a certain stress (force per unit area) and measuring the strain (deformation of the material), then repeating the procedure for a range of stresses. Such measures tell us that tendon typically breaks at a strain of 0.08–0.10, i.e. when it is stretched to a length 8–10% greater than its resting length (Rigby *et al.* 1959; Bennet *et al.* 1986). For a particular strip of tendon connected to a muscle, it is simpler to look at the force the muscle produces and the amount of extension in the tendon this produces, rather than considering stress–strain relationships. Figure 3.9 shows the force–extension curve for a strip of tendon, with the amount of extension of the tendon increasing with increasing force. The low force end of the curve is the so called 'toe' region; here small amounts of force cause the uncrimping of the collagen. This phase of tendon loading causes relatively large amounts of tendon extension. The curve shows both the loading and unloading of the tendon; these two curves do not overlie one another, but demonstrate a hysteresis. This means that not all of the energy stored in the tendon during loading is returned during unloading. The gap between the

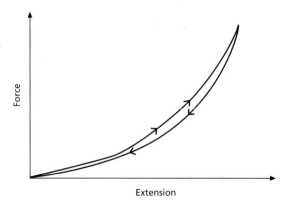

Fig. 3.9 The force–extension curve of a tendon. The arrows reflect the direction of loading and unloading.

two curves indicates the efficiency of tendon as an energy store. For a variety of mammalian tendons the energy loss is between 6% and 11%, indicating it is a very efficient energy store (Bennet *et al.* 1986). The tuning of the properties of tendon to the contractile element with which it lies in series has an important impact on human movement (see 'Interactions in the muscle-tendon complex' below).

The myofibrils in series and parallel comprise the contractile component of the muscle-tendon complex. Tendon is often referred to as a series elastic component because it is an elastic material which lies in series with the contractile component. However, in a muscle the line of action of the muscle fibres is not always coincident with that of the tendon. These elastic properties have important implications for the *in vivo* performance of skeletal muscle.

As well as tendon external to the muscle belly there may also be significant amounts of tendon inside the muscle belly (aponeurotic tendon). The properties of the external and internal tendon are the same (Proske & Morgan 1987). The amount of such tendon depends on the relative arrangement of the muscle fibres and tendon, and this is discussed in the following section.

Muscle pennation

In many human skeletal muscles the fibres may be orientated at an angle to the tendon external to the muscle belly. The angle between the tendon and muscle fibres is called the pennation angle (Fig. 3.10). If the pennation angle is zero then the muscle is said to be parallel fibred or fusiform. There are a variety of types of muscle pennation: principal among these are unipennate, where all the fibres are aligned in one direction, and bipennate, where they are aligned in two directions. Muscle pennation angles vary between individuals. Wickiewicz *et al.* (1983) dissected three cadavers and reported different pennation angles for the same muscle. For example, the vastus intermedius in two of the cadavers had a pennation angle of 5° whilst in the other the angle was 0° (it was parallel fibred). Table 3.1 shows the ranges of angle of pennation for some human muscles.

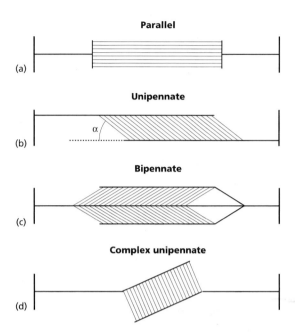

Fig. 3.10 Illustration of different organization of muscle and tendon, including parallel fibred (fusiform), unipennate and bipennate. The angle describing the orientation between the external tendon and muscle fibres is α, the angle of pennation.

The maximum isometric force a muscle belly can produce is a direct function of the number of myofilaments in parallel with one another. If the cross-sectional area (CSA) of a muscle is measured in the plane perpendicular to the long axis of the limb, then for a parallel fibred muscle the force in the tendon is equal to the muscle fibre force and is directly proportional to the cross-sectional area. For a pennated muscle the same relationship does not hold, and account must be taken of the angle of

Table 3.1 The ranges of muscle pennation reported for some human muscles. (Data from Yamaguchi *et al.* 1990.)

Muscle	Pennation angle (deg.)
Gluteus maximus	3.4–5
Gluteus medius	8.0–19.0
Gluteus minimus	5.0–21.0
Biceps femoris	7.0–17.0
Gastrocnemius medialis	6.5–25.0
Gastrocnemius lateralis	8.0–16.0

pennation. For a pennated muscle the following relationship can be stated:

$$F_T = F_F \cos(\alpha) \propto \cos(\alpha) \times \text{PCSA} \qquad (3.1)$$

where F_T is the force in tendon, F_F is the force produced by the muscle fibres, α is the angle of pennation, and PCSA is the muscle's physiological cross-sectional area. (Note the symbol $\propto$ means proportional to.) To allow for the pennation angle the concept of *physiological cross-sectional area* (PCSA) has been introduced. In essence the PCSA is the cross-sectional area of the muscle measured in a plane perpendicular to the line of action of the muscle fibres. For a parallel fibred muscle the following is true:

$$F_T \propto \text{CSA} \quad (\text{CSA} = \text{PCSA}) \qquad (3.2)$$

whilst for a pennated muscle:

$$F_T \propto \text{PCSA} \quad (\text{CSA} < \text{PCSA}) \qquad (3.3)$$

With cadavers the PSCA of a muscle can be measured by a variety of means. *In vivo* medical imaging techniques (e.g. magnetic resonance imaging) can be used to estimate PSCA, usually by taking serial images of the muscle along its length and from these measuring the muscle volume, and then applying the following formula:

$$\text{PCSA} = \frac{\text{Volume} \cos(\alpha)}{\text{FL}} \qquad (3.4)$$

where FL is the fibre length (e.g. Fukunaga *et al.* 1996). For a number of human muscles the PCSA has been measured, and such data permit an evaluation of the individual muscles' potential contributions at a joint. Table 3.2 shows both the CSA and the PCSA of the major ankle plantarflexors—the larger the PCSA the greater the maximum force the muscle can produce.

If the muscle fibres are orientated at an angle α to the tendon then the force in the tendon, which is the same force that is transmitted to the skeletal system, is obtained from

$$F_T = F_F \cos(\alpha) \qquad (3.5)$$

The cosine of zero is one, so for a parallel fibred muscle all of the force is transmitted to the tendon. With increasing angles of pennation the cosine term

Table 3.2 The cross-sectional (CSA) and physiological cross-sectional (PCSA) areas of major human ankle plantarflexors. (Mean data from Fukunaga *et al.* 1992.)

Muscle	CSA (cm^2)	PCSA (cm^2)
Medial gastrocnemius	16.49	68.34
Lateral gastrocnemius	11.24	27.78
Soleus	29.97	230.02
Flexor hallucis longus	4.85	19.32
Tibialis posterior	5.40	36.83
Flexor digitorum longus	1.59	9.12

decreases (e.g. $\cos(10) = 0.98$, $\cos(20) = 0.94$, $\cos(30) = 0.87$) so less force is transmitted to the tendon. Therefore, pennation has an immediate effect on the output of the muscle fibres. For a given force produced by the muscle fibres, less is transmitted to the external tendon. A change in fibre length also results in less change in the muscle belly length, and the velocity of shortening of the muscle fibre length is less than that of the whole muscle belly. The advantage of pennation is that it allows the packing of a large number of fibres into a smaller cross-sectional area. Figure 3.11 illustrates two muscles, both with the same number of fibres of the same thickness, one parallel fibred and the other with a pennation angle of 30°. The parallel fibred muscle is thicker than the pennated muscle, so by increasing the pennation angle, with all other factors being equal, thickness of the muscle belly decreases.

The degree of muscle pennation changes the way muscular mass is distributed along the length of a limb. The pennated arrangement can allow more of the muscle mass to be closer to the joint, compared with the distribution for parallel fibred muscles. This distribution of the muscular mass reduces the segmental moment of inertia about axes of rotation passing through the joint, corresponding to a reduction in the limb's resistance to rotation. Table 3.2 illustrates that the muscles associated with the shank are pennated, thus focusing more muscular mass nearer the proximal joint axes of rotation of the limb than would be achieved if the muscles were all parallel fibred.

Examination of different muscles in terms of their length, pennation and PCSA gives insight into their

Parallel fibred

Unipennate

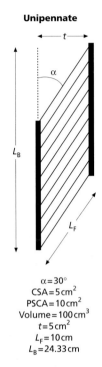

L_B and L_F

t

L_B

α

t

L_B

L_F

$\alpha = 0°$
CSA = 10 cm^2
PSCA = 10 cm^2
Volume = 100 cm^3
t = 10 cm
L_F = 10 cm
L_B = 10 cm

$\alpha = 30°$
CSA = 5 cm^2
PSCA = 10 cm^2
Volume = 100 cm^3
t = 5 cm
L_F = 10 cm
L_B = 24.33 cm

Fig. 3.11 The influence of pennation angle on the thickness of muscle. CSA, cross-sectional area; PSCA, physiological cross-sectional area.

role. For example, the human soleus has relatively high pennation angles, short fibres, and a large cross-sectional area, which means it is well designed to produce large forces. In contrast, the gastrocnemius has longer fibres, a smaller angle of pennation, and a smaller cross-sectional area. In comparison to the soleus the gastrocnemius can produce lower forces but can operate over a greater range and at higher velocities of shortening. Support for the implied functional adaptations of these muscles comes from the data of Johnson *et al.* (1973) who examined the fibre type distribution in these muscles and found the soleus to be composed of predominantly type I (slow) fibres, and both heads of the gastrocnemius to have a homogeneous distribution with equal amounts of type I and type II (fast) fibres.

This architectural property of muscle is not as simple as presented because as a pennated muscle shortens the pennation angle changes. Herbert and Gandevia (1995) used computerized sonography to measure the pennation angle of the human brachialis (an elbow flexor). Their results show that as the muscle shortens its pennation angle increases, in this case from around 9° to 25°. Muscle shortening will occur as muscle fibres shorten to generate force. In addition, as a joint angle reduces from full extension the muscle-tendon complex generally needs to be shorter to be able to actively apply forces to the skeleton, therefore with decreasing joint angle the muscle fibres have to be shorter in order to reduce muscle-tendon complex length. Hence, with muscle shortening, pennation angle increases which in turn means that there is a concomitant change in transfer from the muscle fibres to the external tendon.

With strength training one of the adaptations of muscle is additional muscular mass caused by the fibres becoming thicker (hypertrophy). If a muscle hypertrophies then it would be anticipated that this would be accompanied by the muscle becoming thicker. If great increases in muscle thickness are to be avoided this can be achieved by simultaneously increasing muscle pennation angle. The muscle fibres can become larger but with an increase in pennation angle there need not be a concomitant increase in muscle thickness. Kawakami *et al.* (1993) used ultrasound to measure changes in pennation angle in the human triceps brachii due to strength training. Their results showed a clear increase in pennation angle with strength training. Considering that increasing pennation angle reduces the output from the muscle fibres to the tendon there must be subtle trade-offs occurring when increased pennation is part of the adaptation associated with increased strength.

The representation of muscle architecture shown in Fig. 3.11 serves to illustrate how the key properties of muscle are influenced by pennation. Van Leeuwen and Spoor (1992) demonstrated that the orientation of muscle fibres and aponeurosis as shown in Fig. 3.10 creates muscles which are mechanically unstable. Muscle fibres in pennated muscle do not necessarily run in straight lines and can have curved paths, and the aponeurosis can also be curved. Van Leeuwen and Spoor (1992) identified in the human gastrocnemius curvature of both the muscle fibre paths and the aponeurosis. More realistic representations of muscle pennation therefore have the aponeuroses at an angle to the external tendon (e.g. Fig. 3.10d), and allow for curved muscle fibres and aponeuroses. A complete understanding of muscle *in vivo* will require greater investigation of these phenomena.

Interactions in the muscle-tendon complex

When examining how muscles produce moments at the joints it is important to consider the role of the whole muscle-tendon complex. The forces pro-duced by the muscle fibres are transmitted to the skeleton via tendon. The resulting changes in joint angles and angular velocities will depend on the length and velocity of the muscle-tendon complex (see next section). As tendon is an elastic material, its length changes as forces are applied to it. Tendon compliance has a significant effect on the properties and functioning of the muscle-tendon complex.

As a preliminary illustration of the role of the elastic tendon consider a muscle-tendon complex whose ends are fixed (see Fig. 3.12). As the muscle fibres shorten to generate more force the tendon stretches (albeit somewhat exaggerated in the figure). Therefore, under isometric conditions, where the length of the muscle-tendon complex does not change, the tendon actually lengthens whilst the muscle fibres shorten. The length of the muscle-tendon complex is the sum of the length of the fibres and the length of the external tendon for parallel fibred muscles (similar relationships exist for pennated muscles). This implies that *in vivo* joint angle changes can be achieved by shortening of muscle fibres and lengthening of the tendon. The force–length properties of the muscle-tendon complex are not therefore the same as those of the fibres. The muscle-tendon velocity can be represented by the following equation:

$$V_{MT} = V_F + V_T \qquad (3.6)$$

where V_{MT} is the velocity of the muscle-tendon complex, V_F is the velocity of the muscle fibres, and V_T is the velocity of the tendon. So as the muscle-tendon complex contracts, its velocity is equal to the sum of the tendon and muscle fibre velocities, where these two latter quantities need not be equal. Indeed, the

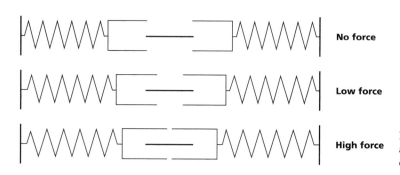

No force

Low force

High force

Fig. 3.12 The extension of tendon and shortening of the muscle fibres during an isometric muscle action.

elasticity of tendon means that it is unusual for tendon and fibre to have the same velocities. In the following paragraphs the extent to which tendon may lengthen is discussed, as well as the influence of this lengthening on muscle-tendon complex properties. The analysis of these properties and those presented to date are for parallel fibred muscles, although the same principles apply with little modification to pennated muscles.

Human tendon is not very compliant, snapping once stretched to 10% of its resting length. Measurements made *in vivo* in humans and other animals typically report that tendon is stretched between 2 and 5% by the maximum isometric force of its muscle fibres (e.g. Morgan *et al.* 1978; Woittiez *et al.* 1984; Bobbert *et al.* 1986a; Loren & Lieber 1995). The maximum forces a tendon will experience will be greater than the maximum isometric force because maximum forces are larger under eccentric conditions, but even so the stretching of tendon seen *in vivo* leaves a significant safety margin between peak strain and breaking strain. Muscles vary in the length of their external tendon, which means they vary in the extent to which the whole muscle-tendon complex length is influenced by tendon extension. To understand these variations it is useful to compare muscles in terms of the ratio of their external tendon length to muscle fibre length. In equation form:

$$\text{ratio } 1 = \frac{L_{\text{TR}}}{L_{\text{F,OPTIM}}} \tag{3.7}$$

where L_{TR} is the resting length of the external tendon, and $L_{\text{F,OPTIM}}$ is the length of the muscle fibres at their optimum length. If the tendon strain due to the maximum force produced by the fibres is the same for all muscles, then the higher this ratio the greater the contribution of tendon stretch to overall muscle-tendon length. In other words, the longer the tendon relative to the muscle fibres the more influence the tendon properties will have. Human muscles typically have ratio-1 values greater than one, indicating that the tendon is longer than the muscle fibres. Figure 3.13 shows four theoretical muscles and the influence of variations in tendon length, fibre length and maximum tendon extension under maximum isometric muscle force on the force–length proper-

ties of the whole muscle-tendon complex. Increasing both tendon extension and tendon length causes a shift of the force–length curve of the whole muscle-tendon complex to the left compared with the curves for the inelastic tendon, therefore increasing the operating range of the muscle-tendon complex. For pennated muscle the length of the muscle belly is the important factor dictating whole muscle-tendon complex force–length curves, but the principles presented still apply.

The stress applied to a tendon is directly proportional to the muscle PCSA, and the strain the tendon experiences is directly proportional to the tendon cross-sectional area (TCSA). The following ratio expresses the relationship between the tendon strain and the muscle stress

$$\text{ratio } 2 = \frac{\text{PCSA}}{\text{TCSA}} \tag{3.8}$$

Tendon does not generally have a cross-sectional area as large as the muscle fibres, with ratio-2 values normally between 10 and 100. The higher this ratio, the more strain the tendon experiences.

These two ratios provide insight into the functional adaptation of muscle designed to utilize the properties of tendon. For example, if both ratios are high then the force produced by the muscle fibres causes larger stretches in long tendons, which causes a large change in muscle-tendon complex length. Conversely, if both ratios are low then the maximum muscle force does not cause much change in the length of the tendon, which is short anyway; therefore tendon extension only causes small changes in muscle-tendon complex length. Table 3.3 presents the ratios for a variety of human muscles. When the ratios are low, the muscle seems well adapted for fine control since when the fibres shorten to produce force there is only a modest change in tendon length. This control of muscle-tendon length (and therefore joint angle and angular velocity) does not require detailed allowance for tendon stretch. For example, the wrist muscles extensor carpi radialis brevis and extensor carpi radialis longus fall into this category. When the ratios are both high, potential changes in tendon length are relatively high. It has been argued that such changes are advantageous in movement because

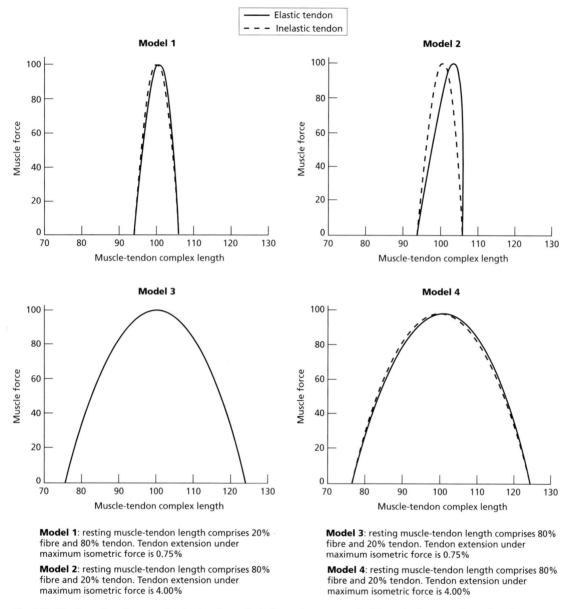

Fig. 3.13 The force–length properties for four hypothetical muscles compared with equivalent muscles with inelastic tendons.

the tendon can act as an energy store. Also, changes in tendon length can allow the muscle fibres to produce more force by enabling them to work for longer periods closer to their optimum length. The human gastrocnemius is an example of a muscle where both ratios are relatively high.

It is methodologically difficult to measure muscle and tendon length changes *in vivo*, but Roberts *et al.* (1997) successfully did this for running turkeys. They showed that during the support phase of running the muscle fibres of the turkey's lateral gastrocnemius remained at the same length whilst the

Table 3.3 The ratio of tendon length (L_{TR}) to muscle fibre length ($L_{F,OPTIM}$), and the ratio of muscle physiological cross-sectional area (PCSA) to tendon cross-sectional area (TCSA) for some human muscles. (Data extracted from Hoy *et al.* 1990; Loren & Lieber 1995; Woittiez *et al.* 1985.)

Muscle	Ratio 1 $= \dfrac{L_{TR}}{L_{F,OPTIM}}$	Ratio 2 $= \dfrac{PCSA}{TCSA}$
Vastii	2.68	–
Lateral gastrocnemius	8.85	96.3
Soleus	11.25	106.0
Hamstrings	3.60	–
Extensor carpi radialis brevis	2.89	16.4
Extensor carpi radialis longus	2.10	9.2
Extensor carpi ulnaris	3.67	13.4
Flexor carpi radialis	3.86	12.0
Flexor carpi ulnaris	4.96	13.3

changes in the length of the gastrocnemius muscle-tendon complex were achieved by the stretching and recoiling of the tendon. They idealized that the muscle fibres acted as rigid struts rather than the active generators of motion. Such an arrangement makes sense because muscles consume less energy when they perform isometric contractions compared with concentric contractions (Ma & Zahalak 1991). Eccentric contractions can be less costly than isometric contractions, but since during a cyclical activity the muscle fibres would have to shorten and lengthen, the net energy cost would be higher than when performing just an isometric contraction. Alexander *et al.* (1982) provide an extreme example of the use of tendon as an elastic energy store. In the camel the plantaris runs from the femur to the toes, with a few millimetres of muscle and over one metre of tendon. Any active changes of length of the muscles will have little effect on overall muscle-tendon length so these tendons act like springs which stretch during landing from a stride and recoil during the push-off. In humans, such extreme examples are hard to find but Alexander (1992) has provided evidence of how the human Achilles tendon functions in a similar fashion during running. The ground reaction forces during the support phase of running are sufficient to stretch the Achilles tendon to such an extent that the stretch and recoil of the tendon can account for most of the motion at the ankle joint during this phase of running.

In humans it is particularly hard to measure the changes in length of the muscle fibres and tendon *in vivo*. One way to circumvent these methodological problems is to use computer models which simulate the motion of interest and estimate muscle fibre and tendon behaviour. Bobbert *et al.* (1986b) simulated the activity of the triceps surae during maximum vertical jumping. Their results show that in both the soleus and gastrocnemius during the final phase of the jump the tendon had a higher velocity of shortening than the muscle fibres. Therefore, the overall velocity of the muscle-tendon complex is greater than that of the muscle fibres. At higher velocities of shortening, the muscle fibres produce less force (Fig. 3.4), so allowing the tendon to shorten at a higher velocity permits the fibres to shorten at a lower velocity but with greater force. This recoiling of the tendon is hypothesized to occur due to stretching of the tendon during the counter-movement phase of the jump.

The muscle cross-bridges do exhibit a degree of elasticity (Huxley & Simmons 1971), but this elasticity is less than that of the tendons and is dependent upon the degree of activity of the fibres and their length. Alexander and Bennet-Clark (1977) have demonstrated that as a general principle, if the tendon is longer than the muscle fibres, the tendon is the predominant site of energy storage.

The aponeurosis in pennated muscle is essentially the same material as the tendon external to the muscle belly; therefore as the muscle fibres generate force the aponeurosis is stretched beyond its resting length. Otten (1988) showed that if the aponeurosis was assumed to be elastic this caused an increase in the active range of the force–length properties of the muscle belly, similar to that illustrated in Fig. 3.13. The stretching of the aponeurosis may be heterogeneous (Zuurbier *et al.* 1994), which probably means that, depending on where they are attached to the aponeurosis, different fibres in a pennated muscle could be operating at quite different lengths. It is also important to consider that the aponeurosis may be an important energy store like the external tendon. Such subtleties of muscle-tendon design have yet to be fully elucidated.

Muscle-tendon line of action

The resultant joint moment is the sum of the moments caused by the muscles crossing the joint, the moment caused by articular contact forces, and the moments due to the ligaments. It is only the muscular moments which are under direct control of the nervous system. In the preceding sections, reference has been made to the factors which dictate muscle forces, but it is also important to consider the translation of these linear forces to the rotational

moments at the joints. The moment for a given muscle is the product of the tendon force and the muscle's moment arm. The moment arm of a muscle depends on its line of action relative to the joint centre of the joint it is crossing. Figure 3.14a shows how the moment arm of the human biceps brachii varies with the elbow joint angle. The relationship is not linear and is influenced by a number of factors including the fact that the joint centre is not normally in a fixed position but changes as the bony structures of the joint rotate about each other. Measurement of the moment arms of a variety of human muscles, both in cadavers and *in vivo*, have shown that they vary in a non-linear fashion with joint angle. Figure 3.14a demonstrates that even if the muscle-tendon complex produced the same forces for all lengths and velocities, there would still be variation in the moments these forces produce at the joint because of the muscle's variable moment arm.

Table 3.4 presents the maximum isometric force and the moment arms of the major elbow flexors for a given joint angle. The brachioradialis can produce less than a third of the force of the biceps but because of its larger moment arm it can produce two-thirds of the moment. Therefore, a large moment arm can compensate for a muscle not

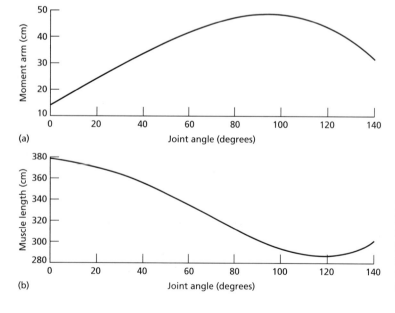

(a)

(b)

Fig. 3.14 For the human biceps brachii (a) the joint angle/muscle moment arm relationship, and (b) the joint angle/muscle length relationship, where 0 degrees is full elbow extension. (Based on the equations of Pigeon *et al.* 1996.)

Table 3.4 The maximum force, moment arm and maximum moment of the major elbow flexors for a given joint angle. (Data obtained from the model of Challis and Kerwin 1994.)

Muscle	Maximum force (N)	Moment arm (m)	Maximum moment (N · m)
Biceps brachii	600.6	0.036	21.6
Brachialis	1000.9	0.021	21.0
Brachioradialis	262.2	0.054	14.2

having a large PCSA and therefore low maximum force-production capacity. Such factors show how it is important not to consider the properties of a muscle-tendon complex in isolation of its moment arm.

As a joint angle changes, so must the muscle-tendon complex length if it is not to become slack; Fig. 14b shows the change in biceps length with joint angle. Muscles do not generally run in straight lines from their origins to their insertions, although this serves as a good first approximation to their line of action. To illustrate the influence of the line of action of a muscle on its properties, two hypothetical muscles are presented in Fig. 3.15. Both muscles are identical except for the locations of their origins and insertions. Varying their origins and insertions changes both the moment arm and muscle-tendon complex length of each of the muscles for a given joint angle. This approximation to reality clearly illustrates how influential this aspect of muscle architecture is on muscle properties.

To further illustrate the influence of the location of the origin and insertion of a muscle on the muscle's potential contribution to the moment at a joint, the two muscles in Fig. 3.15 are examined for a range of joint angles; these results are presented in Fig. 3.16. Muscle B has a larger moment arm than muscle A throughout the range of motion of the joint (Fig. 3.16a). This implies that all other things being equal, it will be able to produce higher joint moments than muscle A. The differences in moment arms of the two muscles also mean that a given change in muscle length will cause a much smaller change in joint angle for muscle A compared with muscle B. Figure 3.16b shows that muscle B is shorter than muscle A throughout the range of motion. How this affects the force-producing capacity of a muscle depends on the muscle's optimum length. For these

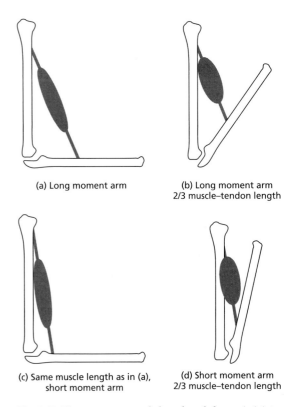

(a) Long moment arm

(b) Long moment arm 2/3 muscle–tendon length

(c) Same muscle length as in (a), short moment arm

(d) Short moment arm 2/3 muscle–tendon length

Fig. 3.15 Moment arm, muscle length and change in joint angle.

simulations it was assumed that their optimum muscle fibre lengths were equal, so for isometric conditions we obtain the curves in Fig. 3.16c. Note the peak isometric muscle force is produced at different joint angles for the two muscles due to their different muscle lengths at the same joint angles. The moment generated at a joint by a muscle is the product of the muscle force and moment arm. For these two muscles the maximum isometric moment

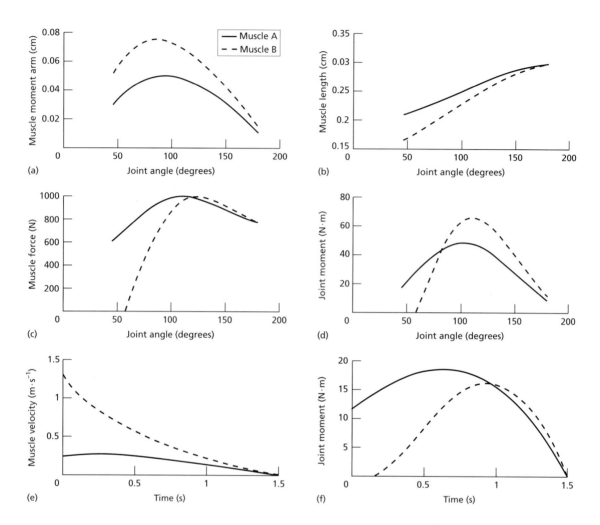

Fig. 3.16 Two theoretical muscles, A and B, have the same properties but different origins and insertions and this gives muscle B the larger moment arm. (a) Joint angle/muscle moment arm relationship. (b) Joint angle/muscle length relationship. (c) Joint angle/muscle force relationship under isometric conditions. (d) Joint angle/muscle moment relationship under isometric conditions. (e) Muscle velocity during joint extension at constant joint angular velocity. (f) Joint moment during joint extension at constant joint angular velocity.

throughout the joint's range of motion is shown in Fig. 3.16d, which illustrates how muscle B produces the largest joint moment throughout most of the joint range of motion, because the larger moment arm of muscle B compensates for its not producing muscle forces as high as muscle A for much of the range of motion.

Much of human movement is dynamic, so the two theoretical muscles were used to simulate an isovelocity joint extension. In these cases the assump-

tion was that the muscles were maximally active throughout the range of motion and the joint angular velocity was a constant $90° \cdot s^{-1}$. Muscle A has the smaller moment arm, which means that for a given change in muscle length this produces a larger change in joint angle than muscle B. Therefore, for this isovelocity joint extension muscle B, due to its large moment, has a greater muscle-shortening velocity throughout the range of motion compared with muscle A (Fig. 3.16e). The forces produced by these muscles were computed allowing for the force–length and force–velocity properties of the muscle fibres, and then their moment was computed by taking the product of their moment arm and muscle force. Under static conditions, muscle B could generally produce higher moments than muscle A; but, under these isovelocity conditions this was not the case as the force–velocity properties of muscle fibres were also important. When the moment generated by each of the muscles is computed, the influence of the force–velocity properties is highlighted. For much of the movement muscle A produces greater moments than muscle B due to its lower shortening velocity, despite muscle A having a smaller moment arm. There are a number of strength testing and training machines which endeavour to force a joint to maintain an isovelocity flexion or extension. These results also demonstrate that although the joints may be operating at constant velocity the muscles are not.

To summarize the results presented above, the location of the origin and insertion of a muscle has a significant effect on the moment-producing capacity of a muscle. If the moment arms are large, the muscle generally operates over a shorter range of motion than a muscle with smaller moment arms. But a muscle with larger moment arms will have to shorten at higher velocities than a muscle with smaller moment arms to produce the same joint angular velocity. These aspects of a muscle's properties are crucial and should be considered when examining the potential role or function of a muscle. For example, if a muscle has to produce a large moment at a joint under static or near static conditions it is possible for that muscle to compensate for not having a large PCSA by having large moment arms. In contrast, even though a muscle may be composed of predominantly type I fibres (slow), it is possible for a muscle to produce rapid joint extensions by having a small moment arm. Clearly the design and specialization of muscle is complex, with a number of important factors interacting with each other.

Summary

The contractile unit is the sarcomere, with muscle composed of many strings of sarcomeres. The force a sarcomere produces changes with its length in a parabolic fashion; it also changes with its velocity of shortening or lengthening. A shortening muscle can produce less force with increasing velocity. A lengthening muscle can produce more force as it yields to the force being applied to it. In whole muscle the more muscle fibres that are arranged parallel to one another, the greater the potential for generating force. In whole muscle, pennation allows for more efficient packing of muscle fibres. If the total range over which a muscle can produce force or maximum velocity of shortening is important then longer muscle fibres are required.

Muscle fibres are connected to the skeletal system via tendon. Tendon has important influences on muscle-tendon output. There are two key properties of tendon which indicate their function: their length relative to the length of the muscle fibres; and their cross-sectional area relative to the muscle's physiological cross-sectional area. There is evidence that having tendons which are relatively long and thin makes movement more efficient. In this case the tendon stretch and recoil can permit the muscle fibres to stay at a constant length, and therefore require less energy, or to shorten at lower velocities, and therefore produce greater force. In contrast, it is possible to have muscle-tendon complexes where the tendon does not exhibit large changes in length because the tendon is short relative to the muscle fibres or because the tendon is thick relative to the muscle fibres, or some combination of both. Such an adaptation is useful if fine control of movement is important because muscle length can be controlled without significant tendon stretch having to be accounted for.

The origin and insertion of a muscle influences the moment arm of the muscle about the joint. This moment arm is important because the forces the muscle-tendon complex produce are transformed into rotational moments, with the net moment being the product of the tendon force and the moment arm of the muscle. Therefore, muscles with larger moment arms produce larger moments than other muscles, all other things being equal. A muscle with a larger moment arm will have to shorten at higher velocities than a muscle with smaller moment arms to produce the same joint angular velocity. So, a muscle with a small moment arm can still produce large moments because during dynamic movements these muscles have the potential to shorten at lower velocities than muscles with large moment arms. Muscles which have fibre type distributions which indicate specialization for slow contractions may actually be capable of producing fast joint movements if the origin and insertion are arranged to give the muscle a small moment arm.

Most muscles in the human musculoskeletal system are designed to fulfil a number of different roles, therefore they are not easily classified as showing one specialization over another. But the preceding review has highlighted some of the ways in which muscle-tendon architecture can influence the forces and moments a muscle can produce and therefore how they influence athletic performance.

References

Alexander, R.M. (1992) *Exploring Biomechanics: Animals in Motion.* Scientific American Library, New York.

Alexander, R.M. & Bennet-Clark, H.C. (1977) Storage of elastic strain energy in muscle and other tissue. *Nature* 265, 114–117.

Alexander, R.M., Maloiy, G.M.O., Ker, R.F., Jayes, A.S. & Warui, C.N. (1982) The role of tendon elasticity in the locomotion of the camel (*Camelus dromidarius*). *Journal of Zoology* 198, 293–313.

Barany, M. (1967) ATPase activity of myosin correlated with speed of muscle shortening. *Journal of General Physiology* 50, 197–218.

Baskin, R.J. & Paolini, P.J. (1967) Volume change and pressure development in muscle during contraction. *American Journal of Physiology* 213, 1025–1030.

Bennet, M.B., Ker, R.F., Dimery, N.J. & Alexander, R.M. (1986) Mechanical properties of various mammalian tendons. *Journal of Zoology* 209, 537–548.

Bobbert, M.F.C., Brand, C., de Hann, A. *et al.* (1986a) Series elasticity of tendinous structures of the rat EDL. *Journal of Physiology* 377, 89P.

Bobbert, M.F., Huijing, P.A. & van Ingen Schenau, G.J. (1986b) A model of the human triceps surae muscle-tendon complex applied to jumping. *Journal of Biomechanics* 19, 887–898.

Challis, J.H. & Kerwin, D.G. (1994) Determining individual muscle forces during maximal activity: Model development, parameter determination, and validation. *Human Movement Science* 13, 29–61.

Close, R. (1964) Dynamic properties of fast and slow skeletal muscles of the rat during development. *Journal of Physiology* 173, 74–95.

Cooper, R.R. & Misol, S. (1970) Tendon and ligament insertion: a light and electron

microscopic study. *Journal of Bone and Joint Surgery* 52A, 1–20.

Dale, W.C. & Baer, E. (1974) Fibre-buckling in composite systems: a model for the ultrastructure of uncalcified collagen tissues. *Journal of Materials Science* 9, 369–382.

Edman, K.A.P. (1979) The velocity of unloaded shortening and its relation to sarcomere length and isometric force in vertebrate muscle fibres. *Journal of Physiology* 291, 143–159.

Edman, K.A.P. & Reggiani, C. (1987) The sarcomere length-tension relation determined in short segments of intact muscle fibres of the frog. *Journal of Physiology* 385, 709–732.

Edman, K.A.P., Mulieri, L.A. & Scubon-Mulieri, B. (1976) Non-hyperbolic force-velocity relationship in single muscle fibres. *Acta Physiologica Scandinavica* 98, 143–156.

Edman, K.A.P., Reggiani, C., Schiaffino, S. & te Kronnie, G. (1988) Maximum velocity of shortening related to myosin isoform composition in frog skeletal muscle fibres. *Journal of Physiology* 395, 679–694.

Engin, A.E. & Chen, S.M. (1986) Statistical data base for the biomechanical properties of the human shoulder complex—II: Passive resistive properties beyond the shoulder complex sinus. *Journal of Biomechanical Engineering* 108, 222–227.

Faulkner, J.A., Clafin, D.R. & McCully, K.K. (1986) Power output of fast and slow fibers from human skeletal muscles. In: *Human Muscle Power* (eds N.L. Jones, N. McCartney & A.J. McComas), pp. 81–94. Human Kinetics Publishers, Champaign, IL.

Feinstein, B., Lindegard, B., Nyman, E. & Wohlfart, G. (1955) Morphologic studies of motor units in normal human muscle. *Acta Anatomica* 23, 127–142.

Fenn, W.O. & Marsh, B.S. (1935) Muscular force at different speeds of shortening. *Journal of Physiology* 85, 277–297.

Fukunaga, T., Roy, R.R., Shellock, F.G. *et al.* (1992) Physiological cross-sectional area of human leg muscles based on magnetic resonance imaging. *Journal of Orthopaedic Research* 10, 926–934.

Fukunaga, T., Roy, R.R., Shellock, F.G., Hodgson, J.A. & Edgerton, V.R. (1996) Specific tension of human plantar flexors and dorsiflexors. *Journal of Applied Physiology* 80, 158–165.

Gordon, A.M., Huxley, A.F. & Julian, F.J. (1966) The variation in isometric tension with sarcomere length in vertebrate muscle fibers. *Journal of Physiology* 184, 170–192.

Harkness, R.D. (1961) Biological functions of collagen. *Biological Review* 36, 399–463.

Hayes, K.C. & Hatze, H. (1977) Passive visco-elastic properties of structures spanning the human elbow joint. *European Journal of Applied Physiology* 37, 265–274.

Herbert, R.D. & Gandevia, S.C. (1995) Changes in pennation with joint angle and muscle torque: in vivo measurements in human brachialis muscle. *Journal of Physiology* 484, 523–532.

Herzog, W., Guimaraes, A.C., Anton, M.G. & Carter-Edman, K.A. (1991) Moment-length relations of rectus femoris muscles of speed skaters/cyclists and runners. *Medicine and Science in Sports and Exercise* 23, 1289–1296.

Hill, A.V. (1938) The heat of shortening and dynamic constants of muscle. *Proceedings of the Royal Society, Series B* 126, 136–195.

Hoy, M.G., Zajac, F.E. & Gordon, M.E. (1990) A musculoskeletal model of the human lower extremity: The effect of muscle, tendon, and moment arm on the moment-angle relationship of musculotendon actuators at the hip, knee, and ankle. *Journal of Biomechanics* **23**, 157–169.

Huijing, P.A. (1985) Architecture of the human gastrocnemius muscle and some functional consequences. *Acta Anatomica* **123**, 101–107.

Huxley, A.F. (1957) Muscle structure and theories of contraction. *Progress in Biophysics and Biophysical Chemistry* **7**, 257–318.

Huxley, A.F. & Simmons, R.M. (1971) Mechanical properties of cross bridges of frog striated muscle. *Journal of Physiology* **218**, 59P–60P.

Johns, R.J. & Wright, V. (1962) Relative importance of various tissues in joint stiffness. *Journal of Applied Physiology* **17** (5), 824–828.

Johnson, M.A., Polgar, J., Weightman, D. & Appleton, D. (1973) Data on the distribution of fiber types in thirty-six human muscles. *Journal of Neurological Science* **18**, 111–129.

Joyce, G.C. & Rack, P.M.H. (1969) Isotonic lengthening and shortening movements of cat soleus. *Journal of Physiology* **204**, 475–491.

Katz, B. (1939) The relation between force and speed in muscular contraction. *Journal of Physiology* **96**, 45–64.

Kawakami, Y., Abe, T. & Fukunaga, T. (1993) Muscle-fiber pennation angles are greater in hypertrophied than normal muscles. *Journal of Applied Physiology* **72**, 37–43.

Lieber, R.L., Loren, G.J. & Friden, J. (1994) *In vivo* measurement of human wrist extensor muscle sarcomere length changes. *Journal of Neurophysiology* **71**, 874–881.

Loeb, G.E., Pratt, C.A., Chanaud, C.M. & Richmond, F.J.R. (1987) Distribution and innervation of short, interdigitated muscle fibers in parallel-fibered muscles of the cat hindlimb. *Journal of Morphology* **191**, 1–15.

Loren, G.J. & Lieber, R.L. (1995) Tendon biomechanical properties enhance human wrist muscle specialization. *Journal of Biomechanics* **28**, 791–799.

Lutz, G.J. & Rome, L.C. (1994) Built for jumping: the design of the frog muscular system. *Science* **263**, 370–372.

Lynn, R. & Morgan, D.L. (1994) Decline running produces more sarcomeres in rat vastus intermedius muscle fibres than does incline running. *Journal of Applied Physiology* **77**, 1439–1444.

Ma, S. & Zahalak, G.I. (1991) A distribution-moment model of energetics in skeletal muscle. *Journal of Biomechanics* **24**, 21–35.

Mashima, H. (1984) Force-velocity relation and contractility in striated muscles. *Japanese Journal of Physiology* **34**, 1–17.

Meijer, K., Bosch, P., Bobbert, M.F., van Soest, A.J. & Huijing, P.A. (1998) The isometric knee extension moment-angle relationship: Experimental data and predictions based on cadaver data. *Journal of Applied Biomechanics* **14**, 62–79.

Morgan, D.L., Proske, U. & Warren, D. (1978) Measurement of muscle stiffness and the mechanism of elastic storage in hopping kangaroos. *Journal of Physiology* **282**, 253–261.

Otten, E. (1988) Concepts and models of functional architecture in skeletal muscle. *Exercise and Sport Sciences Reviews* **16**, 89–137.

Pigeon, P., Yahia, H. & Feldman, A.G. (1996) Moment arms and lengths of human upper limb muscles as functions of joint angles. *Journal of Biomechanics* **29**, 1365–1370.

Proske, U. & Morgan, D.R. (1987) Tendon stiffness: methods of measurement and significance for the control of movement. A review. *Journal of Biomechanics* **20**, 75–82.

Purslow, P.P. (1989) Strain-induced reorientation of an intramuscular connective tissue network: Implications for passive muscle elasticity. *Journal of Biomechanics* **22**, 21–31.

Rigby, B.J., Hirai, N., Spikes, J.D. & Eyring, H. (1959) The mechanical properties of rat tail tendon. *Journal of General Physiology* **43**, 265–283.

Roberts, T.J., Marsh, R.L., Weyand, P.G. & Taylor, C.R. (1997) Muscular force in running turkeys: the economy of minimizing work. *Science* **275**, 1113–1115.

Siegler, S., Moskowitz, G.D. & Freedman, W. (1984) Passive and active components of the internal moment developed about the ankle joint during

human ambulating. *Journal of Biomechanics* **17**, 647–652.

Street, S.F. & Ramey, R.W. (1965) Sarcolemma: Transmitter of active tension in frog skeletal muscle. *Science* **149**, 1379–1380.

Van Leeuwen, J.L. & Spoor, C.W. (1992) Modelling mechanically stable muscle architectures. *Philosophical Transactions of the Royal Society* **336**, 275–292.

Vrahas, M.S., Brand, R.A., Brown, T.D. & Andrews, J.G. (1990) Contribution of passive tissues to the intersegmental moments at the hip. *Journal of Biomechanics* **23**, 357–362.

Walker, S.M. & Schrodt, G.R. (1973) I segment lengths and thin filament periods in skeletal muscle fibers of the rhesus monkey and the human. *Anatomical Record* **178**, 63–82.

Wickiewicz, T.L., Roy, R.R., Powell, P.L. & Edgerton, V.R. (1983) Muscle architecture of the human lower limb. *Clinical Orthopaedics and Related Research* **179**, 275–283.

Wilkie, D.R. (1968) *Muscle.* St. Martin's Press, New York.

Woittiez, R.D., Huijing, P.A., Boom, H.B.K. & Rozendal, R.H. (1984) A three-dimensional muscle model: a quantified relation between form and function of skeletal muscle. *Journal of Morphology* **182**, 95–113.

Woittiez, R.D., Heerkens, Y.F., Holewijn, M. & Huijing, P.A. (1985) Tendon series elasticity in triceps surae muscles of mammals. In *Biomechanics: Current Interdisciplinary Research* (eds S.M. Perren & E. Schneider), pp. 623–628. Martinus Nijhoff Publishers, Dordrecht.

Yamaguchi, G.T., Sawa, A.G.U., Moran, D.W., Fessler, M.J. & Winters, J.M. (1990) A survey of human musculotendon actuator parameters. In: *Multiple Muscle Systems: Biomechanics and Movement Organization* (eds J.M. Winters & S.L.Y. Woo), pp. 717–773. Springer-Verlag, New York.

Zuurbier, C.J., Everard, A.J., van der Wees, P. & Huijing, P.A. (1994) Length-force characteristics of the aponeurosis in the passive and active muscle condition and in the isolated condition. *Journal of Biomechanics* **27**, 445–453.

Chapter 4

Eccentric Muscle Action in Sport and Exercise

B.I. PRILUTSKY

Definitions of eccentric muscle action and negative work and power

In sport and exercise, as well as in daily life, people perform movements by activating skeletal muscles. Depending on whether active muscles shorten, stretch or remain at a constant length, three major types of muscle action can be distinguished: *concentric*, *eccentric* and *isometric*. These three types of muscle action are often called concentric, eccentric and isometric contractions. The latter terminology might be confusing because the word 'contraction' has the meaning of shortening. Therefore in this chapter, the former terminology proposed by Cavanagh (1988)—concentric, eccentric and isometric muscle actions—is adopted.

A muscle is acting eccentrically if it is active (i.e. produces active force as opposed to passive force, see Chapter 2) and its length is increasing in response to external forces (e.g. weight of load, force produced by other muscles, etc.). Correspondingly, muscle is acting concentrically if it is active and shortens. When the length of active muscle is prevented from shortening by external forces and remains constant, the muscle performs isometric action.

Eccentric muscle action takes place in most athletic activities. Therefore, it is important to understand the biomechanical and physiological consequences of eccentric muscle action and how it may affect performance.

To characterize eccentric action in athletic movements and its influence on the physiological systems of the body, a quantitative definition of eccentric action is needed. Consider an isolated muscle with one end fixed and the other end attached to a load (Fig. 4.1). Intensity (or the rate) of eccentric action can be conveniently defined as the product $P_m = F_m \times V_m$, where F_m is muscle force applied to the load, V_m is muscle velocity (or the component of velocity at the point of force application along the line of muscle action), and P_m is power produced by muscle force (or muscle power). If force F_m is smaller than the weight of the load F_e, the load will be moving in the direction opposite to the exerted muscle force (i.e. in a negative direction). In this example, muscle will be performing eccentric action, and muscle power will be negative (Fig. 4.1a). The amount of eccentric action can be defined as the time integral of muscle power P_m, which equals negative work done by the muscle force, W_m. By similar methods, the rate and amount of concentric action can be defined as positive muscle power and positive muscle work, respectively (the product $F_m \times V_m$ is positive because V_m has the same positive direction as F_m; Fig. 4.1b). If muscle force does not produce power and does no work (i.e. the muscle force is equal to weight of the load and $V_m = 0$; Fig. 4.1c), the muscle performs isometric action.

Thus, for quantitative analysis of eccentric action in athletic activities, muscle forces and velocities should be recorded. Forces of individual muscles are typically estimated using mathematical modelling (for reviews, see Crowninshield & Brand 1981; Hatze 1981; Zatsiorsky & Prilutsky 1993; An *et al.* 1995; Herzog 1996; Tsirakos *et al.* 1997), although direct force measurements from selected muscles are also possible (Komi 1990; Komi *et al.* 1996).

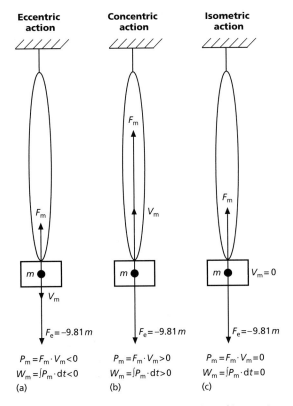

Eccentric action

$P_m = F_m \cdot V_m < 0$
$W_m = \int P_m \cdot dt < 0$
(a)

Concentric action

$P_m = F_m \cdot V_m > 0$
$W_m = \int P_m \cdot dt > 0$
(b)

Isometric action

$P_m = F_m \cdot V_m = 0$
$W_m = \int P_m \cdot dt = 0$
(c)

Fig. 4.1 Definitions of eccentric, concentric and isometric muscle actions and of negative and positive muscle work. (a) Eccentric muscle action takes place when force developed by the muscle, F_m, is smaller than an external force F_e (in this example, weight of mass m, $-9.81 \cdot m$) and the direction of displacement of the point of muscle force application is opposite to the direction of muscle force action. The intensity (or rate) of eccentric action is defined as negative muscle power ($P_m = F_m \times V_m < 0$, where V_m is the velocity component of the point of muscle force application along the line of muscle force action). The integral of P_m over the time of muscle force development defines the amount of eccentric action or negative muscle work, $W_m < 0$. (b) Concentric muscle action takes place when force developed by the muscle, F_m, exceeds an external force and the direction of displacement of the point of muscle force application is the same as the direction of muscle force action. The intensity of concentric action is defined as positive muscle power $P_m = F_m \times V_m > 0$. The amount of concentric action is defined as the time integral of power P_m or positive muscle work, $W_m > 0$. (c) Isometric action takes place when the magnitude of developed muscle force is equal to an external force and the point of muscle force application does not move, $V_m = 0$. The intensity and amount of muscle action is zero: $P_m = 0$ and $W_m = 0$.

Muscle lengths and the rate of their change are obtained from recorded joint angles and a quantitative description of musculoskeletal geometry (Morecki *et al.* 1971; Hatze 1981; Zatsiorsky *et al.* 1981; Delp *et al.* 1990; Pierrynowski 1995). The values of estimated muscle forces and work depend on model assumptions which are difficult to validate.

A more reliable although indirect method for muscle power estimation involves determining power of the resultant joint moment, which reflects the net effect resulting from action of all muscles and passive tissue around the joint: $P_j = M_j \times \omega_j$. In this product, ω_j and M_j are the components of joint angular velocity and the resultant joint moment about the joint axis perpendicular to the plane of interest, and P_j is the power produced by the moment, or joint power. M_j is calculated from recorded kinematics and external forces applied to the body using inverse dynamics analysis (Elftman 1939; Aleshinsky & Zatsiorsky 1978; Winter 1990). The integral of P_j over the time of muscle action yields joint work. The power and work of the joint moment are negative when the directions of M_j and ω_j are opposite (eccentric action, Fig. 4.2a). When M_j and ω_j have the same directions, joint power and work are positive (concentric action, Fig. 4.2b). When $M_j \neq 0$ and $\omega_j = 0$, joint power and work are zero (isometric action, Fig. 4.2c).

Other methods of estimating muscle power and work are more simple and less accurate and include:
• power and work done against external load;
• 'external work';
• 'internal work'; and
• 'total work'.

The latter three indices of work are calculated as the change of external, internal and total energy of the body, respectively (Fenn 1930; Cavagna *et al.* 1964; Pierrynowski *et al.* 1980). It should be mentioned that all the above indices of mechanical work represent work of different forces and moments which related to muscle forces indirectly (Aleshinsky 1986; Zatsiorsky 1986). Therefore, values of different indices of work done in human movements vary greatly (Pierrynowski *et al.* 1980; Williams & Cavanagh 1983; Prilutsky & Zatsiorsky 1992).

In this chapter, different aspects of eccentric muscle action are considered. First, selected facts

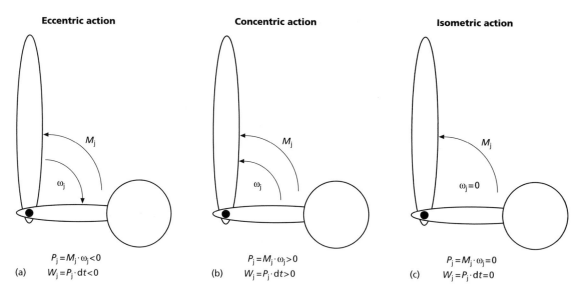

Eccentric action   **Concentric action**   **Isometric action**

$P_j = M_j \cdot \omega_j < 0$ $P_j = M_j \cdot \omega_j > 0$ $P_j = M_j \cdot \omega_j = 0$
(a) $W_j = P_j \cdot dt < 0$ (b) $W_j = P_j \cdot dt > 0$ (c) $W_j = P_j \cdot dt = 0$

Fig. 4.2 Definitions of eccentric, concentric and isometric actions based on negative and positive work of joint moment. (a) The intensity of eccentric action is defined as the negative power of joint moment ($P_j = M_j \times \omega_j < 0$, where M_j is the resultant joint moment and ω_j is the joint angular velocity). Note that M_j and ω_j have opposite directions. The time integral of P_j defines the amount of eccentric action or negative work of joint moment, $W_j < 0$. (b) The intensity of concentric action is defined as the positive power of joint moment ($P_j = M_j \times \omega_j > 0$; M_j and ω_j have the same directions). The time integral of P_j defines the amount of concentric action or positive work of joint moment, $W_j > 0$. (c) Isometric action takes place when the magnitude of the joint moment is equal and opposite to an external moment and there is no joint angle change, $\omega_j = 0$. The intensity and amount of muscle action are zero: $P_j = 0$ and $W_j = 0$.

relevant to the behaviour of isolated muscles during the stretch are reviewed below. Based on these facts, the following section demonstrates how eccentric action may affect various aspects of athletic performance. Comparisons between physiological responses to negative and positive work are then presented in the following section. The final section summarizes quantitative estimates of negative work done by major muscle groups in selected athletic events.

Mechanics and energetics of the isolated muscle during stretch

Muscle mechanical behaviour during and after stretch

While a fully activated muscle or a fibre is being stretched from one constant length to another with moderate speeds, the force recorded on its end

exceeds the maximum isometric force at the same muscle length (Fig. 4.3). At the end of stretch, the force can be two times larger than the maximum isometric force at the same length, so-called 'force enhancement during stretch'. This force enhancement is velocity dependent—force typically increases with the magnitude of stretch velocity (Levin & Wyman 1927; Katz 1939; Edman et al. 1978). When the stretch is completed and the muscle length is kept constant at a new level, force starts decreasing, but is still larger than the force corresponding to isometric action. This so-called 'residual force enhancement after stretch' lasts as long as the muscle is active (Katz 1939; Abbott and Aubert 1952; Edman et al. 1978; Sugi & Tsuchiya 1981; Edman & Tsuchiya 1996). The residual force enhancement after stretch appears when the muscle is stretched above the optimal length L_o (the length at which the muscle develops the maximum force) (Edman et al. 1978; Edman & Tsuchiya 1996).

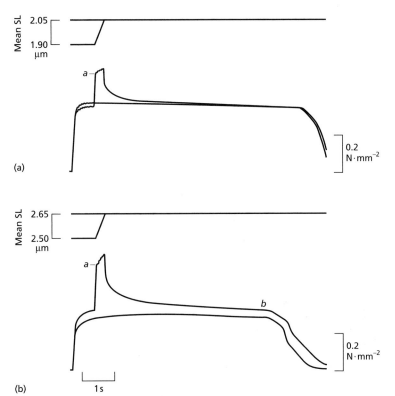

Fig. 4.3 Force and displacement records from a frog single muscle fibre during tetani at two different sarcomere lengths (SL). (a) Stretch during activity from 1.9 to 2.05 μm sarcomere length compared with ordinary isometric tetanus at 2.05 μm. (b) Comparison of stretch from 2.50 to 2.65 μm sarcomere length with isometric tetanus at 2.65 μm. The velocity dependent force enhancement during stretch is denoted by *a*, whereas *b* indicates the residual force enhancement after stretch; the latter appears above optimal sarcomere length L_o. (From Edman & Tsuchiya 1996.)

The force enhancement during stretch is thought to be associated with the increased strain of attached cross-bridges during the stretch (Sugi & Tsuchiya 1988; Lombardi & Piazzesi 1990). The attached cross-bridges (Ford *et al.* 1981) and the tendinous structures (Jewell & Wilkie 1958) constitute the series elastic component (SEC) of the muscle. The force–length (or stress–strain) relationship of the SEC can be determined in quick-release experiments in which a fully activated muscle is suddenly released and allowed to shorten against different constant loads (Jewell & Wilkie 1958). The stress–strain relationship obtained for the SEC is non-linear and monotonic (Fig. 4.4): its instantaneous slope (or stiffness of the series component) is relatively low at low muscle forces and increases with increasing muscle forces. The area under the stress–strain curve equals elastic strain energy stored in the SEC during isometric development of a given force. The elastic energy is released during a release of the muscle. The amount of stored strain energy depends on SEC stiffness, the maximum force the muscle is able to develop at a given length, and the maximum SEC elongation. The SEC elongation in skeletal muscles at maximal isometric force is on average 5% of L_o (Close 1972). As previously mentioned, the muscle stretch can increase developed force by a factor of two. Correspondingly, strain energy stored in the SEC after stretching maximally activated muscle may also increase up to two times (Fig. 4.4). This in turn may contribute to the ability of the muscle to shorten against heavier loads at a given shortening velocity or to shorten faster at a given load compared with a muscle being released from the isometric state (Cavagna & Citterio 1974). The influence of stretch on muscle performance is more pronounced at slow shortening velocities than at fast ones (Fig. 4.5). Release of a fully activated muscle immediately after the muscle is stretched increases positive work done by the muscle up to two times (Cavagna *et al.* 1968). The work enhancement was reported to increase with the velocity of

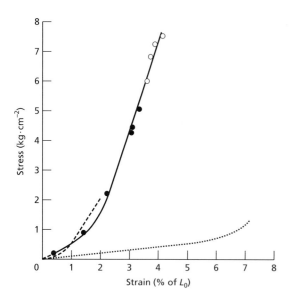

Fig. 4.4 Typical stress–strain curves of the series elastic component of frog gastrocnemius (solid line), of sartorius (dashed line) (data from Jewell & Wilkie 1958), and of rat gracilis anticus (dotted line) (data from Bahler 1967). The open circles refer to data obtained by releasing the muscle immediately after stretching, the filled circles by releasing the muscle in isometric contraction. The stress is expressed in kg · cm^{-2} of muscle cross-section and the strain as a percentage of muscle resting length, L_0. The lengthening of the series elastic component when the stress rises to its full isometric value of 5.2 kg · cm^{-2} is about 3% of the L_0. The elastic energy stored in the series elastic component of frog gastrocnemius (area under solid line) up to P_0 and normalized to muscle mass is on average 55 g · cm · g^{-1}; an additional amount of 63 g · cm · g^{-1} is stored during stretching the active muscle. (From Cavagna 1970.)

the stretch, initial muscle length, and temperature, and to decrease with a pause between the stretch and shortening (Cavagna *et al.* 1968, 1994). The reasons for this enhancement of positive power and work are not clear as the elastic energy stored in the strained cross-bridges is fully discharged by a small muscle release (for further discussion and references, see Edman & Tsuchiya 1996; Edman 1997).

The residual force enhancement after stretch (Fig. 4.3) is observed if the stretch is performed from an initial muscle length exceeding L_0. The mechanisms underlying the residual force enhancement are thought to originate from length non-uniformity

among sarcomeres in series (Julian & Morgan 1979; Morgan 1994; Edman & Tsuchiya 1996). The force–velocity relationship obtained from a muscle developing the residual force enhancement after stretch by releasing it against different constant loads behaves similar to the force–velocity relationship obtained from a muscle demonstrating the force enhancement during stretch (Fig. 4.5): the force–velocity curve shifts to the right with apparently no change in maximum shortening velocity (Edman *et al.* 1978).

Energetics of the muscle during stretch

Metabolic energy expenditure (energy liberated and ~P hydrolysis) of isolated skeletal muscles is lower during stretch of active muscle than during shortening or isometric development of force (Fenn 1923, 1924; Abbot *et al.* 1951; Curtin & Davies 1975). It was also reported that a substantial portion of muscle negative work (work done on the muscle) does not appear in the total muscle heat production (Abbot *et al.* 1951; Hill & Howarth 1959). Abbot *et al.* (1951) suggested three possibilities to explain the above facts:

(a) . . . the work is absorbed in driving backwards chemical processes which have actually occurred as a normal part of contraction; (b) . . . the work is absorbed in some other chemical or physical process at present unknown; and (c) . . . the work is wholly degraded into heat, but that chemical processes normally occurring in contraction are prevented by the stretch.

Evidence for the first and second possibilities was not found (Rall 1985; Woledge *et al.* 1985). It is more likely that the rate of ATP splitting is reduced during stretching of active muscle and the negative work is not utilized in the chemical reactions (Homsher & Kean 1978). The rate of ATP splitting is especially low at low velocities of stretch and can be four times lower compared with isometric force development at the stretch velocity of about $0.2 L_0 \cdot s^{-1}$ (Curtin & Davies 1975). At higher speeds of stretching, metabolic energy expenditure increases. Metabolic energy expenditure approaches the cost of isometric force development at the velocity which corresponds to negative power, the absolute value of which equals the maximum positive power that occurred during shortening of the muscle (Marechal 1964). With increasing stretch velocities further eccentric action becomes more expensive in terms of metabolic energy expenditure compared with isometric action (Marechal 1964), but still cheaper than concentric action (Fenn 1923, 1924).

A low rate of ATP splitting also occurs during the residual force enhancement after stretch (Homsher & Kean 1978; Curtin & Woledge 1979) despite the enhanced forces being produced.

Dissipation of energy

A muscle subjected to periodic stretching and shortening by an attached spring demonstrates damping of imposed oscillations or, in other words, dissipation of energy of oscillations (for terminology, see Zatsiorsky 1997). The ability of the muscle to dissipate energy increases with an increase in activation level (Gasser & Hill 1924) and with the magnitude of length change (Rack & Westbury 1974). For example, the damping of oscillation is approximately 40 times greater in an active muscle compared with a passive one (Fig. 4.6).

A muscle's ability to dissipate mechanical energy of the body seems to have important implications for such athletic activities as landing in gymnastics, where muscles acting eccentrically have to dissipate energy of the body in a short period of time (see 'Dissipation of mechanical energy'). The ability of muscles to dissipate energy is also important for preventing joint angles from reaching the

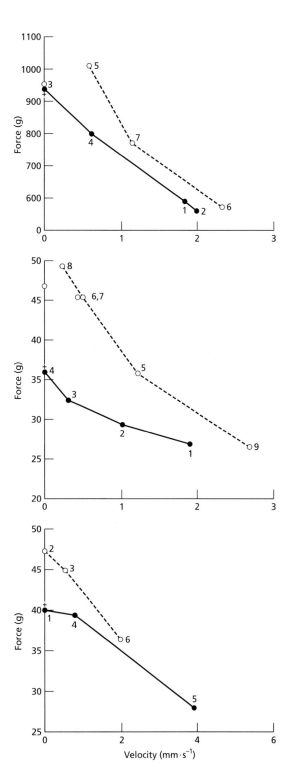

Fig. 4.5 Force–velocity relationships of frog gastrocnemius (top; L_o = 2.5 cm, 0.1–0.2°C), frog semitendinosus (middle; mass = 0.038 g, L_o = 2.5 cm, 0.2–0.6°C), and frog sartorius (bottom; mass = 0.058 g, L_o = 3.25 cm, 0.2–0.7°C). Filled circles and solid line: release from a state of isometric contraction; open circles and dashed line: release at the end of stretching. When the muscle is released immediately after stretching its speed of shortening is greater than when release takes place from a state of isometric contraction. In addition, after stretching the muscle is able to lift a weight greater than the isometric force at the length of release. The force developed by the parallel elastic elements before release was about 25 g for gastrocnemius, and 1 g for semitendinosus and sartorius. (From Cavagna & Citterio 1974.)

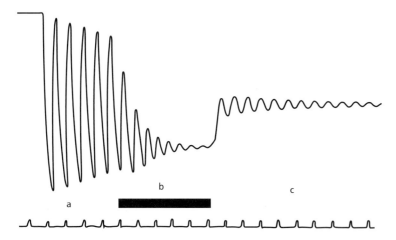

Fig. 4.6 Damping of oscillations in a spring connected to a muscle: (a) unexcited; (b) excited; (c) unexcited again. The damping becomes enormously greater when the muscle is excited. Time marks, 1/5 s. (From Gasser & Hill 1924.)

limits of their range of motion by decelerating body segments.

The data reviewed in this section demonstrate that eccentric muscle action may have important implications for improving athletic performance. First, stretching active muscles may lead to an enhancement of developed force, work and power during subsequent isometric and concentric actions. Second, this enhancement does not require additional metabolic energy expenditure and may increase economy and efficiency of subsequent isometric and concentric actions.

Influence of eccentric action on athletic performance

As previously mentioned, eccentric muscle action can potentially affect performance in athletic activities. A number of studies reviewed in this section support the above expectation.

Maximum moment production and muscle activation

The difference in maximum joint moment between different types of muscle action is clearly seen in moment–angular velocity curves (Fig. 4.7a). These curves are often obtained using isokinetic dynamometers which measure exerted moments at a constant joint velocity. The magnitude of joint moment is highest during eccentric action—the

moment increases with velocity at relatively low velocity values and then it stays at about the same level or declines slightly with velocity (for reviews, see Cabri 1991; Prilutsky 1991). The maximum eccentric moment exceeds the isometric moment by approximately 30–40% (Komi 1973; Barnes 1981; Cabri 1991), which is a smaller difference than seen in experiments on isolated muscles (Cavagna & Citterio 1974; Katz 1939). A smaller enhancement of eccentric moments *in vivo* may be partially explained by the inability of subjects to fully activate their muscles (Westing *et al.* 1990; Westing *et al.* 1991). When subjects' muscles are electrically stimulated, the difference between maximum eccentric and isometric moments increases and resembles results of *in vivo* experiments (Westing *et al.* 1990).

The magnitude of maximum eccentric moments is substantially higher than that of concentric moments (Fig. 4.7a). Since concentric moments sharply decline with angular velocity and eccentric moments do not decrease markedly, the difference in the magnitude between eccentric and concentric moments becomes larger as absolute values of angular velocity increase.

The hypothesis that eccentric exercises require fewer active muscle fibres than concentric exercises with the same resistance (Abbot *et al.* 1952; Asmussen 1953) is supported by lower values of the ratio electromyographic activity (EMG)/force (or the slope of EMG–force relationship) in eccentric action compared with concentric action (Fig. 4.8a;

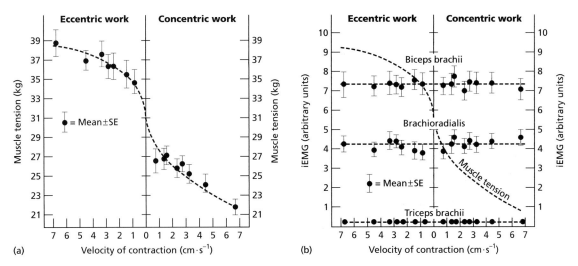

Fig. 4.7 (a) Force–velocity relationship for the human elbow flexor muscles. (b) Integrated EMG (iEMG)–velocity relationship for the human biceps brachii and brachioradialis muscles and their antagonist (triceps brachii). Muscle velocity was estimated from joint angular velocity and muscle moment arm; muscle force was estimated from the measured joint moment and muscle moment arm. (From Komi 1973.)

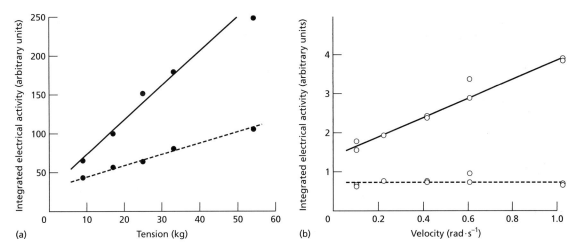

Fig. 4.8 (a) The relation between integrated electrical activity and tension in the human calf muscles. Shortening at constant velocity (solid line) and lengthening at the same constant velocity (dashed line). Each point is the mean of the first 10 observations on one subject. Tension represents weight lifted and is approximately 1/10 of the tension calculated in the tendon. (b) The relation between integrated electrical activity and velocity of shortening (solid line) and lengthening (dashed line) at the same tension (3.73 kg). Each point is the mean of the first 10 observations on one subject. (From Bigland & Lippold 1954.)

see also Asmussen 1953; Komi 1973; Bigland-Ritchie & Woods 1976; Heckathorne & Childress 1981). The EMG magnitude does not appear to depend on the rate of joint angle (or muscle length) changes during eccentric exercise against a constant resistance, whereas EMG in concentric exercises increases with velocity (Fig. 4.8b; see also Eloranta & Komi 1980). These facts are consistent, in general, with the force–velocity relationship (Fig. 4.7a). The EMG magnitude during maximum eccentric and concentric

Table 4.1 The increase in isometric strength after eccentric, concentric and isometric strength training (selected studies).

Subjects	Muscle group(s) (programme length)	Eccentric	Concentric	Isometric	Authors
16 men	Leg flexors Arm flexors (13 weeks, 2 days a week, 2 h a day)	53.6 kg of load 6.4 kg	51.9 kg 8.8 kg		Seliger *et al.* (1968)
26 men	Triceps brachii (30 days, 5 days a week, 2 series of 5 repetitions a day)	10.0 kg of load	8.7 kg		Mannheimer (1969)
21 men and women	Wrist flexors (10 days, 5 max. actions a day)	34.5%		50.2%	Moore (1971)
31 men	Forearm flexors (7 weeks, 4 times a week, 6 max. actions a day)	2.7 kg of load	2.0 kg		Komi and Buskirk (1972)

actions appears to be similar (Fig. 4.7b; Rodgers & Berger 1974; Komi & Viitasalo 1977; Seliger *et al.* 1980; Westing *et al.* 1990; however, see Enoka 1996).

Several authors have reported differences in motor unit behaviour between eccentric and concentric actions (Nordone *et al.* 1989; Howell *et al.* 1995; Enoka 1996): high-threshold motor units seem to be used more extensively in eccentric actions than in concentric actions, and the spike rate of the involved motor units is lower in eccentric actions compared with concentric. A larger involvement of high-threshold motor units in eccentric exercise is supported by the observation that after intensive eccentric exercise, signs of muscle fibre damage are seen more often in type II (fast-twitch) muscle fibres (Friden *et al.* 1983), which are controlled by high-threshold motor units. An alternative explanation for a preferential injury of fast-twitch muscle fibres in eccentric actions is that fast-twitch fibres may be more susceptible to stretch-induced damage because of a less-developed endomysium compared with slow-twitch fibres (Stauber 1989).

Is eccentric action more advantageous for isometric strength training than isometric and concentric actions because higher muscle forces can be produced during eccentric action? In most cases,

eccentric strength training does not lead to higher isometric strength and is comparable with isometric and concentric training (Table 4.1). Even when eccentric training is shown to be more effective for increasing isometric strength, it often has side-effects such as muscle injury and soreness (for reviews, see Armstrong 1984; Prilutsky 1989; Friden & Lieber 1992; see also Chapter 28). Therefore, it appears that combining different types of exercise is a better method for strength training. It should be noted that strength training may be action type specific (Kellis & Baltzopoulos 1995)—eccentric training may improve eccentric strength more than concentric (see e.g. Hortobagyi *et al.* 1996b). Some studies, however, demonstrate similar improvements in eccentric, isometric and concentric strength after eccentric training (Kellis & Baltzopoulos 1995).

Enhancement of positive work and power production

As demonstrated above (see 'Mechanics and energetics of the isolated muscle during stretch'), a preliminary muscle stretch causes a modification of the force–velocity relationship during shortening (Fig. 4.5) and increases strain energy stored in

Table 4.2 Enhancement of athletic performance immediately after eccentric action (selected studies).

Subjects	Movement	Eccentric action	Performance index	Enhancement	Authors
$N = 6$ 22–29 years	Leg extension from a squat position	Countermovement	Mean power	29%	Thys et al. (1972)
$N = 19$	Vertical jump	Countermovement	Jump height	0.02 m	Asmussen and Bonde-Petersen (1974a)
		Drop jump from:			
		0.233 m	Jump height	0.03 m	
		0.404 m	Jump height	0.042 m	
		0.690 m	Jump height	0.023 m	
$N = 5$	Vertical jump; Leg muscle temperature:	Drop jump from 0.4 m	Jump height		Asmussen and Bonde-Petersen (1974a)
	37°C			0.017 m	
	32°C			0.0462 m	
$N = 3$	Elbow flexion	Countermovement	Positive work per unit of EMG	23%	Cnockaert (1978)
	Elbow extensors	Countermovement		111%	
$N = 18$ 18–25 years	Push of pendulum	Countermovement at speed:	Pendulum speed		Bober et al. (1980)
		$0.91 \text{ m} \cdot \text{s}^{-1}$		$0.14 \text{ m} \cdot \text{s}^{-1}$	
		$1.37 \text{ m} \cdot \text{s}^{-1}$		$0.19 \text{ m} \cdot \text{s}^{-1}$	
		$1.82 \text{ m} \cdot \text{s}^{-1}$		$0.21 \text{ m} \cdot \text{s}^{-1}$	
		$2.27 \text{ m} \cdot \text{s}^{-1}$		$0.22 \text{ m} \cdot \text{s}^{-1}$	
		$2.72 \text{ m} \cdot \text{s}^{-1}$		$0.24 \text{ m} \cdot \text{s}^{-1}$	

the SEC (Fig. 4.4). If these changes of muscle mechanical properties take place *in vivo*, they may increase positive work and power production, which would be very useful in many athletic activities. Comparisons between positive work and power (or performance indices related to positive power, i.e. maximum movement velocity, jump height, etc.) obtained with and without preliminary muscle stretch often demonstrate enhancement in performance by the stretch (Table 4.2). The observed enhancement in muscle performance may also be caused by additional activation of muscles being stretched in the stretch–shortening cycle (SSC) (Dietz et al. 1979; Bosco et al. 1981). The nature of this additional activation is unclear, since the gain of stretch reflex may be low during running (Stein et al. 1993) where the enhanced activation occurs (Dietz et al. 1979).

The relative contribution to power enhancement of the above three mechanisms (change in force–velocity curve, increased amount of strain energy in SEC, and stretch reflex) is not known. Some authors question the use of strain energy to enhance positive power in human movements (van Ingen Schenau 1984; van Ingen Schenau et al. 1997) suggesting that its contribution is negligible and the enhancement of muscle performance is the result of a longer time available during the stretch to achieve maximum muscle activation before the concentric phase (van Ingen Schenau 1984; Chapman et al. 1985). Other authors argue, based on their estimations of strain energy stored in human muscle-tendon complexes, that the contribution of SEC can be substantial (see e.g. Hof 1998). In animal locomotion, a substantial (in some cases up to 90%) contribution of SEC strain energy to positive work and power during muscle shortening has been demonstrated using direct *in vivo* measurements of tendon forces (Prilutsky et al. 1996a), muscle fibre length (Griffiths 1991; Gregersen et al. 1998) or both (Biewener et al. 1998; Roberts et al. 1997).

The potential contribution of the stretch reflex to the enhancement of positive power requires metabolic energy consumption due to activation of additional motor units. The energy consumption requirement of the stretch reflex may be used for a separation of its contribution to enhanced performance from the contributions of the other two factors which require less or no additional energy expenditure (see 'Energetics of the muscle during stretch' above). For example, the lowest values of the peak positive power during the stance phase of running long jumps reported in the literature are 3000 W, 1000 W, and 2500 W for the ankle, knee, and hip joints, respectively (Tupa *et al.* 1980; Requejo *et al.* 1998; Stefanyshyn & Nigg 1998). Such high values of positive power do not seem to be accounted for by an estimated peak rate of metabolic power output (about 400 W · kg^{-1} of muscle mass; Hochachka 1985; Wasserman *et al.* 1986) and estimated mass of ankle, knee and hip extensors (from Yamaguchi *et al.* 1990). Thus, it is likely that there is an enhancement of positive mechanical power output in running long jumps that cannot be accounted for without the use of strain energy in SEC and/or the enhancement of the contractile mechanism leading to the shift of the force–velocity relationship.

The peak values of joint positive power in explosive movements performed immediately after the stretch exceed several times the maximum power measured or estimated from the force–velocity or moment–angular velocity curves of the same muscle groups (van Ingen Schenau *et al.* 1985; Edgerton *et al.* 1986; Gregor *et al.* 1988; Prilutsky *et al.* 1992), which is in agreement with the notion of enhancement of positive work and power by the muscle stretch.

Whatever the relative contribution of the three previously described factors to the enhancement of positive power and work in athletic performance might be, their combined effect appears to be substantial (Table 4.2). The performance enhancement depends on the rate of muscle stretch (Asmussen & Bonde-Petersen 1974a; Bober *et al.* 1980; Bosco *et al.* 1981), the time of transition from the stretch to shortening (Thys *et al.* 1972; Bosco *et al.* 1981), the percentage of slow-twitch fibres in the muscle (Viitasalo & Bosco 1982), muscle mechanical properties (Aruin

& Prilutsky 1985), muscle temperature (Asmussen *et al.* 1976), gender (Komi & Bosco 1978; Bosco & Komi 1980), and age (Bosco & Komi 1980).

Economy and efficiency of positive work

Economy of positive work can be defined as positive mechanical work done per unit of metabolic energy spent. Since there are many ways to determine positive mechanical work done (see 'Definitions of eccentric muscle action and negative work and power' above) and metabolic energy spent (Whipp & Wasserman 1969; van Ingen Schenau *et al.* 1997) during human movements, there are many indices of economy of positive work. Efficiency of positive work can be defined (for details, see Prilutsky 1997; Woledge 1997) as: $e_p = W_p/(\Delta E + W_n)$, where e_p is the efficiency of positive work, W_p and W_n are, respectively, the total positive and negative work done by muscles, and ΔE is chemical energy released from the muscles (which can be assessed by measuring the total metabolic energy spent). The term e_p can have different values depending on how W_p, W_n, and ΔE are measured; e_p cannot, however, exceed 1.

Given the facts reviewed in sections above it can be expected that economy and efficiency of positive work performed immediately after negative work (i.e. after muscle stretch) would exceed those of positive work done without a preliminary stretch. First, SEC is able to store more strain energy when the muscle is stretched compared with an isometric force development (Fig. 4.4). This additional energy can potentially be used in the subsequent shortening (see, however, Edman 1997, who questions such a possibility). Second, the shift of the force–velocity curve to the right (Fig. 4.5) does not require additional energy expenditure. Furthermore, energy expenditure required to resist the stretch (to do negative work) is relatively low (see 'Energetics of the muscle during stretch' above; and 'Oxygen consumption during eccentric and concentric exercise' below).

Experimental studies demonstrate that indices of positive work economy in movements where positive work is done immediately after a substantial amount of preliminary muscle stretch—in level running (Lloyd & Zacks 1972; Asmussen & Bonde-Petersen 1974b; Cavagna & Kaneko 1977), in counter-movement jumping (Asmussen & Bonde-Petersen 1974b; Thys *et al.* 1975; Aruin *et al.* 1977; Bosco *et al.* 1982; Kaneko *et al.* 1984; Voight *et al.* 1995), and in squatting (Aruin *et al.* 1979; Thys *et al.* 1972)—have higher values compared with the same indices obtained during walking and running uphill or cycling where muscles supposedly do little or no negative work (Margaria 1938; Whipp & Wasserman 1969). According to estimates of some authors, the contribution of the preliminary stretch to the increase of economy of positive work is 35–53% in running (Cavagna *et al.* 1964; Asmussen & Bonde-Petersen 1974b), 27–34% in squatting (Asmussen & Bonde-Petersen 1974b; Thys *et al.* 1972; Aruin *et al.* 1979), 30–60% in jumping (Bosco *et al.* 1982; Thys *et al.* 1975; Voight *et al.* 1995), and 23% in level walking (Asmussen & Bonde-Petersen 1974b).

Simultaneous *in vivo* measurements of forces and fibre length changes of selected ankle extensor muscles during running in turkey (Roberts *et al.* 1997) and tammar wallabies (Biewener *et al.* 1998) show that most of the positive work done by the studied muscle-tendon complexes resulted from the release of tendon and/or aponeurosis strain energy. As mentioned previously, the contribution of SEC strain energy to positive work in human movements is still under debate.

Dissipation of mechanical energy

In many athletic events which involve landing, the body experiences very high impact forces: the vertical ground reaction force can reach values that exceed body weight by 14 times (Tupa *et al.* 1980; DeVita & Skelly 1992; McNitt-Gray 1993; Simpson & Kanter 1997; Requejo *et al.* 1998), which may result in injuries (Dufek & Bates 1991; Nigg 1985). Two types of injury may occur due to extreme loads: injuries of passive anatomical tissue (ligaments, cartilage, intervertebral discs, etc.) and injuries of muscles. The mechanisms underlying both injury types are not yet precisely understood. If it is proven that the amount of mechanical energy absorbed by the passive tissues during landing impact is a major

contributor to their damage, then the ability of active muscles to dissipate mechanical energy (see 'Dissipation of energy' above) may be very useful in protecting passive anatomical structures.

The amount of mechanical energy passively dissipated can be estimated during barefoot landing on a stiff force plate after a drop jump (Zatsiorsky & Prilutsky 1987). To make this estimation, the percentage of energy dissipated by muscles is obtained as

$$\text{ISL} = \frac{\begin{array}{c}\text{Total negative work of joint}\\ \text{moments during landing}\end{array}}{\begin{array}{c}\text{Reduction in total energy of}\\ \text{the body during landing}\end{array}} \times 100\% \quad (4.1)$$

where ISL is the index of softness of landing (see below). In this approach, it is assumed that the total negative work done by joint moments during the landing is equal to the total negative work done by muscles, and that the nominator and denominator are equal during very soft landings. The latter assumption was verified. In maximally soft landings, the total negative work of joint moments and the reduction in total energy of the body were equal within the accuracy of measurements (Zatsiorsky & Prilutsky 1987; Prilutsky 1990). Note that in walking, running and other activities where power in different joints and changes in kinetic and potential energy of different segments do not always have the same sign, the total work of joint moments and the change in total energy of the body are not equal (Aleshinsky 1986; Zatsiorsky 1986). The index ISL represents the percentage of total energy of the body just before landing, which is dissipated by the muscles. The rest of the body's energy is dissipated by passive structures. In the maximum stiff landings that the subject could perform, up to 30% of the energy was dissipated passively (Zatsiorsky & Prilutsky 1987). If landing is performed on the heels by keeping the legs straight, no joint work will be done and all the energy of the body will be dissipated in the passive anatomical structures. Needless to say it would be very harmful for the body. It appears that athletes are able to regulate muscle behaviour during landing in order to maximize either 'spring' or damping properties of the muscles (Dyhre-Poulsen *et al.* 1991).

The ability of damping high impact accelerations in downhill skiing discriminates well between good and inexperienced skiers (Nigg & Neukomm 1973). Fatigue compromises the ability to attenuate and dissipate impact shock waves during running (Verbitsky et al. 1998; Voloshin et al. 1998), which suggests the involvement of active muscles in damping impact loads. It should be noted here that the enhancement of positive power and economy of positive work immediately after the stretch (see 'Economy and efficiency of positive work' above) and dissipation of energy of the body to protect passive anatomical structures appear to be conflicting demands, and maximizing one property would lead to compromising the other (Dyhre-Poulsen et al. 1991).

In several joints of the swing leg and the upper extremities, negative power is developed prior to their range of motion limit (Morrison 1970; Winter & Robertson 1978; Tupa et al. 1980; Prilutsky 1990, 1991). For example, the knee flexor muscles dissipate energy of the shank and prevent an excessive knee extension in the end of the swing phase during walking and running (see 'Negative work in athletic events' below). Another example of keeping joints within their range of motion by eccentric muscle action is the 'articulation' between the pelvis and the trunk whose relative rotation in the horizontal plane is controlled by muscles developing negative power (Prilutsky 1990). Thus, the muscle's ability for energy dissipation and damping of high-impact forces appears to play an important role not only in attenuating and dissipating impact shock waves, but also in protecting joints from exceeding their range of motion.

Electromechanical delay

The electromechanical delay (EMD) is the interval between the onset of muscle electromyographic activity and developed force or joint moment. According to the literature, EMD ranges from about 30 ms to 100 ms and higher (Cavanagh & Komi 1979; Norman & Komi 1979; Vos et al. 1991) and therefore constitutes a rather large part of the total reaction time, the time interval from the presentation of an unexpected stimulus to the initiation of the response (see e.g. Schmidt 1988). The type of

muscle action affects the duration of EMD. The shortest EMD typically occurs during eccentric action. For example, EMD determined for the biceps brachii during eccentric action is 38 ms (at the slow joint angular velocity) and 28 ms (at the faster velocity), whereas EMD during concentric action is 41 ms and is independent of joint velocity (Norman & Komi 1979). It is thought that a major portion of EMD is associated with the stretch of the SEC to a point where muscle force can be detected (Cavanagh & Komi 1979; Norman & Komi 1979; Grabiner 1986). Therefore, it seems that conditions for a rapid force development are more advantageous during eccentric action (Cavanagh & Komi 1979).

Fatigue and perceived exertion during eccentric action

Two major types of exercise-induced fatigue can be distinguished (Green 1997):

1 Metabolic fatigue, which is related to a failure to maintain desired ATP production rates and tolerate high accumulation of by-products of metabolic reactions.

2 Non-metabolic fatigue, caused by high internal muscle stress, which is believed to be associated with a disruption of internal muscle structures.

Eccentric muscle action is much less metabolically demanding than concentric and isometric actions (see 'Energetics of the muscle during stretch' above; and 'Oxygen consumption during eccentric and concentric exercise' below), and force per number of active muscle fibres is likely to be substantially higher during eccentric action compared with that of concentric and isometric actions (see 'Maximum moment production and muscle activation' above). Therefore, differences in fatigue between eccentric and other types of muscle action can be expected.

Moderate eccentric muscle action appears to cause substantially lower fatigue (smaller declines in developed force and power; Crenshaw et al. 1995; Hortobagyi et al. 1996a) and perceived exertion (Henriksson et al. 1972; Pandolf et al. 1978) compared with concentric action of the same intensity. Note that fewer muscle fibres are activated during eccentric exercise compared with concentric and isometric exercise against the same load.

During eccentric exercise of high intensity (corresponding to 90% of maximum oxygen uptake ($Vo_{2\text{-max}}$) in the corresponding concentric exercise), the subjects are reportedly incapable of continuing exercise for longer than 30 min (Knuttgen 1986). At the point of exhaustion, none of the signs of exhaustion typical for concentric exercise (high values of Vo_2 uptake, heart rate, muscle and blood lactate, etc.) are present (Knuttgen 1986). After 6 weeks of eccentric training with the same intensity, the subjects become able to continue exercise for several hours (Bonde-Petersen *et al.* 1973; Knuttgen *et al.* 1982). It has been thought that inability of untrained subjects to continue eccentric exercise is caused by damage of muscle fibres and inappropriate motor unit recruitment (Knuttgen 1986).

When eccentric and concentric actions are compared at the same oxygen consumption level or when eccentric and concentric exercises are performed with maximum effort, muscles fatigue faster in eccentric exercise (Komi & Rusko 1974; Komi & Viitasalo 1977; Jones *et al.* 1989). Hence, perceived exertion in eccentric exercise is higher than in the corresponding concentric exercise (Henriksson *et al.* 1972; Pandolf *et al.* 1978). Note that muscles develop higher forces in maximum eccentric than in maximum concentric exercise (Fig. 4.7).

Long-lasting SSC exercises (consisting of both eccentric and concentric actions) reduce the enhancement of positive work and power (Gollhofer *et al.* 1987; Avela & Komi 1998).

Physiological cost of eccentric action

In this chapter, we consider differences in physiological responses of the body to negative and positive work (eccentric and concentric actions). Several methods of setting equivalent magnitudes of negative and positive work have been used to study physiological differences between eccentric and concentric exercises. Most of the methods ensure that the subjects produce the same forces or moments at the same absolute values of the rate of muscle length or joint angle change in eccentric and concentric exercise. Three major groups of methods have been used most.

1 Lifting and lowering load (Chauveau 1896b).

2 Going up and down stairs (Chauveau 1896a)

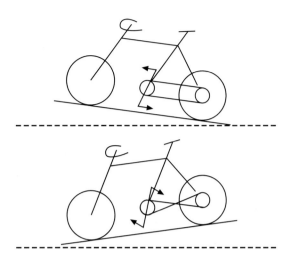

Fig. 4.9 Schematic drawing of a bicycle on the inclined treadmill. Arrangement for uphill and downhill riding. (From Asmussen 1953.)

or walking and running uphill and downhill (Margaria 1938).

3 Cycling forwards and cycling backwards resisting the pedal rotation (Abbot *et al.* 1952; Asmussen 1953) (Fig. 4.9).

Mechanical work performed in the first group of methods is estimated as the product of load weight and the load displacement (upward direction is positive). During walking and running on incline surfaces, work done to raise or lower the centre of mass of the body is determined as $W_{p/n} = \Delta E_{pot} = w \cdot s \cdot \sin \phi$, where $W_{p/n}$ is positive or negative work, ΔE_{pot} is the change of potential energy of the body, w is body weight (body mass in kg times $9.81 \text{ m} \cdot \text{s}^{-2}$), s is the distance travelled on the incline surface (positive for uphill and negative for downhill), and ϕ is the slope of the surface with respect to the horizon (in radians). It should be mentioned that subjects' movements during uphill and downhill walking are not identical. Comparisons between walking uphill forwards and downhill backwards would be better in that sense (Chauveau 1896a; Hill 1965, p. 151). However, the physiological cost of unnatural backward locomotion would likely be altered, which would complicate comparisons of responses to uphill and downhill locomotion (Margaria 1938). In bike ergometer riding, work done is determined from a given resistance. Values of positive and negative work done while moving on inclined surfaces and during cycling, determined as described above, are smaller than values of positive and negative work of joint moments (Williams & Cavanagh 1983; Prilutsky & Zatsiorsky 1992). However, different estimates of muscle work in walking, running and jumping (external work, total work, and total work of joint moments) are correlated (Prilutsky 1990; Prilutsky & Zatsiorsky 1992).

Oxygen consumption during eccentric and concentric exercise

One of the most important variables characterizing physiological responses to exercise is oxygen uptake, which reflects metabolic energy expenditure.

The rate of oxygen uptake ($\dot{V}o_2$) during a 'steady state' exercise (when $\dot{V}o_2$ uptake corresponds to the demands) increases with negative power. The relationship between $\dot{V}o_2$ and $\dot{W}_n$ is linear in the range of 0 to -260 W during cycling (Abbot et al. 1952; Asmussen 1953; Hesser et al. 1977), descending stairs (Kamon 1970; Pandolf et al. 1978), and load lowering by the arm (Monod & Scherrer 1973). During walking and running downhill, the relationship between $\dot{V}o_2$ and $\dot{W}_n$ is not linear (Davies et al. 1974). In the range of negative power of 0 to -260 W, the rate of total oxygen uptake was reported to change from $0.3\,1 \cdot min^{-1}$ to $1.6\,1 \cdot min^{-1}$.

Oxygen uptake during negative work production is lower than that during positive work (Table 4.3). The ratio of oxygen uptake during eccentric and concentric exercise with the same absolute values of work done ($+\dot{V}o_2/-\dot{V}o_2$) always exceeds 1 and depends on exercise (walking, running, cycling, etc.), velocity of movement, and methods of determining $\dot{V}o_2$ (gross oxygen uptake, gross oxygen uptake minus oxygen uptake at rest, etc.). For example, the ratio $+\dot{V}o_2/-\dot{V}o_2$ during cycling exercise increases with cadence from about 2 at 15 r.p.m. to 5.2–10 at 100 r.p.m. (Abbot et al. 1952; Bigland-Ritchie & Woods 1976). Asmussen (1953) reported a ratio of 125 at a cadence of 102 r.p.m. Eccentric training decreases the metabolic cost of performing negative work and increases the ratio $+\dot{V}o_2/-\dot{V}o_2$ up to two times (Davies & Barnes 1972a). Cessation of training for 3–4 months causes $-\dot{V}o_2$ to return to the pretraining values (Klausen & Knuttgen 1971; Knuttgen et al. 1971).

The fact that the ratio $+\dot{V}o_2/-\dot{V}o_2$ exceeds 1 can be explained by the hypothesis that eccentric actions require fewer active fibres compared with the concentric actions against the same load (see 'Maximum moment production and muscle activation' above). The same hypothesis can be used to explain the increase of the oxygen uptake ratio with the speed of movement: the difference in the maximum developed force between eccentric and concentric actions increases with the speed of muscle length change (Fig. 4.7a). In addition, a lower oxygen uptake of eccentric actions per unit of muscle activation can also contribute to the high $+\dot{V}o_2/-\dot{V}o_2$ ratio. According to Bigland-Ritchie and Woods (1976), $\dot{V}o_2$ per unit of integrated EMG of working muscles is about three times lower in eccentric actions compared with concentric.

Pulmonary ventilation in eccentric exercise

The pulmonary ventilation $\dot{V}_E$ per unit of $\dot{V}o_2$ is slightly higher while performing negative work than during positive work (Asmussen 1967; D'Angelo & Torelli 1971; Davies & Barnes 1972b). This fact is probably not related to a change in the sensitivity of chemoreceptors for CO_2 during eccentric actions, which is supported by similar slopes of the relationship $\dot{V}_E$ vs. alveolar partial pressure of CO_2 ($P_A co_2$) during negative and positive work (Davies & Barnes 1972b; Miyamura et al. 1976) and by lower values of $P_A co_2$ during negative compared with positive work (Davies & Barnes 1972b). It was suggested that the increased ratio $\dot{V}_E/\dot{V}o_2$ during negative work is a reflection of a higher neurogenic respiratory drive during eccentric exercise due to larger muscle forces (up to 5–7 times) in eccentric exercise at the same $\dot{V}o_2$ level as in concentric exercise (Asmussen 1967; D'Angelo & Torelli 1971).

Other indices of ventilatory performance, $\dot{V}_E/\dot{V}co_2$, $\dot{V}_E/\dot{V}_T$ ($\dot{V}_T$, the mean expired tidal volume), and $P_V co_2/\dot{V}co_2$, are approximately the same during eccentric and concentric exercise (Davies & Barnes 1972b; Hesser et al. 1977).

Table 4.3 The ratio of oxygen uptake during performing positive and negative work ($+\dot{V}o_2/-\dot{V}o_2$) in equivalent concentric and eccentric exercises (selected studies).

Subjects	Exercise	($+\dot{V}o_2/-\dot{V}o_2$)	Authors
2 men	Cycling, 41–213 W:		Abbott *et al.* (1952)
	25.0 r.p.m.	2.4	
	35.4 r.p.m.	3.7	
	52.0 r.p.m.	5.2	
1 man	Cycling, 25–262 W:		Asmussen (1953)
	45 r.p.m.	5.9	
	68 r.p.m.	7.4	
	85 r.p.m.	13.7	
	92 r.p.m.	44.5	
	102 r.p.m.	125	
2 men	Stair walking, cadence 12 min^{-1} Stair height (m):		Nagle *et al.* (1965)
	0.2	2.9	
	0.3	3.0	
	0.4	3.2	
8 women, 42–51 years	Stair walking, slope 27–40°	1.5–1.8	Richardson (1966)
4 men and women	Walking uphill and downhill	3.7	Kamon (1970)
7 men	Cycling, 48–230 W	2.7	Bonde-Petersen *et al.* (1972)
3 men	Load raising and lowering by the arm, 3.0–9.8 W	3.0	Monod & Scherrer (1973)
4 men and women	Cycling, 25–164 W:		Bigland-Ritchie and Woods (1976)
	30 r.p.m.	4.9	
	50 r.p.m.	6.6	
	80 r.p.m.	8.3	
	100 r.p.m.	10.2	
15 men	Stair walking, slope ± 30°, vertical speed 0.067–0.25 m · s^{-1}	5.3	Pandolf *et al.* (1978)

Heart responses to eccentric exercise

There are varying opinions about differences in the heart rate, cardiac output and stroke volume between eccentric and concentric exercises at the same $\dot{V}o_2$ level (Thomson 1971; Monod & Scherrer 1973). However, many authors agree that the conditions for increasing the stroke volume are more favourable during eccentric exercise than during concentric exercise with the same oxygen uptake.

In eccentric exercise, the venous blood return is larger due to higher muscle forces developed. High muscle forces during eccentric exercise also cause elevated arterial mean pressure and peripheral resistance (Thomson 1971).

Temperature regulation

Heat stress during eccentric exercise is expected to be higher than during concentric exercise with the same oxygen uptake because during eccentric exercise, work done on muscles (i.e. negative work) is dissipated in muscles. To prevent an excessive rise of core temperature during eccentric exercise, the system of temperature regulation provides a higher temperature gradient between muscles and skin, a higher blood flow through the skin, and a more intensive sweat secretion compared with concentric exercise with the same $\dot{V}o_2$ (Nielsen 1969; Smiles & Robinson 1971; Davies & Barnes 1972b; Nielsen et al. 1972). For example, at an air temperature of 20°C, the difference in the sweat secretion between negative and positive work with the same oxygen uptake is about $0.25\,l \cdot h^{-1}$ (Nielsen et al. 1972). In similar conditions, the muscle temperature is about 2°C higher in eccentric than in concentric exercise (Nielsen 1969; Nadel et al. 1972). The latter observation may affect muscle metabolism and the oxygen dissociation curve of the blood in muscles.

Negative work in athletic events

In most of the athletic events, there are phases of movement where the total mechanical energy of the body or some of its segments decreases. This decrease of energy can be caused by external forces (e.g. air or water resistance) and/or by forces developed by muscles and passive anatomical structures such as ligaments, cartilage, etc. In some activities, for example swimming, rowing, road cycling with high speeds, and ergometer cycling against high resistance, the mechanical energy of the athlete is dissipated mostly by external forces, and muscles are likely to do little or no negative work. In activities performed at relatively low speeds on stiff surfaces without slippage, the contribution of external forces to work done on the body is small (for review, see Zatsiorsky et al. 1982; van Ingen Schenau & Cavanagh 1990), and muscles do a substantial amount of negative work. In this section we will analyse events in which muscles do an appreciable amount of negative work: running, normal and race walking, running long and high jumps, and landing. It is assumed here that the work done by the joint moments is the most accurate estimate of muscle work.

Normal and race walking

During walking at constant speeds, absolute values of negative and positive work done in the major joints of the body are approximately the same (Prilutsky & Zatsiorsky 1992). In the cycle of normal walking at speeds of $1.6–2.4\,m \cdot s^{-1}$, estimates of the total negative work summed across the three orthogonal planes and major joints (three joints for each lower and upper extremity, and also trunk and head-trunk articulations) range between −125 and −190 J (Aleshinsky 1978; Zatsiorsky et al. 1982; Prilutsky & Zatsiorsky 1992). Most of the negative work is done (or energy is absorbed) by the joints of the lower extremities (76–88% of the total negative work: Aleshinsky 1978; Prilutsky & Zatsiorsky 1992). Approximately 77–87% of the negative work of the lower extremities is done in the sagittal plane (Aleshinsky 1978; Zatsiorsky et al. 1982; Prilutsky & Zatsiorsky 1992; Eng & Winter 1995).

There are several phases of the walking cycle where moments of the lower extremity absorb mechanical energy (Fig. 4.10; Eng & Winter 1995). After the touchdown during approximately the first 10% of the cycle, the ankle flexors sometimes act eccentrically to decelerate the forward rotation of the foot (this phase is absent in Fig. 4.10). When the distal portion of the foot touches the ground, the ankle extensors start acting eccentrically and absorb energy during 10–40% of the walking cycle (phase A1-S, Fig. 4.10), just before the phase of energy generation by the ankle extensors at the end of the stance phase (40–60%, phase A2-S in Fig. 4.10). The muscles crossing the ankle do −5 to −9 J of negative work, which is 16–19% (or 32–48 J) of the positive work done at the ankle (Winter 1983a; Prilutsky & Zatsiorsky 1992; Eng & Winter 1995). The knee moment produced by the knee extensors mostly absorbs energy during the stance phase (Fig. 4.10). In the second half of the swing phase, knee flexors decelerate forward rotation of the shank by developing negative power, which can exceed 100 W (phase K4-S in Fig. 4.10) (Morrison 1970; Prilutsky & Zatsiorsky 1992; Eng & Winter 1995). Negative work done in the knee during walking with different speeds has been reported to be between −17 and −61 J, whereas positive work values range between 1.4 and

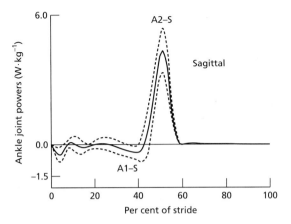

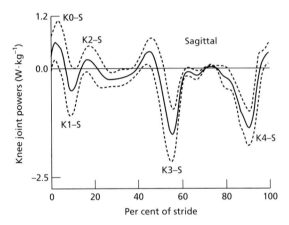

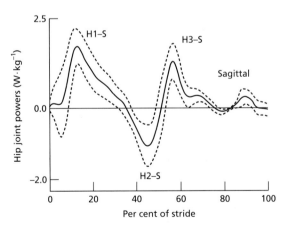

Fig. 4.10 Joint powers normalized to body mass in the sagittal plane during normal walking. The stance phase starts at 0% and ends at about 60% of the stride time. (Adapted from Eng & Winter (1995), pp. 754–56, with permission from Elsevier Science.)

14 J (Winter 1983a; Prilutsky & Zatsiorsky 1992; Eng & Winter 1995). The hip flexor muscles decelerate the thigh extension during approximately the last third of the stance phase (Fig. 4.10, phase H2-S) and do −11 to −60 J of negative work in the sagittal plane (Prilutsky & Zatsiorsky 1992; Eng & Winter 1995).

The conditions for the enhancement of the positive muscle power and work in walking do not appear to be favourable. The phases of positive power generation in the ankle and hip during the stance phase (phases A2-S and H1-S, respectively, Fig. 4.10) are not preceded by a substantial amount of negative work done. Small enhancement of positive power and work may theoretically occur at the ankle during the end of the stance phase and at the hip at the beginning of the swing phase. The knee moment generates little positive work. As mentioned above, the economy of positive work in walking is only slightly higher than that of walking uphill or cycling (Asmussen & Bonde-Petersen 1974b) where presumably little or no negative work is done.

If power produced by each muscle was known, estimates of total negative and positive work done by all muscles could differ from the above values of joint moment work, even if one assumes no coactivation between antagonistic muscles. The presence of two-joint muscles may decrease the negative and positive work required at the joints (Elftman 1940; Morrison 1970; Wells 1988; Prilutsky & Zatsiorsky 1992; Prilutsky *et al.* 1996b) due to opposite angle changes in the adjacent joints and therefore smaller total length changes of two-joint muscles.

In race walking, the amount of negative and positive work done is larger compared with work in normal walking at an average speed. At the race walking speed of 3.2 m · s⁻¹, the total negative work done in 14 joints and three orthogonal planes estimated from Aleshinsky (1978) is 352.1 J. From this amount, 286 J or 81% is done in joints of the lower extremities. Most of the negative work of the lower extremity is done in the sagittal plane (87–89%; Aleshinsky 1978; Zatsiorsky *et al.* 1982). The patterns of power in joints of the lower extremity in the sagittal plane during race walking are somewhat similar to the corresponding patterns in normal walking (Tupa *et al.* 1980; Zatsiorsky *et al.* 1980), despite the fact that the kinetic and potential energy of the body's centre of mass change in phase in race walk-ing and out of phase in normal walking (Zatsiorsky *et al.* 1980, 1982; Cavagna & Franzetti 1981). The magnitude of linear segment and angular joint dis-placements and EMG are greatly exaggerated during race walking as opposed to normal walking (Murray *et al.* 1983; Zatsiorsky *et al.* 1980). Correspondingly, the work of joint moments during race walking is larger. The biggest difference in work between race and normal walking occurs in the elbow and shoulder joints in the sagittal plane (5- to 15-fold), in the 'pelvis-trunk' articulation in the sagittal and frontal planes (threefold), and the knee and hip joints in the sagittal and frontal planes (up to fourfold) (Aleshinsky 1978; Zatsiorsky *et al.* 1982).

It has been suggested, based on in-phase changes in kinetic and potential energy of the centre of body mass in race walking and in running, that the efficiency of race walking should be higher than that of normal walking due to apparently better condi-tions for the use of elastic energy in race walking (Cavagna & Franzetti 1981). The similarity of power patterns in the leg joints between normal and race walking does not support this suggestion.

Pain in the anterior aspect of the lower leg appears to be a common problem among race walkers (Sanzen *et al.* 1986). It is feasible that this syndrome is partly caused by high values of negative power and work produced by the ankle flexors. At the beginning of the stance phase, the ankle is extending (and the ankle flexor muscles are being stretched) after the heel strike and the ankle flexors are active (Zatsiorsky *et al.* 1980; Murray *et al.* 1983; Sanzen *et al.* 1986). The increase in velocity of walking from 1.4 m · s⁻¹ to 3.3 m · s⁻¹ results in the increase of anterior tibial com-partment pressure (and presumably muscle force) by approximately five times (Sanzen *et al.* 1986).

Stair descent

During stair descent, work done by moments at the knee and ankle is mostly negative, whereas very lit-tle negative or positive work is done in the hip joint (Fig. 4.11a; McFadyen & Winter 1988). The ankle

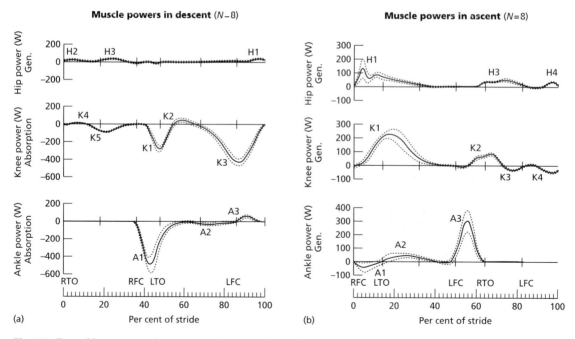

Fig. 4.11 Ensemble average and one standard deviation band of muscle powers at each joint in the sagittal plane during stair descent (a) and ascent (b). RTO, Right toe-off; RFC, right foot contact; LTO, left toe-off; LFC, left foot contact. (Reprinted from McFadyen & Winter (1988), pp. 738–39, with permission from Elsevier Science.)

extensors absorb energy during approximately the first third of the stance (A1; weight acceptance phase). During this phase, the knee extensors are also active and generate negative power (phase K1, Fig. 4.11a). The 'controlled lowering phase' (McFadyen & Winter 1988) lasts from about mid-stance to the beginning of swing and is performed by the knee extensors, which absorb the energy of the body (Fig. 4.11a, phase K3; Morrison 1970; McFadyen & Winter 1988). Thus, during stair descent, most of the work done by joint moments is negative, and the ankle and knee extensors absorb most of the energy. The opposite is true for stair ascent—the knee and ankle extensors do most of the positive work, whereas all three lower-extremity joints absorb little energy (Fig. 4.11b; McFadyen & Winter 1988). These data support the assumption implied in the studies of physiological responses to positive and negative work (see above) that during stair descent and ascent muscles do negative and positive work, respectively. It should be noted that the work estimated from the change in total energy of the centre of mass of the entire body is very close to the work of joint moments during stair walking (assuming the arms do not move much) because, as evident from Fig. 4.11, the power in different joints essentially does not have opposite signs. In movements where the signs of power in different joints are the same, the work of joint moments is similar to the change in total energy of the centre of mass (Aleshinsky 1986; Zatsiorsky 1986).

Level, downhill and backward running

In running at constant relatively low speeds, as in walking, absolute values of the total negative and positive work of joint moments summed across major joints of the body and across three orthogonal planes are approximately the same (Prilutsky & Zatsiorsky 1992). During sprint running with a constant speed, the amount of the total positive work should be slightly higher than the absolute value of the total negative work due to work done against the aerodynamic drag force (Zatsiorsky *et al.* 1982). The total negative work of joint moments per cycle ranges from −241 J to −883 J for speeds of 3.3–6.0 m · s⁻¹ (Aleshinsky 1978; Prilutsky 1990;

Prilutsky & Zatsiorsky 1992). Joint moments of the lower extremity do most of the negative work (80%; Prilutsky & Zatsiorsky 1992). From this amount, lower-extremity moments in the sagittal plane do 82% of negative work (Prilutsky & Zatsiorsky 1992).

Joint moments at the ankle and knee in the sagittal plane (ankle and knee extensors) absorb energy during approximately the first half of the stance phase and generate energy in the second half of the stance phase (Fig. 4.12; Tupa *et al.* 1980; Winter 1983b; Ae *et al.* 1987; Buczek & Cavanagh 1990; Prilutsky &

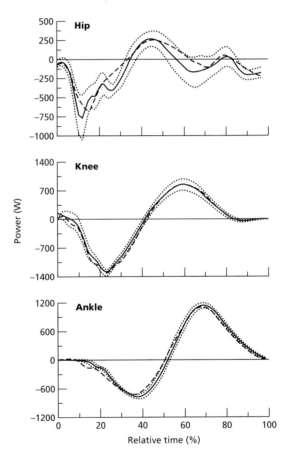

Fig. 4.12 Joint power curves in the sagittal plane from a representative subject during the stance phase of running. Solid line and dotted lines are mean ± 1 standard deviation in normal running. Dashed line is mean in running with a knee brace. Running speed 3.83 m · s⁻¹. (Reprinted from DeVita *et al.* (1996), p. 586, with permission from Elsevier Science.)

Zatsiorsky 1992; DeVita et al. 1996). According to the literature during running at different constant speeds, values of negative and positive work done at the ankle range from −13 to −79 J and from 59 to 106 J, respectively; corresponding values for the knee joint are −30 to −210 J and 25 to 51 J (Buczek & Cavanagh 1990; Winter 1983b; Prilutsky & Zatsiorsky 1992; Stefanyshyn & Nigg 1997). The hip joint power in the stance is more variable and its pattern appears to depend on speed. In the swing phase, the knee joint moments mostly absorb energy—the knee extensors decelerate knee flexion in the first half of the swing, and the knee flexors decelerate knee extension in the second half of the swing. The hip flexors typically absorb energy at the end of the stance phase to decelerate hip extension; during the first part of the swing, the hip flexors accelerate hip flexion; and in the second half of the swing, the hip extensors decelerate hip flexion and accelerate hip extension. Metatarsophalangeal joint moments (plantarflexors) mostly absorb energy during the stance phase of running at 4.0 and 7.1 m · s⁻¹; corresponding values of negative work are −20.9 J and −47.8 J (Stefanyshyn & Nigg 1997).

The fact that the energy-generation phase in the stance of running follows immediately after the energy absorption phase (Fig. 4.12) and that absolute values of the negative and positive work done by the ankle and knee extensors during the stance are similar support the notion that conditions for the enhancement of positive work and work economy are more favourable in running than in walking (Cavagna et al. 1964; Farley & Ferris 1998).

In the stance phase of backward running, the knee extensors are primary generators of energy and do very little negative work (DeVita & Stribling 1991). The ankle extensors still absorb energy in the first half of the stance phase and generate energy in the second half, but the amount of negative and positive work done by them is approximately 50% less than in forward running (DeVita & Stribling 1991). Thus, it can be speculated that the efficiency of positive work in backward running is lower than in forward running, because the major energy generators in backward running, the knee extensors, do not absorb energy prior to the energy-generation phase.

Running downhill at a grade of 8.3% increases negative work done by the ankle extensors from −13 J in level running to −26 J. Corresponding values for the knee extensors are −30 J and −58 J, respectively (Buczek & Cavanagh 1990). Although muscles do relatively more negative work during downhill running, it is not clear why downhill running causes soreness in the leg extensors, whereas level running with comparable values of negative work does not (Buczek & Cavanagh 1990).

Running long and vertical jumps

During the stance phase of maximum running long jumps with the results of 6.1 and 7.0 m, the total negative work done in 15 joints and three orthogonal planes is −878 J (or 130% of the total positive work). From this amount of negative work, −656 J (or 75%) is done in the stance leg joints and −119 J (14%) in the swing leg joints. Most of the negative work of the stance leg is done in the sagittal plane (94%) (Prilutsky 1990). Power patterns and work done in individual joints of the stance leg depend on athlete techniques and the length of the jump. Examples of the powers developed in the stance leg joints during a running long jump are shown in Fig. 4.13 (Tupa et al. 1980). The ankle and knee extensor muscles absorb energy during approximately the first half of the stance, and they generate energy during the rest of the stance. Peaks of negative and positive power at the two joints are very high (Fig. 4.13). Note that peaks of positive power greatly exceed the maximum positive power obtained from the curves of joint moment and joint velocity, measured in maximum concentric actions (van Ingen Schenau et al. 1985; Prilutsky et al. 1992). This observation supports the notion of the enhancement of positive power during the SSC. In addition, some of the power recorded at distal joints may be transferred there from more proximal joints by two-joint muscles (van Ingen Schenau et al. 1985; Prilutsky & Zatsiorsky 1994).

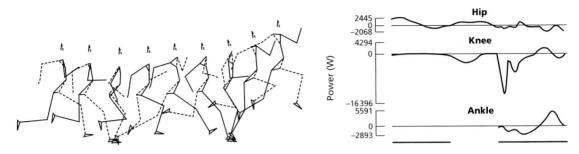

Fig. 4.13 Powers developed by moments at the stance (ipsilateral) leg in the sagittal plane during running long jump. The right horizontal line corresponds to the stance phase of the ipsilateral leg (shown by solid lines on the stick figure); the left horizontal line corresponds to the stance phase of the contralateral leg (shown by dashed lines on the stick figure). The length of the ipsilateral stance phase is 0.148 s; the jump length is 7.2 m. (Adapted from Tupa *et al.* 1980.)

In submaximal running long jumps the amount of negative work done in the sagittal plane is smaller than in maximum jumps: −44, −133, −80 and −28 J for the metatarsophalangeal, ankle, knee and hip joints, respectively; the corresponding values of positive work are 2, 104, 52 and 56 J (Stefanyshyn & Nigg 1998).

Joint power patterns during maximum running vertical jumps are similar, in general, to those in the running long jumps (Fig. 4.14). The peak power values are substantially smaller in the ankle and the knee. The hip extensors do positive work in the first half of the stance, and they mostly absorb energy at the end of the stance phase (Fig. 4.14). However, the hip power is more variable than ankle and knee power in running vertical and long jumps (Stefanyshyn & Nigg 1998). The amounts of negative and positive work done by the extensors of the major leg joints are smaller, in general, during running vertical jumps than during running long jumps (Tupa *et al.* 1980; Stefanyshyn & Nigg 1998).

In standing countermovement vertical and long jumps, the ankle, knee and hip extensors absorb energy of the body to stop the countermovement, and then they generate energy to accelerate the

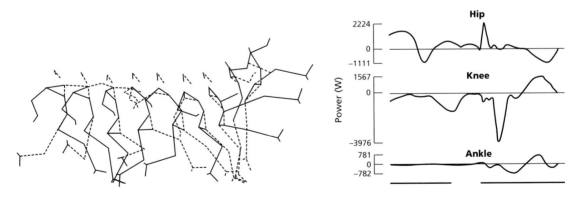

Fig. 4.14 Powers developed by moments at the stance (contralateral) leg in the sagittal plane during running vertical jump. The right horizontal line corresponds to the stance phase of the contralateral leg (shown by dashed lines on the stick figure); the left horizontal line corresponds to the stance phase of the ipsilateral leg (shown by solid lines on the stick figure). The duration of the contralateral stance phase is 0.224 s; the result of the jump is 1.85 m. (Adapted from Tupa *et al.* 1980.)

body (Horita *et al.* 1991; Anderson & Pandy 1993). Despite the fact that the leg extensors experience the SSC and the results of the countermovement jumps are consistently better than squat jumps, where the muscles do not absorb energy prior to the push-off phase (Prilutsky 1990; Bobbert *et al.* 1996), it does not appear that the conditions for the enhancement of positive work due to the preliminary muscle stretch are met in the countermovement jumps. In two computer simulation studies by Anderson and Pandy (1993) and Bobbert *et al.* (1996), the authors demonstrated that elastic energy stored in the muscles prior to the push-off phase was nearly the same in the two types of jump. Bobbert *et al.* (1996) explain a better performance of the countermovement jump compared with the squat jump by a higher muscle force developed at the beginning of the push-off phase in the countermovement jump than in the squat jump. However, since most of the elastic energy in the countermovement jump comes from the decrease in potential energy of the body, and in the squat jump, from work done by the muscle contractile elements on the SEC (Anderson & Pandy 1993), the countermovement jump seems to require less metabolic energy per unit of positive work than the squat jump (Anderson & Pandy 1993; see also 'Economy and efficiency of positive work' above).

Landing

During landings from heights of 0.32–1.28 m, the leg joint moments (leg extensors) do primarily negative work (Prilutsky 1990; DeVita & Skelly 1992; McNitt-Gray 1993; Prilutsky & Zatsiorsky 1994). The amount of work, the relative contribution of different joints to the total work, and patterns of joint powers depend substantially on whether the landing is soft or stiff. In a very soft landing after a jump from 0.5 m (where nearly the entire decrease in the total energy of the body is dissipated by the joint moments (see 'Dissipation of mechanical energy' above), the total negative work done by the leg joints is –592 J; and the ankle, knee and hip moments absorb –159, –248 and –185 J (Prilutsky 1990). In more stiff jumps (where a substantial portion of the

body energy is dissipated in the passive anatomical structures (see 'Dissipation of mechanical energy' above), the negative work done in the joints is typically less (Prilutsky 1990; DeVita & Skelly 1992). Examples of power developed during soft and stiff landings at three leg joints are shown in Fig. 4.15. Peaks of negative power, which are typically greater in stiff landings, can reach –30 to –40 W per unit body mass for landings from 0.32 to 0.59 m, and –150 W per unit body mass for landings from 1.28 m (DeVita & Skelly 1992; McNitt-Gray 1993). For more information about the biomechanics of landing, see Chapter 25.

Cycling

Power and work produced by ankle, knee and hip moments during cycling increase with resistance power and pedalling rate (Fig. 4.16). Most of the work done by the leg moments is positive. For example, according to Ericson (1988), at a resistance power of 120 W and pedalling rate of 60 r.p.m., the total positive work done by moments of one leg in the cycle is 67 J, whereas the corresponding negative work is only –6 J (9%). At a resistance power of 240 W and the same pedalling rate, the values of positive and negative work are 126 J and –7 J (6%), respectively. Almost each major leg muscle acts eccentrically in short periods of the pedal revolution when muscle elongation coincides with the development of muscle forces (Hull & Hawkins 1990; Gregor *et al.* 1991). However, the amount of negative work done by the muscles in cycling is probably small.

Thus, the assumption accepted by many researchers that in normal cycling muscles do primarily positive work seems to be justified.

Acknowledgements

The preparation of this chapter was supported in part by a grant from the Office of Interdisciplinary Programs at Georgia Institute of Technology to the Center for Human Movement Studies (director, Professor Robert J. Gregor). The author thanks Mark A. Broberg for his help in editing the English.

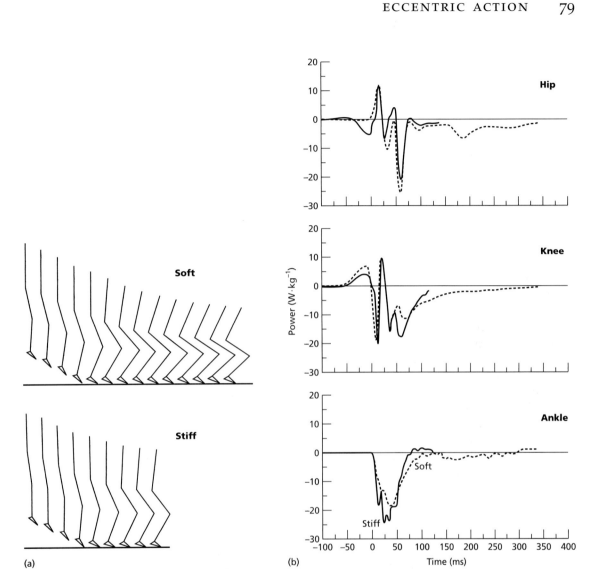

Fig. 4.15 (a) Stick figure representations of typical soft and stiff landings. The stiff landing had a more erect body posture through the landing. (b) Joint power curves normalized to body mass in the sagittal plane from representative soft and stiff landings. Negative and positive times indicate descent and floor contact phases. (From DeVita & Skelly 1992.)

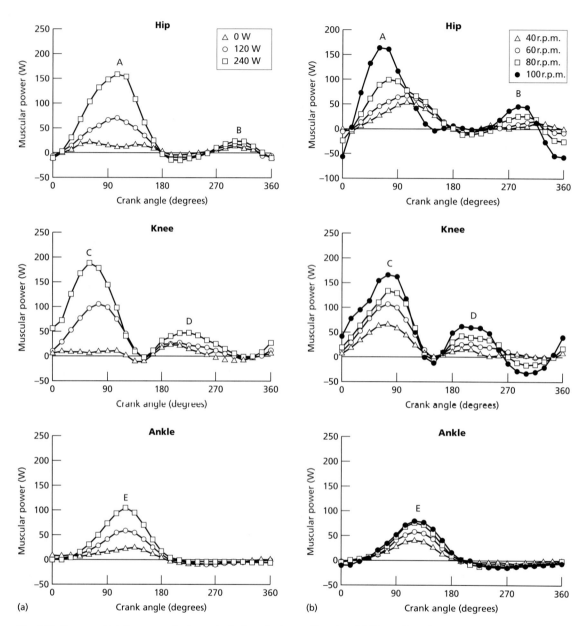

Fig. 4.16 Powers of joint moments in the sagittal plane during cycling: 0 and 360° crank angles correspond to pedal top position, and 180° crank angle to pedal bottom position. A, Positive hip extensor power; B, positive hip flexor power; C, positive knee extensor power; D, positive knee flexor power; E, positive ankle extensor power. (a) Cycling at different resistance powers (0, 120 and 240 W). (b) Cycling at different pedalling rates (40, 60, 80 and 100 r.p.m.) against the same resistance giving power outputs of 80, 120, 160 and 200 W, respectively. (From Ericson 1988; Figs 1 & 2.)

References

Abbott, B.C. & Aubert, X.M. (1952) The force exerted by active striated muscle during and after change of length. *Journal of Physiology* 117, 77–86.

Abbott, B.C., Aubert, X.M. & Hill, A.V. (1951) The absorption of work by a muscle stretched during a single twitch or a short tetanus. *Proceedings of the Royal Society: Biological Sciences* 139, 86–104.

Abbott, B.C., Bigland, B. & Ritchie, J.M. (1952) The physiological cost of negative work. *Journal of Physiology* 117, 380–390.

Ae, M., Miyashita, K., Yokoi, T. & Hashihara, Y. (1987) Mechanical power and work done by the muscles of the lower limb during running at different speeds. In: *Biomechanics X-B. International Series on Biomechanics* (ed. B. Jonsson), pp. 895–899. Human Kinetics Publishers, Champaign, IL.

Aleshinsky, S. Yu. (1978) Mechanical and mathematical modeling of 3D human movements. In: *Biodynamics of Sport Technique* (ed. V.M. Zatsiorsky), pp. 54–117. Central Institute of Physical Culture, Moscow (in Russian).

Aleshinsky, S. Yu. (1986) An energy 'sources' and 'fractions' approach to the mechanical energy expenditure problem. I–V. *Journal of Biomechanics* 19, 287–315.

Aleshinsky, S. Yu. & Zatsiorsky, V.M. (1978) Human locomotion in space analyzed biomechanically through a multi-link chain model. *Journal of Biomechanics* 11, 101–108.

An, K.-N., Kaufman, K.R. & Chao, E.Y.-S. (1995) Estimation of muscle and joint forces. In: *Three-Dimensional Analysis of Human Movement* (eds P. Allard, I.A.F. Stokes & J.-P. Blanchi), pp. 201–214. Human Kinetics Publishers, Champaign, IL.

Anderson, F.C. & Pandy, M.G. (1993) Storage and utilization of elastic strain energy during jumping. *Journal of Biomechanics* 26, 1413–1427.

Armstrong, R.B. (1984) Mechanisms of exercise-induced delayed onset muscular soreness: a brief review. *Medicine and Science in Sports and Exercise* 16, 529–538.

Aruin, A.S. & Prilutsky, B.I. (1985) Relationship between biomechanical properties of muscles and their ability to utilize elastic strain energy. *Human Physiology* 11, 12–16 (in Russian).

Aruin, A.S., Prilutsky, B.I., Raitsin, L.M. & Saveliev, I.A. (1979) Biomechanical properties of muscles and efficiency of movement. *Human Physiology* 5, 426–434.

Aruin, A.S., Volkov, N.I., Zatsiorsky, V.M., Raitsin, L.M. & Shirkovets, E.A. (1977) Influence of elastic forces of the muscles upon efficiency of muscular work. *Human Physiology* 3, 420–426.

Asmussen, E. (1953) Positive and negative muscular work. *Acta Physiologica Scandinavica* 28, 365–382.

Asmussen, E. (1967) Exercise and the regulation of ventilation. *Circulation Research* (Supplement) 20, 132–145.

Asmussen, E. & Bonde-Petersen, F. (1974a) Storage of elastic energy in skeletal muscles in man. *Acta Physiologica Scandinavica* 91, 385–392.

Asmussen, E. & Bonde-Petersen, F. (1974b) Apparent efficiency and storage of elastic energy in human muscles during exercise. *Acta Physiologica Scandinavica* 92, 537–545.

Asmussen, E., Bonde-Petersen, F. & Jorgensen, K. (1976) Mechano-elastic properties of human muscles at different temperatures. *Acta Physiologica Scandinavica* 96, 83–93.

Avela, J. & Komi, P.V. (1998) Interaction between muscle stiffness and stretch reflex sensitivity after long-term stretch–shortening cycle exercise. *Muscle and Nerve* 21, 1224–1227.

Bahler, A.S. (1967) Series elastic component of mammalian skeletal muscle. *American Journal of Physiology* 213, 1560–1564.

Barnes, W.S. (1981) Isokinetic fatigue curves at different contractile velocities. *Archives of Physical Medicine and Rehabilitation* 62, 66–69.

Biewener, A.A., Konieczynski, D.D. & Baudinette, R.V. (1998) In vivo muscle force-length behavior during steady-speed hopping in tammar wallabies. *Journal of Experimental Biology* 201, 1681–1694.

Bigland, B. & Lippold, O.C.J. (1954) The relation between force, velocity and integrated electrical activity in human muscles. *Journal of Physiology* 123, 214–224.

Bigland-Ritchie, B. & Woods, J.J. (1976) Integrated electromyogram and oxygen uptake during positive and negative work. *Journal of Physiology* 260, 267–277.

Bobbert, M.F., Gerritsen, K.G., Litjens, M.C. & van Soest, A.J. (1996) Why is countermovement jump height greater than squat jump height. *Medicine and Science in Sports and Exercise* 28, 1402–1412.

Bober, T., Jaskolski, E. & Nowacki, Z. (1980) Study of eccentric-concentric contraction of the upper extremity muscles. *Journal of Biomechanics* 13, 135–138.

Bonde-Petersen, G., Knuttgen, H.G. & Henriksson, J. (1972) Muscle metabolism during exercise with concentric and eccentric contractions. *Journal of Applied Physiology* 33, 792–795.

Bonde-Petersen, G., Henriksson, J. & Knuttgen, H.G. (1973) Effect of training with eccentric muscle contractions on skeletal muscle metabolites. *Acta Physiologica Scandinavica* 88, 564–570.

Bosco, C. & Komi, P.V. (1980) Influence of aging on the mechanical behavior of leg extensor muscles. *European Journal of Applied Physiology* 45, 209–219.

Bosco, C., Komi, P.V. & Ito, A. (1981) Pre-stretch potentiation of human skeletal muscle during ballistic movement. *Acta Physiologica Scandinavica* 111, 135–140.

Bosco, C., Ito, A., Komi, P.V. *et al.* (1982) Neuromuscular function and mechanical efficiency of human leg extensor muscles during jumping exercises. *Acta Physiologica Scandinavica* 114, 543–550.

Buczek, F.L. & Cavanagh, P.R. (1990) Stance phase knee and ankle kinematics and kinetics during level and downhill running. *Medicine and Science in Sports and Exercise* 22, 669–677.

Cabri, J.M. (1991) Isokinetic strength aspects of human joints and muscles. *Critical Reviews in Biomedical Engineering* 19, 231–259.

Cavagna, G.A. (1970) The series elastic component of frog gastrocnemius. *Journal of Physiology* 206, 257–262.

Cavagna, G.A. & Citterio, G. (1974) Effect of stretching on the elastic characteristics and the contractile component of frog striated muscle. *Journal of Physiology* 239, 1–14.

Cavagna, G.A. & Franzetti, P. (1981) Mechanics of competition walking. *Journal of Physiology* 315, 243–251.

Cavagna, G.A. & Kaneko, M. (1977) Mechanical work and efficiency in level walking and running. *Journal of Physiology* 268, 647–681.

Cavagna, G.A., Saibene, F.B. & Margaria, R. (1964) Mechanical work in running. *Journal of Applied Physiology* 19, 249–256.

Cavagna, G.A., Dusman, B. & Margaria, R. (1968) Positive work done by a previously stretched muscle. *Journal of Applied Physiology* **24**, 21–32.

Cavagna, G.A., Heglund, N.C., Harry, J.D. & Mantovani, M. (1994) Storage and release of mechanical energy by contracting frog muscle fibers. *Journal of Physiology* **481**, 689–708.

Cavanagh, P.R. (1988) On 'muscle action' vs 'muscle contraction'. *Journal of Biomechanics* **21**, 69.

Cavanagh, P.R. & Komi, P.V. (1979) Electromechanical delay in human skeletal muscle under concentric and eccentric contractions. *European Journal of Applied Physiology* **42**, 159–163.

Chapman, A.E., Caldwell, G.E. & Selbie, W.S. (1985) Mechanical output following muscle stretch in forearm supination against inertial loads. *Journal of Applied Physiology* **59**, 78–86.

Chauveau, A. (1896a) La depense energetique respectivement engagec dans le travail positif et dans le travail negatif des muscles, d'après les echanges respiratoires. *Comptes Rendus de l'Academie Des Sciences (Paris)* **122**, 58–64.

Chauveau, A. (1896b) La loi de l'equivalence dans les transformations de la force chez les animaux. *Comptes Rendus de l'Academie Des Sciences (Paris)* **122**, 113–120.

Close, R.I. (1972) Dynamic properties of mammalian skeletal muscles. *Physiological Reviews* **52**, 129–197.

Cnockaert, J.C. (1978) Comparison of the potential energy stored and used by two antagonistic muscular groups. *European Journal of Applied Physiology* **39**, 181–189.

Crenshaw, A.G., Karlsson, S., Styf, J., Backlund, T. & Friden, J. (1995) Knee extension torque and intramuscular pressure of the vastus lateralis muscle during eccentric and concentric activities. *European Journal of Applied Physiology* **70**, 13–19.

Crowninshield, R.D. & Brand, R.A. (1981) The prediction of forces in joint structures: distribution of intersegmental resultants. *Exercise and Sport Science Reviews* **9**, 159–181.

Curtin, N.A. & Davies, R.E. (1975) Very high tension with very little ATP breakdown by active skeletal muscle. *Journal of Mechanochemical and Cell Motility* **3**, 147–154.

Curtin, N.A. & Woledge, R.C. (1979) Chemical change, production of tension and energy following stretch of active

muscle of frog. *Journal of Physiology* **297**, 539–550.

D'Angelo, E. & Torelli, G. (1971) Neural stimuli increasing respiration during different types of exercise. *Journal of Applied Physiology* **30**, 116–121.

Davies, C.T. & Barnes, C. (1972a) Negative (eccentric) work. I. Effects of repeated exercise. *Ergonomics* **15**, 3–14.

Davies, C.T. & Barnes, C. (1972b) Negative (eccentric) work. II. Physiological responses to walking uphill and downhill on a motor-driven treadmill. *Ergonomics* **15**, 121–131.

Davies, C.T., Sargeant, A.J. & Smith, B. (1974) The physiological responses to running downhill. *European Journal of Applied Physiology* **32**, 187–194.

Delp, S.L., Loan, J.P., Hoy, M.G., Zajac, F.E., Topp, E.L. & Rosen, J.M. (1990) An interactive graphics-based model of the lower extremity to study orthopaedic surgical procedures. *IEEE Transactions on Biomedical Engineering* **37**, 757–767.

DeVita, P. & Skelly, W.A. (1992) Effect of landing stiffness on joint kinetics and energetics in the lower extremity. *Medicine and Science in Sports and Exercise* **24**, 108–115.

DeVita, P. & Stribling, J. (1991) Lower extremity joint kinetics and energetics during backward running. *Medicine and Science in Sports and Exercise* **23**, 602–610.

DeVita, P., Torry, M., Glover, K.L. & Speroni, D.L. (1996) A functional knee brace alters joint torque and power patterns during walking and running. *Journal of Biomechanics* **29**, 583–588.

Dietz, V., Schmidtbleicher, D. & Noth, J. (1979) Neuronal mechanisms of human locomotion. *Journal of Neurophysiology* **42**, 1212–1222.

Dufek, J.S. & Bates, B.T. (1991) Biomechanical factors associated with injury during landing in jump sports. *Sports Medicine* **12**, 326–337.

Dyhre-Poulsen, P., Siminsen, E.B. & Voight, M. (1991) Dynamic control of muscle stiffness and H reflex modulation during hopping and jumping in man. *Journal of Physiology* **437**, 287–304.

Edgerton, V.R., Roy, R.R., Gregor, R.J. & Rugg, S. (1986) Morphological basis of skeletal muscle power output. In: *Human Muscle Power* (eds N.L. Jones, N. McCartney & A.J. McComas), pp. 43–64. Human Kinetics Publishers, Champaign, IL.

Edman, K.A.P. (1997) Force enhancement by stretch. *Journal of Applied Biomechanics* **13**, 432–436.

Edman, K.A.P. & Tsuchiya, T. (1996) Strain of passive elements during force enhancement by stretch in frog muscle fibers. *Journal of Physiology* **490**, 191–205.

Edman, K.A.P., Elzinga, G. & Noble, M.I.M. (1978) Enhancement of mechanical performance by stretch during tetanic contractions of vertebrate skeletal muscle fibres. *Journal of Physiology* **281**, 139–155.

Elftman, H. (1939) Forces and energy changes in the leg during walking. *American Journal of Physiology* **125**, 339–356.

Elftman, H. (1940) The work done by muscles in running. *American Journal of Physiology* **129**, 672–684.

Eloranta, V. & Komi, P.V. (1980) Function of the quadriceps femoris muscle under maximal concentric and eccentric contractions. *Electromyography and Clinical Neurophysiology* **20**, 154–159.

Eng, J.J. & Winter, D.A. (1995) Kinetic analysis of the lower limbs during walking: what information can be gained from a three-dimensional model? *Journal of Biomechanics* **28**, 753–758.

Enoka, R.M. (1996) Eccentric contractions require unique activation strategies by the nervous system. *Journal of Applied Physiology* **81**, 2339–2346.

Ericson, M.O. (1988) Mechanical muscular power output and work during ergometer cycling at different work loads and speeds. *European Journal of Applied Physiology* **57**, 382–387.

Farley, C. & Ferris, D.P. (1998) Biomechanics of walking and running: center of mass movements to muscle action. *Exercise and Sport Science Reviews* **26**, 253–285.

Fenn, W.O. (1923) A quantitative comparison between the energy liberated and the work performed by the isolated sartorius of the frog. *Journal of Physiology* **58**, 175–203.

Fenn, W.O. (1924) The relation between the work performed and the energy liberated in muscular contraction. *Journal of Physiology* **58**, 373–395.

Fenn, W.O. (1930) Frictional and kinetic factors in the work of sprint runners. *American Journal of Physiology* **92**, 583–611.

Ford, L.E., Huxley, A.F. & Simmons, R.M. (1981) The relation between stiffness and filament overlap in stimulated frog muscle fibers. *Journal of Physiology* **311**, 219–249.

Friden, J. & Lieber, R.L. (1992) Structural and mechanical basis of exercise-induced muscle injury. *Medicine and Science in Sports and Exercise* **24**, 521–530.

Friden, J., Sjostrom, M. & Ekblom, B. (1983) Myofibrillar damage following intense eccentric exercise in man. *International Journal of Sports Medicine* **4**, 170–176.

Gasser, H.S. & Hill, A.V. (1924) The dynamics of muscular contraction. *Proceedings of the Royal Society: Biological Sciences* **96**, 398–437.

Gollhofer, A., Komi, P.V., Miyashita, M. & Aura, O. (1987) Fatigue during stretch–shortening cycle exercises: changes in mechanical performance of human muscle. *International Journal of Sports Medicine* **8**, 71–78.

Grabiner, M.D. (1986) Bioelectric characteristics of the electromechanical delay preceding concentric contraction. *Medicine and Science in Sports and Exercise* **18**, 37–43.

Green, H.J. (1997) Mechanisms of muscle fatigue in intense exercise. *Journal of Sports Sciences* **15**, 247–256.

Gregersen, C.S., Silverton, N.A. & Carrier, D.R. (1998) External work and potential for elastic storage of energy at the limb joints of running dogs. *Journal of Experimental Biology* **201**, 3197–3210.

Gregor, R.J., Komi, P.V., Browning, R.C. & Jarvinen, M. (1991) A comparison of the triceps surae and residual muscle moments at the ankle during cycling. *Journal of Biomechanics* **24**, 287–297.

Gregor, R.J., Roy, R.R., Whiting, W.C., Lovely, J.A., Hodgson, J.A. & Edgerton, V.R. (1988) Mechanical output of the cat soleus during treadmill locomotion: in vivo vs in situ. *Journal of Biomechanics* **21**, 721–732.

Griffiths, R.I. (1991) Shortening of muscle fibers during stretch of the active cat medial gastrocnemius muscle: the role of tendon compliance. *Journal of Physiology* **436**, 219–236.

Hatze, H. (1981) *Myocybernetic Control Model of Skeletal Muscle*. University of South Africa, Pretoria.

Heckathorne, C.W. & Childress, D.S. (1981) Relationships of the surface electromyogram to the force, length, velocity, and contraction rate of the cineplastic human biceps. *American Journal of Physical Medicine* **60**, 1–19.

Henriksson, J., Knuttgen, H.G. & Bonde-Petersen, F. (1972) Perceived exertion during exercise with concentric and eccentric muscle contractions. *Ergonomics* **15**, 537–544.

Herzog, W. (1996) Force-sharing among synergistic muscles: theoretical considerations and experimental approaches.

Exercise and Sport Science Reviews **24**, 173–202.

Hesser, C.M., Linnarsson, D. & Bjurstedt, H. (1977) Cardiorespiratory and metabolic responses to positive, negative and minimum-load dynamic leg exercise. *Respiration Physiology* **30**, 51–67.

Hill, A.V. (1965) *Trails and Trials in Physiology*. Edward Arnold, London.

Hill, A.V. & Howarth, J.V. (1959) The reversal of chemical reactions in contracting muscle during an applied stretch. *Proceedings of the Royal Society: Biological Sciences* **151**, 169–193.

Hochachka, P.W. (1985) Fuels and pathways as designed systems for support of muscle work. *Journal of Experimental Biology* **115**, 149–164.

Hof, A.L. (1998) In vivo measurement of the series elasticity release curve of human triceps surae muscle. *Journal of Biomechanics* **31**, 793–800.

Homsher, E. & Kean, C.J. (1978) Skeletal muscle energetics and metabolism. *Annual Reviews in Physiology* **40**, 93–131.

Horita, T., Kitamura, K. & Kohno, N. (1991) Body configuration and joint moment analysis during standing long jump in 6-yr-old children and adult males. *Medicine and Science in Sports and Exercise* **23**, 1068–1077.

Hortobagyi, T., Tracy, J., Hamilton, G. & Lambert, J. (1996a) Fatigue effects on muscle excitability. *International Journal of Sports Medicine* **17**, 409–414.

Hortobagyi, T., Hill, J.P., Houmard, J.A., Fraser, D.D., Lambert, N.J. & Israel, R.G. (1996b) Adaptive responses to muscle lengthening and shortening in humans. *Journal of Applied Physiology* **80**, 765–772.

Howell, J.N., Fuglevand, A.J., Walsh, M.L. & Bigland-Ritchie, B. (1995) Motor unit activity during isometric and concentric-eccentric contractions of the human first dorsal interosseus muscle. *Journal of Neurophysiology* **74**, 901–904.

Hull, M.L. & Hawkins, D.A. (1990) Analysis of muscular work in multisegmental movements: application to cycling. In: *Multiple Muscle Systems: Biomechanics and Movement Organization* (eds J.M. Winters & S.L.-Y. Woo), pp. 621–638. Springer-Verlag, Berlin.

van Ingen Schenau, G.J. (1984) An alternative view to the concept of utilisation of elastic energy. *Human Movement Science* **3**, 301–336.

van Ingen Schenau, G.J. & Cavanagh, P.R. (1990) Power equations in endurance sports. *Journal of Biomechanics* **23**, 865–881.

van Ingen Schenau, G.J., Bobbert, M.F., Huijing, P.A. & Woittiez, R.D. (1985) The instantaneous torque-angular velocity relation in plantar flexion during jumping. *Medicine and Science in Sports and Exercise* **17**, 422–426.

van Ingen Schenau, G.J., Bobbert, M.F. & de Haan, A. (1997) Does elastic energy enhance work and efficiency in the stretch–shortening cycle? *Journal of Applied Biomechanics* **13**, 389–415.

Jewell, B.R. & Wilkie, D.R. (1958) An analysis of the mechanical components in frog's striated muscle. *Journal of Physiology* **143**, 515–540.

Jones, D.A., Newham, D.J. & Torgan, C. (1989) Mechanical influences on long-lasting human muscle fatigue and delayed-onset pain. *Journal of Physiology* **412**, 415–427.

Julian, F.J. & Morgan, D.L. (1979) The effect on tension of non-uniform distribution of length changes applied to frog muscle fibers. *Journal of Physiology* **293**, 379–392.

Kamon, E. (1970) Negative and positive work in climbing a laddermill. *Journal of Applied Physiology* **29**, 1–5.

Kaneko, M., Komi, P.V. & Aura, O. (1984) Mechanical efficiency of concentric and eccentric exercises performed with medium to fast contraction rates. *Scandinavian Journal of Sports Sciences* **6**, 15–20.

Katz, B. (1939) The relation between force and speed in muscular contraction. *Journal of Physiology* **96**, 45–64.

Kellis, E. & Baltzopoulos, V. (1995) Isokinetic eccentric exercise. *Sports Medicine* **19**, 202–222.

Klausen, K. & Knuttgen, H.G. (1971) Effect of training on oxygen consumption in negative muscular work. *Acta Physiologica Scandinavica* **83**, 319–323.

Knuttgen, H.G. (1986) Human performance in high-intensity exercise with concentric and eccentric muscle contractions. *International Journal of Sports Medicine* **7**, 6–9.

Knuttgen, H.G., Peterson, F.B. & Klausen, K. (1971) Exercise with concentric and eccentric muscle contractions. *Acta Paediatrica Scandinavica* (Suppl.) **217**, 42–46.

Knuttgen, H.G., Nadel, E.R., Pandolf, K.B. & Patton, J.F. (1982) Effects of training with eccentric muscle contractions on exercise performance, energy expenditure, and body temperature. *International Journal of Sports Medicine* **3**, 13–17.

Komi, P.V. (1973) Measurement of the force-velocity relationship in human muscle under concentric and eccentric contractions. In: *Medicine and Sport* Vol. 8. *Biomechanics* III (eds S. Cerquiglini, A. Venerando & J. Wartenweiler), pp. 224–229. Karger, Basel.

Komi, P.V. (1990) Relevance of vivo force measurements to human biomechanics. *Journal of Biomechanics* 23 (Suppl. 1), 23–34.

Komi, P.V. & Bosco, C. (1978) Utilization of stored energy in leg extensor muscles by men and women. *Medicine and Science in Sports and Exercise* 10, 261–265.

Komi, P.V. & Buskirk, E.R. (1972) Effect of eccentric and concentric muscle conditioning on tension and electrical activity of human muscle. *Ergonomics* 15, 417–434.

Komi, P.V. & Rusko, H. (1974) Quantitative evaluation of mechanical and electrical changes during fatigue loading of eccentric and concentric work. *Scandinavian Journal of Rehabilitation Medicine* (Suppl.) 3, 121–126.

Komi, P.V. & Viitasalo, J.T. (1977) Changes in motor unit activity and metabolism in human skeletal muscle during and after repeated eccentric and concentric contractions. *Acta Physiologica Scandinavica* 100, 246–254.

Komi, P.V., Belli, A., Huttunen, V., Bonnefoy, R., Geyssant, A. & Lacour, J.R. (1996) Optic fibre as a transducer of tendomuscular forces. *European Journal of Applied Physiology* 72, 278–280.

Levin, A. & Wyman, J. (1927) The viscous elastic properties of muscles. *Proceedings of the Royal Society: Biological Sciences* 101, 218–243.

Lloyd, B.B. & Zacks, R.M. (1972) The mechanical efficiency of treadmill running against a horizontal impeding force. *Journal of Physiology* 223, 355–363.

Lombardi, V. & Piazzesi, G. (1990) The contractile response during steady lengthening of stimulated frog muscle fibers. *Journal of Physiology* 431, 141–171.

Mannheimer, J.S. (1969) A comparison of strength gain between concentric and eccentric contractions. *Physical Therapy* 49, 1201–1207.

Marechal, G. (1964) *Le Metabolisme de la Phosphorylcreatine et de l'Adenosine Triphosphate durant la Contraction Musculaire.* Editions Arscia, Brussels.

Margaria, R. (1938) Sulla fisiologia e specialmente sul consumo energetico della marcia e della corsa a varie velocita ed inclinazioni del terreno. *Atti Della Accademie Nazionale Dei Lincei Memorie.* Serie 7, 299–368.

McFadyen, B.J. & Winter, D.A. (1988) An integrated biomechanical analysis of normal stair ascent and descent. *Journal of Biomechanics* 21, 733–744.

McNitt-Gray, J.L. (1993) Kinetics of the lower extremities during drop landing from three heights. *Journal of Biomechanics* 26, 1037–1046.

Miyamura, M., Folgering, H.T., Binkhorst, R.A. & Smolders, F.D. (1976) Ventilatory response to CO_2 at rest and during positive and negative work in normoxia and hyperoxia. *Pflugers Archive* 364, 7–15.

Monod, H. & Scherrer, J. (1973) Equivalence between positive and negative muscular work. In: *Medicine and Sport* Vol 8. *Biomechanics* III (eds S. Cerquiglini, A. Venerando & J. Wartenweiler), pp. 261–267. Karger, Basel.

Moore, J.C. (1971) Active resistive stretch and isometric exercise in strengthening wrist flexion in normal adults. *Archive of Physical Medicine and Rehabilitation* 52, 264–269.

Morecki, A., Fidelus, K. & Ekiel, J. (1971) *Bionika Ruchu.* PWN, Warsaw.

Morgan, D.L. (1994) An explanation for residual increased tension in striated muscle after stretch during contraction. *Experimental Physiology* 79, 831–838.

Morrison, J.B. (1970) The mechanics of muscle function in locomotion. *Journal of Biomechanics* 3, 431–451.

Murray, M.P., Guten, G.N., Mollinger, L.A. & Gardner, G.M. (1983) Kinematic and electromyographic patterns of Olympic race walkers. *American Journal of Sports Medicine* 11, 68–74.

Nadel, E.R., Bergh, U. & Saltin, B. (1972) Body temperatures during negative work exercise. *Journal of Applied Physiology* 33, 553–558.

Nagle, F.J., Balke, B. & Naughton, J.P. (1965) Gradational step tests for assessing work capacity. *Journal of Applied Physiology* 20, 745–748.

Nielsen, B. (1969) Thermoregulation in rest and exercise. *Acta Physiologica Scandinavica* (Suppl.) 323, 1–74.

Nielsen, B., Nielsen, S.L. & Petersen, F.B. (1972) Thermoregulation during positive and negative work at different environmental temperatures. *Acta Physiologica Scandinavica* 85, 249–257.

Nigg, B.M. (1985) Biomechanics, load analysis and sports injuries in the lower extremities. *Sports Medicine* 2, 367–379.

Nigg, B.M. & Neukomm, P.A. (1973) Erschutterungsmessungen beim Shifahren. *Medizinische Welt* 24, 1883–1885.

Nordone, A., Romano, C. & Schieppati, M. (1989) Selective recruitment of high-threshold human motor units during voluntary isotonic lengthening of active muscles. *Journal of Physiology* 409, 451–471.

Norman, R.W. & Komi, P.V. (1979) Electromechanical delay in skeletal muscle under normal movement conditions. *Acta Physiologica Scandinavica* 106, 241–248.

Pandolf, K.B., Kamon, E. & Noble, B.J. (1978) Perceived exertion and physiological responses during negative and positive work in climbing a laddermill. *Journal of Sports Medicine and Physical Fitness* 18, 227–236.

Pierrynowski, M.R. (1995) Analytic representation of muscle line of action and geometry. In: *Three-Dimensional Analysis of Human Movement* (eds P. Allard, I.A.F. Stokes & J.-P. Blanchi), pp. 215–256. Human Kinetics Publishers, Champaign, IL.

Pierrynowski, M.R., Winter, D.A. & Norman, R.W. (1980) Transfers of mechanical energy within the total body and mechanical efficiency during treadmill walking. *Ergonomics* 23, 147–156.

Prilutsky, B.I. (1989) Exercise-induced muscle pain. *Theory and Practice of Physical Culture* N2, 16–21 (in Russian).

Prilutsky, B.I. (1990) Eccentric muscle action in human locomotion. PhD thesis, Latvian Research Institute of Traumatology and Orthopedics, Riga (in Russian).

Prilutsky, B.I. (1991) Eccentric muscle activity in sports locomotion. *Theory and Practice of Physical Culture* N1, 53–61 (in Russian).

Prilutsky, B.I. (1997) Work, energy expenditure, and efficiency of the stretch–shortening cycle. *Journal of Applied Biomechanics* 13, 466–471.

Prilutsky, B.I. & Zatsiorsky, V.M. (1992) Mechanical energy expenditure and efficiency of walking and running. *Human Physiology* 18, 118–127 (in Russian).

Prilutsky, B.I. & Zatsiorsky, V.M. (1994) Tendon action of two-joint muscles: transfer of mechanical energy between joints during jumping, landing, and running. *Journal of Biomechanics* 27, 25–34.

Prilutsky, B.I., Zatsiorsky, V.M., Bravaya, D.Y. & Petrova, L.N. (1992) Maximal power in extending knee joint in one-joint and natural movements. *Human Physiology* 18, 573–583 (in Russian).

Prilutsky, B.I., Herzog, W., Leonard, T.R. & Allinger, T.L. (1996a) Role of the muscle belly and tendon of soleus, gastrocnemius, and plantaris in mechanical energy absorption and generation during cat locomotion. *Journal of Biomechanics* **29**, 417–434.

Prilutsky, B.I., Petrova, L.N. & Raitsin, L.M. (1996b) Comparison of mechanical energy expenditure of joint moments and muscle forces during human locomotion. *Journal of Biomechanics* **29**, 405–415.

Rack, P.M.H. & Westbury, D.R. (1974) The short range stiffness of active mammalian muscle and its effect on mechanical properties. *Journal of Physiology* **240**, 331–350.

Rall, J.A. (1985) Energetic aspects of skeletal muscle contraction: implication of fiber types. *Exercise and Sport Sciences Reviews* **13**, 33–74.

Requejo, P., McNitt-Gray, J.L., Eagle, J., Munkasy, B.A. & Smith, S. (1998) Multijoint load distribution and power generation during high velocity impact. In: *The Third North American Congress on Biomechanics*, pp. 459–460. University of Waterloo, Waterloo.

Richardson, M. (1966) Physiological responses and energy expenditures of women using stairs of three designs. *Journal of Applied Physiology* **21**, 1078–1082.

Roberts, T.J., Marsh, R.L., Weyand, P.G. & Taylor, C.R. (1997) Muscular force in running turkeys: the economy of minimizing work. *Science* **275**, 1113–1115.

Rodgers, K.L. & Berger, R.A. (1974) Motor-unit involvement and tension during maximum, voluntary concentric, eccentric contractions of the elbow flexors. *Medicine and Science in Sports* **6**, 253–259.

Sanzen, L., Forsberg, A. & Westlin, N. (1986) Anterior tibial compartment pressure during race walking. *American Journal of Sports Medicine* **14**, 136–138.

Schmidt, R.A. (1988) *Motor Control and Learning*. Human Kinetics Publishers, Champaign, IL

Seliger, V., Dolejs, L. & Karas, V. (1980) A dynamometric comparison of maximum eccentric, concentric, and isometric contractions using emg and energy expenditure measurements. *European Journal of Applied Physiology* **45**, 235–244.

Seliger, V., Dolejs, L., Karas, V. & Pachlopnikova, I. (1968) Adaptation of trained athletes' energy expenditure to repeated concentric and eccentric contractions. *International Zeitschrift Fur Angewandte Physiologie Einschliesslich Arbeitsphysiologie* **26**, 227–234.

Simpson, K.J. & Kanter, L. (1997) Jump distance of dance landing influencing internal joint forces: I. Axial forces. *Medicine and Science in Sports and Exercise* **29**, 917–927.

Smiles, K.A. & Robinson, S. (1971) Regulation of sweat secretion during positive and negative work. *Journal of Applied Physiology* **30**, 409–412.

Stauber, W.T. (1989) Eccentric action of muscles: physiology, injury, and adaptation. *Exercise and Sport Sciences Reviews* **17**, 157–185.

Stefanyshyn, D.J. & Nigg, B.M. (1997) Mechanical energy contribution of the metatarsophalangeal joint to running and sprinting. *Journal of Biomechanics* **30**, 1081–1085.

Stefanyshyn, D.J. & Nigg, B.M. (1998) Contribution of the lower extremity joints to mechanical energy in running vertical jumps and running long jumps. *Journal of Sports Sciences* **16**, 177–186.

Stein, R.B., Yang, J.F., Belanger, M. & Pearson, K.G. (1993) Modification of reflexes in normal and abnormal movements. *Progress in Brain Research* **97**, 189–196.

Sugi, H. & Tsuchiya, T. (1981) Enhancement of mechanical performance in frog muscle fibers after quick increases in load. *Journal of Physiology* **319**, 239–252.

Sugi, H. & Tsuchiya, T. (1988) Stiffness changes during enhancement and deficit of isometric force by slow length changes in frog skeletal muscle fibers. *Journal of Physiology* **407**, 215–229.

Thomson, D.A. (1971) Cardiac output during positive and negative work. *Scandinavian Journal of Clinical and Laboratory Investigation* **27**, 193–200.

Thys, H., Faraggianna, T. & Margaria, R. (1972) Utilization of muscle elasticity in exercise. *Journal of Applied Physiology* **32**, 491–494.

Thys, H., Cavagna, G.A. & Margaria, R. (1975) The role played by elasticity in an exercise involving movements of small amplitude. *Pflugers Archive* **354**, 281–286.

Tsirakos, D., Baltzopoulos, V. & Bartlett, R. (1997) Inverse optimization: functional and physiological considerations related to the force-sharing problem. *Critical Reviews in Biomedical Engineering* **25**, 371–407.

Tupa, V.V., Aleshinsky, C.Yu., Kaimin, M.A., Pereversev, A.P., Polozkov, A.G. & Fruktov, A.L. (1980) Basic features of the ground interaction in sports locomotion. In: *Biomechanical Basis of Sport Technique in Track and Field Athletics*

(eds V.I. Voronkin & V.M. Zatsiorsky), pp. 4–28. Central Institute of Physical Culture, Moscow.

Verbitsky, O., Mizrahi, J., Voloshin, A., Treiger, J. & Isakov, E. (1998) Shock transmission and fatigue in human running. *Journal of Applied Biomechanics* **14**, 300–311.

Viitasalo, J.T. & Bosco, C. (1982) Electro-mechanical behavior of human muscles in vertical jumps. *European Journal of Applied Physiology* **48**, 253–261.

Voight, M., Bojsen-Moller, F., Simonsen, E.B. & Dyhre-Poulsen, P. (1995) The influence of tendon Youngs modulus, dimensions and instantaneous moment arms on the efficiency of human movement. *Journal of Biomechanics* **28**, 281–291.

Voloshin, A.S., Mizrahi, J., Verbitsky, O. & Isakov, E. (1998) Dynamic loading on the musculoskeletal system—effect of fatigue. *Clinical Biomechanics* **13**, 515–520.

Vos, E.J., Harlaar, J. & van Ingen Schenau, G.J. (1991) Electromechanical delay during knee extensor contractions. *Medicine and Science in Sports and Exercise* **23**, 1187–1193.

Wassermann, K., Hansen, J.E., Sue, D.Y. & Whipp, B.J. (1986) *Principles of Exercise Testing and Interpretation*. Lea & Febiger, Philadelphia.

Wells, R.P. (1988) Mechanical energy costs of human movement: an approach to evaluating the transfer possibilities of two-joint muscles. *Journal of Biomechanics* **21**, 955–964.

Westing, S.H., Seger, J.Y. & Thorstensson, A. (1990) Effects of electrical stimulation on eccentric and concentric torque-velocity relationships during knee extension in man. *Acta Physiologica Scandinavica* **140**, 17–22.

Westing, S.H., Cresswell, A.G. & Thorstensson, A. (1991) Muscle activation during maximal voluntary eccentric and concentric extension. *European Journal of Applied Physiology* **62**, 104–108.

Whipp, B.J. & Wasserman, K. (1969) Efficiency of muscle work. *Journal of Applied Physiology* **26**, 644–648.

Williams, K.R. & Cavanagh, P.R. (1983) A model for the calculation of mechanical power during distance running. *Journal of Biomechanics* **16**, 115–128.

Winter, D.A. (1983a) Energy generation and absorption at the ankle and knee during fast, natural and slow cadences. *Clinical Orthopaedics and Related Research* **175**, 147–154.

Winter, D.A. (1983b) Moments of force and mechanical power in jogging. *Journal of Biomechanics* **16**, 91–97.

Winter, D.A. (1990). *Biomechanics and Motor Control of Human Movement.* John Wiley & Sons, New York.

Winter, D.A. & Robertson, G.E. (1978) Joint torque and energy patterns in normal gait. *Biological Cybernetics* **29**, 137–142.

Woledge, R.C. (1997) Efficiency definitions relevant to the study of the stretch–shortening cycle. *Journal of Applied Biomechanics* **13**, 476–479.

Woledge, R.C., Curtin, N.A. & Homsher, E. (1985). *Energetic Aspects of Muscle Contraction.* Academic Press, London.

Yamaguchi, G.T., Sawa, A.G.U., Moran, D.W., Fessler, M.J. & Winters, J.M. (1990) A survey of human musculotendon actuator parameters. In: *Multiple Muscle Systems: Biomechanics and Movement Organization* (eds J. Winters & L.-Y. Woo), pp. 718–773. Springer-Verlag, Berlin.

Zatsiorsky, V.M. (1986) Mechanical work and energy expenditure in human motion. In: *Contemporary Problems of Biomechanics. Vol 3: Optimization of the Biomechanical Movements* (ed. I.V. Knets), pp. 14–32. Zinatne, Riga (in Russian).

Zatsiorsky, V.M. (1997) On muscle and joint viscosity. *Motor Control* **1**, 299–309.

Zatsiorsky, V.M. & Prilutsky, B.I. (1987) Soft and stiff landing. In: *International Series on Biomechanics, V6B: Biomechanics X-B* (ed. B. Jonsson), pp. 739–743. Human Kinetics Publishers, Champaign, IL.

Zatsiorsky, V.M. & Prilutsky, B.I. (1993) Prediction of forces of individual muscles in humans. In: *Muscle Biomechanics and Movement Structure. Modern Problems of Biomechanics*, Vol. 7 (ed. V.M. Zatsiorsky), pp. 81–123. Institute of Applied Physics, Russian Academy of Sciences, Nizhni Novgorod (in Russian).

Zatsiorsky, V.M., Kaimin, M.A., Tupa, V.V. & Aleshinsky, C.Yu. (1980) *Biomechanics of Race Walking.* Central Institute of Physical Culture, Moscow (in Russian).

Zatsiorsky, V.M., Aruin, A.S. & Seluyanov, V.N. (1981) *Biomechanics of the Human Musculoskeletal System.* FiS, Moscow (in Russian).

Zatsiorsky, V.M., Aleshinsky, S.Yu. & Yakunin, N.A. (1982) *Biomechanical Basis of Endurance.* FiS, Moscow (in Russian).

Chapter 5

Stretch–Shortening Cycle of Muscle Function

P.V. KOMI AND C. NICOL

Introduction

Traditionally muscular exercises have been classified into static and dynamic types. However, even if this classification is further extended into isolated forms of isometric, concentric and eccentric muscle actions, it does not correctly describe the true nature of muscle function and its forms of contraction. Muscular exercises seldom, if ever, involve pure forms of isolated contraction types. This is because the body segments are periodically subjected to impact or stretch forces. Running, walking and hopping are typical examples of how external forces (e.g. gravity) lengthen the muscle. In this particular phase the muscle is acting eccentrically, and concentric (shortening) action follows. According to the

definition of eccentric action, the muscles must be active during stretch. This combination of eccentric and concentric actions forms a natural type of muscle function called the stretch–shortening cycle, or SSC (Norman & Komi 1979; Komi 1984, 1992) (Fig. 5.1).

A particularly important feature of the SSC is that the muscles are preactivated before they are subjected to stretch (eccentric actions). SSC muscle function has a well-recognized purpose: enhancement of performance of the final phase (concentric action) when compared with the isolated action (e.g. Komi 1984). This can be demonstrated in isolated muscle preparations with constant electrical stimulation (e.g. Cavagna *et al.* 1965, 1968), in animal experiments with natural and variable muscle

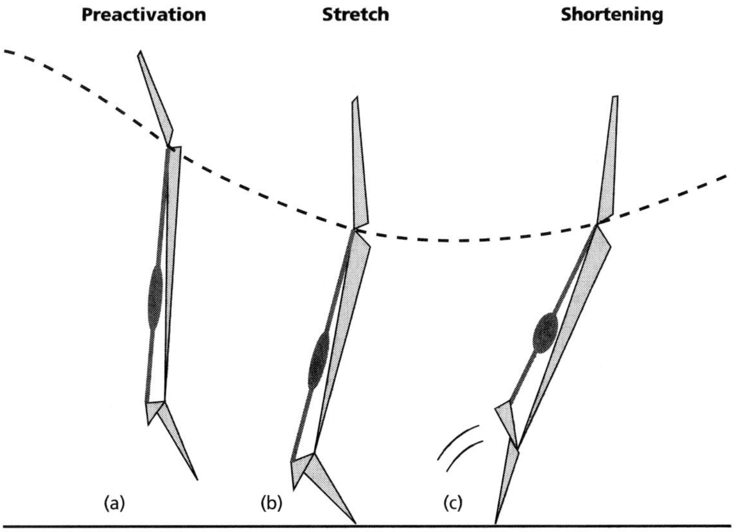

Fig. 5.1 In human walking and running considerable impact loads occur when contact is made with the ground. This requires preactivation of the lower limb extensor muscles before ground contact to prepare them to resist the impact (a) and the active braking (stretch) phase (b). The stretch phase is followed by a shortening (concentric) action (c). (After Komi 1992.)

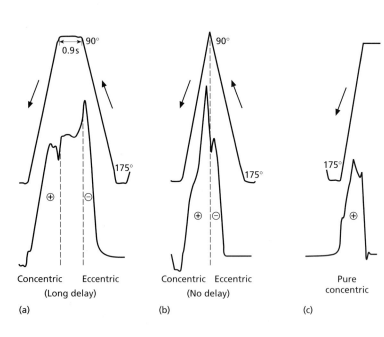

Concentric   Eccentric
(Long delay)

(a)

Concentric   Eccentric
(No delay)

(b)

Pure
concentric

(c)

Fig. 5.2 Demonstration of the importance of the short coupling time between eccentric and concentric phases for performance potentiation in the concentric phase of SSC. (a) Longer delay (0.9 s) was allowed between the eccentric and concentric phases. The potentiation effect on the concentric phase was reduced. (b) Concentric action is preceded by eccentric (–) action, but no delay is allowed when contraction type is changed from stretch to shortening. The eccentric (stretch) phase begins in the middle of the movement from the 175° (knee in an extended position) to the 90° position. Note the clear force potentiation in the concentric phase (+) compared with the condition on the right. (c) Pure concentric contraction of the knee extension from 100° to 175°. (From Komi 1983.)

activation (e.g. Gregor *et al.* 1988), and in maximal effort conditions of human SSC actions (Cavagna *et al.* 1968; Komi 1983). Figure 5.2 demonstrates the force potentiation in SSC in humans where the coupling between the stretch and shortening is varied. Since Cavagna *et al.* (1965) introduced the basic mechanisms of work enhancement when an isolated muscle was subjected to active stretch (eccentric action) prior to its shortening (concentric action), considerable scientific work has been devoted to explain the detailed mechanisms of force and power potentiation in SSC. Cavagna *et al.* (1965) argued that this enhancement is primarily elastic in nature, and although many additional alternative explanations (e.g. Huijing 1992; Komi & Gollhofer 1997; van Ingen-Schenau *et al.* 1997) have been given, no convincing evidence has been presented to refute the notion that elastic potentiation plays an important role in force potentiation during SSC.

At the level of a single muscle group, SSC can be demonstrated well by using direct *in vivo* tendon force measurements, for example during running. The technique used to obtain the Achilles tendon (AT) force curves of Fig. 5.3 involved implanta-

tion of a buckle transducer under local anaesthesia around the AT of a healthy human subject (Komi 1990). This technique allowed the subject to perform unrestricted locomotion, including walking, running at different speeds, hopping, jumping and bicycling. In some cases even maximal long jumps were performed without any discomfort. Figure 5.3 presents typical results of the occurrence of SSC in gastrocnemius and soleus muscles during running at moderate speed. There are several important features to be noted in Fig. 5.3. First the changes in muscle-tendon length are very small (6–7%) during the stretching phase. This suggests that the conditions favour the potential utilization of short-range elastic stiffness (SRES) (Rack & Westbury 1974) in the skeletal muscle. Various length changes are reported in the literature demonstrating that the effective range of SRES in *in vitro* preparations is 1–4% (e.g. Huxley & Simmons 1971; Ford *et al.* 1978). In the intact muscle-tendon complex *in vivo*, this value is increased because series elasticity and fibre geometry must be taken into account. This could then bring the muscle-tendon lengthening to 6–8%. Other findings, in addition to that of Fig. 5.3, indicate that length changes of the triceps

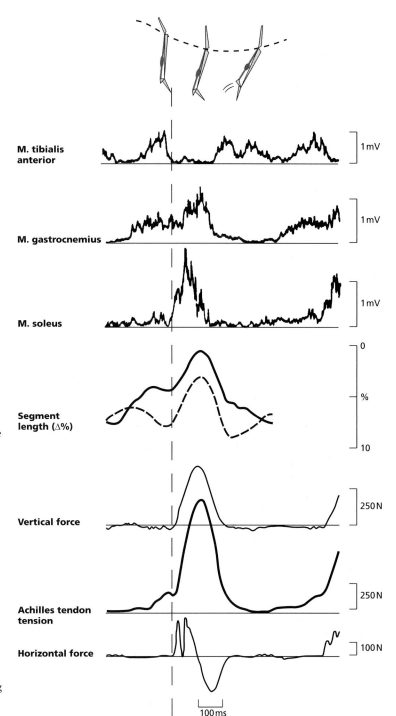

Fig. 5.3 Demonstration of SSC for the triceps surae muscle during the (functional) ground contact phase of human running. *Top*: Schematic representing the three phases of SSC presented in Fig. 5.1. The remaining curves represent parameters in the following order (from the top): rectified surface EMG records of the tibialis anterior, gastrocnemius and soleus muscles; segmental length changes of the two plantar flexor muscles; vertical ground reaction force; directly recorded Achilles tendon force; and the horizontal ground reaction force. The vertical lines signify the beginning of the foot (ball) contact on the force plate and the end of the braking phase, respectively. The subject was running at moderate speed. (From Komi 1992.)

M. tibialis anterior

1 mV

M. gastrocnemius

1 mV

M. soleus

1 mV

Segment length (Δ%)

0

%

10

Vertical force

250 N

Achilles tendon tension

250 N

Horizontal force

100 N

100 ms

surae-Achilles tendon complex are, in running and drop jumps, between 6 and 9% during the functional contact phase. When measurements are made on the muscle fibre level, the values are naturally smaller, as shown by Roberts *et al.* (1997) in turkeys running on level ground.

The second important feature in Fig. 5.3 is that the segmental length changes in these two muscles (gastrocnemius and soleus) take place in phase in both the lengthening and shortening parts of SSC. This is typical for running and jumping, and it has considerable importance because the buckle transducer measures forces of the common tendon for the two muscles. The situation is not so simple in some other activities, such as bicycling (Gregor *et al.* 1991), where the length changes are more out of phase in these two muscles. The third important feature of the example in Fig. 5.3 is that the form of the AT force curve resembles that of a bouncing ball, implying efficient force potentiation.

Muscle mechanics and performance potentiation in SSC

The true nature of force potentiation during SSC can be seen by computing the instantaneous force–length and force–velocity curves from the parameters shown in Fig. 5.3. Figure 5.4 presents the results of such an analysis from fast running; it covers the functional ground contact phase only. It is important to note from this figure that the force–length curve demonstrates a very sharp increase in force during the stretching phase, which is characterized by a very small change in muscle length. The right-hand side of the figure shows the computed instantaneous force–velocity comparison suggesting high potentiation during the shortening phase (concentric action). Figure 5.5, on the other hand, represents examples of electromyographic (EMG)–length and EMG–velocity plots for moderate running. It clearly demonstrates that muscle activation levels are variable and primarily concentrated for the eccentric part of the cycle. This is important to consider when comparing the naturally occurring SSC actions with those obtained with isolated muscle preparations and constant activation levels throughout the cycle.

The force–velocity curve of Fig. 5.4 is a dramatic demonstration that the instantaneous force–velocity curves are very unlike the classical curve obtained for the pure concentric action with isolated muscle preparations (e.g. Hill 1938) or with human forearm

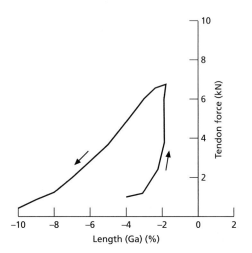
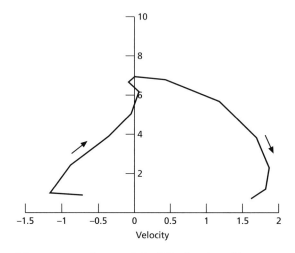

Fig. 5.4 Instantaneous force–length and force–velocity curves of the gastrocnemius muscle for SSC when the subject ran at fast speed (9 m · s⁻¹). The upward deflection signifies stretching (eccentric action) and the downward deflection shortening (concentric action) of the muscle during ground contact. The horizontal axes have been derived from segmental length changes according to Grieve *et al.* (1978). (From Komi 1992.)

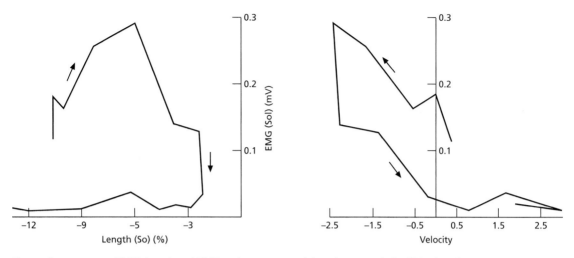

Fig. 5.5 Instantaneous EMG–length and EMG–velocity curves of the soleus muscle for SSC when the subject ran at moderate speed. The arrows indicate how the events changed from stretching to shortening during the contact phase. Please note that the EMG activity is primarily concentrated in the eccentric part of the cycle.

flexors (e.g. Wilkie 1950; Komi 1973). Although Fig. 5.4 does not present directly the comparison of the force–velocity (F–V) curve for the final concentric (push-off) phase with the classical curve, it certainly suggests considerable force potentiation. Unfortunately the human experiment shown in Fig. 5.4 did not include comparative records obtained in a classical way. However, our recent development of *in vivo* measurements with an optic-fibre technique (Komi *et al.* 1995) has now been utilized to obtain these comparisons.

Figure 5.6 shows the instantaneous plots of the force–velocity curve during hopping. The classical type of curve obtained with constant maximal activation for the concentric action of the triceps surae is superimposed in the same graph. The area between the two curves suggests remarkable force potentiation in the concentric part of SSC.

The *in vivo* measurement technique for humans has been developed following reports on animal experiments (e.g. Sherif *et al.* 1983). Many of these animal studies have included similar parameters to

Fig. 5.6 Instantaneous force–velocity curve of the gastrocnemius muscle for the ground-contact phase of hopping. Note that in the concentric phase the force is greater (shaded area) than that of the force–velocity curve measured in the classical way. The data were obtained with the optic-fibre technique (Komi *et al.* 1996) of Achilles tendon force recordings. (From Finni *et al.* in preparation.)

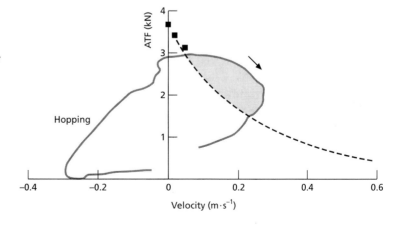

those used in our human studies, such as muscle length, force and EMG. The most relevant report for comparison with present human experiments is that of Gregor *et al.* (1988); these authors measured the mechanical outputs of the cat soleus muscle during treadmill locomotion. In that study the results indicated that the force generated at a given shortening velocity during the late stance phase was greater, especially at higher speeds of locomotion, than the output generated at the same shortening velocity *in situ*. Thus, both animal and human *in vivo* force experiments seem to give similar results with regard to the force–velocity relationships during SSC.

The difference between the force–velocity curve and the classical curve in isolated muscle preparations (e.g. Hill 1938) or in human experiments (e.g. Wilkie 1950; Komi 1973) may be partly due to natural differences in muscle activation levels between the two types of activities. While the *in situ* preparations may primarily measure the shortening properties of the contractile elements in the muscle, natural locomotion, primarily utilizing SSC action, involves controlled release of high forces, caused primarily by the eccentric action. This high force favours storage of elastic strain energy in the muscle-tendon complex. A portion of this stored energy can be recovered during the subsequent shortening phase and used for performance potentiation. Both animal and human experiments seem therefore to agree that natural locomotion with primarily SSC muscle action may produce muscle outputs which can be very different to those of isolated preparations, where activation levels are held constant and storage of strain energy is limited.

The SSC enables the triceps surae muscle to perform very efficiently in activities such as walking, running and hopping. Recent evidence has demonstrated that the gastrocnemius and soleus muscles also function in bicycling in SSC, although the active stretching phases are not so apparent as in running or jumping (Gregor *et al.* 1987, 1991). In contrast to hopping the elastic recoil of the triceps surae muscle plays a much smaller role in countermovement jumps (CMJ) (Fukashiro *et al.* 1993; Finni *et al.* 1998). This is expected because in

CMJ the stretch phase is slow and the reflex contribution to SSC potentiation is likely to be much less than in hopping.

Role of stretch reflexes in force enhancement during SSC

When discussing the possible reflex mechanisms involved in performance potentiation during SSC, the key question is what are the important features of effective SSC function. In our understanding an effective SSC requires three fundamental conditions (Komi & Gollhofer 1997):
1 well-timed preactivation of the muscle(s) before the eccentric phase;
2 a short fast eccentric phase; and
3 immediate transition (short delay) between stretch (eccentric) and shortening (concentric) phases.

These conditions are well met in 'normal' activities such as running and hopping, and seem therefore suitable for possible interaction with stretch reflexes.

Demonstration of short latency stretch reflexes in SSC

Stiffness regulation is a very important concept in the eccentric part of SSC, and stretch reflexes play an important role in this task. Hoffer and Andreassen (1981) demonstrated convincingly that when reflexes are intact, muscle stiffness is greater for the same operating force than in an arreflexive muscle. Thus, stretch reflexes may already make a net contribution to muscle stiffness during the eccentric part of SSC.

In hopping and running, the short-latency stretch reflex component (SLC) can be quite easily observed, especially in the soleus muscle. Figure 5.7 illustrates studies where this component appears clearly in the EMG patterns when averaged over several trials involving two leg hops with short contact times. Also Voigt *et al.* (1997), in a similar study, measured both the origin-to-insertion muscle lengthening and the muscle fibre lengthening. Both measurements showed high stretch velocities in

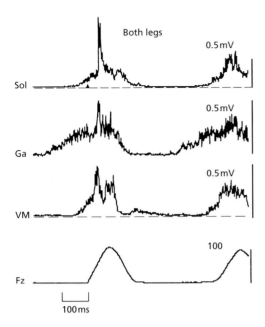

Both legs

0.5 mV

Sol

0.5 mV

Ga

0.5 mV

VM

100

Fz

100 ms

Fig. 5.7 Averaged rectified EMG records of the soleus (Sol), gastrocnemius (Ga), and vastus medialis (VM) muscles in the drop jump from 60 cm height. Note the sharp EMG reflex peak in the soleus muscle during early contact phase. (Reprinted, by permission, from Komi & Gollhofer 1997.) (After Gollhofer *et al.* 1992.)

the early contact phase, which led the authors to conclude that the conditions were sufficient for muscle-spindle afferent activation. The SLC is sensitive to loading conditions as shown in Fig. 5.8, where the stretch loads vary from the preferred submaximal hopping (the records on the top) to drop jumps. In the highest drop jump condition (80 cm) the SLC component becomes less clear, suggesting decreased facilitation from the muscle spindles and/or increased inhibitory drive from various sources (e.g. Golgi tendon organ (GTO), voluntary protection mechanisms, etc.). In cases where the drop jumps have been performed from excessive heights, for example from 140 cm (Kyröläinen & Komi 1995), the subjects had to sustain extreme loads during contact. In these situations, the reduced reflex activation may functionally serve as a protection strategy to prevent muscle and/or tendon injury.

Magnitude of reflex-induced EMG activity

It has been shown during passive dorsiflexion tests that the SLC and the medium latency component (MLC) can be dramatically reduced if the measurements are made during ischaemic blockade of the lower limb (e.g. Fellows *et al.* 1993). This method has been applied to conditions of fast running (Dietz *et al.* 1979), in which the control runs made before ischaemia demonstrated that the gastrocnemius EMG had a clear SLC component during contact. The average peak EMG was at least two times higher than that measured during a maximal voluntary isometric plantar flexion test (Fig. 5.9). When ischaemic blockade was performed, the gastrocnemius EMG during contact was dramatically reduced in the fast running test with the same velocity, but there was no change in preactivation. These results emphasize the potential role of Ia afferent input in SSC-type activities such as running. The ischaemic blockade is used to isolate the Ia afferent information acting on spinal pathways (Fellows *et al.* 1993).

Do reflexes have time to be operative during SSC?

As it has been reportedly questioned and denied that stretch reflexes can operate and contribute to force and power enhancement during SSC (van Ingen-Schenau *et al.* 1997), it is important to examine what role the stretch reflexes may play, if any, during SSC. It is difficult to imagine that proprioceptive reflexes, the existence of which has been known for centuries, would not play any significant role in human locomotion including SSCs. It is true that in normal movements with high EMG activity, the magnitude and net contribution of reflex regulation of muscle force are methodologically difficult to assess. The task becomes much easier when one studies relatively slow (1.2–1.9 rad · s⁻¹) passive dorsiflexions, where the stretch-induced reflex EMG has been reported to enhance AT force by 200–500% over the purely passive stretch without reflex EMG response (Nicol & Komi 1998). Figure 5.10 is an example of

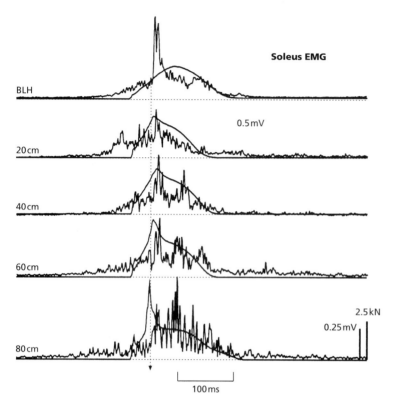

Fig. 5.8 Rectified and averaged EMG-pattern of the soleus muscle and vertical ground reaction force in various stretch–shortening cycle drop jumps with both legs. The figure illustrates the modulation in the pattern and in the force record with increasing stretch load. *From top*: BLH (both legs hopping in place), and 20–80 cm (drop jumps from 20 to 80 cm height, landing with both legs). The dashed vertical line indicates the initiation of the phasic activation with a latency of 40 ms after ground contact. (Reprinted, by permission, from Komi & Gollhofer 1997.)

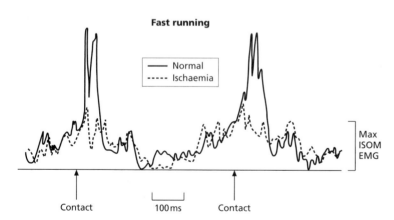

Fig. 5.9 Rectified and averaged EMG activity of the gastrocnemius muscle when the subject was making many steps during fast running on the spot. The control (normal) before ischaemia shows the typical rapid increase of EMG 40 ms after ground contact. The dashed line indicates the same running after 20 min of ischaemia produced by a tourniquet around the thigh. The stretch-induced EMG activity (SLC component) was reduced to the level of Max iISOM EMG (the bar on the right) without reduction in the preactivity before contact. (After Dietz *et al.* 1979.)

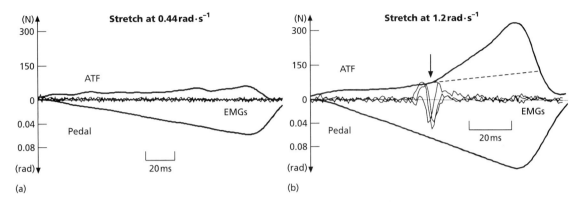

Fig. 5.10 Demonstration of passively induced stretch reflexes on the Achilles tendon force (ATF). (a) Passive dorsiflexion at slow stretch caused no reflex EMG response and led to a small and rather linear increase of the ATF (purely passive response). (b) With faster and larger stretches the reflex contribution to ATF corresponds to the additional ATF response above the purely passive influence represented by the dashed line. (From Nicol & Komi 1998.)

these measurements and it shows a typical delay of 12–13 ms between the onset of reflex EMG and onset of force potentiation.

This time delay is similar to electrical stimulation measurements performed together with fibre-optic recordings of the AT force (Komi *et al.* manuscript in preparation). Considering the duration of the simple stretch reflex loop of 40 ms, the maximum delay between initial stretch and subsequent force potentiation would be around 50–55 ms. When referred to running the first contact on the ground would indicate the point of initial stretch. In marathon running the contact phase usually lasts almost 250 ms implying that this reflex-induced force enhancement would already have functional significance during the eccentric phase of the cycle (Nicol *et al.* 1991c). As the contact phase duration (braking and push-off) decreases as a function of the running speed (Luhtanen & Komi 1978) the net reflex contribution will occur at the end of the eccentric phase at faster speeds, and may be extended partly to the push-off phase in maximal sprinting, where the total contact time is only about 90–100 ms (Mero & Komi 1985). These time calculations certainly confirm that stretch reflexes have ample time to operate for force and power enhancement during SSC, and in most cases during the eccentric part of the cycle. Thus, there are no time restraints for reflexes to be operative in stiffness regulation

during SSC. The large reflex-induced EMG component (see Fig. 5.9) must therefore be regarded as an essential and important contribution to force enhancement in SSC.

Functional significance of stretch reflexes in SSC activities

Some aspects of the functional importance of stretch reflexes during SSC have already been referred to above. It is, however, relevant to emphasize that the reflexes contribute to the efficiency of the motor output by making the force output more powerful. In SSC this can only be accomplished by an immediate and smooth transfer from the preactivated and eccentrically stretched muscle-tendon complex to the concentric push-off, in the case of running or hopping, for example. The range of high stiffness is, however, limited to that of the 'short-range elastic stiffness' (SRES) (Rack & Westbury 1974; Morgan 1977). In this case the stiffness of the muscle-tendon complex depends not only on the range of motion (Kearney & Hunter 1982), but also on the efficiency of the stretch reflex system (Nichols & Houk 1976; Houk & Rymer 1981). High stretch-reflex activity is expected after a powerful stretch of an active muscle (e.g. Dietz *et al.* 1984), and these reflexes are necessary not primarily to enhance SRES, but to linearize the stress-strain characteristics (Nichols

1974; Hufschmidt & Schwaller 1987).

It can be assumed that before ground contact in SSC the initial lengthening of the muscle-tendon complex, shown in Fig. 5.3, occurs in the more or less compliant Achilles tendon. As soon as the 'critical' tension is achieved, which is determined by the amount of activity (preactivation) sent to the muscles prior to contact, the forceful 'yielding' of the cross-links of the acto-myosin complex may take place, with concomitant loss of the potential energy stored in the lengthened cross-bridges (e.g. Flitney & Hirst 1978). From *in vitro* studies it is known that yielding of active cross-bridges can be prevented by intense muscular activation. Such an intense phase-dependent and triggered muscular activation can be provided most effectively by the stretch reflex system, which is highly sensitive to the length and tension changes in the muscle-tendon complex. As discussed earlier, the latencies for the reflex EMG are sufficiently short for it to have functional significance. These latencies (40–45 and 12–14 ms, respectively, for the reflex loop and electromechanical delay) fit well with the occurrence of short- and medium-latency stretch-reflex components (e.g. Lee & Tatton 1982). Our recent data on combined stretch and reflex potentiation are well in agreement with the SRES concept, demonstrating that the cross-bridge force resistance to stretch is particularly efficient during the early part of the cross-bridge attachment (Nicol & Komi 1998). Therefore, the reflex-induced cross-link formation appears to play a very rapid and substantial role in force generation during stretch. Furthermore, as demonstrated by Stein (1982) and Nichols (1987), it is the stretch reflex system that provides high linearity in muscular stiffness. All these aspects may contribute to the observation that mechanical efficiency in natural SSC is higher than that in pure concentric exercise (e.g. Aura & Komi 1986; Kyröläinen *et al.* 1990). The concept of elastic storage favours the existence of reflex activation, and high muscular activation during the eccentric phase of SSC is a prerequisite for efficient storage of elastic energy. Animal studies have shown that an electrically stimulated muscle responds to ramp stretches with linear tension increments, provided the muscle has an intact reflex system (Nichols & Houk 1976; Nichols 1987). This

linearity is restricted to small length changes (e.g. Hoffer & Andreassen 1981) and these small changes are indeed relevant to the SSC exercises referred to in the present discussion (see also Fig. 5.3).

Overall there seems to be enough evidence to conclude that stretch reflexes play an important role in SSC and contribute to force generation during touchdown in activities such as running and hopping. Depending on the type of hopping, for example, the amplitude of the SLC peak and its force-increasing potential may vary considerably. However, the combination of the 'prereflex' background activation and the following reflex activation might represent a scenario that supports yield compensation and a fast rate of force development (Voigt *et al.* 1997). This scenario may be especially effective in a non-fatigued situation, but it can be put under severe stress during SSC fatigue.

Fatigue effects of SSC exercise

Mechanical effects

There are several models for studying exhausting SSC exercise, but they have all given remarkably similar results. A special sledge ergometer developed in our laboratory (Kaneko *et al.* 1984; Komi *et al.* 1987) has been used to perform short-term SSC fatigue in either arm (Gollhofer *et al.* 1987) or leg muscles (Horita *et al.* 1996; Nicol *et al.* 1996). Another possibility is to use long-lasting exercise, such as marathon running, as the SSC fatigue model (e.g. Avela *et al.* 1999a). In these different studies, the immediate changes in mechanical performance reveal clear loss of tolerance to the imposed stretch loads. Figure 5.11 is an example of the arm exercise (Gollhofer *et al.* 1987), in which the repeated 100 SSCs were characterized by progressive increases in the contact time in both braking and push-off phases. More specifically, however, progressive increases in the initial force peak and in the subsequent drop were observed. This phenomenon is similar to that depicted in Fig. 5.8, in which the magnitude of both the impact peak and the subsequent drop was higher with higher dropping height. In the example of Fig. 5.11 the dropping

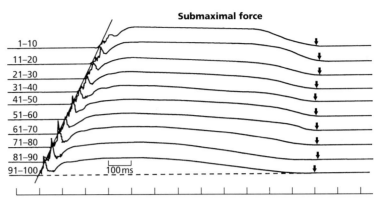

Fig. 5.11 Fatiguing arm SSC exercise resulted in progressive changes in the reaction force record during hand contact with the sledge force plate. The records have been averaged for groups of 10 successive force–time curves. Note the increase in the impact peak with subsequent increase in the force reduction when fatigue progressed. (Adapted from Gollhofer *et al.* 1987.)

height was naturally kept constant, but the subject's ability to tolerate the same stretch load deteriorated considerably with fatigue.

The 'marathon-run' model has also shown similar changes in the ground contact force parameters, either in submaximal running tests (Komi *et al.* 1986) or in tests also including submaximal and maximal SSC tests (Nicol *et al.* 1991a,c). Figure 5.12 is a representative example of such a result, which has been confirmed in subsequent tests with similar marathon-run models (Avela *et al.* 1999). Kinematic analysis has revealed that, both in the short-term

exercise (Gollhofer *et al.* 1987; Horita *et al.* 1996) and long-term SSC fatigue (Nicol *et al.* 1991a), these ground reaction force changes are associated with problems in maintaining a constant angular displacement during contact when fatigue progresses. In a fatigued state the reduction in the force after the impact is likely to be related to the observed faster and longer flexion movement (Nicol *et al.* 1991c; Horita *et al.* 1996). In the case of the arm exercises the dramatic increase in the impact peak results most likely from increased preactivity of the arm extensors, as suggested by Gollhofer *et al.* (1987). The

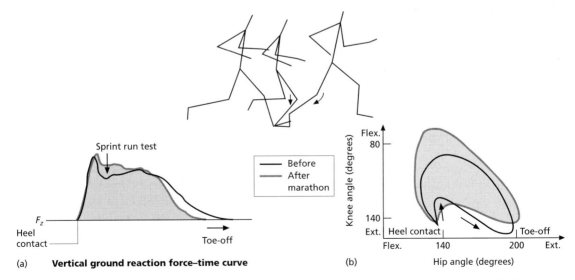

Fig. 5.12 The influence of a marathon run on (a) the vertical ground reaction force and (b) the knee/hip angle diagram. Note a sharp drop in the peak of the sprint force–time curve (a) after the marathon. The angle/angle diagram (b) shows a greater knee flexion immediately after the heel contact in the post-marathon situation. (After Nicol *et al.* 1991a,c.)

decrease in force after impact is, however, probably the main indicator of a reduction in tolerance to repeated stretch loads as fatigue progresses. A logical consequence of this is that in order to maintain the same SSC performance, for example a constant marathon speed, the subject must perform greater work during the push-off phases leading to even faster progression of fatigue.

The mechanical effects of the fatiguing SSC exercise also have long-lasting consequences, which are in many ways similar to purely eccentric exercise. The eccentric fatigue has, however, been referred to more extensively in earlier reviews (e.g. Komi & Nicol 2000; Clarkson et al. 1992), and will therefore not be discussed here in any detail.

In the isometric or concentric fatigue exercises recovery takes place quite rapidly. In SSC exercise, as in eccentric fatigue, both the performance measures (e.g. static and dynamic maximal force test) and the ground reaction force parameters have a recovery phase which may last several days or weeks. In the case of the marathon run, the delayed process takes place in parallel between the maximal EMG activation and maximal force (Fig. 5.13). A more detailed examination of the recovery processes, especially in the short-term intensive SSC exercise, indicates that they take place in a bimodal fashion—showing a dramatic decline immediately after the exercise followed by a short-lasting recovery and a subsequent secondary drop. This second decline in performance may peak either around the

second or third day post-exercise (Nicol et al. 1996; Avela et al. 1999b; Horita et al. 1999). The immediate reduction in performance is naturally related mostly to the metabolic disturbances, whereas the secondary decline must be associated with the well-known inflammatory processes related to muscle damage (Faulkner et al. 1993), which is easily observable after both SSC and eccentric types of fatigue protocols.

Fatigue effects on the stretch reflex-induced force production

Since our earlier reviews (Nicol et al. 1996; Komi & Nicol 2000) considerable evidence has accumulated to indicate that SSC fatigue induces problems in stiffness regulation and that stretch reflexes are major players in this process. Due to the limited space available, the present discussion focuses on the most relevant issues in this regard. The stretch reflex analysis performed either in the passive condition (e.g. Nicol et al. 1996) or during the SSC exercise itself (Horita et al. 1996; Avela & Komi 1998a,b; Avela et al. 1999b) reveal that the stretch reflex amplitude (passive condition) or the short-latency stretch reflex component (SLC) (M_1 amplitude in SSC exercise) are reduced dramatically after the exercise, and their recovery follows the bimodal trend in parallel with the mechanical parameters. Figure 5.14 shows this parallelism as a representative example. The recovery processes are further delayed when the SSC fatigue exercise is repeated, before full recovery, on days 5 and 10 after the first exercise (Nicol et al. 1994). This implies that the stiffness regulation needs a long time to resume its normal state after exhaustive SSC exercise.

There seems to be enough evidence to suggest that coupling could exist also between the performance reduction in SSC and the inflammatory processes resulting from muscle damage. Firstly, decreases in SSC performance are related to increases in an indirect plasma marker (creatine kinase (CK) activity) of muscle damage in the phase corresponding to the secondary injury of Faulkner et al. (1993) and shown in Fig. 5.15a. This coupling concept is further emphasized by Fig. 5.15b, which

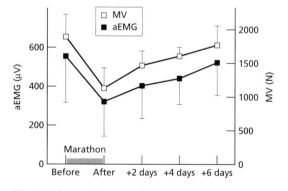

Fig. 5.13 Competitive marathon running causes a dramatic reduction and delayed recovery of maximum EMG and force of the isometric knee extension. (From Pullinen et al. 1997.)

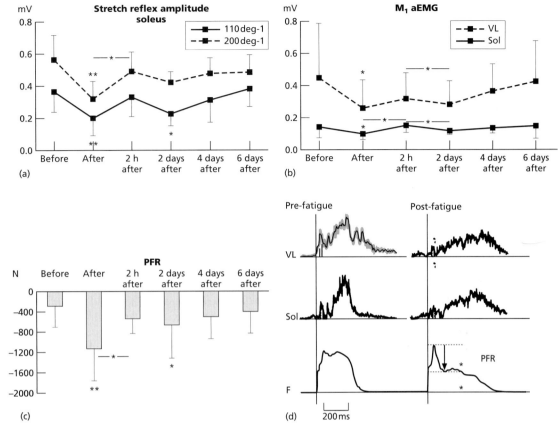

Fig. 5.14 The bimodal trend of recovery of stretch reflexes and ground reaction force on the force plate. The stretch reflexes were measured in two different tests in a group of seven runners before and after a marathon run. (a) Mean changes in the peak-to-peak stretch reflex amplitude of the soleus muscle recorded during 10 mechanically induced passive dorsiflexions (0.17 rad induced at 1.9 and 3.5 rad · s^{-1}). (b) Mean values (±SD) of average area of the SLC component (M$_1$ aEMG) of soleus (Sol) and vastus lateralis (VL) muscles. (c) Peak force reduction (PFR) measured during the standard sledge jump tests. The parameters in (b) and (c) are also shown as pre- and post-marathon comparisons in (d). Note the coupling in the reduction and recovery between reflex parameters and PFR. (From Avela *et al.* 1999b.)

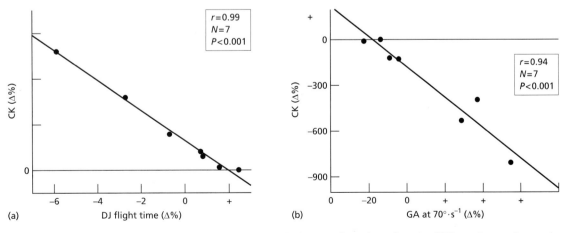

Fig. 5.15 (a) Increase in creatine kinase (CK) activity during the first two days after exhaustive SSC exercise may be associated with decrease in the drop jump (DJ) performance. (b) A similar association is also possible between the recovery of CK activity and stretch reflex amplitude as measured between days 2 and 4 post-SSC fatigue. (Adapted from Nicol *et al.* 1996.)

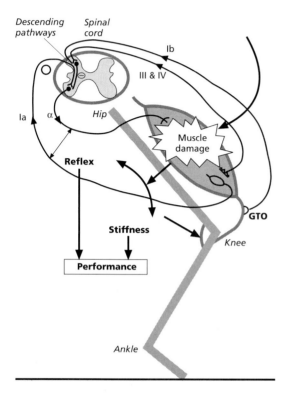

Fig. 5.16 Proposed coupling between SSC exercise-induced muscle damage and performance reduction. Muscle damage changes stiffness regulation through changes in the afferent inputs from the muscle spindle, Golgi tendon organ (GTO) and group III and IV afferent nerve endings. The events occur in the following order. 1. Due to muscle damage the stretch-reflex sensitivity decreases. 2. Muscle (and joint) stiffness regulation becomes disturbed (reduced). 3. The efficiency of SSC function (performance) decreases. The proposed mechanism may be even more apparent in the triceps surae muscle compared with the quadriceps group of the figure. (After Horita *et al.* 1999.)

shows that the subsequent reduction in CK activity between days 2 and 4 post-exercise is also related to the respective recovery of the peak-to-peak stretch reflex EMG amplitude of the examined muscle. This clearly implies that stiffness regulation itself behaves in a similar manner, as Horita *et al.* (1996)

have demonstrated that a parallel exists between the fatigue-induced changes in the stiffness parameters and the short-latency stretch reflex component (SLC).

The coupling concept can be extended also to the discussion of the mechanisms leading to reduced stretch-reflex sensitivity during SSC fatigue. In the case of SSC, however, the observation may not always be uniform, because the intensity and duration of SSC exercise plays an important role in fatiguability of reflex responses (Gollhofer *et al.* 1987).

Figure 5.16 summarizes our current view of the possible interactions between muscle damage, reduced stretch-reflex sensitivity, reduced stiffness regulation, and deterioration in SSC performance. Both presynaptic inhibition (III and IV afferent activation and possibly GTO activation), and several processes of disfacilitation of the alpha motor neurone pool may be involved in the coupling. As regards the latter processes (disfacilitation), our current data rule out the possibility of any significant influence of reduced fusimotor support to the muscle. Instead, however, they strongly suggest that the muscle spindle could be directly or indirectly influenced by exhaustive SSC fatigue (Avela *et al.* 1999a, 2000).

Direct mechanical damage of the intrafusal muscle fibres has been suggested in a previous review (Komi & Nicol 2000). While intrafusal fibres may themselves 'fatigue' in the same manner as the extrafusal fibres, the changes observed in the viscous and elastic properties when the triceps surae muscle was subjected to long-term repeated passive stretches (Avela *et al.* 1998a) strongly suggest that the mechanical stretching of the muscle spindle may be modified in the case of fatiguing SSC exercise as well. Exactly what components are involved in this process has yet to be demonstrated. It has been suggested that deteriorated structural proteins, such as titin and desmin, play a part in the process of muscle damage, and their possible role in SSC fatigue has been discussed (Avela *et al.* 1999a, 2000; Horita *et al.* 1999).

References

Aura, O. & Komi, P.V. (1986) The mechanical efficiency of locomotion in men and women with special emphasis on stretch-shortening cycle exercises. *European Journal of Applied Physiology* **55**, 37–43.

Avela, J. & Komi, P.V. (1998a) Interaction between muscle stiffness and stretch reflex sensitivity after long-term stretch-shortening cycle (SSC) exercise. *Muscle and Nerve* **21**, 1224–1227.

Avela, J. & Komi, P.V. (1998b) Reduced stretch reflex sensitivity and muscle stiffness after long-lasting stretch-shortening cycle (SSC) exercise. *European Journal of Applied Physiology* **78**, 403–410.

Avela, J., Kyröläinen, H. & Komi, P.V. (2000) Neuromuscular changes after long-lasting mechanically and electrically elicited fatigue (submitted for publication).

Avela, J., Kyröläinen, H., Komi, P.V. & Rama, D. (1999a) Reduced reflex sensitivity persists several days after long-lasting stretch-shortening cycle (SSC) exercise. *Journal of Applied Physiology* **86**, 1292–1300.

Avela, J., Kyröläinen, H. & Komi, P.V. (1999b) Altered reflex sensitivity due to repeated and prolonged passive muscle stretching. *Journal of Applied Physiology* **86**, 1283–1291.

Cavagna, G.A., Saibene, F.P. & Margaria, R. (1965) Effect of negative work on the amount of positive work performed by an isolated muscle. *Journal of Applied Physiology* **20**, 157–158.

Cavagna, G.A., Dusman, B. & Margaria, R. (1968) Positive work done by a previously stretched muscle. *Journal of Applied Physiology* **24**, 21–32.

Clarkson, P.M., Nosaka, K. & Braun, B. (1992) Muscle function after exercise-induced muscle damage and rapid adaptation. *Medicine and Science in Sports and Exercise* **24**, 512–520.

Dietz, V., Schmidtbleicher, D. & Noth, J. (1979) Neuronal mechanisms of human locomotion. *Journal of Neurophysiology* **42**, 1212–1222.

Dietz, V., Quintern, J. & Berger, W. (1984) Corrective reactions to stumbling in man. Functional significance of spinal and transcortical reflexes. *Neuroscience Letters* **44**, 131–135.

Faulkner, J.A., Brooks, S.V. & Opiteck, J.A. (1993) Injury to skeletal muscle fibers during contractions: conditions of occurrence and prevention. *Physical Therapy* **73** (12), 911–921.

Fellows, S., Dömges, F., Töpper, R., Thilmann, A. & Noth, J. (1993) Changes in the short and long latency stretch reflex components of the triceps surae muscle during ischaemia in man. *Journal of Physiology* **472**, 737–748.

Finni, T., Komi, P.V. & Lepola, V. (1998) In vivo muscle dynamics during jumping. *Third Annual Congress of the European College of Sport Science, Manchester, UK, 15–18 July, 1998.*

Flitney, F.W. & Hirst, D.G. (1978) Cross-bridge detachment and sarcomere 'give' during stretch of active frog's muscle. *Journal of Physiology* **276**, 449–465.

Ford, L.E., Huxley, A.F. & Simmons, R.M. (1978) Tension responses to sudden length change in stimulated frog muscle fibres near slack length. *Journal of Physiology* **269**, 441–515.

Fukashiro, S., Komi, P.V., Järvinen, M. & Miyashita, M. (1993) Comparison between the directly measured Achilles tendon force and the tendon force calculated from the ankle joint moment during vertical jumps. *Clinical Biomechanics* **8**, 25–30.

Gollhofer, A., Komi, P.V., Fujitsuka, N. & Miyashita, M. (1987) Fatigue during stretch-shortening cycle exercises. II Changes in neuromuscular activation patterns of human skeletal muscle. *International Journal of Sports Medicine* **8**, 38–41.

Gollhofer, A., Strojnik, V., Rapp, W. & Schweizer, L. (1992) Behavior of triceps surae muscle-tendon complex in different jump conditions. *European Journal of Applied Physiology* **64**, 283–291.

Gregor, R.J., Komi, P.V. & Järvinen, M. (1987) Achilles tendon forces during cycling. *International Journal of Sports Medicine* **8**, 9–14.

Gregor, R.J., Roy, R.R., Whiting, W.C., Lovely, R.G., Hodgson, J.A. & Edgerton, V.R. (1988) Mechanical output of the cat soleus during treadmill locomotion in vivo vs. in situ characteristics. *Journal of Biomechanics* **21** (9), 721–732.

Gregor, R.J., Komi, P.V., Browing, R.C. & Järvinen, M. (1991) A comparison of the triceps surae and residual muscle moments at the ankle during cycling. *Journal of Biomechanics* **24**, 287–297.

Grieve, D.W., Pheasant, S.Q. & Cavanagh, P.R. (1978) Prediction of gastrocnemius length from knee and ankle joint posture. In: *Biomechanics VI–A* (eds E. Asmussen & K. Jorgensen), pp. 405–412. University Park Press, Baltimore.

Hill, A.V. (1938) The heat and shortening of the dynamic constant of muscle. *Proceedings of the Royal Society* (London) B **126**, 136–195.

Hoffer, J.A. & Andreassen, S. (1981) Regulation of soleus muscle stiffness in premammillary cats. Intrinsic and reflex components. *Journal of Neurophysiology* **45**, 267–285.

Horita, T., Komi, P.V., Nico, C. & Kyröläinen, H. (1999) Effect of exhausting stretch-shortening cycle exercise on the time course of mechanical behaviour in the drop jump: possible role of muscle damage. *European Journal of Applied Physiology* **79**, 160–167.

Horita, T., Komi, P.V., Nicol, C. & Kyröläinen, H. (1996) Stretch-shortening cycle fatigue: interactions among joint stiffness, reflex, and muscle mechanical performance in the drop jump. *European Journal of Applied Physiology* **73**, 393–403.

Houk, J.C. & Rymer, W.Z. (1981) Neural control of muscle length and tension. In: *Handbook of Physiology. The Nervous System* Vol. II (1) (ed. V.B. Brooks), pp. 257–323. Waverly Press, Baltimore.

Hufschmidt, A. & Schwaller, I. (1987) Short-range elasticity and resting tension of relaxed human lower leg muscles. *Journal of Physiology* **393**, 451–465.

Huijing, P.A. (1992) Elastic potential of muscle. In: *Strength and Power in Sport* (ed. P.V. Komi), pp. 151–168. Blackwell Scientific Publications, Oxford.

Huxley, A.F. & Simmons, R.M. (1971) Proposed mechanism of force generation in striated muscle. *Nature* **233**, 533–538.

van Ingen-Schenau, G.J., Bobbert, M.F. & de Haan, A. (1997) Does elastic energy enhance work and efficiency in the stretch-shortening cycle? *Journal of Applied Biomechanics* **13**, 386–415.

Kaneko, M., Komi, P.V. & Aura, O. (1984) Mechanical efficiency of concentric and eccentric exercise performed with medium to fast contraction rates. *Scandinavian Journal of Sport Science* **6**, 15–20.

Kearney, R.E. & Hunter, I.W. (1982) Dynamics of human ankle stiffness. Variation with displacement amplitude. *Journal of Biomechanics* **15**, 753–756.

Komi, P.V. (1973) Measurement of the force–velocity relationship in human muscle under concentric and eccentric contraction. In: *Medicine and Sport, Biomechanics III* (ed. E. Jokl) Vol. 8, pp. 224–229. Karger, Basel.

Komi, P.V. (1983) Elastic potentiation of muscles and its influence on sport performance. In: *Biomechanik und Sportliche Leistung* (ed. W. Baumann), pp. 59–70. Verlag Karl Hofmann, Schorndorf.

Komi, P.V. (1984) Physiological and biomechanical correlates of muscle function: Effects of muscle structure and stretch-shortening cycle on force and speed. *Exercise and Sports Sciences Reviews/ACSM* **12**, 81–121.

Komi, P.V. (1990) Relevance of in vivo force measurements to human biomechanics. *Journal of Biomechanics* **23** (Suppl. 1), 23–34.

Komi, P.V. (1992) Stretch-shortening cycle. In: *Strength and Power in Sport* (ed. P.V. Komi), pp. 169–179. Blackwell Scientific Publications, Oxford.

Komi, P.V. & Gollhofer, A. (1997) Stretch reflex can have an important role in force enhancement during SSC exercise. *Journal of Applied Biomechanics* **13**, 451–460.

Komi, P.V. & Nicol, C. (2000) Stretch-shortening cycle fatigue. In: *Biomechanics and Biology of Movement* (eds B. McIntosh & B. Nigg). Human Kinetics Publishers, Champaign, IL. (in press).

Komi, P.V., Hyvärinen, T., Gollhofer, A. & Mero, A. (1986) Man-shoe-surface interaction: Special problems during marathon running. *Acta univ. Oul A* **179**, 69–72.

Komi, P.V., Salonen, M., Järvinen, M. & Kokko, O. (1987) In vivo registration of Achilles tendon forces in man. I. Methodological development. *International Journal of Sports Medicine* **8**, 3–8.

Komi, P.V., Belli, A., Huttunen, V. & Partio, E. (1995) Optic fiber as a transducer for direct in-vivo measurements of human tendomuscular forces. In: *Book of Abstracts of the XVth Congress of the International Society of Biomechanics* (eds K. Häkkinen, K.L. Keskinen, P.V. Komi & A. Mero), pp. 494–495. Gummerrus Printing, Jyväskylä, Finland.

Komi, P.V., Belli, A., Huttunen, V., Bonnejoy, R., Geyssaut, A. & Locour, J.R. (1996) Optic fibre as a transducer of tendomuscular forces. *European Journal of Applied Physiology* **72**, 278–280.

Kyröläinen, H. & Komi, P.V. (1995) Differences in mechanical efficiency in athletes during jumping. *European Journal of Applied Physiology* **70**, 36–44.

Kyröläinen, H., Komi, P.V., Oksanen, P., Häkkinen, K., Cheng, S. & Kim, D.H. (1990) Mechanical efficiency of locomotion in females during different kinds of muscle actions. *European Journal of Applied Physiology* **61**, 446–452.

Lee, R.G. & Tatton, W.G. (1982) Long latency reflexes to imposed displacements of the human wrist. Dependence on duration of movement. *Experimental Brain Research* **45**, 207–216.

Luhtanen, P. & Komi, P.V. (1978) Segmental contribution to forces in vertical jump. *European Journal of Applied Physiology* **38**, 181–188.

Mero, A. & Komi, P.V. (1985) Effects of supramaximal velocity on biomechanical variables in sprinting. *International Journal of Sport Biomechanics* **1** (3), 240–252.

Morgan, D.L. (1979) Separation of active and passive components of short-range stiffness of muscle. *American Journal of Physical Medicine* **232**, 45–49.

Nichols, T.R. (1974) Soleus muscle stiffness and its reflex control. PhD thesis, Harvard University, Cambridge, MA.

Nichols, T.R. (1987) The regulation of muscle stiffness. *Medicine and Science in Sports and Exercise* **26**, 36–47.

Nichols, T.R. & Houk, J.C. (1976) Improvement in linearity and regulation of stiffness that results from actions of stretch reflex. *Journal of Neurophysiology* **39**, 119–142.

Nicol, C. & Komi, P.V. (1998) Significance of passively induced stretch reflexes on achilles tendon force enhancement. *Muscle and Nerve* **21**, 1546–1548.

Nicol, C., Komi, P.V. & Marconnet, P. (1991a) Fatigue effects of marathon running on neuromuscular performance I: Changes in muscle force and stiffness characteristics. *Scandinavian Journal of Medicine and Science in Sports* **1**, 10–17.

Nicol, C., Komi, P.V. & Marconnet, P. (1991b) Fatigue effects of marathon running on neuromuscular performance II: Changes in force, integrated electromyographic activity and endurance capacity. *Scandinavian Journal of Medicine and Science in Sports* **1**, 18–24.

Nicol, C., Komi, P.V. & Marconnet, P. (1991c) Effects of marathon fatigue on running kinematics and economy. *Scandinavian Journal of Medicine and Science in Sports* **1**, 195–204.

Nicol, C., Komi, P.V. & Avela, J. (1994) Reduced reflex sensitivity after exhaustive stretch-shortening cycle exercise (abstract). *Symposium on the Neural and Neuromuscular Aspects of Muscle Fatigue, Miami, November 1994.*

Nicol, C., Komi, P.V., Horita, T., Kyrölainen, H. & Takala, T.E.S. (1996) Reduced stretch-reflex sensitivity after exhausting stretch-shortening cycle exercise. *European Journal of Applied Physiology* **72**, 401–409.

Norman, R.W. & Komi, P.V. (1979) Electromechanical delay in skeletal muscle under normal movement conditions. *Acta Physiologica Scandinavica* **106**, 241–248.

Pullinen, T., Leynaert, M. & Komi, P.V. (1997) Neuromuscular function after marathon. *Abstract book of the XVI ISB Congress, August 24–27, Tokyo.*

Rack, P.M.H. & Westbury, D.R. (1974) The short range stiffness of active mammalian muscle and its effect on mechanical properties. *Journal of Physiology* **240**, 331–350.

Roberts, T.J., Marsch, R.L., Weyand, P.G. & Taylor, C.R. (1997) Muscular force in running turkeys: the economy of minimizing work. *Science* **275**, 1113–1115.

Sherif, M.H., Gregor, R.J., Liu, M., Roy, R.R. & Hager, C.L. (1983) Correlation of myoelectric activity and muscle force during selected cat treadmill locomotion. *Journal of Biomechanics* **16**, 691–701.

Stein, R.B. (1982) What muscle variable(s) does the nervous system control in limb movements? *The Behavioral and Brain Sciences* **5**, 535–577.

Voight, M., Dyhre-Poulsen, P. & Simonsen, E.B. (1998) Modulation of short latency stretch reflexes during human hopping. *Acta Physiologica Scandinavica* **163**, 181–194.

Wilkie, D.R. (1950) The relation between force and velocity in human muscle. *Journal of Physiology* **110**, 249.

Chapter 6

Biomechanical Foundations of Strength and Power Training

M.C. SIFF

Introduction

The qualities of strength and power are most popularly associated with sports which require the obvious display of impressive muscular performance such as weightlifting, wrestling and track-and-field events. Consequently, whenever strength training was used as a method of supplementary sports preparation, it was applied most frequently in these types of 'strength' sports and minimally in those sports in which the role of the cardiovascular system was stressed at the expense of almost all other motor qualities.

However, all sports, and indeed all human movements, necessitate the generation of appropriate levels of strength and power in a variety of different applications and situations, as will be discussed later. Several factors have contributed to the prolonged reluctance to accept strength training as a relevant part of the repertoire for preparing all types of international athlete for the rigours of top-level competition, in particular the pre-eminence bestowed by the medical profession on the role of cardiovascular fitness in cardiac and general well-being, the strong scientific focus on metabolic processes as determinants of sporting performance, and the exaggerated condemnation of strength training as a cause of musculoskeletal injury, impaired flexibility and diminished speed of movement.

Biomechanics, the application of mechanics to the understanding of the statics and dynamics of living organisms, appeared to be relegated largely to the analysis of human movement, the aetiology of injuries and the design of equipment for training or competition—an interesting mathematical and computational pursuit playing a somewhat peripheral role compared with the more overt physiological processes which underlie human performance. It is only fairly recently that biomechanics has assumed a prominent position alongside the more traditionally accepted aspects of exercise science. It is now recognized throughout the world as an integral part of exercise science, ergonomics, sports medicine and orthopaedics, with numerous universities offering undergraduate and postgraduate courses in this field.

The contribution of biomechanics to enhancing sporting and industrial efficiency, performance and safety is now well accepted and it is now being applied with great vigour in territory that once seemed largely the preserve of bodybuilders, powerlifters and weightlifters whose pursuit of hypertrophy and strength for many years seemed to be rather irrelevant to other sports.

The reigning belief was—and in some circles still is—that strength, power and all other motor qualities in a sport can be quite adequately developed by means of the sport itself, since this approach ensures that the principle of specificity is exactly adhered to.

Objective

It is the objective of this chapter to apply biomechanics to examine strength and power as motor qualities, and thereby to show how this knowledge may be applied in training to optimize strength and power in a wide range of sporting applications.

The emphasis is on the practical use of this information, i.e. on the value of applied biomechanics, rather than on the predominantly theoretical aspects which often fail to reach the coach and athlete. However, in striving to meet this objective, it does not ignore the fact that biomechanics, like any other component of motor action, does not operate in glorious isolation of the whole gamut of factors which determine human performance.

Scope of biomechanics

Biomechanics as a discipline in its own right is relatively new, but its methods, principles and equations have been used for many years in many other applications. In simple terms, biomechanics is that discipline which borrows mechanics from the world of physics and applies it to living forms in order to understand how they function, with many of the fundamentals in this field being based upon the work carried out by Isaac Newton. This chapter falls into the realm of sports biomechanics, which is that specialization of biomechanics used to analyse how the human body functions in a wide spectrum of sporting activities.

The strengths and weaknesses of sports biomechanics, like that of any other scientific discipline, all lie in the scope and limitations of the paradigms and models used to understand and dissect activity in sport. The dominant paradigm is the widespread use of models which regard the human body as a physical machine and thereby enable us to invoke the powerful physical and mathematical methods which have proved invaluable to the progress of applied mechanics in general. This has enabled scientists to scrutinize the human body in motion far beyond the capabilities of even the most skilled coach and helped sport to refine training methods, competitive techniques, rehabilitation technology and sporting equipment to a degree which seemed the stuff of science fiction less than half a century ago.

At the same time, many issues remain unresolved or controversial, which is a major reason why biomechanics needs to be applied to sport within an integrated framework comprising all possible fields which relate to the structure and function of the human organism in physical action (as is the case in Russia and much of Europe, the word 'organism' is used in preference to 'body', since it refers to all physical and mental aspects of the living human).

Sporting prowess cannot be explained in terms of biomechanics, physiology, motor control, psychology or any single one of the other factors which have become important specializations in the broad field of sports science. Instead, this prowess has to be considered as the result of the synergy of every one of these components acting in a given sport in a given situation for a given individual at any given time. Therefore, although the scope of this chapter lies solidly within the realm of biomechanics, it draws on other relevant components wherever this may be necessary in the interests of providing greater completeness.

In particular, neural processes are a superordinate feature of the biomechanics of strength and power, since they constitute the cybernetic command system which orchestrates the production of human movement. Thus, while it may appear adequate to apply analytical mechanistic methods such as free body diagrams for certain aspects of understanding sporting movement, it is also necessary to comprehend any implications and limitations of this approach in the context of overall control mediated by bioelectrical messages passing between the musculoskeletal and nervous systems of the body. In many respects, relying solely on the methods of biomechanics to analyse human movement is tantamount to analysing a symphony concert by focusing entirely on the resulting sound and the musical instruments involved and ignoring the players and conductor.

For example, it is inadequate to assess the speed and power of athletes by relying entirely on meticulous force plate and high speed video laboratory tests or special field tests without examining the underlying motor control processes. Performance capabilities suggested by outstanding vertical jumps, broad jumps or various agility drills are relatively meaningless if the athlete reacts slowly or inappropriately to sensory stimuli occurring during actual sporting conditions. This is one of the reasons why so-called 'plyometric' or stretch-shortening drills may be of little significant benefit to any athlete.

While these drills may improve speed and power in simple movements, they do not necessarily enhance reaction time, decision time or problem-solving capabilities in complex sporting actions under competitive conditions.

Thus, a basketball player who displays a fairly modest vertical jump, but superior reaction and decision times, may be a far more proficient competitor than a team mate who has a remarkable vertical jump but poor reaction and decision times, or inefficient motor coordination. In other words, isolated biomechanical tests of strength, power and speed may suggest that a player is eminently suited to a given sport, but in the overall context involving vital neural and motor control processes, he or she may be seriously deficient.

Similarly, physiological tests may also yield an incomplete picture of sporting capabilities. For example, muscle biopsies that reveal a high proportion of 'fast twitch' (FT, type IIb) fibres may indicate that an athlete is well suited to activities which require the exhibition of speed, strength or power, but adverse joint leverages, inappropriate force–time curves for given joint actions, and inefficient motor skill may mean that the athlete is a mediocre performer in a given activity, such as sprinting or jumping.

Thus, in striving to apply the methods of biomechanics to sports training, relevant information from allied disciplines will be drawn upon wherever necessary to offer a fuller, more balanced picture of each specific situation.

Objectives of strength and power training

The effective and safe prescription of strength and power training begins with an understanding of force–time and related curves concerning the patterns of force production in sport and resistance training. On this basis we may identify several major objectives of strength training, namely:
- to increase maximal or absolute strength;
- to increase explosive strength;
- to increase the rate of force production;
- to enable the muscles to generate large forces for a given period;

- to enable the muscles to sustain small forces for a prolonged period; and
- to increase muscle and connective tissue hypertrophy.

Then, in using this information to design a suitable training approach, factors such as the following have to be examined:
- the type of strength fitness required;
- the type of muscle contraction involved (isometric, concentric, eccentric);
- the speed of movement over different phases of movement;
- the acceleration at critical points in the movement;
- the rest intervals between repetitions, sets and workouts;
- active vs. passive rest/recuperation intervals;
- the sequence of exercises;
- the relative strength of agonists and antagonists, stabilizers and movers;
- the development of optimal static and dynamic ranges of movement;
- the strength deficit of given muscle groups;
- the training history of the individual;
- the injury history of the individual; and
- the level of sports proficiency of the individual.

The last factor is of exceptional importance because the advanced athlete responds to a given training regime very differently from a novice. For instance, the exact sequencing of strength, strength-speed and hypertrophy methods in a workout or microcycle is of little consequence during the first weeks or months of a beginner's training, but is very important to a more experienced athlete.

The nature of strength

Successful strength and power training depends on a thorough understanding of the factors that influence the development of strength. The next task is to determine which of these factors can be modified by physical training and which methods do so most effectively and safely. Some of these factors are structural while others are functional. Structural factors, however, only provide the potential for producing strength, since strength is a neuromuscular phenomenon which exploits this potential to generate motor activity.

It is well known that strength is proportional to the cross-sectional area of a muscle, so that larger muscles have the potential to develop greater strength than smaller muscles. However, the fact that Olympic weightlifters can increase their strength from year to year while remaining at the same body mass reveals that strength depends on other factors as well.

The most obvious observation is that a muscle will produce greater strength if large numbers of its fibres contract simultaneously, an event which depends on how efficiently the nerve fibres send impulses to the muscle fibres. Moreover, less strength will be developed in a movement in which the different muscles are not coordinating their efforts. It is also important to note research by Vvedensky which has shown that maximum strength is produced for an optimum, not a maximum, frequency of nerve firing (Vorobyev 1978). Furthermore, this optimal frequency changes with level of muscle fatigue (Kernell & Monster 1982).

Determinants of strength

In general, the production of strength depends on the following major structural and functional factors:
- the cross-sectional area of the muscle;
- the density of muscle fibres per unit cross-sectional area;
- the efficiency of mechanical leverage across the joint;
- the number of muscle fibres contracting simultaneously;
- the rate of contraction of muscle fibres;
- the efficiency of synchronization of firing of the muscle fibres;
- the conduction velocity in the nerve fibres;
- the degree of inhibition of muscle fibres which do not contribute to the movement;
- the proportion of large diameter muscle fibres that are active;
- the efficiency of cooperation between different types of muscle fibre;
- the efficiency of the various stretch reflexes in controlling muscle tension;
- the excitation threshold of the nerve fibres supplying the muscles; and
- the initial length of the muscles before contraction.

With reference to the concept of synchronizing action among muscle fibres and groups, it is important to point out that synchronization does not appear to play a major role in increasing the rate of strength production (Miller *et al.* 1981). Efficiency of sequentiality rather than simultaneity may be more important in generating and sustaining muscular force, especially if stored elastic energy and reflexive activity has to be contributed at the most opportune moments into the movement process. Certainly, more research has to be conducted before a definite answer can be given to the question of strength increase with increased synchronization of motor unit discharge.

Specificity in training

Training for enhancing strength and power is not at all straightforward in that strength training displays definite specificity in many respects: all forms of strength training are different and produce significantly different effects on neuromuscular performance.

Fitness training for a given sport is not simply a matter of selecting a few popular exercises from a bodybuilding magazine or prescribing heavy squats, power cleans, leg curls, bench press, circuit training, isokinetic leg extensions or 'cross-training'. This approach may produce aesthetic results for the average non-competitive client of a health centre, but it is of very limited value to the serious athlete. It is not only the exercise which modifies the body, or, more specifically, the neuromuscular system, but the way in which the exercise is performed. In this regard, it is vital to remember that all exercise involves information processing in the central nervous and neuromuscular systems, so that all training should be regarded as a way in which the body's extremely complex computing systems are programmed and applied in the solving of motor tasks (among its many other roles).

For many years, there have been two opposing theories of supplementary strength training in sport. One theory proposes that strength training should simulate the sporting movements as closely as possible with regard to movement pattern, velocity, force–time curve, type of muscle contraction and so forth, whereas the other maintains that it is sufficient to train the relevant muscles with no regard to specificity. Separate practice of technical skills would then permit one to utilize in sporting movements the strength gained in non-specific training. While both approaches to strength training will improve performance, current scientific research strongly supports the superiority of the specificity principle in the following respects:

- type of muscle contraction;
- movement pattern;
- region of movement;
- velocity of movement;
- force of contraction;
- muscle fibre recruitment;
- metabolism;
- biochemical adaptation;
- flexibility; and
- fatigue.

In the context of training, specificity should not be confused with simulation. Specificity training means exercising to improve in a highly specific way the expression of all the above factors in a given sport. While simulation of a sporting movement with small added resistance over the full range of movement or with larger resistance over a restricted part of the movement range may be appropriate at certain stages of training, simulation of any movement with significant resistance is inadvisable since it can confuse the neuromuscular programmes which determine the specificity of the above factors.

Even if one is careful to apply simulation training by using implements or loads that are similar to those encountered in the sport, there will usually be changes in the centre of gravity, moments of inertia, centre of rotation, centre of percussion and mechanical stiffness of the system which alter the neuromuscular skills required in the sport.

Fundamental concepts

The development of strength and power would appear to be a fairly straightforward quest. Since the human constitutes an adaptive and self-regulating organism, the imposition of progressively increasing loads on the musculoskeletal system according to the well-known principle of gradual overload

would be all that is required to achieve this aim. In this context, the load exerts a force on the body, which uses muscle action to stabilize or move that load, thereby giving rise to what we call strength. Once this concept of strength/force has been introduced, we can immediately draw from mechanics a number of other physical definitions which enable us to formulate a scientific framework for analysing sporting action.

Thus, *strength* may be defined as the ability of the body to produce force; *energy* may be understood as that physical quality which imbues an object with the ability to exert a force; *work* may be regarded as the energy involved in moving from one state or position to another; and *power* refers to the rate at which work is done at any instant.

Because force involves the movement of a limb about a joint or fulcrum, the concept of torque (the turning capability of a force) is frequently used in sport biomechanics. *Torque* is defined as product of a force with the perpendicular distance from the line of action of the force to the fulcrum about which it acts (Fig. 6.1). Sometimes, since it is defined in the same way, torque is regarded as synonymous with the *moment* of a force, and in the context of this chapter either term may be used without contradiction.

Even in the most basic applications of resistance training, the concept of torque (or moment) is of great practical value. For instance, the simple act of flexing the elbows will decrease the torque acting about the shoulder during dumbbell side raises, supine dumbbell flyes and bench press by bringing the load closer to the shoulder fulcrum, thereby enhancing the safety of these exercises. Similarly, keeping the line of action of the bar as close as possible to the body during the weightlifting clean or powerlifting deadlift reduces the torque acting

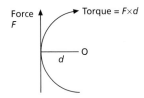

Fig. 6.1 Torque of a force acting at a distance *d* about a fulcrum or joint centre O.

about the lower lumbar vertebrae and the hips, thereby enabling a greater load to be lifted with a greater degree of safety. The common error of swinging the bar away from the body during the later stages of the pull during the Olympic snatch or moving the javelin further away from the shoulder during the wind-up for the throw are examples of the inefficient use of torque.

The obvious implication of an understanding of torque in the case of all joints of the body is that the expression of strength and power is not merely a function of changes in soft tissue structure or neuromuscular efficiency, but also of the optimal use of torque for any sporting movement.

For instance, although the presence of a high percentage of fast-twitch muscle fibres in an athlete may suggest that the latter may be well suited to sports which require production of power and speed, the existence of any inherently disadvantageous limb leverages or techniques which do not optimize torque production in specific complex joint actions may decree that any muscle fibre advantage is of little consequence. Occasionally, however, a disproportionate increase in strength for a given activity may tend to offset these negative factors and enable the athlete to perform very competently, albeit in a less efficient or economic manner.

Later, the issue of torque for activities involving several joints will be examined to caution us against the casual analysis of joint action according to the standard methods of functional anatomy. Hence, we are not necessarily justified in assuming that a given muscle produces the same joint action in a multijoint task because the anatomy charts show that it produces a certain joint action (such as flexion) when only that joint is involved in the movement. Moreover, in multijoint (multiarticular) tasks, a muscle may exert a profound effect over a joint which is not crossed by that muscle.

Contrary to how strength is commonly defined, strength is not the maximal force (or torque) which a muscle can generate; that is actually *maximal strength*. To be consistent with the definition of force according to Newton's Laws (see later), strength is simply the ability to generate force to overcome inertia or a load. Similarly, we can define concepts

such as maximal torque and maximal power, as well as optimal torque and power.

Optimization of force, torque, speed and power or the production of 'just the right amount at the right time' of these motor abilities sometimes seems to be forgotten, especially in the so-called strength, heavy or contact sports. All too often, the solution to most performance problems in such sports seems to be a philosophy of 'the greater the strength and the greater the muscle hypertrophy, the better', despite the fact that one constantly witnesses exceptional performances being achieved in these sports by lighter and less strong individuals.

This identifies a fundamental factor in training for strength and power, namely the importance of developing optimal hypertrophy, strength and power to suit a given individual in a given activity, and avoiding the tendency to develop superfluous hypertrophy or redundant general strength. To identify such inappropriate conditioning, it is helpful to calculate *relative strength* (one's maximal load divided by body mass, in any given lift) and to see how this changes in relation to sport-specific changes in one's chosen sport. If performance remains much the same, while one's relative strength remains the same or decreases along with an increase in overall body mass or lean body mass, then this indicates that the increase in hypertrophy is redundant. If relative strength and maximum strength both increase, but performance remains static, then this suggests that technical skills and psychological factors (such as motivation) need to be carefully scrutinized.

Since bodily motion is the result of muscle action and its underlying metabolic processes, one needs to distinguish between internal and external energy and work. Externally, assuming no losses by heat or sound, mechanical energy generally occurs in the form of potential energy (PE) and kinetic energy (KE), where PE is the energy possessed by a body by virtue of its position and KE is the energy which a body has by virtue of its velocity.

Although external work is defined popularly as the product of the force and the distance through which it is exerted, this definition applies only if the force is constant and acts strictly along the path joining the starting and end points of the movement.

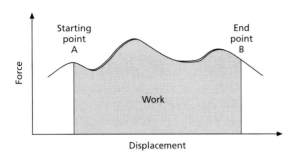

Fig. 6.2 Graphic definition of work as the area under the force–displacement curve.

The mathematical definition based on integral calculus generally is avoided in training texts, because it is felt that it may not be adequately understood by the practitioner, while the popular definition usually attracts the condemnation of the scientist, because of its limited applicability and scope. For this reason, a definition of work in terms of energy changes is given, namely:

work (W) = final energy − initial energy
= final (PE + KE) − initial (PE + KE)

Alternatively, we could draw a graph of how the force varies with displacement; then work would be given by the area under the curve between the starting and end points of the action (Fig. 6.2).

Since some of the fundamental equations used to analyse sporting movements may be expressed in the form of suitable graphs, this same graphic approach may be adopted to enable us to visualize more simply the implications of biomechanics for training and competition.

In this respect, the following relationships will be seen later to play an especially important role in the biomechanics of strength and power in sport:
• force vs. time (or torque vs. time);
• force vs. displacement (and torque vs. joint angle);
• force vs. velocity; and
• rate of force development vs. time.

Initial implications of Laws of Mechanics

Because of their fundamental importance, Newton's three Laws of Motion warrant repetition here:

• Newton I (Law of Inertia): a body will persist in its original state of rest or motion unless acted on by an external agent (i.e. a force).
• Newton II (Law of Acceleration): Newton stated it as 'The change of motion is proportional to the motive force impressed; and is made in the direction of the straight line in which that force is impressed' (Richards *et al.* 1962). In modern terms it may be restated as: the rate of change of velocity (acceleration) is proportional to the resultant force acting on the body and is in the same direction as the force, or, if suitable units are chosen, force = mass × acceleration ($F = m \times a$).
• Newton III (Law of Reaction): for every action there is an equal and opposite reaction.

Despite the familiarity of these laws, some of their implications appear to be forgotten in the practical setting, in particular regarding comparison between machine and free weight training. Some machine manufacturers advertise that their variable resistance machines are superior to free weights, because, in the latter case, the weight remains constant and does not change in response to altering joint leverages throughout range of any movement. Newton's first two laws show clearly that this claim is false, since a load may only be lifted if its weight (due to gravitational acceleration) is overcome by the lifter with an acceleration which exceeds that of gravity.

Furthermore, during the lift, proprioceptive feedback makes the athlete aware that the load is changing and enables him to intervene voluntarily in the loading process by accelerating or decelerating the bar to increase or decrease the force involved. This method is sometimes known as *compensatory acceleration training* (CAT) and can be useful in altering muscle tension or movement velocity to achieve a specific training goal.

Although the role of CAT is well known during concentric movement (in which the load is being overcome), its vital role during eccentric movement (in which the load overcomes the propulsive force) is inadequately appreciated. In non-ballistic eccentric motion in which muscle contraction continues throughout the movement, the muscles try to oppose the effects of the gravity to slow down and ultimately halt the downward motion of the bar. In ballistic motion, in which muscle action is intermittent, so-called antagonistic muscle action comes into play to slow down and halt the limb to ensure that the joint is not dislocated or soft tissues are ruptured.

Even during isometric action (in which no external limb movement is apparent), compensatory processes are at play if no movement is to occur, since neural activation changes due to fatigue, altered mental focus or other physiological processes. This means that the athlete has to maintain adequate muscle tension for the entire duration of the isometric action, either by means of involuntary conditioned reflex action or by voluntary intervention.

The implication for the well-known 'principle of progressive overload' is that 'overload' should refer not simply to the use of progressively greater resistance over a given period, but also to the progressive increase in muscle tension, which may be produced by involuntary or voluntary processes. This change in tension may be produced in ways which relate directly to Newton II and which pose a question of fundamental importance to all strength training. It is relevant to examine this issue before we go any further.

Since force $F = m \times a$, we may apply it to produce the same magnitude of force F in several different ways.

1 $F = M \times a$, where the mass M is large and the acceleration is small.

2 $F = m \times A$, where the mass is small and the acceleration A is large.

3 $F = m \times a$, where both mass and acceleration are moderate.

This might immediately suggest, since the production of an adequate level of muscle tension is necessary for strength training, that all of these methods of 'force training' are entirely the same and it is just a matter of personal choice which method is used. So, the question is: does it make any real difference which method of strength training is used, as long as adequate muscle tension is produced?

If one attempts to answer this question in purely mechanistic terms, one might be tempted to reply 'no' and qualify one's reply with comments about initiating movement against heavy loads with high inertia, possible detrimental effects of sustained loads on the soft tissues of the body, and duration of loading.

Interestingly, practical experience from three different competitive aspects of strength training,

namely Olympic weightlifting, powerlifting and bodybuilding, offers some preliminary information. Option 1, with very heavy loads, is most commonly encountered in powerlifting, whereas the hypertrophy associated with bodybuilding generally is a product of option 3 training, with moderate loads performed for about 8–12 repetitions. Option 2 is characterized by many actions in track-and-field events. Olympic weightlifting, which involves lifting heavy loads rapidly, appears to contradict evidence that velocity decreases with load, but this is because weightlifting is ballistic and relies on the quick movement of the lifter under the bar. It may be concluded that powerlifting is essentially strength generating, while weightlifting is maximum power generating in nature.

The practical evidence shows that the above three ways of generating force do not produce the same results and research reveals that this is because different neural, muscular and metabolic processes are involved in each case. Thus, strength and power training are not simply a matter of using some generalized form of resistance training to produce adequate physical loading and muscle tension; the principle of specificity of training is central to the entire issue.

Some coaches maintain that maximal muscle hypertrophy depends on tension time, with continuous tension times of 30–60 s per set of any exercise being commonly recommended. The observation that the extended use of isometric exercises of this magnitude of duration does not produce the degree of hypertrophy associated with dynamic exercise (which includes eccentric action) militates against this simplistic hypothesis. The fact that tension fluctuates from low to high values throughout a movement also militates against this idea. Clearly, both hypertrophy and strength increase depend on the existence of some minimum level of tension, but nobody has identified what this tension threshold should be in the case of hypertrophy. Moreover, it is well known that novices to resistance training respond to much lower intensities of loading both in terms of hypertrophy and strength gains. It is also known that the development of strength and hypertrophy do not necessitate the induction of fatigue during strength training, but that exercise to momentary failure and at higher percentages of one's 1RM (one repetition maximum) are more relevant in this respect.

Research has shown that the *threshold training stimulus* necessary for increasing muscular strength in the average person should not be less than one-third of the maximal strength (Hettinger & Muller 1953). As strength increases, the intensity of the stimulus required to produce a training effect should be increased, and reach 80–95% of the athlete's maximum. It may be appropriate that the strength of the training stimulus sometimes equals or even exceeds the level of the competition stimulus of the given exercise (Verkhoshansky 1977).

Thus, the development of strength requires that the stimulus intensity be gradually increased. It was discovered that every stimulus has a changing *strengthening threshold*, the achievement of which fails to elicit any further increase in muscular strength (Hettinger 1961). The less trained the muscles, the further the strengthening threshold from the beginning state. The rate at which strength increases from the initial level to the strengthening threshold, expressed as a percentage of the current maximum strength, is independent of sex, age, muscle group and the level of the strengthening threshold. After the strengthening threshold has been reached, strength can be increased only by intensifying the training.

In this regard, according to Korobkov, Gerasimov and Vasiliev (Verkhoshansky 1977), strength increases relatively uniformly during the initial stages of training, independent of how the load is applied in training, whether large or small. Approximately equivalent increases in strength are obtained with loads of 20, 40, 60 and 80% of 1RM. An increase in the intensity of training in the initial stages (e.g. using a heavier load, faster tempo of movement and shorter intervals between sessions) does not always enhance the effectiveness of strength development, this becoming effective only later, as strength increases. This principle is corroborated by the training results of weightlifters (Hettinger 1961; Verkhoshansky 1977).

Specific definitions of strength

Now that some of the fundamental biomechanical aspects of strength and power have been discussed,

we can return to examine the phenomenon of strength more closely.

At the outset, it is vital to remember that strength is the product of muscular action initiated and orchestrated by electrical processes in the nervous system of the body. We have seen that strength is the ability of a given muscle or group of muscles to generate muscular force under specific conditions, while *maximal strength* is the ability of a particular group of muscles to produce a maximal voluntary contraction in response to optimal motivation against an external load. This strength is usually produced in competition and may also be referred to as the *competitive maximum strength*, CF_{max}. It is not the same as *absolute strength*, which usually refers to the greatest force that can be produced involuntarily by a given muscle group by, for example, electrical stimulation of the muscles or recruitment of a powerful stretch reflex by impulsive heavy loading. It should be noted, however, that absolute strength is sometimes used to define the maximum strength which can be produced by an athlete, irrespective of body mass.

It is vital to recognize a *training maximum* (TF_{max}) or training 1RM (single repetition maximum), which is always less than the competition maximum, CF_{max}, in experienced athletes, because optimal motivation invariably occurs under competitive conditions (Fig. 6.3). Zatsiorsky states that the training maximum is the heaviest load that one can lift without substantial emotional excitement, as

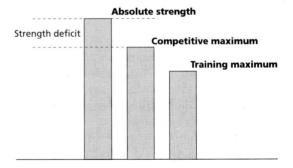

Fig. 6.3 Different types of maximal strength. Absolute strength is produced under involuntary conditions, whereas the other two maxima are the result of voluntary action. The strength deficit is the percentage difference between absolute and maximal strength.

indicated by significant rise in heart rate before the lift (Medvedev 1986). It is noteworthy that, in the untrained person, involuntary or hypnotic conditions can increase strength output by up to 35%, but by less than 10% in the trained athlete. The mean difference between TF_{max} and CF_{max} is approximately 12.5% in experienced weightlifters, with a larger difference being exhibited by lifters in heavier weight classes (Zatsiorsky 1995).

The merit of identifying the different types of strength or performance maxima lies in enabling one to prescribe training intensity more efficiently. Intensity is usually defined as a certain percentage of one's maximum, and it is most practical to choose this on the basis of the competitive maximum, which remains approximately constant for a fairly prolonged period. The training maximum can vary daily, so, while it may be of value in prescribing training for less qualified athletes, it is of limited value for elite competitors. It is relevant to note that competitions involve very few attempts to reach a maximum, yet they are far more exhausting than strenuous workouts with many repetitions, since they involve extremely high levels of psychological and nervous stress. The high levels of nervous and emotional stress incurred by attempting a competitive maximum require many days or even weeks to reach full recovery, even though physical recovery would appear to be complete, so this type of loading is not recommended as a regular form of training.

In other words, any attempt to exceed limit weights requires an increase in nervous excitation and interferes with the athlete's ability to adapt, if this type of training is used frequently. In attempting to understand the intensity of loading prescribed by the apparently extreme Bulgarian coaches who are reputed to stipulate frequent use of maximum loads in training, one has to appreciate that training with a *training maximum* (which does not maximally stress the nervous system) is very different from training with a *competitive maximum* (which places great stress on nervous processes).

Strength is a relative phenomenon depending on numerous factors, so it is essential that these conditions are accurately described when strength is being assessed. For instance, muscular strength varies with joint angle, joint orientation, speed of movement, muscle group and type of movement, so it is largely meaningless to speak of absolute strength without specifying the conditions under which it is generated. Sometimes, the term relative strength is introduced to compare the strength of subjects of different body mass. In this context, *relative strength* is defined as the strength per unit body mass produced by a given individual under specific conditions (e.g. executing a well-defined lift or combination of lifts, such as the squat, snatch or the weightlifting total).

In determining whether an athlete requires a specific type of resistance training, it sometimes is useful to introduce the concept of *strength deficit* (Fig. 6.3), which is defined as the percentage difference between *maximum strength* (voluntary effort) produced in a given action and *absolute strength* (involuntary effort) of which the athlete is capable in that same action. This deficit may be defined under static or dynamic conditions, with the deficit depending on the rate at which force has to be developed in a given joint action. In the laboratory situation, absolute strength may be estimated by subjecting the muscles concerned to the maximum electrical stimulation which can be tolerated.

Strength deficit reflects the percentage of maximal strength potential which is not used during a given motor task, but its accurate measurement is seldom performed in practice, because determination of maximum eccentric strength by electrical stimulation is a difficult and potentially harmful task, and even if this were not the case, most sporting actions involve many muscles and joints, so that measurements of deficits for separate muscle groups would not necessarily relate to performance deficits in complex tasks.

The closest one can approach involuntary recruitment of as many muscle fibres in a given task is to force the body to react by reflex action to a suddenly imposed load. Thus, in a jumping or pulling activity, an approximate measure of strength deficit may be made by comparing the vertical jump achieved from a static start with knees flexed with a vertical jump preceded by a sudden dip. If there is a small difference between the two jumps, this suggests that training focuses more on nervous stimulation via the use of 'shock' and ballistic methods such as plyometrics (stretch-shortening rebound type training). If the deficit is large, then strength and hypertrophy training with 5RM to 8RM loads using methods such as CAT (compensatory acceleration training) is more suitable, with a definite emphasis on the eccentric deceleration phase.

In general, if the strength deficit is large for a given muscle group, an increase in speed-strength may be produced by maximal or near-maximal neuromuscular stimulation (e.g. via weightlifting or plyometric methods). If the strength deficit is small, hypertrophy must be induced by submaximal loading methods as commonly used in bodybuilding, followed by maximal efforts against heavy loads.

Verkhoshansky (1977) has shown that the strength deficit increases as the external resistance and the time of motion decrease, indicating that training to increase maximal strength becomes more important as the time available for a movement becomes longer. Conversely, training to increase rapidity of movement (i.e. nervous system conditioning) becomes more important as the external load decreases. This implies that identification of *explosive strength deficit* is especially important in devising strength training regimes for athletes whose movements allow them little time to produce maximum force, in other words, for actions such as running, jumping, weightlifting and throwing.

Before concerning oneself about strength deficit, it is important to appreciate that superior performance does not depend simply on the ability to produce maximum force, since many sporting actions take place so rapidly that it is impossible to recruit an adequate number of muscle fibres. Presuming that technical skill is adequate, performance may also be limited by the inability to produce the optimal level of strength at any given instant or in a crucial phase of movement (known as the accentuated region of force production). In other words, *rate of force development* (RFD) is another factor vital to sporting prowess. Thus, it is highly relevant to estimate deficits in maximal force production, as well as in the RFD.

Identification of a strength deficit for the most important muscle groups of an athlete enables the coach to design the specific type of strength training more accurately than relying on the more conventional approach of somewhat arbitrarily prescribing a certain number of sets and repetitions of several exercises with a given load. Development of the necessary type of sport-specific fitness entails far more than this: the training programme must also pay careful attention to many other factors including the method of executing each exercise and the manner in which force is displayed relative to time and space.

A more enduring type of strength fitness results from a well-sequenced combination of functional and structural resistance training. However, it is important to monitor regularly any change in relative strength to ascertain if increased hypertrophy is simply adding unproductive tissue bulk without a commensurate increase in functional strength. Other useful measures of training effectiveness are the analysis of injury or soreness patterns, and changes in flexibility, motor skills and reaction time.

Muscle action

All sporting movement is the consequence of muscle action, so an understanding of the different types of muscle action is another basic component of biomechanics.

Traditionally, the following types of muscle contraction are defined: *isotonic* (constant muscle tension), *isometric* (constant muscle length), *isokinetic* (constant velocity of motion) and *isoinertial* (constant load). In addition, movement may occur under *concentric* (muscle shortening) and *eccentric* (muscle lengthening) conditions. Before these terms are unquestioningly applied to exercise, it is important to examine their validity.

Isometric literally means 'same length', a state which occurs only in a relaxed muscle. Actually, it is not muscle length, but joint angle which remains constant. Contraction means 'shortening', so that isometric contraction, like all other forms of muscle contraction, involves internal movement processes which shorten the muscle. Isometric contraction may be defined more accurately to mean muscle contraction which occurs when there is no external movement or change in joint angle. It occurs when the force produced by a muscle exactly balances the resistance imposed upon it and no movement results.

The term *isotonic*, however, should be avoided under most circumstances, since it is very rare for muscle tension to remain the same while joint movement occurs over any extended range. Constancy is possible only over a small range under very slow or quasi-isometric conditions of movement for a limited time (since tension reduces with fatigue or other neuromuscular changes). Whenever movement occurs, muscle tension increases or decreases, since acceleration or deceleration is always involved and one of the stretch reflexes may be activated. European and Russian scientists prefer to use the term *auxotonic*, which refers to muscle contraction involving changes in muscle tension and length. Other authors use the term *allodynamic*, from the Greek *allos* meaning 'other' or 'not the same'. Both terms are more accurate than isotonic in this context.

Isotonic action is most likely to occur under static conditions, in which case we have *isotonic isometric* action. Even then, as is the case with all muscle activation, there is a rise time of tension build-up, an intermediate phase of maximal tension, and a final decay time of tension decrease. For any prolonged action, the tension oscillates irregularly over a range of values. If the load is near maximal, the muscles are unable to sustain the same level of static muscle tension for more than a few seconds and the situation rapidly becomes *anisotonic isometric*.

The word *isokinetic* is encountered in two contexts: firstly, some textbooks regard it as a specific type of muscle contraction, and secondly, so-called isokinetic rehabilitation and testing machines are often used by physical therapists. The term *isokinetic contraction* is inappropriately applied in most cases, since it is impossible to produce a full-range muscle contraction at constant velocity. To produce any movement from rest, Newton's first two Laws of Motion reveal that acceleration must be involved, so that constant velocity cannot exist in a muscle which contracts from rest and returns to that state. Constant velocity can occur only over a part of the range of action.

Similarly, it is biomechanically impossible to design a purely isokinetic machine, since the user has to start a given limb from rest and push against the machine until it can constrain the motion to approximately constant angular velocity over part of its range. The resistance offered by these devices increases in response to increases in the force produced by the muscles, thereby limiting the velocity of movement to roughly isokinetic conditions over part of their range.

One of the few occasions when isokinetic action takes place is during isometric contraction. In this case, the velocity of limb movement is constant and equal to zero. However, it should be pointed out that, even if a machine manages to constrain an external movement to take place at constant velocity, the underlying muscle contraction is not occurring at constant velocity.

Two remaining terms applied to dynamic muscle action need elaboration. *Concentric* contraction refers to muscle action which produces a force that overcomes the load being acted upon; therefore, Russian scientists call it *overcoming* contraction. *Eccentric* contraction refers to muscle action in which the muscle force yields to the imposed load. Thus, in Russia, it is referred to as *yielding* contraction. As with isometric contraction, it has been suggested that unique neural commands may control eccentric contractions, especially since the neural drive to the muscles is reduced, despite maximal voluntary effort under high-tension loading (Westing *et al.* 1988; Westing *et al.* 1991; Enoka 1996).

Since superimposed electrical stimulation was found to increase eccentric torque by more than 20% above voluntary levels and electrically evoked torque alone exceeded voluntary torque by about 12%, it is obvious that the maximum eccentric torque obtained voluntarily does not represent the maximal torque-producing capacity (Westing *et al.* 1990). Interestingly, no corresponding differences were observed between superimposed and voluntary torques under isometric or concentric conditions, so that neural mechanisms may protect against the extreme muscle tension that could otherwise develop under truly maximal eccentric conditions. Comparison between EMG recordings during eccentric and concentric exercise, as well as the magnitude of the training-induced changes in the EMG, also suggest that muscular activity under eccentric loads may be impaired by mental processes (Handel *et al.* 1997).

A little appreciated fact concerning eccentric muscle contraction is that the muscle tension over any full-range movement is lower during the eccentric phase than the isometric or concentric phases, yet eccentric activity is generally identified as being the major cause of delayed-onset muscle soreness (DOMS). Certainly, muscle tension of 30–45% greater than concentric or isometric contraction can be produced by near-maximal eccentric muscle contraction, as when an athlete lowers a supramaximal load in a squat or bench press (but can never raise the same load), but this degree of tension is not produced during the average submaximal training conditions. Interestingly, it has been shown that muscle adaptation to eccentric loading can be achieved by a single session of between 10 and 50 repetitions of submaximal eccentrics, and that increased numbers of repetitions do not increase the protective effect on muscle (Brown *et al.* 1997).

Eccentric training may have special value in enhancing adaptation to strength training, as is suggested by research which revealed that submaximal eccentric exercise encourages faster initial adaptation to strength training than similar training with near maximal concentric loading (Hortobágyi *et al.* 1996). Moreover, greatest concentric muscle EMG and tension has been observed at higher joint velocities, whereas eccentric activity increases as joint velocity decreases (Potvin 1997).

Isometric training

In athletics, isometric exercises were very popular in the mid-1950s as a result of the search for effective methods of developing strength. Hettinger and Muller established that one daily effort of two-thirds of one's maximum exerted for 6 s at a time for 10 weeks will increase strength about 5% per week in the average person (Hettinger 1961), while Clark and colleagues found that static strength continues to increase even after the conclusion of a 4-week programme of isometric training (Verkhoshansky 1977).

The success of isometric training provoked considerable research, much of it being concerned with the question of its effectiveness compared with dynamic training. This research produced rather contradictory data but showed that isometric training can be more effective than dynamic exercises in cases where the specific exercise requires muscle contraction of large magnitude at a certain stage of a movement or during the early stages of injury rehabilitation.

If the sport involves high-speed movement, then sustained isometric training is less effective. Research indicates that there are distinct differences between the training effects of static and dynamic exercises. It is important that muscular tension should be increased slowly and be held for a relatively long time when executing isometric exercises, if the purpose is to develop *absolute strength*. Prolonged maintenance of muscular tension requires an energy expenditure that stimulates adequate adaptation in the neuromuscular system, thereby determining its strength potential. The increase in strength can be more significant than that produced by transient dynamic tension.

A technique known as *oscillatory isometrics* may also be useful in producing powerful contractions over a small range of movement. This is corroborated by research which showed that the maximum tension that can be produced voluntarily during sinusoidally pulsed brief isometric jerks at 5 Hz is the same as the maximum sustained tension (Soechting & Roberts 1975). Basmajian (1978) commented that this emphasizes the importance of muscle fibre recruitment in the gradation of tension and synchronization of motor unit activity during the short bursts of loading.

In other applications, short periods of low-frequency mechanical vibration (10–35 Hz) on the body have been shown to induce faster recovery, have a positive effect on different body systems, modulate muscle activity, elicit a higher stable state of strength and power, lower arterial pressure, and enhance oxidative processes (Kopysov 1978; Lebedev & Peliakov 1991). More recently, it has been found that powerful whole-body vibrations imposed at 26 Hz through the lower extremities produce marked increases in jumping power (Bosco *et al.* 1998).

These findings may relate to a similar impulsive loading process which is associated with the training effects of plyometrics, thereby adding further

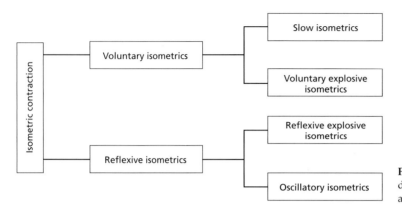

Fig. 6.4 Categorization of the different types of isometric muscle action.

fuel to the debate (van Ingen Schenau *et al.* 1997) about which of the following effects may predominate during plyometrics: elastic energy storage/utilization in the soft tissues, neural facilitation or intrinsic muscle changes.

At this point it must be stressed that isometric training is not simply a matter of holding a static muscle contraction for a given time. Isometric contraction requires a muscle to increase its tension from rest to a maximum or submaximal value over a certain time (the 'rise time'), to sustain this tension for another period (the resistance time) and to decrease this tension to rest or a lower value (the 'decay time'). Consequently, one may distinguish between *explosive isometrics*, which have a very brief rise time, and *slow isometrics*, with a much longer rise time. The isometric contraction may be produced by voluntary contraction or involuntarily by the reflex response of the muscle between the eccentric and concentric phases of plyometric activities such as the depth jump or weightlifting clean-and-jerk. The different types of isometric contraction are categorized in Fig. 6.4.

Each class of isometric training produces its own distinct training effects. If isometric exercises are executed with the accent on the speed of developing force, then they can be as effective for developing explosive strength as dynamic exercises. The steepness of the force–time curve (Fig. 6.5) and the greater magnitude of maximum isometric than dynamic maximum force for equivalent joint angles is the basis for this assertion. In general, the harder the muscles work in overcoming large resistance, the more closely the work becomes isometric, as may be seen from the force–velocity curves of muscle action (see Figs 6.8 & 6.10). In other words, isometric work is really the limiting case of dynamic work as the velocity of movement tends to zero. Furthermore, because the inhibitory effects usually associated with voluntary muscle action are not encountered in reflexive isometric contraction, even greater explosive force can be displayed isometrically than dynamically.

In connection with this, it makes sense to distinguish between isometric training for developing absolute strength and isometric training for developing explosive strength, and to use each of them in the appropriate situation. However, this

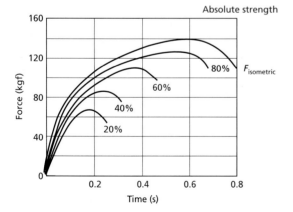

Fig. 6.5 The force–time graph of explosive-isometric tension $F_{isometric}$ and dynamic work with 20, 40, 60 and 80% of maximum strength for a leg-press movement. (From Verkhoshansky 1977.)

still requires detailed experimental corroboration. Nevertheless, isometrics should not be neglected as a means of strength and power development.

If the purpose is to develop *explosive strength*, then the isometric tension should be generated with the maximum speed possible. The reflexive explosive isometric action produced by plyometric movements can be extremely effective in this respect.

Isometric training is reputed to produce maximum strength gains at or very close to the angle at which the isometric exercise is used, so that athletes often avoid this form of training. This observation of specificity must be viewed more critically, since other studies have shown that isometric training also produces strength increases over a range of up to 15° on either side of the training angle (Thepaut-Mathieu *et al.* 1988). This work revealed that this regional specificity of isometric training tends to be exhibited most strongly when the muscle is most shortened and least when the muscle is most lengthened.

In other words, isometric training of muscles in a relatively lengthened state can produce substantial strength increase not only near the region of training, but also throughout the range of movement. This finding, however, should not be interpreted to mean that isometric training can replace other forms of strength training, because the production of a specific type of static or dynamic strength depends on neuromuscular factors which govern the pattern and manner in which muscular force is to be exerted in a given situation.

The difference between static and dynamic muscle contraction lies not in the muscle, but in the nervous system, which controls the intensity, speed, duration, type and pattern of contraction. It is the nervous system which recruits a specific group and number of muscle fibres at a particular rate, time and sequence. It activates prime movers, antagonists, assistant movers, emergency muscles and other groups of muscles to produce the necessary controlled movement of a given joint or series of joints. What needs to be appreciated is that the scope of isometrics is broader than is intimated by most texts on training.

Maintenance of a maximal isometric contraction, however, depends ultimately on autonomic responses produced by muscle fatigue or reflexes elicited in the muscles or connective tissues. Motivation may overcome the negative feedback from these tissues for somewhat longer, but voluntary activation of the muscles eventually becomes impossible and rest becomes necessary.

Isometric contractions may be submaximal or maximal, of short or long duration (depending on the length and frequency of rest intervals), continuous or intermittent, sequenced over a series of different joint angles, alternated between agonist and antagonist, and alternated between different intensities. One can voluntarily oscillate isometric contractions between high and low levels of intensity, thereby prolonging the period of application. Isometrics performed very slowly over a given range of joint action are referred to below as *quasi-isometrics*.

One criticism of traditional training is that it often is believed that muscle action is most efficient if initiated from a completely relaxed state. The justification is that initial tension hinders subsequent action and produces a slower or less-controlled movement. However, isometric contraction released explosively can decrease the reaction response time by as much as 7%, particularly if associated with a strong prestretch. When a movement is produced from a state of complete relaxation, the subsequent action is usually slower and less forceful (Verkhoshansky 1977).

An appreciation of its value and breadth of application should restore isometrics to a place of importance in all training. Since one of the basic principles of PNF (proprioceptive neuromuscular facilitation) is that mobility, or dynamic contraction, is more primitive than stability or isometric contraction, then stability is at a higher level of muscular learning (Knott & Voss 1977). Correct understanding and the use of the isometric state needs to become a vital tool in the repertoire of the scientific coach.

Quasi-isometric contraction

Since any resistance training with heavy loads constrains the athlete to move very slowly, it is relevant to define this type of slow, dynamic isometric action as *quasi-isometric*. Recognition of this discrete type of activity is necessary, because cyclic and acyclic force–velocity curves at near-maximal loads deviate significantly from the hyperbolic relationship displayed at higher velocities (see Fig. 6.10). Unlike isometric activity, which occurs at a fixed joint angle, quasi-isometric activity may be executed over much of the full range of movement. Therefore, its training effects, unlike those of true isometrics, are not produced predominantly close to a specific joint angle. This quasi-isometric activity is highly relevant to training for maximal strength, muscle hypertrophy and active flexibility, rather than maximal power or speed.

One does not necessarily have to try to produce quasi-isometric activity; it is a natural consequence of all training against near-maximal resistance and it takes place with most bodybuilding and powerlifting exercises, provided the lifter avoids any tendency to involve the use of momentum or elastic rebound.

A careful distinction has to be made between the characteristics of the machine or device against which the athlete is working, the external actions produced by muscle contraction and the internal muscular processes. A device may well be designed to constrain its torque or the force in its cables to remain constant over most of its range, but this does not mean that the force or torque produced about a joint by a given muscle group remains the same when working against this machine.

In this respect, it is essential to distinguish clearly between force and torque, since a muscle may produce constant torque about a joint over a certain range, but the force or muscle tension causing the action may vary considerably. Conversely, relatively constant muscle force or tension may produce significantly changing torque. So, if either the force or the lever length change, there will be a change of torque.

The polyphasic nature of muscle action

Dynamic movement is regarded as the result of a *concentric* contraction, in which muscle action overcomes the load, and an *eccentric* contraction, in which muscle action is overcome by the load. Consequently, dynamic muscle action has sometimes been described as biphasic, a term which obscures the fact that all dynamic action involves a static transition phase both at the start and the end of every movement. One cannot initiate, terminate, then repeat any movement without isometric contraction of the muscles involved.

Thus, all dynamic muscle action is polyphasic. The initiating phase from a state of rest is always isometric. This will be followed by either a concentric or eccentric phase, depending on the specific movement. When this phase is completed, the joint will come to rest for a certain period of isometric activity, after which it will be followed by an eccentric or concentric phase to return the joint to its original position.

Clearly, the existence of at least one isometric phase during all joint movement must be recognized in analysing movement and prescribing exercise. Isometric contraction is not simply a separate type of muscle training which occurs only under special circumstances, but a type of muscle action which is involved in all dynamic movement.

Co-contraction and ballistic movement

Sport generally calls upon the muscles to produce two kinds of action: co-contraction and ballistic movement (Basmajian 1978). In *co-contraction*, agonist and antagonist muscles contract simultaneously, with dominance of the former producing the external motion. *Ballistic* movement, which occurs during actions such as running, jumping and throwing, involves bursts of muscular activity followed by phases of relaxation during which the motion continues due to stored momentum. The term 'ballistic' is used, since the course of action of the limb is determined by the initial agonist impulse, just as the flight of a bullet is determined by the initial explosive charge in the cartridge.

Skilled, rapid ballistic and moderately fast continuous movements are preprogrammed in the central nervous system, whereas slow, discontinuous movements are not. The ballistic action rarely involves feedback processes during the movement. *Feedback* from the muscles and joints to the central nervous system permits the ensuing motion to be monitored continuously and to be modified, if necessary. The resulting movement becomes accurately executed and the relevant soft tissues are

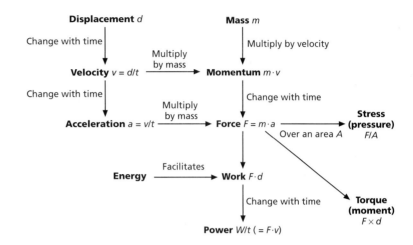

Fig. 6.6 Summary of the major fundamental concepts used in biomechanics.

protected from injury by changes in muscle tension and by the activation of appropriate antagonists to control and terminate the motion.

If no sensory or proprioceptive feedback is implicated, the mode of control is termed *feedforward* or 'open-loop' control (Smith & Smith 1962; Green 1967). Here, control is preprogrammed into the central nervous and neuromuscular systems by the visual and auditory systems before movement begins, so that ongoing monitoring is not involved. The first sign of impending programmed action is the inhibition of antagonist contraction preceding agonist action. Premature activation of the antagonists may not only diminish skill, but it can cause muscle injury. During ballistic and other rapid movement, antagonist contraction is appropriate only to terminate motion of the limb concerned.

Not only is there no continuous antagonist activity throughout ballistic movements, but it is also absent during discontinuous motion (Brooks 1983). The advantage offered by feedforward processes is speed of action, whereas its main disadvantage is the lack of flexibility which can be offered by feedback. Nevertheless, the importance of feedforward processes in human movement should not be underestimated, as revealed by the value of using regimes of visualization and autogenic training in sports preparation.

During ballistic movement, the transition isometric phase between the concentric and eccentric phases is very brief, whereas it may be much

longer during slower maximal efforts produced, for instance, by a powerlifter performing the squat or bench press. The brief isometric contraction between the eccentric and concentric phases of a plyometric movement is of particular importance in speed-strength training. This is one of the ways of producing explosive isometrics, as distinct from slow isometrics. It is associated with the generation of great muscular power during movements such as the weightlifting jerk, shotput or high jump, which combine a maximal voluntary concentric thrust of the knee extensors, in particular, with the reflexive contribution of explosive isometrics produced by the knee dip.

The interrelation between all of the mechanical concepts which have been considered so far may be summarized conveniently in the form of a flow diagram for ease of reference (Fig. 6.6).

The mechanics of movement

The main mechanical concepts introduced above may now be used to analyse sporting movements in more detail. One of the best known relationships concerning muscle action is the hyperbolic curve (Fig. 6.7), which describes the dependence of force on velocity of movement (Hill 1953). Although this relationship originally was derived for isolated muscle, it has been confirmed for actual sporting movement, though the interaction between several muscle groups in complex actions changes some

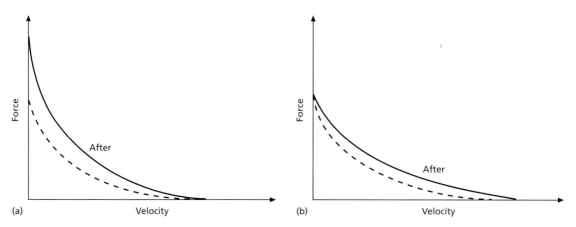

Fig. 6.7 The relationship between force and velocity, based on the work of Hill (1953). (a) The solid curve shows the change produced by heavy strength training. (b) The solid curve shows the change produced by low-load, high-velocity training. (Adapted from Zatsiorsky 1995.)

aspects of the curve (Zatsiorsky & Matveev 1964; Komi 1979).

This curve implies that velocity of muscle contraction is inversely proportional to the load, that a large force cannot be exerted in very rapid movements (as in powerlifting), that the greatest velocities are attained under conditions of low loading, and that the intermediate values of force and velocity depend on the maximal isometric force. The influence of maximal isometric strength on dynamic force and velocity is greater in heavily resisted, slow movements, although there is no correlation between maximal velocity and maximal strength (Zatsiorsky 1995). The ability to generate maximum strength and the ability to produce high speeds are different motor abilities, so that it is inappropriate to assume that development of great strength will necessarily enhance sporting speed.

The effect of heavy strength training has been shown to shift the curve upwards, particularly in beginners (Perrine & Edgerton 1978; Caiozzo *et al.* 1981; Lamb 1984) and light, high-velocity training to shift the maximum of the velocity curve to the right (Zatsiorsky 1995). Since, in both cases, power = force × velocity, the area under the curve represents power, so that this change in curve profile with strength increase means that power is increased at all points on the curve. The term 'strength-speed' is often used as a synonym for power capability in sport, with some authorities preferring to distinguish between *strength-speed* (the quality being enhanced in Fig. 6.7a) and *speed-strength* (the quality being enhanced in Fig. 6.7b).

The graph depicting concentric and eccentric muscle action looks like that depicted in Fig. 6.8. Consequently, muscular power is determined by the product of these changes ($P = FV$) and reaches a maximum at approximately one-third of the maximal velocity and one-half of the maximal force (Zatsiorsky 1995). In other words, maximal dynamic muscular power is displayed when the external resistance requires 50% of the maximal force which the muscles are capable of producing.

The pattern of power production in sporting activities can differ significantly from that in the laboratory, just as instantaneous power differs from average power over a given range of movement. For example, maximum power in the powerlifting squat is produced with a load of about two-thirds of maximum (Fig. 6.9). Power drops to 52% of maximum for a squat with maximal load and the time taken to execute the lift increases by 282%. Power output and speed of execution depend on the load; therefore, selection of the appropriate load is vital for developing the required motor quality (e.g. maximal strength, speed-strength or strength-endurance).

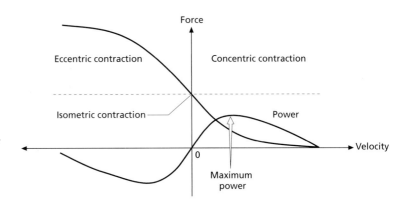

Fig. 6.8 Schematic (not to scale) of the idealized force–velocity curves for concentric and eccentric muscle contraction. The change in muscular power with speed of contraction is also depicted. Note that power is absorbed at negative velocities, i.e. under eccentric conditions.

It is interesting to note that the form of Hill's relationship (Fig. 6.7) has been modified by more recent research by Perrine and Edgerton (1978), who discovered that, for *in vivo* muscle contraction, the force–velocity curve is not simply hyperbolic (curve 2 in Fig. 6.10). Instead of progressing rapidly towards an asymptote for low velocities, the force displays a more parabolic shape in this region and reaches a peak for low velocities before dropping to a lower value for isometric contraction ($V = 0$). In other words, maximum force or torque is not displayed under isometric conditions, but at a certain low velocity. For higher velocities (torque greater than about $200° \cdot s^{-1}$), Hill's hyperbolic relation still applies.

In general, therefore, the picture which emerges from the equation of muscle dynamics is that of an inverse interplay between the magnitude of the load and the speed of movement, except under isometric and quasi-isometric conditions. Although this interplay is not important for the development of absolute strength, it is important for the problem of speed-strength.

The above studies of the relationship between strength and speed were performed in single-jointed exercises or on isolated muscles *in vitro* under conditions which generally excluded the effects of inertia or gravity on the limb involved.

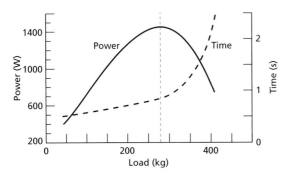

Fig. 6.9 The relationship between power, load and movement time for the powerlifting squat for a group of top + 125 kg lifters whose mean best squat is 407 kg. If a vertical line is drawn at a given load, the intersection with the curves gives the corresponding power and time taken to complete the lift. For example, the line passing through the maximum power of 1451 W occurs for a load of 280 kg moved over a period of 0.85 s.

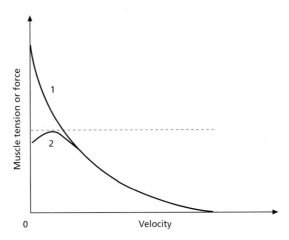

Fig. 6.10 Force–velocity relationship of isolated muscle (curve 1) and *in vivo* human muscles (curve 2) as determined in two separate experiments under similar loading conditions. The hyperbolic curve (1) is based on the work of Hill, while the other curve is obtained from research by Perrine and Edgerton (1978).

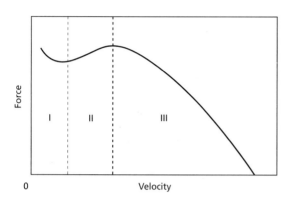

Fig. 6.11 Force–velocity relationship for cyclic activity (based on data of Kusnetsov & Fiskalov 1985).

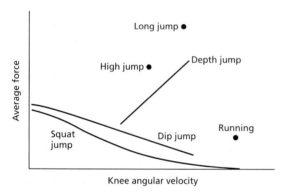

Fig. 6.12 Force–velocity curve for different types of jump. In the squat jump, the contractile component of the muscle is primarily responsible for force production, whereas elastic energy, reflexive processes and other muscle changes play additional roles in dip (countermovement) jumps and depth jumping. The calculated values of F and V for high jump, long jump and sprints are also shown. (Adapted from Bosco 1982.)

Moreover, research has shown that the velocity–time and velocity–strength relations of elementary motor tasks do not correlate with similar relations for complex, multijointed movements. In addition, other studies reveal that there is a poor transfer of speed-strength abilities developed with single-jointed exercises to multijointed activities carried out under natural conditions involving the forces of gravity and inertia acting on body and apparatus. Consequently, Kusnetsov and Fiskalov (1985) studied athletes running or walking at different speeds on a treadmill and exerting force against tensiometers. Their results revealed a force–velocity (F–V) graph (Fig. 6.11) which is very different from the hyperbolic graph obtained by Hill.

This figure also shows that jumping with a preliminary dip (or countermovement) causes the F–V curve to shift upwards away from the more conventional hyperbola-like F–V curve recorded isokinetically or with squat jumps. For depth jumps, the resulting graph displays a completely different trend, where the force is no longer inversely proportional to the velocity of movement. The coordinates describing the more rapid actions of running, high-jumping and long-jumping also fall very distant from the traditional F–V curve (Fig. 6.12).

The reason for these discrepancies lies in the fact that movement under isokinetic and squat jumping conditions involves mainly the contractile component of the muscles, whereas the ballistic actions of the other jumps studied apparently are facilitated by the release of elastic energy stored in the SEC and the potentiation of nervous processes during the rapid eccentric movement immediately preceding the concentric movement in each case.

Studies of F–V curves under non-ballistic and ballistic conditions (Bosco 1982) further reinforce the above findings that the traditional F–V curves (Fig. 6.7) do not even approximately describe the F–V relationship for ballistic or plyometric action. The non-applicability of these curves to ballistic motion should be carefully noted, especially if testing or training with isokinetic apparatus is being contemplated for an athlete.

Other work reveals that the jump height reached and the force produced increases after training with depth jumps (Bosco 1982). Whether this is the result of positive changes in the various stretch reflexes, inhibition of the limiting Golgi tendon reflex, the structure of the SEC of the muscle, or all of these processes is not precisely known yet. What is obvious is that the normal protective decrease in muscle tension by the Golgi tendon organs does not occur to the expected extent, so it seems as if plyometric action may raise the threshold at which significant inhibition by the Golgi apparatus takes place. This has important implications for the concept and practical use of plyometrics.

Speed-strength and strength-speed

The preceding force–velocity curves provide a useful means of distinguishing between the different strength-related fitness qualities. It is tempting to refer simply to speed-strength, but this disguises the fact that certain 'speed-strength' sports require a greater emphasis on speed, while others focus more on strength. This becomes apparent from the force–velocity curve, which enables us to identify various strength-related fitness qualities located between the extremes defined by $V = 0$ (isometric strength) and V = very large (explosive strength).

Examination of this force–velocity curve enables us to recognize five different strength-related qualities (as discussed earlier):
- *isometric strength* at zero velocity;
- *quasi-isometric strength* at very low velocities;
- *strength-speed* at low velocities;
- *speed-strength* at intermediate velocities; and
- *explosive strength* at high velocity.

The distinction between strength-speed and speed-strength is of particular importance in devising conditioning programmes for specific sports. The former is relevant to training where speed development is vital, but strength is more important, whereas the latter refers to training where speed development against resistance is vital, but strength acquisition is somewhat less important. In the competitive setting, speed-strength and strength-speed sports may be divided into the following categories:
- Cyclical, maximum-power, short-duration running, swimming and cycling.
- Maximum power output sprint activities with jumping or negotiating obstacles (e.g. hurdles).
- Maximum power output activities against heavy loads (e.g. weightlifting).
- Maximum power output activities involving the throwing of implements (e.g. shotput, hammer, javelin).
- Jumping activities.
- Jumping activities involving an implement (pole vault).

In the language of physics, the terms speed-strength and strength-speed are synonymous with high *power* (the rate of doing work). This quantity is what clearly distinguishes speed-strength and strength-speed activities from all other types of sport: they both produce a very high power output compared with their longer-duration, lower-intensity counterparts.

Finally, in attempting to analyse speed-strength and strength-speed activities, one must not simply confine one's attention to contractile muscle processes, since these types of rapid action frequently involve some release of stored elastic energy from non-contractile tissues after stretching by preceding eccentric contraction. The role of the myotatic stretch reflex and other neural processes in facilitating powerful involuntary muscle contraction should also be taken into account. It should be noted that the Hill and Perrine–Edgerton curves do not apply to actions which strongly recruit the stretch reflex or involve the release of stored elastic energy.

The interrelation between strength and other fitness factors

Work similar to Hill's has been carried out to examine the relationship between strength and endurance, and speed and endurance. It emerges that the strength–endurance curve is hyperbolic, but the speed–endurance curve is similar to the Perrine–Edgerton force–velocity curve, namely hyperbolic over most of the range, but more parabolic for endurance where speed is high. Figure 6.13 summarizes the interrelation between strength, speed and endurance. Using the same approach as the above section, it enables us to distinguish between the variety of fitness factors involved in all motor activities. If the activities are more cyclic in nature, then the force–velocity curve derived by Kusnetzov and Fiskalov should be applied (Fig. 6.11).

The classical and revised Hill curves are useful for distinguishing between the different strength-related fitness qualities. It is tempting to refer simply to speed-strength, but this disguises the fact that certain 'speed-strength' sports require a greater emphasis on speed and others on strength.

If a movement is to be analysed mathematically, then the force developed at any instant, $F(t)$, may be depicted graphically (Fig. 6.14). In almost all athletic

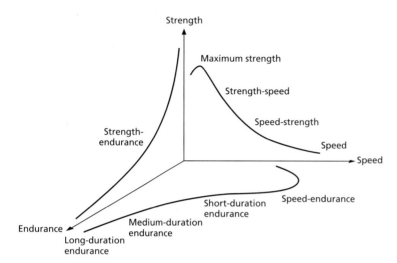

Fig. 6.13 The interdependence of the motor qualities of strength, speed and endurance. The curves (not to scale) are based on the separate data of Hill, Perrine and Edgerton, and Gundlach (Siff & Verkhoshansky 1999).

movements the beginning and end of the force curve lie on the horizontal axis, because the movement begins and ends with zero velocity. The working-effect of the effort is given by the area under the curve $F(t)$ over the time interval t during which the weight W is overcome (the shaded area). An increase in the working-effect of the movement is achieved by increasing this area (i.e. its momentum) and this is one of the major goals for perfecting athletic movements. Other major goals include increasing the maximum force, increasing the rate of force production (the upward slope of the graph), and producing maximum force at the appropriate instant. When a force is applied explosively over a very brief time interval, the resulting rapid change in momentum is known as the *impulse* of the force.

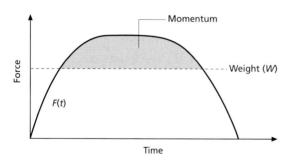

Fig. 6.14 Force–time curve for a load of weight W being overcome by a force $F(t)$.

As sporting performance improves, the structure of the effort produced undergoes specific changes in space and time which can be clearly displayed even within relatively short periods of training, as may be seen from the graphs describing the force profiles, $F(t)$ and $F(s)$, of rapid seated knee extensions, obtained before and after 6 months of training (Fig. 6.15). $F(t)$ refers to the force as a function of time and $F(s)$ denotes the force as a function of displacement. The graphs reveal several features:
- there is an increase in maximum force;
- maximal force is reached more rapidly;
- maximum effort is produced closer to when muscle tension begins;
- the movement time for the effort decreases; and
- the weight of the load is overcome more rapidly.

In exercises involving a combination of muscular work regimes, the working force is preceded by a phase of muscular stretching (e.g. jumping in track-and-field, figure skating and acrobatics). Thus, the perfecting of the movement is achieved by improving the ability of the muscles to generate great force during the transition from eccentric to concentric work (Verkhoshansky 1977). This rapid transition from stretching to contracting causes some decrease in the working amplitude, i.e. there is a decrease in the angle of the working joint during flexion (Fig. 6.16a).

The working-effect in cyclic exercises (e.g. running, swimming and rowing) is increased by

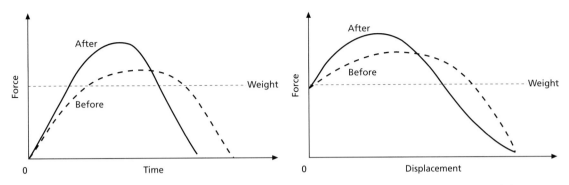

Fig. 6.15 The (*left*) force–time, $F(t)$, and (*right*) force–displacement, $F(s)$, graphs for explosive force, before and after 6 months of strength training. *Weight* refers to the weight of the load being overcome. (Adapted from Verkhoshansky 1977.)

improving the ability to quickly produce maximum force from the state of deep and rapid muscular relaxation during the passive phase of the movement. There is a simultaneous increase in the relative duration of the relaxation phase and a shortening of the absolute duration of the cycle (Fig. 6.16b). Thus, during the course of enhancing sports proficiency, the process of increasing the working-effect of the movement is independent of the regime, while the external work of the motor apparatus displays a specific pattern. This pattern is characterized principally by:

• an increase in maximum force;
• displacement of the instant of maximum force closer to when muscle tension begins;
• an increase in the working amplitude of the movement; and
• a decrease in the time of production of the force.

The magnitude of these changes is specific to the type of sport.

Specific forms of strength expression

Figure 6.14 shows that every sports movement displays several fundamental types of strength expression at different phases of the movement, namely starting-strength, acceleration-strength, explosive strength, absolute strength, and strength-endurance. These strength types may readily be defined by examining the characteristics of this graph and extending its scope by drawing in some of the most important variables, such as slope (Fig. 6.17).

Depending upon the primary coordination structure of the motor activity, muscular strength acquires a specificity which becomes more apparent as the athlete's level of sports mastery grows.

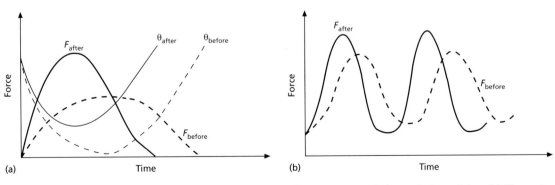

Fig. 6.16 (a) Change in force, F, and joint angle, θ, for reactive-ballistic movements before and after training. (b) Change in force of cyclical movements before and after training. (Adapted from Verkhoshansky 1977.)

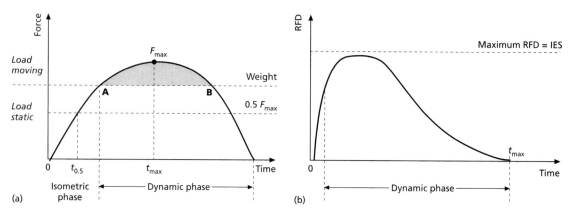

Fig. 6.17 (a) Force–time curve illustrating a method for determining explosive, starting and acceleration strength in lifting a weight. W is the weight being overcome by the force $F(t)$. Movement occurs only when the force exceeds the weight W of the object, namely over the shaded portion of the curve. (b) Rate of force development (RFD) curve obtained by plotting the slope of the force–time graph vs. time. The maximum rate of force development represents the index of explosive strength (IES) (Siff & Verkhoshansky, 1999).

The *relative strength* of an athlete (i.e. force produced per unit body mass) has been defined earlier. This index is sometimes used for comparing the strength of athletes of different body mass, although it is particularly useful for assessing changes in an individual over time. We also defined absolute strength as maximum involuntary strength, while *speed-strength* (power) characterizes the ability to quickly execute an unloaded movement or a movement against a relatively small external resistance.

Explosive strength characterizes the ability to produce maximal force in a minimal time. The index of explosive strength (IES) often is estimated by dividing the maximum force (F_{max}) by the time taken to produce this level of force (t_{max}) (Fig. 6.17a), thus (Zatsiorsky 1995):

$$IES = F_{max}/t_{max}$$

although mathematically it is given by the maximum value of the slope of the force–time curve (Fig. 6.17b).

Explosive force production is also described by another index called the *reactivity coefficient* (RC), which is the explosive strength index relative to body weight or the weight of the object being moved:

$$RC = F_{max}/(t_{max}W) = RFD_{max}/W$$

The most accurate way of assessing force development at any instant is to plot the slope (tan θ) of the force–time graph vs. time, or to use a computer to display simultaneously the curves of force vs. time and the slope of the F–t curve (i.e. the rate of force development) vs. time. The maximum of this rate of force development (RFD) curve gives a precise measure of explosive strength (Fig. 6.17b). In addition it may be noted that the smaller the value of t_{max}, the more explosive the movement. Analysis of the $F(t)$ curve of explosive force reveals three further characteristics of the movement, namely:

• the *maximum strength* of the muscles involved (F_{max});
• the *starting-strength*, or ability of the muscles to develop force during the stage just before external movement occurs (this always occurs under isometric conditions); and
• the *acceleration-strength*, or ability over time to rapidly produce maximal external force while developing muscle tension isometrically or during the primary stages of a dynamic contraction.

The following formula is used to provide an index of starting-strength (ISS, or the S-gradient), which is exhibited during the contraction just preceding movement of the load (Zatsiorsky 1995):

$$ISS = 0.5F_{max}/t_{0.5}$$

where $t_{0.5}$ is the time taken to reach half F_{max}.

The index of acceleration strength (IAS, or the A-gradient), usually used to quantify the rate of force development (RFD) during the late stages of developing muscular force, is described by the formula:

$$IAS = 0.5F_{max} / (t_{max} - t_{0.5})$$

Explosive strength is most commonly displayed in athletic movements when the contraction of the working muscles in the fundamental phases of the exercise is preceded by mechanical stretching. In this instance, the switch from stretching to active contraction uses the elastic energy of the stretch to increase the power of the subsequent contraction. This specific quality of muscle is called its *reactive ability.*

Strength-endurance characterizes the ability to effectively maintain muscular functioning under work conditions of long duration. In sport this refers to the ability to produce a certain minimum force for a prolonged period. There are different types of muscle functioning associated with this ability, such as holding a given position or posture (*static strength-endurance*), maintaining cyclic work of various intensities (*dynamic strength-endurance*) or repetitively executing explosive effort (*explosive strength-endurance*).

Categorization of strength capabilities into four discrete types (absolute strength, speed-strength, explosive strength and strength-endurance), as explained above, can be restrictive in certain ways, because all of them are interrelated in their production and development, despite their inherent specificity. They are rarely, if ever, displayed separately, but are the components of every movement.

Some implications of the laws of dynamics

The force–time curve may be regarded as one of the graphical starting points for sport biomechanics, just as Newton's Second Law of Motion serves as the corresponding mathematical starting point.

Suppose that we wish to use this information to compare the performances of two different athletes in executing the same exercise. They have both been instructed to perform a single maximal repetition of this exercise as rapidly as possible and to hold the

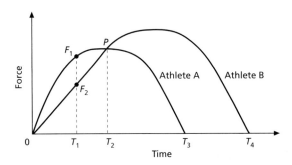

Fig. 6.18 Force curves F_1 and F_2, produced by different athletes in reaching and attempting to maintain their respective maximum forces for as long as possible in a given exercise.

load for as long as possible until fatigue forces them to stop. Their resulting force–time curves (Fig. 6.18) show that athlete B exerts a greater maximal force and continues to produce force for longer than athlete A. However, at any instant T_1 between 0 and time T_2, athlete A is able to exert greater force than athlete B. If the sport concerned requires rapid RFD (rate of force development), then athlete A will have the advantage.

This quality is essential in any sport which involves jumping, striking or throwing, such as basketball, martial arts and track-and-field. In this case, any training aimed at increasing B's maximal strength or bulk will be misdirected, because he or she needs to concentrate on explosive strength (RFD) training. If the sport requires a high maximal force or a large amount of momentum to be exerted irrespective of time, then athlete B will prove to be superior. Athlete A will not improve unless training is directed to increasing maximal strength.

The area under the curve (i.e. the momentum) which describes athlete B's performance is greater than the corresponding area for athlete A, as is the total duration of B's curve (i.e. reflecting muscle endurance), so that B has a distinct advantage in any activity that requires great momentum or great muscle endurance during a single heavy effort. This situation occurs in events such as wrestling, power-lifting and judo.

The informative nature of this type of analysis also reveals the limitations of using isometric or isokinetic dynamometers to assess the muscular strength and performance of any athlete. These devices are unable to measure functional maximal strength, RFD or explosive strength, so it is futile to use them in an attempt to identify functional characteristics or deficiencies to give any accurate bearing on analysing sporting preparedness or progress.

Mechanical position during movement is preserved only within a known range, since the shape of the force–time curve is determined by the characteristics of the neuromuscular system, imparting to it the ability to develop muscular force with the speed necessary to produce the required motor effect. This ability to control muscular activity and movement in space and time is a specific property of the neuromuscular system and requires specialized means of training. A lack of effective neuromuscular training leads to errors and can cost the athlete years of hard and fruitless work.

Most subsequent training and performance errors are caused by inappropriate neuromuscular programming. The above-mentioned motor qualities (force and velocity generation) of the neuromuscular system at a high level of development are inversely proportional to one another. Excessive development of both is not required in athletics because they are not achieved in isolation, but are interrelated aspects of characteristics associated with all motor activity. Depending upon the character and the objective of the movement, one of these qualities achieves greater development but generally displays approximately the same pattern.

Thus, speed-strength, strength-endurance and speed-endurance are not simply derivatives of strength, speed and endurance, but are independent qualities, this being emphasized by the fact that an increase in absolute strength does not necessarily enhance any of these three qualities. They warrant separate recognition alongside other qualities such as absolute strength (Verkhoshansky 1977). However, the first attempts to devise methods for developing these newly recognized qualities reinforced the training method which emphasizes the separate development of each relevant quality.

For instance, this method may prescribe track-and-field exercises for developing speed in weightlifters and gymnasts, weight training for the strength training of track athletes, and prolonged running, swimming and other cyclic exercise for developing general endurance in all athletes. While this may appear to be entirely logical, it is appropriate primarily for the early stages of training and it would be inappropriate for advanced athletes to implement this unifactorial approach exclusively. On the other hand, this does not imply that multifaceted preparation should be the dominant training principle, because this is true only under certain circumstances and does not adequately take into account any interaction among the factors involved. With growth in sporting performance, multifaceted preparation can run counter to the law of gradual development and hinder specific adaptation.

The universal concurrent use of a variety of general training methods or apparently similar sports over the same period to prevent stagnation can be counterproductive and valuable only during particular transitional stages of long-term training. Even then, it is important to combine different training methods or sports according to the most appropriate sequence or combination at each stage of preparation.

It is also not advisable to select strength training methods which simulate sport-specific movements, thereby misapplying the principle of dynamic correspondence and neglecting the value of using a compendium of different methods corresponding to the most important motor characteristics of the given sport. This not only fails to accurately develop the necessary fitness and motor abilities, but also can alter the neuromuscular programmes which control the motor actions. Instead it is important to focus on developing the specific type of fitness and the specific motor characteristics of the sport.

Speed, speed-strength and quickness

In apparent contradiction of the above comments, recent findings show that the judicious superimposition of training of all relevant fitness factors (conjugate training) is sometimes more effective (Verkhoshansky 1977), thereby stressing that the principles of specificity and individuality should play a central role in the design of training programmes. This can be especially important in the development of qualities which relate to the enhancement of speed.

The patterns of sporting movement reflect the complex non-linear sum of many functions of the body, especially the rate of initiating the movement or increasing the speed at any stage of the movement. Regardless of whether the athlete is a sprinter or distance runner, a boxer throwing a punch or a thrower accelerating a projectile, sporting prowess depends upon speed of execution. Nevertheless, this certainly does not mean that a particular speed quality is the sole basis for their success. In its basic forms, speed is displayed in simple, unloaded single-joint movements and involves relatively independent factors such as reaction time, individual movement time, ability to initiate a movement quickly and maximum frequency of movement.

However, developing speed in simple actions does not necessarily enhance the speed of apparently related complex movements. This is emphasized by the lack of correlation between basic forms of speed activity and the speed of movement in cyclic sport locomotion. This is because far more complex neurophysiological control mechanisms and their associated metabolic processes underlie speed in cyclic movements. For example, many motor qualities determine sprinting ability, such as explosive strength, acceleration ability in the start, the development and maintenance of maximum movement speed, and resistance to fatigue (Verkhoshansky 1977).

Speed in sport movements comes primarily from strength and specific types of endurance, although this does not exclude the role of quickness (the ability to initiate movement rapidly from a static state without prestretch), which is just as inherent as strength and endurance, but is displayed fully only when the external resistance of the movement does not exceed 15% of maximal strength (Verkhoshansky 1977).

Speed of movement is associated largely with the fast and slow fibre composition of the muscles, which possess different contractile and metabolic qualities (Komi 1979). It has been fairly well established that athletes who possess a large proportion of fast fibres in their muscles, under equal condi-

tions, display greater movement speed and ability to generate force (Komi 1979).

In addition, excitability of the nervous system is a factor which governs individual speed production, as it has been shown that people with high excitability of the nervous system are distinguished by great speed of movement (Verkhoshansky 1977). Speed apparently has an upper limit that is determined largely by genetics, and lack of improvement in sprinting is not due to the existence of some 'speed barrier', but to limitations imposed by an individual's speed potential. Moreover, all factors determining speed of movement have not been identified yet and further progress will undoubtedly stem from ongoing research.

It is important to point out that maximum speed can be produced only if the corresponding movement receives sufficient energy for its execution. Consequently, in those sports which require the participant to attain high speeds, oppose large resistance, and resist fatigue, it is necessary to examine not only the development of speed, but also those physiological mechanisms involved, such as the contractile potential of the muscles and the underlying metabolic processes. In situations where speed of movement does not require great strength or endurance, it should not be impaired by training with large volumes of redundant work, especially when one notes the relatively low training volumes which are used by top-level sprinters.

Relying on the above background, we may deduce now that quickness and speed of movement are two of the most important independent characteristics in all sport, since, even in apparently less dynamic sports there are always certain stages where effectiveness of speed production can spell the difference between success and failure.

Quickness is a general quality of the central nervous system, being displayed most powerfully during reflexive motor reactions and production of the simplest unloaded movements. The individual characteristics of quickness in all of the forms in which it is displayed are determined by genetic factors, so that the potential for its development is limited. However, reflexes are not immutable, as originally was shown by Pavlov. Indeed, the ability to condition different reflexes and enhance the

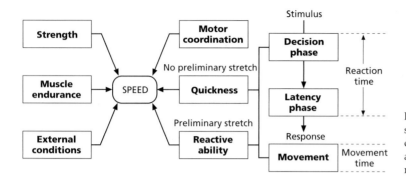

Fig. 6.19 Factors which determine speed of movement. A marked decision phase occurs only if the action is cognitive rather than reflexive.

efficiency of feedforward mechanisms in the brain are integral components of motor proficiency in sport (Siff & Verkhoshansky 1999).

Speed of movement is a function of quickness, reactive ability, strength, endurance and skill to effectively coordinate one's movements in response to the external conditions under which the motor task is to be executed (Fig. 6.19). Compared with quickness, there is far greater potential to enhance speed of movement.

It is important now to recall that different actions in sport rely on the same major motor apparatus and processes. The body does not employ narrow, specialized mechanisms for satisfying each motor demand, such as the production of speed, strength or endurance, but uses a multipurpose system which can control a vast array of different actions. This remarkable ability to adapt to unusual environmental conditions is the result of the functional growth of those systems which resist extreme stresses, such as are encountered in sport.

Thus, an increase in the athlete's special work-capacity is associated not with the development of each fitness quality alone but with the functional specialization of all bodily systems in a manner which produces a high degree of strength, speed or endurance. This information enables one to establish more effective methods for the special physical preparation of athletes.

Conditioning for a given sport requires the development of different types of strength and endurance, a process that begins with the neuromuscular apparatus. It depends on functional hypertrophy of the muscles, enhanced intramuscular and inter-

muscular control, and an increase in metabolic efficiency. Enhancement of muscular potential increases absolute strength, the power of explosive effort and the ability to execute sustained work.

Increased strength occurs by improved functioning of the intramuscular processes via an increase in the number of motor units involved in muscle contraction, via increased motor neurone impulse frequency and via enhanced firing synchronization. This is associated with increased intensity of excitation of the motor neurones from the neurones and receptors of the higher motor levels (the motor cortex, subcortical motor centres and intermediate neurones of the spinal cortex).

Maximum strength is increased chiefly by involving large (high-threshold) motor units in the contraction, whereas endurance work requires the activation of small (low-threshold) units. In the latter case it is possible to alternate the activity of different units, which enables work-capacity to be maintained for longer. Explosive strength is manifested by a rapid increase in muscular tension and is determined to a major extent by the nature of the nervous excitation of the muscles. It is chiefly the initial impulse frequency of the motor neurones and their degree of synchronization that produces faster mobilization of the motor units.

As discussed earlier, the force–time curve of explosive effort is described by qualities of the neuromuscular apparatus such as absolute strength, starting-strength and acceleration-strength. The validity of isolating starting-strength and acceleration-strength has been corroborated by electromyographic research, which reveals differences in their neuromotor patterns, the recruitment of motor units and the firing frequency of the motor neurones during the production of explosive force (Verkhoshansky 1977). This confirms the hypothesis that starting strength is to a certain extent determined by the innate qualities of the neuromuscular apparatus, particularly the ratio of fast- to slow-twitch fibres in the muscles (Viitasalo & Komi 1978).

Specialization of the neuromuscular system to develop absolute, starting and acceleration-strength is determined chiefly by the magnitude of the external resistance overcome. Thus, as the moment of inertia of a rotating mass increases and resists movement, the nature of explosive strength shows that the roles of starting-strength and speed of movement decrease, while the roles of absolute strength and acceleration-strength increase. Thus, the greater the external resistance, the larger the role of absolute strength. The relationship of the latter to body dimensions and phase of training is also well known.

Plyometric training

Research in the direction discussed above led to the development of the so-called 'shock' (plyometric) method of developing explosive strength, reactive ability and power. Essentially, it consists of stimulating the muscles by means of a sudden stretch preceding any voluntary effort. Kinetic energy and not heavy weights should be used for this, where the kinetic energy may be accumulated by means of the body or loads dropping from a certain height. Depth jumps and medicine ball rebounding are two of the exercise regimes commonly used in plyometrics.

The increase in popularity of plyometrics in the West deems it necessary that the concept be more rigorously defined. Plyometrics, or the 'shock method', means precisely that—a method of mechanical shock stimulation to force the muscle to produce as much tension as possible. This method is characterized by impulsive action of minimal duration between the end of the eccentric braking phase and initiation of the concentric acceleration phase. If the transition or coupling phase is prolonged by more than a fraction of a second, the action may be considered to constitute ordinary jumping and not classical training plyometrics.

The activity also is not classically plyometric if the athlete relies upon ongoing feedback processes to control the isometric and concentric actions instead of upon feedforward programmes established before any movement begins. True plyometric training usually involves ballistic rather than co-contraction processes, a concept discussed earlier.

A clear definition of the term 'plyometrics' is essential, because one must distinguish between *plyometric actions*, which occur as part of many running, jumping, hurdling, striking and other rebounding movements in sport, and *plyometric training*, which applies plyometric actions as a distinct training modality according to a definite methodology.

The popular adoption of the term 'plyometrics' in the place of the original Russian term, 'shock method', has produced this confusion. Consequently, plyometric action is often referred to as 'stretch-shortening action' in the scientific literature. Since the word 'pliometrics' (*sic*) originally was coined as a replacement for the term 'eccentric', it might be appropriate to rename plyometric training as *powermetric training* to remove any ambiguity of meaning (Siff 1998).

Plyometric activity is characterized by the following phases of action between initiation and termination of the sequence of events (Fig. 6.20).

1 *An initial momentum phase* during which the body or part of the body is moving because of kinetic energy (KE) it has accumulated from a preceding action.

2 *An electromechanical delay phase*, which occurs when some event, such as contact with a surface, prevents a limb from moving further and provokes the muscles to contract. This delay refers to the time elapsing between the onset of the action potential in the motor nerves and the onset of the muscle contraction. Depending on joint action, this delay varies in magnitude from about 20 to 60 ms (Cavanagh & Komi 1979; Norman & Komi 1979).

3 *An amortization phase* when the KE produces a powerful myotatic stretch reflex which leads to eccentric muscle contraction accompanied by explosive isometric contraction and stretching of connective tissues of the muscle complex. The explosive isometric phase between the end of the

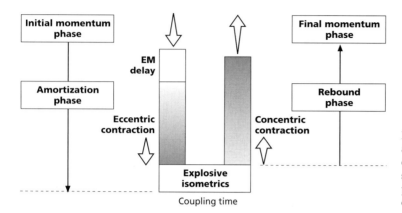

Fig. 6.20 The different phases of a plyometric action. EM delay = electromechanical delay between signal to terminate initial momentum phase and instant when eccentric contraction begins.

eccentric action and the beginning of the concentric action lasts for a period known as the *coupling time* (Fig. 6.20), which will be discussed shortly in greater detail.

4 *A rebound phase* involving the release of elastic energy from connective tissue, together with the involuntary concentric muscle contraction evoked by the myotatic stretch reflex and augmented nervous processes. This phase sometimes may include a timed contribution added by voluntary concentric contraction. The relative contributions to the process by elastic energy and nervous processes is currently a matter of vigorous controversy (e.g. see van Ingen Schenau *et al.* 1997).

5 *A final momentum phase* which occurs after the concentric contraction is complete and the body or limb concerned continues to move by means

including the kinetic energy imparted by concentric contraction, augmentation of nervous processes, and the release of some elastic energy stored in the connective tissues of the muscle complex.

Discussion of coupling time is important because it has a fundamental bearing on whether or not any action may be classified as classical plyometrics. Earlier it was stated that classical plyometrics is characterized by a delay of no more than a fraction of a second between the eccentric and subsequent concentric contractions, a statement which requires some qualification. For instance, research by Wilson *et al.* (1991) examining different delay times in the bench press, showed that the benefits of prior stretch may endure for as long as 4 s, at which stage it is suggested that all stored elastic energy is lost (see Fig. 6.21a).

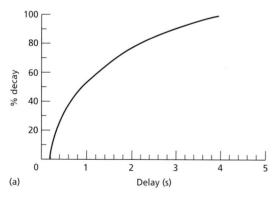

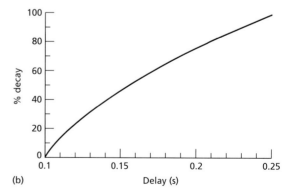

Fig. 6.21 (a) The effect of a time delay on the additional force produced by a preliminary stretch in a bench press (based on the data of Wilson *et al.* 1991). (b) The effect of a time delay on the additional force produced by a preliminary stretch in unloaded rapid elbow flexion (from Siff & Verkhoshansky 1999).

Chapman and Caldwell (1985), on the other hand, found that the benefits of prior stretching during forearm movement were dissipated within 0.25 s, a figure which agrees with other analyses of explosive rebound elbow flexion without additional loading (Fig. 6.21b). Other work by Wilson *et al.* (1991) examining rebound action of the chest/arms concluded that no benefits of prior stretching are evident after 0.37 s.

This research seems to suggest that delays of as long as a second or two can still produce significant augmentation of the subsequent concentric phase for some activities, but delays as short as 0.2 s are sufficient to dissipate the benefits of prior stretch during other activities, probably dependent on factors such as the mass of the limbs and the types of muscle fibre involved. Research by Bosco *et al.* (1983) offers a partial solution to this apparent contradiction. They proposed that individuals with a high percentage of FT (fast-twitch) fibres in the leg muscles exhibit a maximum plyometric effect when the eccentric phase is short, movement range is small and coupling time is brief. On the other hand, subjects with a high percentage of ST (slow-twitch) fibres apparently produce their best jumping performance when the eccentric phase is longer, movement range is greater and the coupling time is longer, since the actin–myosin cross-bridging attachment time is of greater duration.

It is also tempting to attribute these major differences in coupling times to the existence of specific maximum delays for each joint action. While this probably is true for different simple and complex joint actions, it is also important to note that the human body exhibits many different reflexes, each of which acts under different conditions and at different rates.

In particular, there are tonic (static) and phasic (dynamic) stretch reflexes, and very rapid receptors such as Pacinian corpuscles in joint capsules that detect the rates of movement and allow the nervous system to predict where the extremities will be at any precise moment, thereby facilitating anticipatory modifications in limb position to ensure effective control and stability (Guyton 1984). Loss of this predictive function apparently makes it virtually impossible to run, jump, throw or catch. Other receptors such as the Ruffini endings and receptors in the ligaments like the Golgi tendon organs are strongly stimulated when a joint is suddenly moved, and after a slight initial adaptation they transmit a steady response.

In addition, weightlifters and sometimes bodybuilders use the so-called *prestretch principle* to produce a more powerful concentric muscle contraction to enable them to lift heavier loads. In doing so, they begin a movement from a starting position which imposes an intense stretch on the relevant muscles, hold it for a couple of seconds and then thrust as strongly as possible from that position. It would seem that this longer delay would implicate the more tonic type of reflex with a characteristically longer coupling time. The action could certainly not be called plyometric, despite the fact that prior stretch had contributed to the subsequent concentric action. Conversely, phasic reflex activity would more likely be implicated in the explosive movements which typify classical plyometrics and the type of activity depicted in Fig. 6.21.

This explanation also serves to further distinguish between plyometric action and plyometric training, an issue discussed earlier in this section. One cannot simply distinguish between plyometric and non-plyometric solely on the basis of coupling times, otherwise one would have to classify jogging or even brisk walking as classical plyometrics, because the time taken for the ground reaction force to reach a maximum can be less than 0.15 s. One also has to take the force–time pattern and the rate of force development (RFD) into account.

Flexibility and sporting performance

The effective and safe production of appropriate levels of strength and power depends on the range of movement (i.e. flexibility) of every joint involved, the magnitude of this range depending on each specific sporting movement. Thus, the functional production of strength in any sporting activity relies on neuromuscular control and joint stability over a specific range of movement. In other words, the strength and flexibility components of overall fitness must interact in a way which is optimal for each movement and each sporting action. To understand

the training of strength and other fitness qualities which involve range of movement, such as
strength-flexibility, flexibility-speed and flexibility-
endurance, it is necessary to analyse the mechanisms which underlie flexibility and stretching.

Flexibility, or range of movement (ROM), is determined by:

• the structural or architectural limitations of the
relevant joint;
• the mechanical properties of the muscles and
other soft tissues of the joint;
• neuromuscular processes that control muscle
tension and length;
• the level of non-functional muscle tension in the
same or other muscles and soft tissues; and
• the pain threshold of the individual towards the
end of the movement range.

In particular, the location of skeletal prominences,
the length of ligaments, tendons and muscles, and
the sites of attachment and insertion of muscles are
all features which affect the ROM of a joint. In this
respect two types of flexibility are identifiable:
active flexibility and passive flexibility. *Active
flexibility* refers to the maximum ROM that can
be produced under active muscular control for a
particular degree of freedom of any joint, whereas
passive flexibility refers to the maximum ROM that
can be produced passively by imposition of an
external force without causing joint injury.

It should also be remembered that ROM for any
given action (e.g. extension) may be influenced by
simultaneous movement in another direction (e.g.
external rotation). Movement in any given direction
is not necessarily independent of preceding or concurrent movement in other directions, so that laboratory measurements of range of movement may
not be as unequivocal as is intimated by research.
The muscular system is characterized by the integrated action and interaction of many muscles associated with each joint, so that limited flexibility in
a certain direction may not simply be due to the
musculature directly opposing movement in that
direction alone, but also to limitations imposed
by other synergistic muscles and other stabilizing
soft tissues.

Stretching and flexibility training are not necessarily synonymous. Some flexibility exercises are

not stretching exercises although they increase
ROM, because they may focus entirely on modifying neuromuscular processes, in particular the
reflexes that control the functional range of movement. On the other hand, many stretching exercises
do not pay any deliberate attention to neuromuscular processes and tend to concentrate on eliciting
structural changes in the soft tissues. Thus, static
stretches may actually change the length of the
muscle complex, but have an inadequate effect
on the dynamic range of movement required in a
given physical activity. Therefore, it is vitally important to distinguish between the different types of
stretching and flexibility exercises in order to integrate the most appropriate and effective balance of
static and dynamic means of increasing functional
ROM into an overall training programme.

For sports participants active flexibility is by far
the more important, and correlates more strongly
with sporting prowess than passive flexibility
(Iashvili 1982). However, passive flexibility provides a protective reserve if a joint is unexpectedly
stressed beyond its normal operational limits.
Iashvili (1982) also concluded that traditional static
and passive stretching exercises develop mainly
passive flexibility, whereas combined strength and
stretching exercises are considerably more effective in developing active flexibility, particularly if
strength conditioning is applied in the zone of active
muscular inadequacy.

Emphasis on flexibility may neglect the equally
important mechanical qualities of the tissues comprising the joints, in particular their stiffness and
damping ratio. In other words, it is vital that these
tissues offer each joint an effective balance between
mobility and stability under a wide range of operating conditions. For instance, a joint whose tissues
have low stiffness (or high ability to be stretched
easily), but a low damping ratio (or poor ability to
absorb tensile shocks) will be especially susceptible
to overload injuries (Siff 1986).

Limitations in functional ROM should not
automatically be attributed to joint stiffness alone,
because this can lead to an unnecessary emphasis
on stretching. Limitations to full ROM can also
be caused by various forms of spurious or excessive muscle tension such as *coordination tension*,

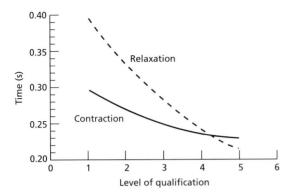

Fig. 6.22 Muscle contraction and relaxation times of athletes of increasing levels of qualification, as measured by electromyography (based on data of Matveyev 1981). Contraction time is the time from the onset of electrical activity in the muscle to the peak force, while relaxation time is the time taken from the signal to disappearance of electrical activity. Level 1 refers to the novice, level 2 is a Class 3 athlete, level 3 is a Class 2 athlete, level 4 is a Class 1 athlete and level 5 is a Master of Sport, according to Russian classification.

which may accompany the appropriate muscle tension required by the given movement. This non-functional tension can occur in both phasic and tonic muscles before, during and after the movement.

The level of proficiency of the athlete has a marked influence on the reflex ability of the muscles to contract and relax (Fig. 6.22). Rapidity of both contraction and relaxation increases with level of mastery, with a decrease in relaxation time becoming especially evident. The importance of teaching athletes to relax the muscles rapidly and efficiently to enhance the functional range of sporting movement then becomes obvious. It is no use having highly flexible joints with well-conditioned, supple connective tissues and a large range of movement, if action is limited by spurious muscle tension.

This is corroborated by the finding that talented sprinters are characterized not so much by large increases in strength, but by an improved ability to relax their muscles during the appropriate phases of movement (Verkhoshansky 1996). Flexibility training therefore should always be combined with neuromuscular training to produce efficient, functional ROM.

Muscle involvement

Standard anatomical textbook approaches describing the action of certain muscle groups in controlling isolated joint actions, such as flexion, extension and rotation, frequently are used to identify which muscles should be trained to enhance performance in sport. Virtually every bodybuilding and sports training publication invokes this approach in describing how a given exercise or machine 'works' a given muscle group, as do most of the clinical texts on muscle testing and rehabilitation.

The appropriateness of this tradition, however, has recently been questioned as a result of biomechanical analysis of multiarticular joint actions (Zajac & Gordon 1989). The classical method of functional anatomy defines a given muscle, for instance, as a flexor or extensor, on the basis of the torque that it produces around a single joint, but the nature of the body as a linked system of many joints means that muscles which do not span other joints can still produce acceleration about those joints.

The anatomical approach implies that complex multiarticular movement is simply the linear superposition of the actions of the individual joints which are involved in that movement. However, the mechanical systems of the body are non-linear and superposition does not apply, since there is no simple relationship between velocity, angle and torque about a single joint in a complex sporting movement. Besides the fact that a single muscle group can simultaneously perform several different stabilizing and moving actions about one joint, there is also a fundamental difference between the dynamics of single and multiple joint movements, namely that forces on one segment can be caused by motion of other segments. In the case of uniarticular muscles or even biarticular muscles (like the biceps or triceps), where only one of the joints is constrained to move, the standard approach is acceptable, but not if several joints are free to move concurrently.

Because joint acceleration and individual joint torque are linearly related, Zajac and Gordon (1989) consider it more accurate to rephrase a statement such as 'muscle X flexes joint A' as 'muscle X acts to

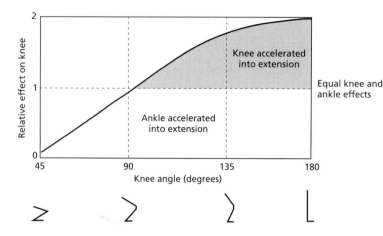

Fig. 6.23 Effect of the soleus muscle on the angular acceleration of the knee relative to the ankle. (Adapted from Zajac & Gordon 1989.)

accelerate joint A into flexion'. Superficially, this may seem a matter of trivial semantics, but the fact that muscles certainly do act to accelerate all joints has profound implications for the analysis of movement. For instance, muscles which cross the ankle joint can extend and flex the knee joint much more than they do the ankle.

Biomechanical analysis reveals that multiarticular muscles may even accelerate a spanned joint in a direction opposite to that of the joint to which it is applying torque.

In the apparently simple action of standing, the soleus, usually labelled as an extensor of the ankle, accelerates the knee (which it does not span) into extension (Fig. 6.23) twice as much as it acts to accelerate the ankle (which it spans) into extension for positions near upright posture (Zajac & Gordon 1989). In work derived from Lombard's Paradox ('antagonist muscles can act in the same contraction mode as their agonists'), Andrews (1985, 1987) found that the rectus femoris of the quadriceps and all the hamstrings act in three different ways during cycling, emphasizing that biarticular muscles are considered enigmatic. This paradox originally became apparent when it was noticed that in actions such as cycling and squatting, extension of the knee and the hip occurs simultaneously, so that the quadriceps and hamstrings are both operating concentrically at the same time. Theoretically, according to the concept of concurrent muscle antagonism, the hamstrings should contract eccentrically while

the quadriceps are contracting concentrically, and vice versa, since they are regarded as opposing muscles.

Others have shown that a muscle which is capable of carrying out several different joint actions does not necessarily do so in every movement (Andrews 1982, 1985). For instance, the gluteus maximus, which can extend and abduct the hip will not necessarily accelerate the hip simultaneously into extension and abduction, but its extensor torque may even accelerate the hip into adduction (Mansour & Pereira 1987).

The gastrocnemius, which is generally recognized as a flexor of the knee and an extensor of the ankle, actually can carry out the following complex tasks (see Fig. 6.24):
1 flex the knee and extend the ankle;
2 flex the knee and flex the ankle; and
3 extend the knee and extend the ankle.

During the standing press, which used to be part of Olympic weightlifting, the back bending action of the trunk is due not only to a Newton III reaction to the overhead pressing action, but also to acceleration caused by the thrusting backwards of the triceps muscle which crosses the shoulder joint, as well as the elbow joint. This same action of the triceps also occurs during several gymnastic moves on the parallel, horizontal and uneven bars. This back-extending action of the triceps is counteracted by the expected trunk-flexing action of the rectus abdominis and the hip extension action of the hip

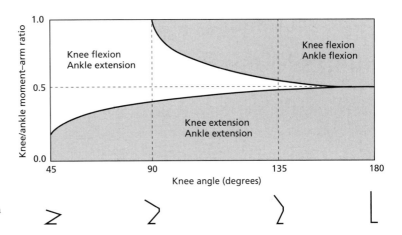

Fig. 6.24 The three possible actions of gastrocnemius revealed by the relative moment-arm ratios of the knee and ankle joints. (Adapted from Zajac & Gordon 1989.)

flexors, accompanied by acceleration of the trunk by the hip flexors.

Appreciation of this frequently ignored type of action by many multiarticular muscles enables us to select and use resistance training exercises far more effectively to meet an athlete's specific sporting needs and to offer superior rehabilitation of the injured athlete.

Finally, because of this multiplicity of actions associated with multiarticular complex movement, Zajac and Gordon stress a point made by Basmajian (1978), namely that it may be more useful to examine muscle action in terms of synergism rather than agonism and antagonism. This is especially important, since a generalized approach to understanding human movement on the basis of breaking down all movement into a series of single joint actions fails to take into account that muscle action is task dependent.

Conclusions

Various biomechanical issues and factors have been covered, and the different types of strength and power introduced, including speed-strength, starting-strength, explosive strength and reactive ability, and how they all relate to the implementation of a suitable training programme for athletes at different stages of proficiency. This discussion, however, should not be regarded as definitive or complete, because of the vast number of issues which concern the wide array of modern sports. Some central issues

have only been touched upon, such as the biomechanics of muscle action, underlying neural programming and the involvement of connective tissue. In addition, despite much research, many questions remain unanswered.

Besides factors such as starting-strength, acceleration-strength, explosive strength and relative strength, most of the other factors which concern the conditioning of the athlete for sport-specific strength and power may conveniently be summarized in the form of a pyramidal model (Fig. 6.25).

In implementing any of the methods suggested by this chapter, it is most relevant to heed the words of N.A. Bernstein about the central role played by efficiency of movement and the situationally appropriate utilization of the forces and different structures of the body involved: 'The movement of the body becomes more economical and consequently more rational, the more the body utilizes reactive and external forces and the less it relies on recruiting active muscles' (Zhekov 1976).

Finally, it is also highly relevant to the application of biomechanics in sport to remember what Roger Bannister said after becoming the first person to run the four-minute mile: 'Though physiology may indicate respiratory and circulatory limits to muscular effort, psychological and other factors beyond the ken of physiology set the razor's edge of defeat or victory and determine how closely an athlete approaches the limits of performance' (Bannister 1956).

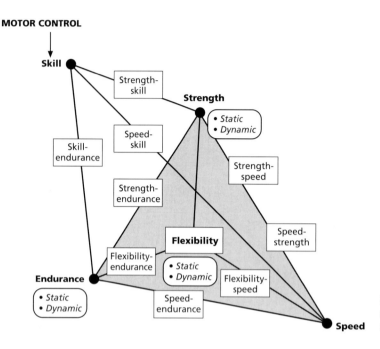

Fig. 6.25 A pyramidal model of some of the important elements of musculoskeletal fitness.

References

Andrews, J.G. (1982) On the relationship between resultant joint torques and muscular activity. *Medicine and Science in Sports and Exercise* **14**, 361–367.

Andrews, J.G. (1985) A general method for determining the functional role of a muscle. *Journal of Biomechanical Engineering* **107**, 348–353.

Andrews, J.G. (1987) The functional role of the hamstrings and quadriceps during cycling: Lombard's paradox revisited. *Journal of Biomechanics* **20**, 565–575.

Bannister, R.G. (1956) Muscular effort. *British Medical Bulletin* **12**, 222–225.

Basmajian, J. (1978) *Muscles Alive*. Williams & Wilkins, Baltimore.

Bosco, C. (1982) Physiological considerations of strength and explosive power and jumping drills (plyometric exercise). In: *Proceedings of Conference '82: Planning for Elite Performance, Canadian Track and Field Association, Ottawa, 1–5 August, 1982*, pp. 27–37.

Bosco, C., Komi, P.V., Tihanyi, J., Fekete, G. & Apor, P. (1983) Mechanical power test and fiber composition of human leg extensor muscles. *European Journal of Applied Physiology* **51**, 129–135.

Bosco, C., Cardinale, M., Colli, R., Tihanyi, J., von Duvillard, S. & Viru, A. (1998) The influence of whole body vibration on jumping ability. *Biology of Sport* **15** (3), 1–8.

Brooks, V. (1983) Motor control: How posture and movements are controlled. *Physical Therapy* **63** (5), 664–673.

Brown, S.J., Child, R., Day, S. & Donnelly, A. (1997) Exercise-induced skeletal muscle damage and adaptation following repeated bouts of eccentric muscle contraction. *Journal of Sports Science* **15** (2), 215–222.

Caiozzo, V.J., Perrine, J.J. & Edgerton, V.R. (1981) Training-induced alterations of the in vivo force-velocity relationship of human muscle. *Journal of Applied Physiology* **51** (3), 750–754.

Cavanagh, P.R. & Komi, P.V. (1979) Electromechanical delay in human skeletal muscle under concentric and eccentric contractions. *European Journal of Applied Physiology* **42** (3), 159–163.

Chapman, A. & Caldwell, G. (1985) The use of muscle strength in inertial loading. In: *Biomechanics IX-A* (eds Winter, D., Norman, D. Wells, R. *et al.*), pp. 44–49. Human Kinetics Publishers, Champaign, IL.

Enoka, R. (1996) Eccentric contractions require unique activation strategies by the nervous system. *Journal of Applied Physiology* **81** (6), 2339–2346.

Green, P. (1967) Problems of organization of motor systems. In: *Progress in Theoretical Biology*, Vol. 2 (eds Rosen, R. & Snell, F.), p. 79–83. Academic Press, New York.

Guyton, A. (1984) *Textbook of Medical Physiology*, 6th edn. W.B. Saunders, Philadelphia.

Handel, M., Horstmann, T., Dickhuth, H. & Gulch, R. (1997) Effects of contract-relax stretching training on muscle performance in athletes. *European Journal of Applied Physiology* **76** (5), 400–408.

Hettinger, T. (1961) *The Physiology of Strength*. 18–30. Charles Thomas, Springfield, IL.

Hettinger, T. & Muller, E. (1953) Muskelleistung and Muskel-training. *Arbeitsphysiologie* **15**, 111–126.

Hill, A.V. (1953) The mechanics of active muscle. *Proceedings of the Royal Society of London (Biology)* **141**, 104–117.

Hortobágyi, T., Barrier, J., Beard, D. *et al.* (1996) Greater initial adaptations to submaximal muscle strengthening than maximal shortening. *Journal of Applied Physiology* **81** (4), 1677–1682.

Iashvili, A. (1982) Active and passive flexibility in athletes specializing in different sports. *Teoriya I Praktika Fizischeskoi Kultury* **7**, 51–52.

van Ingen Schenau, G.J., Bobbert, M. & de Haan, A. (1997) Does elastic energy enhance work and efficiency in the stretch-shortening cycle. *Journal of Applied Biomechanics* **13**, 389–415.

Kernell, D. & Monster, A. (1982) Time course and properties of late adaptation in spinal motoneurons of the cat. *Experimental Brain Research* **46**, 191–196.

Knott, M. & Voss, D. (1977) *Proprioceptive Neuromuscular Facilitation*. Baillière, Tindall & Cassell, London.

Komi, P. (1979) Neuromuscular performance: Factors influencing force and speed production. *Scandinavian Journal of Sports Science* **1**, 2–15.

Kopysov, V. (1978) Vibration massage in the pre-competition conditioning of weightlifters. *Tyazhelaya Atletika* **1**, 52–53.

Kusnetsov, V. & Fiskalov, I. (1985) Correlations between speed and strength in cyclic locomotion. *Teoriya I Praktika Fizischeskoi Kultury (Theory and Practice of Physical Culture)* **8**, 6.

Lamb, D.R. (1984) *The Physiology of Exercise*. MacMillan, New York.

Lebedev, M.A. & Peliakov, A.V. (1991) Analysis of the interference electromyogram of human soleus muscle after exposure to vibration. *Neirofiziologia* **23** (1), 57–65 (article in Russian, summary in English).

Mansour, J.M. & Pereira, J.M. (1987) Quantitative functional anatomy of the lower limb with application to human gait. *Journal of Biomechanics* **20**, 51–58.

Matveyev, L. (1981) *Fundamentals of Sports Training*. Progress Publications, Moscow.

Medvedev, A.N. (1986) *A System of Multi-Year Training in Weightlifting*. Fizkultura i Sport, Moscow.

Miller, R., Mirka, A. & Maxfield, M. (1981) Rate of tension development in isometric contractions of a human hand. *Experimental Neurology* **73**, 267–285.

Norman, R.W. & Komi, P.V. (1979) Electromechanical delay in skeletal muscle under normal movement conditions. *Acta Physiologica Scandinavica* **106** (3), 241–248.

Perrine, J.J. & Edgerton, V.R. (1978) Muscle force-velocity and power-velocity relationships under isokinetic loading. *Medicine and Science in Sports* **10** (3), 159–166.

Potvin, J.R. (1997) Effects of muscle kinematics on surface EMG amplitude and frequency during fatiguing dynamic contractions. *Journal of Applied Physiology* **82** (1), 144–151.

Richards, J.A., Sears, F.W., Wehr, W.R. & Zemansky, M.W. (1962) *Modern College Physics*, pp. 83–84. Addison-Wesley, Harlow.

Siff, M.C. (1986) Ballistic analysis of human knee stability. PhD thesis, University of Witwatersrand, South Africa.

Siff, M.C. (1998) *Facts and Fallacies of Fitness*.

Siff, M.C. & Verkhoshansky, Y.V. (1999) *Supertraining: Strength Training for Sporting Excellence*. Supertraining International, Denver.

Smith, K. & Smith, M. (1962) *Perception and Motion. An Analysis of Space-Structured Behaviour*, pp. 7, 125–147. W.B. Saunders, Philadelphia.

Soechting, J. & Roberts, W. (1975) Transfer characteristics between EMG activity and muscle tension under isometric conditions in man. *Journal of Physiology* **70**, 779–793.

Thepaut-Mathieu, C., Van Hoecke, J. & Maton, B. (1988) Myoelectrical and mechanical changes linked to length specificity during isometric training. *Journal of Applied Physiology* **64** (4), 1500–1505.

Verkhoshansky, Y.V. (1977) *Osnovi Spetsialnoi Silovoi Podgotovki I Sporte (Fundamentals of Special Strength Training in Sport)*. Fizkultura i Sport Publishers, Moscow.

Verkhoshansky, Y.V. (1996) Quickness and velocity in sports movements. *IAAF Quarterly* **2–3**, 29–37.

Viitasalo, J. & Komi, P. (1978) Force-time characteristics and fiber composition in human leg extensor muscles. *European Journal of Applied Physiology* **40**, 7–15.

Vorobyev, A. (1978) *A Textbook on Weightlifting*. International Weightlifting Federation, Budapest.

Westing, S.H., Seger, J., Karlson, E. & Ekblom, B. (1988) Eccentric and concentric torque-velocity characteristics of the quadriceps femoris in man. *European Journal of Applied Physiology* **58** (1–2), 100–104.

Westing, S.H., Seger, J. & Thorstensson, A. (1990) Effects of electrical stimulation on eccentric and concentric torque-velocity relationships during knee extension in man. *Acta Physiologica Scandinavica* **140** (1), 17–22.

Westing, S.H., Cresswell, A. & Thorstensson, A. (1991) Muscle activation during maximal voluntary eccentric and concentric knee extension. *European Journal of Applied Physiology* **62** (2), 104–108.

Wilson, G., Elliot, B. & Wood, G. (1991) The effect on performance of imposing a delay during a stretch-shorten cycle movement. *Medicine and Science in Sports and Exercise* **23** (3), 364–370.

Zajac, F.E. & Gordon, M.F. (1989) Determining muscle's force and action in multi-articular movement. *Exercise and Sport Sciences Reviews* **17**, 187–230.

Zatsiorsky, V.M. (1995) *Science and Practice of Strength Training*. Human Kinetics Publishers, Champaign, IL.

Zatsiorsky, V.M. & Matveev, E.N. (1964) Force-velocity relationships in throwing. *Teoriya I Praktika Fizischeskoi Kultury (Theory and Practice of Physical Culture)* **27** (8), 24–28.

Zhekov, I.P. (1976) *Biomechanics of the Weightlifting Exercises*. Fizkultura i Sport Publishers, Moscow.

PART 2

LOCOMOTION

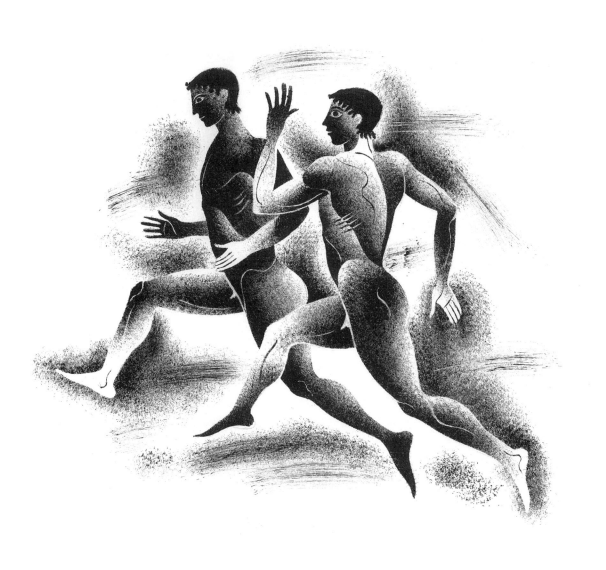

Chapter 7

Factors Affecting Preferred Rates of Movement in Cyclic Activities

P.E. MARTIN, D.J. SANDERSON AND B.R. UMBERGER

Introduction

Many human movements are characterized by the continual repetition of a fundamental pattern of motion (e.g. walking, running, hopping, cycling, swimming, rowing). For cyclic activities, the average speed of progression is defined by the product of the average distance travelled per cycle of motion (e.g. running stride length) and the average rate or cadence at which the cycle of motion is being repeated (e.g. running stride rate or cadence). In normal human movements, these speed, distance and cadence factors are usually freely determined or self-selected by the performer and are rarely fixed or pre-established. In addition, humans have an incredible ability to intentionally alter speed, distance and cadence to meet the demands of the environment. As an example, Nilsson and Thorstensson (1987) observed that over a normal range of walking speeds (1.0–3.0 m · s⁻¹), subjects were able to walk with a lowest possible stride rate of 25 strides · min⁻¹ at the lowest speed and a highest possible rate of 143 strides · min⁻¹ at all speeds. Within a range of running speeds (1.5–8 m · s⁻¹), subjects could run with rates as low as 33 strides · min⁻¹ to as high as 214 strides · min⁻¹. Given this ability to alter cycle cadence and distance factors, how is the preferred cadence chosen, and how does it relate to different optimality criteria? The mechanisms that underlie the selection process leading to a particular cadence-distance combination chosen by a performer for a given activity at a given speed are not clear, although numerous factors have been considered.

While much information has been gained about the neurophysiology of rhythmic movements, especially in lower vertebrates and invertebrates, relatively little attention has been directed to understanding how cycle distance and cadence are determined and controlled by the neuromusculoskeletal system in humans. Nevertheless, it is useful to gain some understanding of how cycle distance and cadence are related, even though available evidence applies primarily to walking. Laurent and Pailhous (1986) had subjects walk overground while imposing only stride rate or stride length by means of auditory or visual cues and allowing all other gait parameters to vary freely. Results revealed that when one parameter (e.g. stride rate) was steadily increased the other parameter (i.e. stride length) remained almost constant despite the lack of constraint imposed on all other parameters. Moreover, Laurent and Pailhous found that stride rate and length were each strongly correlated with speed, but were relatively independent of each other. The authors proposed that speed, not rate or length, is the critical parameter around which locomotion is organized. Indeed, Diedrich and Warren (1995) found that subjects make the transition from a walk to a run at a critical speed (2.2 m · s⁻¹), rather than at a critical stride rate or length, when rate and length are experimentally manipulated. Even if speed is the parameter around which locomotion is ultimately organized, the flexibility with which stride rate and length can be altered implies that the central nervous system (CNS) must have mechanisms for actively controlling these variables.

Because of the lack of dependence between stride rate and length, it has been suggested that rate and length are modulated by two distinct neural control schemes, frequency modulation for rate and amplitude modulation for length (Zijlstra *et al.* 1995). Bonnard and Pailhous (1993) also proposed that stride rate and length are controlled differently by the nervous system. Changes in stride rate are associated with changes in the global stiffness of the lower limb during the swing phase, but not during the stance phase, suggesting that rate is altered by changing the tonic activity of the lower limb muscles during swing. Changing the tonic activity of most or all of the muscles of the limb will alter the resonant frequency of that limb as it swings about the hip joint. Bonnard and Pailhous further suggested that transient changes in stride length are linked to phasic activation of appropriate leg muscles. Patla *et al.* (1989) have shown that transient increases in stride length are indeed produced by phasic increases in the activity of some muscles, and by decreases in the activity of others.

While stride rate and length may follow fairly fixed patterns during unrestrained walking and running, the CNS has the ability to dissociate rate and length if required or desired. Hogan (1984) proposed a physiological mechanism that would allow such a dissociation. When antagonistic muscles are simultaneously active about a joint, the net joint moment is related to the difference between antagonistic muscle forces and joint stiffness is associated with the sum of muscle forces. If the CNS actively modulates the coactivation of antagonistic muscles, stride rate and length can be varied independently within limits. As coactivation is metabolically costly, one might hypothesize that the preferred movement patterns require the least coactivation. This leads to the possibility that cyclic activities are organized to minimize demands placed on the neuromusculoskeletal system (e.g. minimizing energy cost, muscle activation, or muscle stress; or maximizing mechanical efficiency).

This review focuses specifically on the rate or cadence at which cyclic movements are produced and potential factors that influence preferred or self-selected cadences. A wide variety of factors that may be associated with or that directly affect preferred cadence (e.g. energy cost or economy of movement, mechanical work or power, muscular efficiency, muscle stress, inertial characteristics of swinging limbs, movement pattern variability, neuromuscular fatigue, lower extremity stiffness) have been examined over the course of many decades of research in movement science. In addition, research has focused on an equally wide variety of movements or activities. While the majority of studies have investigated walking, running and cycling, there is a more limited number of investigations on other cyclic activities such as hopping, stair climbing, rowing, swimming and wheelchair propulsion that can offer additional insights into cadence determination. Our purpose is to broadly review the existing research literature to consider those factors that may play an important role in establishing preferred cadences and to determine whether selected factors appear to be especially important in influencing fundamental preferred cadences of numerous cyclic activities.

Minimization of movement energy cost

It is intuitively appealing to speculate that submaximal, steady-state cyclic movements are organized such that body mass-specific rate of energy consumption (e.g. $J \cdot kg^{-1} \cdot s^{-1}$) or aerobic demand (e.g. $ml \cdot kg^{-1} \cdot min^{-1}$) is minimized for a given task. Applying this argument specifically to cadence, energy cost for a given activity would be minimized when self-selected or preferred cadences are used. Data for both walking and running lend support to this supposition. Numerous investigators (e.g. Högberg 1952; Zarrugh *et al.* 1974; Cavanagh & Williams 1982; Powers *et al.* 1982; Heinert *et al.* 1988; Holt *et al.* 1991, 1995; Hreljac & Martin 1993) have measured energy cost as stride rate, and thus stride length, were manipulated systematically during constant-speed treadmill walking or running. Results have shown consistently that energy cost reflects a U-shaped relationship with cadence such that as cadence is manipulated both above and below an individual's self-selected or preferred cadence, energy cost rises (Fig. 7.1). As an example, a 5% increase or decrease in stride rate of walking resulted in an 8–10% increase ($1-2 \ ml \cdot kg^{-1} \cdot min^{-1}$)

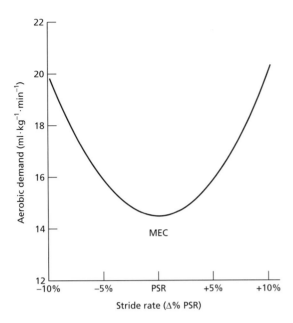

Fig. 7.1 Most economical (MEC) and preferred cadences or stride rates (PSR) are usually closely matched for walking and running at a given speed. Energy cost or aerobic demand tends to be minimized at preferred cadences and increases as stride rate is either increased or decreased from the preferred rate. (Adapted from Hreljac & Martin 1993; Fig. 1.)

in aerobic demand (Holt *et al.* 1991, 1995; Hreljac & Martin 1993). Self-selected cadence and stride length for most individuals usually do not deviate substantially from those that minimize energy cost at a given speed of walking or running. Morgan *et al.* (1994) found that only 20% of a pool of 45 recreational runners reflected a stride length that deviated by more than a few centimetres (5% of leg length) from the most economical stride length and showed a difference in aerobic demand between preferred and most economical conditions that was greater than 0.5 ml · kg⁻¹ · min⁻¹. These results provide convincing evidence that most individuals self-optimize walking and running cadences, and suggest that minimizing energy cost may be an important factor contributing to cadence determination.

Similar responses of energy cost or aerobic demand to cadence changes have been shown for

other activities as well. Seven competitive racewalkers were most economical at their preferred stride rate/stride length combinations and displayed progressively higher energy costs as cadence was either increased or decreased from the preferred rate (Morgan & Martin 1986). In addition, van der Woude *et al.* (1989) studied the effect of cadences ranging from 60 to 140% of preferred cadence on several cardiorespiratory measures during hand-rim wheelchair propulsion on a motor-driven treadmill. Aerobic demand at the preferred cadence was approximately 10% lower than that for cadences either 60% or 140% of the preferred value. U-shaped relationships between aerobic demand and cadence were observed for both experienced and inexperienced wheelchair users at several speeds of progression, although the response of the inexperienced users was less uniform and consistent across speeds. Despite the fact that the preferred cadence of experienced wheelchair users increased systematically by more than 50% (from 0.67 to 1.03 Hz) as speed of progression was increased from 0.55 to 1.39 m · s⁻¹, the preferred cadence at each speed remained the most economical cadence. Considering all of the energy cost or economy research considered thus far, preferred and most economical cadences appear to match well for multiple forms of gait and wheelchair propulsion. A common feature of both types of activities is the presence of distinct propulsion and swing phases, even though magnitudes of muscular and contact forces are substantially different for gait and wheelchair propulsion.

Unfortunately, minimization of energy cost is not generalizable to all cyclic activities. Cycling and arm cranking appear to be two tasks for which preferred and most economical cadences are different. Numerous investigators (e.g. Seabury *et al.* 1977; Jordan & Merrill 1979; Hagberg *et al.* 1981; Böning *et al.* 1984; Coast & Welch 1985; Marsh & Martin 1993, 1997) have examined the effect of pedalling cadence on aerobic demand or energy cost under a variety of power outputs and for subject groups differing in terms of fitness status and experience with the locomotion activity. In general, aerobic demand or energy cost reflects a curvilinear relationship with cadence such that minimum demand occurs at

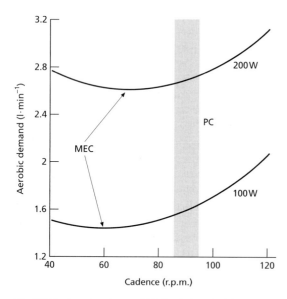

Fig. 7.2 Preferred cadences (PC, shaded region) for cycling at a given power output tend to be substantially higher than most economical cadences (MEC), although some investigators have shown that MEC increases as power output increases. (Adapted from Böning *et al.* 1984.)

about 55–65 r.p.m. (Fig. 7.2). Although preferred cadences have been reported in only a few studies (Hagberg *et al.* 1981; Marsh & Martin 1993, 1997), preferred cadences are normally much higher than the most economical cadences. For example, Marsh and Martin (1997) reported most economical cadences ranging from 53 to 60 r.p.m. for each of three subject groups (highly fit cyclists, highly fit runners, and recreationally active non-cyclists) tested at power outputs ranging from 75 to 250 W. Preferred cadences were approximately 90–95 r.p.m. for the fit cyclists and fit runners and between 80 (at 75 W) and 65 r.p.m. (at 175 W) for a less-fit group of non-cyclists. Similarly, Böning *et al.* (1984) reported most economical cadences ranging from 52 to 67 r.p.m. for a group of fit, amateur road-racing cyclists for power outputs of 50–200 W, respectively. Finally, Seabury *et al.* (1977) found most economical cadences of 44, 54 and 58 r.p.m. for power outputs of 80, 163 and 196 W for two trained distance runners and one recreational cyclist. Only two of the cycling studies cited above report most economical cadences exceeding 70 r.p.m. Coast and

Welch (1985) found that the most economical cadence steadily increases from approximately 50 r.p.m. at 100 W to 78 r.p.m. at 300 W for five trained cyclists, suggesting that exercise intensity may significantly impact the most economical cadence. Although preferred cadences were not measured, they were still likely to be well above most economical cadences for all but the highest power outputs. Only results from Hagberg *et al.* (1981), who studied seven road-racing cyclists at power outputs of about 330 W, have shown a match between the most economical and preferred cadences (91 r.p.m.).

Arm cranking appears to reflect an economy response similar to that observed for cycling, although the phenomenon for arm cranking has received substantially less attention. Powers *et al.* (1984) tested recreational runners at three arm-cranking cadences (50, 70 and 90 r.p.m.) under four power outputs (15, 30, 45 and 60 W). Aerobic demand was lowest at 50 r.p.m. for each power output condition and increased systematically as cadence increased. Unfortunately, Powers *et al.* did not report preferred cadences for their subjects, but other investigators have. Pelayo *et al.* (1997) reported an average preferred cadence of 91 r.p.m. for a group of 20 sedentary subjects exercising at 80% of their maximal arm-cranking aerobic demand, and Weissland *et al.* (1997) found preferred cadence increased from 74 to 81 r.p.m. as exercise intensity increased from 65 to 100% of maximal capacity. Thus, preferred cadences appear to be comparable with, or perhaps slightly lower than, those reported for cycling. Weissland *et al.* also investigated submaximal aerobic demand under three subject-specific cadence conditions: preferred cadence and cadences either 10% greater or 10% lower than preferred. Aerobic demand was significantly higher (approximately 8–13%) under the highest cadence condition relative to preferred cadences. Although aerobic demand differences between the preferred and –10% cadence conditions were not statistically significant, aerobic demand tended to be lower under the preferred cadence condition. Both Weissland *et al.* (1997) and Pelayo *et al.* (1997) observed systematic increases in heart rate as cadence increased. Considering all three arm-cranking studies cited here, the evidence suggests that the most economical cadences for arm cranking are lower than the preferred cadences and that the economy response for arm cranking is similar to that observed in cycling. Nevertheless, much more evidence is needed before any definitive conclusions can be drawn.

Maximizing mechanical efficiency

Mechanical efficiency, which has been defined in several ways (e.g. gross efficiency, net efficiency, work efficiency, delta efficiency; Gaesser & Brooks 1975), has also been proposed as a key element in the processes underlying the selection of preferred rates of movement. Even from the early 1920s it has been known that there is a rate of movement that is most efficient for a given power output (e.g. Hill 1922; Dickinson 1929). An examination of the notion of maximizing efficiency of human movement is not independent of the principle of minimization of the energy cost since an expression of energy cost forms the denominator of an efficiency ratio. More specifically, changes in gross efficiency (total mechanical power output divided by gross rate of energy expenditure) as cadence is manipulated under controlled power conditions are necessarily inversely related to changes in energy cost (e.g. as energy cost rises, gross efficiency falls). Movement efficiency has been investigated in numerous cyclic tasks including running (e.g. Kaneko et al. 1987), walking (Zarrugh et al. 1974), manual working tasks (Corlett & Mahadeva 1970), and cycling (Coast et al. 1986).

Hill (1922), using an elbow flexion task, observed that the efficiency of muscular contractions increased rapidly to a maximum of approximately 26% and then fell more slowly as the duration of contractions increased. Peak efficiency occurred for contraction durations of approximately 1 s. Hill subsequently cited cycling as an activity consistent with this 1 s optimum contraction duration. Benedict and Cathcart (1913) had previously reported a most efficient cadence of 70 r.p.m. for cycling. The significance of Hill's observation, however, is muted when one recognizes that contractions of individual muscles during pedalling rarely last for more than half a pedal cycle. Because of the

shape of the observed muscle efficiency function, Hill also noted that high rates of movement of short duration are likely to result in a substantial loss of efficiency, whereas movement cycles of longer duration suffer from only a small decline in efficiency. This suggests that high cadences may have a more deleterious effect on performance than low rates.

Cavagna and Franzetti (1986) examined the effect of cadence on mechanical power required to sustain constant-speed walking. They noted that maintaining walking speed with long stride lengths and a low cadence increases the magnitude of ground contact forces, whereas use of short stride lengths in combination with a high cadence requires that the limbs be accelerated more frequently. They further suggested that an optimum condition might exist at intermediate cadences that would reduce inefficiencies created by either extreme, and used a mechanical power assessment to test this notion. Two components of mechanical power were quantified as cadence was varied under controlled walking speeds: external power required to lift and accelerate the centre of mass of the body and internal power used to accelerate the limbs relative to the centre of mass. As predicted, external power declined and internal power increased as stride rate increased (Fig. 7.3). The sum of these two power components, which provided an expression of total mechanical power required to sustain walking speed, exhibited a minimum at intermediate cadences of approximately 34, 43 and 52 strides · min^{-1} for walking speeds of 4.6, 5.5 and 6.6 km · h^{-1}, respectively. Assuming that mechanical power is somewhat reflective of demands placed on the musculature, overall muscular effort would be minimized at these minima.

As will be discussed below, Hull and colleagues (Hull & Jorge 1985; Redfield & Hull 1986a) applied a similar concept when using a joint moment cost function to examine the relative demands of generating pedal forces and accelerating the limbs under different cycling cadences. Their quasi-static moment component was a function of external forces applied to the foot via the pedal, and is analogous to Cavagna and Franzetti's external power expression. Their kinematic moment component was related to limb accelerations, which is analogous to internal

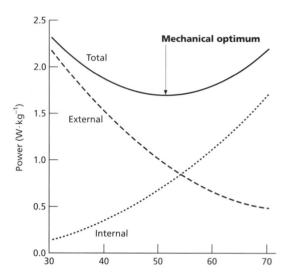

Fig. 7.3 External mechanical power (that associated with motion of the body's centre of gravity) decreases and internal power (that associated with motion of body segments relative to the centre of gravity) increases as cadence increases. Total power, which represents the sum of internal and external components, reflects a minimum at intermediate stride rates. (Adapted from Cavagna & Franzetti 1986.)

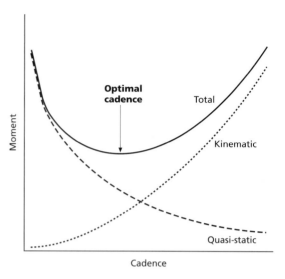

Fig. 7.4 Simulation results from Redfield and Hull (1986a) demonstrated that joint moment contributions associated with acceleration of the limbs (i.e. kinematic component) increase with cadence, and contributions associated with pedal forces acting on the foot (i.e. quasi-static component) decrease with cadence. The sum of these two components (total) reflects a minimum at intermediate cadences (approximately 90–110 r.p.m.). (Reprinted from Redfield & Hull (1986a), pp. 317–329, with permission from Elsevier Science.)

power. The relationships of these variables with respect to cadence or stride rate are strikingly similar in shape (see Figs 7.3 & 7.4) and interpretation. Both approaches predict an optimal rate of movement. Curiously, Cavagna and Franzetti (1986) reported that their calculated mechanically optimal cadence for walking was 20–30% less than self-selected cadences, while Redfield and Hull (1986a) predicted a mechanically optimal cadence approximately 10% higher than typical preferred cycling cadences. Thus, there appear to be other factors not accounted for in these models that influence the determination of self-selected cadences.

Gaesser and Brooks (1975) examined the effect of pedalling cadence and power output on multiple expressions of efficiency. Twelve subjects rode a stationary ergometer at cadences of 40, 60, 80 and 100 r.p.m. at power outputs of 0, 200, 400, 600 and 800 kg m · min⁻¹. The results demonstrated that efficiency tended to increase as power output increased, although the responses varied depending on the efficiency definition that was used. More

importantly, increases in cadence resulted in a decrease in efficiency, regardless of the efficiency expression. Gaesser and Brooks argued that delta efficiency, which is defined as the ratio of a change in power output and the associated change in energy cost, provides the best indicator of true muscular efficiency. Results from Sidossis *et al.* (1992) tend to contradict those of Gaesser and Brooks. In an assessment of the effects of power output (50, 60, 70, 80 and 90% of maximal aerobic capacity) and cadence (60, 80 and 100 r.p.m.) on gross and delta efficiency, Sidossis and colleagues observed that cadence had little effect on gross efficiency. Delta efficiency, however, increased significantly from 20.6 to 23.8% as cadence was increased from 60 to 100 r.p.m. Sidossis *et al.* speculated that the improved delta efficiency reflects an increase in muscular efficiency under higher cadence conditions. Citing fundamental muscle research that demonstrates peak muscular efficiency is achieved when fibre shortening velocity reaches one-third of the maximum velocity of shortening (e.g. Koushmerik & Davies 1969), they speculated that 'by increasing the cadence, the active muscle fibres of the cyclists in the present experiment contracted at velocities closer to the velocity of peak muscular efficiency' (p. 410).

Widrick et al. (1992) argued that accelerations of the limbs, particularly at high cadences, contribute significantly to the muscular effort required to maintain a given cadence and power output. Further, they suggested that exclusion of internal mechanical power (that associated with limb accelerations) from a total power expression 'may confound subsequent conclusions regarding optimal rates of limb movement' (p. 376). Subjects pedalled at 40, 60, 80 and 100 r.p.m. under three external power output conditions (49, 98 and 147 W) established using a Monark bicycle ergometer. Their results demonstrated that internal mechanical power increased systematically as cadence increased for each nominal external power output condition. Thus, total mechanical power (external power plus internal power) also increased as cadence increased. Using energy expenditure estimates computed from aerobic demands for each cycling condition and total mechanical power results, Widrick and colleagues computed mechanical efficiency. Optimal pedalling cadences, defined as the cadence at which mechanical efficiency was maximized, ranged from 82 r.p.m. at 49 W to 101 r.p.m. at 147 W, values that are clearly quite comparable with preferred cycling cadences.

As one final example of the potential relationship between preferred and most efficient rates of movement, Corlett and Mahadeva (1970) developed an instrument to quantify mechanical power during a manual tyre-pumping task. Combining this assessment with measures of oxygen consumption, they were able to quantify the energy expenditure per stroke for different pumping rates. Interestingly, the energy cost per stroke declined as rate of pumping increased from slow (~10 strokes · min^{-1}) to intermediate rates (30–40 strokes · min^{-1}). Energy cost per stroke did not change with further increases in rate (up to 60 strokes · min^{-1}). Further, preferred rates of movement coincided with the minimum

stroke rate at which the energy cost per stroke reached a plateau. Although efficiency was not quantified in this study, this minimum stroke rate corresponds to a rate at which efficiency would be greatest.

From this brief review of mechanical power and efficiency, it can be seen that preferred cadences in several cyclic activities may correspond well with cadences at which efficiency is maximized. Unfortunately, the existing research literature related to human movement efficiency is difficult to interpret because of inconsistencies in the definitions of both mechanical power and energy expenditure expressions used in efficiency ratio calculations. Additionally, mechanical power and energy expenditure can be difficult to quantify and/or control experimentally for many activities. In part because of these difficulties, the number of different activities investigated in efficiency studies is limited.

Mechanical optimization of muscular effort

One approach in the search for an explanation for preferred rates of movement is to use optimization or modelling strategies. These strategies use modifiable characteristics, such as cadence, and kinematic constraints to define muscle action. Such strategies have been used to predict optimal cycling cadence (Redfield & Hull 1986a, 1986b; Hull & Gonzalez 1988; Hull et al. 1988; Kautz & Hull 1993). In cycling, there is an important link between pedalling cadence and performance. Cyclists use the gears of the bicycle to select a particular cadence suited to the riding demands. The traditional approach has been to collect empirical data whereby metabolic cost (e.g. aerobic demand) of riding at particular combinations of cadence and power output have been determined (e.g. Dickinson 1929; Garry & Wishart 1931; Gaesser & Brooks 1975; Seabury et al. 1977; Jordan & Merrill 1979; Hagberg et al. 1981; Böning et al. 1984; Coast & Welch 1985; Marsh & Martin 1993, 1997).

Hull and colleagues have taken a different approach to identifying essential factors that determine optimal pedalling cadence. They argued that physiological cost, which is of considerable importance with respect to overall performance, is directly associated with muscular effort and that mechanical markers (e.g. net joint moments) can provide a reasonable representation of lower-extremity muscular effort (Redfield & Hull 1986a,b). In their earlier efforts, Hull and colleagues (Hull & Jorge 1985; Redfield & Hull 1986a) developed a five-bar linked-segment model that could be used to simulate net joint moment profiles under many different pedalling conditions (e.g. different cadences, power outputs, crank-arm lengths). Inputs for their model included scaled pedal-force profiles, measured crank positions, lower-extremity kinematic data predicted from crank position and anthropometric constraints, and pedal angles derived from a sinusoidal function. In an effort to delineate muscle function more effectively, net joint moments were subsequently divided into a quasi-static component, which was a function of external forces applied to the foot via the pedal, and a kinematic moment related to limb accelerations.

Redfield and Hull (1986a) specifically explored the relationship between net joint moments and pedalling cadence. Net joint moments were simulated for cadences of 63, 80 and 100 r.p.m. at a power output of 200 W. They found that as cadence increased, the kinematic moment increased and the quasi-static moment decreased. The increased kinematic moment was attributed to the increased accelerations of the limbs at higher speeds, whereas the decreased quasi-static moment was a function of the inverse relationship between pedal force and cadence when power output is maintained. When these components are added, a parabolic-like curve representing the total moment is derived (Fig. 7.4). From these results, Redfield and Hull showed that the total joint moment is high at relatively low cadences (< 80 r.p.m.) because of a high quasi-static contribution. At relatively high cadences (> 120 r.p.m.), the total moment is also high because of high kinematic moment contributions. Thus, total joint moment is minimized, suggesting that muscular effort is minimized, at intermediate cadences (105 r.p.m. in their analysis for a 200 W power output). Redfield and Hull concluded that their joint moment cost function provided a valid criterion for assessing optimal cadence for several reasons. First, predicted optimal cadences of the order of 90–110

r.p.m. appear to agree well with preferred cadences of experienced cyclists, rather than with the most economical or efficient cadences (30–60 r.p.m.) reported in the research literature (e.g. Hill 1922; Dickinson 1929; Garry & Wishart 1931; Gaesser & Brooks 1975). Second, predicted optimal cadence rises with increasing power output, and third, optimal cadence appears to be relatively insensitive to pedalling style.

Redfield and Hull (1986b) refined and extended their simulations of optimal cycling cadence by applying a muscle stress-based function that had been used previously in gait research (e.g. Crowninshield & Brand 1981). Their muscle stress-based cost function improved prediction of both propulsive and recovery phase pedal forces as well as net joint moments, compared with their previous moment-based modelling efforts. Hull et al. (1988) subsequently used the muscle stress function to predict the optimal cadence for a 200 W power output and found a minimum in this cost function in the range of 95–100 r.p.m., a value that was consistent with their earlier work using the moment cost function (Redfield & Hull 1986a). Interestingly, the close match between the optimal cadences predicted from the muscle-stress and net joint moment cost functions led Hull et al. to conclude that the moment-based function offered the advantage of greater ease of computation without sacrificing accuracy in predicting optimal cadence.

A crucial feature of any simulation research is the extent to which its results can be supported by empirical data. A fundamental assumption made by Hull et al. (1988) was that pedal forces scale in inverse proportion to the scaling of crank angular velocities as pedalling cadence changes (i.e. as crank velocity increases, pedal forces decrease). MacLean and Lafortune (1991a) showed that while the normal component of the pedal force scaled in proportion to crank velocity during the propulsive phase or downstroke, the reverse was true during the upstroke or recovery phase (i.e. as cadence increased, the normal component increased). Further, shear forces applied to the pedals increased during the downstroke and became smaller in the upstroke as cadence increased. They concluded that scaling of pedal forces in inverse proportion to crank velocity was not acceptable. Thus, use of this assumption may compromise the validity of model predictions.

In a separate presentation, MacLean and Lafortune (1991b) compared optimal cadence determined using five net joint moment-based cost functions with the cadence at which group mechanical efficiency was maximized, the latter being assumed to reflect the optimal cadence criterion. Using a group of 10 experienced cyclists riding at 200 W over five cadences from 60 to 120 r.p.m. (in increments of 15 r.p.m.), they found that only one of their five moment-based cost functions (one based solely on the net moment about the knee) yielded an optimal cadence matching that at which gross mechanical efficiency was maximized (80.4 and 81.3 r.p.m., respectively). The remaining moment-based cost functions yielded optimal cadences that were substantially higher, on average about 100 r.p.m., and much nearer to values reported by Hull and colleagues (Redfield & Hull 1986a; Hull et al. 1988). MacLean and Lafortune suggested that it is not surprising that minimizing the net knee moment will minimize physiological cost and maximize gross mechanical efficiency because of the many muscles acting about the knee in cycling.

Other issues surrounding optimization of cycling cadence, including seat height, foot position, etc., have been explored and are reviewed by Gregor et al. (1991). There remains conjecture regarding the relationships between muscle characteristics and selection of optimal rate (Chapman & Sanderson 1990), and these have yet to be resolved. Currently, there are few or no published empirical data that substantiate the supposed relationship between muscle moments, muscle stress and cadence selection. Clearly, this needs to be a focus of ongoing research.

Minimization of neuromuscular fatigue

Recently, a number of investigators have explored the role of muscle fatigue in determining the optimal cadence for cycling during both steady-state and exhaustive exercise. Sargeant (1994) has defined muscle fatigue as 'the failure to generate or maintain the required or expected force or power output,

resulting from muscle activity, and reversible by rest' (p. 116). In a series of papers, Takaishi, Moritani and colleagues (Takaishi et al. 1994, 1996, 1998) have estimated neuromuscular fatigue, using characteristics of the electromyograph (EMG) signal, to help explain differences between preferred and most energetically optimal cadences in cyclists and non-cyclists. Takaishi et al. (1994) had eight non-cyclists pedal at rates ranging from 40 to 80 r.p.m., at 75% of maximal aerobic power. Not surprisingly, metabolic cost was minimized at the lower cadences, and increased significantly as cadence approached 80 r.p.m. In contrast, the slope of the integrated EMG curve (iEMG) over the course of an exercise bout at a given cadence was significantly lower for the higher cadences. Over time, an increase in the slope of the iEMG is thought to reflect the recruitment of additional motor units, and/or an increase in the firing frequency of previously recruited motor units. As such, the slope of the iEMG is directly related to the intensity of the activity (Takaishi et al. 1994).

Takaishi et al. (1996) also found that the slope of the iEMG was lower at higher cadences (80–90 r.p.m.) in six trained cyclists, whereas metabolic cost was minimized at 60–70 r.p.m. In both cases, the cadences at which the slope of iEMG was found to be lowest were similar to the preferred cadences of the subjects (Takaishi et al. 1994, 1996). As the slope of iEMG was lower at higher cadences, Takaishi et al. (1994, 1996) concluded that the higher cadences chosen by competitive cyclists are selected to help minimize peripheral neuromuscular fatigue. They further noted that the lower iEMG slopes at the higher cadences suggests that fewer type II muscle fibres would be needed to meet the demands of the cycling task.

In support of this contention, Ahlquist et al. (1992) found that glycogen depletion was much greater in type II muscle fibres after cycling at 50 r.p.m. than at 100 r.p.m. at a power output equivalent to 85% of maximal aerobic power. Glycogen depletion was not different in type I fibres between the two cadence conditions. The lower pedal forces required at a higher cadence for a fixed power output (Patterson & Moreno 1990) would require lower muscle forces, and not require the recruitment of as many type II fibres (Ahlquist *et al.* 1992). Patterson and Moreno (1990) noted that the resultant pedal forces were minimized at 90 r.p.m. (at 100 W) and 100 r.p.m. (at 200 W) in a group of 11 recreational cyclists. These values were also very close to the preferred cadences at both power outputs. During steady-state cycling, greater recruitment of type II fibres at lower cadences would presumably lead to more rapid fatigue. At higher cadences, the greater reliance on type I fibres would help prevent the onset of fatigue. Nevertheless, metabolic energy cost will still be higher under high cadence conditions due to the greater number of repetitions performed per unit of time (Takaishi *et al.* 1994, 1996).

Takaishi *et al.* (1996) also noted that non-cyclists showed large increases in the iEMG of the vasti muscles at higher pedalling rates, whereas the trained cyclists did not demonstrate such an increase. The authors suggested that the lack of increase in iEMG for trained cyclists at higher cadences was related to pedalling skill developed by the trained cyclists. In subsequent research, Takaishi *et al.* (1998) demonstrated that while the vasti iEMG did not increase substantially for trained cyclists ($N = 7$) as cadence increased, biceps femoris iEMG did increase dramatically. Trained non-cyclists ($N = 7$) demonstrated a general increase in the iEMG of the vasti muscles as cadence increased, with no increase in biceps femoris activity. In addition, normal pedal forces decreased for both trained cyclists and trained non-cyclists as cadence increased; however, the normal pedal forces were lower for trained cyclists than trained non-cyclists at all but the lowest cadence (45 r.p.m.). The investigators suggested that the trained cyclists had developed a pedalling technique that involved pulling up the leg, via knee flexion, during the recovery portion of the pedal cycle at higher cadences. The speculated technique would allow for the lower pedal force seen in the cyclists, and presumably result in lower muscle stress in the vasti group, and a lower dependence on type II muscle fibres (Takaishi *et al.* 1998).

Some papers in the literature would seem to contradict the findings of the above mentioned studies. Carnevale and Gaesser (1991) found that time to exhaustion was greater at 60 r.p.m. than 100 r.p.m.

in a group of seven untrained subjects at multiple power levels. Similarly, McNaughton and Thomas (1996) reported time to exhaustion was greater at 50 r.p.m. than at 90 or 110 r.p.m. for untrained subjects. These results are consistent with the general finding that metabolic cost is minimized around 50–60 r.p.m. (Seabury *et al.* 1977; Carnevale & Gaesser 1991; Marsh & Martin 1993, 1997; McNaughton & Thomas 1996). While the work of Carnevale and Gaesser, and of McNaughton and Thomas is certainly relevant, it cannot be directly compared with the studies by Takaishi *et al.* (1994, 1996, 1998). The former investigations used power outputs designed to bring about volitional exhaustion in a 1- to 10-min range, while Takaishi *et al.* (1994, 1996, 1998) used power output levels that were designed to allow subjects to cycle for at least 15 min without suffering undue fatigue. Carnevale and Gaesser (1991) and McNaughton and Thomas (1996) also used untrained subjects, while Takaishi *et al.* (1996, 1998) used a combination of untrained non-cyclists, trained non-cyclists, and trained cyclists. A final point not directly addressed by Carnevale and Gaesser (1991) was that while time to exhaustion was substantially greater for 60 r.p.m. vs. 100 r.p.m. at the lowest power output, the time to exhaustion difference between 60 and 100 r.p.m. all but disappeared as power output was increased. With regard to this, Hill *et al.* (1995) suggested that the advantage of decreased metabolic cost at lower cadences may be offset as power output increases, due to the increased muscle force requirements per cycle.

While the data relating to the role of muscle fatigue in setting preferred rate of movement during different modes of cycling are as yet equivocal, the theoretical work of Sargeant (1994) may provide some additional insight. In a muscle of mixed fibre type, the optimal rate of shortening will be a compromise between the power–velocity relationships of type I and type II fibres. During real-world cycling, maximal power output is achieved at approximately 120 r.p.m. (Sargeant 1994). Based on the combined power–velocity relationship of a theoretical whole muscle, and the ability of the CNS to selectively recruit motor units, Sargeant argued that at 80% of maximal power output, pedalling at 120 r.p.m. would result in a reserve of 20% available power, due to the muscle being at the shortening velocity corresponding to the peak of the power–velocity curve. At 60 r.p.m. there would be no power reserve, as the muscle would be on the ascending limb of the power–velocity curve. Pedalling at 120 r.p.m. would also allow the smallest possible contribution from type II fibres to meet the demands of the cycling task (assuming type I fibres were maximally activated). Sargeant additionally contends that having the smallest theoretical contribution from type II fibres requires a progressive increase in cadence as power output is increased. Sargeant's model also predicts that at lower power outputs, the demands are best met at a lower cadence. This would allow a greater reliance on more economical type I fibres than at higher cadences. While the work of Sargeant (1994) is mostly theoretical in nature, at the very least it suggests that the preferred or optimal rate of movement during cycling, and other cyclic activities, may well be determined in large part by underlying mechanical properties of the specific muscles most involved in producing the movements. At present, this notion has not been thoroughly investigated experimentally.

Pendular properties of swinging limbs

Kugler and colleagues (Kugler *et al.* 1980; Kugler & Turvey 1987) noted that limb motions in locomotion are auto-oscillatory and possess mechanically conservative characteristics of a pendular-like mode of organization; in other words, the limbs represent complex pendulum systems. During cyclic activity of an anatomical system (e.g. walking), a certain amount of mechanical energy is dissipated from the system with each cycle of motion. Thus, muscular effort is required to sustain limb pendular-like movements. It has been hypothesized that a resonant frequency for any complex pendulum system can be predicted if the anthropometric and inertial characteristics of the limbs are known. Further, it is suggested that the resonant frequency relates directly to the fundamental rate that minimizes the energy cost associated with sustaining the motion. Holt *et al.* (1990) proposed that walking can be modelled as a force-driven harmonic oscillator (FDHO)

and that the resonant frequency of the FDHO model corresponds to the preferred rate of walking. Results for 24 young adults supported their hypothesis that 'the resonant frequency of a harmonic oscillator can accurately predict that chosen by subjects when appropriate adjustments are made to the formula based on an optimization criterion of minimum force' (p. 64). They concluded that the physical attributes of the lower extremity, more specifically its inertial characteristics, specify the most economical stride rate. In subsequent research, Holt *et al.* (1991) confirmed that preferred stride rate was not different from that predicted from their FDHO model. Subjects walked under eight stride rate conditions (preferred rate, rate predicted using the FDHO model, and rates 5, 10 and 15 strides · min⁻¹ higher or lower than the FDHO rate) as aerobic demand was measured. Both preferred and FDHO predicted stride rates resulted in minimal aerobic demand, lending additional support to the association between preferred stride rate and gait economy. Although the FDHO model has not been applied to activities other than gait, recent research has successfully predicted preferred stride rates for backward walking (Schot & Decker 1998) and for 3- to 12-year-old children (Jeng *et al.* 1997), effectively extending the generalizability of the phenomenon.

The association between the energy cost of walking and running and the inertial characteristics of the lower extremity has been demonstrated in several segment loading studies in which segment inertia has been modified artificially (e.g. Martin 1985; Myers & Steudel 1985; Steudel 1990). In contrasting proximal and distal applications of load, more distally positioned load on the segment produces a larger increase in the moment of inertia of the leg about the hip and a greater increase in the aerobic demand of gait than proximal loading. Less attention has been paid to the effect of load distribution on the temporal features of walking and running. Consistent with the pendular phenomenon, Martin (1985) reported a small (1.2%) but statistically significant decrease in stride rate and increase (2.0%) in swing time when 0.50 kg was added to each foot during treadmill running at 3.33 m · s⁻¹. Recent data from our laboratory have also shown predictable effects of shank and foot loading on walking stride rate in able-bodied (Royer *et al.* 1997) and unilateral below-knee amputees (Mattes *et al.* 2000). Thus, while the FDHO model and pendular mechanics are theoretically sound and appear to apply well to cyclic activities in which the extremities are being oscillated, the magnitude of the effect on cadence is not well substantiated.

Limb stiffness

Recently, Farley, McMahon, and co-workers (Blickhan 1989; McMahon & Cheng 1990; Farley *et al.* 1991; Farley *et al.* 1993; Farley & Gonzalez 1996; Ferris & Farley 1997) have used a simple spring-mass model of the human body to demonstrate that limb stiffness may determine rate of movement in bounding and running gaits. According to this model, the human body is represented as a massless spring (the 'leg spring') and a point mass. It has been shown that the stiffness of the leg spring remains nearly constant as running speed increases in humans and several other animal species (Farley *et al.* 1993; He *et al.* 1991). As running speed increases, the leg spring is swept through a larger angle, increasing the effective stiffness of the overall system, and causing the body to bounce off the ground at a faster rate. During hopping, or at a constant running speed, however, the stiffness of the leg spring appears to be modulated to produce a different hopping rate.

Farley *et al.* (1991) had four subjects hop forwards on a treadmill-mounted force platform at speeds from 0 to 3 m · s⁻¹, and in place on a ground-based force platform. During both hopping conditions, and at all but the fastest treadmill speed, the mean preferred rate was 132 hops · min⁻¹. The body behaved as a simple spring-mass system at the preferred hopping rate and at all rates above preferred. Below the preferred hopping rate, the body did not behave as a simple spring-mass system, implying that the storage and reutilization of elastic energy would be compromised at low rates. At hopping rates above preferred, the stiffness of the leg spring was increased to allow the body still to behave as a simple spring-mass system. As ground contact time decreased with increasing hopping rate, Farley *et al.* (1991) suggested that metabolic cost would increase

at rates above preferred, as the time to generate muscular force would be shortened. A shortened ground contact time has been suggested to require the recruitment of less-economical fast-twitch muscle fibres, and consequently increase metabolic cost (Kram & Taylor 1990). Ferris and Farley (1997) further showed that subjects increase hopping rate by increasing leg-spring stiffness, regardless of surface compliance. However, leg-spring stiffness was increased disproportionately more on compliant surfaces than stiff surfaces, to keep the total vertical stiffness nearly constant at a given rate.

Farley and Gonzalez (1996) had four subjects run on a treadmill-mounted force platform at 2.5 m · s⁻¹, and at stride rates from 26% below to 36% above preferred (preferred stride rate = 79.8 strides · min⁻¹), to see how the behaviour of the spring-mass model was altered to produce different stride rates. While the stiffness of the leg spring has been found to remain constant, and the angle through which the leg spring is swept increases as speed increases (He *et al.* 1991; Farley *et al.* 1993), Farley and Gonzalez found that different stride rates at a constant speed are produced primarily by increasing the leg-spring stiffness. The stiffness of the leg spring was increased over twofold from the lowest stride rate to the highest rate, while the angle swept by the leg spring only decreased slightly at the highest rate. In fact, when stride rate (Farley & Gonzalez 1996) and hopping rate (Farley *et al.* 1991) were each increased by 65%, leg-spring stiffness increased by approximately the same amount (twofold), demonstrating the similarities between these two forms of locomotion.

Farley and Gonzalez (1996) stated that the ability to adjust the leg-spring stiffness is likely to be an important factor in adapting the locomotor system to the demands of the environment. In physiological terms, the stiffness of the leg spring can be adjusted in at least two ways. Changing the orientation of the limbs relative to the ground (McMahon *et al.* 1987), and changing muscle activation patterns (Farley & Gonzalez 1996) will each result in an altered leg-spring stiffness. In summary, Farley *et al.* (1991) suggested their findings help explain why metabolic cost is minimized at the preferred rate of movement in bounding or running gaits. Metabolic cost below the preferred rate will increase due to a loss of elastic strain energy from the system. Above the preferred rate, metabolic cost will increase due to a shorter ground contact time. While the spring-mass model has been valuable in distinguishing important aspects of rate selection in bounding and running gaits, it is not directly applicable to other activities, such as walking, where kinetic energy and gravitational potential energy are 180° out of phase, and the body does not behave as a simple spring-mass system. Interestingly, Bonnard and Pailhous (1993) found that during walking, stride rate is highly dependent on limb stiffness during the swing phase, but independent of limb stiffness during stance. The stiffness changes noted by Farley and co-workers (Blickhan 1989; McMahon & Cheng 1990; Farley *et al.* 1991; Farley *et al.* 1993; Farley & Gonzalez 1996; Ferris & Farley 1997) during running and hopping relate implicitly to the stance phase.

Minimizing movement variability

In addition to metabolic cost, mechanical minimization phenomena and limb inertial properties, movement stability or variability may be another factor that determines the preferred or optimal rate of movement during cyclic activities. The reader should note that high movement stability and low movement variability are synonymous in the present context. Much, if not all, of the literature relating to movement stability during cyclic activities comes out of a dynamical systems approach to movement organization. According to dynamical systems theory, 'behavioural patterns and their dynamics are shown to arise in a purely self-organized fashion from cooperative coupling among individual components' (Kelso & Schöner 1988, p. 27). A primary focus of this theory is the study of stability and the loss of stability. Well-learned or preferred movement patterns are associated with high stability, and a loss of stability is usually indicative of an impending change in behaviour (such as the transition from walking to running).

There is also evidence from more traditional motor behaviour circles that movement variability is an important and relevant issue in control of pre-ferred rate of movement. Smoll (1975), and Smoll and Schutz (1978) found distinct individual differences in preferred cadences and movement variability in a cyclic upper-limb task. They noted that movement variability is uncorrelated with preferred cadence, and is likely to be related to underlying biological variability. According to Smoll (1975), movement variability is indicative of the status of an individual performance, and is an essential component of a complete description of that performance.

Movement variability has previously been characterized as stochastic in nature (Hirokawa 1989). Recent research by Hausdorff and colleagues (Hausdorff *et al.* 1995, 1996), however, has demonstrated that variations in the stride interval during steady-state walking exhibit long-range correlations, such that the fluctuations in stride interval at any point in time are dependent on stride intervals at previous times. The long-term correlations extend as far back as 1000 strides (Hausdorff *et al.* 1996). Interestingly, when subjects walked in time with a metronome set at their preferred stride rate, the long-range correlations disappeared, and the variations in stride interval became random in nature (Hausdorff *et al.* 1996). Hausdorff *et al.* (1995) proposed that chaotic variability is an intrinsic part of the normal locomotor control system. The researchers also suggested that supraspinal centres are responsible for the presence of the long-term correlations. From a control perspective, systems that possess long-range correlations are inherently more resistant to perturbations (Hausdorff *et al.* 1995). Movement variability/stability is clearly a relevant factor for cyclic movement control, and a possible determinant of preferred rate of movement.

One of the most complete accounts of the relationship between movement stability and preferred rate of movement is provided by Holt *et al.* (1995). Their paper is notable because they employed stability, metabolic, mechanical and inertial measures, allowing direct comparisons not usually possible in unifocal studies. They determined three measures of movement stability for eight subjects at their preferred speed as they walked on a treadmill at preferred stride rate, optimal stride rate predicted by a force-driven harmonic oscillator model of the lower

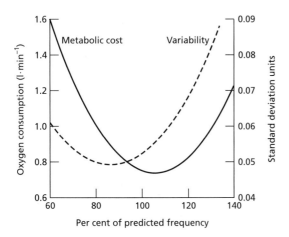

Fig. 7.5 Both aerobic demand and movement variability reflect minima near the resonant frequency or stride rate predicted using a force-driven harmonic oscillator model. This predicted stride also corresponded well with preferred cadences of subjects. (Adapted from Holt *et al.* 1995.)

limb, and ±15, ±25 and ±35% of predicted stride rate. The three stability measures were the standard deviation of the relative phase between the lower limb joints, the standard deviation of a normalized vector length of the phase planes for the head and back, and the magnitude of the spectral power near the predicted and preferred frequencies for the head and joints. They additionally measured metabolic cost and mechanical energy conservation at each stride rate. Holt and colleagues found that movement stability was generally maximized (i.e. variability was minimized) and metabolic cost minimized at the preferred and predicted stride rates, which were not significantly different from each other (Fig. 7.5). Holt *et al.* (1995) noted that the metabolic cost curve was steeper at low stride rates than at high rates, but the reverse was true for the stability curve. The investigators suggested that preferred stride rate may be a compromise between metabolic cost and movement stability.

Maruyama and Nagasaki (1992) measured the variability of many temporal aspects of the stride (stride time, step time, stance time, swing time and double support time) using variable error and coefficient of variation in seven subjects during treadmill walking at speeds ranging from 0.5 to 1.7

m · s⁻¹, and stride rates ranging from 30 to 80 strides · min⁻¹. The two major findings by Maruyama and Nagasaki (1992) were that stride variability for all stride phases decreased as speed increased, and variability was minimized at or near the preferred stride rate at any given speed. In a similar study using 22 subjects walking overground, Sekiya *et al.* (1997) found that spatial variability of stride length was minimized near the preferred stride rate and preferred speed. At the speed most closely approximating the commonly reported energetically optimal speed (1.38 m · s⁻¹), temporal variability was minimized at a stride rate of 58.2 strides · min⁻¹ and spatial variability was minimized at a stride rate of 60.4 strides · min⁻¹. The preferred rates at the same speed were 57.1 strides · min⁻¹ (Maruyama & Nagasaki 1992) and 54.2 strides · min⁻¹ (Sekiya *et al.* 1997). Maruyama and Nagasaki (1992) and Sekiya *et al.* (1997) concluded that preferred stride rate is optimized in terms of metabolic cost and movement stability.

Brisswalter and Mottet (1996) used variability and metabolic cost measures in an analysis of the walk-to-run transition in 10 subjects walking and running on a treadmill. During the preferred transition speed trials, variability increased as walking speed increased in the neighbourhood of the transition speed. After the transition, variability was much lower, consistent with the findings of others (Diedrich & Warren 1995). Brisswalter and Mottet (1996) also expected variability to be lower for walking below the transition speed, and lower for running above the transition speed; however, this was not the case. Variability was lower for running than walking at all common speeds (±0.3 m · s⁻¹ of transition speed). Therefore, below the energetically optimal transition speed, walking is more economical, but also more variable than running. In addressing this paradox, the authors noted the difficulty in associating gross energy cost with movement efficiency, and suggested that metabolic cost alone is not adequate to relate movement efficiency and variability. Another factor not addressed by Brisswalter and Mottet is that at the common speeds, stride rate was higher for running than for walking (1–16%), and variability tended to decrease (up to a point) with increases in rate of movement

(Smoll 1975; Smoll & Schutz 1978), perhaps making the finding of lower variability at all running speeds less surprising. One should keep in mind that the paper by Brisswalter and Mottet dealt with speeds near the preferred transition speed, and did not include data on preferred speed or stride rate for walking or running.

In a paper dealing with the walk-to-run transition, Diedrich and Warren (1998) presented an account of movement stability over a range of walking and running speeds. The walking stability function had a minimum at $1.66 \text{ m} \cdot \text{s}^{-1}$ and $61.8 \cdot \text{strides} \cdot \text{min}^{-1}$. The data from Diedrich and Warren compare favourably with the results from Maruyama and Nagasaki (1992). At a speed of $1.67 \text{ m} \cdot \text{s}^{-1}$, Maruyama and Nagasaki reported minimum variability at $62.0 \text{ strides} \cdot \text{min}^{-1}$, and a preferred rate of $62.4 \text{ strides} \cdot \text{min}^{-1}$. While the stability and metabolic cost relationships were very similar in shape, the respective minima were not coincident (energetically optimal walking speed $\sim 1.3 \text{ m} \cdot \text{s}^{-1}$). Diedrich and Warren (1998) emphasized the similarities between the overall behaviour of the stability and economy functions, and suggested that any minor differences were likely to be related to the fact that global energy expenditure includes costs not associated with the locomotor task. As with research by others (Maruyama & Nagasaki 1992; Holt et al. 1995; Sekiya et al. 1997), the findings of Diedrich and Warren (1995, 1998) point to a strong, if not perfect (Brisswalter & Mottet 1996), relationship between movement stability and economy.

Patla (1985) examined EMG variability at fast, normal and slow stride rates in seven subjects walking on a treadmill at preferred speed. He used a pattern recognition technique to estimate variability. Surprisingly, muscle activity patterns were found to be more variable for the normal stride rate than the slow or fast rates. The author suggested that the attentional demand necessary to walk in a non-preferred manner could account for the lower variability under these conditions. The finding of increased variability for muscle activity at the preferred rate is in direct contrast to the notion that kinematic variability is minimized at the preferred rate (Maruyama & Nagasaki 1992; Holt et al. 1995; Sekiya et al. 1997).

All of the studies reviewed so far have dealt exclusively with adults. A few papers in the literature have dealt with movement variability during locomotion in children. Jeng et al. (1997) determined interlimb and intralimb stability in 45 children aged 3–12 years walking on a treadmill at their preferred stride rates and ±25% of preferred stride rate. In most cases, interlimb and intralimb stability was maximized under preferred stride rate conditions. The authors also noted that by age 7 years, children exhibit a self-optimization pattern similar to adults. Jeng et al. (1997) also observed that 5- to 6-year-olds demonstrated an ability to modulate stride rate not seen in 3- to 4-year-olds, but as a consequence the gait of the 5- to 6-year-olds became more variable. Variability subsequently decreased in the 7- to 12-year-olds. The dramatic differences between the 5- to 6- and 3- to 4-year-olds are possible due to morphological changes that occur between ages 3 and 6; however, they may also be indicative of a transition from a rigid form of control to a more adaptive form of control (Jeng et al. 1997). A more adaptive form of control would by its very nature require more variability in the system. Clark and Phillips (1993) have also suggested that infants also go through a period of stability acquisition during the first 3 months of independent walking. Although the picture is far from complete, locomotion development in children may undergo at least two distinct phases of stability acquisition. One is associated with the initial development of the walking skill, and a second is associated with an increase in the adaptability of stride rate to meet the demands of the environment.

The literature on movement variability at different rates of movement in cyclic activities outside the locomotion arena is sparse. Recently, Dawson et al. (1998) reported changes in temporal variability during rowing on an ergometer and on the water in five competitive rowers, over a range of stroke rates ($18–33 \text{ strokes} \cdot \text{min}^{-1}$). The authors discovered that rowers increase stroke rate primarily by decreasing the duration of the recovery phase, while the duration of the stroke phase changed very little. As stroke rate increased, variability generally decreased for both the recovery phase and the stroke phase. The decreases in variability were most dramatic for the recovery phase, which exhibited considerably higher variability than the stroke phase at the lower rates. Dawson *et al.* (1998) did not determine preferred stroke rate for the rowers in their study. They did note, however, that preferred stroke rate is usually in the range of 30–40 strokes · min^{-1}. This would suggest that movement variability is minimized at or near preferred stroke rates in competitive rowers.

Based on the studies reviewed, movement stability would appear to be a contributing factor to the selection of the preferred cadences during locomotion. Specifically, the results of Holt *et al.* (1995) indicate that stability may cooperate with metabolic cost in setting the preferred stride rate. The findings of Dawson *et al.* (1998) suggest that minimizing variability may be a factor in cadence selection for other activities as well. Many more studies will be needed on other cyclic activities before any far-reaching generalizations can be made regarding the role of movement stability/variability in rate of movement selection.

Summary

The factors that determine the preferred and/or optimal rate of limb movement during any cyclic activity are clearly many. Metabolic cost, mechanical minimization phenomena, muscle mechanical properties, limb inertial parameters, movement stability and limb stiffness all appear to be associated with the preferred rate of movement for one or more activities. The tasks for the future are twofold. For the locomotion arena, well-designed multifactorial studies are needed that will allow us to determine which associated factors are causal, and which are merely related effects. Additionally, many studies are needed using activities other than walking, running and cycling, to determine whether the conclusions reached from the locomotion-based studies have strong generalizability, or are activity specific. Only then will the critical factors underlying the selection of the rate of movement emerge.

References

Ahlquist, L.E., Bassett, D.R., Sufit, R., Nagle, F.J. & Thomas, D.P. (1992) The effect of pedaling frequency on glycogen depletion rates in type I and type II quadriceps muscle fibers during submaximal cycling exercise. *European Journal of Applied Physiology and Occupational Physiology* **65**, 360–364.

Benedict, F.G. & Cathcart, E.P. (1913) *Muscular Work*. Publication no. 187, Carnegie Institute of Washington, Washington, D.C.

Blickhan, R. (1989) The spring-mass model for running and hopping. *Journal of Biomechanics* **22**, 1217–1227.

Böning, D., Gönen, Y. & Maassen, N. (1984) Relationship between work load, pedal frequency, and physical fitness. *International Journal of Sports Medicine* **5**, 92–97.

Bonnard, M. & Pailhous, J. (1993) Intentionality in human gait control: Modifying the frequency-to-amplitude relationship. *Journal of Experimental Psychology: Human Perception and Performance* **19**, 429–443.

Brisswalter, J. & Mottet, D. (1996) Energy cost and stride duration variability at preferred transition gait speed between walking and running. *Canadian Journal of Applied Physiology* **21**, 471–480.

Carnevale, T.J. & Gaesser, G.A. (1991) Effects of pedaling speed on the power-duration relationship for high-intensity exercise. *Medicine and Science in Sports and Exercise* **23**, 242–246.

Cavagna, G.A. & Franzetti, P. (1986) The determinants of the step frequency in walking in humans. *Journal of Physiology* **373**, 235–242.

Cavanagh, P.R. & Williams, K.R. (1982) The effect of stride length variation on oxygen uptake during distance running. *Medicine and Science in Sports and Exercise* **14**, 30–35.

Chapman, A.E. & Sanderson, D.J. (1990) Muscular coordination in sporting skills. In: *Multiple Muscle Systems: Biomechanics and Movement Organization* (eds J.M. Winters & S.L.-Y. Woo), pp. 608–620. Springer-Verlag, New York.

Clark, J.E. & Phillips, S.J. (1993) A longitudinal study of intralimb coordination in the first year of independent walking: A dynamical systems analysis. *Child Development* **64**, 1143–1157.

Coast, J.R. & Welch, H.G. (1985) Linear increase in optimal pedal rate with increased power output in cycle ergometry. *European Journal of Applied Physiology* **53**, 339–342.

Coast, J.R., Cox, R.H. & Welch, H.G. (1986) Optimal pedalling rate in prolonged bouts of cycle ergometry. *Medicine and Science in Sports and Exercise* **18**, 225–230.

Corlett, E.N. & Mahadeva, K. (1970) A relationship between freely chosen working pace and energy consumption curves. *Ergonomics* **13**, 517–524.

Crowninshield, R.D. & Brand, R.A. (1981) A physiologically based criterion of muscle force prediction in locomotion. *Journal of Biomechanics* **14**, 793–801.

Dawson, R.G., Lockwood, R.J., Wilson, J.D. & Freeman, G. (1998) The rowing cycle: Sources of variance and invariance in ergometer and on-the-water performance. *Journal of Motor Behavior* **30**, 33–43.

Dickinson, S. (1929) The efficiency of bicycle-pedalling, as affected by speed and load. *Journal of Physiology* **67**, 242–255.

Diedrich, F.J. & Warren, W.H. (1995) Why change gaits? Dynamics of the walk-run transition. *Journal of Experimental Psychology: Human Perception and Performance* **21**, 183–202.

Diedrich, F.J. & Warren, W.H. (1998) The dynamics of gait transitions: Effects of grade and load. *Journal of Motor Behavior* **30**, 60–78.

Farley, C.T. & Gonzalez, O. (1996) Leg stiffness and stride frequency in human running. *Journal of Biomechanics* **29**, 181–186.

Farley, C.T., Blickhan, R., Saito, J. & Taylor, C.R. (1991) Hopping frequency in humans: a test of how springs set stride frequency in bouncing gaits. *Journal of Applied Physiology* **71**, 2127–2132.

Farley, C.T., Glasheen, J. & McMahon, T.A. (1993) Running springs: Speed and animal size. *Journal of Experimental Biology* **185**, 71–86.

Ferris, D.P. & Farley, C.T. (1997) Interaction of leg stiffness and surface stiffness during human hopping. *Journal of Applied Physiology* **82**, 15–22.

Gaesser, G.A. & Brooks, G.A. (1975) Muscular efficiency during steady-rate exercise: effects of speed and work rate. *Journal of Applied Physiology* **38**, 1132–1139.

Garry, R.C. & Wishart, G.M. (1931) On the existence of a most efficient speed in bicycle pedalling, and the problem of determining human muscular efficiency. *Journal of Physiology* **72**, 426–437.

Gregor, R.J., Broker, J.P. & Ryan, M.M. (1991) The biomechanics of cycling. *Exercise and Sport Sciences Reviews* **19**, 127–169.

Hagberg, J.M., Mullin, J.P., Giese, M.D. & Spitznagel, E. (1981) Effect of pedaling rate on submaximal exercise responses of competitive cyclists. *Journal of Applied Physiology* **51**, 447–451.

Hausdorff, J.M., Peng, C.K., Ladin, Z., Wei, J.Y. & Goldberger, A.L. (1995) Is walking a random act? Evidence for long-range correlations in stride interval of human gait. *Journal of Applied Physiology* **78**, 349–358.

Hausdorff, J.M., Purdon, P.L., Peng, C.K., Ladin, Z., Wei, J.Y. & Goldberger, A.L. (1996) Fractal dynamics of human gait: stability of long-range correlations in stride interval fluctuations. *Journal of Applied Physiology* **80**, 1448–1457.

He, J., Kram, R. & McMahon, T.A. (1991) Mechanics of running under simulated reduced gravity. *Journal of Applied Physiology* **71**, 863–870.

Heinert, L.D., Serfass, R.C. & Stull, G.A. (1988) Effect of stride length variation on oxygen uptake during level and positive grade treadmill running. *Research Quarterly for Exercise and Sport* **59**, 127–130.

Hill, A.V. (1922) The maximum work and mechanical efficiency of human muscles, and their most economical speed. *Journal of Physiology* **56**, 19–41.

Hill, D.W., Smith, J.C., Leuschel, J.L., Chasteen, S.D. & Miller, S.A. (1995) Effect of pedal cadence on parameters of the hyperbolic power-time relationship. *International Journal of Sports Medicine* **16**, 82–87.

Hirokawa, S. (1989) Normal gait characteristics under temporal and distance constraints. *Journal of Biomedical Engineering* **11**, 449–456.

Hogan, N. (1984) Adaptive control of mechanical impedance by coactivation of antagonist muscles. *IEEE Transactions on Automatic Control* **29**, 681–690.

Högberg, P. (1952) How do stride length and stride frequency influence the energy output during running. *Arbeitsphysiologie* **14**, 437–441.

Holt, K.G., Hamill, J. & Andres, R.O. (1990) The force driven harmonic oscillator as a model for human locomotion. *Human Movement Science* **9**, 55–68.

Holt, K.G., Hamill, J. & Andres, R.O. (1991) Predicting the minimal energy costs of human walking. *Medicine and Science in Sports and Exercise* **23**, 491–498.

Holt, K.G., Jeng, S.F., Ratcliffe, R. & Hamill, J. (1995) Energetic cost and stability during human walking at the preferred stride frequency. *Journal of Motor Behavior* **27**, 164–178.

Hreljac, A. & Martin, P.E. (1993) The relationship between smoothness and economy during walking. *Biological Cybernetics* **69**, 213–218.

Hull, M.L. & Gonzalez, H. (1988) Bivariate optimization of pedalling rate and crank arm length in cycling. *Journal of Biomechanics* **21**, 839–849.

Hull, M.L. & Jorge, M. (1985) A method for biomechanical analysis of bicycle pedalling. *Journal of Biomechanics* **18**, 631–644.

Hull, M.L., Gonzalez, H.K. & Redfield, R. (1988) Optimization of pedaling rate in cycling using a muscle stress-based objective function. *International Journal of Sports Biomechanics* **4**, 1–20.

Jeng, S.F., Liao, H.F., Lai, J.S. & Hou, J.W. (1997) Optimization of walking in children. *Medicine and Science in Sports and Exercise* **29**, 370–376.

Jordan, L. & Merrill, E.G. (1979) Relative efficiency as a function of pedalling rate for racing cyclists. *Journal of Physiology* **241**, 49P–50P.

Kaneko, M., Matsumoto, M., Ito, A. & Fuchimoto, T. (1987) Optimum step frequency in constant speed running. *Biomechanics X-B*, (ed. B. Jonsson), pp. 803–807. Human Kinetics Publishers, Champaign, IL.

Kautz, S.A. & Hull, M.L. (1993) A theoretical basis for interpreting the force applied to the pedal in cycling. *Journal of Biomechanics* **26**, 155–165.

Kelso, J.A.S. & Schöner, G. (1988) Self-organization of coordinative movement patterns. *Human Movement Science* **7**, 27–46.

Koushmerik, M.J. & Davies, R.E. (1969) The chemical energetics of muscle contraction. II. The chemistry, efficiency and power of maximally working sartorius muscle. *Proceedings of the Royal Society of London* **1117**, 315–353.

Kram, R. & Taylor, C.R. (1990) Energetics of running: a new perspective. *Nature* **346**, 265–267.

Kugler, P.N. & Turvey, M.T. (1987) *Information, Natural Law, and the Self-Assembly of Rhythmic Movement*. Lawrence Erlbaum Associates, Hillsdale, New Jersey.

Kugler, P.N., Kelso, J.A.S. & Turvey, M.T. (1980) On the concept of coordinative structures as dissipative structures. In: *Tutorials in Motor Behavior* (eds G.E. Stelmach & J. Requin), pp. 3–47. North-Holland, Amsterdam.

Laurent, M. & Pailhous, J. (1986) A note on modulation of gait in man: Effects of constraining stride length and frequency. *Human Movement Science* **5**, 333–343.

MacLean, B.D. & Lafortune, M.A. (1991a) Optimum pedaling cadence determined by joint torque parameters and oxygen cost. In: *XIIIth International Congress on Biomechanics: Book of Abstracts* (eds R.N. Marshall, G.A. Wood, B.C. Elliott, T.R. Ackland & P.J. McNair), pp. 102–104. University of Western Australia, Perth.

MacLean, B.D. & Lafortune, M.A. (1991b) Influence of cadence on mechanical parameters of pedaling. In: *XIIIth International Congress on Biomechanics: Book of Abstracts* (eds R.N. Marshall, G.A. Wood, B.C. Elliott, T.R. Ackland & P.J. McNair), pp. 100–102. University of Western Australia, Perth.

Marsh, A.P. & Martin, P.E. (1993) The association between cycling experience and preferred and most economical cadences. *Medicine and Science in Sports and Exercise* **25**, 1269–1274.

Marsh, A.P. & Martin, P.E. (1997) Effect of cycling experience, aerobic power, and power output on preferred and most economical cycling cadences. *Medicine and Science in Sports and Exercise* **29**, 1225–1232.

Martin, P.E. (1985) Mechanical and physiological responses to lower extremity loading during running. *Medicine and Science in Sports and Exercise* **17**, 427–433.

Maruyama, H. & Nagasaki, H. (1992) Temporal variability in the phase durations during treadmill walking. *Human Movement Science* **11**, 335–348.

Mattes, S.J., Martin, P.E. & Royer, T.A. (2000) Walking symmetry and energy cost in persons with unilateral transtibial amputations: Matching prosthetic and intact limb inertial properties. *Archives of Physical Medicine and Rehabilitation* (in press).

McMahon, T.A. & Cheng, G.C. (1990) The mechanics of running: How does stiffness couple with speed? *Journal of Biomechanics* **23**, 65–78.

McMahon, T.A., Valiant, G. & Frederick, E.C. (1987) Groucho running. *Journal of Applied Physiology* **62**, 2326–2337.

McNaughton, L. & Thomas, D. (1996) Effects of different pedalling speeds on the power-duration relationship of high intensity cycle ergometry. *International Journal of Sports Medicine* **17**, 287.

Morgan, D.W. & Martin, P.E. (1986) Effects of stride length alteration on race-walking economy. *Canadian Journal of Applied Sports Sciences* **11**, 211–217.

Morgan, D.W., Martin, P.E., Craib, M., Caruso, C., Clifton, R. & Hopewell, R. (1994) Effect of step length optimization on the aerobic demand of running. *Journal of Applied Physiology* **77**, 245–251.

Myers, M.J. & Steudel, K. (1985) Effect of limb mass and its distribution on the energetic cost of running. *Journal of Experimental Biology* **116**, 363–373.

Nilsson, J. & Thorstensson, A. (1987) Adaptability in frequency and amplitude of leg movements during human locomotion at different speeds. *Acta Physiologica Scandinavica* **129**, 107–114.

Patla, A.E. (1985) Some characteristics of EMG patterns during locomotion: implications for the locomotor control process. *Journal of Motor Behavior* **17**, 443–461.

Patla, A.E., Armstrong, C.J. & Silveira, J.M. (1989) Adaptation of the muscle activation patterns to transitory increases in stride length during treadmill locomotion in humans. *Human Movement Science* **8**, 45–66.

Patterson, R.P. & Moreno, M.I. (1990) Bicycle pedalling forces as a function of pedalling rate and power output. *Medicine and Science in Sports and Exercise* **22**, 512–516.

Pelayo, P., Sidney, M. & Weissland, T. (1997) Effects of variations in spontaneously chosen rate during crank upper-body and swimming exercise. *Journal of Human Movement Studies* **33**, 171–180.

Powers, S.K., Hopkins, P. & Ragsdale, M.R. (1982) Oxygen uptake and ventilatory responses to various stride lengths in trained women. *American Corrective Therapy Journal* **36**, 5–8.

Powers, S.K., Beadle, R.E. & Mangum, M. (1984) Exercise efficiency during arm ergometry: effects of speed and work rate. *Journal of Applied Physiology* **56**, 495–499.

Redfield, R. & Hull, M.L. (1986a) On the relationship between joint moments and pedalling rates at constant power in bicycling. *Journal of Biomechanics* **19**, 317–329.

Redfield, R. & Hull, M.L. (1986b) Prediction of pedal forces in bicycling using optimization methods. *Journal of Biomechanics* **19**, 523–540.

Royer, T.D., Martin, P.E. & Mattes, S.J. (1997) Perturbability of temporal symmetry of gait by symmetrical and asymmetrical lower extremity inertia changes. *Medicine and Science in Sports and Exercise* **29**, S113.

Sargeant, A.J. (1994) Human power output and muscle fatigue. *International Journal of Sports Medicine* **15**, 116–121.

Schot, P.K. & Decker, M.J. (1998) The force driven harmonic oscillator model accurately predicts the preferred stride frequency for backward walking. *Human Movement Science* **17**, 67–76.

Seabury, J.J., Adams, W.C. & Ramey, M.R. (1977) Influence of pedalling rate and power output on energy expenditure during bicycle ergometry. *Ergonomics* **20**, 491–498.

Sekiya, N., Nagasaki, H., Ito, H. & Furuna, T. (1997) Optimal walking in terms of variability in step length. *Journal of Orthopedic and Sports Physical Therapy* **26**, 266–272.

Sidossis, L.S., Horowitz, J.F. & Coyle, E.F. (1992) Load and velocity of contraction influence gross and delta mechanical efficiency. *International Journal of Sports Medicine* **13**, 407–411.

Smoll, F.L. (1975) Preferred tempo of motor performance: Individual differences in within-individual variability. *Journal of Motor Behavior* **7**, 259–263.

Smoll, F.L. & Schutz, R.W. (1978) Relationship among measures of preferred tempo and motor rhythm. *Perceptual and Motor Skills* **46**, 883–894.

Steudel, K. (1990) The work and energetic cost of locomotion. I. The effects of limb mass distribution in quadrupeds. *Journal of Experimental Biology* **154**, 273–285.

Takaishi, T., Yasuda, Y. & Moritani, T. (1994) Neuromuscular fatigue during prolonged pedalling exercise at different pedalling rates. *European Journal of Applied Physiology and Occupational Physiology* **69**, 154–158.

Takaishi, T., Yasuda, Y., Ono, T. & Moritani, T. (1996) Optimal pedaling rate estimated from neuromuscular fatigue for cyclists. *Medicine and Science in Sports and Exercise* **28**, 1492–1497.

Takaishi, T., Yamamoto, T., Ono, T., Ito, T. & Moritani, T. (1998) Neuromuscular, metabolic, and kinetic adaptations for skilled pedaling performance in cyclists. *Medicine and Science in Sports and Exercise* **30**, 442–449.

Weissland, T., Pelayo, P., Vanvelcenaher, J., Marais, G., Lavoie, J.-M. & Robin, H. (1997) Physiological effects of variations in spontaneously chosen crank rate during incremental upper-body exercise. *European Journal of Applied Physiology* **76**, 428–433.

Widrick, J.J., Freedson, P.S. & Hamill, J. (1992) Effect of internal work on the calculation of optimal pedaling rates. *Medicine and Science in Sports and Exercise* **24**, 376–382.

van der Woude, L.H.V., Veeger, H.E.J., Rozendal, R.H. & Sargeant, A.J. (1989) Optimum cycle frequencies in hand-rim wheelchair propulsion. *European Journal of Applied Physiology* **58**, 625–632.

Zarrugh, M.Y., Todd, F.N. & Ralston, H.J. (1974) Optimizing energy expenditure during level walking. *European Journal of Applied Physiology* **33**, 293–306.

Zijlstra, W., Rutgers, A.W.F., Hof, A.L. & van Weerden, T.W (1995) Voluntary and involuntary adaptation of walking to temporal and spatial constraints. *Gait and Posture* **3**, 13–18.

Chapter 8

The Dynamics of Running

K.R. WILLIAMS

Somewhere near a speed of 2 m · s⁻¹ a walking person will change to a running pattern of movement, with the lack of a period of double support and the presence of a flight phase differentiating running from walking. Over a range of speeds from jogging to sprinting the basic running pattern changes in a variety of ways, generally to optimize movement patterns at the slower speeds typical of distance running, and to maximize power output and speed at sprinting speeds. The changes that occur in the kinematics and kinetics of segmental movements are likely to result from conscious and subconscious efforts to minimize or maximize a variety of specific criteria, such as metabolic energy expenditure, tissue stress, muscle power, fatigue and other factors. For competitive athletes the ultimate goal is to improve performance, while for many others the primary aim is maintaining or improving their state of health and fitness, with performance only a secondary issue.

Biomechanics provides an important adjunct to physiology, psychology and medicine in efforts to better understand why an individual adopts a specific movement pattern. The dynamic characteristics of running will have an effect on metabolic energy expenditure, the fatigue process, susceptibility to injury, and other factors important to both the elite athlete and the weekend jogger. After a short discussion of factors that affect biomechanical measures of running, a variety of topics will be covered that will first present some of the basic information used to describe the dynamics of running, and then highlight some of what is known about the influence mechanical factors have on performance, energy

expenditure, fatigue, footwear and injury. Information specific to sprint speeds will be discussed as appropriate. For additional information, readers are referred to previous reviews of running (Williams 1985a; Nigg 1986; Morgan *et al.* 1989; Putnam & Kozey 1989; Cavanagh 1990; Mero *et al.* 1992; Anderson 1996).

Factors that influence biomechanical measures

Speed of running

Almost all measures of the mechanics of movement in running are affected by speed (Nilsson *et al.* 1985; Frederick & Hagy 1986; Mero & Komi 1986; Munro *et al.* 1987), and for a valid comparison of biomechanical measures between individuals or conditions it is usually necessary to make measurements at the same speed of running. For example, faster sprinters spend a shorter time in contact with the ground during the support period primarily because they are running faster than slower sprinters. Whether a difference in support time might also be related to better performance, beyond the speed-related differences, can only be ascertained by comparing different ability-level sprinters at the same speed. If differences between individuals or conditions are found at different speeds, it is often not possible to distinguish the differences due to speed and the differences due to other factors. Similar concerns are present for distance running. As a result of the influence of running speed on biomechanical measures, almost all comparative studies of running are carried out by controlling or matching speed.

Gender and anthropometric influences

A runner's gender, size and specific anatomical structure may also influence biomechanical variables. Lutter (1985) estimated that out of 3500 injured runners examined over a 7-year period in a sports medicine clinic, only 10% had extremities that would be judged to be biomechanically optimal, making it likely that body structure is partly responsible for differences in the way individuals run. These observations are similar to ones made earlier by James *et al.* (1978) who found that only 22% of 180 subjects had a neutral rearfoot alignment during weight bearing, with 58% pronated and 20% supinated. Biomechanical studies need to consider whether anthropometric factors will affect the measurements being evaluated. For example, since a relationship has been found between the amount of pronation and foot type (Nawoczenski *et al.* 1998), a study evaluating the influence of running shoes on rearfoot pronation should probably also determine each runner's foot type to see if anatomical features confound any effect due to shoes.

Gender may also influence running mechanics. For example, it is often assumed that females have wider pelves relative to height or leg length, and that this causes them to have a greater Q-angle, the angle between a line drawn from the anterior superior iliac spine (ASIS) to the mid-patella and a line from the mid-patella to the tibial tuberosity (Atwater 1990). Individuals with a large Q-angle are often assumed to be more susceptible to certain types of knee injury (Atwater 1990; Messier *et al.* 1991). If a greater Q-angle increases susceptibility to injury, and if females tend to have greater Q-angles than men, then gender may be a risk factor. Messier *et al.* (1991) did find a relationship between Q-angle and patello-femoral pain, but also found that the relationship was similar for both males and females. As a further example, Nelson *et al.* (1977) found that a group of elite male runners took strides longer than those of a group of elite females over a range of speeds when compared in absolute units. When stride length was divided by leg length, relative stride length for females was longer than the same measure for men. This illustrates the importance of looking at both absolute and relative stride length, but since females are on average shorter than males,

it also suggests that caution should be taken to ensure that any differences found are due to gender, and not to differences in size.

Treadmill vs. overground running

Many biomechanical and physiological studies of running are carried out indoors with subjects running on a treadmill since it is much easier to control conditions in the laboratory and the space needed is smaller. Many studies have examined the differences between treadmill and overground running, often with contradictory results, but with a general agreement that there are differences between the two modes (van Ingen Schenau 1980; Nigg *et al.* 1995). Nigg *et al.* (1995) found a systematic difference with subjects landing on the treadmill with a flatter foot position compared with overground running, but also found inconsistent trends among individuals. They concluded that assessing running kinematics on a treadmill may lead to inadequate conclusions about overground running. While overground vs. treadmill differences are usually subtle, and it is typical to apply findings from treadmill running to more general situations, it should be kept in mind that the use of the treadmill may have an influence on results in ways that are not fully understood.

Kinematics of running

Kinematics provides one set of measurements that are often used to identify differences between individual runners, groups of runners, or specified conditions. Of primary interest are measures of the displacement, velocity and acceleration of segments of the body, though there are some areas of study where movements of the centre of mass of the body are of interest.

Whole body kinematics

Stride length (SL) is one of the most frequently studied biomechanical measures. SL here will refer to the distance from one foot contact to the next contact of the same foot, with *step length* defined as the distance between successive footstrikes of different feet. Velocity is determined by both SL and stride rate (SR): $V = SL \times SR$. As shown in the graphs in Fig. 8.1

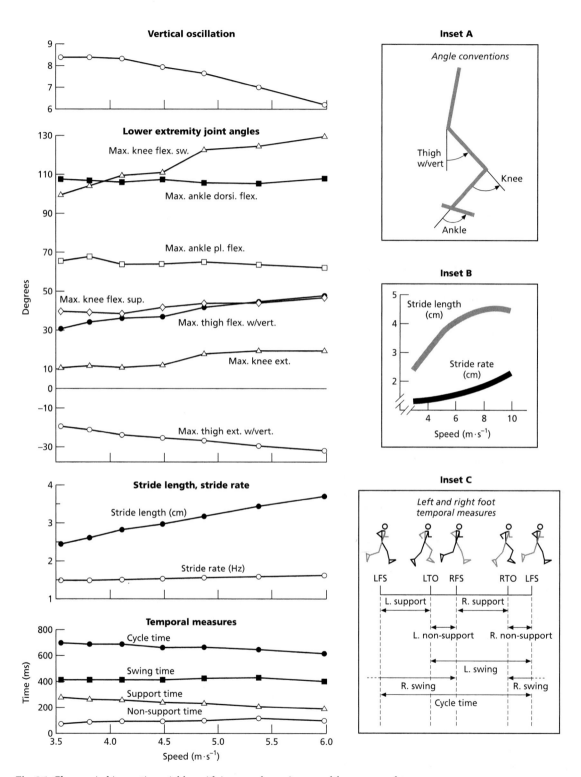

Fig. 8.1 Changes in kinematic variables with increased running speed for an example runner.

for an example runner, both SL and SR increase linearly with speed over a range of distance running speeds (Luhtanen & Komi 1978; Ito *et al.* 1983). Inset B in Fig. 8.1 shows that at higher speeds SL begins to level off, and may decrease, while SR increases proportionately faster than at slower speeds (Dillman 1975; Mero & Komi 1986). Plamondon and Roy (1984) showed that SL, SR and other temporal and spatial parameters were very dependent on speed as sprinters accelerated over the first 18 strides of a 100-m run. Stride length is often put relative to leg length when comparing individuals to reflect the effect body size may have on the length of the stride, but correlational studies have generally shown a weak and non-significant relationship between SL and leg length at distance running speeds (Cavanagh & Kram 1989). Somewhat higher correlations between SL and leg length ($r = 0.70$) and height ($r = 0.59$) have been found for sprinters (Hoffman 1971).

Cycle time, the inverse of SR, decreases with increased running speed, as does both the absolute time and percentage of time spent in support. The change in support time with speed is non-linear in that decreases are greater at slower speeds than at faster speeds. Both relative and absolute non-support times increase with increased running speed, while the time the leg spends in swing increases slightly at lower speeds but decreases slightly at higher speeds (Nilsson *et al.* 1985). For the subject shown in Fig. 8.1 the percentage of time spent in support during a half-cycle decreased from 80% at 3.6 m · s⁻¹ to 66% at 6 m · s⁻¹, with non-support time increasing from 20% to 34%. Ardigao *et al.* (1995) had subjects run using a rearfoot strike in some trials and a forefoot strike in other trials, and found no significant differences in SL or SR based on footstrike position at any speed over the range 3.43–4.04 m · s⁻¹.

Lower-extremity kinematics

THIGH, KNEE AND ANKLE

Figure 8.2 illustrates the patterns of movement that occur in the lower-extremity joints during a running cycle (using the angle convention shown in inset A

in Fig. 8.1). Figures 8.1 and 8.2 show how some of these angles change with speed. The discussion below is based on these and other data (Nilsson *et al.* 1985; Nigg *et al.* 1987). Prior to footstrike, extension of the hip has begun, but there is a slight period of flexion after the foot makes contact due to the forces at impact, and the hip movement quickly resumes extending (Nilsson *et al.* 1985). The knee joint shows two periods of flexion, one during support and the other during swing, with the flexion in swing serving to reduce the leg moment of inertia making it easier to swing the leg through to the next footstrike. Depending on the running style of a particular runner, the ankle may show a rapid plantar flexion following footstrike, for a rearfoot striker, or may begin to dorsiflex, for a midfoot or forefoot striker.

With increasing speed maximal hip flexion and extension angles increase, as does the maximum flexion angle of the knee during both the swing and support periods. The angle of the thigh with the vertical at footstrike increases with increasing running speed, and the angle of the knee at footstrike is less extended at faster compared with slower speeds. There is a less extended angle of the knee prior to footstrike at higher speeds, and while the ankle angle during the pushoff phase becomes slightly more plantarflexed with increased running speed, the maximal dorsiflexion angle during support does not change much. Nigg *et al.* (1987) found that the vertical component of the speed of the heel at footstrike increased with running speed, while the horizontal component showed no change.

REARFOOT PRONATION

The inward rolling motion at the ankle that occurs as the foot goes flat just after footstrike has been studied extensively in distance running because of implied relationships between pronation about the subtalar joint and lower extremity injuries. This motion is often referred to as pronation and supination, as it will be here. Though three-dimensional studies more completely describe the complex movements occurring during pronation (Engsberg 1996; Nawoczenski *et al.* 1998), two-dimensional analyses have been performed most often and the measures obtained would more appropriately be

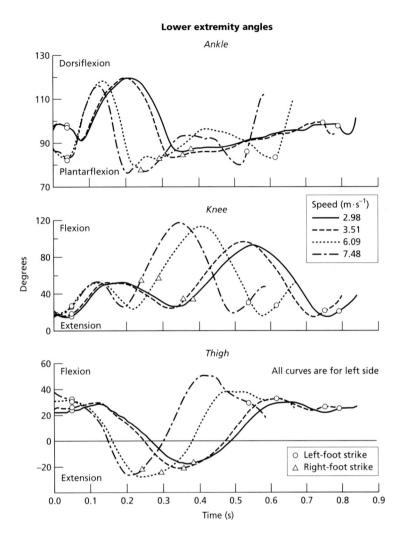

Fig. 8.2 Ankle, knee and thigh angle changes throughout a running cycle at four different running speeds for an example runner.

labelled eversion and inversion rather than pronation and supination (Taunton *et al.* 1985). Figure 8.3 shows typical angles for the leg, heel, and rearfoot during a portion of the support period. The rearfoot angle at footstrike and at maximal pronation, the amount of pronation, and the maximal pronation velocity have all been used to characterize the pronation movement (Nigg 1986).

Table 8.1 shows rearfoot movement data from a group of elite female distance runners and shows the wide range of values that is typical. In this group of runners, the least amount of pronation was for a runner who actually never got beyond a neutral

rearfoot position, with a maximal 'pronation' angle that was still in 3° of supination. At the other end of the spectrum was a maximum pronation value of 18°. In a similar group of elite male runners, running at a slightly faster speed, a maximal pronation angle as high as 24° was found. A variety of factors can influence the amount of pronation that takes place following footstrike, including anatomical structure, footwear, the placement of the foot at contact, and the surface slope. Runners who land with a high amount of supination can be more at risk for inversion sprains. Greater maximal pronation has been associated with a less vertical angle of the leg and a

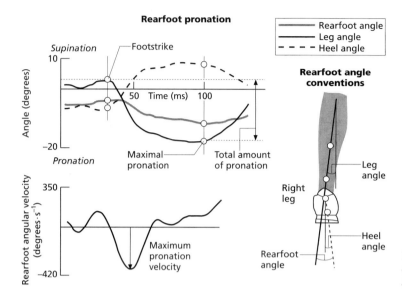

Rearfoot angle conventions

Right leg

Leg angle

Heel angle

Rearfoot angle

Fig. 8.3 Leg, heel and rearfoot angle curves during rearfoot pronation for an example runner.

Table 8.1 Rearfoot pronation values for elite female distance runners at 5.36 m · s⁻¹.

	Angle at footstrike (deg.)	Max. pronation (deg.)	Amount of pronation (deg.)	Max. pronation velocity (deg. · s⁻¹)
Mean	14.5	−8.5	23.0	−902
(SD)	(−6.1)	(4.3)	(5.5)	(280)
Max.	30.2	3.2	38.8	−437
Min.	2.6	−18.6	12.6	−1563
N	47	47	47	26

less supinated rearfoot angle position at footstrike, and greater pronation speed has been associated with a more supinated rearfoot angle and a greater angle of the heel with the vertical at footstrike (Williams & Ziff 1991). Running with a greater stride width—the horizontal distance between successive footstrikes—has been found to reduce pronation (Williams & Ziff 1991).

There is often an association assumed between the nature of the arch of the foot and pronation, with a flat foot assumed to be associated with more pronation and a rigid high-arched foot associated with less pronation. Nawoczenski *et al.* (1998) used three-dimensional methods to assess the relationship between inversion–eversion and tibial medial

and lateral rotation, and found a 'low rearfoot' group (pes cavus) to show relatively more calcaneal eversion compared with a 'high rearfoot' group (pes planus), which showed more tibial rotation. The influence of footwear on pronation, and the effect excessive pronation may have on injuries, is discussed later.

Upper extremity and trunk

Vertical oscillation of the body has been shown to decrease with running speed (Dillman 1975), as shown in Fig. 8.1 for a marker on the head, and has been reported to be as low as 4.7 cm at 9.8 m · s⁻¹ (Mero *et al.* 1992). Runners tend to lean slightly forwards during the run, with values between 4 and 7 degrees for speeds up to 6 m · s⁻¹. The trunk lean angle has been found to increase slightly after foot contact, increasing to as much as 12–13°, and then decrease by the time toe-off occurs (Elliott & Roberts 1980; Elliott & Acklund 1981). Frishberg (1983) reported a forward lean angle of 11.6° for a sprinter at 9.2 m · s⁻¹. Williams found trunk rotation range of motion to average 24.3° at the hip and 26.7° at the shoulder for a cycle of running at 3.6 m · s⁻¹, with considerable variability between subjects (Williams 1982). Lusby and Atwater (1983) found a greater range of motion at the elbow and shoulder joints with increased speed in female runners, with no change in the sequence of movement in relation to foot-ground events. The role of the arms, legs and trunk in rotational movements during running have also been examined using angular momentum measurements (Hinrichs *et al.* 1983). About a vertical axis, the angular momentum of the arms was found to nearly balance the angular momentum of the rest of the body, resulting in relatively low total body angular momentum values throughout the running cycle. Presumably the reciprocal action of the arms in relation to leg motion has a role in optimizing the energy associated with running, and support for this premise comes from a study that showed that $\dot{V}o_2$ (submaximal oxygen consumption rate) increased by 4% when the arms were constrained to remain behind a runner's body (Egbuonu *et al.* 1990).

Kinetics of running

Ground reaction forces and centre of pressure

The greatest musculoskeletal stresses in the lower extremity occur during the support phase of running, and analysis of ground reaction forces can provide insight into the factors that affect these stresses. Figure 8.4 shows vertical, anteroposterior and mediolateral force–time curves that are characteristic of a rearfoot strike and a midfoot or forefoot strike. Table 8.2 shows data for peak forces and the changes in speed, calculated from impulse data for each of the three components of force, for 41 male elite runners. Rearfoot strike patterns typically show two vertical peaks, with the first peak sometimes referred to as the impact peak, influenced primarily by the conditions at footstrike, and the second maximum referred to as the active peak, affected by muscle activity during support (Nigg 1986). Factors such as footwear, running speed, running surface and running style may affect whether the first vertical peak is present or not. Runners who land on the midfoot and forefoot typically show either no vertical force impact peak or a much attenuated peak. During barefoot running Frederick and Hagy (1986) found a greater first vertical force peak to be significantly correlated with faster running

speeds, body mass, stature, step length, leg length, a more plantarflexed ankle position at footstrike, and a greater hip–foot horizontal distance at footstrike. Combined, all these measures accounted for only 52% of the variability in the first vertical peak, indicating that there are other important factors besides the ones they measured. A higher second peak was significantly correlated with most of these same factors, but not with running speed.

Anteroposterior (A-P) forces show a period of braking during the first half of the support phase, when the forward speed of the runner is slowed down, followed by a propulsive phase where forward speed increases. For the speed of 5.96 m · s⁻¹ shown in Table 8.2, the decrease in A-P speed represents a 5% change. The average net change in velocity of 0.03 m · s⁻¹ reflects the extra propulsion needed to overcome air resistance during the flight phase, and these values are similar to values found by others (Munro *et al.* 1987). The net A-P impulse values are also sometimes affected by the somewhat artificial running conditions used in force platform data collection. A sharp rise and fall in the A-P force is often seen in a midfoot or forefoot striker, as shown in Fig. 8.4. It has been more difficult to explain the relationship between patterns of change in the mediolateral forces with movements, though Williams (1982) did find a correlation of 0.71 between the net mediolateral impulse and the position of the foot relative to a midline of progression.

The magnitude of vertical forces varies considerably between runners running at the same speed, as can be seen in the data in Table 8.2. Cavanagh and Lafortune (1980) showed a range of 2nd peak forces from approximately 2.2 to 3.2 × body weight (BW) from a group of 17 runners running at 4.5 m · s⁻¹, with a mean of 2.8 (±0.3) BW for rearfoot strikers and 2.7 (±0.2) for midfoot strikers. When a force platform is used to collect force data, the centre of the pressure distribution under the foot can also be determined. As shown in Fig. 8.4, this has been used to identify the type of landing used by a runner, employing a measure labelled *strike index* (SI), the distance from the back of the heel to the location where the first centre of pressure point is within the shoe contact outline, measured as a percentage of shoe length (Cavanagh & Lafortune 1980).

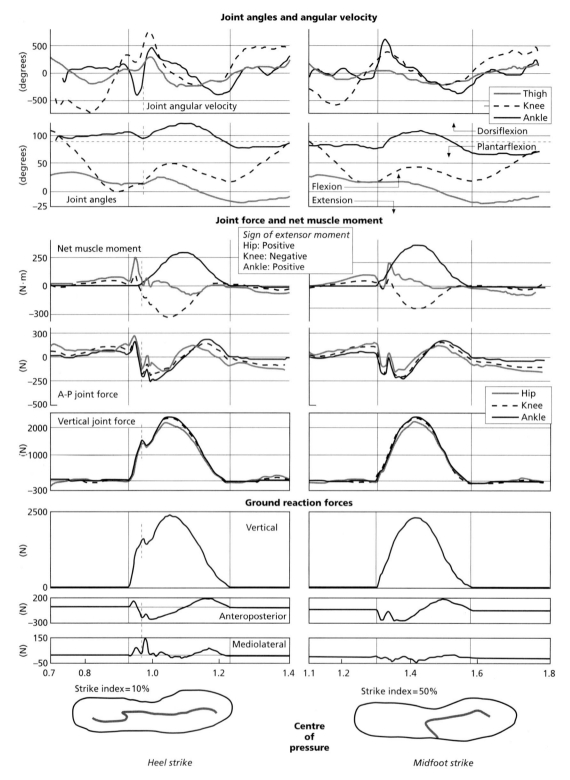

Fig. 8.4 Ground reaction forces, and lower-extremity joint forces, muscle moments, joint angles and joint angular velocity for an example runner.

Table 8.2 Vertical, anteroposterior (A-P) and mediolateral (M-L) ground reaction force peaks and change in velocity data for elite male distance runners at 5.96 m · s⁻¹ (N = 41).

	Vertical 1st peak (BW)	Vertical 2nd peak (BW)	Vertical ΔV (m · s⁻¹)	A-P peak braking (BW)	A-P peak Propulsion (BW)	A-P ΔV braking (m · s⁻¹)	A-P ΔV Propulsion (m · s⁻¹)	M-L peak (medial) (BW)	M-L peak (lateral) (BW)	M-L net ΔV (m · s⁻¹)
Mean	2.83	3.13	1.42	−0.891	0.539	−0.284	0.255	0.344	−0.410	0.049
(SD)	(0.49)	(0.19)	(0.17)	(−0.148)	(0.065)	(−0.044)	(0.050)	(0.117)	(0.316)	(0.072)
Max.	4.16	3.48	1.72	−1.335	0.390	−0.378	0.015	0.620	−0.088	0.275
Min.	1.41	2.72	0.83	−0.630	0.670	−0.185	0.315	0.115	−2.233	−0.145

BW, Body weight.

Cavanagh and Lafortune found 12 of their runners to show a rearfoot strike pattern (SI average = 17%), landing with an average of 10.4° of foot abduction. Similar values for the five midfoot strikers were 50% and 5.3°. The first vertical force peak for the rearfoot strikers averaged 2.2 (±0.4) BW. Unpublished data from the present author show a mean SI of 40.1% (±20.4%) for a group of elite female distance runners running at 5.36 m · s⁻¹, with a range from 6% to 76%.

As running speed increases the magnitude of the vertical ground reaction force increases, as does the rate of loading, and initial contact with the ground tends to occur further forwards on the foot (Frederick & Hagy 1986; Mero & Komi 1986; Munro et al. 1987; Nigg et al. 1987). The magnitude of A-P forces increases with increased running speed, as does the A-P impulse, reflecting a greater decrease and then increase in forward speed during the support phase (Munro et al. 1987).

Joint forces and moments

By combining information from segmental kinematics, ground reaction forces, centre of pressure, and body segment parameters, estimates can be made of the internal joint reaction forces and net muscle moments at each joint in the lower extremity using the methods of inverse dynamics. Examples of these moments and forces during a running cycle for the hip, knee and ankle joints are shown in Fig. 8.4, and other examples are present in the literature (Mann & Sprague 1980; Winter 1983; Putnam & Kozey 1989; Scott & Winter 1990; Prilutsky et al. 1996).

The knee and ankle show extensor moments throughout most of the support period, while the hip moment is extensor in the first half of contact and may become a flexor moment later in support as the leg begins forwards in the swing phase of the running gait. There are a number of differences in the moment patterns immediately after footstrike between rearfoot and midfoot strikers. During the 30 ms after the rearfoot strike shown in Fig. 8.4 the hip shows an extensor moment, the knee a flexor moment, and the ankle a net moment of zero. Absent from this example, but present for some other runners, is a small dorsiflexor ankle moment immediately after footstrike when the tibialis anterior muscle acts eccentrically to ease the foot down. In the midfoot pattern, the extensor hip moment and the flexor knee moment immediately drop towards zero after foot contact, while the ankle shows an immediate extensor moment. Komi (1990) used direct force measures to show that there was a sudden unloading of the Achilles tendon immediately after a heel-first footstrike, with no such change in a midfoot landing, and these results are consistent with the patterns shown in Fig. 8.4. Following footstrike, when the knee flexes as the hip extends, there is likely to be eccentric muscle action in the knee extensors, though the true muscle length changes for multijoint muscles cannot be determined solely from joint angle changes and would have to be estimated from a more sophisticated model than was used here. The small positive spike in the A-P force in Fig. 8.4 following footstrike in the rearfoot strike pattern is reflected in the short positive A-P joint force seen at the hip, knee and ankle following contact. These forces quickly turn negative, but show another sharp change in magnitude a short time later. Vertical joint reaction forces show patterns that parallel vertical ground reaction force changes, with the magnitude of the force gradually decreasing the more proximal the joint. The short dashed vertical lines shortly after footstrike in the rearfoot strike example in Fig. 8.4 designate the time when the foot goes flat, and it can be seen that there is a sharp change in each of the other force and moment curves at this time.

INDIVIDUAL MUSCLE AND SEGMENTAL FORCES

The ability to quantify individual force contributions from muscle and other soft tissues would greatly enhance the ability to identify relationships between movement, force and injury. However, because of the invasive nature of direct measures of muscle force, it is seldom undertaken. Direct measurements have been made using a surgically implanted tendon buckle to measure Achilles tendon forces during running (Komi 1990). For a subject running over a range of speeds, a maximal loading of $12.5 \times$ BW was found for Achilles tendon force at an intermediate speed of $6.0 \text{ m} \cdot \text{s}^{-1}$, with different maximal magnitudes found in other subjects. When given relative to tendon cross-sectional area the resulting stress value was higher than reported values for single-load maximum tendon strength. Komi also found that the rate of loading of the Achilles tendon increased with increased running speed throughout a range of speeds tested up to a maximum speed of $9 \text{ m} \cdot \text{s}^{-1}$.

An alternative method for estimating internal forces is to use musculoskeletal models to predict forces, but these methods may include errors due to the assumptions that have to be made. Forces in the Achilles tendon have been estimated to range from 5 to 10 times BW with ankle bone-on-bone forces ranging from 8.7 to 14 BW (Burdett 1982; Scott & Winter 1990). A model predicting internal forces gave ranges of 4.7–6.9 BW for peak patellar tendon force and 1.3–2.9 BW for plantar fascia force (Scott & Winter 1990). As with individual muscle forces, little information is available identifying direct

bone or joint loading patterns in the lower extremity during running. Burr *et al.* did measure strain and strain rates in the tibia *in vivo* during running (Burr *et al.* 1996), and such studies may provide further insight into the mechanisms of stress-related injuries.

Electromyographic patterns during running

Examples of electromyographic (EMG) activity in several lower-extremity muscles during running are shown in Fig. 8.5, and further examples can be found in the literature (Nilsson *et al.* 1985; Putnam & Kozey 1989; Prilutsky *et al.* 1996). During swing there is steady activity in the tibialis anterior that continues through footstrike, perhaps to provide stability at impact through co-contraction with the triceps surae muscles. The biceps femoris and gluteus maximus both show a period of activity in the time period before footstrike, acting eccentrically to slow the flexion of the hip and extension of the knee. At footstrike there is activity in all the primary muscles that provide extensor support during the contact phase—the gluteus maximus, rectus femoris, vastus lateralis, and gastrocnemius. The gastrocnemius activity during support helps to provide the torque needed to plantarflex the ankle during late support through toe-off, and activity in the biceps femoris in late support may help begin the flexion of the knee that occurs during the flight phase. Rectus femoris activity during the swing phase may help both with flexion of the hip and extension of the knee. At a speed of running of $8 \text{ m} \cdot \text{s}^{-1}$ Nilsson *et al.* found a phase shift in the onset of activity in the gluteus maximus, quadriceps and hamstring muscles, with EMGs turning on sooner in the swing phase before footstrike. Between 4 and $8 \text{ m} \cdot \text{s}^{-1}$ they also found greater rectus femoris activity during swing, aiding in hip flexion, than was found during the support phase.

With increased running speed the magnitude of the EMG signals increases in the lower-extremity muscles (Nilsson *et al.* 1985; Mero & Komi 1986). The absolute duration of activity decreases due to the shorter cycle time associated with increased speed, but peak EMG, overall integrated EMG, and the relative duration of activity as a percentage of cycle time increase with increased speed. van Ingen Schenau *et al.* (1995)

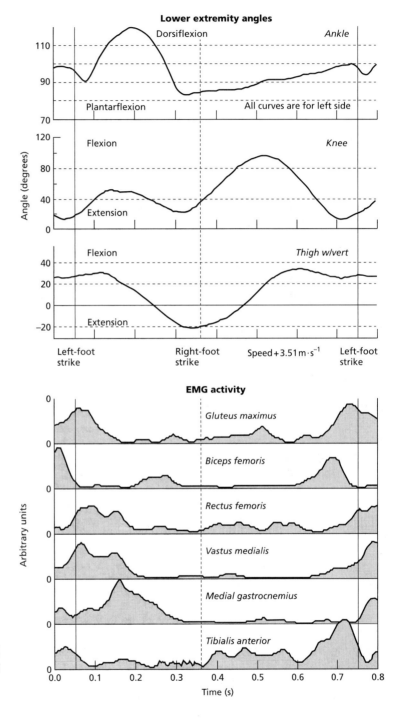

Fig. 8.5 Lower-extremity angles and EMG patterns for six muscles during a cycle of running for an example runner.

examined lower-extremity muscles in running and concluded that monoarticulate muscles show activity primarily during periods when they are shortening, and are not very active in eccentric muscle work, similar to results found for cycling.

Measures of mechanical power

Mechanical power output during running has been measured for many years, but there still is a great deal of confusion over which methods are best to use (Winter 1979; Williams & Cavanagh 1983; Aleshinsky 1986a; van Ingen Schenau & Cavanagh 1990). One of the 'problems' with measuring the external work done in a cyclic activity such as running is that for constant-speed level running the total external work done in a running cycle will be zero, yet there is obvious metabolic energy expenditure involved. The mechanical work done during running has been derived using three general methods, based on:

1 changes in energy levels of the body centre of mass;
2 changes in segmental energy levels derived from kinematics; and
3 changes in segmental power derived from joint forces and moments.

The latter method appears to have advantages over the other two (Aleshinsky 1986a; Putnam & Kozey 1989; van Ingen Schenau & Cavanagh 1990). Different methods of measuring mechanical power during running using a segmental energy approach have yielded results that show up to a 10-fold difference in power for a given level of effort (Williams & Cavanagh 1983).

Aleshinsky (1986b) and van Ingen Schenau and Cavanagh (1990) proposed methods that they believed better addressed some of these methodological problems, but acknowledged that even the proposed methods leave a number of problems unresolved and rely on assumptions that may have major deficiencies. Among the problems (Williams & Cavanagh 1983; Aleshinsky 1986a; van Ingen Schenau & Cavanagh 1990) inherent in calculating mechanical power during a cyclic activity such as running, where the primary work done is to support the body during each foot contact phase, are:

• limitations in identifying the amount of energy transferred between segments;

• inability to determine the exact source of positive mechanical power;
• the capability to calculate only net muscle moments;
• lack of knowledge of the full role of muscles that cross more than one joint; and
• inability to quantify precisely the effect of stretch–shortening cycle contributions on the work done.

The usefulness of measures of mechanical work will be somewhat limited until we better understand some of these factors.

Biomechanics in relation to performance

Most biomechanical studies of running are performed in controlled experimental situations rather than during competition, making the direct association of biomechanical parameters with performance difficult to obtain. Usually it is only possible to obtain kinematic information in competitive situations, limiting the information available, and often the movement patterns in competition are influenced by strategy or the presence of other runners, making it difficult to isolate the importance of biomechanical factors to performance. As a result, most information relating biomechanics to performance comes from either studying factors that are related to performance, such as submaximal oxygen consumption in distance running, or by examining characteristics of different levels of runners in the laboratory and identifying either significant differences in biomechanical measures between groups, or finding strong correlations between performance times and biomechanical indices.

Several studies have compared 'elite' distance runners with 'good' runners, often with equivocal results. Compared with good runners, elite runners have been found to have a longer stride length (SL) at a given speed in distance running (Dillman 1975) and in sprinting (Kunz & Kaufmann 1981), though another study found shorter SLs (Cavanagh *et al.* 1977). Cavanagh *et al.* (1977) found no significant differences in the angles of the thigh with the vertical or the knee angle at various times throughout a running cycle between groups of elite and good male runners. They did find the good runners to plantarflex the ankle 8° more than the elite runners during toe-off. Net muscle torques during the swing phase of running did not show differences between groups, and while there were no differences in vertical oscillation between the groups, the elite athletes did show a more symmetrical vertical oscillation pattern between left and right sides compared with controls.

In another study, an elite group of female runners was found to show a foot contact position further forward on the shoe compared with a control group of good runners at the same speed of running (Williams *et al.* 1987). The elite runners also had lower first and higher second vertical force peaks, a larger change in vertical velocity, a higher peak braking anteroposterior force, higher laterally directed mediolateral forces, and a shorter support time. The elite runners had narrower pelvises than a student population of similar age, and were shorter in stature, lighter and had less iliac crest fat than a typical non-athletic female population.

Biomechanical factors and running economy

Running mechanics are often studied in relation to submaximal oxygen uptake per unit body mass ($\dot{V}o_2$), often termed running economy. Energy expenditure in running will have a direct affect on performance, and anything that will improve economy should have a beneficial effect on performance. If changes in movement patterns result in reduced energy costs, the reduced cost should allow an individual to either maintain a given level of performance for a longer period of time, or to raise the level of effort that can be sustained over a fixed time or distance. In distance running a small improvement in economy can yield substantial benefits. A 1% improvement in a world-class 10 k race yields a 16 s faster time, putting the runner 100 m ahead of where he or she would otherwise finish.

Variations in $\dot{V}o_2$

The variation in economy among runners at the same speed is substantial, with typical variations exceeding 15% and ranging as high as 30% (Williams & Cavanagh 1983; Daniels 1985). Many studies have shown a general linear relationship between economy and speed in running (Daniels 1985; Morgan *et al.* 1989). Economy among a group of subjects running at the same speed is not highly correlated to the stride length (SL) each runner chooses (Brisswalter *et al.* 1996). However, $\dot{V}o_2$ for a given individual does vary with SL, usually being minimum at the freely chosen SL and increasing at shorter or longer SLs (Cavanagh & Williams 1982). Morgan *et al.* (1994) demonstrated that it was possible to train runners who chose an uneconomical SL to run at an SL closer to the one predicted to be optimal, with a concomitant lowering of $\dot{V}o_2$.

To test the sensitivity of economy to changes in biomechanical variables, Egbuonu *et al.* (1990) performed a study where runners deliberately: (i) used increased vertical oscillation; and (ii) ran with their arms behind their backs. While both protocols increased $\dot{V}o_2$ above that for their normal running pattern, by 4% and 4.6%, respectively, the increases were relatively small ($\sim$1.6 ml · kg^{-1} · min^{-1}), and it was suggested that these might be upper limits to changes in economy that result from changes in mechanics. Another study in the same laboratory trained four runners with feedback intended to improve economy (Miller *et al.* 1990). The subjects given feedback significantly reduced $\dot{V}o_2$ compared with pretraining measures, with reductions that were 0.6 ml · kg^{-1} · min^{-1} lower than the reduction found for a control group.

Mechanical power

Submaximal oxygen uptake is a global measure of energy expenditure, and it might be expected to be related to the global measure of total body mechanical work during running. Studies examining the relationship between power and economy across speeds do find strong correlations between metabolic energy costs and mechanical measures of power (Shorten *et al.* 1981). However, strong relationships have not been found between these two measures at any given speed of running, and the lack of a clear association may be in part due to difficulties associated with the methods used to calculate mechanical power, as discussed earlier. At a given running speed, several studies have shown weak trends towards better economy in running being associated with lower mechanical power (Williams & Cavanagh 1987) or total lower body angular impulse (Heise

& Martin 1990), but others have found no specific relationship.

Biomechanical measures

A variety of biomechanical measures describing running mechanics have been identified as being related to better economy, but there are many inconsistencies among studies. Better economy has been associated with:
• less extension at the hip and greater extension at the knee during toe-off, more dorsiflexion, and a greater decrease and subsequent increase in forward velocity during support (Williams et al. 1987);
• a higher first vertical force peak, a greater angle of the shank with the vertical at footstrike, less plantar flexion at toe-off, greater forward trunk lean, and a lower minimum velocity of a point on the knee during foot contact (Williams & Cavanagh 1987);
• a longer support time, lower medially directed ground reaction force, greater extension of the hip and knee at toe-off, and a faster horizontal velocity of a point on the heel at footstrike (Williams & Cavanagh 1986); and
• less arm movement (Anderson & Tseh 1994).
    Ardigao et al. (1995) found no differences in economy in runners when they ran with a rearfoot strike pattern compared with a forefoot strike pattern. Until more consistent relationships are established the relationships described here should be considered tentative and may not be useful as the basis for altering someone's mechanics to improve economy.

Stretch–shortening cycle

A process that has often been cited as a major contributor to the work done in running, and consequently as a mechanism that reduces energy expenditure by muscles, is the stretch–shortening cycle of muscle use involving elastic tissues in the muscle, tendon and arch of the foot (Williams 1985b; van Ingen Schenau & Cavanagh 1990; Taylor 1994; van Ingen Schenau et al. 1997). The work done as a result of the stretch–shortening cycle is often attributed to the storage and reutilization of elastic energy, but there are other factors that have been proposed as being as important or more important, including: increasing the time available for force

production; potentiation of the contractile mechanism during the concentric phase of the movement; and triggering of spinal reflexes (Williams 1985b; van Ingen Schenau & Cavanagh 1990; van Ingen Schenau et al. 1997). Stretch–shortening mechanisms are often used to explain the high (40–70%) efficiency rates often calculated for running (Anderson 1996; Williams & Cavanagh 1983). There seems to be general agreement that economy benefits from stretch–shortening mechanisms, with the mechanical work attributable to stretch–shortening sources reducing the amount of metabolic work done by active muscles (Williams 1985b; van Ingen Schenau & Cavanagh 1990; Taylor 1994). For a more detailed discussion of the issues involving the stretch–shortening cycle see the special issue on the subject in the *Journal of Applied Biomechanics* (Vol. 13, 1997).

Flexibility

Several studies have examined the influence of lower-extremity flexibility on economy. One study found that increased flexibility after a period of flexibility training was associated with better running economy (Godges et al. 1989). However, other studies have shown economy to be better in individuals with less flexibility (Gleim et al. 1990; Craib et al. 1996), with increased contribu-tions from stored elastic energy cited as the likely mechanism.

Body mass and distribution of mass

Measures of $\dot{V}o_2$ are usually given relative to body mass (i.e. as $ml \cdot kg^{-1} \cdot min^{-1}$), but often there is still an influence of size on economy beyond simple scaling to body weight. Moderate correlations have suggested that better economy is associated with runners with greater mass (Anderson 1996; Williams & Cavanagh 1986; Williams et al. 1987; Bergh et al. 1991). Since $\dot{V}o_{2max}$ has also been shown to be lower in runners with greater mass (Bergh et al. 1991), there may be no advantage to the lower $\dot{V}o_2$ in heavier runners since the percentage of $\dot{V}o_{2max}$ may be similar for both light and heavy runners.

    Some have proposed that differences in mass distribution among the segments might be related for the inverse relationship between economy and body weight (Cavanagh & Kram 1985; Pate et al. 1992).

When weights are added to the extremities there is an increase in metabolic energy costs, indicating that mass distribution can affect $\dot{V}o_2$ (Catlin & Dressendorfer 1979; Martin 1985), but any effect due to actual differences in mass distribution among athletes has not been demonstrated. Taylor (1994) found little difference in energy consumption among similar sized animals with very different limb mass distribution.

Air resistance

Air resistance plays a smaller role in the work done during running than in other sports where speed is higher, such as cycling or speed skating. Pugh (1971) found the extra oxygen consumed while running against a wind increased relative to the square of wind velocity. While he predicted the overall energy cost of overcoming air resistance in track running to be approximately 8% at a distance speed of $6\ m \cdot s^{-1}$ and 16% at sprint speeds ($10\ m \cdot s^{-1}$), Davies (1980) predicted somewhat lower values (7.8% at $10\ m \cdot s^{-1}$, 4% at $6\ m \cdot s^{-1}$, and 2% at marathon speeds). Running behind other competitors provides shielding from air resistance and reduces drag and metabolic costs (Kyle 1979). Running in a pack has been predicted to reduce air resistance by 40–80%, depending on how close one runner follows another, lowering oxygen costs by 3–6% (Pugh 1971; Kyle 1979).

Biomechanical factors and injury

As running has increased in popularity over the last 20 years as a form of exercise, so have injuries to runners. The wide variety of methods used to compile injury data make it difficult to identify the true incidence of injury, but van Mechelen (1992) found rates from 37 to 56% in studies of more than 500 subjects. Table 8.3 summarizes the results from several epidemiological studies that attempted to identify the source of lower-extremity injuries in running. It should be noted that the methods used to collect injury statistics and the specific population sampled can have a major effect on results, and such factors may account for some of the large differences seen in the studies in Table 8.3.

Table 8.3 Common injury sites in running.

	Study				
	James *et al.* (1978)	Clement *et al.* (1981)	Ballas *et al.* (1997)	Bennell and Crossley (1996)	Bennell and Crossley (1996)
Type of subjects	Runners	Runners	Runners	Runners	Sprinters
No. of injuries	180	1650	860	39	19
Type of data	Clinic	Clinic	Clinic	Interview	Interview
Site of injury (%)					
Knee pain	29.0	25.8	13.8	15.0	14.0
Shin splints–tibial stress syndrome	13.0	13.2	7.8	13.6	5.0
Achilles tendinitis	11.1	6.0	2.2		
Plantar fasciitis	7.0	4.7	4.0		
Ankle/foot tendinitis				13.9	6.0
Stress fracture	6.0	5.8	9.3	25.1	18.0
Tibial stress fracture		2.6			
Metatarsal stress fracture		3.2			
Iliotibial tract tendinitis	5.0	4.3	3.8		
Patellar tendinitis		4.5	2.2		
Hamstring strain			5.2	4.3	38.0
Adductor strain			6.0		
Ankle lateral ligament sprain			4.9	8.9	3.0
Others			9.4		

This section will consider only scientific studies that have attempted to relate biomechanical and anatomical factors to different types of injury, and will not try to provide a detailed description of typical injuries, nor will it provide information about how best to treat injuries. There are many good articles and books dealing with sports medicine that provide this type of information. There is a paucity of good scientific studies showing definitive relationships between either anatomical factors and injury, or biomechanical measures and injury. The relationships described in the paragraphs below should be viewed as tentative relationships until a stronger body of literature is available to confirm them.

Knee pain

Epidemiological studies of running injuries find the knee to be the most frequent site of injuries (Clement *et al.* 1981; Maughan & Miller 1983) with chondromalacia patella, pain on the undersurface of the patella, as one of the most frequent knee injuries. Rearfoot pronation has often been cited as a primary cause of this type of knee pain, with the internal rotation of the patella that accompanies rearfoot pronation causing the patella to be pulled laterally, increasing the pressure exerted on the undersurface of the patella (James *et al.* 1978). Nigg *et al.* (1984) did find greater pronation in runners with tibial tendinitis compared with runners who felt no pain. However, Landry and Zebas (1985) found no significant relationship between the incidence of knee pain and several different range of motion measurements, including maximal pronation angle, Q-angle and tibial torsion. While Messier *et al.* (1991) also found no relationship with pronation, they did find Q-angle to be a strong discriminator between injured and non-injured subjects, along with several ground reaction force variables.

Shin splints

The term 'shin splints' has been used to describe pain in the anterior or medial portion of the tibia. Several studies (Gehlsen & Seger 1980; Viitasalo & Kvist 1983; Messier & Pittala 1988) have found that runners with a history of shin splints showed greater pronation and/or pronation speed compared with control groups.

Achilles tendinitis and plantar fasciitis

In the foot and ankle, Achilles tendinitis and plantar fasciitis have been associated with both anatomical and movement factors. Excessive pronation has been implicated as a potential causative factor in both these injuries (Clement *et al.* 1984b). Nigg *et al.* (1984) found that runners with Achilles tendon pain had greater maximal pronation angles, as well as higher maximal vertical impact forces, but Messier and Pittala (1988) found no relationship between plantar fasciitis and rearfoot pronation or ground reaction force measures. Training errors have been found to be a primary factor in Achilles tendinitis (in 75% of cases), and the injury is often associated with moderate or severe subtalar or forefoot varus (in 56% of cases) (Clement *et al.* 1984b). Plantar fasciitis has paradoxically been found to be associated with both a flat foot and with a rigid cavus foot, and it has also been linked to a tight Achilles tendon (Warren 1990) and a greater plantarflexion range of motion in the ankle joint (Messier & Pittala 1988).

Stress fractures

Stress fractures result from repetitive loading of bone at levels higher than can be sustained without a gradual breakdown of the involved tissues. Stresses in the bone result from the ground reaction forces applied to the feet, the internal muscle forces caused by muscle contraction, and stress effects resulting from the specific composition and orientation of the bones and joints in the lower extremity. Table 8.4 lists some of the common sites for stress fractures in runners. Ting *et al.* (1988) found no consistent anatomical variations or any ground reaction force patterns that differentiated a relatively small group of runners with previous navicular stress fractures from a control group. Several studies have associated a high-arched foot with a greater incidence of stress fractures (Giladi *et al.* 1985), and one study found more femoral and tibial stress injuries

Table 8.4 Stress fracture sites in runners.

	Study		
	Hulkko and Orava (1987)	Sullivan *et al.* (1984)	Brunet *et al.* (1990)
Type of subjects	Athletes (72% runners)	Runners	Runners
No. of injuries	368	57	139
Type of data	Clinic	Clinic	Self-report
Site of injury (%)			
Tibia*	49.5	43.9	43.9
Metatarsals	19.8	14.0	34.7
Fibula	12.0	21.1	Included in tibial
Femur	6.2	3.5	4.2
Sesamoids	4.1		
Calcaneus		5.3	8.3
Navicular	2.4		
Pelvis	1.9	10.5	9.0
Others	4.1	7.0	–

* Includes fibular stress fractures in Brunet *et al.* (1990).

in high-arched feet and more metatarsal stress fractures in individuals with low arches (Simkin *et al.* 1989).

Muscle activity can modify the stress distribution in the foot. Sharkey *et al.* (1995) hypothesized that a consequence of fatigue during repetitive exercise might be an increase in the loading of the metatarsals, and thus be a factor in the mechanism of stress fractures. Using a cadaveric model they showed that the addition of simulated muscular contributions from the flexor hallucis longus reduced dorsal strain on the 2nd metatarsal, and simulated contraction of the flexor digitorum longus reduced plantar-dorsal bending stress.

Hamstring strain

Another common running injury, particularly for faster sprinting speeds, is the hamstring strain (Agre 1985). The injury is usually assumed to occur near the end of the swing phase when the lengths of the hamstring muscles are near their longest (Frigo *et al.* 1979), and when the muscle action changes from eccentric to concentric (Agre 1985). Agre (1985)

lists a number of factors that have been implicated in the aetiology of hamstring strains but little scientific evidence exists to prove or disprove their involvement. Sprinters with a history of hamstring injuries have been found to have tighter hamstrings compared with runners with no hamstring injuries, as shown by a reduced range of motion at the hip joint (74.1° vs. 67.2°) (Jönhagen *et al.* 1994). They could not identify whether these differences were cause or effect. This study also reported that previously injured sprinters had lower hamstring and quadriceps concentric torques at $30° \cdot s^{-1}$, but not at higher speeds of movement.

Muscle damage and soreness

Runners often experience muscular pain following prolonged downhill running, and the cause of the damage to muscles is thought to be due to the greater amount of eccentric muscle action that occurs when running downhill. Dick and Cavanagh (1987) found a 10% upward drift in $\dot{V}o_2$ during downhill running and a 23% increase in lower-extremity EMG. They hypothesized that damage to muscles and localized muscular fatigue cause the recruitment of more motor units, contributing to the increase in $\dot{V}_{O_2}$. There is evidence that running downhill changes the kinematics of running, as shown by a more flexed knee position at footstrike in downhill compared with level running, and a greater maximal knee angle during support (Eston et al. 1995).

Leg length discrepancy

A difference in length between right and left legs has often been implicated as a factor in running injuries. McCaw (1992) found greater ground reaction force loading in the long leg of a subject who showed a leg length difference. After reviewing the literature, he concluded that while there was no unequivocal demonstration of an association between leg length inequality and increased risk of overuse injuries, neither is there reason to reject the relationship. Friberg (1982) concluded from an epidemiological study that leg length asymmetry predisposed military recruits to stress fractures, but Messier et al. (1991) found no relationship between leg length inequality and patellofemoral pain.

Changes in biomechanics of running with fatigue

As the muscles fatigue during the course of a run, changes often occur in the kinematics, kinetics and patterns of muscle use. A common problem in studies examining fatigue is that running speed usually changes when a runner fatigues, and since most biomechanical variables also change with speed, it can be difficult to identify the changes due to fatigue and those due to the altered speed.

Changes with fatigue have not been consistent among studies. Elliott and Acklund (1981) found a decreased running velocity, a shorter SL, a more extended lower limb, and a slower backward velocity of the foot at footstrike during a fatiguing 10 000 m run. It was not clear whether the biomechanical changes were due to fatigue or the slower speed. In a 3000 m run where speed was controlled, Elliott and Roberts (1980) reported non-significant trends towards decreased SL and increased SR, increased

support time and decreased non-support time, a significantly less vertical lower leg angle at footstrike, a less extended thigh at toe-off, and greater forward lean near the end of the run compared with three other time periods earlier in the run. Others have found SL to increase with fatigue in both overground and treadmill running (Cavanagh et al. 1985; Williams et al. 1991), with most subjects showing a steady increase in SL but some not showing an increase until late in the fatiguing run. One of these studies found only a few trends for changes with fatigue across a group of runners, reporting an increase in maximal knee flexion during the swing phase and greater hip flexion with fatigue (Williams et al. 1991). They also found that changes in specific measures were at times large for individuals.

As with distance running, fatigue studies of sprinters are also complicated by differences in speed, with measures usually collected initially after maximal speed is attained and again near the end of a run. The decreased velocity that usually occurs with fatigue results in a decrease in SL and SR (Bates et al. 1977), and it is also linked to an increase in support time and decreases in the hip and knee range of motion, with the specific changes variable between subjects (Chapman 1982).

Biomechanical factors and footwear/orthotics

During the late 1970s and early 1980s there was a dramatic evolution of the design and materials used in running footwear, and that trend has continued throughout the 1990s as more sophisticated construction techniques have been developed and advances have been made in the materials used in footwear construction. Many of the advances made in footwear design were a consequence of basic information resulting from biomechanical studies of the interaction between running mechanics and footwear.

Running shoes and economy

A number of studies have demonstrated that the design and materials used in footwear construction can affect running economy. While the changes in

$\dot{V}o_2$ are not large, studies have shown a change of from 0.9% to 3.5% in submaximal energy costs. Heavier shoes have been found to increase oxygen cost by 1.9% per 100 g mass difference per shoe (Catlin & Dressendorfer 1979), and when mass is added to shoes, by 1.2% (Frederick et al. 1984) and 1.4% (Martin 1985) per 100 g per shoe.

Shoes with different cushioning properties have also been found to affect $\dot{V}o_2$, with shoes having more cushioning usually being associated with lower oxygen consumption (Frederick et al. 1983), though some contrary results have been found, as in a study where soft-soled inserts with very high-energy-absorption characteristics resulted in increased $\dot{V}o_2$ (Bosco & Rusko 1983). The authors suggested that the increased support time that resulted from the soft inserts may have altered the stretch–shortening cycle of events and reduced elastic contributions to the work done. Frederick et al. (1983) found a significant correlation between $\dot{V}o_2$ and maximum knee flexion velocity following footstrike, with the greater velocities found for harder shoes cited as a possible reason for the increased energy costs. It has been hypothesized that orthotic devices might reduce oxygen consumption by altering lower-extremity mechanics and reducing muscular activity, but the trend across several studies is for a slight increase, perhaps due to the added weight of the orthotics (Clement et al. 1984a).

Jørgensen (Jørgensen 1990) examined $\dot{V}o_2$ and triceps surae and quadriceps muscle EMGs when runners used a regular shoe and an identical shoe with the heel counter cut out, expecting the heel counter to have an effect on foot stability and muscle use. He found reduced oxygen consumption and lower EMG activity at footstrike when the heel counters were in place, providing some support for the hypothesized relationship between stability and economy. In the early 1990s many shoes were touted as having enhanced energy return capabilities, where a runner would take advantage of a spring-like effect as energy stored during foot impact help to propel the runner at toe-off. Shorten (1993) presented convincing data that suggested that the influence this might have on running economy would likely be less than 1%, making it unlikely that energy return by shoes would be a major factor in altering the metabolic costs of running.

Running shoes and running mechanics

The effect of footwear on the biomechanics of running has also been investigated widely. By varying the design and materials in footwear, a variety of changes to running mechanics can be effected. Clarke et al. (1983b) found rearfoot pronation to be greater when softer midsole materials were used and in shoes with less rearfoot flare on the medial side of the shoe, but found heel height to have no effect on pronation. Others found an increase in the amount of pronation going from a softer (25 durometer, shoe A) to a harder (35 durometer) midsole material, and they also showed an increase in pronation velocity in stiffer shoes (Nigg et al. 1986). They suggested that a softer material be placed in the lateral heel to aid in shock absorption and firmer material be used in the medial heel area to help limit pronation, and concluded that increased lateral flare would lead to an increase in pronation. Shoes have also been found to decrease the maximal pronation angle compared with a barefoot condition (Nigg et al. 1984).

While running in racing shoes may have an advantage to oxygen consumption because of the lower $\dot{V}o_2$ associated with a lighter shoe, one of the possible detriments is thought to be less stability. Hamill et al. (1988) found greater pronation in racing shoes (13.4°) compared with training shoes (7.8°), and while running in training shoes caused an average increase of 1.3% in $\dot{V}o_2$, differences were not significant. Orthotics have been found to reduce rearfoot pronation and pronation velocity (Taunton et al. 1985; Smith et al. 1986), but Taunton et al. found no change in knee internal rotation when an orthotic device was used by overpronating runners. Nigg et al. (1986) found the position of a medial support wedge in a shoe could help limit the amount of pronation.

Running shoes and injuries

Many associations have been made between the impact shock that occurs in running and injuries, but there is little, if any, direct evidence that identifies specific mechanisms (Frederick 1986). Some studies have shown a relationship between rearfoot pronation and a variety of knee, leg and foot injuries, as described in an earlier section. There are also studies that have shown how footwear can help control pronation, so it is likely that footwear can have a substantial influence on susceptibility to injury.

Shoe design and materials have an obvious effect on the shock-absorption abilities of shoes, but the wide range often seen in drop-impact tests generally does not correlate well to measures of impact loading on runners assessed using force platform or accelerometer measures (Clarke et al. 1983a; Nigg et al. 1986). This may at least partly be because individual runners may adapt differently to a given shoe. Shoes may cause runners to adjust kinematically, as found in a study by Clarke et al. (1983a), where the ankle was more dorsiflexed at footstrike and knee flexion velocity immediately following heel strike was increased in harder shoes compared with softer shoes. The interaction between the shoe materials, shoe design, and the human runner make it difficult to predict how an individual may react to a given shoe (Frederick 1986). This may also explain why it has been difficult to make direct connections between footwear, impact forces and injuries. Since runners may alter their running mechanics in subtle ways, depending on the shock absorption and stability features in shoes, this may make it more difficult to identify how differences between shoes affect force magnitudes, movement and, indirectly, injury.

Concluding comments

The dynamics of running involve a complex interaction between physiological and mechanical mechanisms. Our understanding of why runners adopt specific movement patterns will mature faster the more we analyse running from a multidisciplinary perspective. A runner is constantly processing a variety of different types of information from both external and internal sources that relate to both the movements involved and the consequences of those movements. Scientists need to process the same diversity of information. Many of the commonly described relationships discussed in the preceding pages between biomechanical parameters and either metabolic energy cost or musculoskeletal injury are still without strong scientific confirmation. Still relatively little is known about the precise mechanisms relating how running movements affect energy consumption or tissue stress, and future efforts should be directed towards identifying such mechanisms. At the same time, much has been learned in the past two decades, and there has been an encouraging trend to more sophisticated studies that go beyond describing 'what' and explores in more detail 'how' and 'why'.

References

Agre, J.C. (1985) Hamstring injuries. Proposed aetiological factors, prevention, and treatment. *Sports Medicine* 2, 21–33.

Aleshinsky, S.Y. (1986a) An energy 'sources' and 'fractions' approach to the mechanical energy expenditure problem—I. Basic concepts, description of the model, analysis of a one-link system movement. *Journal of Biomechanics* 19, 287–293.

Aleshinsky, S.Y. (1986b) An energy 'sources' and 'fractions' approach to the mechanical energy expenditure problem—V. The mechanical energy expenditure reduction during motion of the multi-link system. *Journal of Biomechanics* 19, 311–315.

Anderson, T. (1996) Biomechanics and running economy. *Sports Medicine* 22, 76–89.

Anderson, T. & Tseh, W. (1994) Running economy, anthropometric dimensions and kinematic variables (abstract). *Medicine and Science in Sports and Exercise* 26, S170.

Ardigao, L.P., Lafortuna, C., Minetti, A.E., Mognoni, P. & Saibene, F. (1995) Metabolic and mechanical aspects of foot landing type, forefoot and rearfoot strike, in human running. *Acta Physiologica Scandinavica* 155, 17–22.

Atwater, A.E. (1990) Gender differences in distance running. In: *Biomechanics of Distance Running* (ed. P.R. Cavanagh), pp. 321–362. Human Kinetics Publishers, Champaign, IL.

Ballas, M.T., Tytko, J. & Cookson, D. (1997) Common overuse running injuries: diagnosis and management. *American Family Physician* 55, 2473–2484.

Bates, B.T., Osternig, L.R. & James, S.L. (1977) Fatigue effects in running. *Journal of Motor Behavior* 9, 203–207.

Bennell, K.L. & Crossley, K. (1996) Musculoskeletal injuries in track and field: incidence, distribution and risk factors. *Australian Journal of Science and Medicine in Sport* 28, 69–75.

Bergh, U., Sjodïn, B., Forsberg, A. & Svedenhad, J. (1991) The relationship between body mass and oxygen uptake during running in humans. *Medicine and Science in Sports and Exercise* 23, 205–211.

Bosco, C. & Rusko, H. (1983) The effect of prolonged skeletal muscle stretch-shortening cycle on recoil of elastic energy and on energy expenditure. *Acta Physiologica Scandinavica* **119**, 219–224.

Brisswalter, J., Legros, P. & Durand, M. (1996) Running economy, preferred step length correlated to body dimensions in elite middle distance runners. *Journal of Sports Medicine and Physical Fitness* **36**, 7–15.

Brunet, M.E., Cook, S.D., Brinker, M.R. & Dickinson, J.A. (1990) A survey of running injuries in 1505 competitive and recreational runners. *Journal of Sports Medicine and Physical Fitness* **30**, 307–315.

Burdett, R.G. (1982) Forces predicted at the ankle during running. *Medicine and Science in Sports and Exercise* **14**, 308–316.

Burr, D.B., Milgrom, C., Fyhrie, D. *et al.* (1996) In vivo measurement of human tibial strains during vigorous activity. *Bone* **18**, 405–410.

Catlin, M.J. & Dressendorfer, R.H. (1979) Effect of shoe weight on the energy cost of running. *Medicine and Science in Sports and Exercise* **11**, 80.

Cavanagh, P.R. (ed.) (1990) *Biomechanics of Running*. Human Kinetics Publishers, Champaign, IL.

Cavanagh, P.R. & Kram, R. (1985) Mechanical and muscular factors affecting the efficiency of human movement. *Medicine and Science in Sports and Exercise* **17**, 326–331.

Cavanagh, P.R. & Kram, R. (1989) Stride length in distance running: Velocity, body dimensions, and added mass effects. *Medicine and Science in Sports and Exercise* **21**, 467–479.

Cavanagh, P.R. & Lafortune, M.A. (1980) Ground reaction forces in distance running. *Journal of Biomechanics* **13**, 397–406.

Cavanagh, P.R. & Williams, K.R. (1982) The effect of stride length variation on oxygen uptake during distance running. *Medicine and Science in Sports and Exercise* **14**, 30–35.

Cavanagh, P.R., Pollock, M.L. & Landa, J. (1977) A biomechanical comparison of elite and good distance runners. *Annals of the New York Academy of Sciences* **301**, 328–345.

Cavanagh, P.R., Andrew, G.C., Kram, R., Rodgers, M.M., Sanderson, D.J. & Hennig, E.M. (1985) An approach to biomechanical profiling of elite distance runners. *International Journal of Sport Biomechanics* **1**, 36–62.

Chapman, A.E. (1982) Hierarchy of changes induced by fatigue in sprinting. *Canadian Journal of Applied Sport Science* **7**, 116–122.

Clarke, T.E., Frederick, E.C. & Cooper, L.B. (1983a) Biomechanical measurement of running shoe cushioning properties. In: *Biomechanical Aspects of Sport Shoes and Playing Surfaces* (eds B.M. Nigg & B.A. Kerr), pp. 25–34. University of Calgary, Calgary.

Clarke, T.E., Frederick, E.C. & Hamill, C.L. (1983b) The effects of shoe design parameters on rearfoot control in running. *Medicine and Science in Sports and Exercise* **15**, 376–381.

Clement, D.B., Taunton, J.E., Smart, G.W. & McNicol, K.L. (1981) A survey of overuse running injuries. *Physician and Sports Medicine* **9**, 47–58.

Clement, D.B., Taunton, J. & Wiley, J. P., Smart, G. & McNicol, K. (1984a) The effects of corrective orthotic devices on oxygen uptake during running. In: *Proceedings of the World Congress on Sports Medicine* (ed. L. Prokop), pp. 648–655. World Congress on Sports Medicine, Vienna.

Clement, D.B., Taunton, J.E. & Smart, G.W. (1984b) Achilles tendinitis and peritendinitis: etiology and treatment. *American Journal of Sports Medicine* **12**, 179–184.

Craib, M.W., Mitchell, V.A., Fields, K.B., Cooper, T.R., Hopewell, R. & Morgan, D.W. (1996) The association between flexibility and running economy in sub-elite male distance runners. *Medicine and Science in Sports and Exercise* **28**, 737–743.

Daniels, J.T. (1985) A physiologist's view of running economy. *Medicine and Science in Sports and Exercise* **17**, 332–338.

Davies, C.T.M. (1980) Effects of wind assistance and resistance on the forward motion of a runner. *Journal of Applied Physiology* **48**, 702–709.

Dick, R.W. & Cavanagh, P.R. (1987) An explanation of the upward drift in oxygen uptake during prolonged submaximal downhill running. *Medicine and Science in Sports and Exercise* **19**, 310–317.

Dillman, C.J. (1975) Kinematic analysis of running. *Exercise and Sport Sciences Reviews* **3**, 193–218.

Egbuonu, M.E., Cavanagh, P.R. & Miller, T.A. (1990) Degradation of running economy through changes in running mechanics. *Medicine and Science in Sports and Exercise* **22**, S17.

Elliott, B. & Acklund, T. (1981) Biomechanical effects of fatigue on 10,000 meter running technique. *Research Quarterly for Exercise and Sport* **52**, 160–166.

Elliott, B.C. & Roberts, A.D. (1980) A biomechanical evaluation of the role of fatigue in middle-distance running. *Canadian Journal of Applied Sport Sciences* **5**, 203–207.

Engsberg, J.R. (1996) A new method for quantifying pronation in overpronating and normal runners. *Medicine and Science in Sports and Exercise* **28**, 299–304.

Eston, R.G., Mickleborough, J. & Baltzopoulos, V. (1995) Eccentric activation and muscle damage: biomechanical and physiological considerations during downhill running. *British Journal of Sports Medicine* **29**, 89–94.

Frederick, E.C. (1986) Kinematically mediated effects of sport shoe design: a review. *Journal of Sports Science* **4**, 169–184.

Frederick, E.C. & Hagy, J.L. (1986) Factors affecting peak vertical ground reaction forces in running. *International Journal of Sport Biomechanics* **2**, 41–49.

Frederick, E.C., Clarke, T.C., Hansen, J.L. & Cooper, L.B. (1983) The effects of shoe cushioning on the oxygen demands of running. In: *Biomechanical Aspects of Sports Shoes and Playing Surfaces* (eds B. Nigg & B. Kerr), pp. 107–114. University of Calgary, Calgary.

Frederick, E.C., Daniels, J.T. & Hayes, J.W. (1984) The effect of shoe weight on the aerobic demands of running. In: *Proceedings of the World Congress on Sports Medicine, Vienna.* (eds N. Bachl, L. Prokop & R. Suckert), pp. 616–625. Urban & Schwarzenberg, Wien; Baltimore, MY.

Friberg, O. (1982) Leg length asymmetry in stress fractures. *Journal of Sports Medicine* **22**, 485–488.

Frigo, C., Pedotti, A. & Santambrogio, G. (1979) A correlation between muscle length and EMG activities during running. In: *Science in Athletics* (eds J. Terauds & G.G. Dales), pp. 61–71. Academic Publishers, Del Mar, CA.

Frishberg, B.A. (1983) An analysis of overground and treadmill sprinting. *Medicine and Science in Sports and Exercise* **15**, 478–485.

Gehlsen, G.M. & Seger, A. (1980) Selected measures of angular displacement, strength, and flexibility in subjects with and without shin splints. *Research Quarterly for Exercise and Sport* **51**, 478–485.

Giladi, M., Milgrom, C., Stein, M. *et al.* (1985) The low arch, a protective factor in stress fractures: a prospective study of 295 military recruits. *Orthopaedic Review* **14**, 709–712.

Gleim, G.W., Stachenfeld, N.S. & Nicholas, J.A. (1990) The influence of flexibility on the economy of walking and jogging. *Journal of Orthopaedic Research* **8**, 814–823.

Godges, J.J., Macrae, H., Londgon, C. & Tinberg, C. (1989) The effects of two stretching procedures on hip range of motion and gait economy. *Journal of Orthopaedic and Sports Physical Therapy* **7**, 350–357.

Hamill, J., Freedson, P.S., Boda, W. & Reichsman, F. (1988) Effects of shoe type on cardiorespiratory responses and rearfoot motion during treadmill running. *Medicine and Science in Sports and Exercise* **20**, 515–521.

Heise, G.D. & Martin, P.E. (1990) Inter-relationships among mechanical power measures and running economy. *Medicine and Science in Sports and Exercise* **22**, S22.

Hinrichs, R.N., Cavanagh, P.R. & Williams, K.R. (1983) Upper extremity contributions to angular momentum in running. In: *Biomechanics VIII-B* (ed. H.M.A.K. Kobayashi), pp. 641–647. Human Kinetics Publishers, Champaign, IL.

Hoffman, K. (1971) Stature, leg length, and stride frequency. *Track Technique* **46**, 1463–1469.

Hulkko, A. & Orava, S. (1987) Stress fractures in athletes. *International Journal of Sports Medicine* **8**, 221–226.

van Ingen Schenau, G.J. (1980) Some fundamental aspects of the biomechanics of overground versus treadmill locomotion. *Medicine and Science in Sports and Exercise* **12**, 257–261.

van Ingen Schenau, G.J. & Cavanagh, P.R. (1990) Power equations in endurance sports. *Journal of Biomechanics* **23**, 865–881.

van Ingen Schenau, G.J., Bobbert, M.F. & de Haan, A. (1997) Does elastic energy enhance work and efficiency in the stretch-shortening cycle? *Journal of Applied Biomechanics* **13**, 389–415.

van Ingen Schenau, G.J., Dorssers, W.M., Welter, T.G., Beelen, A., de Groot, G. & Jacobs, R. (1995) The control of mono-articular muscles in multijoint leg extensions in man. *Journal of Physiology (London)* **484** (1), 247–254.

Ito, A., Komi, P.V., Sjödin, B., Bosco, C. & Karlsson, J. (1983) Mechanical efficiency of positive work in running at different speeds. *Medicine and Science in Sports and Exercise* **15**, 299–308.

James, S.L., Bates, B.T. & Osternig, L.R. (1978) Injuries to runners. *American Journal of Sports Medicine* **6**, 40–50.

Jönhagen, S., Nemeth, G. & Eriksson, E. (1994) Hamstring injuries in sprinters. The role of concentric and eccentric hamstring muscle strength and flexibility. *American Journal of Sports Medicine* **22**, 262–266.

Jørgensen, U. (1990) Body load in heel-strike running: the effect of a firm heel counter. *American Journal of Sports Medicine* **18**, 177–180.

Komi, P.V. (1990) Relevance of in vivo force measurements to human biomechanics. *Journal of Biomechanics* **23** (Suppl. 1), 23–34.

Kunz, H. & Kaufmann, D.A. (1981) Biomechanical analysis of sprinting: decathletes versus champions. *British Journal of Sports Medicine* **15**, 177–181.

Kyle, C.R. (1979) Reduction of wind resistance and power output of racing cyclists and runners traveling in groups. *Ergonomics* **22**, 387–397.

Landry, M.E. & Zebas, C. (1985) Analysis of 100 knees in high school runners. *Journal of the American Podiatrics Medicine Association* **75**, 382–384.

Luhtanen, P. & Komi, P.V. (1978) Mechanical factors influencing running speed. In: *Biomechanics VI-B* (eds E. Asmussen & K. Jorgenson), pp. 23–29. University Park Press, Baltimore, MY.

Lusby, L.A. & Atwater, A.E. (1983) Speed-related position-time profiles of arm motion in trained women distance runners. *Medicine and Science in Sports and Exercise* **15**, 171.

Lutter, L.D. (1985) The knee and running. *Clinical Sports Medicine* **4**, 685–698.

Mann, R. & Sprague, P. (1980) A kinetic analysis of the ground leg during sprint running. *Research Quarterly for Exercise and Sport* **51**, 334–348.

Martin, P.E. (1985) Mechanical and physiological responses to lower extremity loading during running. *Medicine and Science in Sports and Exercise* **17**, 427–433.

Maughan, R.J. & Miller, J.D.B. (1983) Incidence of training-related injuries among marathon runners. *British Journal of Sports Medicine* **17**, 162–165.

McCaw, S.T. (1992) Leg length inequality. Implications for running injury prevention. *Sports Medicine* **14**, 422–429.

Mechelen, W. van (1992) Running injuries. A review of the epidemiological literature. *Sports Medicine* **14**, 320–335.

Mero, A. & Komi, P.V. (1986) Force-, EMG-, and elasticity-velocity relationships at submaximal, maximal and supramaximal running speeds in sprinters. *European Journal of Applied Physiology* **55**, 553–561.

Mero, A., Komi, P.V. & Gregor, R.J. (1992) Biomechanics of sprint running. A review. *Sports Medicine* **13**, 376–392.

Messier, S.P., Davis, S.E., Curl, W.W., Lowery, R.B. & Pack, R.J. (1991) Etiologic factors associated with patello-femoral pain in runners. *Medicine and Science in Sports and Exercise* **23**, 1008–1015.

Messier, S.P. & Pittala, K.A. (1988) Etiologic factors associated with selected running injuries. *Medicine and Science in Sports and Exercise* **20**, 501–505.

Miller, T.A., Milliron, M.J. & Cavanagh, P.R. (1990) The effect of running mechanics feedback training on running economy. *Medicine and Science in Sports and Exercise* **22**, S17.

Morgan, D.W., Martin, P.E. & Krahenbuhl, G.S. (1989) Factors affecting running economy. *Sports Medicine* **7**, 310–330.

Morgan, D., Martin, P., Craib, M., Caruso, C., Clifton, R. & Hopewell, R. (1994) Effect of step length optimization on the aerobic demand of running. *Journal of Applied Physiology* **77**, 245–251.

Munro, C.F., Miller, D.I. & Fuglevand, A.J. (1987) Ground reaction forces in running: a reexamination. *Journal of Biomechanics* **20**, 147–156.

Nawoczenski, D.A., Saltzman, C.L. & Cook, T.M. (1998) The effect of foot structure on the three-dimensional kinematic coupling behavior of the leg and rear foot. *Physical Therapy* **78**, 404–416.

Nelson, R.C., Brooks, C.M. & Pike, N.L. (1977) Biomechanical comparison of male and female distance runners. *Annals of the New York Academy of Sciences* **301**, 793–807.

Nigg, B.M. (ed.) (1986) *Biomechanics of Running Shoes*. Human Kinetics Publishers, Champaign, IL.

Nigg, B.M., Luethi, S., Stacoff, A. & Segesser, B. (1984) Biomechanical effects of pain and sportshoe corrections. *Australian Journal of Science and Medicine in Sport* **16**, 10–16.

Nigg, B.M., Bahlsen, A.H., Denoth, J., Luethi, S.M. & Stacoff, A. (1986) Factors influencing kinetic and kinematic variables in running. In: *Biomechanics of Running Shoes* (ed. B.M. Nigg), pp. 139–165. Human Kinetics Publishers, Champaign, IL.

Nigg, B.M., Bahlsen, H.A., Luethi, S.M. & Stokes, S. (1987) The influence of running velocity and midsole hardness on external impact forces in heel-toe running. *Journal of Biomechanics* **20**, 951–959.

Nigg, B.M., De Boer, R.W. & Fisher, V. (1995) A kinematic comparison of over-ground and treadmill running. *Medicine and Science in Sports and Exercise* **27**, 98–105.

Nilsson, J., Thorstensson, A. & Halbertsma, J. (1985) Changes in leg movements and muscle activity with speed of locomotion and mode of progression in humans. *Acta Physiologica Scandinavica* **123**, 457–475.

Pate, R.R., Macera, C.A., Bailey, S.P., Bartoli, W.P. & Powell, K.E. (1992) Physiological, anthropometric, and training correlates of running economy. *Medicine and Science in Sports and Exercise* **24**, 1128–1133.

Plamondon, A. & Roy, B. (1984) Cinématique et cinétique de la course accélérée. *Canadian Journal of Applied Sports Science* **9**, 42–52.

Prilutsky, B.I., Petrova, L.N. & Raitsin, L.M. (1996) Comparison of mechanical energy expenditure of joint moments and muscle forces during human locomotion. *Journal of Biomechanics* **29**, 405–415.

Pugh, L.G.C.E. (1971) The influence of wind resistance in running and walking and the mechanical efficiency of work against horizontal or vertical forces. *Journal of Physiology* **213**, 255–276.

Putnam, C.A. & Kozey, J.W. (1989) Substantive issues in running. In: *Biomechanics of Sport* (ed. C.V. Vaughn), pp. 1–33. CRC Press, Boca Raton, FL.

Scott, S.H. & Winter, D.A. (1990) Internal forces of chronic running injury sites. *Medicine and Science in Sports and Exercise* **22**, 357–369.

Sharkey, N.A., Ferris, L., Smith, T.S. & Matthews, D.K. (1995) Strain and loading of the second metatarsal during heel-lift. *Journal of Bone and Joint Surgery* **77**, 1050–1057.

Shorten, M.R. (1993) The energetics of running and running shoes. *Journal of Biomechanics* **26** (Suppl. 1), 41–51.

Shorten, M.R., Wootton, S. & Williams, C. (1981) Mechanical energy changes and the oxygen cost of running. *Engineering in Medicine* **10**, 213–217.

Simkin, A., Leicher, I., Giladi, M. *et al.* (1989) Combined effect of foot arch structure and an orthotic device on stress fractures. *Foot and Ankle* **10**, 25–29.

Smith, L.S., Clarke, T.E., Hamill, C.L. & Santopietro, F. (1986) The effects of soft and semi-rigid orthoses upon rearfoot movement in running. *Journal of the American Podiatrics Medicine Association* **76**, 227–233.

Sullivan, D., Warren, R.F., Pavlov, H. & Delman, G. (1984) Stress fractures in 51 runners. *Clinical Orthopaedics* **187**, 188–192.

Taunton, J.E., Clement, D.B., Smart, G.W., Wiley, J.P. & McNicol, K.L. (1985) A triplanar electrogoniometer investigation of running mechanics in runners with compensatory overpronation. *Canadian Journal of Applied Sports Science* **10**, 104–115.

Taylor, C.R. (1994) Relating mechanics and energetics during exercise. *Advances in Veterinary Science and Comparative Medicine* **38A**, 181–215.

Ting, A., King, W., Yocum, L. *et al.* (1988) Stress fractures of the tarsal navicular in long-distance runners. *Clinical Sports Medicine* **7**, 89–101.

Viitasalo, J.T. & Kvist, M. (1983) Some biomechanical aspects of the foot and ankle in athletes with and without shin splints. *American Journal of Sports Medicine* **11**, 125–130.

Warren, B.L. (1990) Plantar fasciitis in runners. Treatment and prevention. *Sports Medicine* **10**, 338–345.

Williams, K.R. (1982) Non-sagittal plane movements and forces during distance running (abstract). In: *Sixth Annual Conference of the American Society of Biomechanics.* University of Washington, Seattle, p. 24.

Williams, K.R. (1985a) Biomechanics of running. *Exercise and Sport Sciences Reviews* **13**, 389–441.

Williams, K.R. (1985b) The relationship between mechanical and physiological energy estimates. *Medicine and Science in Sports and Exercise* **17**, 317–325.

Williams, K.R. & Cavanagh, P.R. (1983) A model for the calculation of mechnical power during distance running. *Journal of Biomechanics* **16**, 115–128.

Williams, K.R. & Cavanagh, P.R. (1986) Biomechanical correlates with running economy in elite distance runners. In: *Proceedings of the North American Congress on Biomechanics*, Vol. 2, pp. 287–288. American Society of Biomechanics, Montreal.

Williams, K.R. & Cavanagh, P.R. (1987) Relationship between distance running mechanics, running economy, and performance. *Journal of Applied Physiology* **63**, 1236–1245.

Williams, K.R. & Ziff, K.R. (1991) Changes in distance running mechanics due to systematic variations in running style. *International Journal of Sports Biomechanics* **7**, 76–90.

Williams, K.R., Cavanagh, P.R. & Ziff, J.L. (1987) Biomechanical studies of elite female distance runners. *International Journal of Sports Medicine* **8**, 107–118.

Williams, K.R., Snow, R. & Agruss, C. (1991) Changes in distance running kinematics with fatigue. *International Journal of Sports Biomechanics* **7**, 138–162.

Winter, D.A. (1979) A new definition of mechanical work done in human movement. *Journal of Applied Physiology* **46**, 79–83.

Winter, D.A. (1983) Moments of force and mechanical power in jogging. *Journal of Biomechanics* **16**, 91–97.

Chapter 9

Resistive Forces in Swimming

A.R. VORONTSOV AND V.A. RUMYANTSEV

The nature of hydrodynamic resistance and its components

The body of a swimmer moving through the water experiences a retarding force known as resistance or drag. The nature of hydrodynamic resistance is explained by such physical properties of water as internal pressure, density (responsible for hydrostatic force) and viscosity. While travelling through the water the body will displace some water from its path. The reaction of the water to the moving body appears as: (i) pressure forces perpendicular to its frontal area; and (ii) friction forces acting along the body surface. Since swimming occurs in the state of 'hydrostatic weightlessness' the major part of mechanical work a swimmer performs is directed to overcoming the hydrodynamic resistance. One of the most obvious manifestations of this force is the slowing-down while gliding and then stopping that a swimmer experiences soon after a dive or pushoff. A better understanding of how the swimmer's body interacts with water flow and how hydrodynamic resistance may be reduced using appropriate swimming skills within the framework of the swimming rules should help to increase the swimmer's velocity and maximize swimming achievements.

Hydrodynamic resistance (HDR) may be divided into two categories:
- *passive resistance* (or *passive drag*) is that experienced by a swimmer's body during passive towing, during exposure to water flow in a water flume, and when performing gliding without movements; and
- *active resistance* (or *active drag*) is that experienced by a swimmer during swimming. It incorporates

passive resistance of the core body and additional wave-making and eddies caused by swimming movements (Clarys 1978; Kolmogorov & Duplisheva 1992).

Actually, both active and passive resistance to a swimmer's forward motion have several components:

1 resistance by the air to above-water parts of the body and recovering arms (only while swimming or towing on water surface);
2 friction between water and the surface of the body; and
3 pressure resistance, which includes:
  (a) form resistance caused by eddy formation in the body's wake and behind its segments; and
  (b) wave-making resistance.

The aerodynamic resistance is very small and contributes little to total resistance during swimming since maximum swimming speeds are low compared with locomotion on land, or to rowing, and only relatively little of the body is exposed to the air. Thus, the prime attention of coaches and swimmers should be focused on frictional, wave-making and pressure components of hydrodynamic resistance.

Passive hydrodynamic resistance (passive drag)

Swimmers experience passive drag only during the glide after the start and turns and also possibly during some transitional postures within movement cycles (especially in breaststroke and butterfly). Knowledge of the components constituting passive

184

hydrodynamic resistance and their interaction with the swimmer's body at different flow velocities and body alignments is basic for the development of a proper swimming technique. That is why passive hydrodynamic resistance is one of the favourite research topics in sport swimming.

The magnitude of the passive hydrodynamic resistance (passive drag) may be established experimentally by towing a swimmer in a towing tank or exposing the subject to water flow in a swimming flume. It is described by the formula:

$$F_{DP} = \tfrac{1}{2} C_{DP} \rho V^2 S_M \qquad (9.1)$$

where ρ = water density, V = speed of the water flow interacting with the body, S_M = the area of middle section, and C_{DP} = hydrodynamic coefficient or *drag coefficient*—a dimensionless quantity which is defined as the ratio $F_{DP} / [(\rho V^2 / 2) S_M]$. The drag coefficient is a function of another dimensionless quantity known as the Reynolds number:

$$Re = \rho VL / \mu \qquad (9.2)$$

where ρ = water density, V = flow velocity (towing or gliding speed), L = body length, and μ = coefficient of dynamic viscosity ($\mu = 0.987 \times 10^{-3}$ N · s · m^{-2} at water temp. = 26°C).

Reynolds number (*Re*) in fluid mechanics is a criterion of whether the flow is perfectly steady and streamlined (i.e. laminar flow), or is on average steady with small fluctuations, or is turbulent. The character of water flow around a swimmer's body (i.e. whether it is laminar or turbulent) determines the magnitude of hydrodynamic resistance.

Laminar or *streamlined flow* is flow in which the water travels smoothly and rectilinearly, without any disturbances. The velocity and pressure at each point of such flow remain constant. Laminar flow may be depicted as consisting of thin horizontal layers or *laminae*, all parallel to each other. Laminar flow usually occurs when a body has a streamlined profile and its velocity is low. With increased flow velocity, perturbations and eddy formation occur, until the flow pattern is so disturbed that the flow becomes turbulent.

Turbulence also arises within *boundary layers* around solid objects moving through steady water when the rate of friction within the boundary layer

becomes large enough. It occurs during both active swimming and passive towing. The boundary layer is a thin layer of liquid in contact with the body surface. The fluid in a boundary layer is subject to friction forces, and a range of velocities exists across the boundary layer, from maximum to zero. Boundary layers are thinner at the leading edge of the body and thicker towards the trailing edge. The flow in such boundary layers is generally laminar at the leading or upstream portion of the body and turbulent in the trailing or downstream portion.

According to Clarys (1979) for competitive swimming the Reynolds number (*Re*) is within the range 2×10^5–2.5×10^6. At this high *Re*, the inertial forces dominate, which means that the boundary layer along the rigid body is expected to be turbulent. In contrast to laminar flow the resistance in such flow is increased considerably. A number of experiments with rigid bodies of different shapes over a wide range of *Re* values have shown that the drag coefficient (C_D) is a function of *Re*. From appropriate diagrams C_D can be estimated on the basis of *Re* and incorporated into Eqn. 9.2.

Frictional resistance

Frictional resistance (or *skin resistance* or *skin drag*) is originated in boundary layers. During swimming the water layer in contact with the body surface 'sticks' to it and travels with the same speed as the swimmer. Due to water viscosity this layer interacts with the adjoining external layer and drags it along with it, albeit at a rate slightly slower than the proximal boundary layer (and so on across all components of the boundary layer). The greater the amount of water a swimmer trails behind him, the greater is the frictional resistance.

Smoothness of body surface, skin, hair, and tightness of the swimsuit and nature of its fabric are the main contributors to friction resistance since they increase the formation of eddies in the boundary layer. An increase of turbulence in the boundary layer is accompanied by increased resistance. To form eddies the water molecules take away kinetic energy from the swimmer's body. Thus friction slows down swimming velocity and increases energy losses.

Frictional resistance may be estimated as:

$$F_{fr} = \mu(dV/dZ)S_{fr} \tag{9.3}$$

where μ = coefficient of dynamic viscosity ($\mu = 0.897 \times 10^{-3}$ N · s · m^{-2} at $t = 26°C$), dV = difference between velocity of water layers (d$V = V$), dZ = difference in thickness of water layers, and S_{fr} = wetted body surface area.

Though frictional resistance is considered mainly as a part of passive resistance, it definitely reduces the swimmer's speed during gliding and in some phases of swimming where water flow along the body is laminar. During active swimming at high velocities the formation of eddies in boundary layers diverts some of the body's propulsive energy and thus reduces the efficiency of the swimming technique. That is why smooth body surfaces (skin shaving) and specially designed swimsuits help to reduce the body's surface-to-water friction. These are considered to be important measures for improving swimming performance. High buoyancy reduces the wetted body area and thereby assists in the reduction of friction.

It is still debated whether skin shaving really reduces turbulence in the boundary layer and thereby reduces the frictional resistance, or whether psychological effects are responsible for the improved swimming performance. Sharp and Costill (1989) found that swimmers who shaved their skin before a race demonstrated relatively less energy expenditure, greater stroke distance and faster swimming velocity than those who swam without shaving. Such increased performance may be the result of reduction of skin friction.

Another approach to reducing friction resistance is the development of better designs and fabrics for swimsuits. Modern designs incorporate water-repelling and ultra-thin elastic fabrics to maximize body smoothness, or use fabrics that can 'bind' a thin water film as a lubricant. This is an area of intense competition between swimwear manufacturers.

Pressure resistance (form drag)

A water flow exerts a resistance force F_D on any obstacle in its path. The same force arises when a swimmer moves through stationary water. According to Bernoulli's principle any change in kinetic power of the water flow is accompanied by an opposite proportional change of its pressure on the body surface:

$$pV_i^2/2 + p_i = \text{constant} \tag{9.4}$$

where $pV_i^2/2$ = kinetic energy of a fluid volume and p_i = potential energy of pressure of that volume. It follows from Eqn. 9.4. that the magnitude of pressure forces acting in a direction perpendicular to the body surface changes with the square of the flow velocity.

Pressure resistance is the result of hydrodynamic processes occurring at the front and rear of the moving body. Water pressure in the wake of the body is less then pressure acting on the front. This is due to boundary layers moving relative to the body and each other, thereby performing mechanical work, which slow down and separate from the body surface before they reach the rear portion. Separating water layers form eddies, i.e. rotating water masses with high velocity. Thus behind the point of separation an area of low pressure is formed. The pressure difference between the front and rear of the body—the *pressure gradient*—determines the magnitude of the pressure resistance given the largest cross-sectional area (S_M) perpendicular to the forward motion of the body. Hence, pressure resistance is a result of the pressure gradient created between the high pressure as the swimmer's leading surfaces are propelled through the water, and low pressure in the swimmer's wake caused by eddies.

When a well-streamlined body moves at slow velocity, the boundary layers pass smoothly over the trailing surfaces and very little eddy formation occurs. In this case the pressure resistance will tend to zero and total hydrodynamic resistance will be determined predominantly by friction force. As the swimming velocity increases and the boundary layer around the body decreases in thickness, the effect of the skin friction becomes less and less important compared with the effect of the growing pressure gradient. Eddy formation increases and the point of the boundary layers' separation shifts closer to the front of the body. At near maximal swimming velocities it appears as if a swimmer is surrounded by a 'cloud' of eddies.

Table 9.1 Reynolds numbers and coefficients of form resistance for different body profiles. (After Clarys 1978.)

Body profile	Reynolds number $(Re)\ (= VL/v^*)$	Coefficient of form resistance (C_D)
Form of the droplet	10^4–10^6	0.05
Dolphin	7.5×10^4–7.0×10^7	0.05–0.08
Human body	6.6×10^5–3.5×10^6	0.58–1.04

$^*v = \mu/\rho$

The pressure resistance force changes as:

$$F_P = C_D(\rho V^2/2)S_M \qquad (9.5)$$

where S_M is the maximal cross-sectional area of the body interacting with the water flow, and C_D is the dimensionless coefficient of resistance.

Experimental studies (Karpovich 1933; Onoprienko 1968; Clarys 1978) showed that the form (the profile of the longitudinal section) of the body has the greatest impact upon pressure resistance. The impact of body form finds its manifestation in the magnitude of C_D. Therefore, the pressure resistance is also denoted as *form resistance*, and C_D as the *coefficient of form resistance*.

Fast-swimming fishes and sea mammals (e.g. dolphins) have a well-streamlined form (longitudinal contour) of the body. The body of a human with the same length-to-width ratio as a dolphin experiences much greater hydrodynamic resistance at the same speed. The reason is the existence of a large number of local *pressure resistance centres*—the head, shoulders, buttocks, knees, heels, etc. Clarys (1978) reported significant differences in C_D values for bodies with relatively equal length and cross-sectional area, but different hydrodynamic profiles (Table 9.1).

As form resistance increases with the square of the swimming velocity, its importance in competitive swimming is greater than skin friction, which increases linearly with swimming velocity. It follows from Eqn. 9.5 that the factors affecting the magnitude of form resistance during swimming at the same velocity are shape (C_D) and frontal cross-sectional area. Form resistance also depends upon body buoyancy: high body position relative to the water surface leads to a reduction of the cross-sectional area that is exposed to water flow during swimming.

How large the form drag is and how it may be reduced are questions of practical importance for coaches and swimmers. Sharp edges favour the formation of eddies, and thereby increase the drag. Deviations of a swimmer's body and head from a horizontal alignment as well as body actions that increase the angle of attack (body projection relative to the oncoming water flow) also cause an increase in form resistance and should be avoided. A swimmer is able to reduce form resistance by stretching and streamlining the body, choosing an optimal depth of leg kick, and synchronizing rotation of the hips and shoulders. The main concern for a swimmer is to have streamlining of the body in those phases of the swimming cycle that create maximal propulsive force. This will significantly increase the efficiency of pulling actions (Toussaint & Beek 1992; Maglischo 1993).

Impact of underwater torque upon pressure (form) resistance

Underwater torque is the result of the downward gravitational force and the upward buoyant force acting on the body at different points and thus inducing a couple or *torque*. The gravitational force acts through the body's centre of mass, while the buoyant force acts through the centre of buoyancy. By definition the centre of buoyancy is the centroid of the displaced volume of the water and is dependent on the distribution of the displaced volume of the fluid relative to the body. The resulting torque

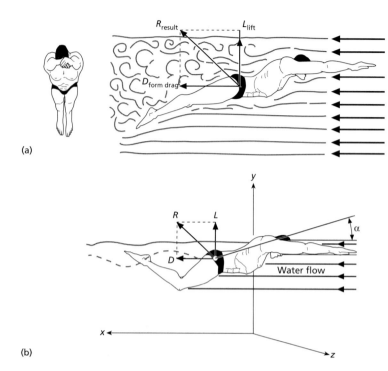

(a)

(b)

Fig. 9.1 The origins of normal (lift) and frontal (drag) components of resultant hydrodynamic resistance (R) due to the angle of attack (α) induced by: (a) underwater torque and (b) deviation of the body from horizontal alignment. D, drag; L, lift; R, resultant resistance; α, angle of attack.

will tend to align the centre of mass and centre of pressure resulting in an upright position in the water. During swimming this torque can influence the hydrodynamic resistance by changing the body orientation relative to the water flow. At zero velocity the swimmer assumes an upright position in the water, hence C_D has its maximal value. During swimming at low and moderate velocities the swimmer's body will adopt an inclined position. The angle between the longitudinal body axis and the velocity (flow) direction is called the *angle of attack* and denoted as α. Since the projection of the body in the direction of gliding/swimming increases with angle of attack it is accompanied by an increase of passive/active pressure resistance acting on the swimmer. The resulting hydrodynamic force has a *normal component* (lift) acting upwards at right angles to the flow/swimming direction, and a *drag force* acting in a direction opposite to the swimming velocity (Fig. 9.1).

With increased towing/swimming velocity the lift created by the oncoming flow raises the legs and lower body of the swimmer and thereby reduces the angle of attack and hence C_D (Alley 1952; Onoprienko 1968; Clarys 1979). When the body reaches a horizontal position, the lift sharply decreases and C_D stabilizes. Experimental studies detected three phases in C_D dynamics with increase of swimming velocity: (i) reduction of C_D due to decrease of the angle of attack; (ii) phase of stabilization; and (iii) increase of hydrodynamic coefficient C_D due to increased wave-making resistance at swimming (towing) velocities of $1.7–1.8 \text{ m} \cdot \text{s}^{-1}$ (Alley 1952; Counsilman 1955; Onoprienko 1968).

To estimate how the resistance increases due to the underwater torque in the glide position usually involves comparing two sets of measurements: one set is made during movement of the passive body in an artificial horizontal position, the other is made in a natural posture. The horizontal body position is created with the help of additional buoyancy. Onoprienko (1968) used for this purpose a set of small spherical floats with very small resistance,

Table 9.2 Impact of underwater torque on hydrodynamic resistance (F_D) during passive towing in streamlined glide position. (From Onoprienko 1968; adapted by Rumyantsev 1982.)

	Towing velocity (m · s⁻¹)			
	0.85	1.1	1.45	1.9
$F_D \pm SD$ (N)				
Towing without additional leg support	3.98 ± 0.48	4.99 ± 0.45	7.17 ± 0.76	13.64 ± 1.0
Towing with additional leg support	3.16 ± 0.27	4.46 ± 0.32	6.90 ± 0.72	13.48 ± 1.0
Difference (%)	$P < 0.01$	$P < 0.05$		

attached between the lower legs of the swimmer. Table 9.2 gives the values of resistance obtained during a towing experiment in the glide position on a water surface with and without additional buoyancy. The results indicate that a high hip position relative to the water surface is an important feature of a rational swimming technique.

One of the distinct biomechanical characteristics of competitive swimming strokes is the magnitude of the angle of attack. It is minimal and relatively constant in the front crawl, then increases progressively through the back crawl, butterfly and breaststroke. Both the butterfly and breaststroke are characterized by angles of attack that are permanently varying during the movement cycle. The angle of attack in these swimming strokes may be positive or negative (depending on whether the shoulder girdle is above or below the hips; see Fig. 9.2). With an increase of the angle of attack from 0 to 5° the hydrodynamic resistance (HDR) increases by up to 15%, while an angle of attack of 18° gives a 50% increase in HDR (Onoprienko 1968). Although intracyclic changes of the angle of attack are inevitable, swimmers should minimize the amplitude of the body's up-and-down movements (and thus minimize the S_M and C_D), especially during the main propulsive phase of the arm-pull. This will help to increase the maximal and average intracycle swimming velocity.

Wave-making resistance

Wave-making resistance is produced when a swimmer moves on or at a small depth under the surface.

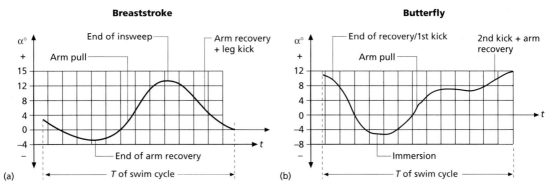

Fig. 9.2 Intra-cyclic change of the angle of attack in (a) breaststroke and (b) butterfly stroke. α, angle of attack; t, time; T, time of swim cycle. (Bulgakova & Makarenko 1996; adapted from Haljand et al. 1986.)

Part of the water displaced by the body along its trajectory moves up from a zone of high pressure to a zone of low pressure (above the non-disturbed water level). Thus prime wave forms. This process is accompanied by mechanical work done by the swimmer against gravity and against the inertia of an amount of water lifted above the surface. The force of wave-making resistance is proportional to the energy, contained within the front or prime wave generated by the body and may be calculated as (Rumyantsev 1982):

$$F_W = \rho(A^3/\lambda^2)(V \sin \alpha)^3 \cos \alpha \, \Delta t \qquad (9.6)$$

where ρ = water density, A = amplitude of the wave, λ = length of the wave, V = wave velocity (= swimming or towing velocity), Δt = time unit, and α = angle between the direction of general centre of mass (GCM) movement and the front of the prime wave.

According to Eqn. 9.6, the wave-making force is proportional to the cube of the swimming (towing) velocity, whereas the form (pressure) resistance increases with the square of the velocity. This means that the relative contribution of the wave-making resistance to the total hydrodynamic resistance becomes significant at near-maximal swimming velocities (Alley 1952; Gordon 1968; Onoprienko 1968) and may be an essential factor limiting increases in swimming speeds.

Two wave patterns are formed:
1 *divergent waves*, namely the 'stern wave' and the 'bow wave', which are pushed out by front and rear parts of the body; and
2 *transverse waves*, which are also formed at the front and rear portions of the body but move at right-angles to the direction of travel.

Parts of the body such as the shoulders and buttocks also generate waves during swimming, as do excessive horizontal and vertical movements of the head and upper body. The waves are visible evidence of energy losses resulting from movements of the body, which require that water is pushed out of the way. A characteristic feature of waves generated by a swimmer's body is that they travel at the same speed as the swimmer and their crest-to-crest length is equal to the distance covered by the swimmer per second. As swimming velocity increases, the crest-to-crest wavelength increases until the swimmer's *waterline length* is the same as the crest-to-crest length of his wave pattern (the point when L_{wave} = waterline length is called the *hull speed*, a term from shipbuilding introduced into sport swimming by Miller (1975)). At that velocity the swimmer is trapped in a self-created hole between crests of waves. The more effort that is applied, the deeper the hole and any further attempts to increase swimming speed simply make it impossible for the swimmer to 'climb out of the hole'. It follows from theoretical assumptions and analogies that it is not possible to travel on the water surface faster than 1 bodylength $\times$ s^{-1}. Even if the arm length is included in the waterline length, the theoretically estimated maximal swimming velocity V_{max} should vary (due to change in body posture) between 1.9 and 2.6 m $\cdot$ s^{-1} for individuals of height 1.95–2.00 m, and between 1.7 and 2.3 m $\cdot$ s^{-1} for individuals of height 1.75–1.85 m. Although unconfirmed by research, there is an opinion among specialists, supported by some sport statistics, that taller swimmers have an advantage over shorter ones in sprint events (Miller 1975; Counsilman 1977; Toussaint *et al.* 1988). This suggestion is based on the Froude number (Fn), a dimensionless criterion of wave-making:

$$Fn = V/\sqrt{(gL)} \qquad (9.7)$$

where V = swimming velocity, g = acceleration due to gravity, and L = swimmer height.

Since low values of Fn are associated with decreased wave-making resistance, an increase in height should result in decreases of Fn and wave-making resistance. Toussaint *et al.* (1990) showed that in children an increase of height from 1.52 to 1.69 m during a 2.5-year longitudinal study resulted in a decrease of Fn from 0.324 to 0.308 at a swimming velocity of 1.25 m $\cdot$ s^{-1} (Table 9.3). Since no significant difference in HDR was found between repeated measurements, Toussaint *et al.* supported the idea that increased pressure drag, caused by a 15% increase in the subjects' body cross-sectional area, was compensated by a decrease in wave-making resistance.

Table 9.3 Effect of a 2.5-year period of growth on different parameters in young swimmers ($N = 13$). (From Toussaint *et al.* 1990.)

	1985 value	±SD	1988 value	±SD	Change in value	±SD	Significance
Anthropometry							
Height (m)	1.52	0.06	1.69	0.08	0.17	0.05	$P < 0.001$
Weight (kg)	40.0	6.8	54.7	7.1	14.7	5.7	$P < 0.001$
Body c/sectional area, S_M (m²)	0.064	0.004	0.074	0.006	0.010	0.005	$P < 0.001$
Dimensionless form indices							
Length/width ratio	4.83	0.29	4.65	0.33	−0.18	0.34	NS
Length/depth ratio	9.35	3.57	39.4	3.04	2.97	3.73	$P < 0.05$
Length/thickness ratio	36.5	3.57	39.4	3.04	2.9	3.73	$P < 0.05$
Width/depth ratio	1.95	0.19	2.13	0.21	0.18	0.24	$P < 0.05$
Drag							
F_D at $V = 1.25$ m · s⁻¹ (N)	30.1	2.37	30.8	4.50	0.7	3.4	NS
Non-dimensional indices							
Reynolds number ($V = 1.25$ m · s⁻¹)	2.2×10^6	0.08×10^6	2.5×10^6	0.12×10^6	0.25×10^6	0.07×10^6	$P < 0.001$
Froude number ($V = 1.25$ m · s⁻¹)	0.324	0.007	0.308	0.006	−0.016	3.8×10^{-4}	$P < 0.001$
C_D ($V = 1.25$ m · s⁻¹)	0.64	0.069	0.54	0.077	−0.089	0.0058	$P < 0.001$
Performance data							
100 m time (s)	72.8	5.84	62.9	3.25	−9.9	3.1	$P < 0.001$
V_{max} (m · s⁻¹)	1.37	0.08	1.53	0.07	0.16	0.05	$P < 0.001$
F_{max} (N)	37.4	6.57	50.2	7.92	12.8	5.84	$P < 0.001$
P_{max} (W)	51.7	11.58	77.2	14.81	25.5	9.66	$P < 0.001$

The influence of depth of submersion upon resistance

If the body moves underwater and waves do not appear on the surface it means that the potential energy of water layers above the body is greater or equal to the energy of high flow pressure of water layers which are in contact with the body. Thus the minimal depth of gliding or swimming, when no waves appear on water surface—the *depth of wave equilibrium*—may be determined as:

$$h_p = V^2/2g \times C_w \qquad (9.8)$$

where V = body velocity, g = acceleration due to gravity, and C_w = non-dimensional wave-making coefficient. In cases where a swimmer may be affected by waves created by his opponents, h_p may be determined as *wave base level*—the depth at which wave energy can no longer affect the body:

$$h_p = \lambda/2 = V/2 \qquad (9.9)$$

where λ = length of the wave, which is equal to the swimming velocity. It seems that the depth at which the wave-making resistance is negligible lies between 0.7 and 1.2 m. When the body moves deeper than h_p body resistance does not change. If the depth of swimming (towing) is less than h_p, body movement through the water is accompanied by the formation of waves, which cause an increase in total hydrodynamic resistance. When part of the body is above the water surface, a reduced frontal area will create pressure resistance and friction becomes much less, but the wave-making resistance will sharply increase. The practical question which arises is whether the total HDR on the surface is greater than that during underwater swimming.

Since wave-making resistance changes with the cube of swimming speed, it becomes a sizeable component of total HDR at maximal speed. As gliding speed after a start and turns is much higher than the average racing speed and waves are not produced

Table 9.4 Relationship of hydrodynamic resistance measured during towing of swimmers using the same gliding postures on and under the water surface.

Authors	Towing connection type	Subjects (number and sex)	Depth of towing (m)	Towing velocity (m · s⁻¹)	Difference on/under surface (%)
Schramm (1959)	Flexible	$N = 2$, males	0.5	1.7	10.5
Ilyin (1961)	Flexible	$N = 1$, male	1	1.4	6
				1.8	4
Onoprienko (1968)	Flexible	$N = 1$, male	0.5	1.1	13
				1.9	9
Gordon (1968)	Flexible	$N = 15$, males	0.5	1.5	15
				1.9	10
Clarys et al. (1974)	Rigid	$N = 53$, males	0.5	1.5	−22
				1.9	−18

* Cited by Rumyantsev (1982).

during a deep glide, it is beneficial to reach and maintain this high gliding speed for a longer time using a leg kick only.

Results of experimental studies on the magnitude of hydrodynamic resistance experienced by swimmers on and under the water surface still remain controversial because of differences in design of towing devices and procedures (posture, depth of towing) employed (Table 9.4). Researchers who found resistance on the surface to be higher than that during underwater towing used flexible connections between the swimmer and the towing device. Such attachments provide higher stability of the body within the water flow during towing underwater than on the surface. This may account for the finding of greater resistance during surface towing than under water. Those authors who found opposite results (Clarys et al. 1978, 1979; Clarys & Jiskoot 1974) used towing devices with a rigid attachment to the swimmer. Thus identical posture and body orientation were provided for both underwater and surface towing.

Phenomenal results have been achieved by some outstanding performers in the backstroke and butterfly disciplines (e.g. D. Berkoff, I. Poliansky, D. Suzuki, D. Pankratov and M. Hyman), who covered up to 50–60% of the competitive distance underwater using only the butterfly kick on the front, back or side. Such performances provide strong grounds for

a re-evaluation of the ratio of hydrodynamic resistance on and under the water. Is underwater swimming really faster than swimming on the surface? Sport practice shows that swimming underwater using kick only *is at least no slower* than swimming on the surface using the full stroke. If one accepts the physiological data showing that the leg kick is much less efficient than the arm pull, it is possible that due to the absence of wave resistance the total hydrodynamic resistance during underwater swimming at high velocity is less than during swimming on the water surface. The record tables of fin swimming support this point of view. The competitive programme in fin swimming includes events both on the surface and underwater. The record times for underwater events are significantly faster than for surface swims (Table 9.5). One more interesting

Table 9.5 World fin swimming records in surface and underwater events.

Event	Surface (only 15 m dive)		Breathhold* or scuba	
	Males	Females	Males	Females
50 m	16.07	18.58	14.83*	16.28*
100 m	36.44	40.96	33.65	36.26
400 m	3.04.58	3.20.37	2.52.65	3.01.84
800 m	6.34.18	6.59.44	6.08.29	6.30.14

fact is that nuclear submarines, using the same engines both on and under the surface, achieve their maximum velocity when submerged (the speed record belongs to Russian submarines—44.5 knots or 82.5 km · h⁻¹). When surfaced, their maximum speed is less than half of that when submerged! This is despite the fact that the friction, form and appendage resistance of submarines is much higher under water than on the surface.

The latest Federation Internationale Natation Amateur (FINA) rules for competitive swimming limit the distance which swimmers are allowed to cover under water to 15 m. However, the nature of the resistance experienced by swimmers on and under the surface requires further investigation since swimmers can still travel significant distances under water after the start and turns.

Total hydrodynamic resistance

It is commonly recognized that total hydrodynamic resistance of the body during passive towing is a sum of its friction, wave-making and form components:

$$F_{total} = F_{friction} + F_{wave-making} + F_{form} \qquad (9.10)$$

The formulas and values used by Rumyantsev (1982) to calculate total hydrodynamic resistance for a swimmer's body are given in Table 9.6. For a flow velocity of 2.0 m · s⁻¹ these components have approximately the following magnitudes:

$F_{form} = 93.5$ N
$F_{friction} = 0.05$ N
$F_{wave-making} = 5$ N

The total hydrodynamic resistance is 98.55 N. These calculations cannot be accepted as precise, but they help to assess the relative contribution of friction, wave-making and form resistance to total resistance at different towing and gliding velocities. Thus the share of wave-making resistance may reach its maximum at a water velocity of 2.0 m · s⁻¹ and above. At lower velocities wave-making resistance is less significant. Calculations show that friction resistance is less than 1–2% of pressure resistance. Since the friction acts along the body surface, it acts most efficiently in laminar flow; transition to turbulent flow is accompanied by predominance of frontal drag forces over friction. The human body is not a perfect hydrodynamic body. It creates a big area of turbulence in the surrounding boundary layers and in the wake at higher towing velocities. This decreases the impact of friction resistance upon total HDR. Nevertheless, some authors still support a prevailing role of friction in total body resistance during swimming. As a rule such conclusions are made on the grounds of results of correlation analysis between total hydrodynamic resistance and body surface area (Karpovich 1933; Onoprienko 1967a, 1968). The fact that the overwhelming majority of studies found a second-degree relationship between swimming (towing) velocity and total hydrodynamic resistance lends

Table 9.6 Formulas and values (ranges) of variables for calculation of contribution of different kinds of resistance into total resistance. (From Rumyantsev 1982.)

Pressure (form) resistance (F_p)	Friction resistance (F_{fr})	Wave-making resistance (F_w)
$F_p = C_x \rho V^2 S_M /2$	$F_{fr} = \mu S_{fr}(dV/dZ)$	$F_w = \rho A^3/\lambda^2 (V \sin \alpha)^3 \cos \alpha$
$C_{DP} = 0.85$ (0.5–1.20)	$\mu = 1 \times 10^{-3}$ N · s · m⁻¹	$A = 0.75$ m (0.05–0.1 m)
$S_M = 0.055$ m² (0.91–0.1 m²)	$S_{fr} = 1.75$ m² (1–2.5 m²)	$\lambda = 4A$ (3–5A)
$\rho = 1000$ kg · m⁻³	$dV = V = 2$ m · s⁻¹	$\alpha = 32.5°$ (20–45°)
$V = 2$ m · s⁻¹	$dZ = 0.55$ m (0.01–0.1m)	$V = 2.0$ m · s⁻¹
		$\rho = 1000$ m³

A = amplitude of wave; C_{DP} = drag coefficient; dV = difference between velocity of water layers; dZ = difference in thickness of water layers; S_{fr} = wetted body surface area; S_M = maximal cross-sectional area of body; V = velocity; α = angle between direction of GCM movement and front of prime wave; λ = length of wave; μ = coefficient of dynamic viscosity; ρ = water density.

support to the predominant role of form (pressure) resistance in swimming. If frictional resistance were predominant, a linear relationship would be expected. Miyashita and Tsunoda (1978) found that the total hydrodynamic resistance of well-trained swimmers is much less than that of novice swimmers despite the fact that the latter had as much as a two times smaller body surface area. It is likely that experienced swimmers may assume a more stream-lined position in the water and thus reduce cross-sectional area and form resistance. (Since the data were obtained in a water flume it seems possible that skilled swimmers can control and reduce the turbulence in the body's wake and pressure gradient by minor leg movements.) In this case an increase of frictional resistance due to a greater surface area does not play a significant role, while a decrease in pressure (frontal) resistance by stream-lining of the body causes reduction of total HDR. The better streamlining is attributed to longer bodies since the point of boundary layer separation is closer to the rear thereby creating less eddy forma-tion than with shorter bodies.

Studies on the influence of body posture and orientation in relation to flow on the magnitude of HDR provide evidence that the form resistance is a major component of total hydrodynamic resistance. It has been shown experimentally (Counsilman 1955; Schramm 1959; Onoprienko 1968; Chernyaev & Maltsan 1974) that the most streamlined posture is the gliding posture in which the body and legs are outstretched, the toes are pointed, the arms are stretched over the head and hands topping one another, and the ears are pressed by the shoulders. Thus the head is efficiently streamlined by the arms to receive the oncoming water flow. Even minor deviations of the head, arms and legs from a stream-lined position during the glide after starts and turns may result in a considerable increase of resistance (Fig. 9.3).

Hydrodynamic resistance during towing on the side or back in a glide position seems to be higher compared with the front glide position (Counsil-man 1955—for towing velocity 0.6–2.2 m · s^{-1}; Clarys & Jiskoot 1974—for $V = 1.9$ m · s^{-1}). These results support the opinion that body form (not body surface area) is a decisive factor in determining the magnitude of the total resistance.

The resistance force changes due to deviation from a streamlined posture and horizontal align-ment. Thus an increase of the angle of attack due to a backward bending in the waist or lifting of the head leads to an increase in resistance of 26, 20 and 12% at $V = 1.1$, 1.45 and 1.9 m · s^{-1} respectively (Onoprienko 1968). At higher velocities the impact of body flexion upon resistance is reduced. As a

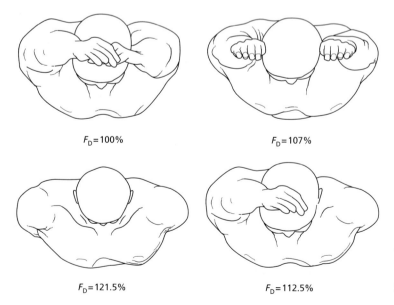

$F_D=100\%$

$F_D=107\%$

$F_D=121.5\%$

$F_D=112.5\%$

Fig. 9.3 Impact of body form upon hydrodynamic resistance during underwater towing (the magnitude of total resistance in glide position conditionally accepted as 100%). (Adapted from Bulgakova & Makarenko 1996.)

Table 9.7 The impact of body posture on passive drag during towing. (From Onoprienko 1968; Makarenko 1996.)

Posture	% Difference in total HDR compared to streamlined glide position
Arms trailing along the body	+37 ($V = 1.1–1.45$ m · s^{-1}) +28 ($V = 1.9$ m · s^{-1})
Arms stretched forwards with hands at shoulder width	+7.7 ($V = 1.1–1.8$ m · s^{-1}) +9.5 ($V = 1.9$ m · s^{-1})
Feet at shoulder width, flexed at $\alpha = 90°$	+26 ($V = 1.9$ m · s^{-1})
One arm along the body, the other stretched forwards	+12.5 ($V = 2.0$ m · s^{-1})

result of the greater lift the body is moved to a higher position relative to the water surface and this tends to counteract the increased resistance. During active swimming a relatively high head position to facilitate breathing should be maintained. It was found that even minor deviations of the head position from a horizontal alignment at flow velocities in the range 1.7–2 m · s^{-1} caused increases of total HDR from 2 to 7% up to 30–40% (Onoprienko 1968; Miyashita & Tsunoda 1978). Table 9.7 demonstrates the impact of swimmer posture upon total HDR (Onoprienko 1968; Chernyaev & Maltsan 1974; Rumyantsev 1982; Makarenko 1996). Analysis of the influence of body build and composition upon hydrodynamic resistance revealed that the most informative characteristics of passive drag are the area of maximal cross-section of the body, and the circumferences of the head and shoulders (Table 9.7). This again emphasizes the importance of pressure resistance in swimming. As a rule cross-sectional dimensions demonstrate a higher correlation with passive resistance than longitudinal ones.

A positive and significant correlation between passive resistance and body weight and volume has been found by Clarys (1978) and others. These characteristics correlate closely with cross-sectional area ($r = 0.9$). Some authors found significant correlation between body surface area and resistance (Clarys *et al.* 1974), while others (Miyashita & Tsunoda 1978)

found no correlation between passive resistance and any anthropometric variable.

In shipbuilding, proportional indexes are widely used to characterize the hydrodynamic qualities of the hull. Numerous attempts have been made to find anthropometric substitutes for hull indexes. Clarys (1978), Miyashita and Tsunoda (1978), Onoprienko (1968) and Safarian (1968) studied the relationship between passive drag and anthropometric indexes of proportionality. They found very few significant ($P < 0.05$) correlation coefficients between total HDR and proportions of the human body. All these authors concluded that anthropometric indexes are useless for characterizing the hydrodynamic qualities of the human body (Table 9.8). In comparison with the relatively smooth ship contours, the human body has a great number of local pressure points. The bony hillocks raised over the surface of the human body (such as knee joints and heel bones) cause increased eddies and thus increase the resistance during swimming. This may distort the influence of body proportions upon total HDR. Skin fat may have some positive impact on hydrodynamic qualities of the human body since it improves buoyancy and smoothness of the body profile. It is presumed that human skin and the subcutaneous fat layer reduce turbulence of the boundary layers and thus decrease resistance. An experiment in which a rigid life-size human body model and a female swimmer with well-developed subcutaneous fat were towed revealed no difference in HDR at a velocity of 1.5 m · s^{-1}. However, at a towing velocity of 1.9 m · s^{-1} the swimmer had 6% less resistance than her own body's model (Onoprienko 1968). Actually, the differences in thickness of skin fat among top swimmers may be too small for this factor to assume significance in reducing the total hydrodynamic force during swimming. It is well known that the swimsuit should be manufactured from smooth, thin, waterproof fabric that tightly fits the body surface. Schramm (1959) found that the resistance of a swimmer wearing a swimsuit two sizes too big increased significantly during towing ($V = 1.7$ m · s^{-1}). Onoprienko (1968) found resistance increased by 3% ($V = 2.0$ m · s^{-1}) during towing of a female swimmer wearing a woollen swimsuit compared with a silk swimsuit (in addition to the

Table 9.8 Correlation of anthropometric characteristics and hydrodynamic resistance.

Author	Clarys (1978)	Safarian (1968)	Onoprienko (1968)	Miyashita & Tsunoda (1978)
Method of towing	Electromechanical with mobile carriage	Electromechanical with stationary platform	Electromechanical with stationary platform	Water flume
Subjects' details	$N = 44$ males Height = 180.9 (± 6.4) cm mg = 73.8 ± 7.3	$N = 77$ males Height = 176.7 (± 6.2) cm mg = 70.8 ± 8.1	$N = 92$ males $N = 67$ females	$N = 8$ females Height = 153.7 cm mg = 46.3 ± 10
Posture	Front glide	Front glide	Front glide	Front glide
Towing velocity (m · s^{-1})	1.5–2.0	1.8	1.9	0.8–1.6
Chest circumference	$P < 0.05$ $r = 0.48$–0.60	$P < 0.05$ $r = 0.84$	–	–
Body surface area	–	–	$P < 0.05$	$P < 0.05$
Weight	$P < 0.05$	$P < 0.05$ 0.85	– –	$P < 0.05$ 0.57
Height	–	$P < 0.05$ 0.62	–	$P < 0.05$ 0.53
Body volume	$P < 0.05$	–	–	–

mg = body weight.

greater frictional resistance, a woollen swimsuit trails a large mass of water behind the swimmer).

Evaluation of passive resistance

It is extremely difficult to determine the frictional, wave-making and/or eddy resistance because the swimmer's propulsion along the water surface is regarded as a collection of numerous travelling pressure points (Miyashita & Tsunoda 1978). Therefore, researchers usually measure the resultant total water resistance of the swimmer in relation to velocity.

The evaluation of passive hydrodynamic resistance is based upon measurements made during towing, or by exposing a fixed body to a water flow. The following conditions must be fulfilled during such experiments.

1 During towing the swimmer should remain in a steady, immobile posture. Even minor changes in posture or in orientation towards water flow may cause significant changes in resistance; the type of towing connection (rigid or flexible connection) has a big impact on the stability of body posture (Table 9.4).

2 The towing force should act parallel to water surface.

3 The towing device should provide uniform velocity throughout the course of towing.

During acceleration and deceleration the gauge will record the inertia of the swimmer's mass as well as the resistance.

Towing devices of the inertial type, where the potential energy of a falling body of fixed weight converts into a towing force, do not provide a constant uniform velocity of towing. The most reliable and precise method of measuring passive drag is by using an electromechanical towing device. This consists of an electric motor of varying power which is used with precise control systems to create the necessary uniform towing velocity. The stationary platform in a water tank and a mobile carriage are used for such experiments.

During measurement of hydrodynamic resistance in a swimming flume the swimmer's body is exposed to an artificial oncoming water flow created by a propeller (Holmer 1974; Miyashita & Tsunoda 1978; Gordon *et al.* 1985). The swimmer is connected to the gauge (on the deck) by a cable. The method is very simple and permits the posture of swimmer to be observed. The absolute values of resistance obtained using this method are slightly lower than values obtained during towing in water tanks. This is due to the effect of lift on the swimmer's body at high flow velocities.

Since different methods and subjects are used in different studies a great variety of data on hydrodynamic resistance is found in the references. Of more practical value may be relative characteristics, i.e. change of resistance with the change of flow velocity, and comparison of resistance magnitudes in the same studies but using different body positions.

Active hydrodynamic resistance (active drag)

If passive drag is the amount of resistance that a human body experiences during towing through stationary water or exposure to mobile water flow in a water tank, in an unchanging posture, the *active drag* is that associated with swimming motions.

While passive drag certainly depends upon body size and shape, active drag has been regarded as a function of the movements as well as a function of the anthropometry and mechanical properties of a rigid core body. Experimental studies based on different measuring techniques are in accord that the relationship between active drag and swimming velocity is quadratical (Di Prampero *et al.* 1974; Clarys 1979; Toussaint *et al.* 1988; Kolmogorov & Duplisheva 1992). This means that the pressure component is the main contributor to active resistance during swimming. The magnitude of active resistance may be established as:

$$F_{DA} = KV^2 \text{ or}$$

$$F_{DA} = \tfrac{1}{2}C_{DA}\rho V^2 A \tag{9.11}$$

where C_{DA} is the coefficient of active drag and A is an anthropometric variable.

Research still leaves open the nature of the relation between active drag and anthropometric characteristics. Clarys (1979) examined the drag of self-propelling bodies and found significantly higher values than those recorded for passively towed bodies. He concluded that neither body shape nor its composition nor skin surface area influences the active drag. It may be considered a product of systematic changes in shape and size (i.e. swimming technique) and is determined by the nature of water flow around the body.

More recently, Huijing *et al.* (1988) found a high correlation between active drag and maximal body cross-section area ($r = 0.87$). Toussaint *et al.* (1988) also related the difference in active drag between male ($F_{DA} = 30V^2$) and female ($F_{DA} = 24V^2$) swimmers to a larger body cross-section in males (0.091 m^2 vs. 0.075 m^2). The greatest difference in active drag between males and females was found for a swimming velocity of 1.0 m · s^{-1}. It reduced sharply with increased swimming velocity. Thus the contribution of anthropometric characteristics (and, hence, the contribution of passive drag) to active resistance decreases at high swimming velocities.

In a 2.5-year longitudinal study of active drag in age group swimmers Toussaint *et al.* (1990) did not find any increase of active drag despite marked increases in body cross-sectional area and skin surface. Although it had been presumed that an increase of both parameters would be accompanied by increases in pressure (form), friction and total resistance, this did not happen.

The most interesting scientific fact is that no correlation has been found between the magnitudes of active and passive drag (Clarys 1978; Kolmogorov & Duplisheva 1992). Moreover, Toussaint *et al.* (1988) and Kolmogorov *et al.* (1997) found the magnitudes of active drag to be 2–3 times smaller than values reported by other authors, who used nondirect measurements. Also, their values were much lower than could be expected if the active drag represents a simple sum of passive drag components and additional wave-making and turbulence resistance caused by a swimmer's movements. In separate individual cases no significant difference between the magnitudes of passive and active drag was detected despite obvious differences in water flow turbulence. Elite swimmers demonstrated a much smaller active drag than average swimmers over the range of swimming velocities.

Measurement of active drag

DIRECT METHODS

Early measurements of active drag (AD) involved indirect calculations based upon changes in oxygen consumption with additional drag loaded onto the swimmer (Di Prampero *et al.* 1974; Clarys 1979). AD found in these studies was much higher than passive drag (PD).

More recently, methods for the direct measurement of active drag have been introduced, namely the 'Measuring Active Drag system' (MAD; Toussaint *et al.* 1988) and the velocity perturbation method (Kolmogorov & Duplisheva 1992). Both the MAD system and velocity perturbation method show that the better technique of elite swimmers gives them much less AD than average swimmers over a range of swimming velocities. Thus the reduction of AD should become a target for stroke development in swimming.

Measuring active drag (MAD) system
(Toussaint *et al.* 1988, 1990)

The MAD system is based on measuring the mean propulsive force *in a swimming-like activity* (this system allows measurement of propulsive force during front crawl swimming only). The swimmer pushes off against grips, which are attached to a tube located 0.8 m under the water surface (Fig. 9.4). The tube is fixed to a force transducer. Thus the force a swimmer applies during pushoff is registered. Since at constant swimming velocity the measured mean propulsive force, F_P, equals the mean active drag force, F_{DA}, this method provides the mean active drag on the swimmer. The authors found that the mean propulsive force (using arm pull only) at a swimming velocity of 1.48 m · s^{-1} appeared to be 53.2 ± 5.8 N, which is 2–3 times smaller than values of active drag reported by other authors. It is, however, in agreement with values reported for passive drag on a towed swimmer.

It was found that F_{DA} in a velocity range of 1.0–1.8 m · s^{-1} is related to the swimming velocity, *V*, raised to the power 2.12 ± 0.20 in males and 2.28 ± 0.35 in females.

The greatest differences in drag force and coefficient of drag between males and females were found for a swimming velocity of 1.0 m · s^{-1}:

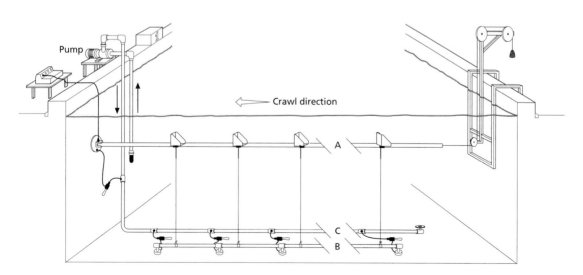

Fig. 9.4 The measuring active drag (MAD) system: general view. (From Hollander *et al.* 1986.)

drag, 28.9 ± 5.1 N and 20.4 ± 1.9 N; drag coefficient, 0.64 ± 0.09 and 0.54 ± 0.07, respectively. These differences become less at higher swimming velocities.

Velocity perturbation method

The velocity perturbation method involves changing the maximal swimming velocity using added drag provided by a hydrodynamic body of known resistance towed by the swimmer (Fig. 9.5). Swimmers performed two maximal-velocity swims of 30 m with and without the hydrodynamic body (HB). The HB was placed at such a distance behind the swimmer that the water was no longer turbu-lent. This critical distance proved to be 3.5–4.5 L (see Fig. 9.5).

Swimming speed, V, and resistance force, F, were measured during both swims. The assumption has been made by authors that the power output (Pto_1) during swimming without the HB is equal to the power output delivered when swimming with the HB (Pto_2): hence, $Pto_1 = Pto_2$. However, not all power generated in swimming can be used to overcome drag. Part of it will be transferred in the form of a flow kinetic energy (P_k). Hence, the equations below are approximations (Toussaint *et al.* 1990). According to Kolmogorov & Duplisheva (1992) the observed difference in velocity (V_2 vs. V_1) should be

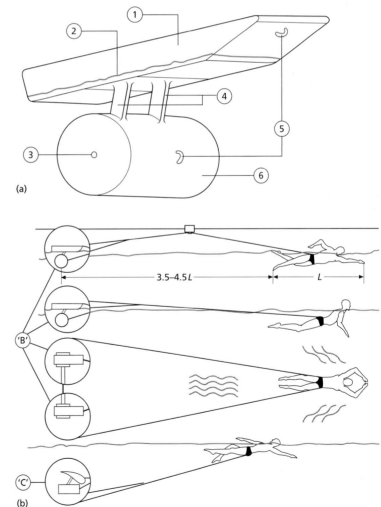

Fig. 9.5 The velocity perturbation method. (a) The structure of the additional hydrodynamic body: 1, carrying body (made of foamplast); 2, water line; 3, a hole for water; 4, kniveposts; 5, fixing hook for ropes; 6, hydrodynamic cylinder (made of light metal). (b) The attachment of an additional hydrodynamic body ('B' and 'C') to the swimmer's body. *L*, body length. (Reprinted from Kolmogorov & Duplisheva (1992), pp. 311–318, with permission from Elsevier Science.)

due to the effect of the added resistance. Hence, in the free swimming conditions power output during free swimming (non-resisted), $Pto_1 = F_{r1}V_1$ and in the added resistance conditions power output during swimming with hydrodynamic body attached to swimmer, $Pto_2 = F_{r2}V_2$, where F_{r1} and F_{r2} are active drag values. Since

$F_{r1} = \frac{1}{2}C_D\rho SV_1^2$ and

$F_{r2} = \frac{1}{2}C_D\rho SV_2^2 + F_b$

and since $P_{to1} = P_{to2}$, $F_{r1}V_1 = F_{r2}V_2$, so it follows that:

$\frac{1}{2}C_D\rho SV_1^3 = \frac{1}{2}C_D\rho SV_2^3 + F_b$ and

$C_D = F_bV_2/\frac{1}{2}\rho S(V_1^3 - V_2^3)$

Substitution of C_D in this equation gives:

$F_{r1} = F_bV_2V_1^2/V_1^3 - V_2^3$.

Since F_b is known the assessment of the magnitude of active drag becomes a very simple procedure of speed measurement during unloaded and loaded swims.

The Kolmogorov–Duplisheva method allows the measurement of active drag during swimming using all four competitive strokes, while the MAD system and indirect methods are applicable only to the front crawl. The estimated error of the method is no higher than 6–8%.

Kolmogorov and Duplisheva made the following conclusions.

1 C_{DA} and C_{DP} do not correlate with each other.
2 A comparison of C_{DA} between male and female revealed no statistically significant differences.
3 Swimming strokes were ranked in terms of resistance (from low to high): freestyle < backstroke (BK) and butterfly (Fly) < breaststroke (BR).
4 Young swimmers have a lower AD than adults.
5 The magnitudes of F_{DA} for men's freestyle were much lower than those predicted previously via indirect methods (Di Prampero 1974; Issurin 1977; Clarys 1979:) or obtained in studies using the MAD system (Toussaint et al. 1988, 1992).
6 Elite swimmers display a biomechanically efficient swimming technique that is characterized by low F_{DA} at maximum V.

The results were in agreement with the ideas of Clarys (1979) and Toussaint et al. (1988) that stroke technique is more important in reducing AD than body composition.

In passive towing C_{DP} depends upon the shape of the swimmer's body and features of the skin and hair. In active swimming C_{DA} quantitatively reflects the interaction of different parts of the moving body with the 'passive' flow of fluid. With the increase in V there is an increase of turbulence in water flow passing the swimmer's body that facilitates the increase in C_{DA}.

INDIRECT METHODS OF ACTIVE DRAG MEASUREMENTS

Bioenergetic methods

These methods are based on re-evaluation of the relationship between the magnitude of towing velocity, additional force and relevant metabolic changes (Di Prampero et al. 1974). During active swimming known horizontal forces are applied to the swimmer by a towing device. The swimmer thus has to generate additional propulsive forces, since the total propulsive force equals the algebraic difference of his own body drag and the known force applied to his body. It is assumed that the concomitant mechanical power (force × velocity) the swimmer has to expend is reflected in the variations of the oxygen intake (Vo_2), which can be measured, and that extrapolation of the linear relationship of active drag and Vo_2 can be used to estimate active body drag. The swimmer is connected to the towing device and performs 5–6 stages of continuous swimming at constant velocity. The design of the towing device allows an additional towing force to be applied along the swimming direction (unloading) as well as in the opposite direction (loading). Each swim is performed in a given time, necessary to establish functional characteristics in a steady state. The theoretical line of regression is constructed, based on the experimental data, and processed using the method of least squares. The regression line is extrapolated towards the relative 'zero' of the physiological parameter. The value of additional

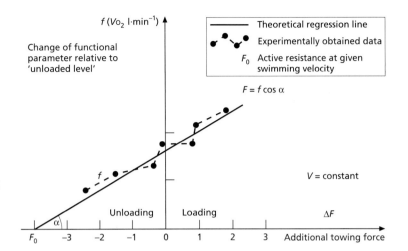

Fig. 9.6 Extrapolation of the active drag based on the relationship between the change in O$_2$ intake and additional towing force during swimming at constant velocity (method of Di Prampero *et al*. 1974). (Adapted from Rumyantsev 1982.)

unloading (F_0) at the point of crossing with the axis of abscissas (axis of ΔF), according to the authors of this method (Di Prampero *et al*. 1974), represents the value of the hydrodynamic resistance which the swimmer overcomes during swimming at a given speed (Fig. 9.6).

Non-direct bioenergetic methods have the following requirements.

1 Swimming should be performed with minimal fluctuations of intracyclic velocity (otherwise the swimmer will have to overcome a water resistance which is significantly higher than the one calculated).

2 The functional criteria chosen should reflect the total increase in energy expenditure caused by the change in the working regimen (intensity of swimming).

3 To provide a more precise evaluation of active resistance, functional changes should be measured during steady-state swimming (one of the limitations of non-direct methods is that they allow the measurements of active drag only for the 'aerobic' range of swimming velocities and are inappropriate for near-maximal and maximal swimming velocities).

A well-argued critique of the bioenergetic methods of determining active drag is presented by Toussaint *et al*. (1992). They showed that the overall work performed by the swimmer is the sum of: (i)

the work to overcome drag; and (ii) the work performed to accelerate a given mass of water backwards, which is due to the fact that in swimming a fixed pushoff point is not available. The propulsive force is generated by pushing against the water and is equal to the impulse ($m \times v$) of the mass of water pushed away. During the pushoff, the energy ($1/2mv^2$) is transferred from the swimmer to the water (Toussaint & Beek 1992).

Hence, measured variations in V_{O_2} reflect not only the concomitant mechanical power due to the added drag, but also the additional power that is dissipated during the production of the kinetic energy in the water that is pushed away. When variations in V_{O_2} are exceptionally attributed to variations in active drag, the active drag is significantly overestimated. Furthermore, it is questionable to use regression equations outside the range in which they were established (Toussaint *et al*. 1990).

Modelling (transitional) method

This method consists of modelling intermediate boundary postures of the phases of swimming motions (swimming cycle) and is based on the evaluation of hydrodynamic coefficients (C_{DP}) for different postures at different towing velocities. Then, during active swimming synchronized video recording and recording of intracyclic velocity are

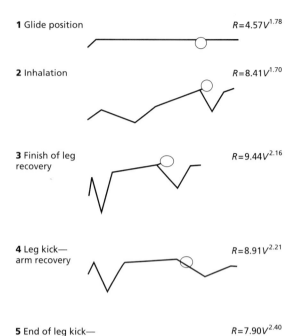

1 Glide position $R = 4.57V^{1.78}$

2 Inhalation $R = 8.41V^{1.70}$

3 Finish of leg recovery $R = 9.44V^{2.16}$

4 Leg kick— arm recovery $R = 8.91V^{2.21}$

5 End of leg kick— beginning of arm pull $R = 7.90V^{2.40}$

Fig. 9.7 The modelling (transitional) method: the relationship between intermediate (boundary) body positions and momentary values of hydrodynamic resistance during breaststroke swimming. R = magnitudes of resistance calculated for distinct boundary postures. (Data from Kent & Atha 1975.)

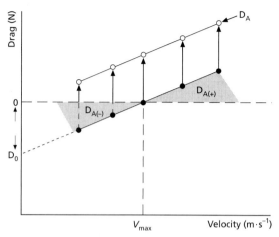

Fig. 9.8 Determination of active drag by extrapolation of the drag ($D_{A(+)}$) and added propulsion ($D_{A(-)}$). (Reprinted from Clarys *et al.* (1985), pp. 11–24, with permission from Elsevier Science.)

performed. The values of the swimming velocity for selected boundary postures are estimated. When the duration and C_{DP} of every phase of the swimming cycle are established, it is possible to calculate the active resistance for a complete swimming cycle (Kent & Atha 1975). The accuracy of this method will depend upon the number of selected boundary postures (Fig. 9.7), but in any case, the resulting magnitude of the hydrodynamic force will differ significantly from its real value. One of the reasons is that when the body moves with acceleration, the real active drag it experiences differs from the values established for uniform swimming velocities. This difference is a result of the inertial force of the added mass of the water acting on the body dur-

ing acceleration. In order to overcome this inertia the swimmer has to expend a significant quantity of energy. In accordance with Newton's Second Law, the full hydrodynamic resistance experienced by the body when it moves with acceleration may be subdivided into two forces:

$$F_{DA} = F_{DP} + \Delta m\, a \qquad (9.12)$$

where F_D = full hydrodynamic resistance, F_{DP} = resistance created by the interaction of the body with oncoming water flow (passive resistance), Δm = added mass of the water, a = acceleration, and hence ma = inertia force of the added water mass. The added mass of the water is determined by the formula:

$$F_t - F_{DP} = (m + \Delta m)a \qquad (9.13)$$

where F_t = towing force, m = body mass of the swimmer, and Δm = added mass of water. Issurin (1977) determined the influence of intracyclic velocity fluctuations and the inertia forces of body mass and added water mass, $(m + \Delta m)a$, on hydrodynamic resistance. He calculated instantaneous values of active resistance and average resistance for half of the cycle (for a front crawl) and found that the values of resistance were 1.5–2 times greater than during passive towing at the same average swimming velocity. This method certainly over-estimates the value of the active drag since the calculation includes the entire magnitude of the passive resistance.

Method of active drag measurement during towed swimming with constant velocity

Clarys *et al.* (1979) used a relatively simple method of measurement of active drag. The swimmer was towed with uniform velocity while performing front crawl swimming movements. The gauge recorded both negative force, $D_{A(-)}$ (due to propulsive force), and positive towing force, $D_{A(+)}$ (the

added drag). The recording was made throughout a range of swimming speeds including the maximal velocity of active swimming. On the graph depicting the relationship 'towing velocity' vs. 'additional towing force' the experimental regression line was extrapolated to 'zero velocity' (Fig. 9.8). The value of the additional towing force at the $x = 0$ point (at zero velocity) added to the original regression line of additional towing force represents the active drag force during swimming at all velocities. The active drag magnitudes obtained with the use of this method are much higher than the magnitude of passive drag in a gliding position and significantly higher than active drag values obtained with the use of direct measurements.

References

Alley, L.E. (1952) An analysis of water resistance and propulsion in swimming crawl stroke. *Research Quarterly* **23**, 253–270.

Bulgakova, N.Zh. & Makarenko, L.P. (eds) (1996) *Sport Swimming*. Physical Culture, Education and Science (Russian State Academy of Physical Education), Moscow.

Chernyaev, E.G. & Maltsan, K. (1974) The investigation of several aspects of front crawl swimming technique. *Plavanie* **2**, 33–36. FiS, Moscow.

Clarys, J.P. (1978) Relationship of human body form to passive and active hydro-dynamic drag. In: *Biomechanics VI-B* (eds E. Asmussen & K. Jorgensen), pp. 120–125. University Park Press, Baltimore.

Clarys, J.P. (1979) Human morphology and hydrodynamics. In *Swimming III* (eds J. Terauds & E.W. Bedingfield), pp. 3–43. University Park Press, Baltimore.

Clarys, J.P. (1985) Hydrodynamics and electromyography: ergonomics aspects in aquatics. *Applied Ergonomics* **16(1)**, 11–24.

Clarys, J.P., Jiskoot, J., Rijken, H. & Brouwer, P.J. (1974) Total resistance in water and its relationship to body form. *Biomechanics IV* (eds R.C. Nelson & C.A. Morehouse), pp. 187–196. University Park Press, Baltimore.

Counsilman, J. (1977) *Competitive Swimming Manual for Coaches and Swimmers*. Counsilman Co, Bloomington, Indiana.

Counsilman, J.E. (1955) Forces in swimming: two types of crawl stroke. *Research Quarterly* **26** (2), 127–139.

Di Prampero, P.E., Pendergast, D.R., Wilson, C.W. & Renny, D.W. (1974) Energetics of swimming in man. *Journal of Applied Physiology* **37**, 1–5.

Gordon, S.M. (1968) Swimming technique (ed. N.A. Butovich). Fizkultura i Sport, Moscow.

Gordon, S., Dmitriev, D. & Chebotareva, I.V. (1985) Dependency of coefficient of resistance on low velocity, age and anthropometric indicators. *Theory and Practice of Physical Culture* **4**, 11–13.

Haljand, R., Tamp, T. & Kaal, R. (1986) *The Models of Swimming Strokes and Methods of Perfection and Control*, 2nd edn. Tallinn Pedagogic Institute, Tallinn.

Hollander, A., De Groot, G., van Ingen Schenau, G.J. & Toussaint, H.M. (1986) Measurement of active drag forces during swimming. *Journal of Sport Sciences* **4**, 21–30. Taylor & Francis Ltd., London: *http://www.tandf.co.uk/journals/*

Holmer, I. (1974) Physiology of swimming man. *Acta Physiologica Scandinavica*, Supplement 407.

Huijing, P.A., Toussaint, H.M., Mackay, R., Vervoorn, K., Clarys, J.P. & de Groot, G. (1988) Active drag related to body dimensions. In: *Swimming Science V*, (eds B.E. Ungerechts, K. Reischle & K. Wilke) pp. 109–113. Human Kinetics Publishers, Champaign, Illinois.

Issurin, V.B. (1977) Evaluation of hydro-dynamic resistance and propelling

forces in swimming. *Theory and Practice of Physical Culture* **9**, 20–21.

Karpovich, P.V. (1933) Water resistance in swimming. *Research Quarterly* **4**, 21–28.

Kent, M.R. & Atha, J. (1975) Intracycle kinematics and body configuration changes in breaststroke. In: *Swimming II* (eds J.P. Clarys & J. Lewillie), pp. 125–129. University Park Press, Baltimore.

Kolmogorov, S. & Duplisheva, A. (1992) Active drag, useful mechanical power output and hydrodynamic force coefficient in different swimming strokes at maximal velocity. *Journal of Biomechanics* **25**, 311–318.

Kolmogorov, S., Rumyantseva, O., Gordon, B. & Cappaert, J. (1997) Hydrodynamic characteristics of competitive swimmers of different genders and performance levels. *Journal of Applied Biomechanics* **13**, 88–97.

Maglischo, E.W. (1993) *Swimming Even Faster*. Mayfield Publishing, Mountain View, California.

Makarenko, L.P. (1996) Fundamentals of swimming technique. In: *Sport Swimming* (eds N. Zh. Bulgakova & L.P. Makarenko), pp. 40–85. Physical Culture Education & Science, Moscow.

Miller, D.I. (1975) Biomechanics of swimming (eds J.H. Wilmore & J.F. Keogh) pp. 219–248. *Exercise and Sport Sciences Reviews*. Academic Press, New York.

Miyashita, M. & Tsunoda, R. (1978) Water resistance in relation to body size. In: *Swimming Medicine IV* (eds B. Eriksson

& B. Firberg), pp. 395–401. University Park Press, Baltimore.

Onoprienko, B.I. (1967a) The influence of anthropometrical data on the swimmer's hydrodynamics. *Theory and Practice of Physical Culture* **4**, 18–23.

Onoprienko, B.I. (1967b) Use of modelling for water resistance to swimmer's body movement research. *Theory and Practice of Physical Culture* **9**, 8–9.

Onoprienko, B.I. (1968) Relationship of hydrodynamic drag and swimmer's body position. *Theory and Practice of Physical Culture* **9**, 12–15.

Rumyantsev, V.A. (1981) *Biomechanics of Swimming*. Central State Institute of

Physical Culture, Moscow.

Rumyantsev, V.A. (1982) *Biomechanics of Sport Swimming*. Central State Institute of Physcial Culture, Moscow.

Safarian, I.G. (1968) Hydrodynamic characteristics of the crawl. *Theory and Practice of Physical Education, USSR* **11**, 18–21.

Schramm, E. (1959) Die Abhangigkeit der Leistungen im Kraulschwimmen vom Kraft-Widerstand verhaltnis. *Wissenschaft Zeitschrift der Deutsche Hochschule Von Korperkultur* 161–180. Leipzig.

Sharp, R. & Costill, D. (1989) Influence of body hair removal on physiological responses during breaststroke swim-

ming. *Medicine and Science in Sports and Exercise* **21**, 576–580.

Toussaint, H.M. & Beek, P.J. (1992) Biomechanics of competitive front crawl swimming. *Sports Medicine* **13**, 8–24.

Toussaint, H.M., De Groot, G., Savelberg, H.H.C.M. *et al.* (1988) Active drag related to velocity in male and female swimmers. *Journal of Biomechanics* **21**, 435–438.

Toussaint, H.M., de Looze, M., van Rossem, B., Leijdekkers, M. & Dignum, H. (1990) The effect of growth on drag in young swimmers. *Journal of Sport Biomechanics* **6**, 18–28.

Chapter 10

Propulsive Forces in Swimming

A.R. VORONTSOV AND V.A. RUMYANTSEV

The nature of propulsive forces in swimming

The aquatic locomotion of a human is a result of the interaction of body segments with the water. On land a human uses the ground surface as a solid and immobile support. Effort is applied against the ground and the ground's reaction transmitted to the body makes the body move. During swimming a swimmer creates the 'immobile support' in the mobile fluid medium, using its density and viscosity, and overcomes opposing resistive forces.

The nature of swimming is that it occurs in water, which resists the swimmer's motion through it. The hydrodynamic resistance (HDR) manifests itself as: (i) the force that slows down and stops the swimmer's motion through the water (see Chapter 9); and (ii) as a *hydrodynamic reaction force* to the movements of the swimmer's limbs through the water. This hydrodynamic reaction force (RF) is the source of propulsion for the swimmer's locomotion.

The swimming velocity depends upon the magnitude and direction of the RF (or *total pulling force*) created by movements of the swimmer's working segments, and the magnitude of the active hydrodynamic resistance. The RF created by the swimmer constantly changes its value and direction during the cycle of swimming motions due to the alteration of working phases and recovery phases. Correspondingly, there are changes in the *effective pulling force*—a component of the resulting RF equal to the projection of the RF vector to the direction of motion. The value of active HDR also changes continuously within the swimming cycle.

The interaction within the swimming cycle of these two horizontal forces (effective pulling force and active hydrodynamic resistance), as a rule not equal at any one moment, may be described by the equation of set non-stationary activity of a swimmer's body in fluid flow (Toussaint *et al.* 1998; Cappaert 1998; Kolmogorov & Lyapin 1998):

$$F_{P(effective)}(t) - F_{DA(frontal)}(t) = (m_0 + \Delta m)dv_{(CM)}/dt \tag{10.1}$$

where $F_{P(effective)}(t)$ = momentary value of total effective propulsive force developed by the swimmer's propelling segments (result of working movements of arms, legs and body); $F_{DA(frontal)}(t)$ = momentary value of frontal component of hydrodynamic resistance affecting the swimmer's body; m_0 = body mass; Δm = added water mass of an inertial origin; and $dv_{(CM)}/dt$ = momentary acceleration of body centre mass.

It follows from Eqn. 10.1 that when $F_{Propulsive} = F_{Drag}$ the swimmer moves with uniform velocity, when $F_P > F_D$ the swimmer accelerates, and when $F_P < F_D$ the swimmer decelerates.

To generate high propulsive force during swimming is not an easy task. Not all components of the resultant RF contribute to an effective RF (*pulling force*) due to deviation of the vector of the reaction force from the swimming direction at certain moments of pulling actions (Schleihauf 1979; Rumyantsev 1982; Cappaert & Rushall 1994). At the same time a substantial part of the mechanical energy of the pulling actions is lost in transfer of kinetic energy to the water mass which the swimmer uses as a support. As a result, only a portion of the

205

mechanical work performed by a swimmer is used effectively to overcome HDR. As we shall demonstrate later in this chapter, it is not enough simply to press against the water as hard as possible. Instead, the aim should be to adroitly change the direction of movement throughout the course of the pull so that the vector of the resulting RF remains as close to the swimming direction as possible.

Biodynamic details of pulling movements

The propulsive forces in swimming originate from muscular contractions (*muscle draught*). When the *biokinematic chains* 'shoulder-forearm-hand' and 'hip-low leg-foot' begin to move they encounter hydrodynamic resistance. When the muscle draught balances the external hydrodynamic RF force and the latter balances the HDR, the body general centre of mass (GCM) begins to accelerate in the direction of locomotion. Thus the hydrodynamic reaction force transforms into a propulsive (pulling) force.

Since the pulling movements are rotational movements of extremities in the joints the system of forces may be expressed by the following equation (the displacement of the axis of rotation conditionally accepted as zero—see Fig. 10.1):

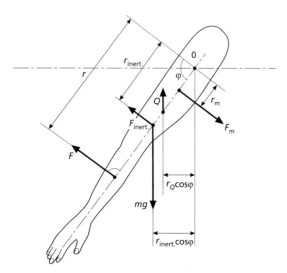

Fig. 10.1 Forces and their levers (relative to the axis of rotation, 0); illustration to Eqn. 10.1.

$$F_m r_m = I \bar{\omega} + Fr - mg r_{inertia} \cos \phi + Q r_Q \cos \phi \quad (10.2)$$

where F_m = resultant force of muscle draught (N); r_m = lever of the resultant muscle force (m); I = moment of the inertia of the arm (kg · m²); F = resultant hydrodynamic reaction force (N); r = lever of the RF (m); mg = gravity (N); $r_{inertia}$ = radius of the arm inertia force (m); Q = hydrostatic force (N); r_Q = lever of the hydrostatic force (m); ϕ = relative angular position of the arm (degrees); and $\bar{\omega}$ = angular acceleration of the arm (± degrees per second per second; may be positive as well as negative).

If we assume that during underwater pull the gravitational and hydrodynamic forces are equal, opposite and colinear the equation is simplified:

$$F_m r_m = I \bar{\omega} + Fr \quad (10.3)$$

It follows from this equation that the reduction of length of the levers of external forces (*inertia* and *hydrodynamic reaction*) by bending the arm at the elbow joint leads to increase of the dynamic and time-spatial characteristics of the arm pull and requires smaller muscle torque. Miller (1975) represented Eqn. 10.2 in the following form:

$$F_m r_m \approx m r_{inertia}^2 \bar{\omega} + C_D r^3 \omega^2 \quad (10.4)$$

where $F_m r_m$ = torque of muscular force; ω = angular acceleration of the arm (or arm segment); m = arm (arm segment) mass (kg); and $C_D r^3 \omega^2$ = torque of the hydrodynamic reaction created by the arm (or arm segment).

If it is assumed that the hand velocity is roughly proportional to the angular velocity in the shoulder multiplied by the distance between hand and shoulder (= r), it follows that the torque of hydrodynamic RF varies as a cube of the length of its lever while the torque of inertia varies as the square of $r_{inertia}$. Miller (1975) supposed that corresponding changes in pulling technique (decrease of $r_{inertia}$ and r and increase of ω) would improve the efficiency of the pulling action. Muscular draught is applied to the shoulder close to the axis of rotation (Fig. 10.2) and the lever of muscle force is small. The resultant RF is applied to the distal portion of the arm and its lever is several-fold longer in respect to the lever of muscle draught. By arm flexion a swimmer changes the ratio of forces applied to opposite ends of the

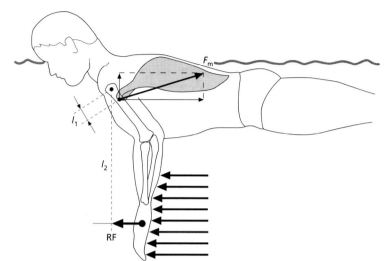

Fig. 10.2 The formation of the muscle draught torque and RF torque during arm pull:

$$I \cdot \omega + RF \cdot l_2 = |-F_{muscle} \cdot l_1|$$

where ω = angular acceleration.

bone lever and is able to balance greater RF torque by smaller muscle torque when the arm is bent. In freestyle and butterfly the elite swimmers demonstrate maximal elbow bending (the angle between shoulder and forearm) in the middle (90–120°) portion of the pull.

As may be seen from Eqn. 10.4, pulling patterns with consecutive flexion–extension of the arm have an obvious biomechanical and hydrodynamic advantage over pulling patterns without movements in the elbow and wrist joints.

1 Movement of the elbow joint allows a selective increase in the angular velocity and acceleration of the hand and forearm without involving the most massive segment of the arm, i.e. the shoulder. Pulling patterns with elbow bending require much less muscle torque to create an equal RF and an effective pulling force than arm pulls without elbow bending.

2 Bending the elbow and wrist joints provides efficient space orientation of the propelling segments (Counsilman 1968; Makarenko 1975; Schleihauf 1979). It increases the working surface area of the pulling segments (projection of these segments to the direction of the pull) and makes it possible to steer the propulsive forces in the direction of swimming.

3 The strength of the arm bent at the elbow joint is significantly higher than that of a straight arm. Measurements of maximal isometric strength in boundary postures, imitating the distinct phases of arm pull, shows that bent arm pull creates on average a 20% greater force than 'straight arm pull' (Butovich & Chudovsky 1968; Vorontsov 1981). It is possible that by bending the elbow, the direction of torque in the shoulder joint changes. This could imply that more muscles can deliver work in the shoulder joint (Toussaint *et al.* 1998).

4 In the course of the arm pull the movements of the arm joints are coordinated in a pattern which provides consecutive achievement of maximal angular velocities in different joints. This avoids excessive loading of the arm muscles, which work in a more economical way. The catch phase is performed by simultaneous extension in the shoulder and flexion in the elbow/wrist joint. At the beginning of the backward pull (*downsweep*) the hand and forearm accelerate due to arm bending in the elbow joint, while the shoulder moves with low angular velocity and gradually passes from a streamlined position to a resistive position.

During the *insweep* the shoulder begins to accelerate its rotation while the angle between the hand and forearm remains relatively constant. Thus the swimmer uses hand and forearm as a single blade. In the main phase, as the shoulder rotation decelerates, the acceleration of the forearm at the elbow joint begins. The forearm performs a fast extension of the elbow joint (*push*), during which the hand slows down its rotation and attains its optimal space orientation. This is the moment when the swimmer's arm delivers the highest magnitude of RF and effective pulling force. After this working part of the pull is completed the exit of the arm from the water is performed by movement at the shoulder joint.

5 The pulling pattern with alternate elbow bending and extension provides a gradual increase of hydrodynamic reaction force and its propulsive component in the initial part of the pull, stabilization in the middle part, and a sharp increase to the maximum force at the end of the pull. In pulling patterns without movements in the elbow and wrist joints the hydrodynamic force decreases significantly after the arm passes the middle of the pull.

Concepts of propulsion in swimming

Theory of the straight 'oar-like' arm pull (OLP)

This theory stems from striving to convert 100% of the hydrodynamic reaction force into effective propulsive force. It follows from Newton's Third Law of Motion that the most efficient types of pull are those employing a straight movement of the hand (and forearm) along the direction of swimming motion under the mid-line axis of the body, with the arm–forearm pitch close to 90° relative to the pulling direction (Fig. 10.3a,b). Thus during the oar-like pull the propulsive force is created almost entirely by pressure (form) resistance. The magnitude of propulsive force (RF) may be derived from Eqn. 9.1: $RF = \frac{1}{2}\rho V^2 C_D S$, where ρ = water density, V = speed of the water flow interacting with the body, C_D = the hydrodynamic coefficient of the propelling segment and S = the surface area of the propelling segment.

For several decades the role of frontal (form) resistance was deemed paramount in describing the origination of propulsive forces in swimming (Cureton 1930; Kiphut 1942; Silvia 1970). The principles of Newtonian mechanics (action-reaction principle, principle of conservation of momentum, principle of proportionality) were employed to prove that straightline arm pull ('oar-like pull'— OLP) is the most efficient, as the direction of the vector of hydrodynamic RF created by the swimmer's

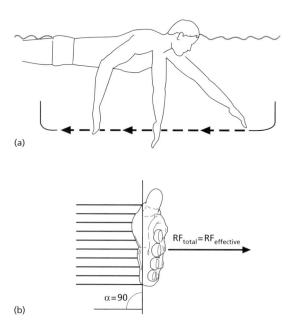

(b)

Fig. 10.3 (a) Oar-like pull (side view). (b) Contribution of the frontal drag force (RF_{total}) on the hand into effective RF.

arm coincides with the direction of swimming motion. It was assumed that in OLP the effort which the swimmer applies to the water maximally transforms into forward propulsion when the direction of the vector of resultant RF maximally coincides with the direction of swimming ($RF_{effective} = RF_{total}$). Any deviation of the swimmer's arms during pull from a straightline direction was interpreted as a technical error or as a movement to compensate for deficiencies in the structure of the human motor apparatus, which is not perfect for aquatic locomotion. This view still has its adherents among scientists and coaches (see, e.g., Rushall et al. 1998).

The lift and lift-and-drag theories: curvilinear (propeller-like) arm pull (PLP)

The theory of OLP presumes that the swimmer should maintain the maximal surface area of the propelling segments ($C_D \cdot S$), and constantly increase the velocity of the pull and pressure created by these segments during the pulling motion. Actually the hand velocity and pulling effort (RF)

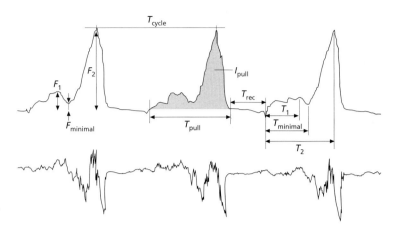

Fig. 10.4 Typical intracycle dynamic of pressure force on swimmer's hand during front crawl.

demonstrates two or three large pulses, with stabilization and even a transient decrease in the middle part of the arm pull. Figure 10.4 shows the typical intracyclic changes of the pressure developed by a swimmer's hand during the front crawl. Such intracyclic pressure dynamics bring into question the importance of the frontal reaction force as the sole or main propulsive force in aquatic locomotion.

The introduction of objective methods of research and biomechanical analysis in the late 1960s and early 1970s revealed significant deviations of the hand trajectory in both vertical and transverse planes from the 'optimal' direction of locomotion in elite swimmers (Fig. 10.5a). These deviations need to be explained.

Opponents of the straight pull used as an argument the principle of 'immobile support', which presumes that efficient pulling actions employ complex trajectories of working movements so that at every point of the pull the working segments of the arms and legs interact with standing, immobile water. As soon as a swimmer begins to apply force against the water the latter starts to move in the direction of the hand motion, leading to a decreased velocity difference between hand and water and decreased efficiency of the pulling action. Therefore, in order to create high RF (to 'find' efficient *supportive reaction*), the pulling segments should interact at every point of the working movement with standing, immobile water. This condition is satisfied when pulling actions are performed not exactly linearly

backwards, but employ a complex curvilinear trajectory. If one considers swimming movements in the orthogonal coordinate system (Fig. 10.5b), it appears that during pulling actions the working segments of the arms and legs accomplish movements not only straight backwards along the x-axis, but also across the transverse (z-y) and vertical (x-y) planes. During the working phase of swimming motions the arm segments interact with three-dimensional (3-D) water flow at some angle of attack and change their leading edge 2–3 times (depending on the swimming stroke). Belokovsky (1971) showed that in synchronized swimming the effective pulling force and high swimming velocity (e.g. 16–17 s for a 25-m swim) may be achieved by using so-called 'standard' figure 8-like sculling patterns without any significant backward displacement of the swimmer's hands. The magnitude of the total and effective propulsive force in this case depends upon the pitch of the hands, the working trajectory, and the velocity of transverse hand movements.

Counsilman (1969, 1971), using an analysis of underwater movies, found that world-class swimmers perform arm pulls as sculling movements with very complex curvilinear trajectories in 3-D space. In these pulling patterns the hand and forearm perform significant vertical and transverse movements and continuously change the direction of the pull and their pitch (the angle of attack and leading edge) relative to the water flow. Counsilman concluded that it is virtually impossible to find

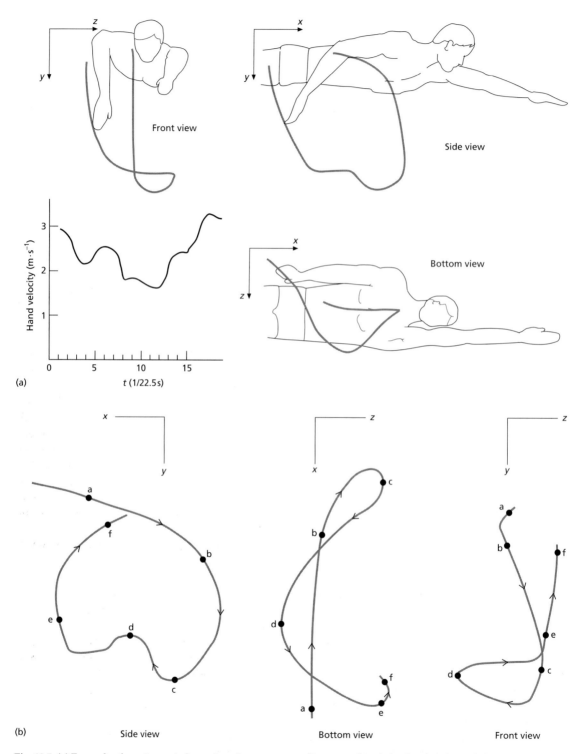

Fig. 10.5 (a) Example of a swimmer's fingertip trajectory pattern (front crawl) and absolute hand speed date.
(b) Trajectory of the hand relative to the system of orthogonal coordinates in front crawl arm pull. (Adapted from Schleihauf 1979.)

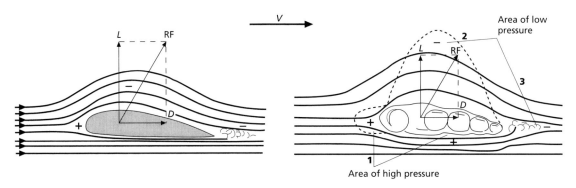

Fig. 10.6 Bernoulli's principle: origin of hydrodynamic lift on (*left*) a hydrofoil and (*right*) the hand (according to Reischle 1979). (1), area of stagnant water—high pressure; (2), area of low pressure above the hand; (3), area of turbulence (low pressure) in the wake of the hand.

instances when the hand and forearm are disposed to the water with an angle of attack exactly 90° to the pulling direction. He made an assumption that the major contributor to human locomotion in water is the hydrodynamic lift force (normal component of resulting hydrodynamic reaction), which originates when the hand and forearm move at an angle of attack to the water flow (to pulling direction). In this case both segments interact with water flow as a hydrofoil.

Counsilman cited Bernoulli's principle to explain the nature of propulsive forces in swimming (Fig. 10.6). According to this principle the hydrodynamic lift originates as the result of the difference between water flow velocities on the upper and lower surfaces of the hand (and forearm). Counsilman estimated that the hydrodynamic profile of the human hand creates a significant lift force. The properties of the hand and forearm as hydrofoils were also studied by Schleihauf (1974), Bartels and Adrian (1974), Reischle (1979), Onoprienko (1981) and Rumyantsev (1982), all of whom shared the opinion that hydrodynamic lift makes a significant contribution to swimming propulsion. Issurin and Kostyuk (1978) found that during swimming at maximal velocity backward displacement of the hand (the projection of its trajectory on the x-axis) comprises only 25% of the length of its absolute trajectory. The average velocity of backward displacement of the hand was found to be less than the average forward velocity of body motion. At the

same time the absolute hand velocity relative to the water flow achieved 3–4 m · s^{-1}. By using transverse and vertical sculling movements, swimmers achieve a high magnitude of lift to create high resulting RF without significant displacement of water mass backwards, and prolong the duration of action of the propulsive force. These theoretical speculations and experimental data formed the basis of the theory of curvilinear, propeller-like pulling patterns (PLP).

Three-dimensional analysis of the absolute movements of limb segments and the core body in relation to orthogonal coordinates has allowed an understanding of the hydrodynamic nature and complexity of propelling forces (Schleihauf 1974, 1979; Wood 1979; Cappaert 1993, 1998). This analysis showed that in sport swimming no examples could be found of pulling patterns in which exclusively the frontal (pressure) or normal (lift) component of hydrodynamic reaction was used to create propelling force.

Propulsive forces are created by contributions of both normal and frontal components of hydrodynamic reaction. The relative contributions of drag and lift forces to a swimmer's propulsion vary significantly between distinct phases and moments, between individuals, and between swimming strokes. By changing the pitch of the hand it is possible to steer the resultant propulsive force in the direction of swimming.

Both drag and lift forces can be derived using the following equations of hydrodynamics:

$F_D = \frac{1}{2}\rho V^2 C_D S$ (see Eqn. 9.1)

$L = \frac{1}{2}\rho V^2 C_L S$ (10.5)

where L = lift force, C_L = coefficient of lift of the propelling segment, S = surface area of the propelling segment, and V = absolute velocity of the propelling segment relative to water flow. It follows from Eqn. 10.5 that to create high total and effective pulling force the following conditions must be satisfied.

1 There should be a high velocity of interaction of the propelling segments with water flow (both frontal and lift forces are proportional to the square of the propelling segment's velocity).

2 There should be optimal hydrodynamic orientation (pitch) of the segments relative to the water flow (selective maximization of C_D and C_L due to the continuously changing direction of the pull).

3 There should be optimal balance between the 'size' of the segment's projection on the pulling trajectory and the 'wing' surface area creating lift.

4 The pulling trajectory should have optimal amplitude and direction.

Counsilman (1977), influenced by the studies of Schleihauf, also came to the conclusion that both drag and lift forces are equally important in creating the effective propulsive force. Thus originated the *lift and drag theory* of swimming propulsion. The results of Schleihauf's studies on the relationship of hydrodynamic drag and lift forces developed by the biokinematic pair 'arm–forearm' facilitated a better understanding of human aquatic locomotion and were used as the basis for subdividing arm pulls into four phases: downsweep, insweep, backsweep and upsweep.

The vortex theory and the complex mechanism theory of swimming propulsion

The vortex theory is widely used for the description and analysis of swimming in fish, and was introduced into sport swimming by Colwin (1984, 1992), who supported his theoretical speculations on vortex theory by some video data obtained in sport swimming. He proposed that part of the kinetic energy lost by swimmers to the water mass could be reabsorbed into pulling action from water vortices.

More recently Toussaint *et al.* (1998) expressed the opinion that neither drag nor lift theories give a complete explanation of the mechanism of pulling, and supported this by successful experiments on visualization of water flow around the swimmer's arm. They assumed that since the pulling segments of arms and legs move in a quasi-steady water flow, the vortex theory may explain better the mechanism of action of the propulsive force. This is especially true for transitional periods of the pull, when the hand and forearm change sharply the direction (leading edge) and velocity of the pull. The mechanism of how the starting vortex and bound vortex (circulation) facilitate the pressure differential and thus increase propulsive force is shown in Fig. 10.7 (the so-called condition of Zhoukovsky).

The latest studies in aerodynamics have disproved the Bernoulli principle as an explanation of lift. This principle assumes equal transit time for particles over and under the aerofoil. In fact, the upper-surface transit time is *always less* than that below (Denker 1998). The generally accepted theory taught that the wing begins to produce lift as result of a 'starting vortex', which is formed behind the trailing edge as the wing moves forward. This vortex causes circulation to appear around the wing. With this circulation superimposed on passing flow, the upper-surface air velocity becomes greater than that below. The flaw in this explanation is that there are no known physical principles to explain how the starting vortex can cause circulation. All that is known is that a starting vortex really does occur, the above-wing flow does have a greater velocity, and the magnitude of the lift force is much greater than would follow from Bernoulli's principle—even a flat aerofoil can create effective lift under certain conditions.

Experiments in water tanks confirm that both lift and drag forces occur when hand and forearm casts are exposed to water flow or are moved relative to standing water (Schleihauf 1974, 1979; Grinev 1977), and both these forces contribute to propulsion in aquatic locomotion. In practice, it is of little concern exactly what is the reason of the lift, and which theory is most accurate.

Recently, the most widely accepted theory of swimming propulsion is the *lift-and-drag theory* of

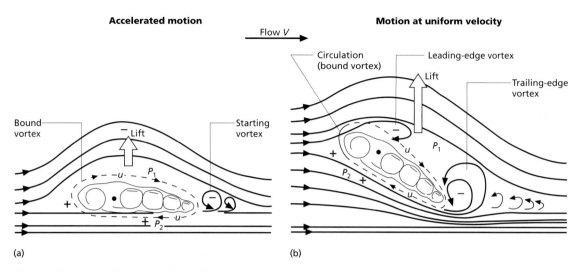

Fig. 10.7 The Vortex Theory: circulation (bound vortex) around the hand and the system of vortices behind the rear surface of the hand create lift (condition of Zhoukovsky). Flow velocity above the 'wing': $V_1 = V - u$. Flow velocity below the 'wing': $V_2 = V + u$. Pressure differential: $P = P_2 - P_1 = 1/2\ (V_1^2 - V_2^2) = 2Vu$ (where u = flow velocity in bound vortex).

propeller-like pull (PLP). Hence, until a better theory of aquatic propulsion is developed, we would like to focus on the lift-and-drag concept in order to discuss the following topics:
• under what conditions does the hydrodynamic reaction force originate on working segments?
• what is the potential of arm and leg segments to create propelling forces? and
• what are the factors determining the efficiency of pulling actions? etc.

Hydrodynamic potential of arm segments

As mentioned above, propulsive forces created by the swimmer are the result of the interaction of arm and leg segments with the water flow during pulling movements. These propulsive forces by their nature are forces of hydrodynamic resistance. The ratio of forces created by distinct segments of limbs is determined as:

$$F_{i+1}/F_i = S_{i+1}\ C_{i+1}\ V_{i+1}^2/S_i\ C_i\ V_i^2 \qquad (10.6)$$

where F_i and F_{i+1} = hydrodynamic forces (N) of segments i and $i + 1$; S_i and S_{i+1} = frontal surface area (m²) of segments i and $i + 1$; C_i and C_{i+1} = non-

dimensional drag coefficients of given segments; and V_i and V_{i+1} = velocities of segments' interaction with water flow. The shoulder has the least $S \times C$ product and least propulsive potential. The forearm and hand have approximately equal $S \times C$ products since the smaller support area of the hand is compensated by a greater drag coefficient C_{Dhand} (Butovich & Chudovsky 1968; Bagrash *et al.* 1973).

A decisive factor in determining the relationship of hydrodynamic forces created by the arm segments is the velocity of their interaction with water flow. The difference in angular and linear velocity of arm segments relative to the axis of the shoulder joint determines the difference in absolute velocity of the segments' interaction with the water flow. Thus it determines the magnitude of total RF created by each arm segment.

The angular and linear velocity increases from shoulder to hand proportionally with the increase in the radius of rotation. Butovich and Chudovsky (1968) and Makarenko (1975) showed that the average intra-cyclic linear velocity of the shoulder and RF created by the shoulder are negligible. Moreover, at some points in the pulling action the shoulder creates a drag to the forward motion. Due

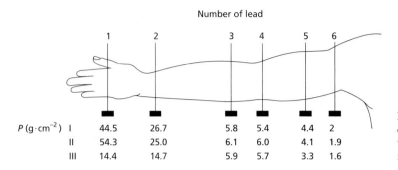

Number of lead

P (g·cm^{-2})						
I	44.5	26.7	5.8	5.4	4.4	2
II	54.3	25.0	6.1	6.0	4.1	1.9
III	14.4	14.7	5.9	5.7	3.3	1.6

Fig. 10.8 Location of the tensioleads on a swimmer's arm and maximal values of the pressure. (Adapted from Rumyantsev 1984.)

to active movements in the elbow and wrist joints the forearm and hand have a significant advantage over the shoulder in terms of angular and linear velocity. Thus only the forearm and hand of a swimmer create significant hydrodynamic reaction forces (i.e. propulsive force).

Miller (1975), using a mathematical model of the front crawl arm pull with bending of the elbow, found that the ratio of hydrodynamic forces of hand and forearm is about 2.5 : 1. Since she used a model which did not include hand movement at the wrist joint, the hand and forearm were assumed to have the same angle of attack relative to the water flow. In reality a swimmer uses minor hand movements at the wrist joint to give the hand the most efficient position (Schleihauf 1979). Thus it may be assumed that the ratio of hydrodynamic forces created by hand and forearm should be greater than the above value.

Bagrash *et al.* (1973), using tensiometry, measured hydrodynamic pressure on distinct arm segments during front crawl swimming (46 male well-trained swimmers). The experiment included:
1 tethered swimming using straight arm pull;
2 tethered swimming using pull pattern with elbow bending; and
3 'natural' swimming.
Figure 10.8 depicts the location of pressure leads and corresponding magnitudes of maximal hydrodynamic pressure during tethered and free swimming (averaged for 20 strokes).

Multiplying the maximal pressure developed by a segment (for hand, readings of lead 1; for forearm, mean value of leads 2 and 3; for shoulder, mean

value of leads 4–6) by the surface area of a segment and corresponding *relative* drag coefficients it is possible to obtain the maximal *relative* hydrodynamic forces of arm segments. The magnitudes of drag coefficients at an angle of attack of 90° were, respectively: for hand 1.0, forearm 0.7, shoulder 0.6 (data obtained during exposure of plaster cast of arm segments to water flow in the water tank; Butovich & Chudovsky 1968).

Table 10.1 gives the values of hydrodynamic forces after correction (Rumyantsev 1982). These measurements show that in conditions of 'natural' swimming (III) the hand creates about 70–75% of the total hydrodynamic force of the arm. A further 20% or so is created by the distal half of the forearm. (N.B. These results were obtained for 'flat' flow using arm casts exposed to water flow at a 90° angle of attack and the sole reaction force acting on the arm segments is frontal (form) resistance.) The conclusion may thus be made that the major propelling

Table 10.1 Maximal intracyclic hydrodynamic force of arm segments during front crawl swimming. (From Bagrash *et al.* 1973; adapted by Rumyantsev 1982.)

Arm segment	S (cm^2)	Relative C_x	F—I (N)	F—II (N)	F—III (N)
Hand	151	1.0	65.8	79.6	61.3
Forearm	221	0.7	24.1	23.6	15.6
Shoulder	217	0.6	5.0	5.1	4.4

C_x = drag coefficient. F—I = force during tethered swimming using straight-arm pull. F—II = force during tethered swimming using elbow bending. F—III = force during 'natural' swimming. S = surface area.

forces during swimming are generated by the hand and distal half of the forearm. It means that in analysing hydrodynamic forces we can neglect any force produced by the shoulder (Schleihauf 1979; Wood 1979). Schleihauf (1979) determined the effective propulsive force delivered by arm segments at a swimming speed of 1.66 m · s^{-1}. The average propulsive force delivered by the hand was 48 N, and the average effective forearm propulsive force was 24 N.

Drag and lift during different phases of pulling actions

Effect of form and orientation of arm segments on hydrodynamic forces

Studies performed in water tanks using casts of the hand with differently shaped palms and finger positions (Counsilman 1968; Makarenko 1975; Onoprienko 1981) show that the most effective combinations for creating a high hydrodynamic reaction are (Fig. 10.9):

1 flat palm with fingers and thumb held together;
2 flat palm with thumb apart; and
3 flat palm with fingers and thumb held slightly apart.

Forms 1 and 2 are more effective for those phases where the hand moves at sharp angles of attack to the pulling direction and works as a hydrofoil. Onoprienko (1981) stressed the important role of the abducted thumb for fixing the hand at the wrist joint and increasing the rigidity of the hand. Form 3 has the advantage for phases where the hand moves relatively straight backwards at an angle of attack > 60° (an increase of the frontal hydrodynamic force despite a decrease of C_{Dx} when the fingers are slightly apart may be attributed to the greater

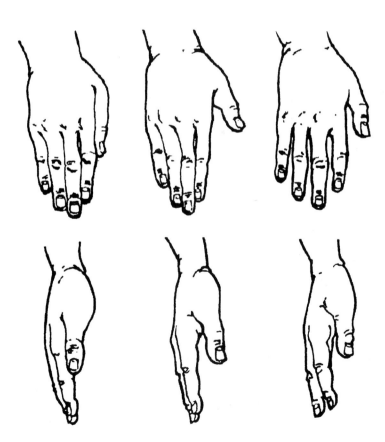

Fig. 10.9 The most efficient hydrodynamic forms of the hand. (From Makarenko 1996.)

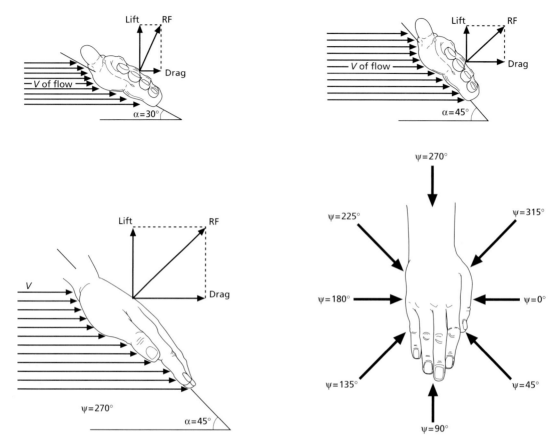

Fig. 10.10 Sweepback angles and angles of attack of the hand.

supporting surface area). Analysis of underwater movies and video recordings (Counsilman 1968, 1977; Haljand 1984; Haljand *et al.* 1986) shows that expert swimmers generally perform pulling actions with some spreading of the fingers. The reason for this is still unknown. It may be that any advantage in hydrodynamic reaction force when the fingers are held tightly together in a strong water flow is cancelled out by the excessive energy spent in keeping the fingers together.

The orientation (*pitch*) of the arm–forearm relative to the 3-D flow is an important factor in determining the ratio of drag and lift forces, the total magnitude of the RF and the effective pulling force. Schleihauf (1974, 1979) exposed plaster casts of the hand to water flow in a tank to analyse the influence

of the pitch of propelling segments on the magnitude of hydrodynamic forces. He considered the arm–forearm model in terms of the characteristics of an aerofoil, namely the angle of attack (α) and *sweepback angle* (ψ; French *tangage*). For a swimmer the angle of attack is the angle formed by the inclination of the propelling surface (arm and leg segments) to the direction of the pull, while sweepback angle defines the leading edge of the propelling segment.

Figure 10.10 depicts the angles of attack and sweepback angles of the hand (arrows show the direction of flow). Analysis of the forces and hydrodynamic (drag and lift) coefficients used a system of coordinates where the *x*-axis related to the flow direction.

Schleihauf (1979) introduces the *lift-to-drag index* to assess the predominant contribution of these two forces in the momentary value of the resultant RF:

$$L/F_D = \tfrac{1}{2}\rho C_{Dy}V^2S / \tfrac{1}{2}\rho C_{Dx}V^2S$$
$$= C_{Dy}/C_{Dx} \qquad (10.7)$$

where C_{Dy} = momentary value of coefficient of lift of the propelling segment, and C_{Dx} = momentary value of the drag coefficient.

This formula may be used to determine the lift and drag ratio in resultant RF for distinct phases of the arm pull and for the entire pull. If the value of the index > 1, then lift predominates; if < 1 then the drag component is greater.

Frontal component of the hydrodynamic RF (frontal drag, F_D)

In experiments involving streamlining the hand casts and increasing the angle of attack the co-efficient of the frontal force, C_{Dx}, increases exponentially and achieves its maximum at an angle of 90°. The form of the propelling segment and the sweepback angle also influence the magnitude of C_{DX} and F_D at different angles of attack (Table 10.2).

Normal component of hydrodynamic reaction—hydrodynamic lift (*L*)

Streamlining of the hand by water flow creates a small ($|C_{Dy}| < 0.2$) normal force even at $\alpha = 0°$ and $\psi = 90°$ (Reischle 1979; Schleihauf 1979). With increased angle of attack (α) up to its critical value (30–35°) the coefficient of normal reaction (C_{Dy}) also increases, but beyond these critical values of α it again decreases to 0 at a 90° angle of attack.

Changes in the form of the propelling segments, angle of attack and sweepback angle cause much greater variation in the normal component of the hydrodynamic reaction than the frontal component (Table 10.3). The greatest variation of C_{Dy} due to changes of magnitude of the sweepback angle was found for angles of attack below 60°. For angles of attack greater than 60° the absolute values and dynamics of C_{Dy} become very similar at different sweepback angles.

Separation of the fingers significantly decreases the normal component (lift), while thumb abduction increases the lift. The maximal value of C_{Dy} for the hand occurred with the thumb abducted to 75% of its maximal amplitude (Schleihauf 1979). It may be concluded that when it is necessary to create significant lift, as in sculling movements ($\alpha < 35°$), the most efficient hand position is with the fingers held together and the thumb apart.

Table 10.2 The impact of the form of the propelling surface and sweepback angles on the magnitude of frontal reaction at given angles of attack.

Authors	Method	Position of fingers	$\psi°$	$\alpha°$	$C_{x'maximal}$
Schleihauf (1979)	Hand casts exposed to flow in water channel	Thumb apart from fingers	0	75–90	1.35
			90	90	1.40
			180	80–90	1.30
			270	70–80	1.40
		Fingers 4–6 mm apart, thumb apart	0	85	1.15
Wood (1979)	Hand casts, aerochannel, $V = 40$ m · s^{-1}	Fingers together	90	90	1.10
		Fingers tightly adducted, palm concave	90	90	1.07
		Fingers apart	90	90	1.07

$\psi°$ = sweepback angle; $\alpha°$ = angle of attack; $C_{x'}$ = hydrodynamic coefficient of frontal RF.

Table 10.3 Impact of the form of the propelling surface and its sweepback angle on the maximal normal component of hydrodynamic reaction at given angles of attack.

Authors	Form of propelling segment and finger positions	$\psi°$	$\alpha°$	$C_{y'\text{maximal}}$
Schleihauf (1979)	Hand cast			
	Fingers together, thumb abducted 90°	0	15	0.85
		90	55	0.65
		180	30	0.85
		270	35	1.10
	Fingers together, thumb abducted 67.5°	0	40–45	0.80
	Fingers 3.2 mm apart, thumb at 67.5°	0	45–50	0.70
	Fingers 6.4 mm apart, thumb at 67.5°	0	45–55	0.50
	Fingers together, thumb at 45°	0	50	0.70
Wood (1979)	Hand-forearm cast			
	Fingers together	0	55	0.60
		90	50	1.07
		180	35	0.46
	Fingers together, hand concave	0	55	0.68
		90	50	1.01
		180	35	0.57
	Fingers apart	0	60	0.53
		90	55	0.88
		180	15	0.44

$\psi°$ = sweepback angle; $\alpha°$ = angle of attack; $C_{y'}$ = coefficient of the lift (normal force).

The resulting hydrodynamic reaction force (RF)

The momentary magnitude of the resulting hydrodynamic force created by the hand and forearm is determined by the form of the 'hand–forearm' connection, angle of attack, sweepback angle and absolute velocity of the arm and forearm in respect to 3-D water flow.

In the course of the pull a swimmer varies α and ψ of the hand and forearm in order to use effectively both drag and lift forces to create a high resulting RF and effective pulling force. With an angle of attack (α) between 10 and 35° the resulting hydrodynamic force is created predominantly by the normal (lift) component ($C_{Dy}/C_{Dx} \geq 1.33$). Within the range 35–55° the RF of the hand is formed by equal contributions of normal and frontal (drag) components ($C_{Dy}/C_{Dx} = 0.75$–1.33). With angles of attack of the hand >55° the RF is formed predominantly by the drag ($C_{Dy}/C_{Dx} \leq 0.75$). When the angle of attack is greater than 75° the resulting hydrodynamic reaction force is formed almost exclusively by the drag.

It should be stressed that most effective coefficients of hydrodynamic reaction (C_D) occur when the angle of attack of the arm–forearm $\geq 30°$. Swimmers strive for this degree of flow streamlining during the main phase of the pull. According to the data of Schleihauf (1979) and Cappaert (1998) the angle of attack of the hand and forearm at the instant when they develop maximal RF and effective pulling force is within the range 60–75°. However, during the initial (insweep) and transitional phases of the pull swimmers use sharp angles of attack (Schleihauf 1979).

Much smaller hydrodynamic reaction is produced when the angle of attack of the propelling segments is ≤ 10–$15°$. Values in this range are used by swimmers during the parts of the recovery that are performed under water (arm entry and exit in front and back crawl and butterfly, forward sweep in breaststroke).

It is worth mentioning the strong relationship between the RF and sweepback angle of the hand. Thus a hand orientation with $\alpha = 15°$ and $\psi = 0°$

gives 31% greater RF than with $\alpha = 15°$ and $\psi = 45°$. Increasing the angle of attack by $10°$ ($\alpha = 25°$) at $\psi = 0°$ creates 8% less RF than at $\alpha = 25°$ and $\psi = 45°$ (Schleihauf 1979; Rumyantsev 1982).

Comparison of the oar-like pull (OLP) and curvilinear pull (CLP)

It is now firmly established that efficient arm pull patterns begin with active 'overtaking' rotational movements of the hand and forearm at the elbow and wrist joints with respect to the shoulder (Counsilman 1968, 1977; Makarenko 1975; Haljand et al. 1986). This technique is characterized by a gradual increase of the hydrodynamic RF and its effective component (Counsilman 1977; Schleihauf et al. 1979; Haljand et al. 1986; Maglischo 1993). It helps to avoid significant angular accelerations of the arm segments and sudden changes in intracycle velocity of the swimmer. Unskilled swimmers have been found to have a rapid increase of hydrodynamic reaction at the beginning of the pull followed by chaotic changes (Counsilman 1977; Schleihauf 1979).

During the preliminary phase the total RF and effective pulling force increase gradually with an increase of the angle of attack and velocity of the hand and forearm. At the moment of entry into the water the hand with fingers together creates a minor resistive force. At the same time extension of the arm over the head improves the streamlining of the head and shoulders and reduces total HDR. This effect is facilitated by the positive vertical component of the RF created by the hand.

During the transitional phase there is a gradual decrease of the angle of attack of the hand and forearm, and the magnitude of RF and effective pulling force also decreases.

In the middle part of the arm pull the propulsive force is created by roughly equal contributions of the normal and frontal components of RF. An optimal relationship of these two components is determined by a number of factors. The most important are as follows.

1 Rules for particular swimming disciplines limit the direction and amplitude of movements, and their timing.

2 The relationship of the velocity of a swimmer's GCM motion to the relative velocity of the propelling segments (V_{GCM}/V_{hand}). The closer to 1 is this ratio, the greater the advantage in velocity of interaction with water flow, the *better support reaction* attains the swimmer.

3 Speed-strength abilities and strength endurance of the swimmer. These determine the changes in kinematic and dynamic characteristics of the pulling actions during an entire race (angle of arm flexion in elbow joint, stroke rate, stroke distance, etc.).

4 The range of movement and flexibility of the joints, which limit the possible variations in the position of the pulling segments relative to the water flow and direction of locomotion.

5 Development of the kinesthetic sense ('feeling for water'), allowing manipulation of the parameters of pulling actions. Schleihauf (1979) assumed that CLP requires more perfect 'feeling for the water' than OLP.

Schleihauf (1979) showed that in elite swimmers the propulsive part of the arm pull in every stroke shows the following.

1 Patterns with exaggerated curvilinear trajectory of arm–forearm movement:

   (a) pulls with predominantly transverse movements of the hand and forearm; and

   (b) pulls with significant change of the depth of the pull.

In these pulling patterns the propulsive force is created predominantly by the normal (lift) component of hydrodynamic reaction and efficient propulsive force may be created in all phases of the pull.

2 Patterns with a relatively straight trajectory. Here the propelling force is created predominantly by the frontal pressure force, mainly in the middle part of the pull while the hand moves backwards.

The CLP has some advantages over the OLP. Thus in order to achieve an equal absolute velocity of interaction with water flow the CLP utilizes a lower *relative* backward velocity of the arm segments and requires much less effort to overcome their inertia than OLP (Table 10.4 gives mass-inertial characteristics of the propelling segments). This advantage of the CLP depends upon swimming velocity. During swimming at low velocities a

Table 10.4 Relative mass (% of total body mass) of arm and leg segments in adult males. (From Zatsiorsky *et al.* 1981.)

Segment	Mass of segment/body mass × 100%
Hand	0.61
Forearm	1.62
Upper arm	2.71
Foot	1.37
Lower leg	4.33
Upper leg	14.17

swimmer using OLP is able to achieve (by increasing relative arm velocity) the same velocity of arm–forearm interaction with water flow as in CLP. So the advantage of CLP will be only in the smaller effort needed to overcome the inertia of the pulling segments. At maximal swimming velocity, when the relative backward velocity of the pulling segments is limited by the speed-strength abilities of an athlete, the OLP does not allow such a high velocity of arm–forearm interaction with the flow as in CLP. As the external load increases with increased swimming velocity the angle of arm bending at the elbow joint also increases (Butovich & Chudovsky 1968; Counsilman 1977). This movement is aimed at utilizing the angles of maximal force (AMF) and is accompanied by a deviation of the arm–forearm trajectory from the direction of motion.

Apart from the advantage in velocity of interaction of the propelling segments with the water flow, the CLP allows the pulling segments to find 'still water' and thus increase the stroke distance while maintaining the optimal stroke rate. Moreover, the longer duration of arm interaction with the flow (longer pulling trajectory) of CLP may create a greater impulse of RF than OLP.

The main advantage of OLP is the utilization of most effective coefficients of hydrodynamic reaction due to high angles of attack ($\alpha = 55$–$75°$), while CLP achieves lower values of C_{Dx} as it utilizes much smaller angles of attack. Thus a smaller velocity of arm interaction with water flow in OLP may be compensated by a greater C_{Dx}. Due to effective arm–forearm orientation and direction of pull the

OLP allows greater transformation of the hydrodynamic reaction force into an effective propulsive force during swimming.

Thus it may be concluded that both pulling patterns have high propulsive potential. However, the use of OLP and CLP in individuals will depend on a number of hydrodynamic and biomechanical (anatomical) factors.

Normal and frontal components of propulsion in different swimming strokes

The amount by which the hydrodynamic reaction force may deviate from the direction of propulsion depends on the swimming stroke. In *synchro-symmetrical* swimming strokes (e.g. breaststroke and butterfly) transverse components of the hydrodynamic force are mutually discharged and vertical components are used efficiently for body support. In swimming strokes with alternate arm and leg movements (front and back crawl) it is necessary to avoid significant deviation of the hydrodynamic reaction force from the swimming direction, since this may cause undesirable sideways and vertical deviation of the body and thus increase the hydrodynamic resistance. It follows that during butterfly and (especially) breaststroke swimming, the pulling action may be closer to a CLP and even a propeller-like pulling pattern than occurs during front and back crawl. Assessment of the relative contribution of the lift and drag in the resultant RF and effective pulling force may be made on the basis of the data given in Table 10.5. For different swimming strokes the combination of drag and lift force and the distribution of total and effective hydrodynamic force within the swimming cycle will vary significantly.

The *lift-and-drag index, diagonality index* and *force distribution index* show that lift predominates over drag force in breaststroke. In freestyle and butterfly lift and drag forces appear to be about equally important during the major portion of the propulsive phases of the pull. In backstroke, swimmers use drag force more than lift force (i.e. sculling movements are less important for backstroke than for breaststroke, butterfly or freestyle).

Table 10.5 Characteristics of pulling motion curve-linearity in four competitive swimming strokes.

Stroke	Diagonality index*	Lift-and-drag index†	Force distribution index‡
Freestyle	59 ± 13	1.04 ± 0.28	0.82 ± 0.07
Butterfly	44 ± 21	0.95 ± 0.39	0.81 ± 0.06
Backstroke	47 ± 17	0.77 ± 0.21	0.58 ± 0.13
Breaststroke	81 ± 9	1.25 ± 0.21	0.65 ± 0.13

* The diagonality index is the average angle of the negative hand line of motion and the forward direction at the points of first, second and third maximal RF production.
† The lift-and-drag index is the average ratio of lift and drag forces (C_L/C_D) at the three largest occurrences of RF.
‡ The force distribution index is the average location of the three largest occurrences of RF expressed as a percentage of the total duration of the underwater phase of the arm pull.

Figure 10.11a–d shows a hand propulsive force diagram (combination of lift and drag force into resultant RF), intracyclic dynamics and impulse of total and effective propulsive forces in four swimming strokes (Schleihauf 1979). These graphs characterize the rhythmical structure of the pull and values of forces applied by swimmers in distinct phases of the pull. The largest effective propulsive forces in freestyle and butterfly occur near the end of the arm pull (after the hand passes two-thirds of the pull). In breaststroke the largest effective propulsive force occurs at the midpoint of the inward sculling motion of the hands.

The cycle of arm movements and phases of arm pull

The *swimming cycle* or *cycle of swimming movements* as a multiple repeated system of movements consists of a preliminary part (*recovery*) and a working part (*pull*). The recovery is aimed at restoring the working posture of the arms or legs, while the pull creates the propulsive force.

A single cycle is characterized by a beginning and end, and intervening *phases* which differ in their kinematic and dynamic characteristics and have distinct motor objectives. The optimal duration of each phase within the swimming cycle is necessary for the effective coordination of swimming movements and maintenance of high and relatively uniform intracyclic velocity.

Table 10.6 shows the phases of the arm cycle in all swimming strokes. The main feature of such a subdivision of the cycle into phases is the prevailing direction of the vector of hand velocity within the system of immobile orthogonal coordinates (Schleihauf 1979).

The objective of the initial phase is to prevent any decrease of intracyclic velocity, start acceleration of the body, and move the pulling segments to their most effective position in readiness for the main part. In this phase the hand and forearm work as hydrofoils. The acceleration of the body GCM during the initial pulling phase is created in breaststroke and butterfly by leg kick (the transfer of the pulling effort from legs to arms). In front and back crawl this initial acceleration is accomplished by the main phase of pull of the opposite arm (transfer of the pulling effort from one hand to another) and also by utilization of kinetic energy (inertia) of the entire system.

The objective of the main phase is to achieve maximal intracyclic velocity. During the main phase the hand and forearm maintain an optimal orientation relative to the water flow and direction of motion. From an anatomical point of view the main phase can be subdivided into two parts: pull and push. The boundary point between these parts is the

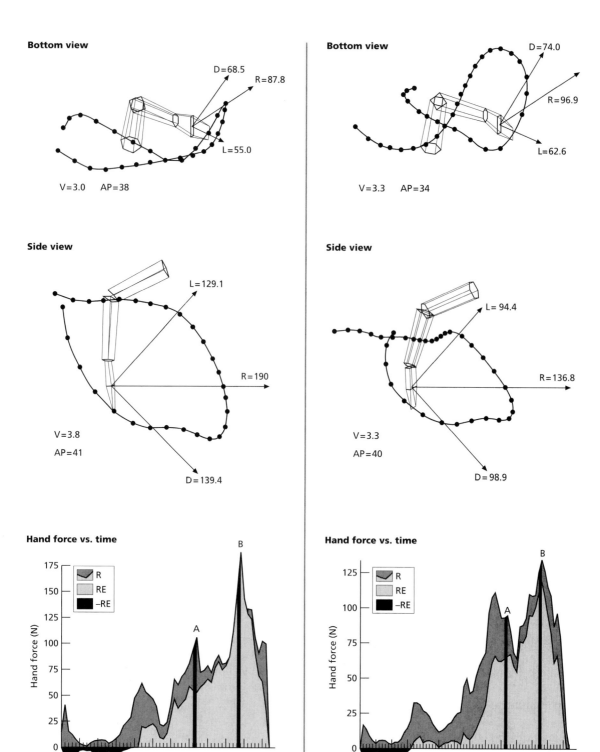

Bottom view

D=68.5
R=87.8
L=55.0
V=3.0   AP=38

Bottom view

D=74.0
R=96.9
L=62.6
V=3.3   AP=34

Side view

L=129.1
R=190
V=3.8
AP=41
D=139.4

Side view

L=94.4
R=136.8
V=3.3
AP=40
D=98.9

Hand force vs. time

R
RE
−RE

B
A

Hand force (N)

175
150
125
100
75
50
25
0

Time (1/66 s)

Hand force vs. time

R
RE
−RE

B
A

Hand force (N)

125
100
75
50
25
0

Time (1/66 s)

(a)

(b)

Fig. 10.11 Impulse of resultant and effective reaction force in four competitive swimming strokes: (a) freestyle; (b) butterfly; (c) backstroke; and (d) breaststroke. AP, angle of pitch (degrees); V, absolute hand velocity relative to water flow (m · s⁻¹); D, frontal drag component; L, lift component; RF, resultant reaction force. (a) *bottom view*, middle of stroke; *side view*, finishing sweep motion; *hand force vs. time*, R, resultant force; RE, resultant effective force. (b) *bottom view*, inward

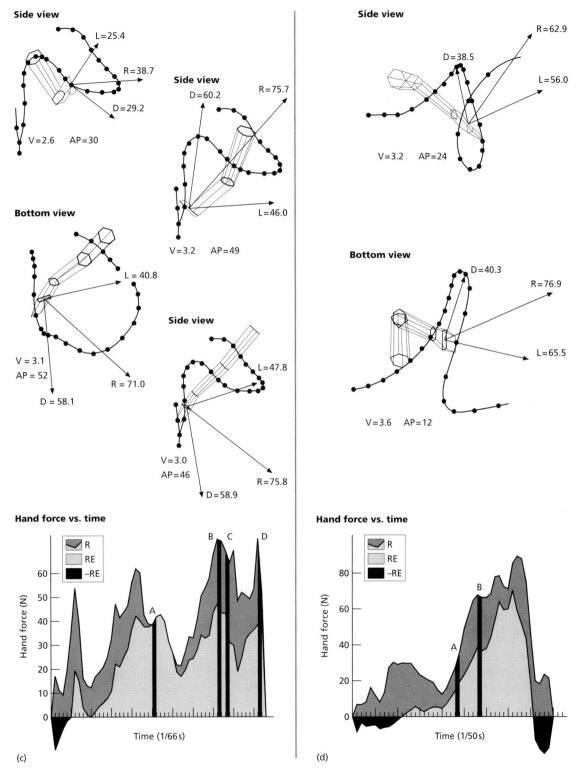

scull motion; *side view*, finishing sweep motion. (c) *side view*: midstroke; *side view*, downward sweep; *bottom view*, inward sweep; *side view*, upward sweep. (d) *side view*, downward sweep; *bottom view*, inward scull motion. (From Schleihauf 1979.)

Table 10.6 The structure of the arm cycle in competitive swimming strokes.

	Phases of cycle				
	Pull (working part)				
Swimming stroke	Initial	Main	Transitional	Preliminary part (recovery)	
Front crawl ⎫ Back crawl ⎬ Butterfly ⎭	Downsweep	Insweep-outsweep	Upsweep	Exit and movement above water	Entry and extension forwards
Breaststroke	Outsweep	Insweep		Arm stretch	

moment when the hand crosses the transverse plane (y-z) passing through the shoulder joint. The push is the most vigorous, decisive part of the pull, and maximal intracycle swimming velocity occurs during the last two-thirds of the push.

In the course of the transitional phase (end of the pull) the hand and forearm create mostly vertical and lateral reaction forces to lever out the negative forces (gravity, inertia). Another motor objective of the transitional phase in front crawl, backstroke and butterfly is to achieve arm exit with minimal resistance to forward motion of the body.

The objective of the recovery phase is to restore the initial position of the arm for the start of the next cycle with minimal effort. The inertia of the arm segment (in butterfly and breaststroke inertia of the upper body as well) may be utilized to minimize the fluctuation of the intracyclic velocity.

Biodynamics of leg movements in swimming

The role of leg movements in propulsion

Leg actions are able to create greater hydrodynamic forces than arm actions (Butovich & Chudovsky 1968; Bagrash *et al.* 1973; Belokovsky & Kuznetsov 1976; Haljand 1984, 1986). There are several reasons for this.

1 Legs possess significantly greater propelling surface area.

2 The relative movement of the feet during the working phase has no backward part (except in breaststroke). This allows a high velocity of interaction with the water flow to be developed at any swimming velocity.

3 The muscle groups of the legs are significantly stronger than those of the arms (Onoprienko 1981).

In sport swimming these features play a minor role for creating effective propulsive forces. In fin-swimming the propelling surface area of the lower extremities is increased more than twofold, giving a three- to fourfold increase in hydrodynamic RF and a 1.5- to 2-fold increase in swimming velocity (Onoprienko 1981).

Due to the orientation of the foot and lower leg relative to the water flow and direction of motion these high hydrodynamic forces act mostly in a vertical direction and only a small fraction of them acts straightforwards in the direction of motion. Consequently, leg kick creates a smaller effective propulsive force than arm pull. In front and back crawl about 15% of the total propulsive force is created by leg kick. In butterfly stroke the contribution of leg kick propulsion is greater, maybe up to 20–25%. The exception is breaststroke, in which approximately equal proportions of the total propulsive force are created by leg and arm movements.

Despite the limitations of legs as propelling agents, leg movements create useful propulsive forces in every swimming stroke at any swimming velocity (Persyn *et al.* 1975; Onoprienko 1981). Besides contributing to propulsion, leg movements also perform several very important compensatory functions (Butovich & Chudovsky 1968; Makarenko

1975; Persyn *et al.* 1975; Haljand *et al.* 1986). They serve to:
• neutralize the negative forces (gravity and inertia) and transverse components of hydrodynamic reaction force made by pulling actions;
• smooth the intracycle fluctuations of swimming velocity;
• maintain a high and streamlined body position;
• regulate the velocity and amplitude of body rotation around the longitudinal axis in front and back crawl and around the transverse axis during breaststroke and butterfly;
• facilitate the propulsive phases of arm pull; and
• unify all movements in a single system, the swimming cycle.

Hydrodynamic potential of leg segments

The contribution of leg segments to propulsion is determined by the velocity of their interaction with the water flow, their surface area and their hydrodynamic coefficients. Bagrash *et al.* (1973) used tensiometry to measure hydrodynamic pressure experienced by distinct leg segments during front crawl swimming under the following conditions, denoted I–III:
I—during tethered swimming using straight leg kick without noticeable knee flexion;
II—during tethered swimming with 'natural' leg kick;
III—during free swimming.

Figure 10.12 shows the location of tensioleads on a swimmer's leg and the corresponding maximal values of hydrodynamic pressure (average for 20 cycles) in conditions I, II and III.

The values of the maximal intracycle pressure forces for distinct leg segments are given in Table 10.7. Calculations were based on: (i) for foot—readings of lead 1; (ii) for lower leg—average readings of leads 2 and 3; (iii) for upper leg—average readings of leads 4, 5 and 6.

It was found that in 'natural' swimming the foot created about 70% of the leg's hydrodynamic reaction. Another 20% of RF is created by the lower leg. The foot's contribution to propulsion appears more significant if one takes into consideration its advantage in space orientation in water flow (Counsilman 1977). The intracyclic dynamics of the hydrodynamic reaction force vary significantly from stroke to stroke and from individual to individual. It may be concluded that the main propelling segments of the leg are the foot and distal half of the lower leg.

Table 10.7 Maximal intracyclic hydrodynamic forces developed by the leg segments during front crawl swimming. (From Bagrash *et al.* 1973; adapted by Rumyantsev 1982.)

Leg segments	S (cm²)	Relative C_D	F—I (N)	F—II (N)	F—III (N)
Foot	185	1.0*	94.1	126.0	110.4
Lower leg	301	0.7	33.1	46.7	38.3
Upper leg	580	0.7	7.5	11.8	9.4

C_D = coefficient of hydrodynamic resistance. F—I = force during tethered swimming using straight leg kick without noticeable knee flexion. F—II = force during swimming with 'natural' leg kick. F—III = force during free swimming. S = surface area.
* C_D of the foot was conditionally accepted as 1.0.

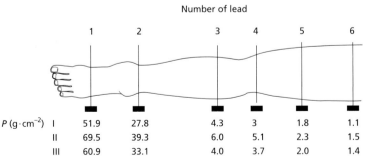

Number of lead

	1	2	3	4	5	6
P (g·cm⁻²) I	51.9	27.8	4.3	3	1.8	1.1
II	69.5	39.3	6.0	5.1	2.3	1.5
III	60.9	33.1	4.0	3.7	2.0	1.4

Fig. 10.12 Location of tensioleads on swimmer's leg. (Data from Bagrash *et al.* 1973.)

The form and orientation of the leg (foot) in water flow and 3-D space

The question of the influence of the form and orientation of the leg on hydrodynamic forces remains open. Onoprienko (1981) studied the influence of the limited range of angle of attack on frontal resistance of the foot at a flow velocity of $2.0 \text{ m} \cdot \text{s}^{-1}$. He found that during interaction of water flow with the frontal surface of feet in the range of angles $60-90°$ ($\psi = 90°$) there was moderate increase of frontal drag ($F_{X' \text{ at } \alpha = 90°}/F_{X' \text{ at } \alpha = 60°} = 1.08$) due to an increase in the propelling surface of the foot. When water flow interacts with the internal surface of the foot ($\psi = 90°$) at a $90°$ angle of attack ($\alpha = 90°$) there is much less hydrodynamic reaction than at $\psi = 0°$ ($F_{X \text{ at } \psi = 0°}/F_{X \text{ at } \alpha = 90°} = 1.28$). The reduction of frontal hydrodynamic reaction was a result of reduction of C_D with change of flow direction relative to the foot ($C_{D \text{ at } \psi = 0°}/C_{D \text{ at } \psi = 90°} = 1.13$) due to a decrease in the supporting area. The change of ψ from $45°$ to $90°$ ($\alpha = 90°$) gives an increase of supporting area (from 200 to 223 cm^2) and decrease of hydrodynamic pressure from 0.32 to 0.28 N $\cdot$ cm^{-2}. As a result F_X varied insignificantly.

Though leg movements are able to create a high resultant hydrodynamic RF, due to space orientation of the foot and lower leg, the major component of the hydrodynamic reaction is directed along the vertical axis downwards (upwards in backstroke). The transverse component is also significant while the component of hydrodynamic reaction in the direction of locomotion is small.

Since during natural swimming at high velocity the foot of a skilled swimmer does not move backwards relative to the system of immobile coordinates (Makarenko 1975; Reischle 1979), propulsive forces are delivered predominantly by the normal component of hydrodynamic reaction. Consequently, leg actions develop a much smaller effective propulsive force than arm actions (except in breaststroke and butterfly).

Coordination of joint movements of the leg segments during leg kick

The most effective kicking patterns use movements in all leg joints. The advantage of leg kick with knee flexion–extension over straight leg kick corresponds to the advantage of arm pull with flexion in elbow and wrist over the straight arm pull.

A selective increase in the angular velocity of the proximal segments (upper leg) has a fundamental impact on leg kick due to the mass-inertial characteristics of the leg segments (see Table 10.4). Transition from the distal to the proximal segment of the leg involves a much greater increase in muscle mass compared with a similar transition along the arm. The muscles of the upper leg begin acceleration of the leg during the working phase. Coordination of the joint movements of the leg segments is characterized by an *overtaking movement* of the upper leg relative to the lower leg and foot. During the crawl and butterfly the hip begins an upward movement while the lower leg and foot are still accelerating downwards. This pattern of leg movement has been called 'whip-like' movement. Thus during a leg kick there is consecutive transformation of the torque of internal and external forces from the hip joint to the knee joint and ankle joint, with a gradual increase of amplitude and angular velocity of segments from the hip to the foot (Haljand 1986; Table 10.8).

The maximal intracyclic value of the leg kick's propelling force is recorded, as a rule, during the second quarter of leg extension at the knee joints (Haljand 1984). This is delivered by effective space orientation and high angular velocity of the foot. After this moment, if there is no need to create significant vertical force, the swimmer can decrease the relative velocity of knee extension and finish the movement using leg inertia. This technique facilitates the efficiency of the leg kick. With

Table 10.8 Angular amplitude (φ) and velocity (ω) of leg kick in hip joint and knee joint during butterfly swimming in skilled swimmers. (From Haljand 1974; adapted by Vorontsov 1981.)

Joint	Type of movement	φ ($\bar{X} \pm \text{SD}$)	ω ($\bar{X} \pm \text{SD}$)
Hip	Extension	24 ± 3	140 ± 43
	Flexion	30 ± 7	151 ± 64
Knee	Flexion	67 ± 19	261 ± 39
	Extension	62 ± 14	420 ± 101

increased swimming velocity kicking movements with reduced amplitude and high tempo are more efficient. A fast and narrow leg kick provides a high velocity of foot interaction with the water flow and reduces the negative effect of resistance and inertia forces during leg recovery.

Contribution of the core body in swimming propulsion

Since a swimmer's body is subject to hydrodynamic resistance it is important that it undergoes *locomotor reconfiguration*—the ability to change its form and rigidity in order to reduce hydrodynamic resistance (HDR) and transfer the effort from segment to segment. Of course, this ability is developed in humans much less than in sea mammals and fishes. Nevertheless, it is commonly held that one of the fundamental differences between the elite and ordinary swimmer is the ability to reduce HDR during swimming (Counsilman 1968; Toussaint & Beek 1992; Maglischo 1993).

Colwin (1984, 1992) has introduced into swimming theory the term *kinematic streamlining*. Referring to the swimmer, this term perhaps has a narrower meaning than locomotor reconfiguration. It presumes the synchronization of body and limb alignment with peaks of arm–forearm acceleration during the pull in order to reduce: (i) the frontal surface area exposed to water flow and turbulence in body wake; and (ii) wave resistance. Hence, propulsive forces will predominate over resistive ones (see Eqn. 10.1) and swimming velocity will increase significantly.

The body of a swimmer can contribute directly to propulsion with undulating movements, especially in the butterfly and breaststroke (Persyn *et al.* 1992; Coleman *et al.* 1998). Coleman *et al.* (1998) came to the conclusion that in breaststroke the forces calculated on the basis of instantaneous velocity and acceleration of the body, differ in timing and amount from the forces due to hand motion, calculated accordingly to the algorithms of Schleihauf using drag and lift coefficients. They used visualization of water flow in the body wake to show that *added water mass* may contribute to stabilization and even increase the velocity of the body GSM.

Rolling of the body along its longitudinal axis in the front and back crawl helps the swimmer to utilize the massive and strong muscles of the back and breast and, thus, increase the muscle draught and resultant RF. This rotation also assists recovery of the opposite arm over the water and reduces transverse movements of the arms.

Characteristics of a rational swimming technique

Countless attempts to quantify the 'average' values of spatial, time-spatial and dynamic (kinetic) characteristics of pulling and kicking patterns in world-class swimmers have failed due to the huge variability of these parameters (Counsilman 1968, 1977; Makarenko 1975; Schleihauf 1979; Schleihauf *et al.* 1988; Maglischo 1993). This variability stems from the significant differences demonstrated by world-class swimmers in body type and composition, level of basic and complex physical abilities (flexibility, maximal strength, rapidity, speed-strength, explosive strength, etc.). Nevertheless, it is possible to establish certain principles and qualitative characteristics of a rational swimming technique. Individual techniques should satisfy these principles in order to develop a highly effective propulsive force and achieve high swimming velocities.

Effective use of lift and drag to create a high supportive RF

Effective pulling patterns employ complex curvilinear or diagonal motions in the course of which a swimmer constantly changes the pitch of the arm–forearm and the direction of motion. Thus, lift and drag forces are combined in a high resultant RE and effective pulling force. At every point of the curvilinear pulling trajectory the propelling segments interact with the standing undisturbed water and shift a larger mass of the water over a shorter distance. The smaller the backward displacement of the propelling segments in respect to the immobile system of orthogonal coordinates, the higher the efficiency of the working movements. In the front crawl, top-class swimmers demonstrate a backward displacement of the hand within the range 0.4–0.5 m while less skilled swimmers have hand displacements of 0.6–0.7 m and more (Issurin & Kostyuk 1978).

'High elbow' position during arm pull

One of the distinct features of a rational swimming technique is an arm pull with a high elbow position relative to the hand. From the point of view of hydrodynamics, an overtaking rotational movement of the arm–forearm relative to that of the shoulder (elbow bending) gives working segments their most efficient form and position (increase of $C_{D\ hand}$, S_{hand} and $C_{D\ forearm}$, $S_{forearm}$) in the water flow and provides high resultant RF. The movement of the elbow joint also facilitates muscle draught to balance the high value of hydrodynamic reaction.

Using angles of maximal force during pulling actions: coordination of joint movements

The biomechanical chains of the human motor apparatus are able to exert maximal joint torque in isolated movements when the limb's segments occupy a particular position relative to each other and the core body. In this position the direction of muscle draught and the starting length of the muscles are optimal for delivering the maximal effort. The angles at which segments are disposed relative to each other when the maximal force (muscle torque) is generated are called the *angles of maximal force* (AMF). During locomotion in water the swimmer is trying to perform a significant part of the working movements within the range of AMF in the elbow, shoulder, hip and knee joints, to create maximal torque at the appropriate instants.

Arm pull in the front and back crawl and butterfly is a complex movement. It consists of two parts: (i) pulling—consecutive flexing of the arm at the wrist and elbow joints and extension at the shoulder joint; and (ii) pushing, performed by continuous extension at the shoulder joint accompanied by extension at the elbow and wrist joints. Each part has its own zone of AMF. The two largest pulses of the RF during arm pull (Fig. 10.12) are the result of the consecutive utilization of the AMF and highly precise timing of joint movement in three joints. Swimmers increase and decrease hand and forearm velocity

with every change of pulling direction. Correspondingly, intracyclic propulsive force changes in pulses. The first largest peak of muscle effort occurs during the *pulling part of* underwater movement when the angle between the forearm and the direction of motion is about 45°, and the angle between the forearm and shoulder is approximately 160°.

The final part of the pulling phase and first half of the push phase is performed by active extension of the shoulder with utilization of the hand and forearm as a supporting surface. Shoulder extension gradually slows during the latter half of the push phase, and active extension of the elbow take place. The second largest pulse of RF occurs during the last third of the push.

Maintaining uniform high intracyclic swimming velocity

Swimming is a cyclical locomotion during which the working phases alternate with preliminary movements needed to recover the initial working posture of the limbs. During the recovery phase propulsive forces do not act on the swimmer's body and it is the subject of hydrodynamic drag and inertia. Hence the swimming velocity decreases until the working phase of the next swimming cycle begins, when it starts to increase again.

Fluctuations of intracyclic swimming velocity are inevitable since a significant part of pulling action is performed beyond the range of AMF and recovery is necessary. The fluctuations necessitate additional effort to accelerate the body's GCM and overcome the inertia of the body and added mass of the water (Issurin 1977). Thus velocity fluctuations increase the energy cost of swimming.

The magnitude of intracyclic velocity fluctuations may be reduced and average swimming velocity increased by shortening the duration of recovery, increasing the amplitude and frequency of the pulling actions, and improving the timing of arm and leg movements.

Reduction of hydrodynamic resistance and action of negative forces

The position of the head relative to the water level

and the horizontal alignment of the body affect the magnitude of frontal resistance (wave-making resistance + form resistance) experienced by the swimmer. The swimmer should maintain the most streamlined position and keep the angle of attack within a given range.

When a swimmer adopts a prone, streamlined position in the water the gravity force is balanced by the upthrust (buoyancy force). During active swimming he/she needs to periodically lift the head and part of the upper body to perform recovery and inhalation. During these auxiliary movements the weight of the 'out of the water' body parts may increase from 5 to 15 kg, giving rise to the sinking force. To compensate for this sinking force the swimmer must apply an additional upwardly directed force. Skilled swimmers usually perform the recovery and auxiliary movements rapidly with minimal lifting of body parts out of the water. The timing of arm and leg movements as well as transverse arm movements during the pull is partly designed to compensate or eliminate the negative action of this sinking force.

Optimal ratio of stroke rate to stroke distance

The *stroke rate* is the number of strokes or complete swimming cycles performed per unit time (usually per second). *Stroke distance* is the distance covered by a swimmer per stroke or per complete swimming cycle. Swimming velocity usually equates to the product of stroke rate and stroke distance:

$$V = SR \times SD \qquad (10.8)$$

where SR = stroke rate (pulls · s^{-1}), and SD = stroke distance (m).

It follows from Eqn. 10.8 that different ratios of SR and SD may result in the same swimming velocity, although an individual swimmer achieves a maximal swimming velocity only at one particular ratio of SR and SD. Too high a stroke rate disturbs the coordination of the swimming movements since the muscles are not able to relax during recovery and thus fatigue sets in very rapidly. During swimming with a low SR and high SD the swimmer has to make an excessive effort in every stroke, which may increase the anaerobic fraction of total energy

supply. The consequent accumulation of lactic acid decreases the swimmer's working capability.

During training every swimmer selects the most effective individual ratio of SR and SD. The 'comfortable' stroke rate seems to be the most stable individual characteristic, depending probably on the nature of the individual's nervous system and muscle fibre composition. It changes very little over multiyear training periods. The objective of technical training is to develop maximal SD for a given individual's comfortable stroke rate.

The value of stroke distance and its dynamics during competitive racing are the important criteria of stroke quality. It depends upon technical and physical training (muscle power) and an individual's 'feeling for the water'.

Conservation of mechanical energy within the system of swimmer's movements

Efficient conservation of kinetic energy within the swimming cycle is achieved by the following.
1 Relatively rigid fixation of segments in joints during pulling actions (e.g. fixation of the shoulder at the beginning of the downsweep) altered by fixation of the hand and forearm in the elbow and wrist joints at the end of insweep-beginning of outsweep).
2 Locomotor reconfiguration of the body in order to store elastic energy, dampen oscillations of propulsive force, and reduce HDR via:
  (a) optimal level of tension of body muscles creating a relatively rigid frame on which are transmitted the forces of hydrodynamic reaction developed by the arm and leg movements;
  (b) relaxation of non-active muscles; and
  (c) kinematic streamlining—ideal alignment of the body at the instants of peak propulsive force.
3 Use of the kinetic energy (inertia) of the recovering segments to increase propulsive momentum.
4 Transfer of the kinetic energy of the moving segments into potential energy of elastic deformation of muscles and tendons.

Acknowledgement

The authors are grateful to P. Brown for help in editing the manuscript.

References

Bagrash, L.F., Minenkov, V.V. & Chubarov, M.M. (1973) Tensiometrical studies of swimmers' efforts. *Theory and Practice of Physical Culture* **4**, 27–31.

Barthels, K. & Adrian, M.J. (1974) Three-dimensional spatial hand patterns of skilled butterfly swimmers. In: *Swimming II* (eds P.J. Clarys & L. Lewillie), pp. 154–160. University Park Press, Baltimore.

Belokovsky, V.V. (1971) Analysis of standard sculling patterns in synchronised swimming. Presentation at the Annual Scientific Session of Swimming Department of the Central State Institute of Physical Culture, Moscow, June 1971.

Belokovsky, V.V. & Kuznetsov, V.V. (1976) Analysis of dynamic forces in crawl stroke swimming. In: *Biomechanics V-B* (ed. P.V. Komi), pp. 235–242. University Park Press, Baltimore.

Butovich, N.A. & Chudovsky, V.D. (1968) *Sport Swimming*. Fizkultura i Sport, Moscow.

Cappaert, J. (1993) 1992 Olympic report. Limited circulation communication to all.

Cappaert, J.M. (1998) Biomechanics of swimming as analysed by 3 D technique. In: *Abstract Book of VIII International Symposium 'Biomechanics and Medicine in Swimming', Jyuvaskyla, Finland, 28 June–2 July 1998* (eds K.L. Keskinen, P.V. Komi & A.P. Hollander), p. 41. Jyuvaskyla University Publishers, Jyuvaskyla, Finland.

Cappaert, J. & Rushall, B.S. (1994) *Biomechanical Analysis of Champion Swimmers*. Sport Science Associates, Spring Valley, CA.

Coleman, V., Persyn, U. & Ungerechts B. (1998) A mass of water added to the swimmer's mass to estimate the velocity in dolphin-like swimming below water surface. In: *VIII International Symposium on Biomechanics and Medicine in Swimming, Jyväskylä, Finland, 28 June–2 July 1998*, p. 49. Gummerus Printing, Jyväskylä, Finland.

Colwin, C.M. (1984) Fluid dynamics: Vortex circulation in swimming propulsion. In: *ASCA World Clinic Yearbook*, pp. 38–46. American Swimming Coaches Association, Fort Lauderdale, FL.

Colwin, C.M. (1992) *Swimming Into the 21st Century*. Human Kinetics Publishers, Champaign, IL.

Counsilman, J.E. (1968) *The Science of Swimming*. Prentice Hall, Englewood Cliffs, NJ.

Counsilman, J.E. (1969) The role of sculling movements in the arm pull. *Swimming World* **10**, 6–7.

Counsilman, J.E. (1971) The application of Bernoulli's principle to human propulsion in water. In: *Swimming I* (eds L. Lewillie & J.P. Clarys), pp. 59–71. Université Libre de Bruxelles, Brussels.

Counsilman, J.E. (1977) *Competitive Swimming Manual for Coaches and Swimmers*. Counsilman Co., Bloomington, IN.

Cureton, T.K. (1930) Mechanics and kinesiology of swimming. *Research Quarterly* **1**, 87–121.

Denker, J.S. (1998) See how it flies. A new spin on the perceptions, procedures and principles of flight. http://www.monmouth.com/~jsd/how/htm/title.html.

Grinev, V.G. (1977) Utilisation of lift and drag forces in swimming propulsion. PhD thesis (abstract), State Central Institute of Physical Culture, Moscow.

Haljand, R. (1984) A new scientific approach to analysing swimming technique. In: *How to Develop Olympic Level Swimmers: Scientific and Practical Foundations* (ed. J.L. Cramer), pp. 72–105. International Sport Media, Helsinki.

Haljand, R., Tamp, T. & Kaal, R. (1986) *The Models of Swimming Strokes Technique and Methodics of its Perfection and Control*, 2nd edn. Tallinn Pedagogic Institute, Tallinn.

Hollander, P.A., de Groot, G., van Ingen Schenau, G.J., Kahman, R. & Toussaint, H.M. (1988) Contribution of the legs in front crawl swimming. In: *Swimming V* (eds B.E. Ungerechts, K. Reischle & K. Wilke), pp. 39–43. Human Kinetics Publishers, Champaign, IL.

Issurin, V.B. (1977) Evaluation of hydrodynamic resistance and propelling forces in swimming. *Theory and Practice of Physical Culture* **9**, 20–21.

Issurin, V.B. & Kostuk, Yu.I. (1978) Underwater kinematic characteristics of front crawl arm pull. *Theory and Practice of Physical Culture* **9**, 13–15.

Kiphut, R.J.H. (1942) *Swimming*. Barnes, New York.

Kolmogorov, S.V. & Lyapin, S.H. (1998) Biomechanics of a set unstationary active motion of biological objects in water environment. In: *Abstract Book of VIII International Symposium 'Biomechanics and Medicine in Swimming', Jyuvaskyla, Finland, 28 June–2 July 1998*, p. 82. Jyuvaskyla University Publishers, Jyuvaskyla, Finland.

Maglischo, E.W. (1993) *Swimming Even Faster*. Mayfield Publishing Co., Mountain View, CA.

Makarenko, L.P. (1975) *Technical Skill of a Swimmer*. Fiskultura i Sport, Moscow.

Makarenko, L.P. (1996) Fundamentals of swimming technique. In: *Sport Swimming* (eds N.Zh. Bulgakova & L.P. Makarenko), pp. 40–129, Fiskultura, Obrazovanie i Nauka, Moscow.

Miller, D.I. (1975) Biomechanics of swimming. In: *Exercise and Sport Sciences Reviews* (eds J.H. Willmore & J.F. Keogh), pp. 219–248. Academic Press, NY.

Onoprienko, B.I. (1981) *Biomechanics of Swimming*. Zdorov'ya, Kiev.

Persyn, U., De Maeyer, J. & Vervaeke, H. (1975) Investigation of hydrodynamic determinants of competitive swimming strokes. In: *International Series on Sport Sciences*, Vol. 2, *Swimming II* (eds L. Lewillie & J.P. Clarys), pp. 214–222. University Park Press, Baltimore.

Persyn, U., Coleman, V. & Van Tilborg, L. (1992) Movement analysis of the flat and the undulating breaststroke pattern. In: *Biomechanics and Medicine in Swimming* (eds D. MacLaren, T. Reilly & A. Lees), pp. 75–80. E. & F.N. Spon, London.

Reischle, K. (1979) A kinematic investigation of movement patterns in swimming with pro-optical methods. In: *Swimming III* (eds J. Terauds & E.W. Bedingsfield), pp. 127–136. University Park Press, Baltimore.

Rumyantsev, V.A. (1984) *Bio-dynamical Principles of Pulling Technique in Human Swimming*. Central State Institute of Physical Culture, Moscow.

Rumyantsev, V.A. (1982) *Biodynamic Principles of Propulsion in Swimming*. Central State Institute of Physical Culture, Moscow.

Rushall, B.S., Springings, E.J., Holt, L.E. & Cappaert, J.M. (1998) Forces in swimming – a re-evaluation of current status. In: *Swimming Science Bulletin*, No. 19 (ed. B.S. Rushall), pp. 1–36. San Diego State University, San Diego, CA.

Schleihauf, R.E. (1974) A biomechanical analysis of freestyle. *Swimming Technique* **11**, 89–96.

Schleihauf, R.E. (1979) A hydrodynamic analysis of swimming propulsion. In: *Swimming III* (eds J. Terauds & E.W. Bedingsfield), pp. 70–109. University Park Press, Baltimore.

Schleihauf, R.E., Higgins, J.R., Hinrichs, R. *et al.* (1988) Propulsive techniques: front crawl stroke, butterfly, backstroke and breaststroke. In: *Swimming V* (eds B. Ungerechts, K. Reischle & K. Wilke), pp. 53–59. Human Kinetics Publishers, Champaign, IL.

Silvia, C.E. (1970) *Manual and Lesson Plans for Basic Swimming, Water Stunts, Life-saving, Springboard Diving, Skin and Scuba Diving*. C.E. Silvia, Springfield, MA.

Toussaint, H.M. & Beek, P.J. (1992) Bio-mechanics of competitive front crawl swimming. *Sports Medicine* **13** (1), 8–24.

Toussaint, H.M., Hollander, A.P., van den Berg, C. & Vorontsov, A. (2000) Mech-anics and energetics of swimming. In: *Biomechanics of Swimming, Exercise and Sport Science* (eds W.E. Garrett & D.T. Kirkendall), pp. 639–660. Lippincott, Williams & Wilkins, PA.

Vorontsov, A.R. (1981) *Biomechanical Foundations of Swimming Technique*.

Central State Institute of Physical Culture, Moscow.

Wood, T.C. (1979) A fluid dynamic analysis of the propulsive potential of the hand and forearm in swimming. In: *Swimming III* (eds J. Terauds & E.W. Bedingsfield), pp. 62–69. University Park Press, Baltimore.

Zatsiorsky, V.M., Aruin, A.S. & Seluyanov, V.N. (1981) *Biomechanics of Human Motor System*. Fizkultura i Sport, Moscow.

Chapter 11

Performance-Determining Factors in Speed Skating

J.J. DE KONING AND G.J. van INGEN SCHENAU*

Introduction

Speed skating can be described by an energy flow model. Such a model includes expressions that describe both the generation of mechanical energy from chemical substrates and the destination of the flow of energy. These models are useful for the quantitative evaluation of the influence of technical, physiological and environmental variables on speed skating performance. The objective of this chapter is to explain the peculiar nature of speed skating technique and to demonstrate the effects of several performance-determining factors for speed skating by means of a model based on the flow of energy.

Speed skating technique

In most patterns of locomotion, humans generate propulsive forces by pushing against the environment in a direction opposite to the direction of movement. A runner, for example, pushes backwards against a fixed location on the ground to propel himself in a forward direction (Fig. 11.1a). Even in cycling, where it looks as if there is no rigid contact with the ground, forces are directed via the tyre to fixed locations on the road. In speed skating, however, something essentially different occurs. Due to the peculiar qualities of ice, skaters are able to glide with relatively high velocities in the desired forward direction. Skaters make use of the so-called

'gliding technique', which means that the propulsive movements against the ice are made while the skate continues to glide forward (van Ingen Schenau et al. 1987; de Koning et al. 1995). However, when a skate is gliding forward, it is impossible for it to generate propulsive forces by pushing in a backward direction. The only possible direction for an effective pushoff is at right angles relative to the gliding motion of the skate (Fig. 11.1b). The difficulty of the skating technique lies in the transformation of the sideward pushes into a forward velocity. This transformation can best be explained by reference to Fig. 11.1b and Fig. 11.2.

The pushoff force (F_p) generated by the skater has a horizontal (F_x) and a vertical component (F_z). The magnitudes of these components depend on the angle between the force vector F_p and the horizontal, the so-called pushoff angle, α. The horizontal component F_x of the pushoff force causes acceleration in a direction perpendicular to the gliding skate, from right to left, or with a push from the other leg, from left to right. The resulting sideward velocity (v_2 in Fig. 11.2) can be added to the gliding velocity (v_1) in a more or less forward direction. These two velocities result in a new velocity (v_3) with a slightly changed direction in, again, a more or less forward direction. When this is done alternately by the right and left leg, the skater makes a sinusoidal motion.

During the skating cycle the trunk must be kept almost horizontal to minimize frontal area and hence air frictional losses (van Ingen Schenau 1982). At the same time, on conventional skates, powerful plantarflexion needs to be suppressed to prevent

*Prof. G.J. van Ingen Schenau passed away on 2nd April 1998.

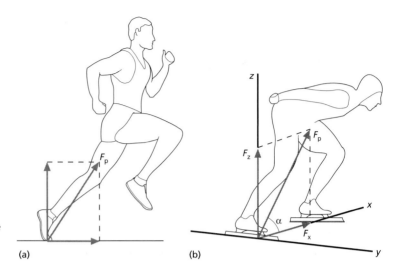

Fig. 11.1 There are big differences between running and skating in the way in which propulsive forces are generated. This largely explains the differences in speed attained by these forms of locomotion. (Adapted from Gemser *et al.* 1999.)

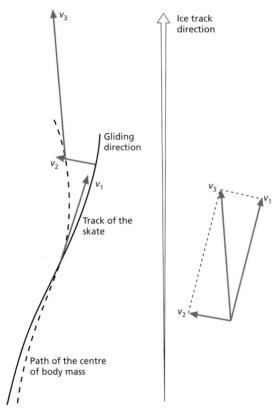

Fig. 11.2 The pushoff results in a velocity (v_2) of the body's centre of mass with respect to the skate. Together with v_1 this determines the new magnitude and direction of velocity (v_3) of the body's centre of mass. (Adapted from Gemser *et al.* 1999.)

the front of the blade from scratching the ice and causing ice frictional losses and disturbances in balance. The absence of trunk rotation and foot rotation results in a pushoff which is mainly done by rotation of only the upper and lower leg. This means that for a proper gliding technique on conventional skates, the pushoff is mainly caused by knee extension.

During the gliding phase of the skating cycle the knee angle is more or less constant. During the pushoff a rapid knee extension occurs. A closer look at the knee angle during the pushoff shows that the knee is not fully extended when the skate is lifted from the ice (Fig. 11.3). This happens at a knee angle of 160°. This early termination of the pushoff is caused by the above-mentioned absence of trunk extension and plantarflexion (van Ingen Schenau *et al.* 1996). Due to this absence the acceleration of the heavy trunk relative to the gliding pushoff skate depends mainly on the velocity at which the hip moves away from the ankle (pushoff velocity V_{ha} in Fig. 11.3). The peak in this velocity is reached far before full extension, at a knee angle of 140°. Soon after the instant that the velocity V_{ha} reaches its maximum, the inertia of the relatively heavy trunk and contralateral leg pulls the skate from the ice and brings the pushoff to an end. With instrumented conventional skates we were able to measure pushoff forces as well as ice friction forces during skating. From the force signals we learnt that the

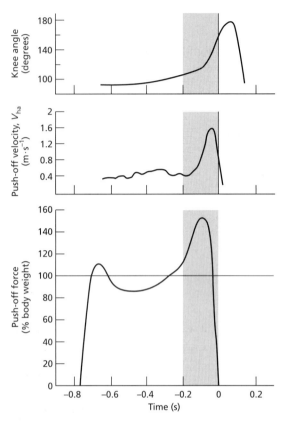

Fig. 11.3 The knee angle, pushoff velocity (V_{ha}) and pushoff force while skating on conventional skates. These are averaged values, measured in five elite speed skaters. In the last 0.2 s of the skating stride the pushoff takes place. (Adapted from Gemser *et al.* 1999.)

peak in pushoff force is reached at a knee angle of 130°. The maximal force was equivalent to 150% of body weight and dropped sharply when the pushoff velocity was over its maximum (Fig. 11.3).

On the basis of the observations described above and a comparison with results from experiments on vertical jumping (Bobbert & van Ingen Schenau 1988), our research group constructed in the mid-1980s a skate which permits the shoe to rotate in a hinge relative to the blade of the skate (van Ingen Schenau *et al.* 1996). We called this skate the 'klap-skate'. The skate allows for a plantarflexion without the drawbacks described before. Skating with this type of skate results in an increase in average power

output of the athlete. Recently all international-level speed skaters have changed to these new skates. All participants of the speed skating disciplines at the 1998 Winter Olympics in Nagano were using these skates, resulting in new world records at each skated distance. The introduction of this new skate by the late Gerrit Jan van Ingen Schenau has changed competitive speed skating forever. The results of biomechanical and physiological research into the exact mechanism behind the increase in perform-ance achieved with this skate will be published soon (Houdijk *et al.* in preparation).

Power in speed skating

Performance in speed skating depends strongly on the power production capacity of the skater. This power is primarily used to overcome the air and ice friction and to increase the kinetic energy of the skater. When a skater is skating at a constant velo-city, there is no change in kinetic energy, so power produced is equal to power dissipated by air and ice friction. In such a particular case there is a balance between power production and power dissipation. In competition such situations are rare. In most cases the generation of mechanical power by the aerobic and anaerobic energy systems will not equal the power necessary to overcome air and ice fric-tion. When the energy systems are producing more mechanical power than is required to overcome air and ice friction the skater will accelerate, and when the energy produced is less than required the skater will decelerate. This will result in a certain velocity profile over the course of the race. With the help of models incorporating power production and power dissipation, it is possible to simulate a race and pre-dict the velocity profile and performance time. This approach was used by van Ingen Schenau *et al.* (1990, 1991, 1992, 1994), de Koning *et al.* (1992a) and de Koning and van Ingen Schenau (1994) to simu-late performances in speed skating, running and cycling.

A model based on the described power equation can be used to investigate the relative importance of factors such as energy production and skating posture and so guide training. For instance, it would be interesting to know how speed skating performance is influenced by training-induced changes in physical parameters, such as oxygen consumption and anaerobic capacity, and by technical parameters, such as trunk position and knee angle. From previous studies it is known that factors like skating posture and distribution of power during the race have a strong effect on performance. Besides the athletic ability of the skaters, environmental factors such as wind (van Ingen Schenau 1982) and ice conditions (de Koning *et al.* 1992b) also strongly affect performance.

The remaining part of this chapter will focus on the use of a power equation applied to speed skating as a tool to demonstrate the relative influence of several performance-determining factors. An experimental analysis of technical and physiological variables was carried out and calculations were made to predict the influence of each variable of interest on performance in the 500, 1000 and 1500 m races of particular skaters. The predicted performances were compared with actual performances of the skaters during their national championships. The variables of interest were the aerobic energy production, anaerobic energy production, race strategy, skating position and environmental factors.

Modelling of speed skating

Power equation

A model (van Ingen Schenau *et al.* 1990) for speed skating based on a power equation that includes expressions for power production and expressions for power dissipation can be written as:

$$P_o = P_f + \frac{dE_{mcb}}{dt} \quad (11.1)$$

where P_o is the average total power output (the mean generated power) of the skater, P_f is the average power loss to air and ice friction, and dE_{mcb}/dt is the average rate of change of the kinetic, rotational and potential energy of the body. The rate of change of mechanical energy of the body averaged over multiple cycles is in speed skating predominantly determined by the rate of change of kinetic energy of the mass centre:

$$\frac{dE_{mcb}}{dt} = \frac{d(\frac{1}{2}mv^2)}{dt} = mv\frac{dv}{dt} \quad (11.2)$$

with v the cycle averaged speed. The rate of change of kinetic energy can thus be calculated by:

$$P_o - P_f = \frac{d(\frac{1}{2}mv^2)}{dt} \quad (11.3)$$

To perform valid simulations of speed skating performance it is necessary to have valid expressions for P_o and P_f.

Determination of power production (P_o)

The metabolic power production of the athlete is the sum of the power produced by the aerobic and anaerobic energy production systems. At the beginning of a maximal exercise bout, the external power output can be considerably higher than that which can be generated later during the exercise. This is due to the immediate availability of energy-rich phosphates and anaerobic glycolysis for the generation of muscle power output (e.g. Åstrand & Rodahl 1986; Serresse *et al.* 1988; Davies & Sandstrom 1989). Due to the limited phosphate pool, the time taken for the aerobic system to develop maximal aerobic power, and the lower maximum value of this aerobic power, a large decrease in power output can be observed during the course of maximally performed exercises.

To model aerobic and anaerobic power production as a function of time, we had 12 male speed skaters, all participants of the Calgary Olympic Oval Program, perform two cycle ergometer tests on a mechanically braked ergometer: a 30 s all-out sprint test and a 2.5 min supramaximal test according to a protocol by de Koning *et al.* (1994).

The 30 s sprint test was a Wingate-type test which the subjects had to perform in an all-out fashion right from the start. The 2.5 min test was preceded by 6 min of submaximal cycling directly followed by the 2.5 min test period. The subjects had to perform the test at an intensity higher than their maximal level, which was predicted on the basis of body mass and power output values in a comparable population of skaters (van Ingen Schenau *et al.* 1988; de Koning *et al.* 1994).

The mechanical power output was determined by the product of the measured pedalling rate and the measured braking force on the flywheel of the ergometer. The results where corrected for the energy flow to and from the flywheel of the cycle ergometer.

The total metabolic power output during the cycle ergometer tests has an aerobic (P_{aer}) and an anaerobic (P_{an}) component:

$$P_o = P_{an} + P_{aer} \tag{11.4}$$

For the estimation of the aerobic power the kinetics of the oxygen consumption ($\dot{V}o_2$) was modelled with:

$$\dot{V}o_2 = \dot{V}o_{2\text{-max}}(1 - e^{-\lambda t}) \tag{11.5}$$

with λ a time constant. On the assumption that 1 litre of O_2 consumed liberates 20.9 kJ of metabolic energy (Åstrand & Rodahl 1986) and with the gross efficiency calculated from the power output and oxygen consumption measured during the sub-maximal exercise preceding the 2.5 min test, the mechanical aerobic power kinetics was modelled as:

$$P_{aer} = P_{aer\text{-max}}(1 - e^{-\lambda t}) \tag{11.6}$$

with $P_{aer\text{-max}}$ the maximal mechanical aerobic power contribution. The value for the time constant λ (0.1069 s^{-1}) was obtained from literature (de Koning et al. in preparation).

To determine the mechanical equivalent of the anaerobic part of the total mechanical power measured during the 30 s sprint test, the aerobic contribution in the total mechanical power output was subtracted from the total mechanical power:

$$P_{an} = P_o - P_{aer} \tag{11.7}$$

The resulting anaerobic power could properly be described by a first-order system:

$$P_{an} = P_{an\text{-max}} e^{-\gamma t} \tag{11.8}$$

with $P_{an\text{-max}}$ the maximal mechanical anaerobic power at $t = 0$ and γ a time constant. Values for $P_{an\text{-max}}$ and γ were obtained by fitting Eqn. 11.8 to Eqn. 11.7. The expression for the anaerobic power output is extrapolated to calculate the total power output during the speed skating races (Fig. 11.4).

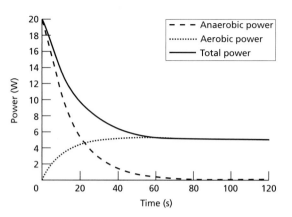

Fig. 11.4 Aerobic and anaerobic energy kinetics during high-intensity exercise. (Adapted from Gemser et al. 1999.)

As extensively discussed for running, the stroke (or cycle) averaged value for the rate of change of segmental energy in cyclic movements is equal to the rate of change of mechanical energy of the mass centre of the body only (e.g. Williams & Cavanagh 1983; Aleshinsky 1986a,b). The amount of power associated with the acceleration and deceleration of body segments is thus not accounted for in the power equation. In comparison to cycling the power associated with acceleration and deceleration of body segments will be substantial in speed skating (de Boer et al. 1986). This means that P_o will be smaller during skating than the mechanical power actually liberated in the contracting muscles. It is known from previous work that external mechanical power and oxygen consumption during maximal skating are lower than during maximal cycling (van Ingen Schenau & de Groot 1983). It is assumed that the difference in P_o during cycling and skating can be approximated by one parameter expressing a certain (constant) fraction f_r of the measured external power in cycling. The value of this parameter, f_r, is estimated on the basis of actual 1500 m performances. The 1500 m event is often judged as a key distance in all-round speed skating since performance at this distance strongly relies on both the aerobic and anaerobic pathways in power production. The parameter f_r is defined as:

$$f_r = \frac{W_{1500\,m}}{E_{1500\,m}} \qquad (11.9)$$

with $W_{1500\,m}$ the sum of the kinetic energy and the calculated work done against friction during the 1500 m race, and $E_{1500\,m}$ the available mechanical energy equivalent of the metabolic processes, as measured on the cycle ergometer, during the time of a 1500 m race.

To determine f_r, the velocity and duration of the 1500 m skating performance were obtained from the seasonal best times of the skaters in this study. $W_{1500\,m}$ was calculated with the equations for air and ice friction. The available mechanical energy equivalent of the metabolic processes ($E_{1500\,m}$) was determined by integration of the equations for the anaerobic and aerobic energy kinetics, as measured during cycling, over the time needed to cover the 1500 m.

The total power output (P_o) during speed skating is now described by:

$$P_o = f_r(P_{an} + P_{aer}) \qquad (11.10)$$

It should be noted that f_r is the only parameter that is estimated from actual speed skating performances of the athletes. Moreover, f_r does not influence the time constants and thus the kinetics of the aerobic and anaerobic pathways.

Determination of power dissipated to friction (P_f)

In speed skating the skater has to overcome ice- and air-frictional forces. Air friction has two components, friction drag and pressure drag. Friction drag is caused by friction in the layers of air along the body and is dependent on, for example, the roughness of the suit. In speed skating, friction drag is relatively small with respect to pressure drag. According to Bernoulli's law, the pressure in the front of the skater is higher than the pressure behind the skater. This is a result of a difference in the relative velocity of the air with respect to the front and back the body. This pressure difference is mainly determined by the dynamic pressure $1/2\rho v^2$ where ρ is the density of the air and v the velocity of the air with respect to the body. Given a cross-sectional area (the surface within the contour of a frontal picture) A_p, the pressure drag equals $1/2\rho v^2 A_p$. This relationship, however, does not account for the influence of streamlining, and the contribution of friction drag. Therefore, a dimensionless coefficient C_d is added to this equation and is called the drag coefficient. This drag coefficient can only be determined experimentally. Total air friction force F_{air} thus equals:

$$F_{air} = 1/2\rho v^2 A_p C_d \qquad (11.11)$$

Wind tunnel experiments on speed skaters (van Ingen Schenau 1982) showed a strong dependency of C_d on velocity, v. With these wind-tunnel experiments relations between air friction and anthropometric variables as well as skating position were made. For a steady speed v the air frictional force (F_{air}) and air frictional power (P_{air}) has been modelled as:

$$F_{air} = k_1 e^{-0.000125h} v_1^2 l^3 \sqrt{m} F(\theta_1) G(\theta_0) H(v_1) \qquad (11.12)$$

$$P_{air} = F_{air} v \qquad (11.13)$$

with $k_1 = $ constant; $h = $ altitude; $v_1 = $ velocity of the air relative to the skater; $l = $ body height; $m = $ body mass; $F(\theta_1)$ and $G(\theta_0) = $ expressions which account for trunk position and knee angle, respectively; $H(v) = $ influence of the velocity on the drag coefficient; and $v = $ velocity of the skater relative to the ice. Since velocity variations within a stroke are small in speed skating, the influence of these within-stroke variations in v on the calculation of P_{air} (and P_{ice}) is ignored.

The ice frictional force (F_{ice}) and ice frictional power loss (P_{ice}) is assumed to be equal to:

$$F_{ice} = \mu m g \qquad (11.14)$$

$$P_{ice} = F_{ice} v \qquad (11.15)$$

with μ the ice friction coefficient and g the gravitational acceleration.

To obtain values associated with speed skating techniques, the skaters were filmed during 1500 m races at the Canada Cup and Olympic Oval Finale in the indoor speed skating oval in Calgary. The subjects were filmed in the sagittal plane with a 16 mm high-speed film camera operated at a frame rate of 100 Hz. To define the positions of the lower leg, upper leg and upper body, points on the body

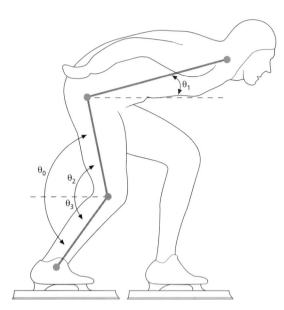

Fig. 11.5 The most important angles for describing the skating position. The common values for these angles in all-round speed skaters are: θ_1: 10–30°; θ_0: 100–130°; θ_3: 60–80°. (Adapted from Gemser *et al.* 1999.)

corresponding with the lateral malleolus, knee joint, greater trochanter and neck were digitized using a motion analyser (Fig. 11.5). Each film frame was digitized three times to improve the accuracy of determination of the body segmental positions. From these positions the average trunk angle (θ_1) and knee angle (θ_0) during the gliding phase of the stroke were obtained. These trunk and knee angles were used to calculate the air frictional forces as described above.

Simulations

For each step in the simulation, the rate of change of kinetic energy was calculated with:

$$P_o(t) - P_{air}(v) - P_{ice}(v) = \frac{d(\tfrac{1}{2}mv^2)}{dt} \qquad (11.16)$$

The time history of the kinetic energy of the mass centre of the body, and therewith the velocity, was acquired by simultaneous integration of this equation with a variable step size second-order predictor, third-order corrector integration algorithm

using the Runge–Kutta method. The simulations were performed for the 500, 1000 and 1500 m events.

The input parameters for the simulation model consist of subject-specific data, group averaged data and data from the literature.

Factors that influence performance

Results from physiological testing and film analysis

The primary purpose of collecting the anthropometric, physiological and movement analysis data was to acquire parameter values for the simulation model described above. Table 11.1 shows the mean values of the relevant test parameters. Individual parameter values were used in the model calculations.

Simulation results

Typical examples of a velocity–time curve obtained from simulation, time histories of power output and frictional power losses are shown in Fig. 11.6. According to the power equation described above, the skating velocity increases as long as the power output exceeds the power losses to friction. The velocity decreases when these frictional losses are larger than the power output.

The mean times necessary to cover the 500, 1000 and 1500 m derived by simulation are presented in Table 11.2. The simulations appear to show a close

Table 11.1 Results from physiological testing and film analysis.

Parameter*	Mean (SD)
$\dot{V}O_2$max (l · min^{-1})	4.57 (0.43)
Gross efficiency	0.21 (0.02)
P_{an-max} (W · kg^{-1})	17.83 (1.89)
γ (s^{-1})	0.0347 (0.008)
Ratio skating/cycling f_r	0.55 (0.06)
Length (m)	1.81 (0.02)
Mass (kg)	74.0 (4.4)
Trunk angle θ_1	13.7° (4.1)
Knee angle θ_0	106.0° (5.5)

* For explanation of symbols see text.

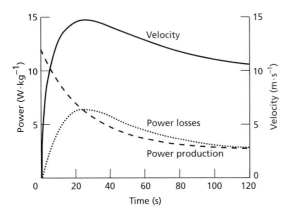

Fig. 11.6 Simulated pacing pattern of a 1500 m race. The skating velocity increases as long as the power output exceeds the power losses to friction. The velocity decreases when these frictional losses are larger than the power output. (Adapted from Gemser *et al.* 1999.)

Table 11.2 Mean results from simulations and actual speed skating.

Distance	Speed skating*	Simulation*	Difference (%)
500 m	0:39.18 (1.33)	0:39.16 (1.32)	0.11 (3.13)
1000 m	1:18.08 (2.05)	1:16.30 (1.59)	2.33 (1.72)
1500 m	1:58.97 (2.04)	1:59.58 (1.92)	0.51 (0.22)

* 'Stopwatch' times, in minutes and seconds.
Values in ( ) denote standard deviation.

fit to the actual mean skating times. On average the times derived from simulation are 1% different from the actual times of the speed skaters in this study. These results indicate that good predictions of speed skating performances can be made with a power equation model.

The good performance of the model gives us the opportunity to carry out simulations in which we systematically change different input variables of the model. These changes in input variables will give changes in simulated speed skating times and hence demonstrate the relative importance of the input variables on speed skating performance. In the remaining part of this chapter we will focus on variables that influence power production and variables that influence power losses to friction.

Power production

The energy for muscular contraction comes immediately from adenosine triphosphate (ATP). ATP is split into adenosine diphosphate (ADP) and a free phosphate group during the process of resetting the myosin cross-bridge. There are three energy systems that counteract the decrease in ATP concentration during muscular contraction. They are the phosphagens, the lactate-producing energy system and the aerobic energy system.

The phosphagen energy system includes the ATP within the muscle cell and a related compound, creatine phosphate (CP), which is capable of rapidly converting ADP to ATP. The lactate-producing energy system produces ATP at a high rate by degrading glycogen to lactic acid. This system works well except that lactate is an acid which exerts several negative effects in the muscle cell. The aerobic energy system produces ATP by oxidizing carbohydrates and free fatty acids (FFA). This system depends upon the availability of oxygen delivered from the circulatory system. In most energy-demanding sports (running, cycling, swimming, skiing) the aerobic energy system is of primary importance. In speed skating, however, the characteristic crouched posture and deeply bent knee position interfere with blood flow to the leg and hip muscles and increase the importance of the lactate-producing energy system.

During high-intensity exercise, the oxygen uptake increases rapidly to near maximal values (Fig. 11.4). In contrast, the kinetics of the anaerobic energy supply shows, after an initial peak at the onset of exercise, a decrease as time progresses. The decrease in anaerobic power output is larger than the increase in aerobic power output, resulting in a gradually decreasing total power output in time (Fig. 11.4). The percentage aerobic vs. anaerobic energy metabolism changes rapidly as the length of the event increases. Table 11.3 presents the relative contributions of the aerobic and anaerobic pathways to the total energy production per distance. One should be careful when interpreting these figures. The relative contributions include the large amount of anaerobic work necessary to accelerate during the start. When this part is covered, the

Table 11.3 Relative contribution in total work done by the anaerobic and aerobic energy system.

Energy system	Speed skating discipline		
	500 m	1000 m	1500 m
Anaerobic	70%	49%	36%
Aerobic	30%	51%	64%

skaters will have to rely on aerobic power to a greater extent than is suggested by the figures in Table 11.3. Even at 1000 m one has to cover the last lap predominantly on the basis of aerobic power. During the last lap of a 1500 m race the energy supply is > 90% aerobic.

Higher values for $\dot{V}o_{2\text{-max}}$ will only have small effects on the relative contributions of the aerobic and anaerobic energy systems at the different distances, but considerable effect on skating speed, and thus on final times. Table 11.4 presents the difference in speed skating performance as a result of changes in $\dot{V}o_{2\text{-max}}$. The mean $\dot{V}o_{2\text{-max}}$ as measured during the cycle ergometer tests is used as reference. The variation in maximal oxygen uptake over which the simulations are performed is close to the range in maximal oxygen uptake as found for the speed skaters. This means that the variation in the maximal oxygen uptake can be judged as a 'physiological range'.

The same type of calculations can be done with the anaerobic energy system. If we take the anaerobic capacity (the area under the anaerobic power output curve, Fig. 11.4) as the variable to alter over the range as observed in the group of athletes in this

Table 11.4 Effect of simulated changes in maximal oxygen uptake ($\dot{V}o_{2\text{-max}}$) on performance time.*

Event	−10%	−5%	$\dot{V}o_{2\text{-max}}$	+5%	+10%
500 m	0:39.29 (+0.8%)	0:39.13 (+0.4%)	0:38.98	0:38.83 (−0.4%)	0:38.68 (−0.8%)
1000 m	1:17.31 (+1.5%)	1:16.71 (+0.7%)	1:16.15	1:15.60 (−0.7%)	1:15.07 (−1.4%)
1500 m	2:02.70 (+2.5%)	2:01.15 (+1.2%)	1:59.69	1:58.34 (−1.1%)	1:57.06 (−2.2%)

* 'Stopwatch' times, in minutes and seconds.

Table 11.5 Effect of simulated changes in anaerobic capacity (P_{an}) on performance time.*

Event	−15%	−7.5%	P_{an}	+7.5%	+15%
500 m	0:41.03 (+5.3%)	0:39.97 (+2.5%)	0:38.98	0:38.07 (−2.3%)	0:37.24 (−4.5%)
1000 m	1:19.80 (+4.8%)	1:17.92 (+2.3%)	1:16.15	1:14.49 (−2.2%)	1:12.94 (−4.2%)
1500 m	2:04.56 (+4.1%)	2:02.08 (+2.0%)	1:59.69	1:57.44 (−1.9%)	1:55.32 (−3.6%)

* 'Stopwatch' times, in minutes and seconds.

study we see even larger effects on skating speed (Table 11.5). This stresses the importance of the anaerobic energy system for speed skating.

In most of the metric style speed skating events there is a regularly observed tendency for the athlete to decelerate during the latter 30–50% of the event. In the longer events (5 km and 10 km), the pace tends to be relatively more even, while some contemporary athletes even have a 'negative split' (skating the second half faster than the first).

Tactical considerations aside, the primary issue that determines the pacing strategy is, on the one hand, the velocity of the skater when passing the finish line (this velocity is useless after the finish line, and thus represents a waste of kinetic energy) and, on the other hand, the risk of a massive slowdown late in the race due to fatigue. In longer events or in conditions with a greater potential for slowing down if power output is decreasing (e.g. bad ice, low altitude, windy conditions), a more conservative use of the athlete's energetic resources is often chosen. However, in shorter events or in events with less potential for slowing down (e.g. high altitude, good ice) the athlete and his or her coach often choose a more aggressive strategy.

Performances in speed skating events depend on the time taken to cover a certain distance. At the start, it takes a considerable time to cover the first few metres. This means that high acceleration at the beginning of the race is beneficial. This is illustrated by high coefficients of correlation between 100 m split times and 500 m final times during major (sprint) competitions. In a study during the 1988 Winter

Table 11.6 Results (race times*) from simulation with three different strategies.

Strategy	Event		
	500 m	1000 m	1500 m
1. 'All-out'	0:38.98	1:16.15	1:59.69
2. 'Super-sprint'	0:37.59	1:14.92	1:59.40
3. 'Constant-power'	0:39.37	1:17.36	2:00.56

* 'Stopwatch' times, in minutes and seconds.

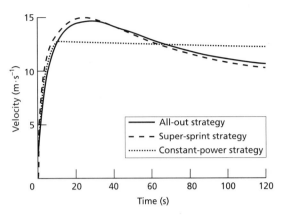

Fig. 11.7 Pacing patterns during simulated 1500 m races with an 'all-out' strategy, a 'super-sprint' strategy and a 'constant-power' strategy. (Adapted from Gemser *et al.* 1999.)

Olympics, velocity patterns of a large group of skaters during starts in the 500 m event were obtained (de Koning *et al.* 1989). The average acceleration in the first second of the race, calculated from the increase in velocity, showed a strong relation with the 100 m and 500 m distance times. The coefficients of correlation between the average initial acceleration and 100 and 500 m times were −0.76 and −0.75, respectively. This means that a large part of the very small range in final times of these highly trained Olympic skaters could be explained by differences in acceleration during the first second of the start. Fast acceleration at the start of the sprint is only possible when large amounts of anaerobic energy are available in the first few pushoffs of the race. This is supported by significant correlations between peak anaerobic power output measured on cycle ergometers and personal best times in 500 m skating races.

With the simulation model some interesting calculations can be made to mimic different possible strategies for pacing, and thus for spending the available anaerobic energy during the race. When we assume that a skater can spend a certain amount of anaerobic energy (his anaerobic capacity) during the race and he is free in the distribution of that energy, different pacing strategies can be employed. Three additional simulations were performed with the following three strategies.
1 Strategy 1: the 'all-out' strategy, where the skater was skating according to the anaerobic kinetics as measured on the cycle ergometer.
2 Strategy 2: the 'super-sprint' strategy, where the skater has a 20% increased anaerobic peak power output but an unchanged anaerobic capacity.

3 Strategy 3: the 'constant-power' strategy, where the skater is producing a constant power output after a 15 s 'all-out' start.
In all three simulations the energy spent during the different races is equal. Results of these simulations are summarized in Table 11.6.

The times in Table 11.6 show that the best results are obtained when the power output at the onset of the race is highest. These results show that the anaerobic capacity in itself is not a decisive factor for sprinting events. It rather appears that sprinting performances are strongly influenced by the rate of liberation of anaerobic energy at the very onset of a race.

The results of the simulations of the 1500 m event show that the most 'sprinter-type' strategy (strategy 2) only gives a small advantage. The strategy with a constant power output after an all-out start of 15 s is slower than the 'all-out' and 'super-sprint' strategies. The velocity patterns of the 1500 m skated according to the different strategies are shown in Fig. 11.7. The more uniform velocity pattern of the 'constant-power' strategy results in lower air frictional forces but has the disadvantage that the skater is passing the finish with a high velocity and thus a high content of kinetic energy. This kinetic energy has its origin from the energy systems but is not used to overcome friction, and in that sense is useless. For best results there is an optimal distribution between energy used to overcome friction and kinetic energy left at the end of the race. It should be noted that for 1500 m races, strategies 1 and 2 could create big problems for the athlete because of the accumulated muscle lactate and associated reduction in power generation. Needless to say, this phenomenon is not incorporated in the simulations given here. It is likely that during actual 1500 m races skaters will make use of a combined strategy 1 and strategy 3 approach.

Power losses to friction

Coaches and scientists are well aware of the powerful impact that skating posture has on air friction. All skaters are instructed to skate with a trunk position that is as horizontal as possible and with a knee angle that, during the gliding phase, is as small as possible. The effect on performance of a number of these factors has been calculated, which gives an indication of the magnitude of their influence. In these calculations one single factor is varied at a time, assuming that all other circumstances remain the same. This is the only way in which an impression can be obtained of the relative importance of such a factor. This does not mean that immediate conclusions can be drawn regarding individual skaters. For example, it will be shown that skating just a few degrees lower will lead to a considerable gain in time. But the posture of a skater cannot be changed easily, since this has a major influence on the force level at which, especially, the knee extenders have to work. However, this kind of knowledge does make clear that, besides technical reasons relating to pushoff, a deeper skating posture is an important factor that should be addressed during the development of a speed skater. This example will hopefully sufficiently clarify what this section deals with, namely indicating the relative importance of a number of factors that influence friction and thus performance.

Some of these factors influence not only friction but also the glide and pushoff techniques. Here also, the focus in this section will be on the effects on friction and frictional losses.

SKATING POSTURE

Figure 11.5 shows some important angles that describe the skating posture. These angles are: (i) the angle that records the position of the trunk with respect to the horizontal (θ_1); and (ii) the angle at the knee joint during the gliding phase (θ_0). This latter angle is equal to the sum of θ_2 and θ_3, which are the angles that record the positions of the upper and lower leg. The angles θ_1 and θ_0 have a big influence on friction, and their influence on performance is shown in Tables 11.7 and 11.8, respectively.

The results in Table 11.7 and Table 11.8 show that the trunk angle especially is an extremely important factor. One can state that skaters who have their trunk in a relatively horizontal position have an extremely large advantage compared to skaters with a more inclined trunk position. With a trunk angle only 5° smaller skaters are able to skate the 1500 m in 3 s less. When viewing recordings of

Table 11.7 Effect of simulated changes in trunk angle (θ_1) on performance time.*

Event	+5°	+2.5°	$\theta_1 = 13.7°$	−2.5°	−5°
500 m	0:39.42 (+1.1%)	0:39.20 (+0.6%)	0:38.98	0:38.76 (−0.6%)	0:38.54 (−1.1%)
1000 m	1:17.65 (+2.0%)	1:16.89 (+1.0%)	1:16.15	1:15.40 (−1.0%)	1:14.64 (−2.0%)
1500 m	2:02.78 (+2.6%)	2:01.24 (+1.3%)	1:59.69	1:58.16 (−1.3%)	1:56.63 (−2.6%)

* 'Stopwatch' times, in minutes and seconds.

Table 11.8 Effect of simulated changes in knee angle (θ_0) on performance time.*

Event	+10°	+5°	$\theta_0 = 106°$	−5°	−10°
500 m	0:39.50 (+1.3%)	0:39.24 (+0.7%)	0:38.98	0:38.72 (−0.7%)	0:38.47 (−1.3%)
1000 m	1:17.88 (+2.3%)	1:17.01 (+1.1%)	1:16.15	1:15.28 (−1.1%)	1:14.40 (−2.3%)
1500 m	2:03.26 (+3.0%)	2:01.49 (+1.5%)	1:59.69	1:57.92 (−1.5%)	1:56.14 (−3.0%)

* 'Stopwatch' times, in minutes and seconds.

skaters in the 1960s and 1970s, it is clear that the tremendous improvement in speed skating performances during the last decades is due largely to an improvement in the trunk position. The same recordings show that the current high-performance speed skaters have smaller knee angles than the skaters of former decades, but these differences are not very large. This is understandable since the knee angle in particular has a strong influence on the force of the muscles that have to do external work. This force level of the hip and knee extensor muscles is to a large extent determined by the position of the upper leg. Due to anatomical limitations, the skater is not entirely free to choose each knee and trunk position without changing the horizontal position of his centre of gravity with respect to his ankle joint. This might explain why, especially over short distances, not all high-performance skaters can be trained to hold their trunk in a horizontal position.

ICE FRICTION AND ALTITUDE

The ice friction coefficient can vary greatly between tournaments, but also during tournaments. The first is not really disturbing. As long as all competitors have good or bad ice the average times may exceed expectations or be disappointing, but the ice conditions do not affect the competition. But when ice quality changes during a tournament, a tournament could very well turn into a lottery.

Measurements have shown that, especially on outdoor tracks, the ice friction coefficient may increase by more than 50% between ice preparations. An ice

friction coefficient of 0.004 can be judged as good ice; values in the range 0.005–0.006 indicate wet ice or ice with frost on it, whereas values in the range 0.002–0.003 indicate ice of superior quality. The effect of a 50% increase in this coefficient on a 1500 m time would be 2.8 s. The final times for longer distance races (5 and 10 km) are even more sensitive to such a change in ice quality (because the relative contribution of ice friction is higher). Such influences justify the use of the word 'lottery'. The effect of ice friction, expressed as the coefficient of ice friction, on performance is shown in Table 11.9.

The air friction a skater is subjected to is directly proportional to the density of the air, and air density markedly decreases at higher altitudes. However, air density can also vary notably at the same location. The air density is approximately proportional to air pressure. The most extreme readings that can be made from a barometer at sea level (970–1040 millibar) could already account for a 7% difference in air density. Expressed in terms of performance time this means a maximal calculated difference of approximately 0.8 s per lap as a result of changes in air pressure alone. Of course, this holds true only if all other circumstances remain equal, but this is often not the case on outdoor tracks. High barometer readings are often coupled to fine and freezing weather, while the advantage of low barometer readings is often nullified by the concomitant presence of wind and high humidity. Still, such variations in air pressure will often be the prime explanation for performances that are below expectations despite apparently optimal conditions.

Table 11.9 Effect of ice friction coefficient (μ) on performance time.*

Event	$\mu = 0.006$	$\mu = 0.005$	$\mu = 0.004$	$\mu = 0.003$	$\mu = 0.002$
500 m	0:39.44 (+1.1%)	0:39.18 (+0.5%)	0:38.98	0:38.79 (−0.5%)	0:38.57 (−1.1%)
1000 m	1:17.60 (+1.8%)	1:16.80 (+0.9%)	1:16.15	1:15.44 (−0.9%)	1:14.76 (−1.8%)
1500 m	2:02.97 (+2.7%)	2:01.06 (+1.1%)	1:59.69	1:58.16 (−1.3%)	1:56.69 (−2.5%)

* 'Stopwatch' times, in minutes and seconds.

Table 11.10 Effect of (standardized) local barometric pressure on performance time.*

Event	+30 mB	+15 mB	P = 1010 mB	−15 mB	−30 mB
500 m	0:39.18 (+0.5%)	0:39.09 (+0.3%)	0:38.98	0:38.88 (−0.3%)	0:38.79 (−0.5%)
1000 m	1:16.80 (+0.9%)	1:16.47 (+0.4%)	1:16.15	1:15.81 (−0.4%)	1:15.48 (−0.9%)
1500 m	2:01.06 (+1.1%)	2:00.38 (+0.6%)	1:59.69	1:59.02 (−0.6%)	1:58.34 (−1.1%)

* 'Stopwatch' times, in minutes and seconds.

Table 11.11 Effect of altitude on performance time.*

	Location (altitude above sea level)				
	Hamar (126 m)	Nagano (375 m)	Inzell (690 m)	Calgary (1035 m)	Salt Lake City (1305 m)
Air pressure 0 m = 1000 mbar	984	954	917	879	849
500 m	0:39.70 (+1.8%)	0:39.49 (+1.3%)	0:39.25 (+0.7%)	0:38.98	0:38.81 (−0.4%)
1000 m	1:18.53 (+3.1%)	1:17.84 (+2.2%)	1:17.02 (+1.1%)	1:16.15	1:15.56 (−0.8%)
1500 m	2:04.41 (+3.9%)	2:03.05 (+2.8%)	2:01.43 (+1.5%)	1:59.69	1:58.55 (−1.0%)

* 'Stopwatch' times, in minutes and seconds.

The influence of air pressure is much more obvious on indoor tracks, but here too disappointing times are often attributed to the ice conditions. For example, when shortly after the opening of the first 400 m indoor track in the world (Thialf in Heerenveen, The Netherlands) many world records were broken on that track while the air pressure was (very) low. This led to unjustly high expectations during later tournaments, simply because the air pressure was not taken into account. Many skaters, reporters and sometimes even coaches tend to doubt the skills of the local ice resurfacers. By systematically measuring the air pressure, coaches can assure themselves that the variable times in Heerenveen are mostly due to changes in air pressure. During sprint tournaments, when the same distances are skated on both days, even small differences in air pressure from one day to the next can often account for small differences in average times. As Table 11.10 shows, it is therefore always important to keep an eye on the barometer when judging the performances on ice.

The air pressure and therefore the air density decrease significantly at increasing altitudes above sea level, as can be seen in Table 11.11. This means that at high-altitude tracks, in principle, faster times may be expected than at sea level. With the aid of the simulations it has been calculated what the advantages of skating on higher-altitude tracks would be at several distances if all other circumstances were identical. The results are shown in Table 11.11, where the altitude of Calgary is used as reference.

However, a number of marginal notes should be made in this regard. First of all, the advantage of decreased air resistance may be partly nullified by a lower aerobic capacity, which is the result of the decreased oxygen concentration in the air concomitant with decreased air pressure. This could result in a lower oxygen consumption. Measurements have shown, however, that, especially after a period of acclimatization, the maximally generated power on a cycle ergometer will hardly, if at all, decrease at the altitudes which are mentioned in Table 11.11. In addition, oxygen consumption is especially limited on the muscular level in speed skating and thus the influence of a decreased oxygen concentration in the air will presumably affect performance at even higher altitudes than it does in cycling or running. Regarding this aspect one would expect faster times, even at longer distances, if tracks were constructed at even higher altitudes.

A second aspect that should be considered when interpreting the predictions of Table 11.11 is the previously mentioned effect of changes in air pressure as a result of high- and low-pressure areas. If, for example, one skates a personal best time in Hamar or Heerenveen at relatively low pressure, a performance in Calgary can be really disappointing if the race coincides with a high-pressure area. The chances of this happening are rather high since the average winter air pressure in Calgary, if converted to sea level, is higher than in, for example, The Netherlands or Norway. Therefore, the average differences in performance between Calgary and Heerenveen or Hamar are smaller than the model predicts. This holds especially true for skaters who

often skate in Heerenveen or Hamar (they have a higher chance of coming across low-pressure areas). This unevenly distributed game of chance also holds true for skaters who often skate in Calgary: their performances in Hamar or Heerenveen can be very disappointing in comparison with their own personal best times.

Conclusions

From the issues that have been the focus of this chapter a number of conclusions can be drawn that may be of great importance to speed skaters in competition.

As has been stated, the optimal performance of the competitive skater depends on both the minimization of frictional losses and the maximization of power. Regarding friction, the most important factors are body position and air density. On the power generation side it is clear that for short distances the distribution of available energy is of great importance. Obviously, there must be caution in translating simulation results for practical applications. Still, to summarize this chapter, it is possible to create a picture of the mechanically 'ideal speed skater' on the basis of this simulation approach. The ideal skater skates low, keeps his or her trunk in a good horizontal position, and generates a high amount of power. This high power is generated predominantly by a large amount of work at pushoff. The skater should use klapskates and pushoff correctly sideways, which theoretically makes every pushoff optimally effective.

References

Aleshinsky, S.Y. (1986a) An energy 'sources' and 'fractions' approach to the mechanical energy expenditure problem-I. Basic concepts, descriptions of the model, analysis of a one-link system movement. *Journal of Biomechanics* **19**, 287–293.

Aleshinsky, S.Y. (1986b) An energy 'sources' and 'fractions' approach to the mechanical energy expenditure problem-II. Movement of the multi-link chain model. *Journal of Biomechanics* **19**, 295–300.

Åstrand, P.O. & Rodahl, K. (1986) *Textbook of Work Physiology*. McGraw-Hill, New York.

Bobbert, M.F. & van Ingen Schenau, G.J. (1988) Coordination in vertical jumping. *Journal of Biomechanics* **21**, 249–262.

de Boer, R.W., de Groot, G. & van Ingen Schenau, G.J. (1986) Specificity of training in speed skating. *Biomechanics X-B* (ed. B. Jonsson). Human Kinetics Publishers, Champaign. IL.

Davies, C.T.M. & Sandstrom, E.R. (1989) Maximal mechanical power output and capacity of cyclists and young adults. *European Journal of Applied Physiology* **58**, 838–844.

Gemser, H., de Koning, J.J. & van Ingen Schenau, G.J. (eds) (1999) *Handbook of*

Competitive Speed Skating. International Skating Union, Lausanne.

van Ingen Schenau, G.J. (1982) The influence of air friction in speed skating. *Journal of Biomechanics* **15**, 449–458.

van Ingen Schenau, G.J. & de Groot, G. (1983) Differences in oxygen consumption and external power between male and female speed skaters during supra maximal cycling. *European Journal of Applied Physiology* **51**, 337–345.

van Ingen Schenau, G.J., de Boer, R. & de Groot, G. (1987) On the technique of speed skating. *International Journal of Sport Biomechanics* **3**, 419–431.

van Ingen Schenau, G.J., de Boer, R.W.,

Geysel, J.S.M. & de Groot, G. (1988) Supramaximal test results of male and female speed skaters with particular reference to methodological problems. *European Journal of Applied Physiology* **57**, 6–9.

van Ingen Schenau, G.J., de Koning, J.J. & de Groot, G. (1990) A simulation of speed skating performances based on a power equation. *Medicine and Science in Sports and Exercise* **22**, 718–728.

van Ingen Schenau, G.J., Jacobs, R. & de Koning, J.J. (1991) Can cycle power predict sprint running performance? *European Journal of Applied Physiology* **63**, 255–260.

van Ingen Schenau, G.J. (1992) The distribution of anaerobic energy in 1000 and 4000 metre cycling bouts. *International Journal of Sports Medicine* **13**, 447–451.

van Ingen Schenau, G.J., de Koning, J.J. & de Groot, G. (1994) Optimisation of sprinting performance in running,

cycling and speed skating. *Sports Medicine* **17**, 259–275.

van Ingen Schenau, G.J., de Groot, G., Schreurs, A.W., Meester, H. & de Koning, J.J. (1996) A new skate allowing powerful plantar flexions improves performance. *Medicine and Science in Sports and Exercise* **28**, 531–535.

de Koning, J.J. & van Ingen Schenau, G.J. (1994) On the estimation of mechanical power in endurance sports. *Sport Science Reviews* **3**, 34–54.

de Koning, J.J., de Groot, G. & van Ingen Schenau, G.J. (1989) Mechanical aspects of the sprint start in Olympic speed skating. *International Journal of Sport Biomechanics* **5**, 151–168.

de Koning, J.J., de Groot, G. & van Ingen Schenau, G.J. (1992a) A power equation for the sprint in speed skating. *Journal of Biomechanics* **25**, 573–580.

de Koning, J.J., de Groot, G. & van Ingen Schenau, G.J. (1992b) Ice friction during

speed skating. *Journal of Biomechanics* **25**, 565–571.

de Koning, J.J., Bakker, F.C., de Groot, G. & van Ingen Schenau, G.J. (1994) Longitudinal development of young talented speed skaters: physiological and anthropometric aspects. *Journal of Applied Physiology* **77**, 2311–2317.

de Koning, J.J., Thomas, R., Berger, M., de Groot, G. & van Ingen Schenau, G.J. (1995) The start in speed skating: from running to gliding. *Medicine and Science in Sports and Exercise* **27**, 1703–1708.

Serresse, O., Lortie, G., Bouchard, C. & Boulay, M.R. (1988) Estimation of the contribution of the various energy systems during maximal work of short duration. *International Journal of Sports Medicine* **9**, 456–460.

Williams, K.R. & Cavanagh, P.R. (1983) A model for the calculation of mechanical power during distance running. *Journal of Biomechanics* **16**, 115–128.

Chapter 12

Cross-Country Skiing: Technique, Equipment and Environmental Factors Affecting Performance

G.A. SMITH

Introduction

Relatively few sports have gone through revolutionary technique changes without abandoning the old techniques. For example, in high-jumping, the 'Fosbury flop' has completely displaced older techniques. Virtually no one high-jumps with the straddle or the western roll techniques any more. In cross-country skiing, the revolutionary development of skating as a racing technique occurred in the early 1980s. The performance advantages of ski-skating became readily apparent within one or two seasons, and by 1985 skating had come to dominate elite ski racing. In an effort to salvage traditional skiing technique, the International Ski Federation (FIS) decreed that World Cup events were to be divided into 'classic' and 'free technique' races. Classic races would be skating-restricted while the free technique races were unrestricted. The half classic, half skating split to the World Cup schedule which was suggested by the FIS has been maintained since then and is matched by equal emphasis given to classical and skating in national and even most regional ski racing.

The 'split personality' of cross-country skiing which has resulted from the maintenance of traditional and newer skating techniques provides a wide variety of movement patterns which are commonly used in ski racing (see Fig. 12.1). The almost infinite variations of technique that can be observed in any ski race illustrate the daunting nature of undertaking generalizations aimed at the relationship of technique to performance. Nevertheless, cross-country skiing is a technical as well as an endurance sport, where race performance is not completely determined by physiology. Mechanical factors clearly affect how skiers move over snow—understanding those factors has challenged sport biomechanists for several decades.

The development of biomechanical understanding of ski technique has followed a predictable course from kinematics to kinetics. Early studies of both classical (Dillman 1979; Martin 1979; Gagnon 1981; Dal Monte et al. 1983) and skating techniques (Gervais & Wronko 1988; Smith et al. 1988) were largely descriptive in nature and provided some insights into the movement pattern characteristics. Subsequent kinetic analyses have provided a starting point for explaining the observed kinematics, though to date these explanations are quite incomplete. A review of this literature spanning more than two decades encounters a large body of physiological and biomechanical writing devoted to understanding cross-country skiing performance. In that somewhat confusing array of studies, one relationship has been clearer than most others: whether skating or striding or double-poling, faster skiers with better race performance tend to ski with greater cycle length than do slower skiers (Bilodeau et al. 1996). Figure 12.2 illustrates this relationship for the double-poling technique with 20 skiers competing in the women's 30 km race from the Lillehammer Winter Olympics. While this relationship has not been observed for all terrain and conditions, the frequency with which something like Fig. 12.2 has been seen suggests that top-performing ski racers are often able to glide further per cycle than slower skiers.

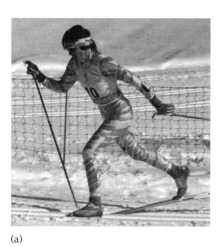
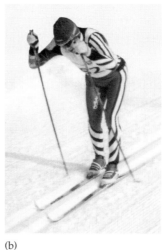
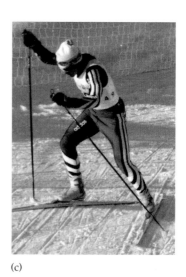

(a)   (b)   (c)

Fig. 12.1 Classic and skating techniques of cross-country skiing. Races are designated as 'free technique', in which skating is permitted, and 'classical' in which it is restricted. Diagonal stride (a) is the fundamental classical technique, while double-poling (b) is used in both disciplines. A variety of skating techniques (c) are used as terrain and conditions affect ski glide characteristics.

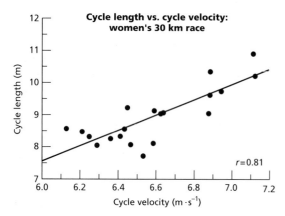

Fig. 12.2 Cycle length and race performance. Double-poling cycle length and race time data from the women's 30 km race of the Lillehammer Winter Olympics (from Smith *et al.* 1996). Faster skiers are often able to generate greater cycle lengths than slower skiers while maintaining similar cycle rates.

The remainder of this chapter will address factors which allow top-performing skiers to generate greater cycle lengths than others. As a mechanical system, a skier moving over snow is driven by the forces acting on the system thus the focus of the following will be largely on kinetic characteristics.

Forces acting on the skier

Cross-country skiing performance is affected by a wide range of factors that determine a skier's speed. Unlike an endurance sport such as running, where physiological capacities are the major determinants of performance, and where environmental conditions, equipment and technique have relatively little effect, skiing performance is often influenced by mechanics. Across the wide range of skiing techniques, several general factors can be described which directly determine a skier's motion. These are illustrated in Fig. 12.3 and can be collectively grouped into forces which are resistive and those which are propulsive in nature. This section will describe various methods of force measurement, gravitational and inertial mass effects on skiing, and the origins of snow and air drag forces. Following sections of this chapter will focus on minimization of drag forces acting against a skier and on optimization of propulsive forces which drive the motion.

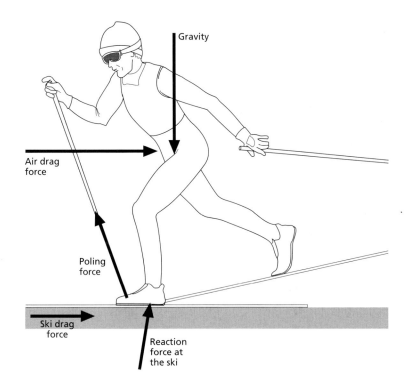

Fig. 12.3 Forces acting on a skier.

Reaction forces at the skis and poles

Skier-generated forces applied through the skis and poles are probably the most easily adjusted of the kinetic factors determining a skier's performance. In both classical and skating races, competitors commonly employ a variety of techniques which affect the distribution of forces and the metabolic costs to the skier (Hoffman 1992). Measurement of the ski and pole reaction forces is of considerable interest for understanding ski technique as it can shed light on the relative importance of the upper body to the legs in propulsion; it can illustrate characteristic differences between techniques; and it can be used to detect individual skier weaknesses in technique. Despite this potential, such force measurements are rarely done and a rather incomplete picture of ski and pole forces currently exists.

Undoubtedly, the difficulty of measuring ski and pole forces in the natural environment has been a major obstacle to advanced understanding of cross-country skiing mechanics. Several research groups have developed instrumentation and measurement methods for obtaining skiing forces. In classical skiing, the skis are constrained to run in two parallel tracks; the various classical techniques being relatively planar, they can be reasonably analysed using two-dimensional methods (Ekstrom 1981; Komi 1985, 1987). In contrast, the more recently developed skating techniques involve three-dimensional motion, which complicates the process of force component determination (Smith 1989; Street & Frederick 1995).

Two general approaches to ski force measurement have been used: the traditional force plate embedded in a surface and portable force measurement systems attached to skis and poles. For skiing, both approaches are difficult to implement and involve serious obstacles to measurement without adversely affecting technique and equipment characteristics. In classical skiing, several devices have been used to measure ski and pole reaction forces. For example, Komi (1987) reviewed both the fixed and the portable plate approaches, showing his current designs in 1987 (Fig. 12.4). Because of the extended glide phases which characterize skiing

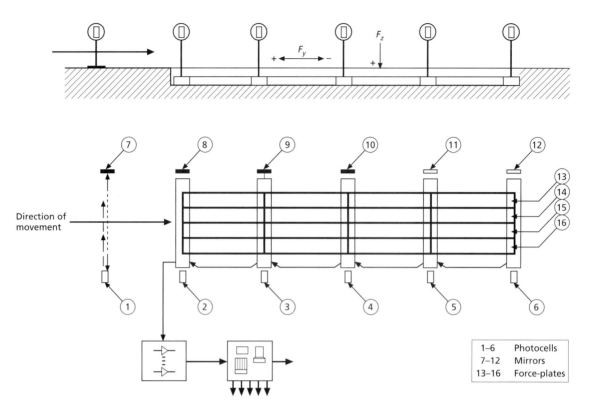

Fig. 12.4 Force plate with fixed positioning. This plate was designed for measuring pole and ski reaction forces in diagonal stride technique and was mounted in a fixed position under snow. (From Komi 1987.)

strides, to measure a complete cycle requires an unusually large force plate array compared with other locomotion research. The 6 m-long plate created by the Finnish researchers was adequate for slower skiing conditions, such as on uphill terrain, where a full cycle with both right and left kick and poling forces could be obtained (Fig. 12.5). The plate was approximately 60 cm wide in the mediolateral direction with four independent sections being separately measured. These allowed for independent analysis of each ski and pole reaction force. Force components in the vertical and anterior-posterior propulsive direction were directly outputted from the configuration and did not require additional kinematic information.

In contrast, the skating techniques which became popular in the succeeding decade are non-planar three-dimensional movement patterns for which the fixed force plate design would be inadequate.

Portable force plates attached to the ski when combined with telemetry equipment or with portable data-logging computers allow the measurement of ski reaction forces without the constraints imposed by a fixed plate. Several examples of such portable plates have been developed (Ekstrom 1981; Komi 1987; Smith 1989; Street & Frederick 1995) and have been used for assessment of both classical striding and skating techniques. However, the force components which can be obtained in this manner are local to the coordinate system of each ski and pole rather than the global system defined by the ski track. To obtain meaningful force components requires the additional measurement of ski and pole positions and orientations synchronized with the force data (Fig. 12.6). The three-dimensional motion analysis required to obtain these kinematic data is a time-consuming process which makes obtaining force components for the skating techniques a considerably

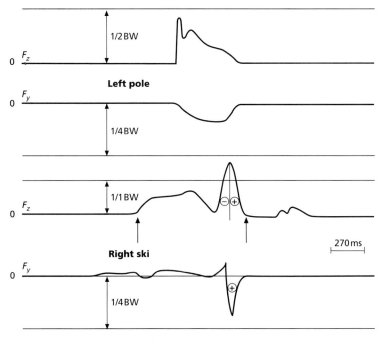

Fig. 12.5 Pole and ski reaction forces. Forces were measured using the force plate array of Fig. 12.4 and have been normalized to body weight (BW). (From Komi 1987.)

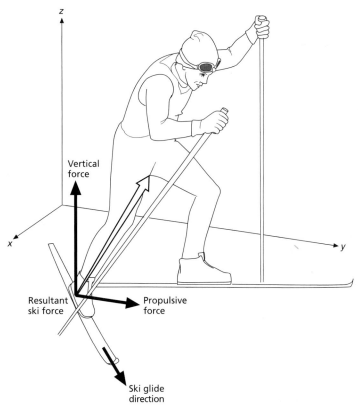

Fig. 12.6 Force components in skating. To obtain three-dimensional force components in skating, the resultant force applied normal to the ski surface is resolved into a vertical, a propulsive and a mediolateral component. These are determined from the ski orientation and edging angles synchronized with resultant reaction forces on the ski.

more difficult undertaking than for the relatively planar classical techniques. Later in this chapter results from the few studies which have reported skiing force data will be discussed in the context of optimizing the propulsive forces from the skis and poles.

Snow drag forces

Sliding of skis on snow is a relatively complex physical phenomenon which is at best only partially understood (Colbeck 1994b). In cross-country ski racing, the snow surfaces are prepared mechanically with large grooming machines, which leave a relatively smooth and firm surface behind. In classical races, parallel tracks are also set and used for most portions of the course. Except when fresh snow falls during races, skis generally glide on firm surfaces into which they dig relatively little. The efforts made in race course preparation are directly aimed to reduce one aspect of ski drag forces—those associated with a ski's penetration into loose snow. The energy lost to moving loose snow as a ski ploughs through it slows ski glide. While this is a recognized resistive force affecting ski performance, little test information is available publicly (see Lind & Sanders (1997) for general discussion). It is probably safe to assume that ski manufacturers expend some efforts in understanding the specific characteristics which allow a ski to ride over soft snow without much ploughing to reduce glide speed; however, such studies are usually proprietary and not readily available.

In contrast to the macroscopic forces involved in ploughing through snow, several microscopic effects which are thought to control the drag forces acting on a sliding ski have been well researched and are available in the general scientific literature. Several characteristics of sliding surfaces affect the resistive forces acting against a ski. These include the ski surface materials, the smoothness of the sliding surface ('structure'), the temperature of the snow and ski surface, and electrical charge distribution on the ski. Except in extremely cold conditions, ski sliding is lubricated by meltwater from slight amounts of heating of the surface. While generally serving to decrease frictional forces for a ski sliding on snow, in some situations excessive meltwater may increase drag forces due to capillary action of the water,

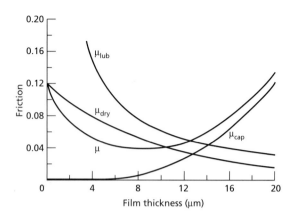

Fig. 12.7 Coefficient of friction (μ) and the effect of meltwater film thickness. Total coefficient of friction is influenced by dry friction, meltwater lubrication and capillary drag. (From Colbeck 1992.)

snow crystals and ski base. Figure 12.7 illustrates the relative contributions to the co-efficient of friction as a function of the amount of meltwater on a sliding surface (Colbeck 1992). Under very wet conditions, capillary action may account for the largest proportion of the drag force while under dry (cold) conditions, limited melt-water lubrication affects the frictional forces. Lind and Sanders (1997) include a general discussion of these relationships; see Colbeck (1992) for a more comprehensive analysis.

Snow and air temperatures have considerable effects on the drag forces acting on a ski. A qualitative observation easily made while ski skating on shaded snow and nearby sunny snow is the difference in drag force. Ski glide often can be dramatically decreased under cold conditions. These effects are well known and have been addressed by ski wax manufacturers whose products when matched to snow conditions may decrease the snow drag forces to some extent. Less well understood is how ski temperature influences drag forces and how it is affected by base composition, ski design and environmental conditions. Colbeck (1994a) instrumented skating skis with an array of thermocouples along the base and measured ski temperature during short periods of ski-skating. Temperatures along the base showed clear periodic oscillations corresponding to the skating cycle (Fig. 12.8). Local fluctuations of less than 1°C were typical during the glide and subsequent recovery phases. Ski base temperature displayed a

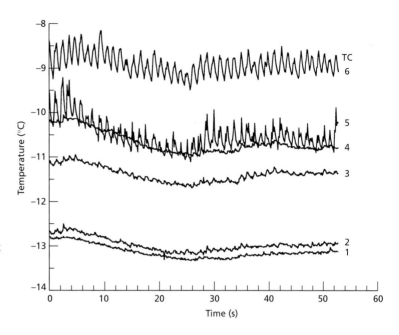

Fig. 12.8 Ski base temperatures during skating. Thermocouples (TC) along the ski base responded to frictional heating during each skating stroke. During recovery while the ski was in the air and off the snow surface, the temperature dropped to ambient levels. (From Colbeck 1994a.)

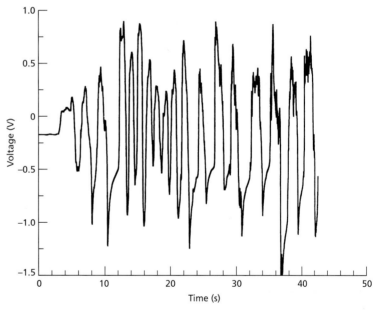

Fig. 12.9 Electrostatic charge on skis during skating. As skis move over snow charge build-up can be detected as a voltage across the top and bottom surfaces of the ski. Electrostatic charge on the ski is thought to attract dirt to the ski base, which affects ski glide by increasing snow drag forces. (From Colbeck 1995.)

progressive increase from ski tip to tail and was found to be sensitive to ski speed as well as environmental conditions (sun/shade and temperature). Much is not understood about the relationship of ski temperature to drag force. It is likely that surface waxing and structuring as well as overall ski flexion characteristics affect surface temperature. How these affect performance is unknown.

Ski drag is also thought to be affected by electrical charging of ski surfaces. While the origins of such charging are not clear, its magnitude can be measured directly by treating top and bottom surfaces of a ski as a large capacitor. Colbeck (1995) described this process with instrumented alpine skis; several illustrations from that paper are relevant to cross-country skiing. In Fig. 12.9, voltage fluctuations of

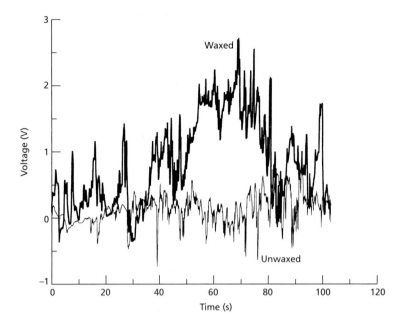

Fig. 12.10 Electrostatic charging with different waxes. Some additives to ski waxes are touted as being 'antistatic' supplements. In the case illustrated here, the additive increased rather than decreased charge build-up on the ski. (From Colbeck 1995.)

about ±1 V were found during skating. Discussion in the popular skiing literature connects electrical charging on skis to the pickup of dirt onto the sliding surface which in turn increases the snow drag force (Brown 1989). Various 'antistatic' additives are available as supplements to ski waxes. Figure 12.10, from Colbeck (1995), compared an unwaxed alpine ski base with an antistatic waxed surface and shows how under some conditions such an additive may be detrimental.

Air drag forces

Movement of a skier through the atmosphere results in drag forces which are dependent on the relative velocity of the skier and air. Except in the case of strong tailwinds, such forces oppose a skier's motion. The well-known relationship from fluid mechanics determines the magnitude of 'profile' drag forces which depend on air density (ρ), skier frontal area (A), shape (C_D, drag coefficient), and relative velocity (V):

$$\text{drag force} = 1/2\rho A C_D V^2 \qquad (12.1)$$

This relationship emphasizes that two factors under a skier's control affect the air resistance opposing motion: frontal area and shape. When skiing at slow

speeds such as on uphill terrain, air drag forces are relatively small. But on downhill sections and on fast snow, skiing speeds may easily reach 10–20 m · s⁻¹, where such forces may be substantial. Skier adjustment of technique and body positioning can reduce both the frontal area and drag coefficient. Svensson (1994) included graphs illustrating the variation of air drag force as a function of body position and speed (Fig. 12.11). On downhills, tucked vs. upright body positions can reduce drag forces by half or more; however, for the range of skating and striding techniques, drag forces at a given speed differ by relatively small amounts. Other mechanical and physiological factors probably affect technique choice more than aerodynamics for the moderate speeds typical of many parts of race courses.

While cross-country ski racing is an individual sport, often skiers may be in a position to ski close behind other competitors. In such circumstances, air drag forces can be slightly reduced on the trailing skier. The magnitude of the effect depends on the skier speeds relative to the air and on how closely the second skier is following. Bilodeau *et al.* (1994) completed physiological measurements on leading and trailing skiers following closely behind. At similar speeds, a skier 'drafting' behind a leader maintained heart rates about 5% lower than the leader.

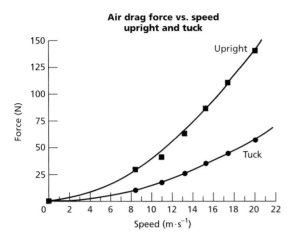

Fig. 12.11 Air drag force vs. speed for various skier positions. Wind tunnel testing of skier positioning showed that drag force is substantially different for tucked positions in comparison to more upright postures. (Data from Svensson 1994.)

Gravitational force and body mass

In hilly terrain, gravitational forces may be resistive or propulsive in direction. The magnitude of the force depends on the slope involved and is mathematically a function of the sine of the angle. On downhills steeper than some minimum angle (which depends on snow drag forces), a skier will accelerate until reaching a terminal velocity where gravitational force, ski/pole propulsive forces and drag forces are in equilibrium. When simply gliding down such a hill, the equilibrium is reached between gravity propelling the skier and snow and air drag resisting the motion. Under fast snow conditions and on slopes where air drag is considerably greater than snow drag this equilibrium is approximated by equating the gravitational force component with air drag force:

$$mg\ \sin\theta = {}^{1}\!/_{2}\rho AC_{D}V^{2} \tag{12.2}$$

where m is a skier's mass, g is the acceleration of gravity at the earth's surface, and θ is the angle of the downhill slope. This equation can be rearranged to solve for velocity V. The equation includes both mass and area terms which relate to a skier's physical characteristics and allows some estimation of the effect of body mass on terminal velocity. Because

body mass is mainly a function of volume, as body mass increases, frontal area (A) also increases, but not linearly with mass. Area changes approximately as mass to the 2/3 power. Hence as body mass increases, the ratio of body mass to frontal area does not hold constant but increases. Terminal velocity changes as the square root of the mass to area ratio and thus increases with body mass. This well-known result gives larger, more massive skiers an advantage on downhill terrain.

On uphill terrain, drag forces are relatively small and a skier's mechanical work is mainly against gravity. While more massive skiers must do more work in hill climbing they also tend to have greater metabolic capacities for work. Bergh (1987) has argued that this balance of physical capacity vs. work against gravity tips mainly in the favour of larger skiers. On flat terrain and moderate uphills, more massive skiers may have a slight advantage over smaller skiers; on steep uphills, low mass is a definite advantage. Hoffman *et al.* (1990) tested the relationship of body mass to energy cost in roller skiing. While they found the frictional characteristics of roller skiing to be slightly different than skiing on snow, other relationships were reasonably matched to the theoretical predictions of Bergh (1987). The advantages for skiers of large mass are slight and the ranks of elite cross-country skiers span a wide range of body sizes (Bergh & Forsberg 1992). Using data from Olympic races, Street and Gregory (1994) have shown that despite a large mass range for male competitors (58–85 kg), no relationship of mass to 50 km race performance was observed.

Minimizing drag forces

While skiing performance is influenced by all of the kinetic factors discussed in the previous sections, drag force acting on the skis is probably the focus of more effort than the other forces affecting motion. After training preparations are complete, skiers have little control over kinetic factors affecting performance like air drag, body mass and snow surface conditions. But considerable effort is put into ski preparation in hopes of minimizing the drag forces which slow ski gliding. The magnitude of performance differences due to these forces is not well known.

Ski glide speed and performance

Differences in glide characteristics between skis and between ski base preparations are often detectable by even casual recreational skiers. But at the elite level of international competition, most teams have professional technicians who specialize in ski preparation and maintenance. Therefore, one would expect to find relatively homogeneous glide characteristics within such competitors. There are numerous stories within the nordic skiing community about races where strong teams have been handicapped by poor choices of wax and ski preparation for difficult conditions. But excluding these unusual situations, many skiers suspect that glide characteristics remain a distinguishing advantage of the very fastest skiers. In a study designed to test this assumption and carried out during the 1992 Winter Olympic Games at Albertville, glide speed measurements were recorded during the men's 50 km race (Street & Gregory 1994).

The 50 km race at the 1992 Olympics involved three laps of about 17 km. Near the 15 km point (32 km at the second lap), a moderately steep downhill of about 150 m length descended to a flat of about 40 m. The downhill was of sufficient length that skiers approached terminal velocity for that slope and conditions. All descended using a tight, tucked position. Video records were made of the skiers gliding through the flat region after the hill during the first and second laps and their velocities through a 20 m mid-section on the flat were determined. Glide speed on a downhill is affected by skier mass,

air drag, snow drag and the initial velocity at the top of the hill and was distributed quite widely (Fig. 12.12). Street and Gregory systematically analysed each factor through modelling of skier motion down such a slope given the range of body sizes and initial velocities at the top of the hill. Initial velocity and air drag characteristics (A and C_D) probably had relatively smaller influences on the variability of glide speed observed at the bottom of the hill while skier mass and snow drag were found to have considerably more influence on ultimate glide speed. However, mass of the skiers in the study was not related to overall performance ($r = 0.12$), or to glide speeds in lap 1 ($r = 0.24$) or lap 2 ($r = 0.16$). Hence, mass explains very little of the variability of glide speed observed in this race. The frictional forces of the ski sliding over snow were probably the largest determinant of glide speed in this situation.

In a skating race such as the Olympic 50 km analysed by Street and Gregory (1994), glide characteristics of the ski affect every stride a skier takes as the skating techniques involve pushing from a moving ski. On fast downhills such as that analysed, snow drag and air drag forces both are important, but on flats and uphills where speed is considerably less, snow drag force is a dominant factor. While it is more difficult to assess the influence of snow drag on performance in these slower environments, it is likely that a substantial fraction of race performance is explained by this factor. Of course on uphill and flat terrain, physiology and technique characteristics have considerable effects on performance as well.

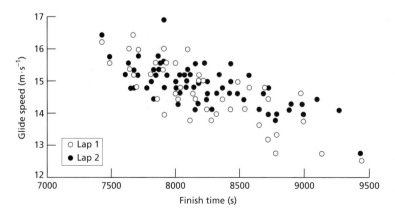

Fig. 12.12 Glide speed vs. race time. Top finishers in the men's 50 km race (Albertville Olympic Winter Games 1992) were faster through a test area following a 150 m downhill. Snow drag was found to account for much of this relationship. Skier mass, initial velocity and aerodynamic characteristics had less effect on glide speed variability across skiers. (Data from Street & Gregory 1994.)

Ski pressure distribution

The importance of glide to ski performance has stimulated efforts to measure various characteristics which affect snow drag forces. Of most importance is probably a ski's pressure distribution under load (Brown 1989). Qualitatively, a match of snow firmness, skier weight and ski stiffness must be made so that the ski tip does not plough through the snow (too stiff) or the mid-section of the ski does not drag (too soft). A ski designed to optimize glide will distribute the skier-applied forces in a smooth pattern without local fluctuations, which are thought to increase drag. Unfortunately, other factors complicate ski design. Skating skis must also be stable and track well and they must be torsionally stiff to allow edging. Classical skis are designed primarily to glide in tracks and must be capable of dramatically different pressure distributions under varying loads. A classical ski must be able to flex sufficiently to press the mid-section firmly against the snow for wax grip-

ping yet glide smoothly on the tip and tail regions when moderately loaded. Typical pressure distributions for skating and classic skis are illustrated in Fig. 12.13. While the skating ski pressure distribution results in relatively low pressure mid-ski at full body weight, the classic ski exhibits large mid-ski pressures at full body weight (see Ekstrom 1981).

The pressure distributions illustrated in Fig. 12.13 show the general response of the example skis to loading, and where available for individual skis this may provide a useful means of matching skis with skier. However, very little careful research is available in the public domain about how pressure distribution affects ski glide. Ski manufacturers may have proprietary information detailing such relationships but little is available in the scientific literature. Further, the pressure distribution information that is available (like Fig. 12.13) suffers from the difficulty of generalizing to real skiing conditions. Dynamic loading of skis, particularly when edged as in skating, is likely to generate different pressure

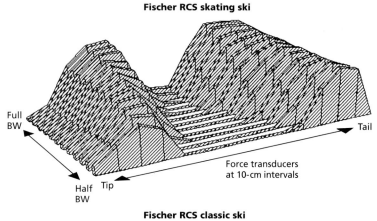

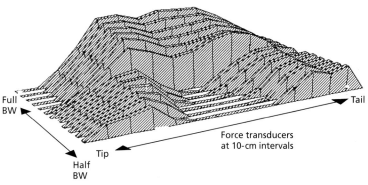

Fig. 12.13 Pressure distribution under skating and classic skis. Characteristic pressure distribution patterns were measured for a range of forces. At full body weight (BW) classic skis must allow the ski mid-section with grip wax to press against the snow, while skating skis under similar load distribute the force quite differently. (Adapted from pressure distribution graphics from Eagle River Nordic: www.ernordic.com/FischerRCSSkt.htm and www.ernordic.com/FischerRCSCapPlus.htm.)

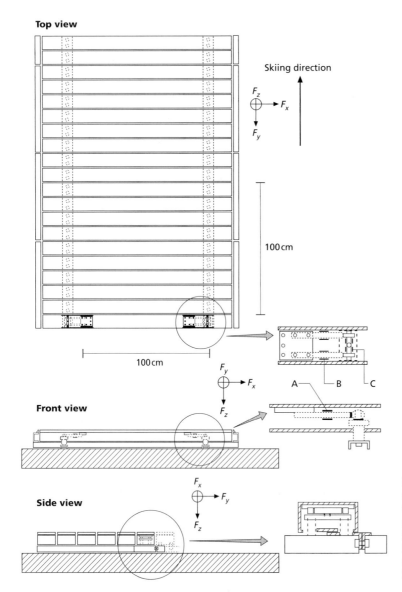

Fig. 12.14 Force plate composed of multiple instrumented beams. This unusual design allowed not only determination of three-dimensional forces in skating but also the dynamic force distribution under the ski during a skating stroke. (From Leppävuori *et al.* 1993.)

distribution patterns than the flat, static loadings typically measured. While portable instrumentation for dynamic measurement of ski pressure has not been currently developed, a fixed force plate design described by Leppävuori *et al.* (1993) allows some assessment of pressure distribution under a ski. This unusual force plate (Fig. 12.14) was composed of 20 beams of 10 cm width and more than a metre length. Each was instrumented for measurement of three-dimensional force components. The array of beams was configured for placement under snow cover which allowed measurement of ski reaction force components by summing the 20 beam outputs (Fig. 12.15). Unfortunately, the overall length of the plate (2.2 m) is not much longer than typical cross-country skis, which during a single skating stroke or single step in classical skiing may easily glide through several metres. These limitations hinder full stance phase ski reaction force measurement but do provide some insights into force under regions of the ski. Figure 12.16, from the paper by Leppävuori *et al.*, compares two force distributions during mid-

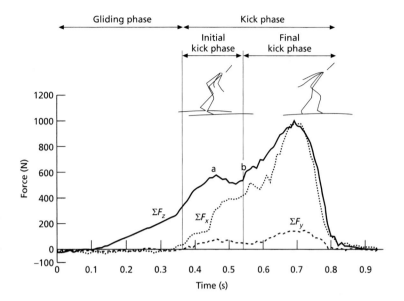

Fig. 12.15 Ski reaction force in skating. Due to the relatively short force plate length, the ski was only partially on the force plate as skating began. Thus, the early phases of the force–time record are much less than observed with other measurement systems. (From Leppävuori *et al.* 1993.)

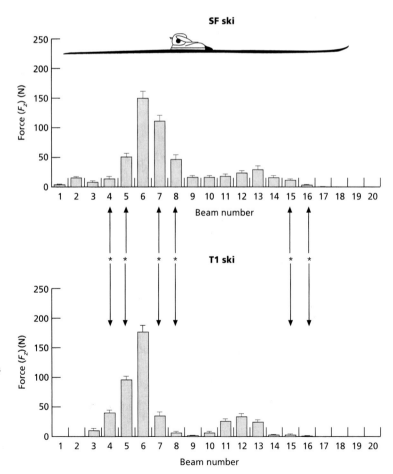

Fig. 12.16 Force distribution underneath skis in skating. Two ski designs were measured for force distribution near the middle of the skating stroke. The peak forces were located just behind the heel of the boot. Note that the pattern is quite different from the static measurements of Fig. 12.12. (From Leppävuori *et al.* 1993.)

stance when ski loading is probably about body weight. Both skis exhibit considerably different patterns from that shown in Fig. 12.13, which was measured statically. Whether this was due to a true difference in dynamic vs. static loading of skis or if it was due to skier technique or perhaps to some instrumentation idiosyncrasy is unknown.

While we currently recognize that ski flex and the pressure distribution pattern are probably very important factors affecting ski glide, additional instrumentation for dynamic measurement will probably be required before the subtle relationships between ski glide and ski design will be thoroughly explored and understood.

Ski surfaces and friction

Snow drag forces result from a combination of ploughing of a ski and of surface interactions with snow. Ploughing is largely a function of ski stiffness characteristics while surface friction depends on ski base material, wax on the surface, roughness of the surface, snow grain size, temperature, and other physical conditions. Figure 12.7 (Colbeck 1992) illustrates the coefficient of friction of a ski as a function of meltwater film thickness, which in turn depends on various snow and ski characteristics. At very low temperatures very little melting is thought to occur as a ski slides over snow. The dry frictional forces of low-temperature sliding tend to be quite large. In Fig. 12.17a,b the direct interaction of snow crystals and ski surface can be seen. Sliding under such conditions requires either deformation or fracturing of the snow crystals (Colbeck 1994b). In contrast (Fig. 12.17c), under warmer, wetter conditions where meltwater is created, sliding may be accomplished with at least partial separation of the ski surface from snow crystals. Whether some direct ski to crystal interaction exists under these conditions depends on how much meltwater is generated, which depends on temperature and frictional heating.

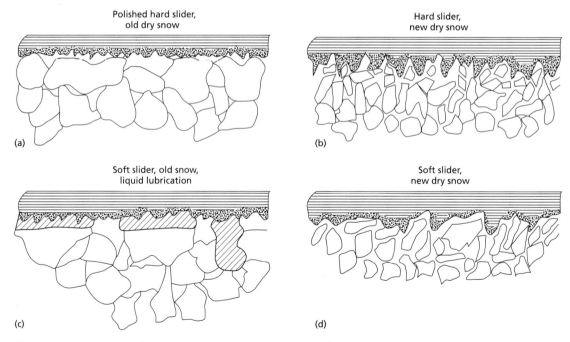

Fig. 12.17 Snow–ski surface interactions. Ski surfaces may be prepared with hard or soft waxes which will interact with wet and dry snow in different ways. New dry snow tends to have small fine crystals which 'catch' in the small surface roughnesses of the ski and wax. Older dry snow is more rounded and may produce less snow drag than newer snow. Wet snow may have free water which creates drag on the ski through capillary action. (From Lind & Sanders 1997; Fig. 8.3.)

Meltwater interaction between ski and snow crystals serves to lubricate sliding but also introduces capillary drag, which has a magnitude dependent on the contact angle of water with the ski surface (Colbeck 1994b). Contact angle is affected by the thin film of wax normally applied to ski surfaces. Various wax compositions allow for the 'tuning' of ski surface to the snow characteristics. These compositions range from relatively hard waxes, which are generally used in cold conditions with little meltwater generation, to quite soft waxes for wet snow with considerable meltwater affecting sliding. Wax hardness is thought to affect the penetration of snow asperities into the wax, which in turn affects melting. Too little penetration into a very hard wax generates little heating of the surface and little meltwater generation. Too soft a wax may result in wax deformation rather than snow crystal melting. In addition to crystal penetration, wax composition affects water contact angle. While it is generally assumed that warmer glide waxes are in part composed to decrease contact angle, no published data exist to support this expectation.

Ski wax chemistry is largely a proprietary science hidden to the public. While the past decade has seen the introduction of numerous fluorinated 'waxes' for skis, little has been published on the physical processes which influence their sliding characteristics. Traditional waxes have been more thoroughly explained chemically and physically (see Street & Tsui 1986). Other additives to ski wax (such as graphite) are touted as having antistatic characteristics. Sliding skis do generate small surface voltages such as that shown in Figs 12.9 and 12.10 (Colbeck 1995). However, the extent to which such charge build-up attracts dirt (Brown 1989) and how substantially it may affect ski glide is unknown.

Surface roughness characteristics (referred to as structure) are also known to affect ski sliding over snow. The effects involve complex interactions of pore size between snow crystals, amount of meltwater and direction of the roughness elements (Colbeck 1994b). Under warm conditions with abundant water lubrication, the ski surface may be separated by meltwater from the snow crystals. With minimal separation, snow crystals may 'catch' in surface roughnesses, but with thick meltwater layers, appropriately sized roughness is thought to break up water droplet attachments between ski and snow. At the same time, surface smoothness is important as it enhances water slippage. The direction of surface roughness may also affect snow drag. Colbeck (1994b) suggested that structure orientated along the ski is advantageous under wetter/warmer conditions, while transverse orientated structure may work better under colder conditions when less melting occurs. Unfortunately, determining the effect of structure size and orientation under various snow conditions is still a matter of experiment. While there are many coaching suggestions for ski base preparation, these are largely based on collective wisdom rather than systematic, controlled invest-igation aimed to advance theoretical understanding.

Optimizing propulsive forces

Motion of a skier is determined by the sum of the forces acting on the body (Fig. 12.3). While minimizing drag forces is an important component of optimizing performance, it is skier-generated propulsive forces which directly cause forward motion. These propulsive forces are one component of the three-dimensional resultant reaction force at each pole and each ski (Fig. 12.6). An earlier section of this chapter reviewed some of the instrumentation that has been developed for force measurement in skiing. This section will focus on the components of force and the factors affecting optimization of propulsion.

Classic technique forces

The vertical and propulsive components of force shown in Fig. 12.5 (Komi 1987) represent the relatively little that is known about diagonal stride forces (see also Ekstrom 1981). This classic technique involves 'kicking' from a momentarily stationary ski onto the other gliding ski, which in the next half cycle slows to a stop allowing the skier to kick from it. During the very brief stationary period of the ski's motion, a large vertical force compresses the mid-section of the ski against the snow. With appropriate wax on the ski, the mid-section momentarily sticks to the snow due to the large normal force and high pressure in that region (Fig. 12.13). The static frictional force is large enough during the kicking phase that a brief propulsive component of force in the forward direction can be generated. The magnitude of this force depends on the frictional characteristics during kick. This can vary widely depending on snow conditions, ski stiffness and wax properties. While vertical forces during this kick phase easily exceed body weight, the propulsive forces are much smaller (approxim-ately 10–20% of body weight) and are of very short duration—less than 0.1 s (Ekstrom 1981; Komi 1987). In contrast, skating forces (discussed below) are applied over a considerably longer time interval.

Generating propulsive force during the kick phase of diagonal stride requires careful timing of the vertical and horizontal forces matched to the glide speed of the ski. As the ski slows to a stop, the large vertical force must quickly compress the cambered mid-section of the ski to the snow surface, which momentarily creates a large static frictional force. Optimal technique directs the ski reaction force vector at an angle such that the propulsive force component matches the maximum frictional force attainable for the conditions. An early kicking motion will compress the ski mid-section while the ski is moving and tend to decrease the glide unnecessarily. A late kick will compress the ski camber after the ski has momentarily stopped and will decrease the vertical force component, which will in turn decrease the static frictional force from which propulsive force is generated.

In both classical and skating techniques, poling forces are mainly axial in direction and have been measured using both under-snow force plates and instrumented poles. If instrumented poles are used, the pole orientation in space can be used along with the axial force to determine force components. In classical ski techniques like diagonal stride and double poling, the poles move mainly in a sagittal plane and forces can be resolved into vertical and propulsive components. For a given poling force, the propulsive component increases as the pole is angled in the forward direction and away from vertical. Specifically, the vertical and propulsive

components are functions of the angle θ (with respect to vertical):

$$\text{propulsive component} = F_{\text{pole}} \sin\theta \qquad (12.3)$$

$$\text{vertical component} = F_{\text{pole}} \cos\theta \qquad (12.4)$$

where F_{pole} is the resultant force along the longitudinal axis of the pole. Thus when the poles are vertical (zero angle), no propulsive force is generated. As poling angle from vertical increases, the proportion of propulsive force increases. While vertical poling forces do not contribute to propulsion, they may act to decrease the vertical reaction forces on the ski(s) and potentially diminish snow drag forces. (This effect has not been measured and we can only conjecture that the vertical poling forces would decrease ski reaction forces by perhaps 20% of body weight during the glide phase of diagonal stride.)

From the relationship of pole angle to propulsive force component, a superficial assessment would suggest that skiers should plant the pole at an angle well beyond vertical to maximize propulsive force throughout the poling phase. However, most elite skiers do not follow this pattern. In a study of double-poling technique, Smith et al. (1996) found that under relatively fast conditions skiers planted the poles at about 15° and that faster skiers tended to plant the pole closer to vertical. Mechanically this makes sense as it allows for a longer period of poling—more vertically planted poles tend to be planted further forwards and are in contact with the snow for a longer time period. With this pattern, the pole is initially relatively vertical as forces generated by elbow and shoulder extensor activity build toward peak values. As poling progresses and the poling angle becomes more effective, poling forces peak. Later in the poling phase, as resultant forces diminish, the pole angle continues to increase away from the vertical enhancing the effectiveness of the poling force. These effects can be seen in the F_y force curve of Fig. 12.5, where a relatively sustained plateau of propulsive force was observed.

A more vertically planted pole may also place the arm in a more advantageous position for sustained extension activity in a stretch–shortening cycle. Figure 12.18 illustrates the elbow angle to pole angle relationship for several top finishers in the women's

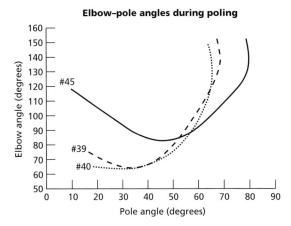

Fig. 12.18 Elbow and pole angles during double-poling. Beginning at the left of each curve, poling began with the poles about 10–15° from vertical and proceeded to more inclined poling positions. Elbow positionings varied across subjects. Mean elbow angle at pole plant was about 106°; however, some, like skier #45 (the race winner), used a considerably more extended elbow positioning initially. Most skiers had considerable elbow flexion near the beginning of poling, which probably involved preloading of the triceps brachii prior to elbow extension. (From Smith *et al.* 1996.)

30 km race at the Lillehammer Olympics (Smith *et al.* 1996). These (and most other) skiers of the study planted the pole at about 10–15°. Initial arm motion involved flexing of the elbow followed only later, when the poles were inclined at 40 or 50° from vertical, by a rapid elbow extension. It is likely that some preloading of triceps brachii muscles occurred early in poling followed by elbow extension and active muscle shortening later when pole angles were most effective. From Fig. 12.18, it is apparent that a somewhat more extended elbow position at pole plant may allow for a longer period of preloading with greater flexion preceding elbow extension at pole angles greater than 45°. These assessments are based on pole–arm–trunk kinematics in double-poling. While it is likely that the segmental relationships will be slightly different in diagonal stride where trunk flexion is minimal, the principle of planting the pole in a manner that enhances preloading and takes advantage of the stretch–shortening cycle for most effective poling angles must still be advantageous.

Skating forces

Ski reaction forces in the skating techniques are orientated approximately perpendicular to the ski surface. Because skating skis are prepared with glide wax and are without the grip waxes required for classical skiing, there is no means of using static friction to generate propulsive force. In a manner similar to speed skating, the ski is set down at an angle to the forward direction and while gliding it is placed on edge. The edged platform of the ski resists forces perpendicular to it as these simply compress the snow under the ski. Forces in other directions cannot be generated as the frictional forces are insubstantial. Figure 12.6 illustrates the resultant ski reaction force perpendicular to the ski surface; components can be determined if the ski positioning with respect to the snow surface (edging angle) and with respect to the forward direction are known.

While there are various ski reaction force patterns which characterize each of the skating techniques (Fig. 12.19), the generation of propulsive force involves similar relationships in each case. The propulsive force component from a skating ski depends on the ski's edging angle and on its orientation with respect to the forward direction. With the resultant ski force (F_{ski}) normal to the ski surface, each of these angles affects the propulsive component as the sine of the angle. Thus propulsive force component from a skating ski can be calculated from:

$$F_{propulsive} = F_{ski} \sin\alpha \sin\beta \qquad (12.5)$$

where α is the edging angle of the ski surface with respect to the snow surface (0° being flat) and β is the orientation angle (0° being straight ahead). From this equation it is obvious that propulsive force increases (for a given resultant ski force) as either the orientation angle or the edging angle increases.

A common observation in skating is the relationship of ski orientation angle to skiing speed. On flat and fast terrain, the skis are angled away from the forward direction a relatively small angle, while under slower conditions and on uphill terrain the ski angles increase substantially. For example, on flat terrain used during the 1992 Olympic races, ski angles were about 6–8° (men; Smith & Heagy 1994)

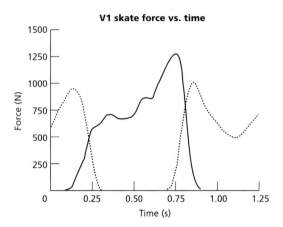
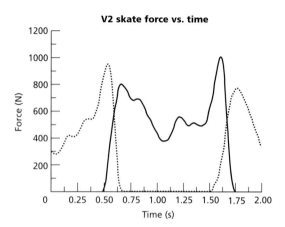

Fig. 12.19 Resultant ski reaction forces during skating. In skating, the resultant force is approximately perpendicular to the ski surface. Subtle differences of timing exist for the various skating techniques (see Fig. 12.20). Each graph begins the cycle at pole plant. V1 involves one poling action while V2 technique has two poling actions per cycle. Cycle times for V2 are typically longer than for V1.

and 10–12° (women; Gregory *et al.* 1994). In contrast, skiers on uphill terrain of the Calgary Olympic races skated with a much greater angle of skis to the forward direction (means about 28–30°) (Smith *et al.* 1988). Mechanically, this response would be expected based on the relationship of ski angle to propulsive force component expressed in Eqn. 12.5. On the flat, only air and snow drag forces resist a skier's motion, requiring relatively modest propulsive forces to maintain skiing speed. On uphill terrain, gravity is an additional force against which a skier is working. This requires greater propulsive forces to maintain uphill skiing speed. These greater propulsive forces can be generated either by increasing the resultant ski reaction forces, by increasing the ski angle with respect to forward direction (β in Eqn. 12.5 above) or by increasing the ski edging angle on the snow surface (α). While no force comparison of flat to uphill skiing is available, on grades of 9 and 14% ski forces have been measured (Smith 1989). For these moderate and steep uphills, average forces were similar while ski orientation angles changed with grade. Based on this evidence, it is likely that skiers maintain similar skating force magnitudes on different terrain but generate greater propulsive force mainly through adjustment of ski orientation and edging angles.

Ski orientation angle interacts with other kinematic characteristics of a skating stroke. As ski angles increase away from the forward direction, a skier's lateral displacement during the stroke increases and displacement in the forward direction may decrease. The changing orientation angle of a ski from flat to uphill terrain also results in a modification to the effective slope up which the ski is gliding. By angling the ski laterally, a skier can increase the glide distance during a skating stroke and the glide time before the ski speed decreases substantially. Thus increased orientation angle of the ski can accomplish two things—the propulsive force component can be increased and uphill ski glide can be enhanced. These come at the expense of increased lateral motion, which may be constrained by topology of the surroundings. As displacement in the forward direction during a cycle decreases with increased ski angle, a skier must increase the skating stroke rate to maintain speed but this would come at the expense of glide on each ski. At some point, stroke rate limitations combined with race course width limits restrict a skier's ability to use greater ski angles to increase propulsive force without exceeding physiological optima.

Ski edging angle is a measure of a ski's flatness to the snow surface. It affects performance by in

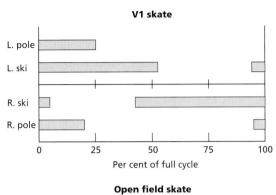

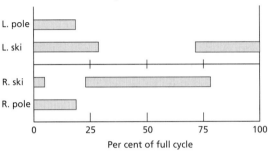

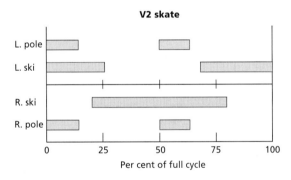

Fig. 12.20 Skating phase diagrams. Timing of the poling and skating phases are shown for the V1, 'open field' (V2alt) and V2 skating techniques. (Data from Bilodeau *et al.* 1992.)

part determining the propulsive force component during a skating stroke and also by affecting ski penetration into surface snow layers, which may increase snow drag force while providing a firm platform from which skating forces are generated. Conventional wisdom from ski coaches suggests that a 'flat ski' will glide faster than an edged ski. In skating, glide directly affects cycle length. As faster skiers tend to ski with greater cycle lengths it is a common connection to relate ski edging to glide and to performance. While it is reasonable to expect snow drag forces to be greater on an edged ski than on one that is flat (due to deeper penetration and increased ploughing), this has not been demonstrated and the magnitude of the increased drag is unknown. The typical description of fast skating techniques like the V2 and the V2alt (open field) includes a long glide phase on each ski prior to pushing off with a vigorous knee extension. This timing can be seen in the phase plots of Fig. 12.20 (Bilodeau *et al.* 1992). The implication of some coaching suggestions is that a relatively static flat ski position be maintained during the early parts of each skating stroke where the ski is mainly gliding.

However, this static flat ski emphasis is not typical of elite skiers (Smith & Heagy 1994). Figure 12.21 illustrates mean ski edging angles during fast skating on flat terrain during the men's 50 km race at the 1992 Olympics. None of the 17 elite skiers analysed in that study exhibited a ski edging phase where a flat ski was statically maintained. Most skiers set the ski down on the snow initially with it being flat to the surface and all moved away from the initial positioning immediately. Static posturing to enhance ski glide has not been observed for elite skiers and it is likely to be a disadvantageous skating technique. This observation must not be misunderstood to mean that ski edging and a flat ski are unimportant characteristics for ski glide. Note in Fig. 12.21 that despite smoothly increasing edging angles on the strong side skate over the last 30% of the cycle, the ski is only 10° from flat. This modest amount of edging may have little effect on ski glide while allowing a skier to dynamically stroke from side to side. It is only later in each skating stroke (Fig. 12.19), when ski reaction forces are largest, that the skis are substantially edged. Several skiers of this sample were observed to set the ski down on the lateral edge (negative ski angle), rotate through flat and onto the medial ski edge during the glide phases on each side. This technique may be advantageous on flat, fast terrain as it may prolong the time where the ski is within a few degrees of flat while promoting a continuous dynamic movement toward the next skating stroke.

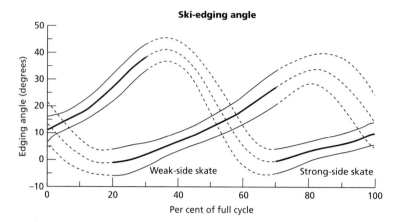

Fig. 12.21 Edging angle during open field skating on flat terrain. Skating phases are indicated by the heavy lines; recovery phases (when the ski is not in snow contact) by the thin lines. Plots are mean ±SD throughout a full cycle. Note that no plateau region of near-zero angle was observed. Skiers continuously change edging angle throughout the whole skating stroke. (From Smith & Heagy 1994.)

Technique and equipment choices

In both classic and skating races, skiers employ a variety of techniques in traversing the length of typical race courses. Technique choice in skiing is similar to gearing choices that cyclists make in riding over variable terrain. On downhills, high gears allow the continuation of pedalling without exceeding a cyclist's cadence maximum. On flat terrain, moderate gearing is used which allows riding at optimal pedalling rates. On steep uphills, low gears are used to minimize pedalling force demands and to maintain cadence near optimal levels. Just as cycling cadence is affected by gearing, in skiing, ski-cycle rates are affected by technique. And just as cadence is affected by cycling speed and by terrain, skiing speed and technique affect ski-cycle rate. Similar factors probably influence a racer's decisions about technique choices and about gearing. While these have not been well researched, one can conjecture that muscle strength and composition in conjunction with cardiovascular characteristics enter into the internal calculus of technique/gearing choice.

In classic skiing, typical techniques include double-poling, kick double-pole, diagonal stride, ski running, and herringbone (high to low 'gearing', respectively). Skating technique can be similarly ordered: V2, open field (V2alt), V1 and diagonal skate. Cycle characteristics of the three primary skating techniques and how these change with terrain have been most clearly researched (Boulay *et al.*

1995). Figure 12.22 shows the typical decrease of skiing speed as slope increases. This response derives almost completely from cycle length decreases while cycle rates are almost constant for each technique across a range of slopes. With cycle rates of about 0.6 Hz, the V2 technique is much like a high gear where the slow cadence goes with a greater displacement per cycle. In contrast, V1 is a higher frequency (about 1 Hz), shorter cycle length technique rather like a lower gear. Open field skate is somewhere in between these 'gearings.'

The observations illustrated in Fig. 12.22 represent kinematic characteristics under near-maximal skiing speed for each slope condition. Curiously, skiing speeds on slight downhills or moderate uphills were quite similar for the three techniques. Only on more demanding uphills did the rate/length differences in technique translate into advantages for the 'lower gear' V1 technique. As skiing speed increases beyond the $7 \text{ m} \cdot \text{s}^{-1}$ level observed in the study by Boulay *et al.*, it is likely that V1 would become disadvantageous compared with V2 and open field. While this comment is just conjecture, it is an easily measured relationship which skiers can individually test.

Under racing conditions, very little time is spent skiing at the maximal rates of the Boulay *et al.* (1995) study. When skiing at submaximal speeds during a race, performance is optimized in part by using techniques which most economically match the mechanical to the metabolic costs. While comprehensive physiological measurements have been

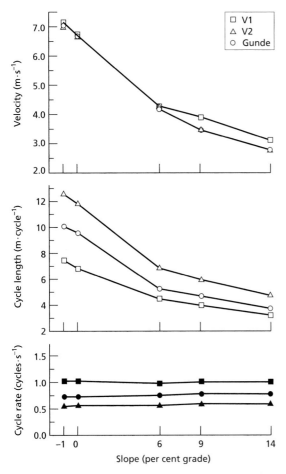

Fig. 12.22 Skating cycle characteristics as a function of slope. The decreased speed observed as slope increases is mainly due to cycle length changes while cycle rate stays nearly constant. (Note: Gunde skate, open field and V2alt are synonymous.) (From Boulay *et al.* 1995.)

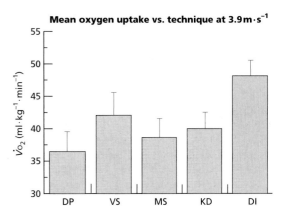

Fig. 12.23 Submaximal $\dot{V}o_2$ for double-poling (DP), skating (VS), marathon skate (MS), kick double-pole (KD), and diagonal stride (DI). (Data from Hoffman & Clifford 1990.)

3.9 m · s^{-1} on flat snow surface). Across several studies, double-poling has consistently been more 'economical' than other techniques but has also involved operating at greater percentages of technique-specific maximal oxygen uptake (Hoffman *et al.* 1994) and at greater lactate levels (Mittelstadt *et al.* 1995). This suggests that factors other than just aerobic cost of a technique may affect performance.

Pole length

Double-poling relies strictly on the upper body to generate propulsive force through the poles. It has been extensively studied in recent years because of the importance of poling to the skating techniques. In classical diagonal stride, no systematic analysis of pole vs. ski contributions to propulsion has been published, but from Komi's (1987) representative graphs (Fig. 12.5) it appears that poling forces contribute modestly to diagonal stride performance. In V1 skating uphill, poling forces have been found to contribute about two-thirds of the propulsive impulse driving a skier's motion (Smith 1989). This substantial component of skating makes optimizing poling kinematics and kinetics an important aspect of preparation. Skiers typically use poles for skating which are 10–15 cm longer than those used for classical races. Little systematic investigation is

completed for a variety of ski techniques (Hoffman & Clifford 1990; Hoffman 1992; Hoffman *et al.* 1998), no direct comparisons of metabolic costs of the primary skating techniques are available (see Bilodeau *et al.* (1991) for estimates based on heart rate response). In classic skiing, relative economy of diagonal stride, kick double-pole and double-poling have been measured on flat and uphill terrain (Hoffman & Clifford 1992; Hoffman *et al.* 1994, 1998). Figure 12.23 illustrates the technique—oxygen uptake response at constant velocity (about available comparing the effects of pole length on performance. In double-poling, Gibbons *et al.* (1992) found no difference in physiological characteristics in comparisons of long and short poles (about 89 and 83% of body height) for treadmill rollerskiing. In contrast, Siletta (1987) simulated race conditions on snow and compared performance with three pole lengths (100, 105 and 110% of shoulder height). The longest poles were overall advantageous for seven of the nine skiers tested. All skiers were faster skating uphill with the longest poles. The elbow angle–pole angle relationship (Fig. 12.18) is likely to be affected by the length of the pole. The nature of this interaction is unknown currently. In the decade since the study by Siletta, considerable fluctuation of 'recommended' pole lengths has been distributed by coaches and equipment suppliers. While skating pole lengths even longer than the 110% (of shoulder height) were popular for a few years, current conventional wisdom has moderated that recommendation somewhat. Without the results of a systematic test of the effect of pole length on kinematic, kinetic and performance characteristics, we can only speculate about how pole length influences those characteristics.

Mechanical characteristics of poles change with length. The most important of these characteristics deal with mass and its distribution. While manufacturers of ski equipment take great pains to reduce the mass of skis and poles, these items contribute a small but not negligible proportion of the overall energy cost of motion. Ski mass is lifted and accelerated with each stride or each skating stroke, requiring energy to accomplish the demands of each technique. However, ski motion involves little rotation. In contrast, ski poles are rotated about an axis near the handle during each cycle and pole moment of inertia is a critical factor in pole design. Pole mass (excluding basket and handle) may be less than 100 g in typical lengths and have a moment of inertia as little as 0.06 kg m^2. Adding a basket to the shaft may increase overall mass by 15% or more and increase moment of inertia by 32–49% (Street & Tsui 1987)!

With longer ski poles, mass and especially moment of inertia increase. These mechanical characteristics directly affect the energy costs and perhaps the kinematics of poling. The greater moment of inertia of long poles will tend to increase the time required to swing the pole forwards during recovery, directly decreasing cycle rate. During the poling phase, a longer pole may potentially increase poling time, during which greater propulsive impulse *may* be generated but also decreasing cycle rate as well. These competing advantages/ disadvantages change with pole length and suggest that some optimizing principle is involved. Unfortunately, the details of that relationship are not clearly understood at present.

Summary

Performance in cross-country skiing is affected by ski and pole reaction forces, by snow and air drag forces, and by gravity. Each of these resistive and propulsive forces may be influenced by skier technique, body characteristics, equipment and environmental conditions. A general relationship of ski racing which has been observed under many conditions of terrain and technique is that faster skiers move with greater cycle lengths but similar cycle rates to slower skiers. This chapter has addressed some of the factors which elite skiers use to advantage and which allow them to ski faster than others.

Propulsive forces from skis and poles counter the resisting forces of air and snow drag to maintain constant velocity. Skiing optimally must involve minimizing drag forces without degrading technique. Glide speed measurements clearly demonstrate that the fastest skiers start with the fastest skis.

Ski reaction forces generate a major fraction of propulsive force in diagonal stride. Timing of the kick phase in diagonal technique generates an optimal vertical force which produces a momentarily large static friction and very brief propulsive impulse. In contrast, skating strokes are of considerably greater duration and depend on ski angles with respect to the surface and to the forward direction to create propulsive force. Edging of the ski probably increases snow drag force. Optimal ski handling involves sufficient edging of the ski to generate some propulsive force without producing substantially larger drag force. However, because the propulsive component is a small fraction of the resultant forces applied to a skating ski, poling forces play a larger role in propelling a skater than is true in diagonal stride. Measurements on uphill terrain suggest that poling is the major contributor to skating propulsion.

Equipment characteristics can have a substantial impact on skier technique and on performance. Ski stiffness, pressure distribution and surface preparation affect how a ski interacts with a snow surface. Pole characteristics can affect technique cycle rates, propulsive components of force, and the energy requirements to maintain skiing speeds. Optimal ski performance involves all these factors to minimize the mechanical costs of skiing at maximally sustainable metabolic rates.

References

Bergh, U. (1987) The influence of body mass in cross-country skiing. *Medicine and Science in Sports and Exercise* **19**, 324–331.

Bergh, U. & Forsberg, A. (1992) The influence of body mass in cross-country ski racing. *Medicine and Science in Sports and Exercise* **24**, 1033–1039.

Bilodeau, B., Roy, B. & Boulay, M.R. (1991) A comparison of three skating techniques and the diagonal stride on heart rate responses and speed in cross-country skiing. *International Journal of Sports Medicine* **12**, 71–76.

Bilodeau, B., Boulay, M.R. & Roy, B. (1992) Propulsive and gliding phases in four cross-country skiing techniques. *Medicine and Science in Sports and Exercise* **24**, 917–925.

Bilodeau, B., Roy, B. & Boulay, M.R. (1994) Effect of drafting on heart rate in cross-country skiing. *Medicine and Science in Sports and Exercise* **26**, 637–641.

Bilodeau, B., Rundell, K.W., Roy, B. & Boulay, M.R. (1996) Kinematics of cross-country ski racing. *Medicine and Science in Sports and Exercise* **28**, 128–138.

Boulay, M.R., Rundell, K.W. & King, D.L. (1995) Effect of slope variation and skating technique on velocity in cross-country skiing. *Medicine and Science in Sports and Exercise* **27**, 281–287.

Brown, N. (1989) *Nordic Update Ski Prep and Wax Guide.* Timberline Publishing, Bellevue, WA.

Colbeck, S.C. (1992) A review of the processes that control snow friction. *CRREL Monograph 92–2.* Cold Regions Research and Engineering Laboratory, Hanover, NH.

Colbeck, S.C. (1994a) Bottom temperatures of skating skis on snow. *Medicine and Science in Sports and Exercise* **26**, 258–262.

Colbeck, S.C. (1994b) A review of the friction of snow skis. *Journal of Sports Sciences* **12**, 285–295.

Colbeck, S.C. (1995) Electrical charging of skis gliding on snow. *Medicine and Science in Sports and Exercise* **27**, 136–141.

Dal Monte, A., Fucci, S., Leonardi, L.M. & Trozzi, V. (1983) An evaluation of the diagonal stride technique, in cross country skiing. In: *Biomechanics VIII-B* (eds H. Matsui & K. Kobayashi), pp. 851–855. Human Kinetics Publishers, Champaign, IL.

Dillman, C. (1979) Biomechanical evaluations of cross-country skiing techniques. *Journal of the United States Ski Coaches Association* **2** (4), 62–66.

Ekstrom, H. (1981) Force interplay in cross country skiing. *Scandinavian Journal of Sports Science* **3** (2), 69–76.

Gagnon, M. (1981) *A Kinematic Analysis of the Alternate Stride in Cross-Country Skiing.* In: *Biomechanics VII-B* (eds A. Morecki, K. Fidelus, K. Kedzior & A. Wit), pp. 483–487. Polish Scientific Publishers, Warsaw, Poland.

Gervais, P. & Wronko, C. (1988) The marathon skate in nordic skiing performed on roller skates, roller skis, and snow skis. *International Journal of Sport Biomechanics* **4**, 38–48.

Gibbons, T., Drobish, K., Watts, P. *et al.* (1992) The effects of two different pole lengths on the physiological responses during double pole roller skiing. *Medicine and Science in Sports and Exercise* **24**, S162.

Gregory, R.W., Humphreys, S.E. & Street, G.M. (1994) Kinematic analysis of skating technique of Olympic skiers in the women's 30-km race. *Journal of Applied Biomechanics* **10**, 382–392.

Hoffman, M.D. (1992) Physiological comparisons of cross-country skiing techniques. *Medicine and Science in Sports and Exercise* **24**, 1023–1032.

Hoffman, M.D. & Clifford, P.S. (1990) Physiological responses to different cross country skiing techniques on level terrain. *Medicine and Science in Sports and Exercise* **22**, 841–848.

Hoffman, M.D. & Clifford, P.S. (1992) Physiological aspects of competitive cross-country skiing. *Journal of Sports Sciences* **10**, 3–27.

Hoffman, M.D., Clifford, P.S., Bota, B., Mandli, M. & Jones, G.M. (1990) Influence of body mass on energy cost of roller skiing. *International Journal of Sport Biomechanics* **6**, 374–385.

Hoffman, M.D., Clifford, P.S., Watts, P.B. *et al.* (1994) Physiological comparison of uphill roller skiing: diagonal stride versus double pole. *Medicine and Science in Sports and Exercise* **26**, 1284–1289.

Hoffman, M.D., Clifford, P.S., Snyder, A.C. *et al.* (1998) Physiological effects of technique and rolling resistance in uphill roller skiing. *Medicine and Science in Sports and Exercise* **30**, 311–317.

Komi, P. (1985) Ground reaction forces in cross-country skiing. In: *Biomechanics IX-B* (eds D. Winter, R. Norman, R. Wells, K. Hayes & A. Patla), pp. 185–190. Human Kinetics Publishers, Champaign, IL.

Komi, P.V. (1987) Force measurements during cross-country skiing. *International Journal of Sport Biomechanics* **3**, 370–381.

Leppävuori, A.P., Karras, M., Rusko, H. & Viitasalo, J.T. (1993) A new method of measuring 3-D ground reaction forces under the ski during skiing on snow. *Journal of Applied Biomechanics* **9**, 315–328.

Lind, D. & Sanders, S.P. (1997) *The Physics of Skiing.* American Institute of Physics, Woodbury, NY. Springer-Verlag, New York.

Martin, P. (1979) Diagonal stride on uphill terrain. Master's thesis, University of Illinois at Urbana-Champaign.

Mittelstadt, S.W., Hoffman, M.D., Watts, P.B. *et al.* (1995) Lactate response to uphill roller skiing: diagonal stride versus double pole techniques. *Medicine and Science in Sports and Exercise* **27**, 1563–1568.

Siletta, T. (1987) The effects of pole length variation on the skiing performance of elite cross-country skiers using V-skating techniques. *Proceedings of 1987 FIS Trainers Seminar*. Cross-Country Canada, Ottawa.

Smith, G.A. (1989) The effect of velocity and grade on the kinematics and kinetics of V1 skating in cross country skiing. Doctoral dissertation, The Pennsylvania State University, University Park, PA.

Smith, G.A. & Heagy, B.S. (1994) Kinematic analysis of skating technique of Olympic skiers in the men's 50-km race. *Journal of Applied Biomechanics* **10**, 79–88.

Smith, G.A., McNitt-Gray, J. & Nelson, R.C. (1988) Kinematic analysis of alternate stride skating in cross-country skiing. *International Journal of Sport Biomechanics* **4**, 49–58.

Smith, G.A., Fewster, J.B. & Braudt, S.M. (1996) Double poling kinematics and performance in cross-country skiing. *Journal of Applied Biomechanics* **12**, 88–103.

Street, G.M. & Frederick, E.C. (1995) Measurement of skier-generated forces during roller-ski skating. *Journal of Applied Biomechanics* **11**, 245–256.

Street, G.M. & Gregory, R.W. (1994) Relationship between glide speed and Olympic cross-country ski performance. *Journal of Applied Biomechanics* **10**, 393–399.

Street, G.M. & Tsui, P. (1986) *Compositions of Glide Waxes Used in Cross Country Skiing*. Unpublished manuscript. Biomechanics Laboratory, Pennsylvania State University.

Street, G.M. & Tsui, P. (1987) *Evaluation of Competition Cross Country Ski Poles 1986–87*. Unpublished manuscript. Biomechanics Laboratory, Pennsylvania State University.

Svensson, E. (1994) *Ski Skating with Champions, How to Ski with Least Energy*. Svensson, Seattle, WA.

PART 3

JUMPING AND AERIAL MOVEMENT

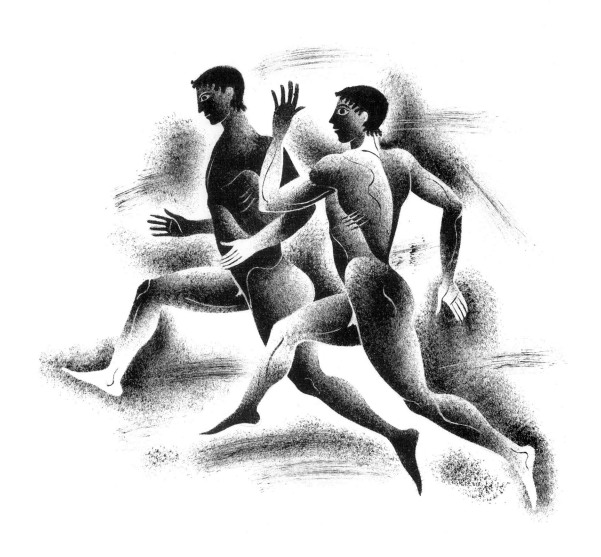

Chapter 13

Aerial Movement

M.R. YEADON

Introduction

Most sports movements have an aerial phase. In sprinting the runner spends less than half of the time in contact with the ground (Hopper 1973), while in the triple jump the aerial phases are much longer than the contact phases (Hay & Miller 1985). Typically tennis players are off the ground when the ball is played (Elliott 1989) and basketball players release the ball while airborne (Hay 1993). The same is true for the release in the discus and shot events (Hay 1993). In jumping activities it is the aerial phase that is evaluated to give a score for the performance. In the long jump and high jump events the horizontal and vertical displacements during the aerial phase are used as measures of performance, while in trampolining and diving rotation and aesthetics are also included in the evaluation.

In an aerial phase of a sports movement the athlete is freely falling under gravity. In freefall the balance mechanisms of the inner ear do not operate normally since they too are in freefall (Graybiel 1970). The otolith and semicircular canals can no longer provide information on the orientation of the head relative to the vertical direction. They do, however, give information on linear and angular accelerations (Wendt 1951) which can be used by athletes to help control aerial movements (Yeadon & Mikulcik 1996).

Motion of the mass centre

In the aerial phases of most sporting movements, air resistance has little effect and the path of the mass centre follows a parabola that is determined by the position and velocity of the mass centre at takeoff. In the competition performance shown in Fig. 13.1 the height of the mass centre at takeoff is 1.31 m while the horizontal and vertical velocities are 4.7 m · s⁻¹ and 4.5 m · s⁻¹. During the aerial phase the horizontal velocity of the mass centre remains constant since there are no horizontal forces acting (if air

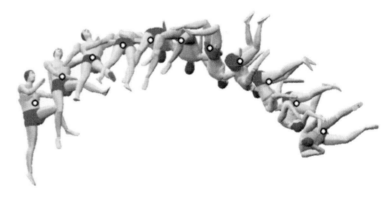

Fig. 13.1 The flight phase of a high-jump performance showing the parabolic path of the mass centre.

resistance is neglected) while the vertical motion has a constant downwards acceleration of 9.81 m · s⁻² due to the weight of the body. The vertical take-off velocity of 4.5 m · s⁻¹ determines that the mass centre rises to a peak height of 2.34 m in a time of 0.46 s. The horizontal takeoff velocity of 4.7 m · s⁻¹ determines that the mass centre covers a horizontal distance of 2.16 m during this time.

In the case of ski jumping, however, the takeoff parameters do not completely determine the path of the mass centre during flight since air resistance produces drag and lift forces which can be used by the skilled jumper to maximize the distance of the jump (Denoth *et al.* 1987; Hubbard *et al.* 1989).

Rotation during flight

In running jumps, the takeoff phase typically produces rotation even where this is disadvantageous to the performance. In long-jumping undesirable forward angular momentum is produced during the takeoff and a hitch-kick, involving arm and leg rotations, is often used to minimize the forward rotation in the aerial phase (Hay 1975; Herzog 1986). In high-jumping, both twist and somersault rotations are produced during takeoff and these are used to advantage in clearing the bar (Hopper 1963; Dapena 1980, 1995). In gymnastics skills, the somersault is initiated during the takeoff phase, while twist may be initiated either during the takeoff or during the aerial phase (van Gheluwe 1981). Although the movement of the mass centre is predetermined at takeoff (so long as air resistance can be neglected) the athlete has considerable control over rotational motion during the aerial phase.

At takeoff a gymnast has a certain quantity of angular momentum about the mass centre and this remains constant during the aerial phase since the only force acting is the weight of the gymnast and this force acts through the mass centre. For the simple case in which the body rotates about a single axis the angular momentum is the product of moment of inertia and angular velocity. A ballet dancer or a figure skater takes off for a twisting jump with arms wide and subsequently brings the arms close to the body. The effect of this is to reduce the moment of inertia about the twist axis and to increase the speed

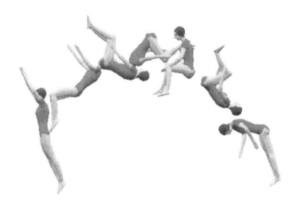

Fig. 13.2 A double backward somersault from a floor exercise showing the increased speed of somersault rotation when the body is tucked.

of rotation. In the double somersault shown in Fig. 13.2 taken from a floor exercise at the 1996 Olympic Games, the gymnast is initially in an extended configuration and is somersaulting relatively slowly, whereas subsequently the gymnast adopts a tucked position which has a smaller moment of inertia so that the somersault rate increases. By extending again at an appropriate time the gymnast can land the skill on the feet and maintain balance. For twisting somersaults in which rotations take place about more than one body axis, the situation is more complex but the same principle of angular momentum conservation governs the motion (Yeadon 1993a).

Somersaulting

While a gymnast has considerable control over the rotation in the aerial phase the angular momentum for a specific skill is often quite tightly constrained by the requirements for the good performance. Figure 13.3 depicts a good performance of a double somersault dismount from the high bar in a straight or extended position. Since the gymnast must remain extended throughout the aerial phase he has only a limited ability to adjust his moment of inertia, primarily by changing arm position. As a consequence the angular momentum generated prior to release must lie within fairly tight limits in order for a good performance to be possible. The angular

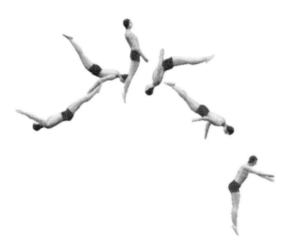

Fig. 13. 3 A double somersault dismount from the high bar with a straight body.

Fig. 13.4 A triple somersault dismount from the high bar with the body tucked.

momenta in four double somersault dismounts from the high bar in Olympic competition varied by as much as 16% although only one of the dismounts could be considered to demonstrate a good straight position during flight (Kerwin *et al.* 1990).

For body positions other than straight there is more freedom for the gymnast to adjust the somersault rate. In the tucked triple somersault dismount from high bar shown in Fig. 13.4 there is sufficient angular momentum to allow the movement to be completed successfully. If there were slightly less angular momentum than this, the gymnast could compensate by adopting a tighter tucked position. There could, however, be considerably more angular momentum without this being detrimental to a good performance. With more angular momentum the gymnast could delay the movement into the tucked position and could extend earlier prior to landing. In fact the angular momentum of the straight double somersault shown in Fig. 13.3 is 18% greater than the angular momentum of the tucked triple somersault shown in Fig. 13.4. This indicates that a gymnast who can do a straight double somer-

sault dismount from high bar should be able to generate ample angular momentum for a tucked triple somersault dismount. Some gymnasts have employed a split tuck technique in which the knees are pulled wide to reduce the moment of inertia about the somersault axis, but this technique is a break in form and only marginally increases the somersault rotation (Kerwin *et al.* 1990).

Twisting

To understand the mechanics of a multilink system performing somersaults with twist, it is helpful to look at the rotational motion of a rigid body. There are only two general types of motion that a rigid body can exhibit (Yeadon 1993a). The first of these is the *wobbling somersault* in which the body somersaults about a horizontal axis but also has an oscillating motion in which it twists one way and then the other (Fig. 13.5). During this motion the body also tilts first one way and then the other so that the head is to one side of the feet and then later to the other (see the first and last images in Fig. 13.5).

Fig. 13.5 During a wobbling somersault the twist oscillates left then right.

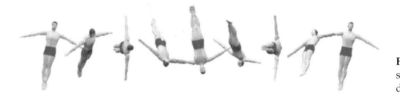

Fig. 13.6 During a twisting somersault the twist continues in one direction.

The second type of motion is the *twisting somersault* in which the twist is always in the same direction (Fig. 13.6). During this motion the body is always tilted in the same direction away from the somersault plane (the plane normal to the angular momentum vector). This tilt varies with the twist and is smallest for an even number of quarter twists (images 1, 6 and 11 of Fig. 13.6) and greatest for an odd number of quarter twists (images 3 and 9 of Fig. 13.6). This variation in the tilt angle is known as *nutation* from the theory of spinning tops (Synge & Griffith 1959) and is important for the understanding of how aerial twist is produced (Yeadon 1993c).

Since there are two quite different types of rigid body motion it might be possible that a multilink system such as the human body could change its motion from one type to the other merely by changing body configuration.

Contact twist

Angular momentum is built up while the body is in contact with the diving board or gymnastics apparatus so that it is somersaulting at takeoff. Twist may be initiated in a similar way by turning the arms and trunk in the direction of the twist while the feet are in contact with the takeoff surface. If the body is extended at takeoff this will produce a twisting somersault in which the body is tilted away from the vertical after half a somersault (Eaves 1969; Biesterfeldt 1974). Because this tilt disappears of its own accord after a complete somersault, it does not pose a problem in tumbling skills in which the gymnast takes off and lands on the feet. In twisting dives, however, there is a potential problem since entry is made into the water after one and a half somersaults. In the computer simulation shown in Fig. 13.7 the body maintains left–right symmetry throughout (upper sequence in Fig. 13.7) and overcomes this potential problem by adopting a piked position as the required number of twists nears completion. This causes the motion to change from a twisting somersault to a wobbling somersault. While the body is in the wobbling mode of motion the tilt angle is allowed to oscillate so that when the body extends it is almost vertical. This technique has its limitations since for large amounts of twist the wobble in the piked position becomes excessive and the twist is much harder to control (Yeadon 1993b).

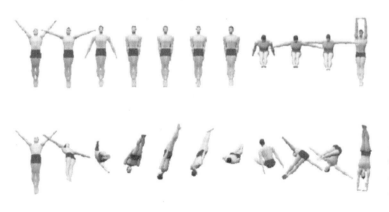

Fig. 13.7 A computer simulation of a backward 1½ somersault dive with 1½ twists in which the twist is produced during the takeoff.

Aerial twist

The way in which a cat rights itself by producing a half twist in mid-air after being dropped in an inverted position has been studied for more than a century (Marey 1894; McDonald 1960). Some coaches have thought that this is the main mechanism that divers use to produce twist (Rackham 1960; Eaves 1969). The twist is produced by using a hula-hoop circling movement of the hips during the aerial phase. If the initial angular momentum is zero it must remain so during flight and so the angular momentum associated with the hip circling produces a twisting of the whole body in the opposite direction (Kane & Scher 1969). A simulation of this movement is shown in Fig. 13.8 in which the hips circle to the right producing a twist to the left. The body moves from a forward flexed position through a side arch over the right hip, into a back arch,

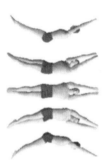

Fig. 13.8 Computer simulation of an aerial half twist using the 'hula' or 'cat' technique.

through a side arch over the left hip and ends in a forward flexed position again, having completed a half twist. A skilled trampolinist can produce a full twist using two cycles of such a movement while airborne.

It is evident that gymnasts, trampolinists and divers do not use this hula technique to produce multiple twists during the aerial phase of a somersault since the body typically remains straight during the twist. If somersault is present then any technique that tilts the body away from the somersault plane will result in twist in order to maintain constant angular momentum (Frolich 1980). The most obvious way of producing tilt during freefall is to raise one arm laterally while lowering the other. In a plain jump there is no angular momentum and this arm movement will produce a tilting of the whole body in order to maintain zero angular momentum (upper sequence of Fig. 13.9). If the same arm movements are made during a plain somersault, a similar amount of tilt (8°) results and the body automatically twists in order to maintain constant angular momentum (Yeadon 1990).

Any movement in which left–right symmetry is not maintained is likely to produce some twist. In the simulation shown in Fig. 13.10 the body makes a partial hula movement while extending from a piked to a straight position. In a plain jump this hula movement with wide arms produces tilt while the body is in a side arch configuration due to a reorientation of the principal axes of inertia (Yeadon & Atha 1985). Once the body extends, however, the

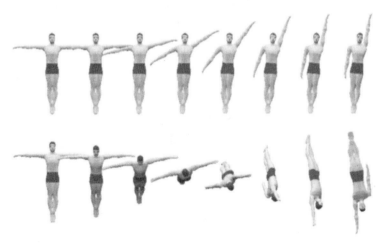

Fig. 13.9 Aerial twist in a somersault resulting from tilt produced by asymmetrical arm movement.

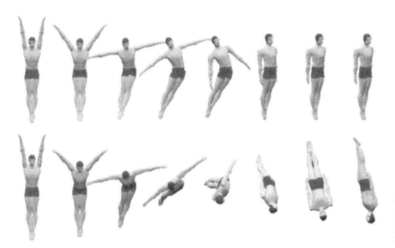

Fig. 13.10 Aerial twist in a somersault resulting from tilt produced by asymmetrical hip movement.

final tilt is only 3° (upper sequence of Fig. 13.10). If the same movements are made during a somersault the situation is somewhat different. Once the body is in a side arch position with wide arms there is considerable tilt (10°) of the principal axis corresponding to minimum moment of inertia and so the body starts to twist in order to maintain constant angular momentum. As the twist increases up to a quarter twist, the tilt angle also increases due to the nutation effect. When the body extends to a straight position the tilt angle is not reduced in the same way as for a plain jump with a hula movement since this extension is made at around the quarter twist position and any reorientation therefore changes the somersault rather than the tilt. As a consequence this technique produces considerable tilt (11°) in a somersault and is a viable method of producing aerial twist.

It is fortuitous that the hula movement that produces a twist to the left in a jump also produces tilt which will result in a twist to the left in a forward somersault. During the takeoff for a forward somersault from the floor or trampoline or diving board the body flexes at the hips so that initially it is in a piked position which is suitable for this technique. For a backward somersault the body is initially arched and use of a partial hula movement while extending again produces tilt which results in twist in the same direction as the hula twist. If the body is rotating backwards in a piked position, however, the tilt produced by a hula movement results in twist in the opposite direction to the hula twist. This conflict greatly reduces the effectiveness of the technique (Yeadon 1993c) and it is preferable to use asymmetrical arm movement to produce aerial twist from a piked configuration when rotating backwards.

The tilt produced by an asymmetrical arm movement will be greater when the arms move through a large angle. In order to achieve this in a computer simulation, the left arm is first lowered to the side of the body together with some adduction and abduction so that it passes in front of the body (upper sequence of Fig. 13.11). This minimizes the negative tilt produced by the initial arm movement and places the arms in an asymmetrical position from which each arm may be rotated through half a revolution. This produces twice the tilt (16°) of the arm movement shown in Fig. 13.9 since the arms move through twice the angle. When the same arm movements are made during a somersault a similar amount of tilt results and a rapid twist ensues (lower sequence of Fig. 13.11). As the twist nears three revolutions the body flexes at the hips and the arms are spread wide. This removes the tilt so that a one and a half somersault dive with three twists can be completed. It is important that the left arm initially sweeps across the body as it is lowered to the side as otherwise the body becomes tilted in the opposite direction and twists to the right while the arm is being lowered. In this case the double

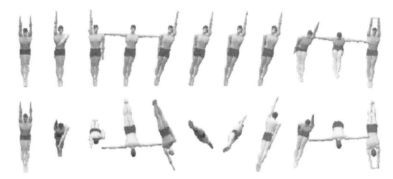

Fig. 13.11 Simulation of a forward 1½ somersault dive with three twists using asymmetrical movements of the arms.

arm movement occurs around the quarter twist position and produces little change in the tilt angle since the reorientation of the body manifests itself mainly as a change in somersault rotation.

The asymmetrical hip technique shown in Fig. 13.10 may be used to produce one and a half twists in a single or double somersault. In Yeadon (1997a) a progression based on computer simulations is described for learning a double somersault with one and a half twists in the second somersault (Fig. 13.12). In the first somersault the body is flexed into a piked position and then moves through a side arch position with wide arms while extending. The arms are then adducted to accelerate the twist and as the one and a half twists are completed first the right arm and then the left arm is abducted to help remove the tilt. The body also moves through a side arch position while flexing in order to use the asymmetrical hip technique to help remove the tilt. The asymmetrical hip technique is capable of producing tilt when the somersault is forwards and of removing tilt when the somersault is backwards. It is not effective in removing the tilt in a dive such as in

Fig. 13.11 where the final somersault direction is forwards.

Stopping the twist

In the simulation shown in Fig. 13.11 tilt was removed using a reversal of the initial asymmetrical arm movement that was used to produce the tilt. This technique may be used in dives with an even number of half twists. For an odd number of half twists a reversal of the initial arm movement would increase the tilt and speed up the twist. In such a case it is necessary to reverse the arm positions during the twist without affecting the tilt so that they are in a suitable position for removing the tilt prior to entry. In backward and reverse twisting dives there are typically 1½, 2½ or 3½ twists, and this technique is often used. The lower sequence of Fig. 13.13 is taken from a performance of a backward 1½ somersault dive with 1½ twists. The upper sequence shows the body configurations used in the dive. After takeoff the left arm is lowered and the right arm is held high producing tilt that results in a

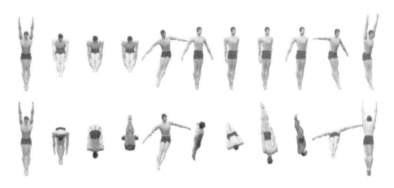

Fig. 13.12 A double somersault with 1½ twists in the second somersault produced using asymmetrical hip movement.

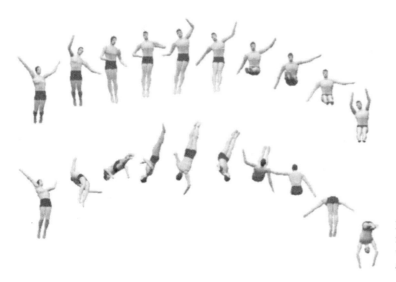

Fig. 13.13 Stopping the twist by removing the tilt in a backward 1½ with 1½ twists using asymmetrical arms.

twist to the left. During the twist the arm positions are reversed while keeping the arms close to the body so as not to slow the twist. As the 1½ twists near completion the diver first pikes and then lowers his left arm while raising his right arm so as to remove the tilt. By first flexing at the hips the moment of inertia about the frontal axis is reduced so that more tilt can be removed by the asymmetrical arm movement.

Contributions of twisting techniques to tilt and twist

The simulation model of Yeadon *et al.* (1990a) has been used to determine the contributions of the various twisting techniques to the production of tilt and hence twist in actual performances by using modifications of the body configurations used by the athlete. To determine the contribution of asymmetrical arm movement, for example, a modified simulation can be carried out in which the right arm mirrors the original left arm movement so that the arms move symmetrically. The difference in the tilt

angles produced in this simulation and the original simulation based on the actual arm movement gives a measure of the contribution to the tilt angle from asymmetrical arm movement (Yeadon 1993d). Other contributions can be determined in a similar manner.

Figure 13.14 depicts a performance of a double somersault from trampoline with a full twist in the second somersault. In such a movement, where almost a complete somersault occurs prior to the initiation of twist, it is to be expected that little contact twist is used and that aerial techniques are responsible for the production of twist. Prior to twisting the body is piked and since it is rotating backwards asymmetrical hip movement is unable to produce much tilt since the directions of hula twist and tilt twist are in conflict. As a consequence it might be expected that the twist is produced by asymmetrical arm movement in the aerial phase, and a simulation analysis yields just this result (Yeadon 1993d). Such simulation analyses have shown that the greatest contributions are made by asymmetrical arm and hip techniques in the aerial phase in springboard diving (Yeadon 1993e), in single somersault

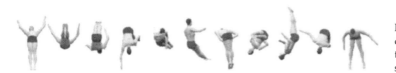

Fig. 13.14 Performance of a double backward somersault from trampoline with one twist in the second somersault.

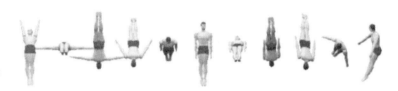

Fig. 13.15 Simulation of an unstable double backward somersault leading to a quarter twist.

dismounts with one twist from high bar (Yeadon *et al.* 1990b) and in double somersault dismounts with one twist from the rings (Yeadon 1994). There is some evidence, however, that major contributions are made by contact techniques in multiple somersaults with twist when there is substantial twist in the first somersault in, for example, high bar dismounts (Yeadon 1997b) and freestyle aerial skiing (Yeadon 1989).

Control of aerial movement

If a rigid body is somersaulting about its intermediate principal moment of inertia the motion is unstable in the sense that twist will build up exponentially until the body completes a half twist (Marion 1965; Hinrichs 1978). In practice this will pose a potential problem for somersaults about a lateral axis when the body is held straight. Figure 13.15 depicts a hypothetical simulation of a double somersault in which slight arm asymmetries lead to a quarter twist towards the end of the movement. Nigg (1974) suggested that the arms could be extended laterally during a straight somersault in order to minimize the effect of this instability. Yeadon and Mikulcik (1996) showed that this strategy will not decrease the build-up of twist. An alternative strategy of asymmetrical arm adduction and

abduction based upon the twist angular velocity and acceleration is capable of preventing the build-up of twist providing that the time delay in the feedback loop is less than a quarter of a somersault. There is evidence that the inner ear organs normally used for balance provide the required feedback data on twist velocity and acceleration rather than the visual system (Yeadon & Mikulcik 1996). The main function of the eyes may be to obtain angular information on body orientation in space in order to make in-flight adjustments for correct landing orientation (Rezette & Amblard 1985).

In actual performances of straight double somersaults such asymmetrical arm movements are not readily apparent to an observer or to the performer making the corrective adjustments. This is probably because the corrective movements made are small and the build-up of twist is small. Occasionally, however, the build-up of twist may be corrected somewhat late and a larger arm asymmetry will be required. An example of such a case is shown in Fig. 13.16 which depicts an actual performance of a double straight somersault on trampoline in which considerable arm asymmetry is evident after 1½ somersaults.

The build-up of twist can be used to good effect to produce an aerial twist using only a small asymmetry in the arm positions. Figure 13.17 depicts

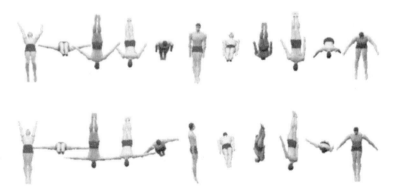

Fig. 13.16 A performance of a double straight somersault in which corrective arm asymmetry is apparent late in the movement.

Fig. 13.17 Simulation of a double backward somersault with one twist in the second somersault arising from slight arm asymmetry in the first somersault.

a theoretical simulation of a double somersault with one twist in the last $1\frac{1}{4}$ somersaults. During the first three-quarters of a somersault the arms are spread wide but with a small (5°) asymmetry. This leads to a slow build-up of tilt and twist during the first somersault. The twist is accelerated by adducting both arms towards the end of the first somersault. As one revolution of twist nears completion, first the right arm is adducted and then the left arm in order to remove the tilt and stop the twist. Since this asymmetrical arm movement for stopping the twist comprises exactly the same technique as that for preventing the build-up of twist in a straight somersault it is likely that learning this type of control in a twisting somersault is carried over into the control of non-twisting somersaults or vice versa.

Summary

Most sports movements contain an aerial phase during which the body loses contact with the ground or apparatus. While the path of the mass centre during flight is determined by its location and velocity at takeoff, the amount and type of rotation of the body is largely under the control of the athlete. Somersault rotation is a consequence of the angular momentum generated during takeoff. Twist rotations may be initiated during takeoff or during the aerial phase by means of asymmetrical arm or hip movements. Asymmetrical arm movements may be used to stop the twist in a twisting somersault or to prevent the build-up of twist in a non-twisting somersault. The control of the twist in this way is possible using feedback via the inner ear balance mechanisms, provided that the somersault rate is not too high.

References

Biesterfeldt, H.J. (1974) Twisting mechanics I. *Gymnast* **16** (6,7), 46–47.

Dapena, J. (1980) Mechanics of rotation in the Fosbury-flop. *Medicine and Science in Sports and Exercise* **12**, 45–53.

Dapena, J. (1995) The rotation over the bar in the Fosbury-flop high jump. *Track Coach* **132**, 4201–4210.

Denoth, J., Luethi, S.M. & Gasser, H.H. (1987) Methodological problems on optimization of the flight phase in ski jumping. *International Journal of Sport Biomechanics* **3**, 404–418.

Eaves, G. (1969) *Diving: the Mechanics of Springboard and Firmboard Techniques.* Kaye & Ward, London.

Elliott, B.C. (1989) Tennis strokes and equipment. In: *Biomechanics of Sport* (ed. C.L. Vaughan), pp. 263–288. CRC Press, Boca Raton.

Frolich, C. (1980) The physics of somersaulting and twisting. *Scientific American* **242**, 112–120.

van Gheluwe, B. (1981) A biomechanical simulation model for airborne twist in backward somersaults. *Journal of Human Movement Studies* **7**, 1–22.

Graybiel, A. (1970) Vestibular problems in prolonged manned space flight. In: *Vestibular Function on Earth and in Space* (ed. J. Stahle), pp. 9–25. Pergamon Press, Oxford.

Hay, J.G. (1975) Biomechanical aspects of jumping. *Exercise and Sport Sciences Reviews* **3**, 135–161.

Hay, J.G. (1993) *The Biomechanics of Sports Techniques,* 4th edn. Prentice-Hall, Englewood Cliffs, NJ.

Hay, J.G. & Miller, J.A. (1985) Techniques used in the triple jump. *International Journal of Sport Biomechanics* **1**, 185–196.

Herzog, W. (1986) Maintenance of body orientation in the flight phase of long jumping. *Medicine and Science in Sports and Exercise* **18**, 231–241.

Hinrichs, R.N. (1978) Principal axes and moments of inertia of the human body: an investigation of the stability of rotary motions. MA thesis, University of Iowa.

Hopper, B.J. (1963) Rotation—a vital factor in athletic technique. *Track Technique* **12**, 356–361.

Hopper, B.J. (1973) *The Mechanics of Human Movement.* Crosby, Lockwood, Staples, London.

Hubbard, M., Hibbard, R.L., Yeadon, M.R. & Komor, A. (1989) A multisegment dynamic model of ski jumping. *International Journal of Sport Biomechanics* **5**, 258–274.

Kane, T.R. & Scher, M.P. (1969) A dynamical explanation of the falling cat phenomenon. *International Journal of Solids and Structures* **5** (7), 663–670.

Kerwin, D.G., Yeadon, M.R. & Lee, S.-C. (1990) Body configuration in multiple somersault high bar dismounts. *International Journal of Sport Biomechanics* **6**, 147–156.

Marey, E.-J. (1894) Mécanique animale: Des mouvements que certains animaux exécutent pour retomber sur leurs pieds lorsqu'ils sont précipités d'un lieu élevé. *La Nature* 10 November 1984, 369–370.

Marion, J.B. (1965) *Classical Dynamics of Particles and Systems.* Academic Press, New York.

McDonald, D. (1960) How does a cat fall on its feet? *New Scientist* **7** (189), 1647–1649.

Nigg, B.M. (1974) Analysis of twisting and turning movements. In: *Biomechanics IV* (eds R.C. Nelson & C.A. Morehouse), pp. 279–283. Macmillan, London.

Rackham, G. (1960) The origin of twist. *Swimming Times* **47** (6), 263–267.

Rezette, D. & Amblard, B. (1985) Orientation versus motion visual cues to control sensorimotor skills in some acrobatic leaps. *Human Movement Science* **4**, 297–306.

Synge, J.L. & Griffith, B.A. (1959) *Principles of Mechanics,* 3rd edn. McGraw-Hill, New York.

Wendt, G.R. (1951) Vestibular functions. In: *Handbook of Experimental Psychology* (ed. S.S. Stevens), pp. 1191–1223. Wiley, New York.

Yeadon, M.R. (1989) Twisting techniques used in freestyle aerial skiing. *International Journal of Sport Biomechanics* **5**, 275–284.

Yeadon, M.R. (1990) The simulation of aerial movement—III. The determination of the angular momentum of the human body. *Journal of Biomechanics* **23**, 75–83.

Yeadon, M.R. (1993a) The biomechanics of twisting somersaults. Part I: Rigid body motions. *Journal of Sports Sciences* **11**, 187–198.

Yeadon, M.R. (1993b) The biomechanics of twisting somersaults. Part II: Contact twist. *Journal of Sports Sciences* **11**, 199–208.

Yeadon, M.R. (1993c) The biomechanics of twisting somersaults. Part III: aerial twist. *Journal of Sports Sciences* **11**, 209–218.

Yeadon, M.R. (1993d) The biomechanics of twisting somersaults. Part IV: Partitioning performance using the tilt angle. *Journal of Sports Sciences* **11**, 219–225.

Yeadon, M.R. (1993e) Twisting techniques used by competitive divers. *Journal of Sports Sciences* **11** (4), 337–342.

Yeadon, M.R. (1994) Twisting techniques used in dismounts from rings. *Journal of Applied Biomechanics* **10**, 178–188.

Yeadon, M.R. (1997a) The biomechanics of the human in flight. *American Journal of Sports Medicine* **25** (4), 575–580.

Yeadon, M.R. (1997b) Twisting double somersault high bar dismounts. *Journal of Applied Biomechanics* **13**, 76–87.

Yeadon, M.R. & Atha, J. (1985) The production of a sustained aerial twist during a somersault without the use of asymmetrical arm action. In: *Biomechanics IX-B* (eds D.A. Winter, R.W. Norman, R.P. Wells, K.C. Hayes & A.E. Patla), pp. 395–400. Human Kinetics Publishers, Champaign, IL.

Yeadon, M.R. & Mikulcik, E.C. (1996) The control of non-twisting somersaults using configurational changes. *Journal of Biomechanics* **29**, 1341–1348.

Yeadon, M.R., Atha, J. & Hales, F.D. (1990a) The simulation of aerial movement—IV. A computer simulation model. *Journal of Biomechanics* **23**, 85–89.

Yeadon, M.R., Lee, S. & Kerwin, D.G. (1990b) Twisting techniques used in high bar dismounts. *International Journal of Sport Biomechanics* **6**, 139–146.

Chapter 14

The High Jump

J. DAPENA

Introduction

This chapter describes the mechanics of the Fosbury-flop style of high jumping, and explains a rationale followed for the evaluation of the techniques used by individual elite high jumpers.

Since 1982, our laboratory has studied the techniques of the best high jumpers in the USA. This work is part of the Scientific Support Services programme sponsored by USATF (USA Track and Field, the governing body for track and field athletics in the USA) at several biomechanics laboratories. The goal of the programme is to give the best US athletes biomechanical information to help improve their performance through changes in technique.

Personnel from our laboratory generally film the top American high jumpers every year at the final of the USATF Championships or at some other major competition. The films are subsequently analysed using three-dimensional biomechanical research

Table 14.1 General information on the analysed jumpers, and meet results.

Athlete	Country	Standing height (m)	Mass (kg)	Personal best mark* (m)	Best height cleared at the meet† (m)
Men					
Gennadiy Avdeyenko	USSR	2.02	82	2.38	2.38 (W87)
Hollis Conway	USA	1.84	68	2.40	2.34 (O92)
Tim Forsyth	Australia	1.97	75	2.34	2.34 (O92)
Igor Paklin	USSR	1.91	72	2.41	2.38 (W87)
Artur Partyka	Poland	1.91	73	2.37	2.34 (O92)
Patrik Sjöberg	Sweden	2.00	82	2.42	2.34 (O92)
Javier Sotomayor	Cuba	1.94	82	2.44	2.34 (O92)
Dwight Stones	USA	1.95	82	2.34	2.34 (T84)
Jan Zvara	Czechoslovakia	1.91	85	2.36	2.34 (W87)
Women					
Amy Acuff	USA	1.88	64	1.98	1.96 (U97)
Galina Astafei	Romania	1.84	65	2.00	2.00 (O92)
Susanne Beyer-Helm	East Germany	1.78	58	2.02	2.02 (W87)
Emilia Dragieva	Bulgaria	1.69	55	2.00	2.00 (W87)
Heike Henkel	Germany	1.82	63	2.07	2.02 (O92)
Stefka Kostadinova	Bulgaria	1.80	60	2.08	2.05 (W87)
Ioamnet Quintero	Cuba	1.80	60	1.98	1.97 (O92)
Coleen Sommer	USA	1.76	58	2.00	1.96 (U87)

* By the end of the meet in which the jumper was analysed.
† T84 = 1984 US Olympic Trials; W87 = 1987 World Indoor Championships; U87 = 1987 USATF Championships; O92 = 1992 Olympic Games; U97 = 1997 USATF Championships.

methods. Reports and videotapes containing mechanical data, computer graphics and interpretations are then prepared, and sent to the coaches and athletes. The reports and videotapes evaluate the advantages and disadvantages of the present techniques of the athletes, and suggest how to correct some of the technique problems. The rationale used for the technique evaluations stems from a comprehensive interpretation of the Fosbury-flop style of high jumping based on the research of Dyatchkov (1968) and Ozolin (1973), on basic research carried out by the author and collaborators (Dapena 1980a,b, 1987, 1995a,b, 1997; Dapena & Chung 1988; Dapena *et al.* 1990, 1997c), and on the experience accumulated through the analysis of US and other high jumpers at our laboratory since 1982 in the course of service work sponsored by USATF, the USOC (United States Olympic Committee), and the IOC (International Olympic Committee) (e.g. Dapena *et al.* 1993a,b, 1997a,b).

The main purpose of this chapter is to describe this interpretation of the Fosbury-flop style of high jumping, and to explain the rationale followed in the reports for the evaluation of technique. The discussions are illustrated with data from the highest jumps by men and women in our database. Table 14.1 shows general information on these athletes, and their results in the analysed competitions. They all used the Fosbury-flop style.

Phases of a high jump

A high jump can be divided into three parts: the run-up phase, the takeoff phase and the flight or bar clearance phase. The purpose of the run-up is to set the appropriate conditions for the beginning of the takeoff phase. During the takeoff phase, the athlete exerts forces that determine the maximum height that the centre of mass (COM) will reach after leaving the ground and the angular momentum (or 'rotary momentum') that the body will have during the bar clearance. The only voluntary movements that can be made after leaving the ground are internal compensatory movements (e.g. one part of the body can be lifted by lowering another part; one part of the body can be made to rotate faster by making another part slow down its rotation).

The run-up serves as a preparation for the takeoff phase, the most important phase of the jump. The actions of the athlete during the bar clearance are less important: Most of the problems found in the bar clearance actually originate in the run-up or takeoff phases.

General characteristics of the run-up

The typical length of the run-up for experienced high jumpers is about 10 steps. In most athletes who

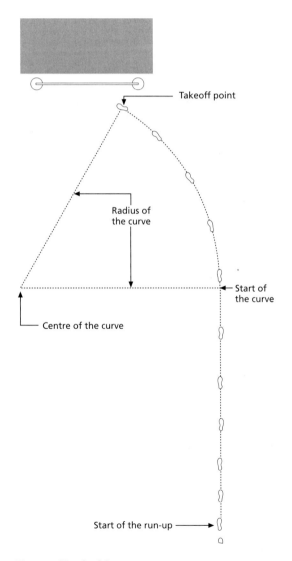

Fig. 14.1 Sketch of the run-up.

use the Fosbury-flop technique, the first part of the run-up usually follows a straight line perpendicular to the plane of the standards, and the last four or five steps follow a curve (Fig. 14.1). One of the main purposes of the curve is to make the jumper lean away from the bar at the start of the takeoff phase. The faster the run-up or the tighter the curve, the greater the lean towards the centre of the curve.

Approach angles

Figure 14.2 shows an overhead view of the footprints and of the COM path during the last two steps of the run-up, the takeoff phase and the airborne phase. Notice that the COM path is initially to the left of the footprints. This is because the athlete is leaning towards the left during the curve. The path then converges with the footprints, and the COM is almost directly over the takeoff foot at the end of the takeoff.

Figure 14.2 also shows angles t_1, p_2, p_1 and p_0: t_1 is the angle between the bar and the line joining the last two footprints; p_2 and p_1 are the angles between the bar and the path of the COM in the airborne phases of the last two steps; p_0 is the angle between the bar and the path of the COM during the airborne phase that follows the takeoff. The angles are smaller in athletes who move more parallel to the bar. The values of these angles are shown in Table 14.2.

Progression of the run-up

To start the run-up, the athlete can either walk a few steps and then start running, or make a standing start. In the early part of the run-up, the athlete should follow a gradual progression in which each step is longer and faster than the previous one. After a few steps, the high jumper will be running rather fast, with long, relaxed steps similar to those of a 400-metre or 800-metre runner. In the last two or three steps of the run-up the athlete should gradually lower the hips. This has to be done without a significant loss of running speed.

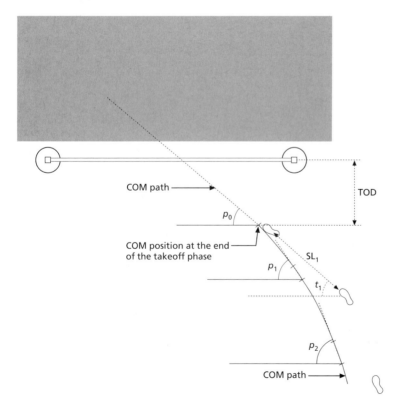

Fig. 14.2 Footprints and centre of mass (COM) path.

Table 14.2 Direction of the footprints of the last step (t_1), direction of the path of the centre of mass (COM) in the last two steps (p_2 and p_1) and after takeoff (p_0), direction of the longitudinal axis of the foot with respect to the bar (e_1), with respect to the final direction of the run-up (e_2) and with respect to the horizontal force made on the ground during the takeoff phase (e_3), length of the last step (SL$_1$, expressed in metres and also as a percentage of the standing height of the athlete), and takeoff distance (TOD).

Athlete	t_1 (°)	p_2 (°)	p_1 (°)	p_0 (°)	e_1 (°)	e_2 (°)	e_3 (°)	SL$_1$ (m)	SL$_1$ (%)	TOD (m)
Men										
Avdeyenko	33	54	44	39	23	21	25	2.27	112	0.96
Conway	15	47	30	34	−9	39	36	2.11	115	0.94
Forsyth	26	46	39	38	17	21	22	2.18	111	0.91
Paklin	32	50	40	33	4	36	43	2.16	113	0.86
Partyka	28	51	41	33	16	25	35	1.83	96	1.01
Sjöberg	26	48	37	29	11	26	35	2.10	105	0.77
Sotomayor	31	–	41	31	11	30	40	2.31	119	0.84
Stones	32	55	44	38	−5	50	56	2.00	102	0.99
Zvara	33	55	43	44	23	20	20	2.11	111	0.67
Women										
Acuff	23	50	36	33	18	18	22	1.69	90	0.53
Astafei	32	–	39	34	21	18	24	2.00	109	0.88
Beyer-Helm	29	50	42	40	24	18	20	1.80	101	1.04
Dragieva	33	47	41	40	31	10	11	1.85	109	0.82
Henkel	30	55	41	38	42	−1	4	1.91	105	0.94
Kostadinova	34	51	43	37	26	16	24	2.06	114	0.98
Quintero	30	51	42	34	27	14	24	1.91	106	0.75
Sommer	23	44	36	33	30	6	11	1.72	98	0.90

Note: Some of the values in this table may not fit perfectly with each other, because of rounding off.

Horizontal velocity and height of the COM at the end of the run-up

The takeoff phase is defined as the period of time between the instant when the takeoff foot first touches the ground (touchdown) and the instant when it loses contact with the ground (takeoff). During the takeoff phase, the takeoff leg pushes down on the ground. In reaction, the ground pushes up on the body through the takeoff leg with an equal and opposite force. The upward force exerted by the ground on the athlete changes the vertical velocity of the COM from a value that is initially close to zero to a large upward vertical velocity. The vertical velocity of the athlete at the end of the takeoff phase determines how high the COM will go after the athlete leaves the ground, and is therefore of great importance for the result of the jump.

To maximize the vertical velocity at the end of the takeoff phase, the product of the vertical force exerted by the athlete on the ground and the time during which this force is exerted should be as large as possible. This can be achieved by making a large vertical force while the COM travels through a long vertical range of motion during the takeoff phase.

A fast approach run can help the athlete to exert a larger vertical force on the ground. This can occur in the following way. When the takeoff leg is planted ahead of the body at the end of the run-up, the knee extensor muscles resist the flexion of the leg, but the leg is still forced to flex because of the forward momentum of the jumper. In this process the extensor muscles of the knee of the takeoff leg are stretched. It is believed that this stretching stimulates the muscles, which in turn allows the foot of the takeoff leg to exert a larger force on the ground.

Table 14.3 Height of the centre of mass (COM) at the start of the takeoff phase (h_{TD}, expressed in metres and also as a percentage of the standing height of the athlete), horizontal velocity in the last two steps of the run-up (v_{H2} and v_{H1}), horizontal velocity after takeoff (v_{HTO}), change in horizontal velocity during the takeoff phase (Δv_H), vertical velocity at the start of the takeoff phase (v_{ZTD}), and vertical velocity at the end of the takeoff phase (v_{ZTO}).

Athlete	h_{TD} (m)	(%)	v_{H2} (m · s⁻¹)	v_{H1} (m · s⁻¹)	v_{HTO} (m · s⁻¹)	Δv_H (m · s⁻¹)	v_{ZTD} (m · s⁻¹)	v_{ZTO} (m · s⁻¹)
Men								
Avdeyenko	0.92	45.5	8.1	7.9	3.7	−4.2	−0.3	4.50
Conway	0.78	42.5	7.4	7.4	3.4	−4.0	−0.6	4.65
Forsyth	0.95	48.5	7.2	7.3	3.8	−3.4	−0.6	4.55
Paklin	0.85	44.5	8.1	7.7	3.9	−3.9	−0.5	4.55
Partyka	0.93	48.5	7.6	7.4	4.1	−3.3	−0.6	4.50
Sjöberg	0.98	49.0	7.2	7.5	4.0	−3.5	−0.6	4.25
Sotomayor	0.89	46.0	–	8.0	4.0	−4.0	−0.7	4.60
Stones	0.92	47.0	7.0	7.1	3.5	−3.5	−0.4	4.40
Zvara	0.89	46.5	6.9	6.6	2.6	−4.0	−0.6	4.65
Women								
Acuff	0.92	49.0	6.3	6.3	3.5	−2.8	−0.2	3.80
Astafei	0.88	48.0	–	7.2	4.1	−3.1	−0.7	3.95
Beyer-Helm	0.86	48.0	6.9	7.2	3.8	−3.4	−0.5	4.00
Dragieva	0.81	47.5	6.9	7.2	3.5	−3.7	−0.8	4.10
Henkel	0.89	49.0	7.4	7.2	4.3	−2.9	−0.5	3.90
Kostadinova	0.90	50.0	7.5	7.3	4.2	−3.1	−0.5	4.00
Quintero	0.84	46.5	7.3	6.7	3.8	−2.9	−0.8	3.90
Sommer	0.87	49.5	6.9	7.1	4.3	−2.8	−0.6	3.85

Note: Some of the values in this table may not fit perfectly with each other, because of rounding off.

In this way, a fast run-up helps to increase the vertical force exerted during the takeoff phase. (For a more extended discussion of the mechanisms that may be involved in the high jump takeoff, see Dapena & Chung 1988.) Table 14.3 shows the values of v_{H2}, the horizontal velocity of the athlete in the next-to-last step of the run-up, and of v_{H1}, the horizontal velocity of the athlete in the last step of the run-up, just before the takeoff foot is planted on the ground. The value of v_{H1} is the important one.

To maximize the vertical range of motion through which force is exerted on the body, the centre of mass needs to be in a low position at the start of the takeoff phase and in a high position at the end of it. The COM of most high jumpers is reasonably high by the end of the takeoff phase, but it is difficult to have the COM in a low position at the start of the takeoff phase. This is because in such a case the body has to be supported by a deeply flexed non-takeoff leg during the next-to-last step of the run-up, which requires a very strong non-takeoff leg; it is also difficult to learn the appropriate neuromuscular patterns that will permit the athlete to pass over the deeply flexed non-takeoff leg without losing speed. Table 14.3 shows the value of h_{TD}, the height of the COM at the instant that the takeoff foot is planted on the ground to start the takeoff phase. It is expressed in metres, but also as a percentage of the standing height of each athlete. The percentage values are more meaningful for comparing athletes.

It is possible to achieve an approach run that is fast and low in the last steps. However, it requires considerable effort and training. If an athlete has learned how to run fast and low, a new problem could occur: The athlete could actually be too fast and too low. If the takeoff leg is not strong enough, it will be forced to flex excessively during the takeoff phase, and then it may not be able to make a forceful

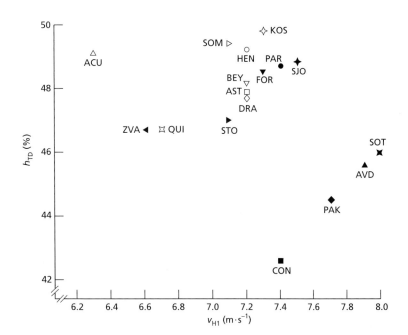

Fig. 14.3 Horizontal velocity at the end of the run-up (v_{H1}) and height (h_{TD}) of the centre of mass (COM) at the end of the run-up.

extension in the final part of the takeoff phase. In other words, the takeoff leg may suffer partial or complete collapse (buckling) under the stress, and the result will be an aborted jump. Therefore, it is important for a high jumper to find the optimum combination of run-up speed and COM height. We will now see how this can be done.

Figure 14.3 shows a plot of h_{TD} vs. v_{H1}. Each point represents one jump by one athlete. (A different symbol has been assigned to each athlete in Fig. 14.3; the same symbol will be used in subsequent graphs.) This kind of graph permits one to visualize simultaneously how fast and how high an athlete was at the end of the run-up. For instance, a point in the upper right part of the graph would indicate a jump with a fast run-up but high COM at the end of the run-up.

Let us consider what would happen if all the athletes shown in Fig. 14.3 had similar dynamic strength in the takeoff leg. In such a case, the athletes in the upper left part of the graph would be far from their limit for buckling, the athletes in the lower right part of the graph would be closest to buckling, and the athletes in the centre, lower left or upper right parts of the graph would be somewhere

in between with respect to buckling. Therefore, if all the athletes shown in Fig. 14.3 had similar dynamic strength, we would recommend the athletes in the upper left part of the graph to learn how to run faster and lower, and then experiment with jumps using run-ups that are faster and/or lower than their original ones. Athletes in the centre, lower left and upper right parts of the graph would also be advised to experiment with faster and lower run-ups, possibly emphasizing 'faster' for any jumpers in the lower left part of the graph, and 'lower' for jumpers in the upper right part of the graph. The athletes in the lower right part of the graph would be cautioned against the use of much faster and/or lower run-ups than their present ones, because these athletes would already be closer to buckling than the others.

The procedure just described would make sense if all the jumpers in Fig. 14.3 had similar dynamic strength in the takeoff leg. However, this is unlikely. Some high jumpers will be more powerful than others. Since stronger athletes can handle faster and lower run-ups without buckling, it is possible that an athlete in the upper left part of the graph might be weak, and therefore close to buckling, while an

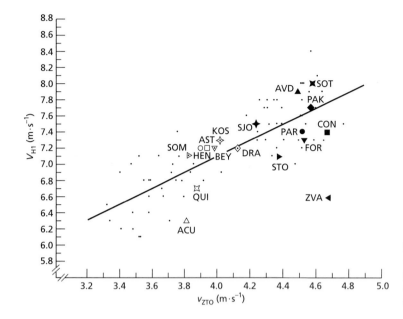

Fig. 14.4 Relationship between the vertical velocity at the end of the takeoff (v_{ZTO}) and the horizontal velocity at the end of the run-up (v_{HI}).

athlete farther down and to the right in the graph might be more powerful, and actually farther from buckling. The optimum combination of run-up speed and COM height will be different for different high jumpers.

High jumpers with greater dynamic strength in the takeoff leg will be able to handle faster and lower run-ups without buckling during the takeoff phase. However, it is not easy to measure the 'dynamic strength' of a high jumper's takeoff leg. The personal record of an athlete in a squat lift or in a vertical jump-and-reach test are not good indicators. This is because these tests do not duplicate closely enough the conditions of the high-jump takeoff. Therefore, we used instead the vertical velocity of the high jumper at the end of the takeoff phase (v_{ZTO}—see below) as a rough indicator of the dynamic strength of the takeoff leg. In other words, we used the capability of a high jumper to generate lift in a high jump as a rough indicator of the athlete's dynamic strength or 'takeoff power'.

To help us predict the optimum horizontal speed at the end of the run-up, we made use of statistical information accumulated through film analyses of male and female high jumpers in the course of Scientific Support Services work in the period 1982–87 (Dapena *et al.* 1990). The athletes involved in these studies were all elite high jumpers filmed at the finals of national and international level competitions (USATF and NCAA Championships, US Olympic Trials, World Indoor Championships).

Each small dot in Fig. 14.4 represents one jump by one of the athletes in our statistical sample. The other symbols show the athletes used here for illustration purposes. The horizontal axis of the graph shows vertical velocity at takeoff (v_{ZTO}): The most powerful high jumpers are those able to generate most lift, and they are to the right in the graph; the weaker jumpers are to the left. The vertical axis shows the final speed of the run-up (v_{HI}). The diagonal 'regression' line shows the trend of the statistical data. The graph agrees with our expectations: The more powerful jumpers, those able to generate more lift (v_{ZTO}), can also handle faster run-ups (v_{HI}) without buckling.

So, what is the optimum run-up speed for a given high jumper? It seems safe to assume that high-jumpers will rarely run so fast that the takeoff leg will buckle. This is because it takes conscious effort to use a fast run-up, and if the athlete feels that the leg has buckled in one jump, an easier (slower) run-up will be used in subsequent jumps. Since partial

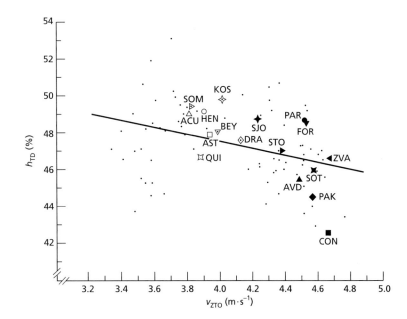

Fig. 14.5 Relationship between the vertical velocity at the end of the takeoff (v_{ZTO}) and the height of the COM at the end of the run-up (h_{TD}, expressed as a percentage of standing height).

buckling will begin to occur at run-up speeds immediately faster than the optimum, few high jumpers would be expected to regularly use run-ups that are faster than their optimum. We should expect a larger number of high jumpers to use run-up speeds that are slower than their optimum. This is because a fair number of high jumpers have not learned to use a fast enough run-up. Therefore, the diagonal regression line which marks the average trend in the graph probably marks speeds that are somewhat slower than the optimum. In summary, although the precise value of the optimum run-up speed is not known for any given value of v_{ZTO}, it is probably faster than the value predicted by the diagonal regression line; athletes near the regression line or below it were probably running too slowly at the end of the run-up.

A similar rationale can be followed with the graph of h_{TD} vs. v_{ZTO}, shown in Fig. 14.5. Each small dot in Fig. 14.5 represents one jump by one of the athletes in our statistical sample. The horizontal axis of the graph again shows vertical velocity at takeoff (v_{ZTO}): the most powerful high jumpers are those able to generate more lift, and they are to the right in the graph; the weaker jumpers are to the left. The vertical axis shows the height of the COM at the

start of the takeoff phase (h_{TD}). Although the data are more 'noisy' than in the previous graph (there is a wider 'cloud' around the regression line), the graph in Fig. 14.5 also agrees with our general expectations: The more powerful jumpers (larger v_{ZTO} values) can be lower at the end of the run-up (smaller h_{TD} values) without buckling. In Fig. 14.5, jumpers on the regression line or above it have defective techniques, and the optimum will be somewhere below the regression line.

When Figs 14.4 and 14.5 are used as diagnostic tools, it is necessary to take into consideration the information from both graphs. For instance, if a given athlete is near the regression lines in Figs 14.4 and 14.5, or below the regression line in Fig. 14.4 and above the regression line in Fig. 14.5, we should presume that this athlete is not near the buckling point. Therefore the athlete should be advised to increase the run-up speed and/or to run with lower hips at the end of the run-up. However, if an athlete is slightly below the regression line in Fig. 14.4, but markedly below it in Fig. 14.5, the situation is different. Since the COM was very low during the run-up, maybe the athlete was close to the buckling point, even though the run-up speed was not very fast. In this case, it would not be appropriate to advise an increase in run-up speed, even if the athlete was running somewhat slower than we would expect.

Some caution is needed here. The use of a faster and/or lower run-up will put a greater stress on the takeoff leg, and thus may increase the risk of injury if the leg is not strong enough. Therefore, it is important to use caution in the adoption of a faster and/or lower run-up. If the desired change is very large, it would be advisable to make it gradually, over a period of time. In all cases, it may be wise to further strengthen the takeoff leg, so that it can withstand the increased force of the impact produced when the takeoff leg is planted.

Vertical velocity of the COM at the start of the takeoff phase

The vertical velocity at the end of the takeoff phase, which is of crucial importance for the height of the jump, is determined by the vertical velocity at the start of the takeoff phase and by the change that takes place in its value during the takeoff phase. In normal high jumping, at the end of the run-up (i.e. at the start of the takeoff phase) the athlete is moving fast forwards, and also slightly downwards. In other words, the vertical velocity at the start of the takeoff phase (v_{ZTD}) usually has a small negative value. It is evident that for a given change in vertical velocity during the takeoff phase, the athlete with the smallest amount of negative vertical velocity at touchdown will jump the highest. The values of v_{ZTD} are shown in Table 14.3. The jumpers with the best techniques in this respect are those with the least negative v_{ZTD} values.

In each step of the run-up the COM normally moves up slightly as the athlete takes off from the ground, reaches a maximum height, and then drops down again before the athlete plants the next foot on the ground. In the last step of the run-up, if the takeoff foot is planted on the ground early, the takeoff phase will start before the COM acquires too much downward vertical velocity. To achieve this, the athlete has to try to make the last two foot contacts with the ground very quickly one after the other. In other words, the tempo of the last two foot supports should be very fast.

If the length of the last step is very long, it could contribute to a late planting of the takeoff foot, and therefore to a large negative value for v_{ZTD}. Table 14.2 shows the length of the last step of the run-up (SL_1). This length is expressed in metres, but to facilitate comparisons among athletes it is also expressed as a percentage of the standing height of the athlete.

Another factor that influences the vertical velocity at the start of the takeoff phase is the way in which the COM is lowered in the final part of the run-up. High-jumpers can be classified into three groups, depending on the way in which they lower the COM. Many athletes lower their COM early (two or three steps before the takeoff), and then move more or less flat in the last step. These athletes typically have a moderate amount of downward vertical velocity at the instant that the takeoff phase starts. The second group of athletes keep their hips high until almost the very end of the run-up, and then they lower the COM in the last step. These athletes have a large negative vertical velocity at the start of the takeoff phase, regardless of how early they plant the takeoff foot on the ground. A third group of athletes lower the COM in the same way as the first group, but then raise it again quite a bit as the non-takeoff leg pushes off into the last step. These athletes typically have a very small amount of downward vertical velocity at the start of the takeoff phase, which is good, but they also waste part of their previous lowering of the COM.

The first and the third techniques have both advantages and disadvantages, but the second technique seems to be less sound than the other two, because of the large downward vertical velocity that it produces at the instant of the start of the takeoff phase.

Orientation of the takeoff foot and potential for ankle and foot injuries

At the end of the run-up, the high jumper's COM is moving at an angle p_1 with respect to the bar (see 'Approach angles' above). During the takeoff phase, the athlete pushes on the ground vertically downwards, and also horizontally. The horizontal force that the foot makes on the ground during the takeoff phase points forwards, almost in line with the final

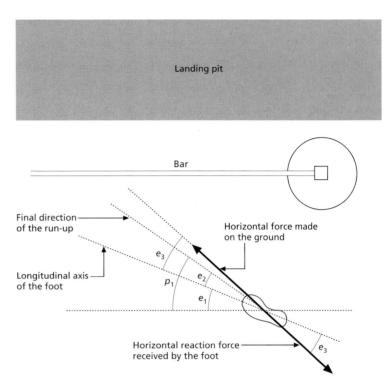

Fig. 14.6 Angles of foot, of run-up direction, and of horizontal force (see text).

direction of the run-up, but usually it is also deviated slightly towards the landing pit (see Fig. 14.6).

Most high jumpers plant the takeoff foot on the ground with its longitudinal axis pointing in a direction that generally is not aligned with the final direction of the run-up nor with the horizontal force that the athlete is about to make on the ground: It is more parallel to the bar than either one of them. Since the horizontal reaction force that the foot receives from the ground is not aligned with the longitudinal axis of the foot, the force tends to make the foot roll inwards. (See the sequence in Fig. 14.7, obtained from a high-speed videotape taken during the 1988 International Golden High Jump Gala competition in Genk, Belgium—courtesy of B. Van Gheluwe.) In anatomical terminology, this rotation is called 'pronation of the ankle joint'. It stretches the medial side of the joint, and produces compression in the lateral side of the joint. If the pronation is very severe, it can lead to injury of the ankle. It also means that the foot becomes supported less by its outside edge, and more by the longitudinal

(forward–backward) arch on the medial side of the foot. According to Krahl and Knebel (1979), this can lead to injury of the foot itself.

Pronation of the ankle joint occurs in the takeoffs of many high jumpers. However, it is difficult to see without a very magnified image of the foot. Because of this, pronation of the ankle joint generally is not visible in our standard films or videotapes of high-jumping competitions (and therefore it does not show in our computer graphics sequences either). This does not mean that there is no ankle pronation; we just cannot see it.

In an effort to diagnose the risk of ankle and foot injury for each high jumper, we measure angles e_1 (the angle between the longitudinal axis of the foot and the bar), e_2 (between the longitudinal axis of the foot and the final direction of the run-up) and e_3 (between the longitudinal axis of the foot and the horizontal force) in each jump (see Fig. 14.6). The values of these angles are reported in Table 14.2. For diagnosing the risk of injury, e_3 is the most important angle. Although the safety limit is not known with certainty at this time, anecdotal evidence suggests that e_3 values smaller than 20° are reasonably safe, values between 20 and 25° are somewhat risky, and values larger than 25° are dangerous.

Trunk lean

Figure 14.8 shows BFTD, BFTO, LRTD and LRTO, the backward/forward and left/right angles of lean of the trunk at the start and the end of the takeoff phase, respectively. The values of these angles are given in Table 14.4. The trunk normally has a backward lean at the start of the takeoff phase (BFTD). Then it rotates forwards, and by the end of the takeoff it is close to vertical, and sometimes past the vertical (BFTO). Due to the curved run-up, the trunk normally has also a lateral lean towards the centre of the curve at the start of the takeoff phase (LRTD). During the takeoff phase, the trunk rotates towards the right (towards the left in athletes who take off from the right foot), and by the end of the takeoff it is usually somewhat beyond the vertical (LRTO)—up to 10° beyond the vertical (LRTO = 100°) may be considered normal. Table 14.4 also shows the values of ΔBF and ΔLR. These are the changes that occur during the takeoff phase in the backward/forward and left/right angles of tilt of the trunk, respectively.

Statistical information (Dapena, unpublished observations) shows a relationship of the trunk lean angles with the vertical velocity of the athlete at the end of the takeoff phase, and consequently with the peak height of the COM. If two athletes have similar run-up speed, height of the COM at the end of the run-up and arm actions during the takeoff phase (see below), the athlete with smaller BFTD, ΔBF, LRTD and ΔLR values generally obtains a larger vertical velocity by the end of the takeoff phase. This means that athletes with greater backward lean at the start of the takeoff phase and greater lateral lean towards the centre of the curve at the start of the takeoff phase tend to jump higher. Also, for a given amount of backward lean at the start of the takeoff phase, the athletes who experience smaller changes in this angle during the takeoff phase generally jump higher, and for a given amount of lateral lean at the start of the takeoff phase, the athletes who

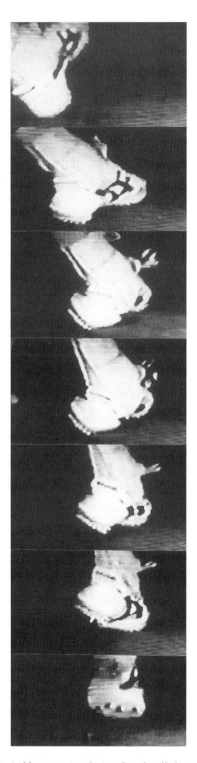

Fig. 14.7 Ankle pronation during the takeoff phase. (Videotape courtesy of B. Van Gheluwe.)

Side view

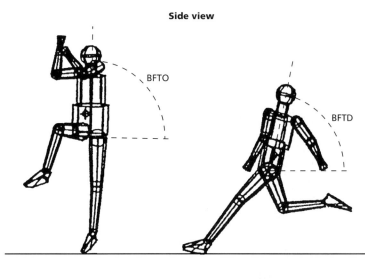

Back view

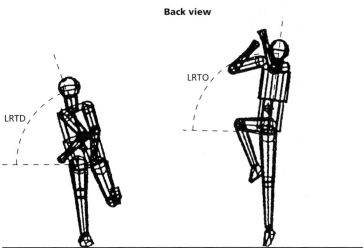

Fig. 14.8 Backward/forward (BF) and left/right (LR) tilt angles of the trunk at the start (TD) and at the end (TO) of the takeoff phase.

experience smaller changes in this angle during the takeoff phase also tend to jump higher.

However, before jumping to conclusions and deciding that all high jumpers should lean backwards and laterally as much as possible at the start of the takeoff phase, and then change those angles of lean as little as possible during the takeoff phase itself, it is necessary to take two points into consideration. Firstly, small values of BFTD, ΔBF, LRTD and ΔLR are not only statistically associated with larger vertical velocities at the end of the takeoff phase (which is good), but also with less angular

momentum (see below), and therefore with a less effective rotation during the bar clearance.

Also, we cannot be completely certain that small values of BFTD, ΔBF, LRTD and ΔLR *produce* a takeoff that generates a larger amount of vertical velocity and therefore a higher peak height for the COM We do not understand well the cause–effect mechanisms behind the statistical relationships, and it is possible to offer alternative explanations, such as the following. Weaker athletes are not able to generate much lift, mainly because they are weak. Therefore, they are not able to jump very high. This

Table 14.4 Angles of tilt of the trunk [backward/forward at the start of the takeoff phase (BFTD) and at the end of the takeoff phase (BFTO) and the change in this angle during the takeoff phase (ΔBF); left/right at the start of the takeoff phase (LRTD) and at the end of the takeoff phase (LRTO), and the change in this angle during the takeoff phase (ΔLR)], activeness of the arm nearest to the bar (AAN) and of the arm farthest from the bar (AAF), summed activeness of the two arms (AAT), activeness of the lead leg (LLA), and summed activeness of the three free limbs (FLA).

Athlete	BFTD (°)	BFTO (°)	ΔBF (°)	LRTD (°)	LRTO (°)	ΔLR (°)	AAN (mm · m⁻¹)	AAF (mm · m⁻¹)	AAT (mm · m⁻¹)	LLA (mm · m⁻¹)	FLA (mm · m⁻¹)
Men											
Avdeyenko	71	92	21	76	104	28	4.3	10.5	14.8	24.0	38.7
Conway	76	83	7	79	95	16	6.7	12.2	18.9	21.2	40.2
Forsyth	71	86	15	76	104	28	10.0	10.7	20.8	24.9	45.6
Paklin	77	81	5	77	99	22	5.3	8.9	14.2	14.1	28.2
Partyka	75	89	14	76	92	16	3.3	7.1	10.4	15.4	25.8
Sjöberg	74	88	15	75	98	23	6.7	10.0	16.7	18.7	35.4
Sotomayor	71	77	5	79	101	22	5.9	10.8	16.7	24.5	41.2
Stones	74	90	16	73	91	19	3.4	8.3	11.7	18.3	30.0
Zvara	68	83	15	77	95	18	9.0	13.3	22.3	41.7	64.0
Women											
Acuff	73	87	14	78	92	14	0.5	7.1	7.5	19.1	26.6
Astafei	77	82	5	84	102	18	3.6	6.6	10.2	13.5	23.7
Beyer-Helm	79	94	15	74	96	23	2.3	7.0	9.3	15.6	24.9
Dragieva	76	82	6	80	92	12	1.3	7.3	8.5	21.8	30.4
Henkel	82	90	8	75	97	22	5.9	8.3	14.2	19.3	33.4
Kostadinova	73	84	12	77	93	17	−0.4	6.2	5.8	21.0	26.8
Quintero	73	91	18	79	104	26	4.4	10.0	14.4	18.2	32.7
Sommer	80	90	10	81	99	18	2.2	4.9	7.1	17.8	24.9

Note: Some of the values in this table may not fit perfectly with each other, because of rounding off.

makes them reach the peak of the jump relatively soon after takeoff. Consequently, they will want to rotate faster in the air to reach a normal horizontal layout position at the peak of the jump. For this, they will generate more angular momentum during the takeoff, which in turn will require larger values of BFTD, ΔBF, LRTD and ΔLR. We cannot be sure which interpretation is the correct one: does the trunk tilt affect the height of the jump, or does the weakness of the athlete affect the height of the jump and (indirectly) the trunk tilt? Or are both explanations partly correct? At this point, we do not know for sure.

Arm and lead leg actions

The actions of the arms and of the lead leg during the takeoff phase are important for the outcome of the jump. As these free limbs are accelerated upwards during the takeoff phase, they exert by reaction a compressive force downwards on the trunk. This helps the takeoff leg to exert a larger force on the ground. The increased downward vertical force exerted on the ground evokes by reaction an increased upward vertical force exerted by the ground on the athlete. This produces a larger vertical velocity of the COM of the athlete by the end of the takeoff phase, and consequently a higher jump.

There is no perfect way to measure how active the arms and the lead leg are during the takeoff phase of a high jump. Currently, we express arm activeness as the vertical range of motion of the COM of each arm during the takeoff phase (relative to the upper end of the trunk), multiplied by the fraction of the whole body mass that corresponds to the arm, and divided by the standing height of the subject. The activeness of the lead leg is similarly measured as the vertical range of motion of the COM of the lead leg during the takeoff phase (relative to the lower end of the trunk), multiplied by the fraction of the whole body mass that corresponds to the lead leg, and divided by the standing height of the subject. In effect, this means that the activeness of each free limb is expressed as the number of millimetres contributed by the limb motion to the lifting of the COM of the whole body during the takeoff phase, per metre of standing height. Defined in this way, the activeness of each free limb takes into account the limb's mass, its average vertical velocity during the takeoff phase, and the duration of this vertical motion. It allows the comparison of one jumper with another, and also direct comparison of the lead leg action with the arm actions.

Table 14.4 shows the activeness of the arm nearest to the bar (AAN) and of the arm farthest from the bar (AAF), the summed activeness of the two arms

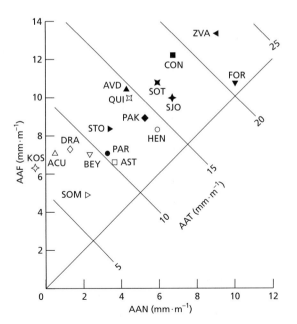

Fig. 14.9 Activeness of the arm nearest to the bar (AAN), of the arm farthest from the bar (AAF), and combined activeness of both arms (AAT).

(AAT), the activeness of the lead leg (LLA) and the combined activeness of all three free limbs (FLA). Larger values indicate greater activeness of the limbs during the takeoff.

Figure 14.9 shows a plot of AAF vs. AAN for the sample jumps. The ideal is to be as far to the right and as high up as possible on the graph, as this gives the largest values for the total arm action, AAT, also shown in the graph.

For a good arm action, both arms should swing strongly forwards and upwards during the takeoff phase. They should not be too flexed at the elbow during the swing—a good elbow angle seems to be somewhere between full extension and 90° of flexion.

The diagonal line going from lower left to upper right in Fig. 14.9 indicates the points for which both arms would have equal activeness. The positions of the points above the diagonal line reflect a well-established fact: high jumpers are generally more active with the arm that is farthest from the bar.

Some high jumpers (including many women) fail to prepare their arms correctly in the last steps of the run-up, and at the beginning of the takeoff phase the arm nearest to the bar is ahead of the body instead of behind it. From this position the arm is not able to swing strongly forwards and upwards during the takeoff, and these jumpers usually end up with small (or even negative) AAN values. These athletes should learn to bring both arms back in the final one or two steps of the run-up, so that both arms can later swing hard forwards and up during the takeoff phase. Learning this kind of arm action will take some time and effort, but it should produce a higher jump. If an athlete is unable to prepare the arms for a double-arm action, the forward arm should be in a low position at the start of the takeoff phase. That way, it can be thrown upwards during the takeoff, although usually not quite as hard as with a double-arm action.

Figure 14.10 shows a plot of LLA vs. AAT for the trials in the sample. The ideal is to be as far to the right and as high up as possible on the graph, as this gives the largest values for the total free limb action, FLA, also shown in the graph.

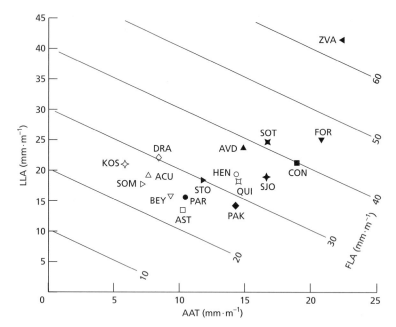

Fig. 14.10 Combined activeness of both arms (AAT), activeness of the lead leg (LLA), and total activeness of the free limbs (FLA).

Takeoff time

The duration of the takeoff phase (T_{TO}) is shown in Table 14.5. (Due to the slow camera speeds used, the value of T_{TO} can easily be in error by 0.01 s, and sometimes by as much as 0.02 s.) This 'takeoff time' is influenced by a series of factors. Some of them are beneficial for the jump; others are detrimental. Short takeoff times go together with a strong action of the takeoff leg (good), but also with weak arm actions and with a high COM position at the start of the takeoff phase (bad). In summary, takeoff times are informative, but the length of the takeoff time by itself does not necessarily indicate good or bad technique.

Change in horizontal velocity during the takeoff phase

It was explained before that the athlete should have a large horizontal velocity at the instant immediately before the takeoff foot is planted on the ground to start the takeoff phase, and that therefore no hori-

zontal velocity should be lost before that instant. However, the horizontal velocity should be reduced considerably during the takeoff phase itself. The losses of horizontal velocity that all high jumpers experience during the takeoff phase (see Δv_H in Table 14.3) are due to the fact that the jumper pushes forwards on the ground during the takeoff phase, and therefore receives a backward reaction force from the ground. These losses of horizontal velocity during the takeoff phase are an intrinsic part of the takeoff process, and they are associated with the generation of vertical velocity. If an athlete does not lose much horizontal velocity during the takeoff phase, this may be a sign that the athlete is not making good use of the horizontal velocity obtained during the run-up. We could say that the athlete should produce a lot of horizontal velocity during the run-up so that it can then be lost during the takeoff phase while the athlete obtains vertical velocity. If not enough horizontal velocity is produced during the run-up, or not enough is lost during the takeoff, the run-up is not being used appropriately to help the athlete to jump higher.

Table 14.5 Takeoff time (T_{TO}), height of the bar (h_{BAR}), maximum height of the centre of mass (COM) (h_{PK}), clearance height in the plane of the standards (h_{CLS}), absolute clearance height (h_{CLA}), effectiveness of the bar clearance in the plane of the standards (Δh_{CLS}), and absolute effectiveness of the bar clearance (Δh_{CLA}); twisting angular momentum (H_T), forward somersaulting angular momentum (H_F), lateral somersaulting angular momentum (H_L) and total somersaulting angular momentum (H_S) during the airborne phase.

Athlete	T_{TO} (s)	h_{BAR} (m)	h_{PK} (m)	h_{CLS} (m)	h_{CLA} (m)	Δh_{CLS} (m)	Δh_{CLA} (m)	H_T (*)	H_F (*)	H_L (*)	H_S (*)
Men											
Avdeyenko	0.21	2.38	2.46	2.41	2.42	−0.05	−0.04	40	75	80	110
Conway	0.18	2.34	2.41	2.33	2.35	−0.08	−0.06	45	40	85	90
Forsyth	0.17	2.34	2.44	2.35	2.39	−0.09	−0.05	45	60	80	100
Paklin	0.20	2.38	2.41	2.40	2.41	−0.01	0.00	45	75	80	110
Partyka	0.15	2.34	2.39	2.36	2.36	−0.03	−0.03	40	80	90	120
Sjöberg	0.16	2.34	2.33	2.35	2.35	0.02	0.02	40	70	85	110
Sotomayor	0.17	2.34	2.44	2.36	2.39	−0.08	−0.05	60	5	100	100
Stones	0.17	2.34	2.36	2.29	2.29	−0.07	−0.07	35	60	85	105
Zvara	0.23	2.34	2.46	2.36	2.36	−0.10	−0.10	75	50	80	95
Women											
Acuff	0.18	1.96	2.07	1.97	1.97	−0.10	−0.10	30	95	80	125
Astafei	0.15	2.00	2.09	2.00	2.01	−0.09	−0.08	50	35	90	100
Beyer-Helm	0.16	1.97	2.06	2.00	2.03	−0.06	−0.03	45	80	85	115
Dragieva	0.15	2.00	2.06	2.00	2.00	−0.06	−0.06	40	95	70	115
Henkel	0.14	2.02	2.06	2.05	2.05	−0.01	−0.01	45	80	85	120
Kostadinova	0.14	2.05	2.09	2.09	2.09	0.00	0.00	60	90	100	135
Quintero	0.17	1.97	2.04	1.97	1.97	−0.07	−0.07	40	55	90	105
Sommer	0.14	1.96	1.99	1.94	1.95	−0.05	−0.04	45	105	85	130

Note: Some of the values in this table may not fit perfectly with each other, because of rounding off.

* Angular momentum units: $s^{-1} \times 10^{-3}$.

Height and vertical velocity of the COM at the end of the takeoff phase

The peak height that the COM will reach over the bar is completely determined by the end of the takeoff phase. It is determined by the height and the vertical velocity of the COM at the end of the takeoff phase.

At the instant that the takeoff foot loses contact with the ground, the COM of a high jumper is usually at a height somewhere between 68% and 73% of the standing height of the athlete. This means that tall high jumpers have a built-in advantage: their centres of gravity will generally be higher at the instant that they leave the ground.

The vertical velocity of the COM at the end of the takeoff phase (v_{ZTO}, shown in Table 14.3) determines how much higher the COM will travel beyond the takeoff height after the athlete leaves the ground.

Height of the bar, peak height of the COM, and clearance height

The height of the bar (h_{BAR}) and the maximum height reached by the COM (h_{PK}) are shown in Table 14.5. All of the jumps shown here were successful clearances.

The true value of a high jump generally is not known: If the bar is knocked down, the jump is ruled a foul and the athlete gets zero credit, even though a hypothetical bar set at a lower height would have been cleared successfully; if the bar stays up, the athlete is credited with the height at which the bar was set, ignoring whether the jumper

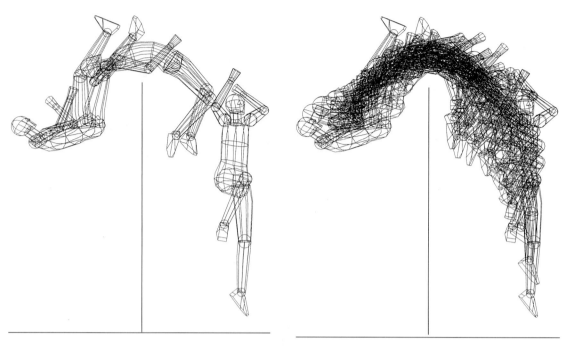

Fig. 14.11 Three images of a bar clearance.

Fig. 14.12 All the images of a bar clearance available from film analysis.

had room to spare over it or whether the jumper depressed the bar during the clearance.

Using computer modelling and graphics, it is possible to estimate the approximate maximum height that an athlete would have been able to clear cleanly without touching the bar in a given jump ('clearance height'), regardless of whether the actual jump was officially a valid clearance or a foul. Figure 14.11 shows three images of a high jumper's clearance of a bar set at 2.25 m. Figure 14.12 shows all the images obtained through film analysis of the bar clearance. In Fig. 14.13 the drawing has been saturated with intermediate positions of the high jumper, calculated through a process called curvilinear interpolation. The scale in the 'saturation drawing' shows that in this jump the athlete would have been able to clear a bar set in the plane of the standards at a height of 2.34 m (h_{CLS}) without touching it. A closer examination of Fig. 14.13 also shows that the maximum height of the 'hollow' area below the body was not perfectly centred over the bar: If this athlete had taken off closer to the plane of the standards,

he would have been able to clear a bar set at an absolute maximum height of 2.35 m (h_{CLA}) without touching it.

Due to errors in the measurements taken from the films or videotapes, in the thicknesses of the various body segments of the computer graphics model and in the degree of curvature of the trunk in the drawings, the value of the clearance height in the plane of the standards (h_{CLS}) and the value of the absolute clearance height (h_{CLA}) obtained using this method are not perfectly accurate. A test showed that the true value of h_{CLS} will be over- or underestimated on average by between 0.02 m and 0.03 m. Therefore, the calculated clearance height values should be considered only rough estimates. Another point to consider is that high jumpers can generally depress the fibreglass bar by about 0.02 m (and sometimes by as much as 0.04 or even 0.06 m) without knocking it down.

Table 14.5 shows the maximum height that the athlete would have been able to clear without touching the bar in the plane of the standards (h_{CLS})

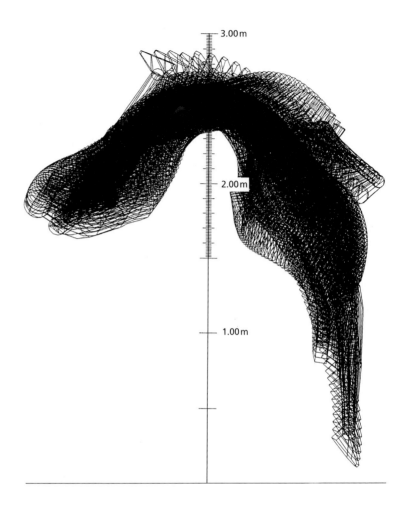

3.00 m

2.00 m

1.00 m

Fig. 14.13 Graph of a bar clearance produced through saturation with interpolated images.

and the absolute maximum height that the athlete would have been able to clear without touching the bar (h_{CLA}).

The differences between the clearance heights and the peak height of the COM indicate the effectiveness of the bar clearance in the plane of the standards ($\Delta h_{CLS} = h_{CLS} - h_{PK}$) and the absolute effectiveness of the bar clearance ($\Delta h_{CLA} = h_{CLA} - h_{PK}$). Table 14.5 shows their values in the sample trials. Larger negative numbers indicate less effective bar clearances.

The main reasons for an ineffective bar clearance are: taking off too close or too far from the bar, insufficient amount of somersaulting angular momentum, insufficient twist rotation, poor arching, and bad timing of the arching/un-arching process. These aspects of high jumping technique will be discussed next.

Takeoff distance

The distance between the toe of the takeoff foot and the plane of the bar and the standards is called the 'takeoff distance' (TOD in Fig. 14.2). The value of this distance is shown in Table 14.2, and it is important because it determines the position of the peak of the jump relative to the bar: If an athlete takes off too far from the bar, the COM will reach its maximum height before crossing the plane of the standards, and the jumper will probably fall on the bar; if the athlete takes off too close to the bar, there will be a large risk of hitting the bar while the COM is on the way up, before reaching its maximum height. Different athletes usually need different takeoff distances. The optimum value for the takeoff distance of each athlete is the one that will make the COM of the jumper reach its maximum height more or less directly over the bar, and it will depend primarily on the final direction of the run-up and on the amount of residual horizontal velocity that the athlete has left after the completion of the takeoff phase.

In general, athletes who travel more perpendicular to the bar in the final steps of the run-up (indicated by large p_2 and p_1 angles in Table 14.2) will also travel more perpendicular to the bar after the completion of the takeoff phase (indicated by large p_0 angles in Table 14.2), and they will need to take off farther from the bar. In general, athletes who run faster in the final steps of the run-up (indicated by large values of v_{H2} and v_{H1} in Table 14.3) will also have more horizontal velocity left after takeoff (indicated by large values of v_{HTO} in Table 14.3); thus, they will travel through larger horizontal distances after the completion of the takeoff than slower jumpers, and they will also need to take off farther from the bar in order for the COM to reach its maximum height more or less directly over the bar.

High jumpers need to be able to judge after a miss whether the takeoff point might have been too close or too far from the bar. This can be done by paying attention to the time when the bar was hit. If the bar was hit a long time after the takeoff, this probably means that the bar was hit as the athlete was coming down from the peak of the jump, implying that the athlete took off too far from the bar, and in that case the athlete should move the starting point of the run-up slightly closer to the bar; if the bar was hit very soon after takeoff, this probably means that the bar was hit while the athlete was still on the way up towards the peak of the jump, implying that the takeoff point was too close to the bar, and in that case the athlete should move the starting point of the run-up slightly farther from the bar.

Angular momentum

Angular momentum (or 'rotary momentum') is a mechanical factor that makes the athlete rotate.

High jumpers need the right amount of angular momentum to make in the air the rotations necessary for a proper bar clearance. The athlete obtains the angular momentum during the takeoff phase, through the forces that the takeoff foot makes on the ground; the angular momentum cannot be changed after the athlete leaves the ground.

The bar clearance technique of a Fosbury-flop can be described roughly as a twisting somersault. To a great extent, the twist rotation (which makes the athlete turn his or her back to the bar during the ascending part of the flight path) is generated by swinging the lead leg up and somewhat away from the bar during the takeoff, and also by actively turning the shoulders and arms during the takeoff in the desired direction of the twist. These actions create angular momentum about a vertical axis. This is called the twisting angular momentum, H_T. The H_T values of the analysed athletes are shown in Table 14.5. (To facilitate comparisons among athletes, the angular momentum values have been normalized for the mass and standing height of each athlete.) Most high jumpers have no difficulty obtaining an appropriate amount of H_T. (However, we will see later that the actions that the athlete makes in the air, as well as other factors, can also significantly affect whether the high jumper will be perfectly face-up at the peak of the jump, or tilted to one side with one hip lower than the other.)

The somersault rotation, which will make the shoulders go down while the knees go up, results from two components: a forward somersaulting component and a lateral somersaulting component.

Forward somersaulting angular momentum (H_F)

During the takeoff phase, the athlete produces angular momentum about a horizontal axis perpendicular to the final direction of the run-up (see Fig. 14.14a and the sequence at the top of Fig. 14.15). This forward rotation is similar to the one produced when a person hops off from a moving bus facing the direction of motion of the bus: After the feet hit the ground, the tendency is to rotate forward and fall flat on one's face. It can be described as angular momentum produced by the checking of a linear motion.

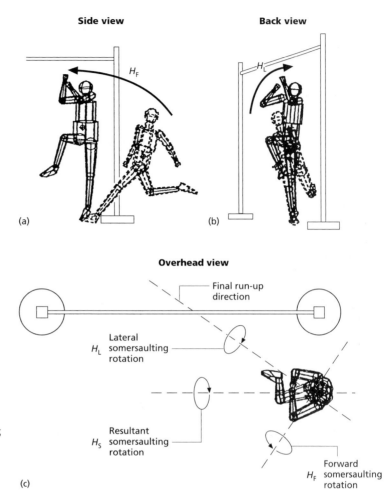

Side view   **Back view**

H_F H_L

(a)   (b)

Overhead view

Final run-up direction

H_L Lateral somersaulting rotation

H_S Resultant somersaulting rotation

H_F Forward somersaulting rotation

Fig. 14.14 (a) Forward somersaulting angular momentum; (b) lateral somersaulting angular momentum; (c) resultant somersaulting angular momentum.   (c)

The tilt angles of the trunk at the start and at the end of the takeoff phase (see 'Trunk lean' above) are statistically related to the angular momentum obtained by the athlete (J. Dapena, unpublished observations). Large changes of the trunk tilt from a backward position towards vertical during the takeoff phase are associated with a larger amount of forward somersaulting angular momentum. This makes sense, because athletes with a large amount of forward somersaulting angular momentum at the end of the takeoff phase should also be expected to have a large amount of it already during the takeoff phase, and this should contribute to a larger forward rotation of the body in general and of the trunk during the takeoff phase.

Statistics show that jumpers with a very large backward lean at the start of the takeoff phase (small BFTD angles) do not get quite as much forward somersaulting angular momentum as other jumpers. The reasons for this are not completely clear.

The forward somersaulting angular momentum can also be affected by the actions of the arms and lead leg. Wide swings of the arms and of the lead leg during the takeoff can help the athlete to jump higher (see 'Arm and lead leg actions' above). However, in a view from the side (top sequence in Fig. 14.16) they also imply backward (clockwise) rotations of these limbs, which can reduce the total forward somersaulting angular momentum of the body.

Side view

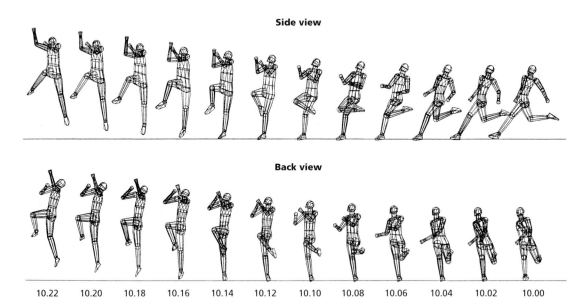

Back view

10.22   10.20   10.18   10.16   10.14   10.12   10.10   10.08   10.06   10.04   10.02   10.00

Fig. 14.15 Side and back views of the takeoff of a standard jump. To facilitate the comparison of one jump with another, the value $t = 10.00$ s is arbitrarily assigned in all jumps to the instant at which the takeoff foot first makes contact with the ground to start the takeoff phase.

Side view

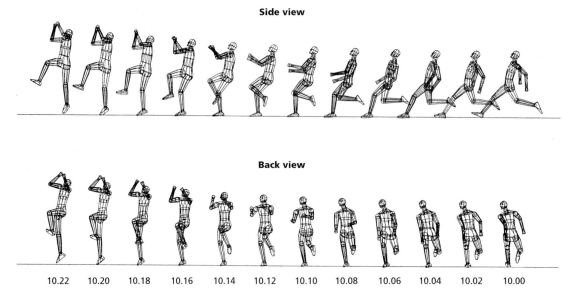

Back view

10.22   10.20   10.18   10.16   10.14   10.12   10.10   10.08   10.06   10.04   10.02   10.00

Fig. 14.16 Side and back views of the takeoff of a jump with direct forward arm swing.

To lessen this problem, some high jumpers turn their back partly towards the bar in the last step of the run-up, and then swing the arms diagonally forwards and away from the bar during the takeoff phase (see Fig. 14.17). Since this diagonal arm swing is not a perfect backward rotation, it interferes less with the generation of forward somersaulting angular momentum.

Side view

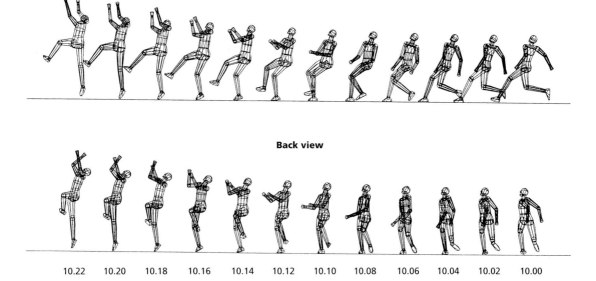

Back view

10.22   10.20   10.18   10.16   10.14   10.12   10.10   10.08   10.06   10.04   10.02   10.00

Fig. 14.17 Side and back views of the takeoff of a jump with diagonal arm swing.

Lateral somersaulting angular momentum (H_L)

During the takeoff phase, angular momentum is also produced about a horizontal axis in line with the final direction of the run-up (see Fig. 14.14b and the bottom sequence in Fig. 14.15). In a rear view of an athlete who takes off from the left leg, this angular momentum component appears as a clockwise rotation.

If the jumper made use of a straight run-up, in a rear view the athlete would be upright at touchdown, and leaning towards the bar at the end of the takeoff. Since a leaning position would result in a lower height of the COM at the end of the takeoff phase, the production of angular momentum would thus cause a reduction in the vertical range of motion of the COM during the takeoff phase. However, if the athlete uses a curved run-up, the initial lean of the athlete to the left at the end of the approach run may allow the athlete to be upright at the end of the takeoff phase (see Fig. 14.14b and the bottom sequence in Fig. 14.15). The final upright position contributes to a higher COM position at the end of the takeoff phase. Also, the initial lateral tilt contributes to a lower COM position at the start of the takeoff phase. Therefore the curved run-up,

together with the generation of lateral somersaulting angular momentum, contributes to increase the vertical range of motion of the COM during the takeoff phase, and thus permits greater lift than if a straight run-up were used. (However, some caution is necessary here, since statistical information suggests that jumpers with an excessive lean towards the centre of the curve at the start of the takeoff phase tend to generate a smaller amount of lateral somersaulting angular momentum than jumpers with a more moderate lean. The reasons for this are not clear.)

There is some statistical association between large changes in the left/right tilt angle of the trunk during the takeoff phase and large amounts of lateral somersaulting angular momentum at the end of the takeoff phase (J. Dapena, unpublished observations). This makes sense, because athletes with a large amount of lateral somersaulting angular momentum at the end of the takeoff phase should also be expected to have a large amount of it already during the takeoff phase, which should contribute to a larger rotation of the trunk during the takeoff phase from its initial lateral tilted position toward the vertical.

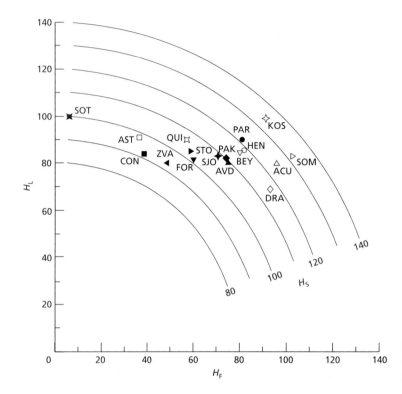

Fig. 14.18 Forward (H_F), lateral (H_L) and total (H_S) somersaulting angular momentum.

The reader should be reminded at this point that although large changes in tilt during the takeoff phase and, to a certain extent, small backward and lateral leans of the trunk at the start of the takeoff phase (i.e. large BFTD and LRTD values) are associated with increased angular momentum, they are also statistically associated with reduced vertical velocity at the end of the takeoff phase, and therefore with a reduced maximum height of the COM at the peak of the jump. This supports the intuitive feeling of high jumpers that it is necessary to seek a compromise between the generation of lift and the generation of rotation.

The bottom sequence in Fig. 14.17 shows that in an athlete who takes off from the left leg a diagonal arm swing is associated with a clockwise motion of the arms in a view from the back, and therefore it contributes to the generation of lateral somersaulting angular momentum.

High jumpers usually have more lateral than forward somersaulting angular momentum. The sum of these two angular momentum components adds up to the required total (or 'resultant') somersaulting angular momentum, H_S (Fig. 14.14c).

The forward (H_F), lateral (H_L) and total (H_S) somersaulting angular momentum values of the analysed athletes are shown in Table 14.5, and in graphical form in Fig. 14.18. In general, athletes with more angular momentum tend to rotate faster.

Female high jumpers tend to acquire more angular momentum than male high jumpers. This is because the women do not jump quite as high, and therefore they need to rotate faster to compensate for the smaller amount of time available between the takeoff and the peak of the jump.

Adjustments in the air

After the takeoff is completed, the path of the COM is totally determined, and there is nothing that the athlete can do to change it. However, this does not mean that the paths of all parts of the body are determined. What cannot be changed is the path of the point that represents the average position of all the

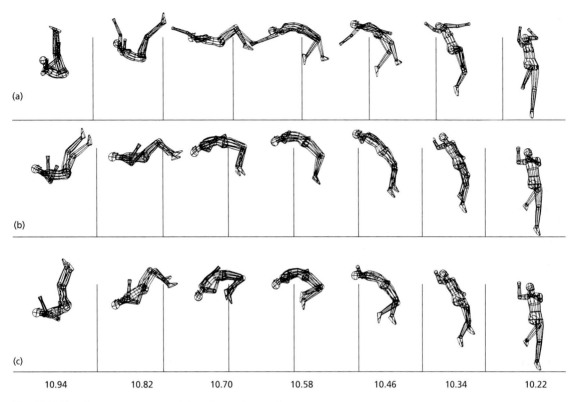

Fig. 14.19 Bar clearance sequences of three jumps (see text).

body parts (the COM), but it is possible to move one part of the body in one direction if other parts are moved in the opposite direction. Using this principle, after the shoulders pass over the bar the high jumper can raise the hips by lowering the head and the legs. For a given position of the COM, the farther the head and the legs are lowered, the higher the hips will be lifted. This is the reason for the arched position on top of the bar.

To a great extent, the rotation of the high jumper in the air is also determined once the takeoff phase is completed, because the angular momentum cannot be changed during the airborne phase. However, some alterations of the rotation are still possible. By slowing down the rotations of some parts of the body, other parts of the body will speed up as a compensation, and vice versa. For instance, the athlete shown in Fig. 14.19a slowed down (and even reversed) the counterclockwise rotation of the take-

off leg shortly after the takeoff phase was completed, by flexing at the knee and extending at the hip ($t = 10.34$–10.58 s). In reaction, this helped the trunk to rotate faster counterclockwise, and therefore contributed to produce the horizontal position of the trunk at $t = 10.58$ s. Later, from $t = 10.58$ to $t = 10.82$ s, the athlete slowed down the counterclockwise rotation of the trunk, and even reversed it into a clockwise rotation; in reaction, the legs simultaneously increased their speed of rotation counterclockwise, and thus cleared the bar ($t = 10.58$–10.82 s).

The principles of action and reaction just described both for translation and rotation result in the typical arching and un-arching actions of high jumpers over the bar. The athlete needs to arch in order to lift the hips, and then to un-arch in order to speed up the rotation of the legs. As the body un-arches, the legs go up, but the hips go down.

Therefore, timing is critical: If the body un-arches too late, the calves will knock the bar down; if the body un-arches too early, the athlete will 'sit' on the bar and will also knock it down.

Another way in which rotation can be changed is by altering the 'moment of inertia'. The moment of inertia is a number that indicates whether the various parts that make up the body are close to the axis of rotation or far from it. When many parts of the body are far from the axis of rotation, the moment of inertia of the body is large, and this decreases the speed of turning about the axis of rotation. Vice versa, if most parts of the body are kept close to the axis of rotation, the moment of inertia is small, and the speed of rotation increases. This is what happens to figure skaters in a view from overhead when they spin: as they bring their arms closer to the vertical axis of rotation, they spin faster about the vertical axis. In high jumping, rotation about a horizontal axis parallel to the bar (i.e. the somersault) is generally more important than rotation about the vertical axis, but the same principle is at work. The jumps shown in Fig. 14.19b and c both had the same amount of somersaulting angular momentum. However, the athlete in Fig. 14.19c somersaulted faster: both jumpers had the same tilt at $t = 10.22$ s, but at $t = 10.94$ s the athlete in Fig. 14.19c had a more backward-rotated position than the athlete in Fig. 14.19b. The faster speed of rotation of the jumper in Fig. 14.19c was due to a more compact body configuration in the period between $t = 10.46$ s and $t = 10.70$ s. It was achieved mainly through a greater flexion of the knees. This configuration of the body reduced the athlete's moment of inertia about an axis parallel to the bar, and made him somersault faster. (The jumps shown in Fig. 14.19b and c were artificial jumps generated using computer simulation. This ensured that the athlete had exactly the same position at takeoff and the same amount of angular momentum in both jumps.)

The technique used by the athlete in Fig. 14.19c can be very helpful for high jumpers with low or moderate amounts of somersaulting angular momentum. Both jumps shown in Fig. 14.19b and c had the same amount of angular momentum ($H_S = 110 \cdot 10^{-3}$ s^{-1}), and the centre of mass reached a peak height 0.07 m higher than the bar in both jumps. While the athlete in Fig. 14.19b hit the bar with his calves ($t = 10.82$ s), the faster somersault rotation of the athlete in Fig. 14.19c helped him to pass all parts of the body over the bar with some room to spare.

In the rare cases in which a high jumper has a very large amount of angular momentum, the technique shown in Fig. 14.19c could be a liability, because it might accelerate the rotation so much that the shoulders would hit the bar on the way up. For athletes with a very large amount of somersaulting angular momentum, it would be better to keep the legs more extended on the way up to the bar, following the body configuration pattern shown in Fig. 14.19b. This will temporarily slow down the backward somersault, and thus prevent the athlete from hitting the bar with the shoulders on the way up to the bar. (Of course, the athlete will still need to arch and un-arch with good timing over the bar.)

The twist rotation: problems in its execution

It was pointed out earlier that the twist rotation in high jumping is produced to a great extent by the twisting component of angular momentum, H_T. But it was also mentioned that other factors could affect whether the jumper would be perfectly face-up at the peak of the jump, or rotated to one side with one hip lower than the other. One of the most important of these factors is the relative sizes of the forward and lateral components of the somersaulting angular momentum. We will now see how this works.

Figure 14.20 shows sketches of a hypothetical high jumper at the end of the takeoff phase and after three pure somersault rotations in different directions (with no twist), all viewed from overhead. For simplicity, we have assumed that the final direction of the run-up was at a 45° angle with respect to the bar. A normal combination of forward and lateral components of somersaulting angular momentum would produce at the peak of the jump the position shown in Fig. 14.20b, which would require in addition 90° of twist rotation to generate a face-up orientation. If instead an athlete generated only

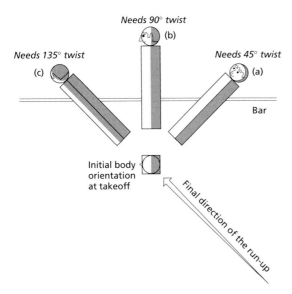

Fig. 14.20 Sketch showing the relationship between the direction of the somersaulting rotation and the amount of twist rotation needed to reach a face-up position at the peak of the jump.

lateral somersaulting angular momentum, the result would be the position shown in Fig. 14.20a, which would require only about 45° of twist rotation to achieve a face-up orientation; if the athlete generated only forward somersaulting angular momentum, the result would be the position shown in Fig. 14.20c, which would require about 135° of twist rotation to achieve a face-up orientation. It is very unusual for high jumpers to have only lateral or forward somersaulting angular momentum, but many jumpers have much larger amounts of one than the other. The example shows that jumpers with particularly large amounts of forward somersaulting angular momentum and small amounts of lateral somersaulting angular momentum will need to twist more in the air if the athlete is to be face-up at the peak of the jump. Otherwise, the body will be tilted, with the hip of the lead leg lower than the hip of the takeoff leg. Conversely, jumpers with particularly large amounts of lateral somersaulting angular momentum and small amounts of forward somersaulting angular momentum will need to twist less in the air than other jumpers in order to be perfectly

face-up at the peak of the jump. Otherwise, the body will be tilted, with the hip of the takeoff leg lower than the hip of the lead leg.

Another point that needs to be taken into account is that, while the twisting component of angular momentum (H_T) is a major factor in the generation of the twist rotation in high jumping, it is generally not enough to produce the necessary face-up position on top of the bar. In addition, the athlete also needs to use rotational action and reaction about the longitudinal axis of the body to increase the amount of twist rotation that occurs in the air. In a normal high jump, the athlete needs to achieve about 90° of twist rotation between takeoff and the peak of the jump (see Fig. 14.20b). Approximately half of it (about 45°) is produced by the twisting angular momentum; the other half (roughly another 45°) needs to be produced through rotational action and reaction. Rotational action and reaction is sometimes called 'catting' because cats dropped from an upside-down position with no angular momentum use a mechanism of this kind to land on their feet.

The catting that takes place in the twist rotation of a high jump is difficult to see, because it is obscured by the somersault and twist rotations produced by the angular momentum. If we could 'hide' the somersault and twist rotations produced by the angular momentum, we would be able to isolate the catting rotation, and see it clearly. To achieve that, we would need to look at the high jumper from the viewpoint of a rotating camera. The camera would need to somersault with the athlete, staying aligned with the athlete's longitudinal axis. The camera would also need to twist with the athlete, just fast enough to keep up with the portion of the twist rotation produced by the twisting component of angular momentum. That way, all that would be left would be the rotation produced by the catting, and this rotation is what would be visible in the camera's view. It is impossible to make a real camera rotate in such a way, but we can use a computer to calculate how the jump would have appeared in the images of such a camera if it had existed. This is what is shown in Fig. 14.21. The sequence in Fig. 14.21 covers the period between takeoff and the peak of the jump, and progresses from left to right. All the images are viewed from a direction aligned with the

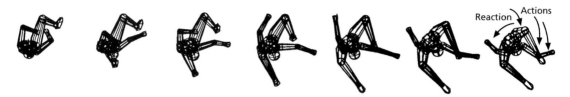

Fig. 14.21 Catting: use of clockwise rotations of the right leg and arm to produce counterclockwise twist rotation of the rest of the body (see text).

longitudinal axis of the athlete. (The head is the part of the athlete nearest to the 'camera'.) As the jump progressed, the camera *somersaulted* with the athlete, so it stayed aligned with the athlete's longitudinal axis. The camera also *twisted* counterclockwise with the athlete, just fast enough to keep up with the portion of the twist rotation produced by the twisting component of angular momentum. Figure 14.21 shows a clear counterclockwise rotation of the hips (about 45°) between the beginning and the end of the sequence. This implies that the athlete rotated counterclockwise faster than the camera, i.e. faster than the part of the twist rotation produced by the twisting component of angular momentum. The counterclockwise rotation of the hips visible in the sequence is the amount of twist rotation produced through catting. It occurred mainly as a reaction to the clockwise motions of the right leg, which moved towards the right, and then backwards. (These actions of the right leg are subtle, but nevertheless visible in the sequence.) In part, the counterclockwise catting rotation of the hips was also a reaction to the clockwise rotation of the right arm. Without the catting, the twist rotation of this athlete would have been reduced by an amount equivalent to the approximately 45° of counterclockwise rotation visible in the sequence of Fig. 14.21.

Some jumpers emphasize the twisting angular momentum more; others tend to emphasize the catting more. If not enough twisting angular momentum is generated during the takeoff phase, or if the athlete does not do enough catting in the air, the athlete will not twist enough in the air, which will make the body adopt a tilted position at the peak of the jump, with the hip of the lead leg lower than the hip of the takeoff leg. This will put the hip of the lead leg (i.e. the low hip) in danger of hitting the bar.

There are other ways in which problems can occur in the twist rotation. If at the end of the takeoff phase an athlete is tilting backwards too far, or is tilting too far towards the right (too far towards the left in the case of a jumper who takes off from the right foot), or if the lead leg is lowered too soon after takeoff, the twist rotation will be slower. This is due to interactions between the somersault and twist rotations which are too complex to explain here; for more details see Dapena (1997).

According to the previous discussion, a tilted position at the peak of the jump in which the hip of the lead leg is lower than the hip of the takeoff leg can be due to a variety of causes: an insufficient amount of twisting angular momentum; a much larger amount of forward than lateral somersaulting angular momentum; insufficient catting in the air; a backwards tilted position of the body at the end of the takeoff phase; a position that is too tilted towards the right at the end of the takeoff phase (towards the left in the case of jumpers taking off from the right foot); and premature lowering of the lead leg soon after takeoff.

When this kind of problem occurs, it is necessary to check the cause of the problem in each individual case, and then decide the easiest way to correct it.

Acknowledgements

The research that led to the findings presented here was funded in part by grants from the United States Olympic Committee, USA Track & Field, and the International Olympic Committee.

References

Dapena, J. (1980a) Mechanics of translation in the Fosbury-flop. *Medicine and Science in Sports and Exercise* **12**, 37–44.

Dapena, J. (1980b) Mechanics of rotation in the Fosbury-flop. *Medicine and Science in Sports and Exercise* **12**, 45–53.

Dapena, J. (1987) Basic and applied research in the biomechanics of high jumping. In: *Current Research in Sports Biomechanics* (eds B. Van Gheluwe & J. Atha), pp. 19–33. Karger, Basel.

Dapena, J. (1995a) How to design the shape of a high jump run-up. *Track Coach* **131**, 4179–4181.

Dapena, J. (1995b) The rotation over the bar in the Fosbury-flop high jump. *Track Coach* **132**, 4201–4210.

Dapena, J. (1997) Contributions of angular momentum and catting to the twist rotation in highjumping. *Journal of Applied Biomechanics* **13**, 239–253.

Dapena, J. & Chung, C.S. (1988) Vertical and radial motions of the body during the take-off phase of high jumping. *Medicine and Science in Sports and Exercise* **20**, 290–302.

Dapena, J., McDonald, C. & Cappaert, J. (1990) A regression analysis of high jumping technique. *International Journal of Sport Biomechanics* **6**, 246–261.

Dapena, J., Angulo-Kinzler, R.M., Caubet, J.M. *et al.* (1993a) Track and field: high jump (Women). In: *Report for 1992 Summer Olympic Games Biomechanics Projects* (IOC: Medical Commission/ Biomechanics Subcommission). International Olympic Committee, Lausanne.

Dapena, J., Angulo-Kinzler, R.M., Turró, C. *et al.* (1993b) Track and field: high jump (Men). In: *Report for 1992 Summer Olympic Games Biomechanics Projects* (IOC: Medical Commission/ Biomechanics Subcommission). International Olympic Committee, Lausanne.

Dapena, J., Gordon, B.J., Hoffman, L. & LeBlanc, M.K. (1997a) High jump, #15 (Women). In: *Report for Scientific Services Project* (USATF). USA Track & Field, Indianapolis.

Dapena, J., Hoffman, L., Gordon, B.J. & LeBlanc, M.K. (1997b) High jump, #16 (Men). In: *Report for Scientific Services Project* (USATF). USA Track & Field, Indianapolis.

Dapena, J., Ae, M. & Iiboshi, A. (1997c) A closer look at the shape of the high jump run-up. *Track Coach* **138**, 4406–4411.

Dyatchkov, V.M. (1968) The high jump. *Track Technique* **34**, 1059–1074.

Krahl, H. & Knebel, K.P. (1979) Foot stress during the flop takeoff. *Track Technique* **75**, 2384–2386.

Ozolin, N. (1973) The high jump takeoff mechanism. *Track Technique* **52**, 1668–1671.

Chapter 15

Jumping in Figure Skating

D.L. KING

Introduction

The sport of figure skating is an intricate blend of artistry and athleticism. Of the many athletic skills performed by singles skaters, perhaps the most spectacular are the jumps. The first section of this chapter will familiarize the reader with the various jumps performed in figure skating. Next, the primary biomechanical principles important to jumping in skating will be introduced, followed by the techniques by which skaters utilize these principles during a jump. Lastly, a discussion of hypothetical techniques that could possibly maximize the utilization of biomechanical principles will be presented.

Review of skating jumps

To date, there are six standard jump types that figure skaters regularly perform during competition. These jumps are the Salchow, Loop, Toe Loop, Lutz, Flip and Axel. The differences between these jumps are most apparent in the takeoff phase, which can be described by:

1 the direction the skater is facing during the glide into the takeoff;

2 the foot upon which the skater is gliding;

3 the edge of the blade which the skater uses; and

4 the part of the blade (edge or toe-pick) the skater uses for the takeoff.

Thus, to properly understand each jump, the anatomy of a figure-skating boot and blade will be reviewed.

The blade on a figure-skating boot is usually 3–4 mm wide and is bevelled to produce an outside and inside edge (Fig. 15.1a). The blade also has a rocker, or is curved slightly from front to back as viewed

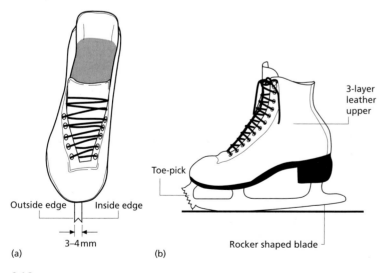

Outside edge | Inside edge

3–4mm

(a)

Toe-pick

Rocker shaped blade

3-layer
leather
upper

(b)

Fig. 15.1 (a) Front view of figure-skating boot showing bevelled blade and inside and outside edges. (b) Side view of skating boot showing blade rocker and toe-pick.

from the side (Fig. 15.1b). Different skills, such as the takeoffs of different jumps, require a skater to hold a glide on either the inside or outside edge of the blade. The front of the blade has a jagged toe-pick with 6–7 teeth approximately 7 mm long (Fig. 15.1b). The toe-pick is used in several of the jumping techniques, when the skater firmly plants the toe-pick into the ice and then springs (or vaults) into the air from this toe-pick plant.

The Salchow, Loop and Axel are edge jumps during which a skater either takes off the back inside (Salchow), back outside (Loop) or forward outside (Axel) edge of the skate blade. Assuming the skater rotates counterclockwise in the air, skaters glide into both the Salchow and Loop backwards. However, the takeoff leg for the Salchow is the left leg, and the takeoff leg for the Loop is the right leg. The Axel, another edge jump, is the only jump for which skaters glide into the jump facing forwards. Again, assuming a counterclockwise rotation in the air, the takeoff for the Axel would be from the left leg.

The Toe Loop, Lutz and Flip are all jumps during which the skater springs off the toe-pick during the takeoff of the jump. These three jumps are distinguished by both the foot used for the toe-pick and the edge upon which the skater glides into the takeoff. During the Toe Loop, the skater holds a back outside edge on the right foot, assuming the counterclockwise rotation in the air, prior to picking with the left toe-pick at takeoff. During the Flip and Lutz, the skater glides into the takeoff on the left foot, holding a back inside edge (Flip) or back outside edge (Lutz). For both jumps, the skater picks with the toe of the right foot to spring into the air, again assuming a counterclockwise rotation. For counterclockwise rotation in the air, all jumps are landed with the skater facing backwards on the outside edge of the right foot. The tracings left on ice from the different approach patterns easily illustrates the differences in these six jumps. Figure 15.2 presents a schematic of typical tracings of each jump, assuming counterclockwise rotation in the air. A summary of these jumps is also presented in Table 15.1.

All of these jumps can be performed with various degrees of difficulty by increasing the number of revolutions completed in the air. The simplest jumps

are singles, during which one revolution is completed in the air. The exception to this is the single Axel, which has an extra half-revolution in the air due to the forward facing takeoff (Fig. 15.3). With the added half-revolution in Axel jumps, and the premise that it is harder to control a forward edge than a backward edge whilst skating, the Axel is considered to be the most difficult of the six jumps described here. Accordingly, the predominant amount of research conducted on jumping in skating has focused on the Axel, and the preponderance of information presented in this review will address the Axel jump.

The most difficult Axel jump performed to date is the triple Axel, which has been a mainstay in men's single competitions since the 1980s. However, many of the most elite male skaters are now performing quadruple jumps. While, though a few female skaters have also completed triple Axels, no female skater has yet completed a quadruple jump.

Another method by which skaters add difficulty to a jump is to perform a series of jumps in a row—a jump combination. In other words, the landing of one jump is immediately followed by the takeoff of another jump. Since all landings are on the right foot, assuming a counterclockwise rotation in the air, the only two jumps which could immediately follow a landing are the Loop, which takes off from the back outside edge of the right foot, or Toe Loop, which is essentially a Loop with a pick of the left toe at takeoff. Both male and female skaters are able to perform many different triple-triple combination jumps.

Biomechanical principles

Two of the more obvious quantities that determine (at least partially) if a skater completes a given jump are flight time and angular velocity about the longitudinal axis of the skater. In other words, a skater must have appropriate angular velocity to complete the required number of revolutions in the given time; or, conversely, a skater must have sufficient time to complete the required number of revolutions given the angular velocity. Accordingly, the generation of vertical velocity, generation of angular momentum about the longitudinal axis, and control of moment of inertia about the longitudinal

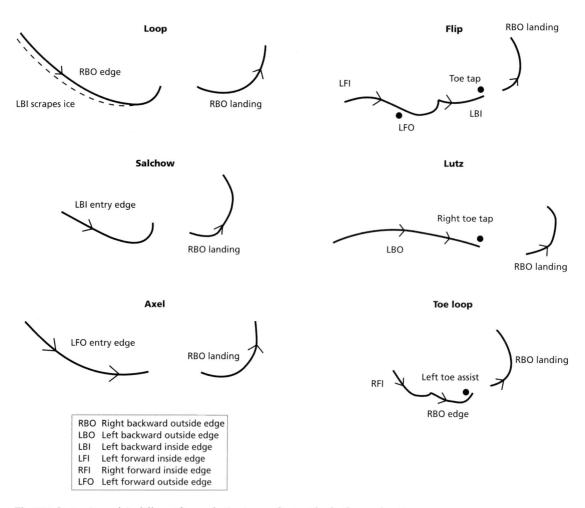

Fig. 15.2 Ice tracings of six different figure-skating jumps. See text for further explanation.

Table 15.1 Description of figure-skating jumps for a skater who rotates counterclockwise in the air.

Jump type	Approach	Takeoff	Landing
Flip	Backwards left inside edge	Right toe-pick	Backwards right outside edge
Lutz	Backwards left outside edge	Right toe-pick	Backwards right outside edge
Salchow	Backwards left inside edge	Left edge	Backwards right outside edge
Loop	Backwards right outside edge	Right edge	Backwards right outside edge
Toe Loop	Backwards right outside edge	Left toe-pick	Backwards right outside edge
Axel	Forward left outside edge	Left edge	Backwards right outside edge

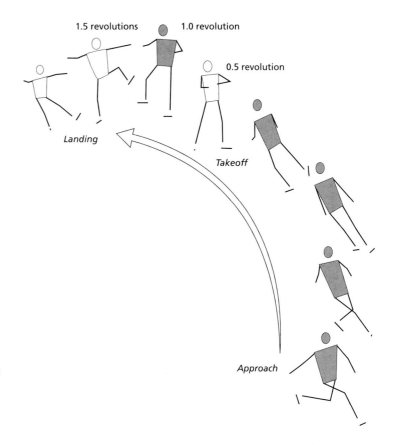

Fig. 15.3 Stick figure representation of an actual single Axel jump showing the forward takeoff and one-and-a-half revolutions in the air. Notice that the skater is facing forwards at takeoff and backwards at landing. The shaded body represents the back of the skater, and the open body represents the front of the skater.

axis are three very important concepts to jumping in skating.

Vertical velocity

The vertical velocity at takeoff will determine how high a skater jumps and to some extent this will also determine flight time. The greater the vertical velocity at takeoff, the greater is the time to peak of flight—time up. However, since skaters do not necessarily take off and land with their centres of mass (COM) at the same vertical position, time up may not equal time down. The COM is a theoretical point representing the centre of mass distribution of a person. In various double and triple jumps, many skaters exhibit longer time dropping down from peak of flight than time moving up to peak of flight. Thus, many skaters actually land with their COM

lower than at takeoff (Lockwood 1996; King 1997).

To generate vertical velocity, a vertical impulse must be created. Since impulse depends both on the magnitude and direction of force production and the time of force application (Eqn. 15.1), the skaters must generate a vertical ground reaction force to gain vertical velocity for takeoff. Initially, as a skater approaches a jump, he or she is travelling horizontally across the ice. At this point during the takeoff, the skaters possess zero vertical velocity. Based on the impulse momentum relationship (Eqn. 15.2), the vertical impulse—calculated as the area under the force–time curve from the point of zero velocity during the takeoff until last contact with the ice, divided by the mass of the skater—will be equal to the vertical velocity of the skater at takeoff. A hypothetical illustration of this concept is illustrated in Fig. 15.4.

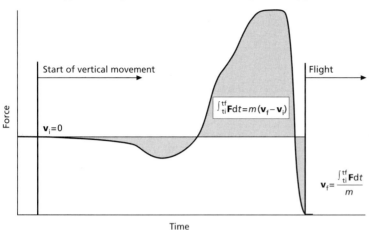

Hypothetical ground reaction force during a skating jump

Start of vertical movement

Flight

$$\int_{ti}^{tf}\mathbf{F}dt=m(\mathbf{v}_f-\mathbf{v}_i)$$

$\mathbf{v}_i=0$

$$\mathbf{v}_f=\frac{\int_{ti}^{tf}\mathbf{F}dt}{m}$$

Force

Time

Fig. 15.4 Hypothetical ground reaction force data for a figure-skating takeoff, demonstrating the impulse momentum relationship. **F** is the net external force acting on the subject in the vertical direction and is equal to the ground reaction force of the skater minus the skater's body weight.

$$I=\int_{t_i}^{t_f}Fdt \tag{15.1}$$

where I = impulse, F = force, t_f = final time and t_i = initial time.

$$\int_{t_i}^{t_f}Fdt=p_f-p_i \tag{15.2}$$

$$\int_{t_i}^{t_f}Fdt=m(v_f-v_i) \tag{15.3}$$

$$v_f=\frac{\int_{t_i}^{t_f}Fdt}{m}+v_i \tag{15.4}$$

where p_f = final momentum, p_i = initial momentum, v_i = initial velocity, v_f = final velocity and m = body mass.

To analyse the techniques with which skaters create a vertical impulse, it is useful to break the jump takeoff into separate phases. The takeoff of the Axel jump has been previously divided into three separate phases, which are useful for describing the generation of vertical impulse (Albert & Miller 1996). These phases are:
• *glide*—defined as the free running of the takeoff skate on the forward outside edge;
• *transition*—defined from the beginning of the upward movement of the COM to the instant before the skater begins to rock forwards on the skate blade; and

• *pivot*—defined as the period of time between when the skater begins to rock forwards onto the toe-pick until last contact with the ice (Fig. 15.5).

During the glide phase of the Axel takeoff, skaters have small negative vertical velocities (Albert & Miller 1996). The vertical velocity remains negative, despite an extension of the takeoff leg due to the forward rotation of the shank about the ankle joint (Albert & Miller 1996). Since the transition period is operationally defined as the initiation of upward motion, it is during this phase when the skaters begin to generate positive vertical velocity. The transition phase is characterized by knee extension of the support leg; however, the extension is not continuous and there is often a period of either zero knee angular velocity or slight knee flexion (Albert & Miller 1996).

In addition to generating a vertical impulse from the extension of the takeoff leg during the transition phase, skaters gain considerable vertical velocity by rotating forwards over their skate boot (Aleshinsky 1987; Albert & Miller 1996). At the end of the transition phase, many skaters perform a 'skid', which seems to contribute to the forward rotation, and has thus has been credited with helping to generate vertical velocity (Aleshinsky 1987). A skid is characterized by the skate scraping across the ice as the blade is turned perpendicular to the direction of motion of the skater. The impetus behind this hypothesis is

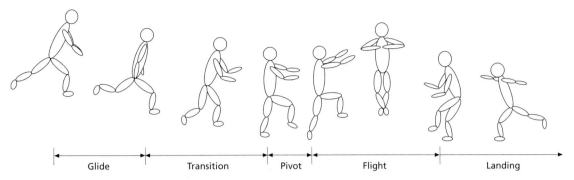

Fig. 15.5 Schematic of the takeoff phases of the Axel jump as defined by Albert and Miller (1996). (Adapted from King 1997.)

that as the skid slows the skate, horizontal velocity is 'transferred' to vertical velocity as the body rotates forwards over the slowing foot. This forward rotation provides the centre of mass with a tangential component of velocity about the axis of rotation. The skaters also possess a radial component of velocity, due primarily to the extension (or flexion) of their takeoff leg, which is represented by the centre of mass moving radially away from (or towards) the axis of rotation. A schematic of the tangential and radial components of velocity is presented in Fig. 15.6.

During the last stages of the glide and throughout the first half of the transition phase, the tangential contribution to the skater's vertical velocity is positive (Albert & Miller 1996). Concurrently, the radial contribution to vertical velocity is usually negative as the radius of the COM to the ankle continues to decrease. This is primarily due to ankle dorsiflexion,

but also to the downward motion of the shank foot and skate segments of the free leg. The motion of the free leg during this time typically consists of hip flexion and knee extension. Simultaneously, the upper extremities are in the upward half of their swing during the transition phases, but their masses are not large enough to counteract the negative motion of the more massive lower extremities (Albert & Miller 1996).

During the second half of the transition, the tangential contribution to vertical velocity gradually decreases to zero while the radial component becomes positive (Albert & Miller 1996). At this time, all segments are displacing in the upward direction. It is during this phase of the takeoff that the skater powerfully extends the takeoff leg creating a large vertical ground reaction force which dramatically increases the vertical velocity of the skater. As is expected, this propulsive phase of

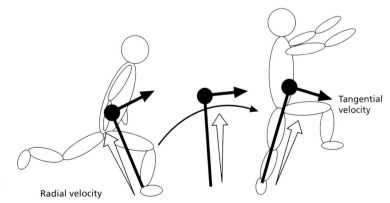

Fig. 15.6 Schematic of tangential and radial components of velocity during an Axel takeoff.

the takeoff is characterized by concentric activity of the leg extensor muscles. The quadriceps and gastrocnemius—responsible for knee extension and ankle plantarflexion, respectively—are highly activated during the takeoff of the Loop jump (Kho & Bishop 1996). It is likely that the major hip extensor is the gluteus maximus, although this has yet to be experimentally confirmed in figure-skating jumps.

By the end of the transition phase, the radial contribution to vertical velocity is responsible for the entire positive vertical velocity of the skater (Albert & Miller 1996). Interestingly, no apparent relationship has been found between the presence of a skid and the contribution of the tangential component of velocity to the vertical velocity of the skater (Albert & Miller 1996). In retrospect, this is not surprising, since the major contribution of the tangential component to vertical velocity occurs during the first half of the transition phase, while the skid, when present, occurs during the second half of the transition phase. During the second half of the transition, skaters are driving their arms and free leg upwards and extending the hip, knee and ankle of their supporting leg, which contributes to the large positive radial component of vertical velocity. In fact, there are significant correlations between knee extension strength and shoulder abduction strength and jump height in single and double Axels (Podolsky et al. 1990).

During the pivot phase, skaters rotate past vertical, which causes the tangential component of velocity to become negative (Albert & Miller 1996). The radial contribution to the vertical velocity of skaters is positive during this phase, although it typically decreases slightly nearing the later stages of the pivot (Albert & Miller 1996). An example graph of the time progression of the tangential and radial components to vertical velocity are provided for a single Axel performed by an elite female skater (Fig. 15.7).

Characteristic vertical velocities for the Axel jumps are in the range 2.5–3.0 m · s⁻¹. On the lower end, average vertical takeoff velocities are around 2.6 m · s⁻¹ for accomplished male skaters performing double Axels (Albert & Miller 1996), while on the high end average vertical velocities can be up to 3.3 m · s⁻¹ for elite male skaters performing double Axels (King et al. 1994). Differences observed

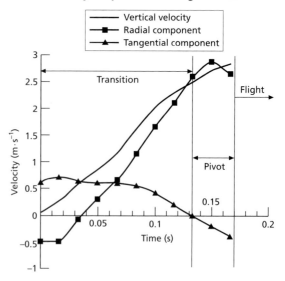

Fig. 15.7 Vertical takeoff velocity and the radial and tangential velocity components of the centre of mass of an elite female skater performing a single Axel. (Data from King 1997.)

amongst various skaters are likely to be attributed to the differing skill levels of the skaters and the intention of the skaters, as the artistic impression of a jump cannot be ignored.

Interestingly, rarely have significant differences been observed in vertical velocity between single, double and triple Axels (King 1997). More typically, skaters exhibit similar vertical velocities at takeoff (and flight times) for single, double and triple Axels (Aleshinsky 1986; King et al. 1994; Albert & Miller 1996). However, there are significant differences in vertical velocity (or jump height) for male and female skaters performing the same jumps. As might be anticipated, male skaters tend to have significantly higher vertical velocities in both single and double Axels (Albert & Miller 1996; King 1997).

Likewise, male skaters tend to outjump their female counterparts in off-ice vertical jump testing. An elite group of junior male skaters jumped 19% higher than their female counterparts off ice, which compares favourably with the same male skaters jumping 22% higher than the same female skaters during single and double Axels performed on ice (King 1997).

The ground reaction force of skaters performing jumps off ice also tends to be quite different between male and female skaters, with male skaters demonstrating higher vertical impulses than female skaters of similar ability (Dainty 1979). The higher impulse was attributed primarily to greater time of force production rather than higher peak force. The male skaters actually exhibited a 'double peaked' force profile, which was hypothesized to have been generated from a more forceful extension of the takeoff leg just prior to takeoff compared with the female skaters (Dainty 1979). This suggests that female skaters could potentially benefit from creating a more sustained 'push' from the ice during takeoff, though further research is mandated due to the small homogeneous subject pool of 10 very select skaters.

Flight time, which as previously mentioned is dependent on vertical velocity and the difference in COM height at takeoff and landing, is generally between 0.5 and 0.7 s for most jump types (Aleshinsky 1986; King et al. 1994; King 1997). The lower landing position, or a 'seated' position at landing, is observed most often in multirevolution jumps (Lockwood 1996; Richards & Henley 1996). While delaying the landing allows the required revolutions to be completed, the increased flight time results from flexing the hip and knee joint whilst in the air. Thus, the resulting landing has been described as a 'collision' landing instead of a 'soft' landing (Lockwood 1996). With the hip and knee already flexed, little additional flexion is available in these joints to absorb the landing and spread the force over a longer impact time. Confounding the lower landing position and limited hip and knee flexion during landing, is the reasonably stiff skating boot. The average ankle range of motion (ROM) in a traditional skating boot, typically composed of three layers of leather for an elite skater, is approximately 17° (Richards & Henley 1996). Due to the limited ankle ROM, dorsiflexion of the ankle joint is unlikely to play a major role in reducing impact forces upon landing. (Lockwood 1996; Richards & Henley 1996). A typical in-skate pressure pattern for a skater is high pressure under the toe immediately

upon first contact with the ice land on the front of the blade followed almost immediately (< 0.1 s) by a weight transfer to the heel of the boot (D. King, unpublished data collected at 1998 USFSA/USOC Sports Medicine and Science Camp, Colorado Springs).

Angular momentum

Very generally, the angular momentum of a rotating body remains constant until a force couple or eccentric force acts upon it. This is the analogue equivalent of Newton's First Law. Since a force couple or eccentric force can only act on a skater whilst the skater is still on the ice, skaters must generate the total required angular momentum for the jump during takeoff. This angular momentum about the longitudinal axis through COM of the skater allows the skater to complete the required revolutions in the air.

Skaters can generate an eccentric force through the movement of their free leg and arms. By definition, an eccentric force is a force whose line of action does not pass through the axis of rotation of the body on which it acts. The movement of the free leg and arms produces a horizontal ground reaction force which acts on the blade of the takeoff leg. Thus, the ground reaction force produced by the skater causes an external torque which produces angular momentum about the longitudinal axis through the COM of the skater.

Based on the definition of torque (Eqn. 15.3), the magnitude of the torque will depend on the magnitude of the horizontal ground reaction force and the moment arm of that torque (the perpendicular distance from the line of action of the force to the axis of rotation). While few, if any, studies have examined the production of horizontal ground reaction force during a figure skating takeoff, it is possible to perform a theoretical analysis of the likely line of action and moment arm length of the ground reaction force during the takeoff of a jump (Albert & Miller 1996).

$$T = r \times F \quad \text{or} \quad T = F r_{\perp} \quad (15.5)$$

where T = torque vector; F = force vector; r = distance from axis to point of application of force;

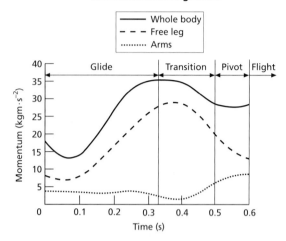

Segmental contributions to whole body angular momentum in a single Axel

Fig. 15.8 Angular momentum about the vertical axis for the whole body, arms and free leg of a skater performing a single Axel. (Adapted from Albert & Miller 1996.)

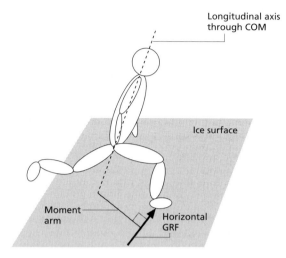

Fig. 15.9 Schematic of proposed mechanism for generating an external torque during takeoff. The movement of the arms and free leg produces a horizontal ground reaction force presumably directed inwards towards the centre of the skater's approach circle. This eccentric force has a large moment arm due to the position of the skate relative to the longitudinal axis through the COM of the skater.

T = torque (magnitude only); F = force (magnitude only); $r_\perp$ = force moment arm (perpendicular distance from axis to line of action of force).

During the glide phase of the Axel takeoff, the predominant contribution to angular momentum about the vertical axis is from the movement of the free leg, as illustrated in Fig. 15.8 (Albert & Miller 1996). The movement of the free leg causes a ground reaction force whose horizontal component is most likely perpendicular to the long axis of the blade and directed towards the centre of the skater's approach pattern (Albert & Miller 1996). Since the whole body COM of the skater is behind the skate during this period, the ground reaction force is an eccentric force and causes an external torque about the longitudinal axis through the COM of the skater (Fig. 15.9). The direction of this external torque is consistent with the direction of the skater's intended rotation once in the air. During this time period, skaters lean inwards, rotate their hips forwards, and begin to swing their free leg forwards. By the end of the glide phase, skaters typically have gained between 58 and 100% of their total angular momentum for flight (Albert & Miller 1996).

As skaters enter the transition phase of the Axel, their angular momentum continues to increase slightly, again primarily due to the horizontal ground reaction forces produced by the movement of their free leg (Albert & Miller 1996). However, as the skaters progress through the transition phase, their angular momentum about the longitudinal axis through their COM tends to plateau or even decrease (Albert & Miller 1996). As no information is currently available on the horizontal ground reaction forces during takeoff, the decrease in total body angular momentum could be due to a decrease in the magnitude of the horizontal ground reaction force, a reduction in the moment arm of this eccentric force, or a combination of both.

Additionally, as previously noted, the latter portion of the transition phase is often signified by a skidding action. During this time period, skaters are generally in a more upright posture and are extending the knee of their supporting leg. As a result, the COM is farther forward or closer to the toe of the takeoff foot. This position, combined with the turning of the skate during the skidding action, would theoretically reduce the moment arm of the horizontal ground reaction force (Albert & Miller 1996). A decreased moment arm could account for the observed decrease (or constant) total body angular moment. Hypothetically, even if the skidding action were to cause an increase in the horizontal reaction force (about which no information is available in the literature), a significantly reduced moment arm could easily account for angular momentum about the longitudinal axis remaining constant or decreasing.

During the pivot phase, the angular momentum of the whole body about the longitudinal through the COM of the skater typically continues to decrease (Albert & Miller 1996). It is likely that the combined movements of the free leg and arms result in a reduction of the magnitude of the horizontal ground reaction force during this phase; however, the horizontal ground reaction force has not been experimentally measured. Simultaneously, based on the position of the COM of the skater in relation to the takeoff foot, it would appear that the moment arm of the horizontal ground reaction force is also decreasing.

Interestingly, there does not appear to be any statistical difference between the total body angular momentum for single and double Axels at the instant of takeoff (Albert & Miller 1996). Typical whole body angular momentum and moment of inertia values for skaters performing Axel jumps are presented in Table 15.2 (Albert & Miller 1996). The obvious conclusion is that for single and double Axels, skaters do not rely on generating greater angular momentum to gain the increase in angular velocity needed to complete the double Axel.

Moment of inertia

The moment of inertia of the whole body about the vertical axis of a skater usually reaches a maximum near the end of the glide phase (Albert & Miller 1996). After this point, the moment of inertia decreases through the end of the glide phase and into the transition. The decrease in moment of inertia of the skaters continues throughout the transition and pivot phases. Average moments of inertia of skaters at takeoff during single and double Axels are reported in Table 15.3.

As mentioned previously, angular momentum values are generally quite similar between single and double Axels; however, there is usually a significant difference in the moments of inertia of the skaters at takeoff for these jumps (Albert & Miller 1996). Typically, skaters possess smaller moments of inertia about their vertical axis at takeoff in higher revolution jumps (Aleshinsky 1986, 1987; Albert & Miller 1996). For example, it is quite common for a skater to have a smaller moment of inertia at the instant of takeoff for a double Axel compared with a single Axel.

The combination of similar angular momentum values with smaller moments of inertia corresponded to higher angular velocities at takeoff in multirevolution jumps. The increased angular velocity observed at takeoff during the higher revolution Axels likely results from skaters initiating their rotation while still on the ice (Aleshinsky 1986). Most skaters demonstrate significantly greater on-ice prerotation at takeoff during high-revolution jumps as compared with single jumps, with some skaters completing between 90 and 180

Table 15.2 Angular momentum about the longitudinal axis at takeoff for single and double Axel jumps. (Adapted from Albert & Miller 1996.)

	Angular momentum (kg · m² · s⁻¹)	
	Males	Females
Single Axel	28.6 ± 8.8	16.5 ± 3.1
Double Axel	29.6 ± 11.1	16.2 ± 2.9

Table 15.3 Moment of inertia about the longitudinal axis at takeoff for single and double Axel jumps. (Adapted from Albert & Miller 1996.)

	Moment of inertia (kg · m²)	
	Males	Females
Single Axel	4.3 ± 1.1	2.9 ± 0.8
Double Axel	3.7 ± 1.1	2.5 ± 0.6

degrees of the rotation whilst still on the ice (King *et al.* 1994; King 1997).

Additionally, skaters generally possess smaller moments of inertia in the air during higher revolution jumps, due to tighter rotating positions in the air, which result in faster peak angular velocities during flight (Aleshinsky 1986). Thus, when faster angular velocities at takeoff are coupled with faster maximum angular velocities during flight, the result is greater overall *average* angular velocities for the flight phase of the jump. Recalling that many skaters do not jump higher in multirevolution Axels than in single Axels (Aleshinsky 1986; King *et al.* 1994; Albert & Miller 1996), it can be concluded that most skaters complete the additional revolution by increasing their average angular velocity through prerotation on the ice and smaller moments of inertia.

Summary

Again, limiting the discussion of the biomechanics of figure-skating jumps to Axel jumps, several general conclusions are warranted. Vertical velocity is gained through both tangential and radial motion of the centre of mass of the skater. Initially, the primary gain in vertical velocity is from tangential motion as the skater rotates forwards over the boot. Concurrently, the radial contribution is usually negative, due to dorsiflexion of the ankle of the takeoff leg and downward motion of the free leg. These movements are followed by upward motion of the free leg and arms and powerful extension of the takeoff leg, which cause an upward radial motion of the centre of mass. The skid, which often occurs in multirevolution jumps at the end of the transition phase, does not seem to be related to the contribution of tangential motion to vertical velocity. Since the skid typically occurs well after skaters have taken advantage of the tangential component of vertical velocity, the skidding action does not appear to aid the transfer of horizontal motion to vertical motion of the centre of mass.

Skaters generate the majority of their angular momentum needed for flight during the glide phase of the takeoff. The angular momentum is generated primarily from the rotation of the hips and move-

ment of the free leg, which create a horizontal ground reaction force. This eccentric force presumably has a reasonably large moment arm due to the skate being well ahead of the whole body COM during this phase. Thus, a relatively large external torque is created about the longitudinal axis through the COM of the skaters which produces the desired angular momentum for the jump. Throughout the transition and pivot phases, angular momentum remains fairly constant or may even decrease. It is not known if this decrease is due to a reduction in the horizontal ground reaction force, moment arm, or both.

Skaters do not appear to generate greater angular momentum in double Axels compared with single Axels. Instead the jumps are completed with both similar angular momentum values and similar jump heights. To complete more revolutions in the Axel jumps, skaters rely on increasing average angular velocity. This is accomplished through:

1 greater angular velocity during takeoff—due to a prerotation on the ice and a smaller moment of inertia during takeoff; and

2 greater angular velocity during flight—due to attaining a small minimum moment of inertia more quickly once in the air.

Some skaters do delay the landings of their jumps by flexing their hips and knees just prior to landing to enable the completion of the last revolution. This technique is most common in multirevolution jumps.

It is likely that many of these result could be extrapolated to other figure-skating jumps. For example, it is quite conceivable that similar findings in jump height, angular momentum and moment of inertia would be observed across all the jump types. However, it is also likely that the toe-jumps, or even the other edge jumps, rely on different mechanisms for generating vertical velocity and angular momentum given the different mechanics of the free leg when approaching a jump backwards and vaulting off a toe-pick. Theoretically, when using the toe-pick to vault off the ice, skaters may create an external force couple (from the separate ground reaction forces acting on each blade) which could also contribute to the generation of angular momentum.

Theoretical techniques

At first impression, relying on decreases in moment of inertia instead of increases in angular momentum to complete multirevolution jumps may seem counterintuitive to basic scientific principles (Aleshinsky 1986, 1987; Aleshinsky *et al.* 1988; Albert & Miller 1996). It has been theorized that a better technique to complete a maximum number of revolutions in a jump (or merely to increase the number of revolutions in a jump) would be to have a large angular momentum and moment of inertia at takeoff (Aleshinsky 1986). The large moment of inertia about the longitudinal axis would serve two purposes: (i) to generate larger angular momentum at takeoff; and (ii) to provide the skater with the opportunity to greatly reduce the moment of inertia in flight resulting in a dramatic increase in angular velocity. In order to complete a jump in this manner, a skater would need to maximize moment of inertia about the longitudinal axis at takeoff, quickly reduce this moment of inertia in air resulting in a radical increase in angular velocity, and then reverse this procedure upon preparation for landing (Aleshinsky 1986). Whilst in flight, the skater would try to maintain a minimal moment of inertia for as long as possible, which would then maximize average angular velocity. This hypothetical technique is based on the theories of conservation of angular momentum and generation of angular momentum (using a large moment of inertia during takeoff to generate great angular momentum for flight). Since angular momentum remains constant during the flight phase, once in the air the only technique skaters have to increase their angular velocity is to pull their arms and legs into a tight body posture and minimize their moment of inertia.

One of the practical advantages of the theoretical technique vs. the observed technique for completing maximum (or greater) revolutions in the air, includes the ability to maintain the body in an open position during takeoff. Accordingly, the whole body moment of inertia about the longitudinal axis would be quite large at takeoff. This would not only allow for potentially greater generation of angular momentum, but consequently implies that the skater would be able to perform the jump without prerotating on the ice. Many skaters increase angular velocity at takeoff during multirevolution jumps, at least the Axel, by 'transferring' horizontal velocity to rotational velocity with the braking force associated with the skid (Aleshinsky 1986). It is conceivable that if a skater could reduce this braking force, he or she would save energy, and thus allow more energy to be spent in the generation of greater vertical velocity (Aleshinsky 1986).

It must be remembered, however, that skaters are currently increasing jump revolutions without using the 'hypothetically' best technique (King *et al.* 1994; Albert & Miller 1996; King 1997). Accordingly, there must be several disadvantages to this hypothetical technique which cause the skaters to employ other techniques whilst performing multirevolution jumps. While taking off from the ice in an open body position with a large moment of inertia may be aesthetically appealing, the cost is undoubtedly the great strength and power needed to quickly reduce the moment of inertia by pulling in the arms and legs to a tight rotating position. Thus, the importance of adductor strength in skating to counteract centrifugal force experienced by the skater during fast rotations in the air cannot be emphasized enough (Aleshinsky 1986).

Focusing only on the Axel jump, recall that skaters often utilize a skid during takeoff, which seems to result in greater prerotation on the ice and higher angular velocities at takeoff. The down side to the skid is a reduction in horizontal speed and seemingly no gain in angular momentum. However, the benefits of being able to take off with higher angular velocities and smaller moments of inertia appear to outweigh the costs (Aleshinsky 1986; Albert & Miller 1996).

Despite these results, it is conceivable that if skaters were to concentrate on increasing adductor strength and utilizing the hypothetically best technique, further increases in jump revolutions, beyond the levels which have thus far been achieved, might be feasible (Aleshinsky 1986). Indeed, comparing more highly rated jumps to lowly rated jumps of a single jump type, for example double Axels, the more highly rated jumps are closer in appearance to the 'theoretically' best technique. Specifically, highly rated double Axels performed by junior

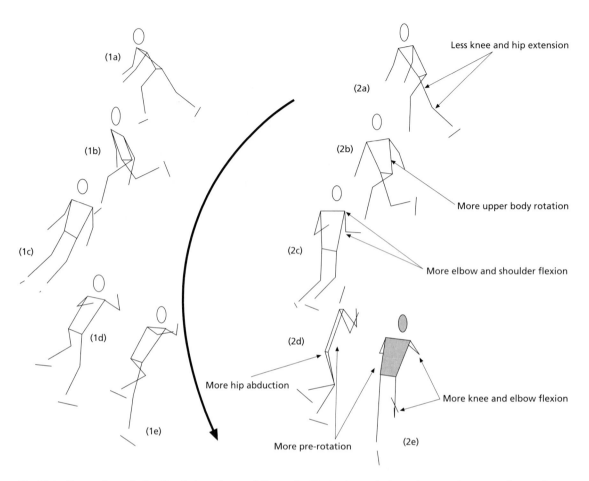

Fig. 15.10 Comparison of takeoff techniques in two different double Axels. Axel 1 (1a–1e) received a rating of 8 out of 10, and Axel 2 (2a–2e) received a rating of 5 out of 10 by two figure-skating coaches. Picture 'a' is the beginning of the transition phase and picture 'e' is last contact with the ice. Both jumps were successfully landed.

elite skaters were characterized by greater vertical and horizontal takeoff velocities, less prerotation at takeoff, and lower angular velocities at takeoff and in flight compared with more lowly rated double Axels (King 1997). Figure 15.10 illustrates some of the differences in the takeoffs of a highly and more lowly rated double Axel.

However, it is unclear whether skaters employing this technique were at an advantage because the technique is theoretically superior for achieving higher revolution jumps or whether they were scored highly due to the aesthetics of the jump. Most people would agree that jumps which are both high and long, and during which the skater undergoes a dramatic increase in angular velocity in the air, are most impressive. Thus, skaters employing the hypothetically best technique, by maintaining a large moment of inertia at takeoff, are going to exhibit these characteristics and are more likely to achieve high ratings (when the jumps are rated individually as opposed to a component of an entire programme). Since figure skating is a subjective sport where both technical and artistic merit determine a skater's marks, striving for the hypothetically best technique may be a good goal for skaters—whether it is to create a dramatic appearance to their jumps or to try to attain more revolutions.

Conclusions

Currently there is a solid base of knowledge regarding the biomechanics of skating jumps, although much of the available information concerns only the Axel jumps. From these data, two of the more interesting biomechanical characteristics concerning the performance of Axels are:

1 that many skaters do not use additional jump height to complete higher revolution jumps; and

2 that angular momentum is generally not greater for higher revolution jumps.

However, the Axel is unique compared with other jumps in that it is forward-facing at takeoff and requires an extra half-revolution in the air. Thus, it may not be prudent to make general assumptions about other skating jumps from data collected on the Axel. Accordingly, more definitive information is needed about the techniques employed by skaters in other types of jumps to develop a complete picture of the biomechanics of skating jumps. Additionally, with advances in technology, information is becoming available on both takeoff and landing forces during skating jumps (Foti 1990; Kho & Bishop 1996; Lockwood 1996; Richards & Henley 1996; Kho 1998). The interpretation of these data tends to suggest that skating boots are not optimally designed for jumping. While there has been significant research in the area of boot design (Foti 1990; Richards & Henley 1996), this line of research needs continued pursuance to take advantage of new information and ongoing advances in materials science and technology.

References

Albert, W. & Miller, D. (1996) Takeoff characteristics of single and double Axel figure skating jumps. *Journal of Applied Biomechanics* **12**, 72–87.

Aleshinsky, S. (1986) What Biomechanics can do for figure skating part II. *Skating* December, 11–15.

Aleshinsky, S. (1987) A biomechanical report of USFSA/USOC/PSGA junior elite camp participants. *Professional Skater* **18**, 24–28.

Aleshinsky, S., Smith, S., Jansen, L. & Ramirez, F. (1988) Comparison of biomechanical parameters demonstrated by Brian Boitono in triple and double Axel jumps. In: *Proceedings of 12th Annual Meeting of American Society of Biomechanics, University of Illinois, Champaign, IL*, p. 201.

Dainty, D. (1979) The importance of impulse production in jumping. *Circle: Figure Skating Coaches of Canada* **11**, 7–8.

Foti, T. (1990) The biomechanical evaluation of landings in an articulated boot figure skate. Master's thesis, University of Delaware.

Kho, M. (1998) Ground reaction forces in simulated figure skating jump takeoffs and landings. In: *Proceedings from North American Congress on Biomechanics, Waterloo, Ontario, Canada*, pp. 431–432.

Kho, M. & Bishop, P. (1996) Muscle activation patterns in simulated loop jumps. In: *Proceedings from International Congress on the Sports Medicine and Sports Science of Skating, San Jose, California.*

King, D. (1997) A biomechanical analysis of the Axel: critical parameters for successful jumps. *Professional Skater* January/February, 10–12.

King, D., Arnold, A. & Smith, S. (1994) A kinematic comparison of single, double, and triple axels. *Journal of Applied Biomechanics* **10**, 51–60.

Lockwood, K. (1996) Kinetic and kinematic characteristics of impact upon landing single, double, and triple revolution jumps in figure skating. In: *Proceedings from International Congress on the Sports Medicine and Sports Science of Skating, San Jose, California.*

Podolsky, A., Kaufman, K., Cahalan, T., Aleshinsky, S. & Chao, E. (1990) The relationship of strength and jump height in figure skaters. *American Journal of Sports Medicine* **18**, 400–405.

Richards, J. & Henley, J. (1996) Effects of ankle mobility on landing forces in skating. In: *Proceedings from International Congress on the Sports Medicine and Sports Science of Skating, San Jose, California.*

Chapter 16

Springboard and Platform Diving

D.I. MILLER

This chapter focuses upon selected mechanical aspects of elite diving performance within the context of the rules governing international competition. After a consideration of the influence of characteristics of the takeoff surfaces, the functional components of both platform and springboard dives are discussed. Examples of these components, namely preparation, takeoff, flight and entry, are taken from the performances of Olympic medallists and finalists.

Competition overview

Diving became an Olympic event for men in 1904 and for women in 1912. Between 1928 and 1936, there were High Diving and Springboard Diving competitions for both men and women. Since 1948, these events have been referred to as Platform Diving and Springboard Diving (Henry & Yeomans 1984). The most recent addition to international competition, and introduced into the Olympics in 2000, is synchronized diving. Separate contests on the 3 m springboard and the 10 m platform involve dives being performed by two divers simultaneously.

Dive designations

The Federation International de Natation Amateur (FINA), the governing body for all aquatic sports including competitive diving, identifies all dives with a unique number–letter code. This dive code, consisting of three or four numbers and a letter, surpasses language barriers and is readily interpreted by divers

and their coaches. For the sake of brevity, FINA dive designations will be employed in this chapter.

In the FINA coding system, dives are identified first by group:

front = 1;
back = 2;
reverse = 3;
inward = 4;
twist = 5; and
armstand = 6.

Second, dives from the first four groups are categorized as non-flying (0) or flying (1). A flying dive is one in which the first half-somersault is done in the straight position. Most dives performed in competition are non-flying.

Third, dives are identified by the number of half-somersaults executed during the flight (3 being a $1\frac{1}{2}$, 7 being a $3\frac{1}{2}$ and so on). If a dive involves a twist, the number of half-twists are specified next (2 being a full twist, 5 being a $2\frac{1}{2}$ twist, etc.).

Finally, dives are categorized by the body position in which they are executed: straight (i.e. layout) = A; pike = B; tuck = C; and free = D.

Non-twisting dives are identified by three numbers followed by a letter. Thus a 205C is a back $2\frac{1}{2}$ tuck; a 101A is a front dive straight; a 113B is a flying front $1\frac{1}{2}$ pike; and a 307C is a reverse $3\frac{1}{2}$ tuck. Because few flying dives are performed, the flying designation is only included in the verbal description if it is present.

Since twisting dives can be done from the front, back, reverse, inward or armstand groups, they are identified by four numbers followed by a letter. Thus a 5152D is a front $2\frac{1}{2}$ somersaults with a full twist in free position; a 5237D is a back $1\frac{1}{2}$ with $3\frac{1}{2}$ twists free; and a 5111A is a front dive with a half-twist straight. With the exception of dives (i.e. $\frac{1}{2}$ somersault), most twisting somersaults are executed in the free (D) position.

Although dives from the first five groups are done from both springboard and platform, armstands are only performed from the platform. Their identification code begins with a 6 and is followed by whether the somersault is front (1), back (2) or reverse (3), then by the number of half-somersaults and finally by the number of half twists executed during the flight. This number code is followed by the dive position (A, B or C). Thus a 631B is an armstand cut-through in the pike position (i.e. reverse rotation); a 600A is an armstand dive straight (i.e. no rotation); 616C is an armstand triple somersault tuck; and a 624B is an armstand back double somersault pike.

Degree of difficulty

Each dive has a degree of difficulty (DD). The simplest dive with a 1.2 DD is the front dive tuck (101C) from a 1 m springboard or 5 m platform. At the opposite extreme are dives such as those performed by male competitors in the 1996 Olympic Games: a 307C from 3 m and a 109C from 10 m with DDs of 3.5; and a 207B and 5239D from 10 m with DDs of 3.6. The DD of a dive increases as more somersaults and twists are added. Body position is another factor. The diver's moment of inertia about the somersaulting axis through the centre of gravity (CG) in flight is related to the square of the distance of the various body segments from that axis. Therefore, dives executed in the straight position are more difficult than those done in pike, and dives executed in the pike position are in turn more difficult than those done in tuck. The DD formula also takes into account the height from which a dive is executed, the type of approach used and whether or not the diver can see the water before the somersaulting action is nearly completed.

International competition

International springboard and platform competi-

tions currently require divers to perform a set number of dives with a limited total DD and another specified number of dives without any limit on DD. The former, comprising simpler dives referred to as 'dives with limit', are performed in the semifinal round. Each dive must be selected from a different dive group. On springboard, both men and women do five of these dives with limit. On platform, the women do four and the men five. In the preliminary and final rounds, divers must execute their most difficult dives, termed 'dives without limit'. On springboard, women perform five and men six of these dives, with at least one being selected from each of the first five dive groups. On platform, women perform four and men six dives without limit, each from a different dive group (FINA Handbook 1998–2000).

Judging

According to FINA rules, each dive is judged on a scale from 0 to 10 based on the grace and technique of the starting position, run, takeoff, flight and entry. Neither the approach to the starting position nor any movements beneath the water are to be taken into consideration. Disregarding the difficulty of the dive, judges award points and half-points according to the following guidelines:
completely failed = 0;
unsatisfactory = $\frac{1}{2}$–2;
deficient = $2\frac{1}{2}$–$4\frac{1}{2}$;
satisfactory = 5–6;
good = $6\frac{1}{2}$–8; and
very good = $8\frac{1}{2}$–10.

To determine the total award for the dive, the highest and lowest scores are always eliminated and the remainder summed. With five judges, the middle three scores are summed and then simply multiplied by the DD. When there are seven judges, the sum is multiplied by $\frac{3}{5}$ and then by the DD for the dive.

Approach to analysis

Figure 16.1 provides a schematic representation of the interrelationships among dives from the first four groups. In the front and back groups, the

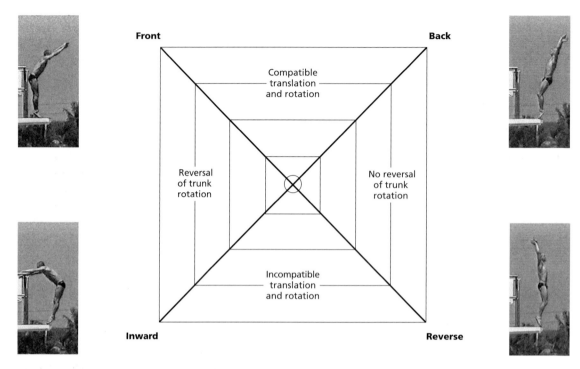

Fig. 16.1 Interrelationships among the first four dive groups with positions at last contact for the 107B, 207C, 307C and 407C demonstrated by 1996 Olympic platform gold medallist Dmitry Sautin.

direction of translation or linear motion and the direction of somersaulting are compatible whereas in the inward and reverse groups the diver is travelling in one direction and somersaulting in the other. In dives from the back and reverse groups, there is a consistent motion into the somersault throughout the takeoff whereas in dives from the front and inward groups, the upper body must change its rotational direction. And finally, dives from the front and reverse groups on springboard are classified as running dives because they have a moving approach. By contrast, dives from the back and inward groups are termed standing dives. On platform, it is common for divers also to use a standing approach when executing one or more somersaults from the reverse group. While front dives and $1\frac{1}{2}$ somersaults on platform may begin with a standing approach, most multiple somersaulting dives from the front group are initiated with a running approach.

Dives can be analysed in terms of functional components that are common to many jumping type activities, namely: preparation, takeoff, flight and entry. Operational definitions of these and related terms as they apply specifically to competitive diving are as follows.

• *Approach*—the walking or running steps preceding the hurdle in running dives.

• *Hurdle*—the jump upwards (springboard) or leap forwards (platform) immediately preceding the takeoff in running dives.

• *Preparation*—the diver's movements that precede the takeoff. In running dives, they include the approach steps and hurdle. In standing dives on springboard, these motions encompass initial activation of the board (equivalent to approach steps). In standing dives on both springboard and platform, preparation incorporates the diver's upward motion and drop back towards the takeoff surface (equivalent to the hurdle). The end of the preparation phase is marked by a change in the diver's vertical acceleration from down to up. The location of this transition cannot be located precisely for platform dives without the benefit of output from a force plate. For springboard dives, however, it coincides with the start of downward board tip motion at the beginning of final board depression.

• *Takeoff*—the period of two-foot contact with the springboard or the period of one- or two-foot contact with the platform following the preparation and immediately prior to flight. For a springboard dive, it includes both the final depression and recoil of the board. For a platform dive, it begins during the diver's final drop towards the surface of the platform.

• *Flight*—the free-fall period from last contact with the takeoff surface until initial contact with the water.

• *Entry*—the interval between the diver's initial contact with the water and the point at which the diver begins to return to the surface.

Characteristics of diving surfaces

Competitive dives are performed from two different surfaces: a springboard that is compliant and a platform that is rigid (formerly referred to as a firmboard). While platform heights are 1, 3, 5, 7.5 and 10 m above the water, only the highest three are used in competition. In world-class meets, such as the Olympic Games, all platform dives must be executed from the 10 m level. The lower platforms are used for practising line-ups as well as for lead-ups related to executing more difficult dives or dives from greater heights.

Springboards are 1 m and 3 m above the water.

The board currently used in competition is the Maxiflex 'B' (Fig. 16.2). It is constructed of a basic single-piece extrusion of aluminium alloy, is 4.88 m (16 ft) in length and has a mass of approximately 54 kg. From a 0.584 m region near the middle that allows for fulcrum adjustment, the board is double tapered: back to the anchor end as well as forward to the tip. The inclusion of 189 diagonal perforations within 0.7 m of the tip makes this part of the board the most compliant (Sprigings *et al.* 1990). Beneath the surface of the board and running its entire length to reinforce it are its two sides, six ribs and a torsion box. This springboard and its precursors, the Maxiflex and Duraflex developed by Ray Rude and manufactured by Arcadia Air Products (Sparks, NV), have been used in the Olympic Games since 1960 (McFarland 1997–98).

Although an extremely complex system (Kuipers & Van de Ven 1992; Kooi & Kuipers 1994), the competitive springboard acts like a linear spring with a small mass on top (Sprigings *et al.* 1989, 1990). From the standpoint of diving performance, the influence of damping is negligible. When a load is applied to a springboard, the board tip will move down in proportion to the load as would a linear spring (e.g. Lanoue 1936; Darda 1972; Stilling 1989; Boda 1992). The greater the load, the greater the deflection. Thus, the springboard obeys Hooke's Law. The relationship between load and deflection is given by the spring constant, k, which has units of $N \cdot m^{-1}$. Consequently, a board with a spring constant of 5000 $N \cdot m^{-1}$ will require a force or load of 5000 N to deflect it 1 m.

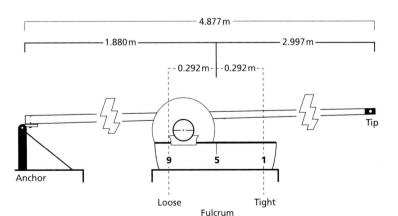

Fig. 16.2 Dimensions and fulcrum positions of the Maxiflex B springboard used in competition.

When a load is applied to the board between the fulcrum and the board tip and then removed quickly, the board tip will oscillate. This is also similar to the response of a linear spring. If the board is released from a small deflection, it will remain in contact with the fulcrum and oscillate in a regular fashion with the oscillations becoming progressively smaller. If the board is released from a large deflection such as in the support phases of the hurdle and takeoff, the board will lose contact with the fulcrum as it rides up. During the sub-sequent downward motion, it will collide with and bounce off the fulcrum. Con-sequently, the vertical oscillation of the board tip will be irregular until it again regains continuous contact with the fulcrum. From that time onward, its vertical pattern of motion will approximate a damped sine wave (Miller *et al.* 1998).

The deflection and oscillation characteristics of the board are influenced by the position of the fulcrum. The latter is designated by a number from 1 to 9 that can be read from a tape fixed to the board surface (Fig. 16.2). When the fulcrum is closer to the free end (lower fulcrum numbers), the board is said to be stiff or hard. Its spring constant is in the range of 5500–6500 N · m^{-1} (Sprigings *et al.* 1990; Miller & Jones 1999). When the fulcrum is closer to the hinged anchor end (higher fulcrum numbers), the board is described as being loose, soft or compliant, with reported spring constants ranging from 4000 to 5000 N · m^{-1}. The difference in stiffness between the tightest and loosest fulcrum settings is approxim-ately 1500 N · m^{-1}. If the fulcrum is moved closer to the board tip, effectively making the spring stiffer, the board tip will oscillate more rapidly. Conversely, if the fulcrum is moved back closer to the hinged end, as is the practice of most elite divers, the spring is more compliant. This means that when it is loaded and then released it will oscillate more slowly.

For a given fulcrum setting and all else being equal, the board deflection and oscillation char-acteristics are also affected by the location and magnitude of any load that is applied to the board. A board that is loaded, as occurs when the diver is in contact with it, will oscillate more slowly than if it is free. And a particular load will deflect the board more if it is applied closer to the board tip than if it is applied nearer the fulcrum. Therefore, a diver who lands back from the end of the board in a takeoff will not be able to push the board down as far as a diver who lands on the end. Similarly, a diver with a long hurdle will not push the board down as far during hurdle support as a diver with a shorter hurdle because the force applied during hurdle support will be further back from the board tip.

Most divers rely on experience and 'feel' for the board when deciding where to set the fulcrum with respect to the hinged anchor end of the board. While all Maxiflex boards used in competition are similar, elite divers are able to discern variations in spring-board response due to minor differences in mass, installation and/or age of the board. On average, semifinalists in the 1996 Atlanta Olympics set their fulcrums at 6.3 ± 1.7 (men) and 6.1 ± 1.8 (women) for standing dives and 7.8 ± 0.9 (men) and 7.2 ± 1.4 (women) for running dives.

Preparation for takeoff

Preparation for the takeoff of a dive differs between standing and running dives and between spring-board and platform. These motions, however, serve a single purpose. Whether they involve approach steps and hurdle, setting the board in motion and/or reaching a stretched position and then dropping down towards the takeoff surface, they are designed to lay the groundwork for an effective takeoff. This is the criterion against which differing preparatory techniques must be assessed.

Starting position for standing dives

At the beginning of dives from the back and inward groups, the diver's weight is on the balls of the feet with the heels raised and extended beyond the edge of the takeoff surface. This position increases the range over which the heels can drop at the beginning of the takeoff. It thereby allows a greater stretch to be imposed on the calf muscles, facilitating the production of plantar flexion force. For standing reverse dives from platform, the diver's toes are at or near the edge of the platform.

In achieving a balanced position in preparation

for an armstand takeoff, the palmar surfaces of the diver's hands are in contact with the platform. The fingers are spread to enlarge the base of support. Maintaining balance in this inverted position is more difficult than in standing dives (McNitt-Gray & Anderson 1993; Slobounov & Newell 1996). The base of support is smaller, and the CG is higher above the platform surface. The upper extremities supporting the diver's weight are not as strong as the lower extremities. Balance control is critical, however, as there is a 1–3 point deduction for inability to demonstrate a balanced position prior to takeoff.

Board activation

In back and inward rotating dives from springboard, the board is initially depressed slightly by the diver's weight. Divers then set the board in motion by a subtle alteration in their ankle position. The amplitude of the rocking or pumping motion gradually increases due to repeated impulses applied through the diver's feet. These repeated impulses overcome the inertia of the diver and of the board and produce a greater oscillation than would be possible with only a single impulse (Eaves 1969). During the final pump, the heels of elite divers drop below the surface of the board. From this instantaneous position of maximum dorsiflexion, the ankle rapidly moves towards maximum plantar flexion with the toes also extending (Fig. 16.3).

As the diver reaches the highest position and then begins to the drop to initiate the takeoff, the acceleration of the body is negative or downward. As a result the board is unweighted and moves up to approximate its unloaded horizontal position. The subsequent downward motion of the board tip that signals the start of standing springboard takeoffs can be detected using the single frame advance feature on a VCR.

Standing dive preparation on platform

This distinction between the end of the preparation and the start of the takeoff phase is not as clear in platform dives because the takeoff surface is rigid.

To be consistent with its use in springboard dives, however, the preparatory motion is considered complete once the diver begins to accelerate up. On platform reaction force records, this instant can be readily identified as the final time at which the vertical platform reaction force exceeds body weight prior to the flight of the dive. Following from Newton's Second Law, the sum of the forces (ΣF) acting on the diver equals the diver's mass × acceleration of the diver's CG or mass centre ($m \times a$). In the vertical direction, weight (W) and the vertical component of the platform reaction (VPRF) are the only external forces acting on the diver. Therefore, when the VPRF exceeds W, the vertical acceleration (a_v) must be positive.

$$\Sigma F = ma \tag{16.1}$$

$$VPRF - W = ma_v \tag{16.2}$$

$$VPRF = ma_v + W \tag{16.3}$$

Running dive preparation

Preparation for running dives on platform characteristically involves approach steps that increase in speed followed by a long, low hurdle. This is in distinct contrast to the generally slower approach steps and shorter, higher hurdle associated with the preparation for front and reverse springboard dive takeoffs. The reason for the difference in the characteristics of the approach steps lies in the differing function that they serve as a result of the nature of the respective takeoff surfaces. The platform approach and hurdle are similar to what might be seen in a tumbling run leading up to the execution of one or more forward somersaults. The long, low hurdle sets the stage for a braking or 'blocking' reaction force elicited at the beginning of the takeoff to facilitate forward rotation. In the case of the hurdle on springboard, height is important. The greater the height, the greater the diver's downward velocity at the beginning of the takeoff and the more kinetic energy available to aid in deflecting the springboard.

Most divers at the elite level have a brief period of flight in the step that immediately precedes the hurdle support phase on springboard. During

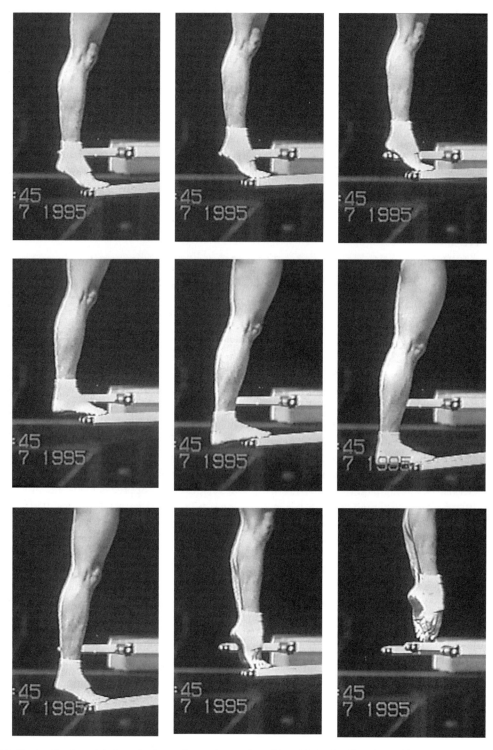

Fig. 16.3 Final activation of the board prior to depression and recoil in a 407C takeoff performed by 1992 and 1996 Olympic gold medallist, Xiong Ni.

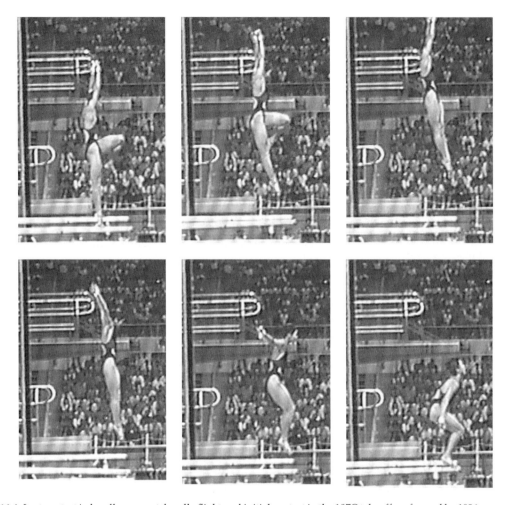

Fig. 16.4 Last contact in hurdle support, hurdle flight and initial contact in the 107C takeoff performed by 1996 springboard gold medallist, Fu Mingxia.

hurdle support the board is depressed to almost half the extent of its maximum depression during the takeoff. The time required for springboard depression and recoil in hurdle support is comparable to the time required for the takeoff (Miller 1984).

The height of the diver's CG at the beginning of hurdle flight in springboard is higher than when the diver contacts the board to begin the takeoff. For semifinalists at the 1995 World Diving Cup and 1996 Olympics, this difference averaged 0.34 m for the men and 0.29 m for the women. Although some of the difference is due to the fact that the arms are

stretched above the head at the start of hurdle compared with being at or below hip level on landing, a more influential factor is the difference in the position of the lower extremities at the start and end of hurdle flight (Fig. 16.4).

Video analysis reveals that the board tip oscillates between $2\frac{1}{4}$ and $2\frac{1}{2}$ cycles while the diver is in the hurdle flight (Jones & Miller 1996). For elite divers, the time it takes for the board to complete these cycles depends much more upon the extent to which the board rebounds from the fulcrum than where the fulcrum is set (Miller *et al.* 1998). In most cases during hurdle flight, some degree of rebound will be superimposed on the natural frequency of the board, thereby slowing the oscillations. This influence, which is more pronounced for men than women and for senior than junior divers, turns out to be somewhat of a compensatory mechanism. The higher divers jump in the hurdle, the more the board rebounds from the fulcrum and the longer the board takes to complete the oscillations. But since the divers have more time in the air in the hurdle, they may still be able to manage the split-second timing required to 'catch' the board effectively as it moves down.

As the diver drops back to the board to prepare for landing, both lower extremities are together. By the time contact is made, the ankles are dorsiflexed and the knees and hips are flexed (Fig. 16.4). This precontact joint flexion can serve two purposes. First, it extends the duration of hurdle flight allowing the board more time to complete its oscillations so that the diver can catch it when it is moving down. Second, it may increase joint stiffness on landing, so limiting the amount of energy-absorbing flexion at the beginning of the takeoff.

Takeoffs

The importance of the takeoff phase in both springboard and platform dives cannot be overemphasized. In less than half a second, competitors must produce sufficient vertical momentum for the flight of the dive; adequate horizontal momentum to clear the takeoff surface; and enough angular momentum to execute the required number of twists and/or somersaults. It is not the diver's position at last contact with the takeoff surface that determines the relative success of the dive but rather the magnitude and direction of the forces that have been applied throughout the takeoff period.

The production of linear and angular motion for the flight of the dive can be approached from the standpoints of direct or inverse dynamics. These represent two sides of the same equation (i.e. two sides of the same coin). In the case of straight-line motion or translation, linear impulse (the influence of the resultant force acting over a designated time) equals the change in linear momentum (quantity of

linear motion) over that same time period. In the case of rotation, angular impulse with respect to the CG is equal to the change in angular momentum with respect to the CG. Angular impulse represents the influence of the resultant torque or moment of force acting over a designated time period. Angular momentum indicates the quantity of angular motion.

Since reaction force data are available for platform takeoffs, the direct route will be travelled in the discussion of platform takeoffs. For springboard takeoffs, inverse dynamics will be used in examining individual segment contributions to changes in momentum.

Springboard

DEPRESSION

When the board is depressed during the support phase of the takeoff (as well as the hurdle), elastic strain energy is stored in the board (Sanders & Wilson 1988). This is similar to what happens when a spring is compressed. The amount of energy stored depends upon the stiffness of the spring/board and how much it is compressed or depressed. Much of the energy stored in the springboard at maximum depression should be available to help project the diver up into the flight of the dive (or the hurdle).

Assuming the diver can catch the board effectively, the higher the hurdle, the greater the diver's downward velocity on contact with the board and the more kinetic energy that can be transferred to the board to aid in its depression. This is, however, only a part of the picture (Lanoue 1936; Sanders & Wilson 1988). The fact that there is a substantial increase in the magnitude of the vertical velocity between the beginning and end of the takeoff indicates that the diver is interacting with the board during the takeoff. Consequently, the board tip is depressed further than would be possible as the result of kinetic energy contributed by the hurdle. Male medallists at the 1996 Olympic Games increased the magnitude of their vertical velocity in absolute terms by approximately $2 \, \text{m} \cdot \text{s}^{-1}$ from the beginning to the end of the takeoff. For example, Mark

Lenzi changed his vertical velocity from -4.0 m · s^{-1} to 5.9 m · s^{-1} for his 307C and from -2.3 m · s^{-1} to 4.5 m · s^{-1} for his 405B. It should also be noted that the diver has already started to move up when the board tip reaches its maximum deflection.

To supplement board depression resulting from the diver's kinetic energy at the beginning of the takeoff, divers employ their knee extension, trunk rotation and armswing to accelerate upwards with respect to the board. Because the board is compliant, this relative acceleration assists in pushing the board down. Divers have a definitive period of upward acceleration with respect to the board during the initial half of springboard depression (Miller & Munro 1984; Sanders & Wilson 1988).

The contribution of the upper extremities to board deflection appears to be small (~10%). It generally occurs within the first half to two-thirds of the springboard depression phase when the upper extremities accelerate up with respect to the shoulders (Miller & Munro 1984). This relative upward acceleration occurs as a result of the arms slowing their downward velocity at the end of the downswing and then increasing their upward velocity at the beginning of the upswing (Fig. 16.5). The arms therefore push down against the shoulders during this period. If the diver is in contact with the board and the segment link system of the diver's body is sufficiently rigid, this relative arm force will be transmitted down through the body to help depress the diving board (Sprigings *et al.* 1987).

The lower extremities account for approximately 75% of the initial relative vertical acceleration, in no small measure due to the fact that they accelerate the large mass of the trunk. Examination of reverse dives pike (301B) executed by semifinalists in the 1996 Olympics (Miller 1998), however, suggests that this initial relative upward acceleration may be related to the board tip's continued downward acceleration immediately after contact by the diver. Therefore, the initial relative acceleration is necessarily high and may be less important than what occurs when the board approaches its maximum deflection.

The 301B analysis (Miller 1998) indicated that, following a brief period of continued lower extremity joint flexion after contacting the board, the majority of male divers and many of the top female divers employed a two-phase pattern of knee extension to aid in depressing the board (Fig. 16.6). This two-phase extension pattern was also evident in dives from the back group and was used by a number of

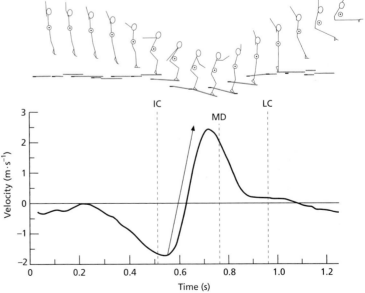

Fig. 16.5 Relative vertical velocity of the centre of gravity of the upper extremities with respect to the shoulders during the performance of a 301B by 1992 and 1996 Olympic silver medallist, Irina Lashko. The arrow indicates the region of upward acceleration of the upper extremities with respect to the shoulders. IC, initial contact; MD, maximum board depression; and LC, last contact.

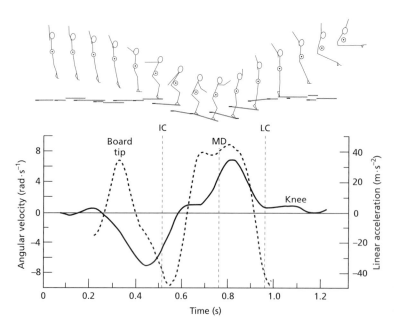

Fig. 16.6 Angular velocity of the knee joint and vertical acceleration of the board tip during the execution of a 301B by Irina Lashko. Positive angular velocity indicates knee extension, and negative angular velocity indicates knee flexion.

competitors in their execution of forward rotating dives. The slowing of the initial period of knee extension consistently occurred when the diving board tip began to accelerate up. This upward acceleration of the board tip indicated that the force exerted by the board as a function of its spring constant or stiffness and deflection had exceeded the downward force applied by the diver. Thus, at this point, the diver began to encounter noticeable resistance to deflecting the board tip. Consequently, the speed of knee extension slowed as evidenced by the reduced slope of the angular velocity against time curve for this joint. There followed an increase in knee angular velocity that continued through maximum depression of the springboard. In effect, these elite divers were pushing through maximum depression. This action should result in greater depression of the board or in keeping the board in a maximally or near maximally deflected position longer than otherwise would be the case.

RECOIL

It is during recoil of the springboard that ankle plantarflexion occurs and when most of the angular momentum necessary for the flight is generated.

The latter is evident in Fig. 16.7, which shows the total body angular momentum as a function of time for dives without limit from all four non-twisting groups performed by 1992 Olympic gold and 1996 Olympic bronze springboard medallist, Mark Lenzi. During dive preparation, there is little if any total body angular momentum with respect to the CG (Miller & Munro 1985b; Sanders & Wilson 1987). As the takeoff proceeds, the total body angular momentum is in the intended direction of rotation for almost the entire time for dives from the back and reverse groups since the rotational direction of the trunk and arms does not change. The most substantial increase, however, occurs just after the board begins to recoil. By contrast, in dives from the forward and inward group in which the direction of trunk rotation must be reversed, the direction of total body angular momentum does not become consistent with the direction of the somersault until after recoil of the board has begun.

Contributions of the lower extremities, upper extremities and trunk–head that sum to the total are illustrated in Fig. 16.8. In all four dive groups, angular momentum of the lower extremities continued to increase during the latter part of recoil right through

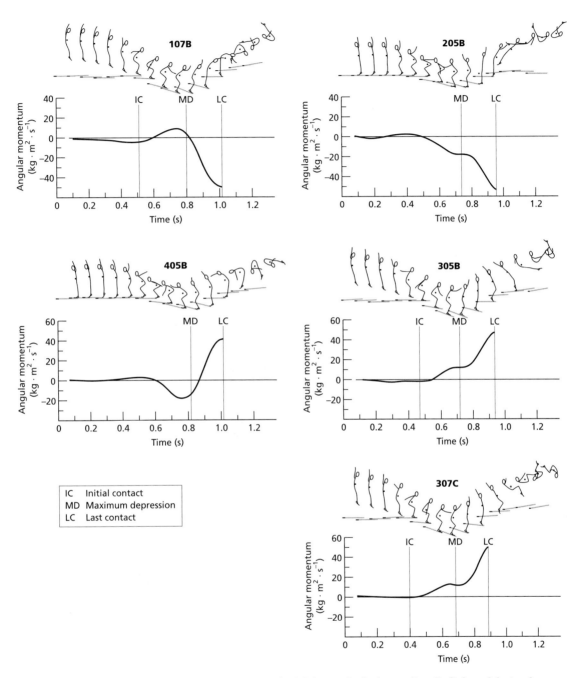

Fig. 16.7 Total body angular momentum with respect to the CG during the final part of hurdle flight and during the takeoff of springboard dives without limit performed by Mark Lenzi in the 1996 Olympics springboard finals.

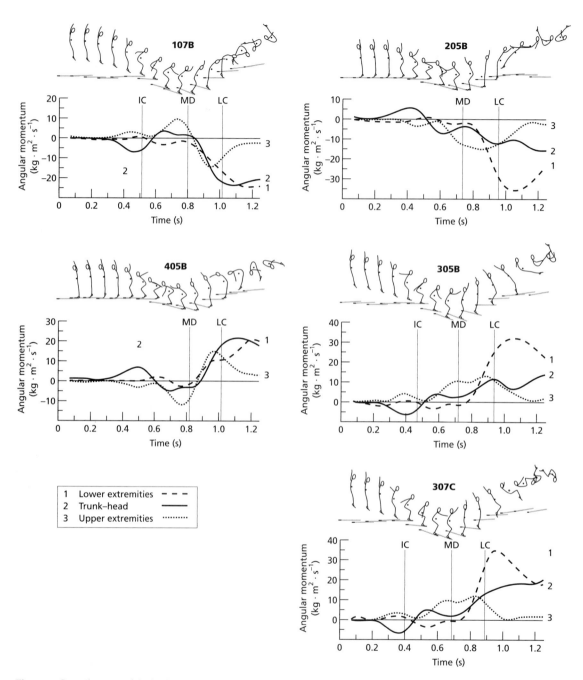

Fig. 16.8 Contributions of the body segments to angular momentum of the total body with respect to the CG at the end of hurdle flight, during the takeoff and at the start of dive flight for springboard dives performed by Mark Lenzi. Refer to Fig. 16.7 for the total angular momentum patterns for these dives.

the end of the takeoff. The fact that the upper extremities appear to be responsible for approximately 25–50% of the angular momentum at last contact with the board underlines the importance of a fast, reasonably straight armswing in the plane of the somersault during recoil in dives without limit (Miller & Munro 1985b).

Research by Golden (1981, 1984), in which he filmed the front (101B, 103B, 105B, 107B) and inward (401B, 403B, 405B) takeoffs, revealed similar patterns of somersault initiation. Dives from the inward group resembled those of the front group with one more somersault. Thus, the 401B and 103B were comparable, as were the 403B and 105B. Because of the increased speed of arm and trunk rotation in the direction of the somersault during recoil to build up the additional angular momentum required, divers assumed their pike position progressively earlier for each additional somersault that had to be performed during the flight. As a result, marked differences were evident in the diver's body position at last contact with the board. Golden confirmed that as the number of somersaults to be executed in flight increased, the diver's vertical velocity at the end of the takeoff decreased thereby reducing the dive height.

DURATION

The duration of running springboard takeoffs is generally less than half a second. Averages for 301B takeoffs of male and female competitors in the 1995 World Diving Cup and 1996 Olympic Games were 0.49 s and 0.44 s, respectively. During the finals of National Sports Festival V in 1983, Greg Louganis had a contact time of 0.49 s for his 301B. Louganis, diving from a Duraflex board less compliant than the Maxiflex currently in use, averaged takeoff times of 0.45 ± 0.1 s for dives with and without limit from the front and reverse groups (Miller & Munro 1985a). He spent $56 \pm 2\%$ of his takeoff time depressing the board.

It is not surprising that the time devoted to board depression exceeds that of recoil. To some extent in all dives, more energy is absorbed by divers during the recoil period. As they prepare for the required number of somersaults, divers tend to accelerate downwards with respect to the board. This 'unweighting', which permits the board to recoil faster, is even more marked when a takeoff is rushed. The accompanying absorption of energy from the board leads to a reduction in the diver's vertical velocity at the end of the takeoff (Miller & Munro 1985a).

Takeoff duration can also be influenced somewhat by fulcrum position. When the fulcrum is set further back (i.e. looser board, higher fulcrum numbers), divers will depress the board further and be in contact with the board longer. The increased duration of the takeoff may give them more time to complete the armswing and the trunk rotation needed to build up somersaulting angular momentum. However, with the softer board, the diver's knees will tend to flex more at the beginning of the takeoff before the diver experiences sufficient resistance from the board to begin knee extension (Jones & Miller 1996). If divers lack the strength to control this additional knee flexion, their knees may buckle.

Platform

Takeoff duration is considerably shorter for platform than springboard dives. For standing takeoffs, the time from the start of final upward acceleration until last contact with the platform is about a third of a second (Miller et al. 1989a, 1990). In running dives, contact time is approximately 0.15 s (Shapiro et al. 1993).

TRANSLATION

During the takeoff, the diver pushes against the platform and the platform pushes back or reacts with a force equal in magnitude but opposite in direction (Newton's Third Law). The force transmitted though the feet (or hands) to the platform (and responsible for generating the reaction force) depends on acceleration of all the diver's body segments, each contributing in proportion to its mass. Since muscles pulling across joints causing segments to rotate produce most of this acceleration, platform reaction force (PRF) has its basis in muscle force. The harder the diver pushes against the platform, the greater will be the PRF that acts through the centre of pressure (i.e. point of application) on the diver's feet or hands.

Unlike body weight, the magnitude and direction of the PRF do not remain constant during the take-off. Therefore, it is convenient to divide PRF into vertical and horizontal components so that the focus can be upon the change in magnitude in a given direction. The *vertical* component always acts in an upward direction. It is responsible for the diver's vertical velocity and ultimately for the height of the dive and its flight duration. The *horizontal* PRF contribution can be subdivided into one component directed forwards or back and another side-to-side. All platform takeoffs will have the *forward–back* component. In standing and armstand dives, it will be directed primarily away from the platform in a propulsive direction since it is responsible for generating sufficient horizontal velocity to carry the diver safely away from the edge of the platform during the flight. In running dives, this component will be directed predominantly back towards the base of the tower in a braking direction to slow the diver's forward momentum and promote forward somersaulting angular momentum. Twisting dives from the back, reverse and armstand groups as well as dives with asymmetrical takeoff actions resulting from bilateral differences in anatomical structure, injury, or technique may also elicit a significant *side-to-side* component of PRF (Miller *et al.* 1989b).

Characteristic vertical and horizontal PRF–time histories exerted in standing takeoffs of dives with and without limit as executed by 1984 and 1988 double Olympic gold medallist Greg Louganis are illustrated in Fig. 16.9. It is convenient to describe these platform reaction patterns with reference to weight since such divisions have functional significance with respect to the performance (Miller *et al.* 1989a). As described earlier in relation to standing dive preparation on platform, when the vertical PRF exceeds the magnitude of body weight, vertical acceleration must be positive or upward. During this period, termed weighting, vertical velocity increases. When the vertical PRF is less than body weight, referred to as unweighting, vertical acceleration is negative and vertical velocity decreases.

At the start of standing dives, the vertical component of PRF is equal to the diver's body weight just as if the diver were standing on a set of weight scales. Body weight magnitude is indicated by the horizontal dashed line in each of the force records shown in Fig. 16.9. The vertical PRF may then briefly move slightly above and/or below the body weight value. Next follows an unmistakable period of unweighting when by definition the vertical PRF is less than body weight as the result of the diver's downward acceleration. Most of this period is associated with the diver's CG dropping towards the platform.

As the downward velocity slows and the diver begins to move in an upward direction, both of which cause upward or positive acceleration, the vertical PRF increases rapidly above body weight. This final weighting phase is marked by a maximum force that is several times greater than the diver's body weight. During takeoffs for dives from the back and reverse groups, the maximum vertical PRF is between three and four times body weight (Miller *et al.* 1989a, 1990; Shapiro *et al.* 1993). The region of the highest vertical PRF coincides with the diver's lowest body position when the diver's velocity is changing direction from down to up. Eccentric hip and knee extensor muscle activity must therefore play an important role in the generation of the vertical PRF for the first third to half of the major weighting phase. It is during final weighting that vertical momentum required for the flight is developed. It is also during final weighting when most of the horizontal momentum and angular momentum are generated for the flight of the dive (Miller *et al.* 1989a, 1990).

The diver's highest vertical velocity coincides with the point at which the vertical PRF equals body weight as it drops towards zero signifying the start of flight. During the very brief final unweighting phase when the vertical PRF is less than body weight and the diver's vertical acceleration is therefore negative, the vertical velocity of the diver's CG decreases slightly.

The takeoff time for executing inward somersaults from the platform is the shortest of any of the standing dives. To partially compensate, the vertical PRF reaches maximum values of approximately five to six times body weight (Shapiro *et al.* 1993). In spite of the higher force, the vertical impulse (area

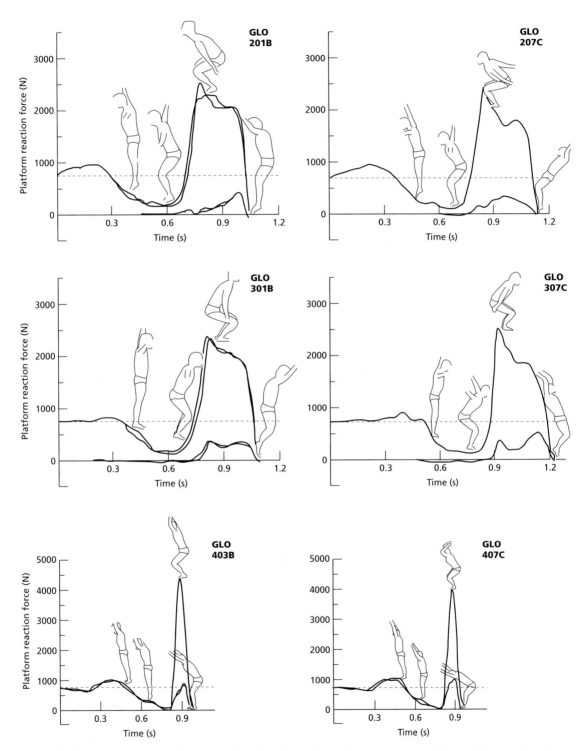

Fig. 16.9 Vertical and horizontal platform reaction force–time histories for back, reverse and inward dives performed by Greg Louganis in the 1986 World Championships. Double lines indicate that the records for the preliminary and final rounds have been superimposed.

Table 16.1 Maximum platform reaction force (body weights) and change in CG velocity during Greg Louganis' 10 m takeoffs in the 1986 World Diving Championships.

Dive	Round	Score	Max. reaction force (BW)		Change in velocity (m · s⁻¹)*	
			Horizontal	Vertical	Horizontal	Vertical
113B†	Final	8.9	−1.8	9.1	−1.0	4.9
107B†	Final	8.9	−1.8	7.9	−0.9	4.4
201B	Prelim.	7.9	0.5	3.2	0.6	3.9
207C	Prelim.	8.5	0.4	3.4	0.9	3.2
301B	Prelim.	8.3	0.4	3.3	0.9	3.3
307C	Final	8.6	0.6	3.5	1.0	2.6
403B	Prelim.	8.9	1.1	6.0	0.9	2.5
407C	Final	7.1	1.4	5.5	1.1	1.5

* For dives with standing takeoffs, the change in velocity corresponds closely to the velocity at last contact with the platform.
† Running dive.

between the force curve and the zero line) is less than achieved in back and reverse takeoffs (Table 16.1). Consequently, the diver's upward velocity at the start of the flight for platform dives from the inward group is also notably less.

During the brief time interval associated with running takeoffs, the vertical PRF either directly or following an impact peak reaches a maximum of approximately six times body weight before falling back to zero. The horizontal component of PRF is also higher than in standing takeoffs, with peaks ranging from 1.5 to 5 times body weight being reported (Shapiro *et al.* 1993). While the horizontal (braking) PRF continues to slow the diver's forward motion during almost if not all of the takeoff, the diver still has more horizontal velocity at the end of the takeoff in running (~1.7 m · s⁻¹) than in standing dives (~1.0 m · s⁻¹).

ROTATION

Although horizontal and vertical translation are necessary for the flight of a dive, the essence of the performance lies in the somersaults and/or twists that are executed as the diver's CG follows its predetermined parabolic flight path. Consequently, the way in which the PRF acts upon the diver during the takeoff to influence angular momentum with respect to the diver's CG must be taken into consid-

eration. Whether the PRF tends to produce somersaulting angular momentum in one direction or the other (if at all) depends entirely on its line of action with respect to the CG. If it passes directly through the CG (as frequently occurs during the early part of the takeoff), it (like the weight) will have zero moment of force or torque and will not be able to produce any change in angular momentum with respect to the CG. The line of action of the PRF must pass at some distance from the CG if it is to have an influence on rotation. The perpendicular distance from the CG to the line of action of the force is known as the moment arm. The moment of force, or torque, is the product of the magnitude of the force and its moment arm. Consequently, the larger the force and/or the longer the moment arm, the more the diver's angular momentum will be changed.

During most platform takeoffs, although the line of action of the PRF may pass first on one side of the CG and then on the other, there will be a predominant pattern that is consistent with building up angular momentum in the direction of the somersault to be executed. Overall, the moment of force or torque produced by the PRF must promote rotation in the direction of the somersault. For dives from the back and reverse groups, the line of action of the PRF must pass in front of the CG throughout most of the takeoff. For dives from the front and inward groups, it must pass behind the CG (Fig. 16.10).

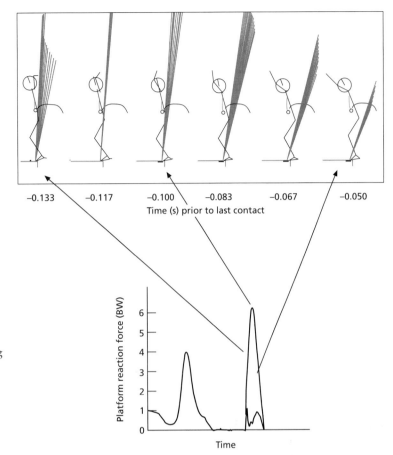

Fig. 16.10 Platform reaction force during an inward takeoff. During the final weighting phase of 1992 and 1996 Olympic gold medallist Fu Mingxia's 407C takeoff, the line of action of the PRF passes behind her CG promoting inward somersaulting angular momentum. The curve line behind the CG indicates its path in the initial stages of flight. On the PRF record (below), the horizontal component is substantially smaller than the vertical and is most noticeable during final weighting.

As in springboard dives, angular momentum with respect to CG at last contact in the takeoff of platform dives is positively related to the number of somersaults being executed. Everything else being equal, the greater the number of somersaults, the larger the angular momentum. In a comparison of takeoffs for dives from the first four groups performed in the pike position and involving progressively increasing numbers of somersaults, Hamill *et al.* (1986) found that the maximum angular momentum contribution of the upper extremities and lower extremities occurred at the end of the takeoff. With the exception of the front dive pike, the angular momentum of the upper extremities exceeded that of the lower extremities and accounted for roughly half the total angular momentum by this point in the takeoff. As the number of rotations to be executed in flight increased, the percentage of angular momentum contributed by the upper extremities decreased although it continued to exceed that of the lower extremities. The important role of the armswing in generating angular momentum for the flight was clear.

When the diver's position is inverted in armstand takeoffs, it is the lower extremities that must take the leading role in generating angular momentum for the flight. For example, at last contact with the platform in the takeoff for the reverse triple somersault tuck (636C), Dmitry Sautin's lower extremities accounted for 75% of the total angular momentum with respect to the CG (Murtaugh & Miller 1998).

Crowhop

Careful examination of vertical platform reaction force–time histories during takeoffs for inward somersaulting dives reveals that many divers actually lose contact with the platform during the major unweighting phase of the takeoff. This is evidenced by the fact that the platform reaction force goes to zero as the divers drop from their extended preparatory position. It is extremely difficult if not impossible for a judge sitting on an elevated chair on the deck to see this loss of contact. When it occurs during a 3 m springboard takeoff, however, it is more evident.

It would seem logical to assume that this loss of contact between the feet and the takeoff surface, known as a crowhop, would provide an advantage. In the past, however, divers using this technique were seldom penalized by the officials. Although rule D.1.8 in the FINA 1988–92 Handbook stated that 'When executing a standing dive, the diver must not bounce on the board before the take-off or the referee shall declare it a failed dive', few referees were willing to classify the crowhop as a double bounce and make such a call in international competition. Another rule (D.6.2) indicated 'where a diver, preparing for a backward take-off, lifts his feet slightly off the board, that shall not be considered a bounce, but an involuntary movement, and each judge shall deduct from his award according to his individual opinion' and provided considerable leeway for the judges. Consequently, in 1992 an investigation was undertaken to document potential advantages furnished by the crowhop to provide a scientific basis for changes in the FINA rules governing standing springboard takeoffs.

An analysis of 3 m springboard back and inward takeoffs performed by 65 women in international competition between 1989 and 1992 showed that the crowhop was a well-established pattern employed by certain divers in all their standing takeoffs (Miller 1994, 1995). Not unexpectedly, divers employing this technique had significantly greater downward velocities at the beginning of springboard depression resulting in increased kinetic energy available to transfer to the board to aid in its depression. Further, divers who crowhopped did not damp the activation of the board immediately prior to final depression in the takeoff as was the case with divers who maintained contact with the board. Finally, there was an over-representation of divers employing the crowhop in dives with the highest DDs, namely the back $2\frac{1}{2}$ pike (205B) and the inward $2\frac{1}{2}$ pike (405B). Therefore, it appeared that divers were able to do more difficult dives if they used a crowhop at the start of their takeoffs.

After several years of discussion on this issue, the Technical Diving Committee of FINA modified the rules regarding standing springboard takeoffs. Currently, Rule D.6.3.4 in the 1998–2000 FINA Handbook indicates 'When executing a standing dive the diver must not bounce on the board or platform before the take-off or the referee shall declare a maximum of $4\frac{1}{2}$ points.' And Rule D.3.5 further states that 'When a diver, when executing a standing dive, lifts his feet slightly off the board or platform, each judge shall deduct one or two points from his award according to his individual opinion.' These rules should now make it easier to deal with divers who might otherwise gain an unfair advantage through the inclusion of a crowhop in their standing takeoffs.

Flight

For all practical purposes, air resistance is negligible in springboard diving. It is also frequently ignored in platform competitions although it may have an influence on performance under windy conditions. During the flight of a dive (when air resistance is neglected), the only external force acting on the diver is the body weight directed down from the CG. Consequently, the diver's horizontal velocity remains constant. The vertical velocity becomes progressively less, decreasing from positive at last contact with the takeoff surface to zero at the peak of the flight. It then becomes more and more negative until the diver contacts the water for the entry. As a result, the trajectory followed by the CG in flight is parabolic.

Velocities at the start of dive flight are higher for springboard than platform dives and for running than standing dives (Tables 16.1 & 16.2). Everything else being equal, dives requiring fewer somersaults will have larger vertical velocities when leaving the

Table 16.2 Vertical velocities (m · s⁻¹) of the centre of gravity at the beginning of flight of non-twisting springboard dives without limit of five male divers placed in the top eight in the 1996 Olympics.

Dive	Diver				
	ZYU	MLE	SDO	MMU	FPL
107B	5.7	5.7	5.2	5.2	5.4
305B	5.7	5.7	5.0	5.8	5.6
307C	5.8	5.9	–	–	5.7
205B	4.9	4.8	4.5	4.4	4.6
405B	–	4.5	3.9	4.0	3.9
407C	4.7	–	–	–	–

takeoff surface and consequently will go higher. Likewise the same dive performed under identical conditions in a tuck position will achieve greater height than when done in the pike position, and a dive performed in pike in turn will be higher than if it were executed in a straight position. In general, the vertical velocities of women at the beginning of flight of springboard dives are approximately 1.0 m · s⁻¹ less than those of their male counterparts performing the same dives (Miller 1981). Horizontal velocities for both springboard and standing platform dives during flight tend to vary from approximately 0.7 m · s⁻¹ to 1.2 m · s⁻¹.

Again, assuming air resistance is negligible, the angular momentum (i.e. quantity of angular motion) of the diver with respect to the CG remains constant throughout the flight as the diver rotates about an axis through the CG. While the speed of the somersault or twist (i.e. angular velocity) can be increased by bringing the body segments closer to the axis of rotation (i.e. reducing the moment of inertia), the magnitude and direction of the angular momentum with respect to the CG remains constant (Frohlich 1979, 1980; Kuipers 1987). Likewise, the speed of the somersault can be decreased by moving from a tuck to a pike position or from a pike to a straight position, but the total angular momentum is not changed.

At the beginning of flight, considerable effort is required to assume and hold a compact tuck or a tight pike position. The greater the angular velocity, the greater the force required. Although the vertical velocity and magnitude of the angular momentum with respect to the CG for 2½ pike and 3½ tuck dives are comparable (for a given diver and dive group; cf. Table 16.2 and Fig. 16.7), the force necessary to maintain a compact body position during flight is significantly higher in the latter case. Data from medallists in the 1996 Olympics men's springboard competition indicate that a maximum centripetal force equivalent to two additional body weights (BW) is required to hold the quasi-rigid position during the 3½ tuck (~6–7 BW compared with ~4–5 BW). This may be a key factor in a diver's ability to execute higher DD dives that have additional rotational requirements.

Additional details concerning the mechanics of the human body somersaulting and twisting in flight can be found in Chapter 13.

Entries

Although divers may enter the water either feet or head first, the latter is much more common. There is little question that the entry makes a lasting impression upon spectators and judges alike. Since divers strike the water at speeds in excess of 50 km · h⁻¹ from the 10 m platform and in the neighbourhood of 30 km · h⁻¹ from the 3 m springboard, safety as well as performance factors must be taken into consideration during this final phase of the dive.

Divers strive to 'rip' their entries, disappearing beneath the water with a minimum of splash to the accompaniment of a characteristic ripping sound. According to Brown (1982), who has carried out the most definitive work in this area, the rip technique was first identified by US divers performing armstand cut-through dives from the platform. When they flattened their feet immediately prior to contacting the water, the surface of the water was disturbed but the usual accompanying splash was minimized or eliminated. Prominent among divers who perfected and popularized the rip entry was Klaus DiBiasi from Italy. DiBiasi won Olympic silver in 1968 and gold in 1972 and 1976 for his 10 m performances.

Brown and colleagues (Brown & Abraham 1981, 1983; Brown et al. 1984) described the fixed sequence of events that occur as a result of the diver's entry into the water. As the diver contacts the water and passes through the free surface, a cavity is created and an air–water mixture is dragged down with the diver. Since the diver's velocity is high, the velocity of the air–water mixture in the diver's wake will be considerably higher than that of the surrounding water. In accordance with Bernouilli's Principle (i.e. high velocity associated with low pressure and vice versa), the cavity produced by the diver's entry will be a region of low pressure. According to Brown *et al.* (1984), the density of the air–water mixture comprising the cavity and the velocity of its leading edge will influence the up-jet of water accompanying surface closure. They suggested that turbulence in the cavity may cushion the closing and thereby lessen the up-jet. They also speculated that the up-jet, which is significantly lower and of shorter duration in rip entries, could be the result of early surface closure. Following the up-jet, cavity turbulence returns to the surface resulting in seething. A late splash that sometimes occurs in conjunction with this seething would seem to come too late to influence the judge's award (Brown & Abraham 1981). Judges focus on the water for only about 1.6 s after the appearance of the initial splash (i.e. up-jet). By the time any late splash appears, the award has been entered and the judges are no longer attending to the entry point.

To facilitate rip entries that earn the highest scores, divers currently employ a 'flat-hand' technique (Fig. 16.11). The fingers and wrists are extended, and forearms rotated inwards with the hands grasping one on top of the other so that the palms are towards the water (le Viet *et al.* 1993). Divers also tend to 'swim' their entries moving their arms laterally or in front once their hands penetrate the water. The swim is often followed by a somersaulting or a scooping action (Brown *et al.* 1984; Carter 1986). Both the flat-hand and early swim techniques have been suggested as possible causative factors in shoulder and wrist injuries experienced by platform divers.

The magnitude of the force encountered upon entry depends upon the diver's velocity just prior to contact with the water and how quickly that velocity is reduced as the diver passes below the surface. Rapid deceleration associated with a flat body entry

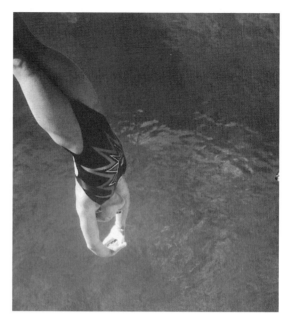

Fig. 16.11 The flat hand position in preparation for entry is shown by Jenny Keim, 1996 Olympic springboard finalist. (Photo courtesy of Ken Redmond.)

results in a much higher force than the more gradual reduction in velocity accompanying an entry in which the body is well aligned and slips through the break in the water's surface made by the hands or feet. Even in the case of these so-called 'clean' entries, however, maximum forces appear to be in the range of 16–25 times body weight for 10 m platform dives (Stevenson 1985).

It is important to recognize that the diver's rotational motion does not stop when the hands (or feet, in the case of foot-first entries) contact the water. The remainder of the body continues in the direction of the somersault. This motion has the potential for creating whiplash if the trunk and hips are not stabilized through muscle contraction. In addition, the whipping action creates splash, detracting from the aesthetics of the entry and reducing the award for the dive. The extent to which somersaulting velocity is altered on entry will determine whether the diver's path beneath the surface is vertical or angled forwards or backwards (Brown & Abraham 1983).

Considering that platform divers execute 24–30 dives from 10 m for two to three days each week, making a career total averaging over 29 000 entries (Anderson *et al.* 1993), the importance of developing and employing an entry technique that is both safe and effective is evident. In addition to the necessity of statically contracting the muscles of the trunk during entry, the upper extremities must also be stabilized to prevent the hands being driven back against the head and possibly resulting in shoulder dislocation. Although judges are not to consider what the diver does beneath the surface when making their awards, the underwater movements have a definite influence on the appearance of the entry, the subsequent splash or absence thereof, and the potential for developing acute or chronic injury of the upper extremities or spinal column.

Acknowledgements

The author is indebted to United States Diving for its continuing support for research into the biomechanical aspects of diving. Much of the information included in this chapter will be found in a more extensive form in the upcoming U.S. Diving publication, *Biomechanics of Competitive Diving*. Appreciation is also expressed to the Medical Commission of the IOC for its sponsorship of diving biomechanics projects at the 1996 Olympic Games.

References

Anderson, S.J., Gerard, B. & Ziatkin, M. (1993) Cervical spine problems in competitive divers. In: *US Diving Sport Science Seminar 1993 Proceedings* (eds R. Malina & J.L. Gabriel), pp. 144–157. United States Diving Publications, Indianapolis, IN.

Boda, W.L. (1992) Modelling the springboard and diver as an oscillating spring system. PhD thesis, University of Massachusetts.

Brown, J.G. (1982) Biomechanical analysis of the rip entry in competitive diving. MA thesis, University of Texas at Austin.

Brown, J.G. & Abraham, L.D. (1981) Characteristics of entries in competitive diving. In: *Proceedings of the 1981 United States Diving Sport Sciences Seminar* (ed. D. Golden), pp. 109–117. United States Diving Publications, Indianapolis, IN.

Brown, J.G. & Abraham, L.D. (1983) The role of whip in rip entries. In: *Proceedings of the 1983 United States Diving Sport Sciences Seminar* (ed. D. Golden), pp. 3–14. United States Diving Publications, Indianapolis, IN.

Brown, J.G., Abraham, L.D. & Bertin, J.J. (1984) Descriptive analysis of the rip entry in competitive diving. *Research Quarterly for Exercise and Sport* **55**, 93–102.

Carter, R.L. (1986) Prevention of springboard and platform diving injuries. *Clinics in Sports Medicine* **5**, 185–194.

Darda, G.E. (1972) A method of determining the relative contributions of the diver and springboard to the vertical ascent of the forward three and one-half somersaults tuck. PhD thesis, University of Wisconsin.

Eaves, G. (1969) *Diving. The Mechanics of Springboard and Firmboard Techniques.* Kaye & Ward, London.

Frohlich, C. (1979) Do springboard divers violate angular momentum conservation? *American Journal of Physics* **47**, 583–592.

Frohlich, C. (1980) The physics of somersaulting and twisting. *Scientific American* **242** (3), 154–164.

Golden, D. (1981) Kinematics of increasing rotation in springboard diving. In: *Proceedings of the 1981 United States Diving Sports Science Seminar* (ed. D. Golden), pp. 55–81. United States Diving Publications, Indianapolis, IN.

Golden, D.M. (1984) A comparison of the translational and rotational kinematics of increasing rotation in springboard diving. PhD thesis, Southern Illinois University.

Hamill, J., Ricard, M.D. & Golden, D.M. (1986) Angular momentum in multiple rotation nontwisting platform dives. *International Journal of Sport Biomechanics* **2**, 78–87.

Henry, B. & Yeomans, P.H. (1984) *An Approved History of the Olympic Games.* Alfred Publishing, Sherman Oaks, CA.

Jones, I.C. & Miller, D.I. (1996) Influence of fulcrum position on springboard response and takeoff performance in the running approach. *Journal of Applied Biomechanics* **12**, 383–403.

Kooi, B.W. & Kuipers, M. (1994) The dynamics of springboards. *Journal of Applied Biomechanics* **10**, 335–351.

Kuipers, M. (1987) A note on somersaulting and twisting. *Journal of Engineering Mathematics* **21**, 253–260.

Kuipers, M. & Van de Ven, A.A.F. (1992) Unilateral contact of a springboard and a fulcrum. *Transactions of the American Society of Mechanical Engineers* **59**, 682–684.

Lanoue, F. (1936) Mechanics of fancy diving. Master of Education thesis, Springfield College, Springfield, MA.

McFarland, S. (1997–98) Thanks a million. *Inside USA Diving* **5** (4), 3, 11.

McNitt-Gray, J.L. & Anderson, D.D. (1993) Balance control strategies of collegiate divers during the take-off phase of platform dives. In: *US Diving Sport Science Seminar Proceedings* (eds R. Malina & J.L. Gabriel), pp. 121–128. United States Diving Publications, Indianapolis, IN.

Miller, D.I. (1981) Body segment contributions of female athletes to translational and rotational requirements of nontwisting springboard dive takeoffs. In: *The Female Athlete. A Socio-Psychological and Kinanthropometric Approach* (eds J. Borms, M. Hebbelinck & A. Venerando), pp. 206–215. Karger, Basle.

Miller, D.I. (1984) Biomechanical characteristics of the final approach step, hurdle and take-off of elite American springboard divers. *Journal of Human Movement Studies* **10**, 189–212.

Miller, D.I. (1994) The crowhop: technique fault or unfair advantage. *Journal of Biomechanics* **17**, 597 (abstract).

Miller, D.I. (1995) The crowhop: nature, extent and significance. *Inside USA Diving* **3** (1), 20–21.

Miller, D.I. (1998) Pushing through maximum depression to increase springboard dive height. In: *Proceedings of NACOB '98*, pp. 443–444. University of Waterloo, Ontario.

Miller, D.I. & Jones, I.C. (1999) Characteristics of Maxiflex springboards revisited. *Research Quarterly for Exercise and Sport* **70**, 395–400.

Miller, D.I. & Munro, C.F. (1984) Body segment contributions to height achieved during the flight of a springboard dive. *Medicine and Science in Sports and Exercise* **16**, 234–242.

Miller, D.I. & Munro, C.F. (1985a) Greg Louganis' springboard takeoff: I. Temporal and joint position analysis. *Journal of Sport Biomechanics* **1**, 209–220.

Miller, D.I. & Munro, C.F. (1985b) Greg Louganis' springboard takeoff: II. Linear and angular momentum considerations. *Journal of Sport Biomechanics* **1**, 288–307.

Miller, D.I., Hennig, E., Pizzimenti, M.A., Jones, I.C. & Nelson, R.C. (1989a) Kinetic and kinematic characteristics of 10-m platform performances of elite divers: I. Back takeoffs. *International Journal of Sport Biomechanics* **5**, 60–88.

Miller, D.I., Pizzimenti, M.A. & Jones, I.C. (1989b) Taking off: biomechanics research applied to elite diving performance. In: *Proceedings of the First IOC World Congress on Sport Sciences*, pp. 249–253. U.S. Olympic Committee, Colorado Springs.

Miller, D.I., Jones, I.C., Pizzimenti, M.A., Hennig, E. & Nelson, R.C. (1990) Kinetic and kinematic characteristics of 10-m platform performances of elite divers: II. Reverse takeoffs. *International Journal of Sport Biomechanics* **6**, 283–308.

Miller, D.I., Osborne, M.J. & Jones, I.C. (1998) Springboard oscillation during hurdle flight. *Journal of Sports Sciences* **16**, 571–583.

Murtaugh, K. & Miller, D.I. (1998) The golden armstand. In: *Proceedings of NACOB '98*, pp. 449–450. University of Waterloo, Ontario.

Sanders, R.H. & Wilson, B.D. (1987) Angular momentum requirements of the twisting and nontwisting forward 1 1/2 somersault dive. *International Journal of Sport Biomechanics* **3**, 47–62.

Sanders, R.H. & Wilson, B.D. (1988) Factors contributing to maximum height of dives after takeoff from the 3m spring-board. *International Journal of Sport Biomechanics* **4**, 231–259.

Shapiro, R., Stine, R.I., Oeffinger, D., Horstman, B. & Keller, L. (1993) Investigation of selected kinetic parameters of 10 meter platform diving performance. In: *US Diving Sport Science Seminar Proceedings* (eds R. Malina & J.L. Gabriel), pp. 80–91. United States Diving Publications, Indianapolis, IN.

Slobounov, S.M. & Newell, K.M. (1996) Postural dynamics in upright and inverted stances. *Journal of Applied Biomechanics* **12**, 185–196.

Sprigings, E.J., Paquette, S.E. & Watson, L.G. (1987) Consistency of the relative vertical acceleration patterns of a diver's armswing. *Journal of Human Movement Studies* **13**, 75–84.

Sprigings, E.J., Stilling, D.S. & Watson, L.G. (1989) Development of a model to represent an aluminum springboard in diving. *International Journal of Sport Biomechanics* **5**, 297–307.

Sprigings, E.J., Stilling, D.S., Watson, L.G. & Dorotich, P.D. (1990) Measurement of the modeling parameters for a Maxiflex 'B' springboard. *International Journal of Sport Biomechanics* **6**, 325–335.

Stevenson, J.M. (1985) The impact force of entry in diving from a ten-meter tower. In: *Biomechanics IX-B* (eds D.A. Winter, R.W. Norman, R.P. Wells, K.C. Hayes & A.E. Patla), pp. 106–111. Human Kinetics Publishers, Champaign, IL.

Stilling, D.S. (1989) Improving springboard diving through biomechanical analyses and knowledge based expert system application. Master of Science thesis, University of Saskatchewan.

le Viet, D.T., Lantieri, L.A. & Loy, S.M. (1993) Wrist and hand injuries in platform diving. *Journal of Hand Surgery* **18A**, 876–880.

Chapter 17

Determinants of Successful Ski-Jumping Performance

P.V. KOMI AND M. VIRMAVIRTA

Introduction

Ski-jumping is an exciting sport requiring complex skills and involving several phases—inrun, takeoff, flight and preparation for landing—each of which has importance to the length of the jump. In general the performance includes both ballistic and aerodynamic factors (Fig. 17.1). The ballistic factors include release velocity and release position from the takeoff table, whereas aerodynamic factors during takeoff and flight influence the gliding properties of the jumper/ski system (velocity, suit design, surface area, posture of the jumper/ski system, turbulence, and resisting and lifting forces). It is important to realize that both ballistic and aerodynamic factors place special demands on the jumper so that he can optimally maximize the vertical lift and minimize the drag forces.

Takeoff is probably the most crucial phase for the entire ski-jumping performance. The purpose of the takeoff is to increase the vertical lift and simultaneously maintain or even increase the horizontal release velocity. It is therefore important to emphasize that it is the jumper and his or her ability to perform a skilful takeoff and the subsequent flight phase, which finally determines the length of the jump. For this reason great demand is placed on the jumper's neuromuscular system, especially because of the unusually short time available for execution of the takeoff.

This chapter makes an attempt to review factors that are involved in ski-jumping performance.

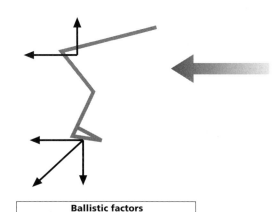

Aerodynamic factors
• Gliding properties of the jumper/skis system (e.g. resisting and lifting aerodynamic forces)

Ballistic factors
• Velocity, position of the jumper at the release instant from the takeoff table

Fig. 17.1 Schematic illustration of the aerodynamic and ballistic features influencing ski-jumping performance.

Special effort will be made to characterize the takeoff action and link this to the relevant neuromuscular functions of the jumper. Techniques of measurement of the actual takeoff forces have improved considerably during the last two decades. These aspects are also described, both methodologically and also with respect to the neuromuscular requirements and especially how

349

they are related to the length of the jump. Integration of muscle activation patterns with the takeoff technique is also relevant for an understanding of ski-jumping performance. The present review is a follow-up of a previous article on the same topic (Komi & Virmavirta 1997).

Characteristics of the takeoff performance

Ski-jumping takeoff is performed from a crouch position (Fig. 17.2) during a very short time, ranging from 0.25 to 0.30 s (Komi *et al.* 1974b; Schwameder & Müller 1995). This time period covers, on average, 7.1 m from the takeoff table. Thus the first takeoff movements are initiated during the transition phase from the end of the inrun curve to the flat table. This phase is crucial for the timing and coordination of the movements due to sudden disappearance of the centrifugal force at the end of the inrun curve. Kinematically the rapid takeoff movement can then be characterized by changes in two major angles: hip and knee. The hip angle displacement is, on average, from 40° to 140° (Arndt *et al.* 1995; Schwameder & Müller 1995), emphasizing that the hip extension continues in the air after the takeoff edge has been passed (Fig. 17.2). Similarly knee joint extension (from 70° to 140°) is not completed while on the takeoff table. However, the knee extension velocity reaches a very high

value of over 12 rad · s⁻¹ (Virmavirta & Komi 1993b), which is usually reached a few milliseconds before passing the takeoff edge. In an optimal takeoff the hip extension velocity is also relatively high (≈10 rad · s⁻¹) (Virmavirta & Komi 1994), which is caused mainly by the thigh movement but with a smaller upper body extension (Arndt *et al.* 1995). Thus the upper body is maintained in a lower position to reduce the drag forces (Virmavirta & Komi 1993a). This adds to the lift forces with a resulting reduction in the load for the extension movement. According to the force–velocity relationships of the muscle the light load can be moved with higher movement velocity (Wilkie 1950; Komi 1973). The knee extension velocity is reportedly the highest correlating factor of all takeoff parameters to the distance jumped (Arndt *et al.* 1995). The powerful knee extension movement results therefore in a surprisingly high vertical velocity (V_v, normal to the takeoff table) of the centre of mass of the jumper/ski system. Velocities in the range 2.3–3.2 m · s⁻¹ are not unusual (Komi *et al.* 1974b; Virmavirta & Komi 1993a; Schwameder & Müller 1995).

In addition to high vertical and horizontal velocities the purpose of the takeoff movement is also to produce angular momentum. The somersault angle, defined as the angle between a line connecting the knee and shoulder joint centre to the global longitudinal axis, has been used to describe

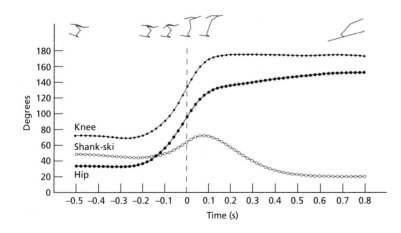

Fig. 17.2 Progression of the knee, hip and shank-ski angles before and after the takeoff instant. The takeoff movement begins, on average, 0.28 s before the release instant (dashed vertical line). (From Schwameder & Müller 1995.)

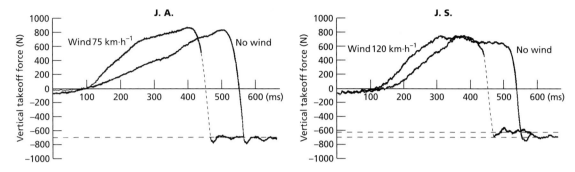

Fig. 17.3 Vertical force–time curves of the simulated ski-jumping takeoffs of two different jumpers in wind and non-wind conditions during wind tunnel experiments. The force plate in the wind tunnel was level with the tunnel floor.

the production of forward momentum in ski-jumping takeoff (Arndt *et al.* 1995). A greater angular velocity enables the jumper to prepare for and subsequently assume the flight position as rapidly as possible from the takeoff.

To obtain maximal height the jumper's centre of mass (COM) must be located along the line of action of the vertical ground reaction force, whereas the production of angular momentum requires the COM to be located anterior to this line. Evidence has been presented that the more successful jumps are characterized by higher knee extension velocities and simultaneously by a more rapidly decreasing somersault angle towards the takeoff edge (Arndt *et al.* 1995).

Wind tunnel experiments

The wind tunnel has usually been used to examine the aerodynamic features of the flight phase. Our recent study (Virmavirta *et al.*, in preparation) has, however, focused on the takeoff action in the wind tunnel. This allows the possibility of characterizing how aerodynamic lift influences the force–time characteristics of the takeoff. It has been speculated (Virmavirta & Komi 1993a) that this aerodynamic lift could considerably increase the takeoff velocity compared with the non-wind condition in the laboratory. Figure 17.3 is a demonstration of this effect, as measured in the wind tunnel. The take-off time becomes considerably shorter and the rate

of force production greater in the simulated wind conditions. Figure 17.3 is then a good demonstration why the actual takeoff can be performed in a short period of time. This is well in agreement with the general knowledge of the force–velocity characteristics of the human skeletal muscle. This aspect is discussed further below (see 'Force–velocity relationship').

Optimal aerodynamic position after the takeoff

When a Swedish ski-jumper, Jan Boklöv, introduced the so-called V-style technique at the end of the 1980s no evidence existed regarding the possible superiority of this technique over the traditional position of the jumper/ski system during the flight phase. Since then considerable scientific effort has been devoted to studying this new technique, both in wind tunnels and during normal ski-jumping situations. Mahnke and Hochmuth (1990) were among the first to undertake a comprehensive series of wind-tunnel experiments investigating the benefits of the V-style compared with the traditional style. Figure 17.4 summarizes the advantages of the modern V-style. The V-style ski position is usually adopted progressively so that the takeoff perform-ance can be executed without additional difficulty. Figure 17.5 demonstrates flight positions of the 15 best jumpers during the different flight phases in the Ski-Flying

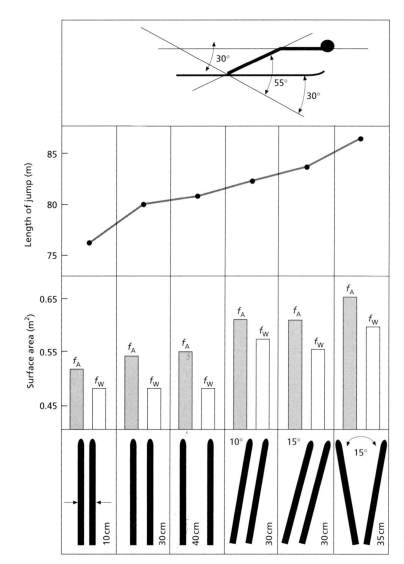

Fig. 17.4 Influence of ski position on the lift (f_A) and drag (f_W) area and on the length of the jump in simulated ski-jumping conditions when the position of the jumper/ski system was fixed as shown above. (From Mahnke & Hochmuth 1990).

World Championships of 1994 (mean flight distance 186.7 m and flight time 6.3 s). The lower part of Fig. 17.5 shows that the V angle increases during the first part of the flight, as has also been reported by Arndt *et al.* (1995). However, the great variability in different parameters among the good jumps of Fig. 17.5 demonstrates that no single fixed model exists to characterize the optimal performance.

The ideal flight position of the jumper/ski system has usually been described using the parameter of the ratio of the aerodynamic lift to drag. It is now known, however, that the development of ski-jumping aerodynamics, especially in big hills, has approached the situation where the resultant aerodynamic force almost equals the weight of the jumper (Fig. 17.6). Due to this development computer simulations have been used quite

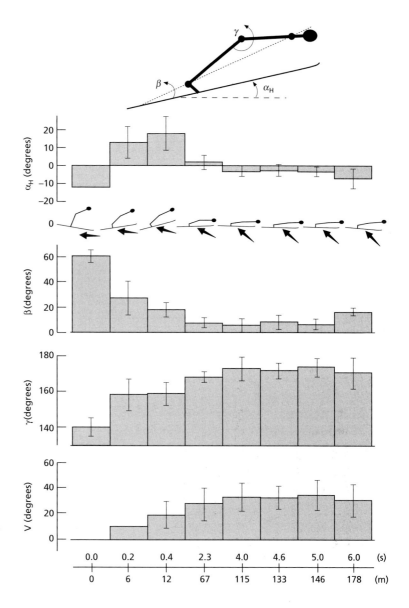

Fig. 17.5 Mean values and standard deviations of the position angles of the 15 best jumps in the 13th World Championships in Ski Flying. (From Müller *et al.* 1996.)

successfully to estimate how the different aerodynamic factors play a role in influencing the flight distance. For details, the reader is referred to Müller *et al.* (1995, 1996), who have well demonstrated how the various aerodynamic factors together with the wind and jump profile influence the flight distance. These measurements have also revealed the interesting feature that the landing is usually safe with low impact forces provided that landing takes place before the critical point where the landing slope begins to curve.

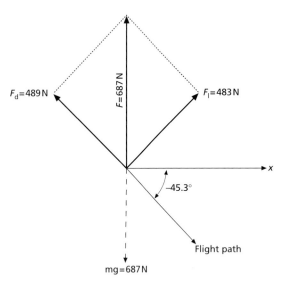

Fig. 17.6 The resultant force compensates for the weight of the jumper ($m = 70$ kg) during the flight phase (see text for explanation). F, Aerodynamic force (resultant); F_l, lift force; F_d, drag force. (From Müller 1997.)

and in actual jumping hill conditions (Table 17.1). The incentive for force measurements in ski-jumping has been a basic assumption that by recording the takeoff forces it is possible to explore factors that influence the final result (i.e. the length of the jump). Correlation between the force parameters and length of the jump has been found for individual jumpers as well as for a certain group of jumpers (Fig. 17.7). By complementing the force measurements with the synchronized motion analysis it is possible to examine in more detail how the force production influences the jumpers' capabilities to obtain a proper flight position (Fig. 17.8).

The preceding description of the takeoff parameters is naturally selective and somewhat simplified. Its serves, however, to highlight those factors which can then be related to and interpreted by the functioning of the jumper's neuromuscular system. Short takeoff time, high knee angular velocity and low upper body position are special requirements and very specific to ski-jumping. Clarifications to the problems from the point of view of neuromuscular limiting factors can be looked from the well-known force–time and force–velocity curves as well as the force–length relationships of isolated human skeletal muscles as well as muscle groups. The possibility of utilizing muscle elasticity for enhancing takeoff must also be examined.

Limiting neuromuscular factors in ski-jumping takeoff

Since Hochmuth's classical studies (1958–59) the takeoff forces exerted by ski-jumpers have been studied both in simulated laboratory conditions

Table. 17.1 Force measurements made in actual ski-jumping conditions.

Reference	Venue	Transducer type	Inrun conditions
Sobotka & Kastner (1979)	Seefeld (AUT)	Force plate	Snow
Troxler & Rüegg (1979)	St. Moritz (SUI)	Force plate	Snow
Tveit & Pedersen (1981)	Hurdal (NOR)	Ski binding	Snow
Virmavirta (1988)	Jyväskylä (FIN)	Force plate	Snow
Vaverka (1987)	Frenstat p.R. (TCH)	Force plate	Plastic
Virmavirta & Komi (1989)	Calgary (CAN)	Force plate	Snow
Jost (1993)	Oberwiesenthal (GER)	Force plate	Plastic
Virmavirta & Komi (1993a,b)	Jyväskylä (FIN)	Force bar	Frost rail
Virmavirta (1993)	Jyväskylä (FIN)	Force bar	Frost rail
Schwameder & Müller (1995)	Stams (AUT)	EMED insole	Porcelain
Yamanobe et al. (1997)	Hakuba (JPN)	Force bar	Porcelain

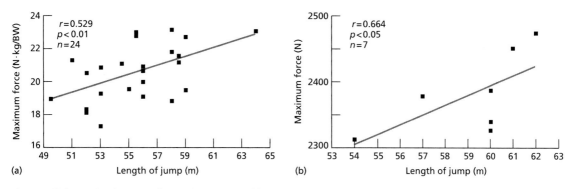

Fig. 17.7 Relationship between the maximum normal force and the length of the jump: (a) among a group of ski-jumpers; and (b) for the individual jumper. (From Virmavirta & Komi 1993b; Komi & Virmavirta 1997.)

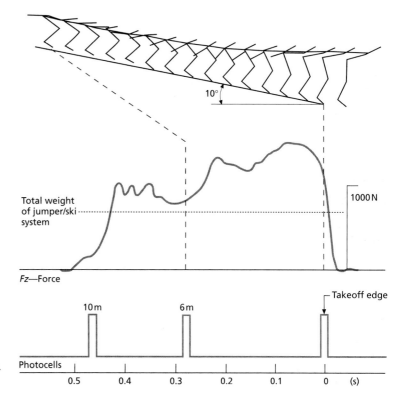

Fig. 17.8 The takeoff technique and force curves of the jumper, M. Nykänen, measured on the small jumping hill (critical point K = 65 m). (After Virmavirta & Komi 1993a.)

Force–time curve

In isometric conditions, when the muscle is maximally activated the force production to the peak force level requires in human leg extension 600–1200 ms (Fig. 17.9). When this is compared to the time available for the takeoff movement (280 ms), one can understand that the time to produce force is indeed a limiting factor in ski-jumping.

The importance of the short takeoff time can be characterized by comparing schematically the takeoff forces between actual ski-jumping and simulated ski-jumping takeoffs (Fig. 17.10). It is interesting to note that ski-jumpers have more favourable isometric

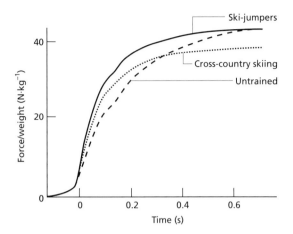

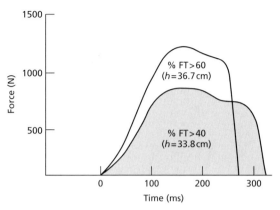

Fig. 17.9 Force–time characteristics of bilateral isometric leg extension among ski-jumpers, untrained controls (policemen) and cross-country skiers. Note that the trained ski-jumpers are able to exert a greater force in a shorter time compared to the other groups. (From Viitasalo & Komi 1978.)

Fig. 17.11 Average vertical force–time (FT) curves for vertical jumps made by two groups of subjects with different muscle fibre compositions on a force platform. The jumps were performed from a starting position with a relatively extended knee angle. (From Bosco & Komi 1979.)

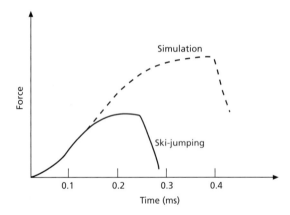

Fig. 17.10 Schematic presentation of the vertical force–time relationships in an actual ski-jumping takeoff and in a simulated ski-jumping takeoff in the laboratory. This suggests that the time is a limiting factor in actual ski-jumping takeoff.

force–time curves than controls (Fig. 17.9) or, for instance, endurance athletes. This may be due to adaptation to training *per se* and/or to the more favourable muscle fibre composition of the ski-jumpers. It is well known that skeletal muscle contains muscle fibres that have different mechanical characteristics. Fast-twitch (FT) (or type II) fibres have a shorter force rise time and if a majority of the fibre population of a

specific muscle is type II it is very likely that the force–time characteristics favour rapid force production. Ski-jumpers are reportedly fast type in their muscle fibre composition (Komi *et al.* 1977). In a vertical jump test those subjects having more FT fibres are superior to those having a majority of slow-twitch (type I) fibres in their vastus lateralis muscle (Bosco & Komi 1979) (Fig. 17.11). It is perhaps not a coincidence that Figs 17.3 and 17.11 have similar features with regard to the duration of the force production.

Force–velocity relationship

The average knee extension velocity of over 12 rad · s^{-1} found during takeoff also implies a more favourable use of the FT fibre population. Tihanyi *et al.* (1982) have studied the maximal knee extension movement with varying loads and discovered, in addition to the conventional force–velocity (F–V) dependence, a clear shift to the right and up of the F–V curve at higher velocities (and lighter loads) among subjects having a majority of FT fibres in the vastus lateralis muscle. Velocities of over 12 rad · s^{-1} rely certainly on the contractile performance of the FT fibres. Thus it is very likely that good ski-jumping takeoff action with high knee-extension velocity can be performed only if the jumper's knee-extension muscles have sufficient proportions of the FT muscle fibres.

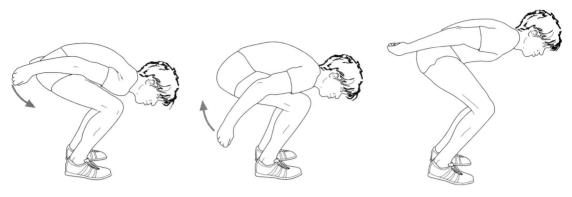

Fig. 17.12 A proposed arm action to produce sudden unweighting (and possible takeoff potentiation) during ski-jumping takeoff. The amplitude of the quick arm action downwards is slightly exaggerated here. (From Komi 1980.)

Force–length (force–angle) relationship

Assuming again that the knee-extension muscles are mostly involved in the ski-jumping takeoff, the performance of these muscles is limited also by the initial muscle lengths (joint angle). If the inrun position is too deep (small knee angle), the force production capability is drastically limited compared with the more extended (e.g. 75–80°) knee angle (Eloranta & Komi 1981). Timing is also critical here: a deep crouch position with small knee angle may produce high extension velocity but to attain it may require more time than is available on the takeoff table.

Possible use of muscle elasticity

It is well known that when an active muscle is prestretched prior to its shortening the final power (and velocity) can be higher than that attained in a purely shortening muscle action (Cavagna *et al.* 1968). When applied to a vertical jump (Komi & Bosco 1978) the jumps performed with a preliminary countermovement will attain higher takeoff velocity compared with a jump performed without countermovement. This phenomenon can be well demonstrated in a simulated ski-jumping takeoff in the laboratory (Komi *et al.* 1974a). A takeoff performed with a preparatory countermovement can reach a vertical takeoff velocity that is 10–20% greater than in jumps without countermovement. Despite these relatively clear differences in the laboratory tests

the use of the preliminary countermovement has not gained uniform acceptance among coaches and jumpers. The major problem arises when the countermovement is performed too excessively and timed improperly with the transition from the inrun curve to the flat table. Successful ski-jumpers perform the countermovement often intuitively with rapid arm movements. As proposed in Fig. 17.12 this very short but quick arm movement downwards will cause a short but quick unweighting action with the resulting prestretch in the knee-extensor muscles. Sometimes it is also possible to see this phenomenon as a quick but short-amplitude knee flexion movement. It must be emphasized, however, that any efforts to amplify the countermovement will very likely result in an uncontrolled takeoff motion. This is probably the reason why some athletes and coaches have not favoured the use of the countermovement.

Use of electromyography during ski-jumping

Only a few electromyograph (EMG) studies in ski-jumping have been reported (Watanabe *et al.* 1972; Virmavirta & Komi 1991; Schwirtz *et al.* 1996). In these measurements the main concern has been to describe certain muscle activities during the ski-jumping performance. Figure 17.13 presents examples of the rectified EMG activities for one jumper during ski-jumping performance. Figure 17.14 shows the mean integrated EMG activities for a group of

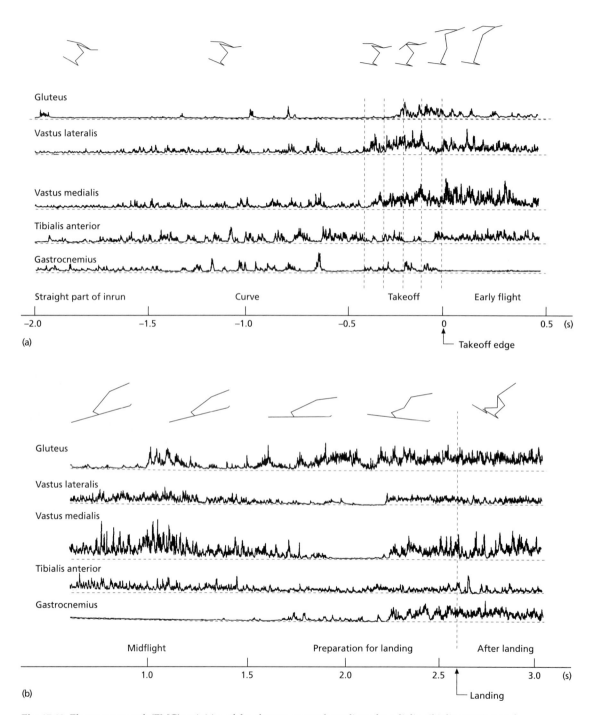

Fig. 17.13 Electromyograph (EMG) activities of the gluteus, vastus lateralis and medialis, tibialis anterior, and gastrocnemius muscles with corresponding positions of a single jumper during an entire ski-jump, starting from the preparation for takeoff (a) and ending at landing (b). (From Virmavirta & Komi 1991.)

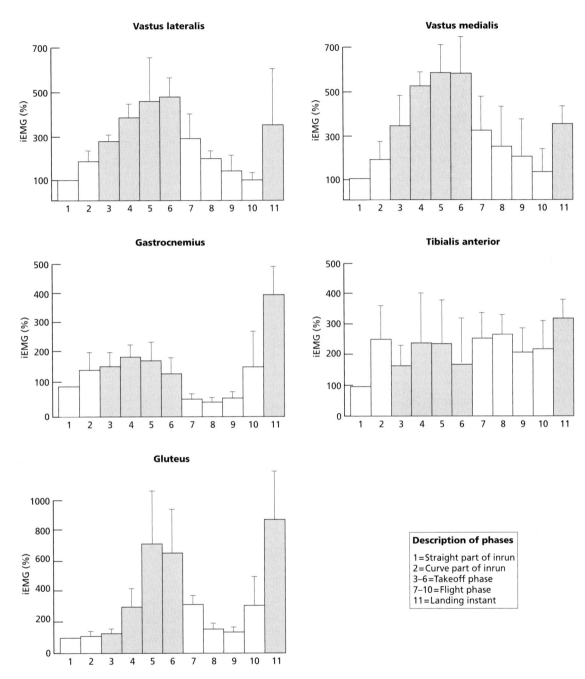

Fig. 17.14 Mean integrated EMG (iEMG) activities of different muscles for a group of jumpers from different phases of a ski-jump. (From Virmavirta & Komi 1991.)

jumpers from the different phases of the jump. From these illustrations it can be observed that the leg-extensor muscles are mainly responsible for the execution of the takeoff. Strong action in the hip joint is demonstrated by the increase in the activity of the gluteus muscle at the end of takeoff. Characteristically for a ski-jumping takeoff, the gastrocnemius muscle is only weakly active. Utilization of the gastrocnemius, especially during the last phase of takeoff, is much different from the takeoff action in vertical jumps, where plantarflexion is important. The quick lifting of skis does not allow effective use of the gastrocnemius (i.e. plantar-flexion) and thus the takeoff is performed more with the knee-extensor muscles. On the other hand, the structure of the ski boots limits the possibility for efficient plantar-flexion during the take-off. On the basis of the above mentioned facts the use of the simulation takeoffs with training shoes may have a negative transfer to the real performance.

Concluding remarks

Although much is known about the takeoff action in ski-jumping the ideal or individually optimal take-off performance has not yet been described. Research can help in this process, and the comprehensive use of kinematic, kinetic and EMG techniques may prove useful in this regard. Figure 17.15 shows, schematically, our latest attempts (in progress) to achieve this goal and collect numerous different parameters with modern recording techniques (e.g. 40-channel data logger). The preliminary data obtained with this approach (Virmavirta *et al.*, in preparation) emphasize that the takeoff action is very similar regardless of the size of the jumping hill (Fig. 17.16).

Takeoff action can be regarded as successful only if, in addition to high vertical and horizontal velocities, it achieves an optimal aerodynamic position. Future research should therefore concentrate also on this transition phase from takeoff to early flight. Isolated studies with the flight aerodynamics are not always useful unless they are combined with the takeoff kinetics and the associated requirements of the jumper's neuromuscular function.

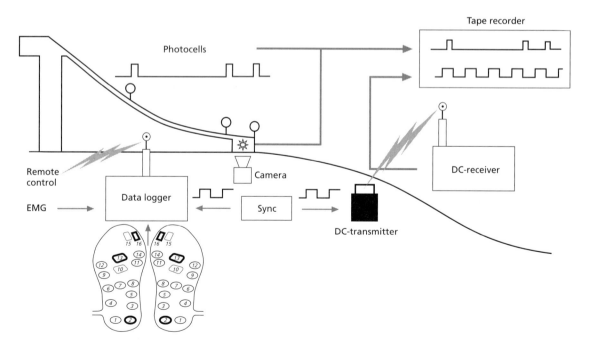

Fig. 17.15 Schematic presentation of the various methods currently used by the authors to study ski-jumping takeoff and early flight phases.

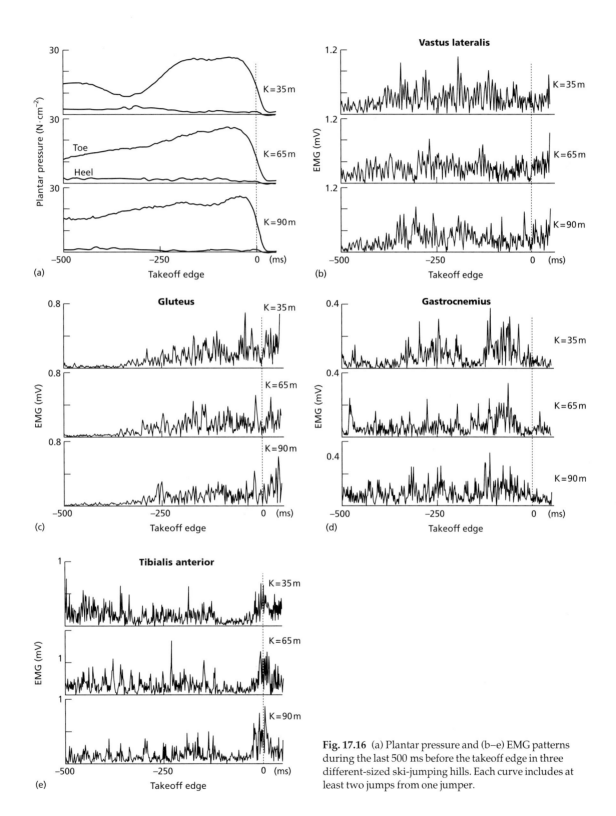

Fig. 17.16 (a) Plantar pressure and (b–e) EMG patterns during the last 500 ms before the takeoff edge in three different-sized ski-jumping hills. Each curve includes at least two jumps from one jumper.

References

Arndt, A., Brüggemann, Virmavirta, M. & Komi, P.V. (1995) Techniques used by Olympic ski jumpers in the transition from takeoff to early flight. *Journal of Applied Biomechanics* **11**, 224–237.

Bosco, C. & Komi, P.V. (1979) Mechanical characteristics and fibre composition of human leg extensor muscles. *European Journal of Applied Physiology* **41**, 275–284.

Cavagna, G.A., Dusman, B. & Margaria, R. (1968) Positive work done by the previously stretched muscle. *Journal of Applied Physiology* **24**, 31–32.

Eloranta, V. & Komi, P.V. (1981) Function of the quadriceps femoris muscle under the full range of forces and differing contraction velocities of concentric work. *EMG and Clinical Neurophysiology* **21**, 419–431.

Hochmuth, G. (1958–59) Untersuchungen über den Einfluss der Absprungbewegung auf die Sprungweite beim Skisprung. [Investigation of the effect of takeoff on jump length in ski jumping.] *Wissenschaft Z DHFK, Leipzig* **1**, 29–59.

Jost, B. (1993) Performance success in ski jumping related to vertical take-off speed. In: *Proceedings of the XIth Symposium of the International Society of Biomechanics in Sports* (eds J. Hamill, T. Derrick, E.H. Elliot *et al.*). Amherst, MA.

Komi, P.V. (1973) Relationship between muscle tension, EMG and velocity of contraction under concentric and eccentric work. In: *Developments in Electromyography and Clinical Neurophysiology* (ed. J.E. Desmedt), pp. 596–606. Karger, Basle.

Komi, P.V. (1980). Lihaksiston elastisuus ja sen merkitys liikuntasuorituksen kannalta. [Muscle elasticity and its importance for sport performance]. *Liikunta Ja Tiede* **1**, 14–17.

Komi, P.V. & Bosco, C. (1978) Utilization of elastic energy in jumping and its relation to skeletal muscle fiber composition in man. In: *Biomechanics VIA* (eds E. Asmussen & J. Jörgensen), pp. 79–85. University Park Press, Baltimore.

Komi, P.V. & Virmavirta, M. (1997) Ski-jumping take-off performance: Determining factors and methodological advances. In: *Science and Skiing* (eds E. Müller, H. Schwameder, E. Kornexl & C. Raschner), pp. 36–48. Chapman & Hall/Cambridge University Press, Cambridge.

Komi, P.V., Luhtanen, P. & Viljamaa, K. (1974a) Hetkellinen kontaktivoimien mittaaminen voimalevyanturilla. [Measurement of instantaneous contact forces on the force platform.] *Research Reports from the Department of Biology of Physical Activity* 5. University of Jyväskyla, Jyväskyla, Finland.

Komi, P.V., Nelson, R.C. & Pulli, M. (1974b) *Biomechanics of ski-jumping*. Studies in Sport Physical Education and Health, No. 5. University of Jyväskylä.

Komi, P.V., Rusko, H., Vos, J. & Vihko, V. (1977) Aerobic performance capacity in athletes. *Acta Physiologica Scandinavica* **100**, 107–114.

Mahnke, R.-D. & Hochmuth, G. (1990) *Neue Erkenntnisse zur Luftkraftwirkung beim Skispringen*. [*New understanding of the aerodynamic forces in ski jumping*.] Research report from Forschungsinstitut für Körperkultur und Sport, Leipzig.

Müller, W. (1997) Biomechanics of ski jumping – scientific jumping hill design. In: *Science and Skiing* (eds E. Müller, H. Schwameder, E. Kornexl & C. Raschner), pp. 36–48. Chapman & Hall/Cambridge University Press, Cambridge.

Müller, W., Platzer, D. & Schmöltzer, B. (1995) Scientific approach to ski safety. *Nature* **375**, 455.

Müller, W., Platzer, D. & Schmöltzer, B. (1996) Dynamics of human flight on skis: Improvements on safety and fairness in ski jumping. *Journal of Biomechanics* **29** (8), 1061–1068.

Schwameder, H. & Müller, E. (1995) Biomechanische Beschreibung und Analyse der V-technik im skispringen. *Spectrum der Sportwissenschaft* **7** (1), 5–36.

Schwirtz, A., Gollhofer, A., Schwitzer, L. & Mross, H. (1996) Diagnosis of jumping and neuromuscular coordination in ski jumping. In: *1st International Congress on Skiing and Science. Abstract Book*, pp. 36–37. St Christhof, Austria.

Sobotka, R. & Kastner, J. (1979) Registrierung des Kraftimpulses beim Skiabsprung. [Measurement of the takeoff forces in ski jumping.] In: *Zur Biomechanik Des Skilaufs* (ed. F. Fetz), pp. 90–97. Inn-Verlag, Innsbruck.

Tihanyi, J., Apor, P. & Fekete, Gy. (1982) Force-velocity-power characteristics and fiber composition in human knee extensor muscles. *European Journal of Applied Physiology* **48**, 331–343.

Troxler, G. & Rüegg, P. (1979) Kraftmes-sung auf dem Schanzentisch. [Force measurement on the takeoff table in ski jumping.] Semesterarbeit in Elektrotechnik an der ETH, Zürich.

Tveit, P. & Pedersen, P.O. (1981) Forces in the take-off in ski jumping. In: *Biomechanics VII-B* (ed. E. Morecki, K. Fidelus, K. Kedzior & A. Wit), pp. 472–477. University Park Press, Baltimore.

Vaverka, F. (1987) *Biomechanika skoku na lyzích*. Univerzita Palackéhov Olomouc, Czechoslovakia.

Viitasalo, J. & Komi, P.V. (1978) Force-time characteristics and fiber composition in human leg extensor muscles. *European Journal of Applied Physiology* **40**, 7–15.

Virmavirta, M. (1988) Biomechanics of ski jumping. MSc thesis, Department of Biology of Physical Activity, University of Jyväskylä.

Virmavirta, M. (1993) The take-off forces in ski jumping. Licentiate thesis, Department of Biology of Physical Activity, University of Jyväskylä.

Virmavirta, M. & Komi, P.V. (1989) Takeoff forces in ski jumping. *International Journal of Sport Biomechanics* **5**, 248–257.

Virmavirta, M. & Komi, P.V. (1991) Electromyographic analysis of muscle activation during ski jumping performance. *International Journal of Sports Biomechanics* **7**, 175–182.

Virmavirta, M. & Komi, P.V. (1993a) Measurement of take-off forces in ski jumping. Part I. *Scandinavian Journal of Medicine and Science in Sports* **3**, 229–236.

Virmavirta, M. & Komi, P.V. (1993b) Measurement of take-off forces in ski jumping. Part II. *Scandinavian Journal of Medicine and Science in Sports* **3**, 237–243.

Virmavirta, M. & Komi, P.V. (1994) Takeoff analysis of a champion ski jumper. *Coaching and Sport Science Journal* **1** (1), 23–27.

Watanabe, T., Kasaya, A. & Kawahara, Y. (1972) Kinematic studies on ski jumping. In: *Proceedings of the International Congress of Winter Sports Medicine*, pp. 98–105, Sapporo.

Wilkie, D.R. (1950) The relation between force and velocity in human muscle. *Journal of Physiology* **110**, 249–280.

Yamanobe, K., Tamura, K. & Watanabe, K. (1997) A research of forces and their timings of ski jumping. In: *ISB XVI*[th] *Congress, Tokyo, Japan* (eds M. Miyashita, F. Fukanaga & S. Fukashiro). *Abstract book*, 87.

PART 4

THROWING AND HITTING

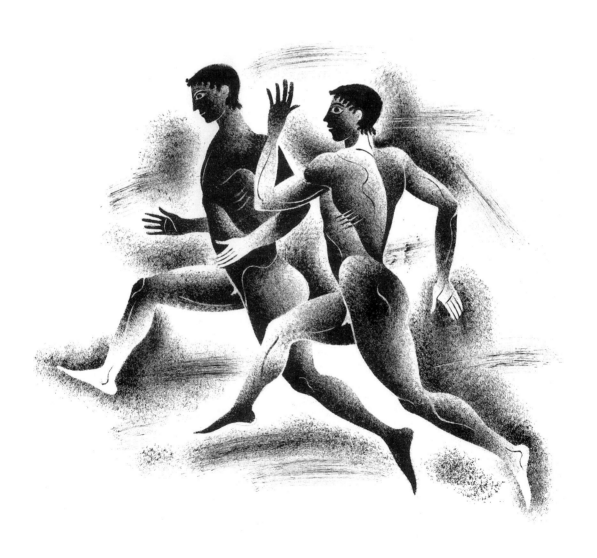

Chapter 18

Principles of Throwing

R. BARTLETT

Throwing skills

What is throwing?

The New Shorter Oxford English Dictionary defines the verb 'throw' (in its meaning in the context of this chapter) as: 'Project or propel through the air, cast, drive, shoot. . . . Project (something) through the air or space with usually sudden force, from the hand or arm; cast, hurl, fling. Hurl or fling something, as a missile' (Brown 1993; p. 3296). In line with this definition, this chapter focuses on the principles of those sports or events in which the participant throws, passes, bowls or shoots an object from the hand or, in the case of lacrosse, from an implement. Some, or all, of these principles relate to: throws from a circle—hammer (see also Chapter 22) and discus throws, shot put (see also Chapter 21); cross-over skills—javelin throw (see also Chapter 20) and cricket bowling; pitching in baseball and softball; shooting and passing movements in basketball, net-ball, handball, water polo and lacrosse; throwing-to skills in baseball, cricket, soccer, rugby, American and other variants of football; underarm bowling; and dart throwing. Many of these are used as examples

throughout the chapter. The chapter excludes any striking skills, in which an object is moving when intercepted by the hand or hand-held implement.

Classification of throwing skills

Throwing movements are often classified as underarm, overarm or sidearm (e.g. Adrian & Cooper 1989; Luttgens *et al.* 1992). The last two of these can be viewed as diagonal movement patterns, with trunk lateral flexion being mainly responsible for determining whether they are overarm or sidearm (Atwater 1979). In the overarm pattern, the trunk laterally flexes away from the throwing arm, while in a sidearm pattern the trunk laterally flexes towards that arm.

UNDERARM THROWS

These are characterized by the shoulder action, which is predominantly flexion from a hyper-extended position above the horizontal (Fig. 18.1). In the preparation phase, the weight transfers to the rear foot and the front foot steps forwards. This step is longer for skilled throwers (Adrian & Cooper

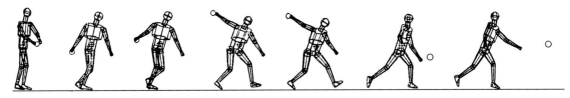

Fig. 18.1 Underarm throwing pattern. (Adapted from Adrian & Cooper 1989.)

365

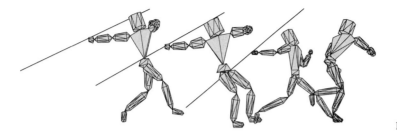

Fig. 18.2 Javelin throw.

1989). Weight transfers onto the front foot during the action phase, as the pelvis and trunk rotate to the left (for a right-handed thrower). The elbow extends during the action phase and, at release, the throwing arm is parallel to, or slightly in front of, the line of the trunk. Curling and softball pitching are underarm throws, as are ten-pin and various other bowling actions, used, for example, in crown green bowling and skittles.

OVERARM THROWS

These are characterized by lateral rotation of the humerus in the preparation phase and its medial rotation in the action phase (e.g. Dillman *et al.* 1993). This movement is one of the fastest joint rotations in the human body. Many of the other joint movements are similar to those of the underarm throw (Adrian & Cooper 1989). The sequence of movements in the preparation phase of a baseball pitch,

for example, include, for a right-handed pitcher, pelvic and trunk rotation to the right, horizontal extension and lateral rotation at the shoulder, elbow flexion and wrist hyperextension (Luttgens *et al.* 1992). These movements are followed, sequentially, by their anatomical opposite at each of the joints mentioned plus radio-ulnar pronation.

Baseball pitching, javelin throwing (Fig. 18.2), throwing from the outfield in cricket, and passing in American football are classic examples of one-arm overarm throws. The mass (inertia) and dimensions of the thrown object—plus the size of the target area and the rules of the particular sport—are constraints on the movement pattern of any throw. Bowling in cricket (Fig. 18.3) differs from other similar movement patterns, as the rules do not allow the elbow to extend late in the delivery stride. The predominant action at the shoulder is therefore circumduction. The soccer throw-in uses a two-handed overarm throwing pattern. The shot put combines overarm

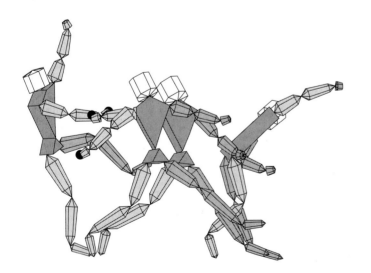

Fig. 18.3 Cricket fast bowling. (From Bartlett 1997a.)

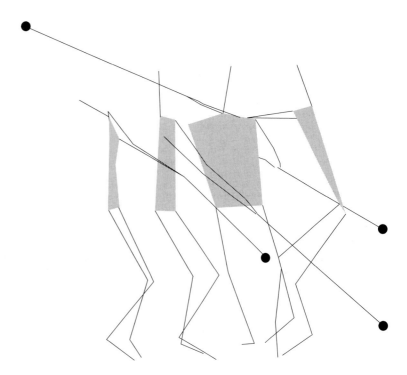

Fig. 18.4 Hammer throw. (From Bartlett 1997a.)

throwing with a pushing movement, because of the event's rules and the mass of the shot. Basketball shooting uses various modifications to the overarm throwing pattern, depending on the rules of the game and the circumstances and position of the shot—including release speed and accuracy requirements. Passing in basketball, in which accuracy is also crucial, varies from the overarm patterns of the overhead and baseball passes to the highly modified pushing action of the chest pass. In dart throwing, the dominant requirement for accuracy restricts the action phase movements to elbow extension with some shoulder flexion-abduction.

SIDEARM THROWS

These throws are sometimes considered to differ from underarm and overarm throws, mainly by restricted action at the shoulder joint. The dominant movement is rotation of the pelvis and trunk with the arm abducted to a position near the horizontal (Adrian & Cooper 1989). Unlike the other two

throwing patterns, in which the movements are in the sagittal, or a diagonal plane, frontal plane movements dominate in sidearm throws. The discus throw, the baseball throw and some shots in handball are of this type. The hammer throw (Fig. 18.4) is probably best characterized as a sidearm throw (Kreighbaum & Barthels 1990) rather than an underarm throw (Adrian & Cooper 1989).

Goal orientation

The goal of a throwing movement will generally be distance, accuracy or some combination of the two. The goal is important in determining which of the movement principles discussed below are more, and which are less, applicable. Some authors (e.g. Kreighbaum & Barthels 1990) distinguish between throw-like movements for distance, in which segmental rotations occur sequentially, and push-like movements for accuracy, in which segmental rotations occur simultaneously. However, few throws in sport have no accuracy requirements. Even those, such as javelin, discus and hammer throwing and shot putting, in which the distance of the throw is predominant, have to land in a specified area and have rules that constrain the throwing technique. In throws for distance, the release speed—and therefore the force applied to the thrown object—is crucial.

In some throws, the objective is not to achieve maximal distance; instead, it may be accuracy or minimal time in the air. The latter will be particularly important in throws from the outfield in baseball and to the wicketkeeper in cricket. In such throws, the release speed, height and angle need to be such that the flight time is minimized within the accuracy and distance constraints of the throw. In accuracy-dominated skills, such as dart throwing, or in some passes and set shots in basketball, the release of the object needs to achieve accuracy within the distance constraints of the skill. The interaction of speed and accuracy in these skills is often expressed as the speed-accuracy trade-off. This has been investigated particularly thoroughly for basketball shooting (e.g. Brancazio 1992). The shooter has to release the ball with speed and accuracy to pass through the basket. This is discussed at the end of the next section.

Optimizing the release of a thrown object

Bodies launched into the air that are subject only to the forces of gravity and air resistance are termed projectiles. Projectile motion occurs frequently in sport; it is covered in more detail in Chapter 19.

Release parameters

There are three parameters, in addition to gravitational acceleration (g), which determine the trajectory of a simple projectile, such as a ball, shot or hammer. These are the release speed, angle and height (Fig. 18.5).

RELEASE ANGLE (θ)

This is defined as the angle between the projectile's velocity vector and the horizontal at the instant of release. The size of the release angle depends on the

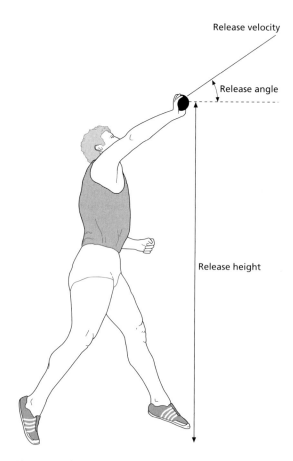

Fig. 18.5 Release parameters. (Adapted from Bartlett 1997a.)

purpose of the activity. In the absence of aerodynamic forces, all projectiles will follow a flight path that has a parabolic shape, which depends upon the magnitude of the release angle (Fig. 18.6).

RELEASE SPEED (v_0)

This is defined as the magnitude of the projectile's velocity vector at the instant of release. When the release angle and height are held constant, the release speed will determine the magnitude of a projectile's maximum vertical displacement (its apex) and its range (maximum horizontal displacement). The greater the release speed, the greater are the apex and range. It is common practice to resolve

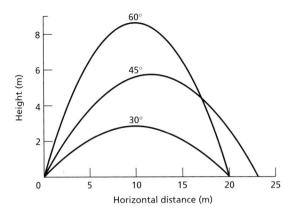

Fig. 18.6 Effect of release angle on shape of parabolic trajectory for a release speed of 15 m · s⁻¹ and zero release height. (From Bartlett 1997a.)

a projectile's velocity into its horizontal and vertical components and then to analyse these independently. Horizontally, a projectile is not subject to any external forces (ignoring air resistance) and will therefore maintain constant horizontal velocity during its airborne phase. The range travelled by a projectile is the product of its horizontal velocity and its time of flight. The release speed is by far the most important of the release parameters in determining the range achieved, because the range is proportional to the square of the release speed. Doubling the release speed would increase the range fourfold.

RELEASE HEIGHT (y_0)

This is not equal to zero if the projectile lands at a level higher or lower than that at which it was released. This is the case with most sports projectiles, for example in a shot put or a basketball shot. For a given release speed and angle, the greater the relative release height, the longer is the flight time, and the greater are the range and maximum height.

Optimal release and the interaction of release parameters

In many throws, the objective is to maximize, within certain constraints, the range achieved by the projectile. Any increase in release speed (v_0) or release height is always accompanied by an increase in the range. If the objective of the throw is to maximize range, it is important to ascertain the best (optimum) release angle to achieve this. The optimum angle for maximum range for zero relative release height is 45°. For the more general case of non-zero release height (y_0), the optimum release angle (θ) can be found from:

$$\cos 2\theta = g y_0 / (v_0^2 + g y_0) \tag{18.1}$$

For a good shot putter, for example, this would give a value around 42°.

Although optimum release angles for given values of v_0 and y_0 can easily be determined mathematically, they do not always correspond to those recorded from the best performers in sporting events. This is even true for the shot put (Tsirakos *et al.* 1995), in which the object's flight is the closest to a parabola of all sports objects. The reason is that the calculation of an optimum release angle assumes, implicitly, that the release speed and release angle are independent of one another. For a shot putter, the release speed and angle are, however, not independent, because of the arrangement and mechanics of the muscles used to generate the release speed of the shot. A greater release speed, and hence range, can be achieved at an angle (about 35°) that is less than the optimum release angle for the projectile's flight phase. If the shot putter seeks to increase the release angle to a value closer to the optimum angle for the projectile's flight phase, the release speed decreases and so does the range.

In javelin throwing, there has been some research to assess the interdependence or otherwise of the various release parameters. The two for which an interrelationship is known are release speed and angle. Two groups of researchers have investigated this relationship, one using a 1 kg ball (Red & Zogaib 1977) and the other using an instrumented javelin (Viitasalo & Korjus 1988). Surprisingly, they obtained very similar relationships over the relevant range, expressed by the equation:

release speed = nominal release speed
  − 0.13 (release angle − 35)   (18.2)

where the angles must be in degrees and the speed in m · s⁻¹. The nominal release speed is defined as the maximum speed at which a thrower is capable of throwing for a release angle of 35°.

Another complication arises when accuracy becomes crucial to successful throwing, as in shooting skills in basketball (Brancazio 1992). A relationship between release speed and release angle is then found that will satisfy the speed-accuracy trade-off. For a given height of release and distance from the basket, a unique release angle exists for the ball to pass through the centre of the basket for any realistic release speed. Margins of error for both speed and angle exist about this pair of values. The margin of error in the release speed increases with the release angle, but only slowly. However, the margin of error in the release angle reaches a sharp peak for release angles within a few degrees of the minimum-speed angle (the angle for which the release speed is the minimum to score a basket). This latter consideration dominates the former, particularly as a shot at the minimum speed requires the minimum force from the shooter. The minimum-speed angle is therefore the best one (Brancazio 1992).

Aerodynamic effects

In some throwing events, such as the javelin and discus throws, and throws of a spinning or seamed ball, the aerodynamic characteristics of the projectile can significantly influence its trajectory. It may travel a greater or lesser distance than it would have done if projected in a vacuum, and it may swerve (or laterally deviate). Under such circumstances, the calculations of range and of optimal release parameters need to be modified considerably to take account of the aerodynamic forces acting on the projectile. Furthermore, more release parameters (e.g. Fig. 18.7) are then important. These include the angular velocities of the object at release—such as ball or discus spin and the pitching and yawing angular velocities of a javelin—and the 'aerodynamic' angles—the angles of pitch and yaw of a javelin or discus and the seam angle on a single-seamed ball. The effects of some of these are touched on later in this chapter and dealt with more comprehensively in Chapter 19.

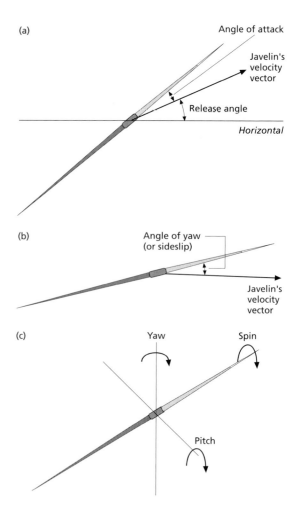

Fig. 18.7 Aerodynamic angles: (a) side view; (b) plan view; and (c) angular velocities for a javelin.

Principles of throwing skills

Skilful throwing should follow the biomechanical principles of coordinated movements: 'general laws based on physics and biology which determine human motion' (Bober 1981). These principles are subdivided into (see e.g. Bartlett 1999):
• universal principles, which are valid for all activities, including throwing;
• principles of partial generality, valid for large groups of activities, for example, throws for distance or those requiring precision or accuracy; and
• particular principles, valid for specific throws.

The coordination of joint and muscle actions is often considered to be crucial to the successful execution of throwing movements. However, it should be noted that not all of the underlying assumptions have been rigorously tested (Bartlett 1997b). For example, the transfer of angular momentum between body segments is often proposed as a feature of vigorous sports movements, including throws. Several investigators (e.g. Putnam 1983; Sørensen et al. 1996) have shown that, in kicking, angular momentum is not transferred from the thigh to the shank when the thigh decelerates. Instead, the performance of the kick would be improved if the thigh did not decelerate. Its deceleration is caused by the motion of the shank through inertia coupling between the two. As kicking has much in common with throwing—Kreighbaum and Barthels (1990) characterize kicking as a 'throw-like' movement—we might expect similar distal-to-proximal behaviour for the arm segments in throwing. This has been confirmed for the interaction of the upper arm and forearm in overarm pitching (Putnam 1993).

Furthermore, the role of movement variability—both intraindividual and interindividual (Hore et al. 1996)—in distance-and accuracy-dominated throws has not been fully explained to date. The shortage of systematic research into the applicability to throwing of some of the principles of coordinated movement should be borne in mind when reading and applying the following sections.

Universal principles

USE OF PRESTRETCH

This principle relates to the stretch–shortening cycle of muscular contraction (Hatze 1983). In performing most throws, a segment often moves in the opposite direction to the one intended: this is considered further in the section on phase analysis below. This initial countermovement is often necessary simply to allow the subsequent movement to occur. Other benefits arise from the increased acceleration path and the various phenomena of the stretch–shortening cycle. The latter involve initiation of the stretch reflex; storage of elastic energy; and stretching the muscle to optimal length for forceful contraction—

the last of these relates to the muscle's length–tension curve.

MINIMIZATION OF ENERGY USAGE

This principle relates to the metabolic energy used to perform a specific task; it is also known as the 'principle of limitation of excitation of muscles' (Bober 1981). Some evidence supports this as an adaptive mechanism in skill acquisition, for example, the reduction in unnecessary movements during the learning of throwing skills (e.g. Higgins 1977). The large number of multijoint muscles in the body supports the importance of energy efficiency as an evolutionary principle.

PRINCIPLE OF MINIMUM TASK COMPLEXITY

This principle relates to the control of redundant degrees of freedom in the kinematic chain (Higgins 1977). The kinematic chain (now more commonly referred to as the kinetic chain, and this term will be used throughout the rest of this chapter) proceeds from the most proximal to the most distal segment. Coordination of that chain becomes more complex as the degrees of freedom—the possible axes of rotation plus directions of linear motion at each joint—increase. A kinetic chain for throwing, from shoulder girdle to fingers, contains about 17 degrees of freedom. Obviously many of these need to be controlled to permit any degree of movement replication (see e.g. Hore et al. 1994). For example, in a basketball set shot the player keeps the elbow well into the body to reduce the redundant degrees of freedom. The forces need to be applied in the required direction of motion. This principle explains why skilled movements, including throws, look so simple.

Principles of partial generality

SEQUENTIAL ACTION OF MUSCLE

This principle has several alternative expressions: the summation of internal forces; serial organization; and the transfer of angular momentum along the kinetic chain. It is most important in throws for distance, such as discus throwing. It involves the recruitment of body segments into the movement at the correct time. Movements are generally initiated by the large muscle groups, which are usually pennate and which produce force to overcome the inertia of the whole body plus the object being thrown. The sequence is continued by the faster muscles of the extremities. These not only have a larger range of movement and speed but also improved accuracy, owing to the smaller number of muscle fibres innervated by each motor neurone (the innervation ratio). In correct sequencing, proximal segments move ahead of distal ones, which ensures that muscles are stretched to develop tension when they contract.

Throwing generally involves an open kinetic chain—one with a free end (Fig. 18.8). It is then possible for a distal segment to rotate without any muscle action at its proximal joint (see also Kreighbaum & Barthels 1990). This can occur if the movement of a proximal segment is decelerated, by an antagonist muscle for example, and momentum is transferred along the chain. This is often associated with ballistic throwing movements, and some supportive electromyographic evidence does exist. This evidence can be used to support the principles of minimization of energy usage and the sequential action of muscles. Little or no activity of the triceps brachii muscle is usually found, for example, during the action phase of the baseball pitch by skilled pitchers, despite the extension of the elbow during that phase (e.g. Atwater 1979). However, as we noted above, little research has been reported into such fundamental questions as 'is there a distal-to-proximal transfer, as in kicking where the distal segment causes the deceleration of the proximal segment rather than the latter transferring momentum to the former?'

A similar comment applies to other issues, such as whether throwing is a whip-like or flail-like action. When a whip is cracked, a bending wave travels along it, transferring kinetic energy from the proximal to the distal end. Although it has been postulated that this principle is used by skilled throwers, there is little empirical evidence to support this assumption. In a simple computer simulation model of throwing, with one knee muscle and one elbow muscle, Alexander (1991) showed that sequential

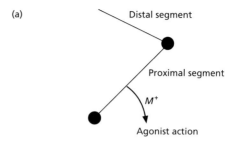

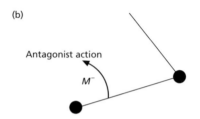

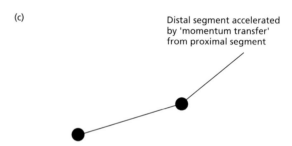

Fig. 18.8 Open kinetic chain: (a) moment ($M+$) of agonists of proximal joint; (b) moment ($M-$) from antagonists of proximal joint; (c) transfers momentum to segment distal to the distal joint. (From Bartlett 1999.)

activation of the two muscles resulted in a longer throw than achieved with simultaneous activation. This is in accord with the principle of this section, and was also reported by Herring and Chapman (1992) for a three-segment model. Alexander also found that a unique delay period between the activation of the two muscles maximized the total work done by them. However, a longer delay period increased the proportion of the work done that was converted into kinetic energy of the thrown object. This suggests that the whip explanation of throwing movements is both oversimplified and misleading (Alexander 1992).

MINIMIZATION OF INERTIA

This is most important in throws requiring a large release speed. Movements at any joint should be initiated with the distal joints in a position that minimizes the moment of inertia, to maximize rotational acceleration. For example, in the javelin throw, the delivery phase begins with the elbow flexing to reduce the moment of inertia of the arm and javelin about the shoulder. This principle relates to the generation and transfer of angular momentum, which are affected by changes in the moment of inertia.

PRINCIPLE OF IMPULSE GENERATION

This principle is, again, mainly important in throws for distance. It relates to the impulse–momentum equation:

$$\text{impulse} = \text{change of momentum}$$
$$= \text{average force} \times \text{time force acts} \qquad (18.3)$$

This equation shows that a large impulse is needed to produce a large change of momentum. This requires either a large average force or a long time of action. In impulse generation, the former must predominate because of the explosive short duration of many sports movements, such as a shot put, which requires power, i.e. the rapid performance of work.

MAXIMIZING THE ACCELERATION PATH

This principle arises from the work–energy relationship ($\Delta E = \bar{F}s$), which shows that a large change in mechanical energy (ΔE) requires either a large average force ($\bar{F}$) or maximization of the distance (s) over which we apply force. This is an important principle in throws requiring a large release speed, for example, a shot-putter making full use of the width of the throwing circle. In ballistic movements, which are fast, muscles function mainly as accelerators. In such movements, the use of electromyography can only tell us when a muscle is contracting—if we account for the electromechanical delay—rather than what the muscle is doing. To understand the latter more fully, further detailed information on the kinematics of each of the segments and the forces and torques (moments) at the joints is needed. This becomes increasingly complex as the length of the kinetic chain increases, although the muscles will still generate joint torques. The torques at any joint will depend not only on the accelerating effects at that joint by the muscles that cross it, but also on accelerations at other joints in the kinetic chain (see e.g. Zajac & Gordon 1989).

STABILITY

A wide base of support is needed for stability; this applies not only for accuracy-dominated throws, such as darts, but also in many throws for distance, where sudden changes in the momentum vector occur. The horizontal component of the ground reaction force, particularly that on the thrower's front foot, is important in establishing a firm support base and eliminating sliding in vigorous throws. Cleated or spiked shoes are normally used to achieve this increased traction force.

CHECKING OF LINEAR MOTION

This principle (also called the hinged-moment principle) is sometimes evoked to explain movements in throws involving a run-up (e.g. Dyson 1978). The ground contact forces in the delivery stride cause the whole body to decelerate. However, this principle states that these forces cause the upper part of the body, and the object to be thrown, to rotate around the support foot and accelerate. For the principle to be valid, the forces on the feet should act behind the body's centre of mass, not in front of or through it (Alexander 1992). The few force-platform studies of these throws suggest this not to be the case for those parts of the delivery stride for which the ground contact forces are largest (e.g. Deporte & van Gheluwe 1988). Again, there is a lack of empirical research to support this principle.

Phases of a throw

The first step in the analysis of a motor skill is often the timing of the duration of the phases of the movement (e.g. Bartlett 1999). This is sometimes referred to as segmentation of the movement (e.g. Kanatani-Fujimoto *et al*. 1997). The division of a throwing movement into separate, but linked, phases is also useful because of the sheer complexity of many throwing techniques. The phases of the movement should be selected so that they have a biomechanically distinct role in the overall movement, which is different from that of preceding and succeeding phases. Each phase then has a clearly defined biomechanical function and easily identified phase boundaries, often called key moments or key events. Although phase analysis can help the understanding of throwing movements, the essential feature of these movements is their wholeness; this should always be borne in mind when undertaking any phase analysis of a throw.

Phases of ballistic movements

'Ballistic' movements are considered, kinesiologically, to be ones that are initiated by agonist muscle activity, continued by a 'coasting' period with no muscle activation, and terminated by deceleration by the antagonistic muscles or by passive tissue structures (e.g. Rasch & Burke 1978). These movements are generally fast. Many ballistic sports movements, including throws, can be subdivided biomechanically into three phases: preparation; action; and recovery (follow-through). Each of these phases has specific biomechanical functions. The later phases depend upon the previous phase or phases. It should be noted that, when recording the durations of these phases, a suitable definition of the phase boundaries needs to be chosen. For example, in a lacrosse shot, the end of the backward movement of the stick might be chosen as defining the end of the preparation phase and start of the action phase. However, at that instant, the legs and trunk will be in their action phase, while the distal joints of the throwing arm may not yet have reached the end of their preparation phase. This is reflected in the principle of sequential action of muscles (see above). This indicates one drawback of phase analysis, a certain arbitrariness in the selection of the key events.

PREPARATION PHASE

This phase has the following biomechanical functions.
• It puts the body into an advantageous position for the action phase.
• It maximizes the range of movement of both the implement and the thrower's centre of mass; i.e. it increases the acceleration path.
• It allows the larger segments to initiate the throw (sequential action of muscles).
• It puts the agonist muscles on stretch (stretch–shortening cycle) 'thus increasing the output of the muscle spindle to reinforce gamma discharge and increasing impulse through afferent neurones to the motor pools of functional muscle' (Gowitzke & Milner 1980). If the goal of the throwing movement is distance, then a fast backswing will gain the advantage of an increased phasic (speed-dependent) discharge, while a long backswing will increase the tonic (position-dependent) response. A fast backswing will promote a greater rise in spindle frequency leading to a stronger action, while a minimum hesitation between the preparation and action phases will allow full use of the phasic response. If the goal of the movement is distance, but the preparatory position must be held, as in a discus throw, then the phasic response cannot be used. To make full use of the tonic response, it is then necessary to use the longest possible backswing consistent with other requirements. If accuracy is the main goal, then a short and slow preparation is needed to control both the phasic and tonic spindle output so as to produce only the small forces needed. A short hesitation at the end of the preparation allows the phasic response to subside to the tonic level and aids accuracy; this is evident in the techniques of skilful dart throwers.
• It makes use of the length–tension relationship of the agonist muscles by increasing the muscle length to that at which maximum tension is developed (about 1.2 times the resting length).
• It allows the storage of elastic energy in the series elastic and parallel elastic elements of the agonist muscles. This energy can then be 'repaid' during the action phase.

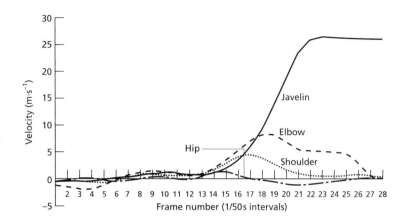

Fig. 18.9 Time series of segment and implement speeds relative to the centre of mass for the javelin throw. (From Best *et al*. 1993; with permission from E. & F.N. Spon, London).

• It provides Golgi-tendon organ facilitation for the agonists in the action phase by contraction of the antagonist muscles.

ACTION PHASE

Many of the general biomechanical principles of coordinated movement (see above) become evident here. In skilful throwers, we observe the sequential action of muscles as segments are recruited into the movement pattern at the correct time. Movements are initiated by the large muscle groups and continued by the faster, smaller and more distal muscles of the limbs. This increases the speed throughout the movement as the segmental ranges of movement increase (Fig. 18.9). The accuracy of movement also increases through the recruitment of muscles with a progressively decreasing innervation ratio. The segmental forces are applied in the direction of movement, and movements are initiated with minimum inertia as the movement proceeds along the kinetic chain. Finally, redundant degrees of freedom are controlled. The movements should be in accordance with these biomechanical features if the movement pattern is correct. In throws for distance, where release speed is usually the predominant requirement, all these principles should be evident, whereas in accuracy-dominated throws, one or more principles may be of lesser importance.

RECOVERY PHASE

This involves the controlled deceleration of the movement by eccentric contraction of the appropriate muscles. A position of temporary balance (stability) may be achieved. For a learner, the follow-through may require a conscious effort to overcome the Golgi-tendon organ inhibition that is reinforced by antagonistic muscle spindle activity.

Phases of other throwing movements

Some throwing movements do not easily fit the above pattern. For example, the following phases are normally defined for the javelin throw:
1 run-up: generation of controllable speed;
2 withdrawal: increase of acceleration path of javelin;
3 cross-over stride;
4 delivery stride: the action phase; and
5 recovery.

The first three of these together fulfil most of the functions of the preparatory phase of a three-phase throwing pattern. For a detailed evaluation of the biomechanical functions of these phases of the javelin throw, see Bartlett and Best (1988) or Morriss and Bartlett (1996). For a similar phase analysis of cricket bowling see Bartlett *et al*. (1996), and for discus throwing see Bartlett (1992).

Biomechanics of throwing injury

Throwing injuries, as other injuries, occur when the load applied to a tissue exceeds its failure tolerance. The occurrence and types of throwing injuries to the musculoskeletal system depend on the following factors. The influence of technique on throwing injuries will be the main focus of this section.

Load characteristics

The load characteristics can be divided into the following categories:
- type of load;
- magnitude of load;
- load rate; and
- frequency of load repetition.

Injuries are often divided into traumatic and overuse injuries. Traumatic, or acute, injury has a rapid onset often caused by a single external load. Overuse injuries result from repetitive trauma preventing tissue from self-repair and may affect bone, tendons, bursae, cartilage and the muscle-tendon unit (Pecina & Bojanic 1993); they occur because of microscopic trauma (or microtrauma). Overuse injuries are associated with repetitive loading of a joint, or other structure, at loads below those that would cause traumatic injury (Andriacchi 1989).

For example, bone injuries are mostly fractures; these are traumatic when associated with large loads. 'Stress' fractures are overuse injuries sustained at loads that are within the normal tolerance range for single loading, but that have been repeated many times, as in throwing training. The fractures are microscopic and should, more correctly, be termed fatigue fractures: all fractures are caused by stresses in the bone. Fractures are usually caused by various combinations of compression, bending and torsion that lead to various basic patterns of fracture (Gozna 1982). Fractures are not all that common in throwing.

Characteristics of loaded tissues

All injuries in sport and exercise involve failure of a biological material. To understand how injury to the musculoskeletal system occurs, it is necessary to know the loads and properties that cause specific tissues to fail. These relate to the material and structural properties of the various tissues of the musculoskeletal system—cortical and cancellous bone, cartilage, muscles, fascia, ligaments and tendons (see Bartlett 1999, for further consideration). The biological material properties that are important in this context include: density, elastic modulus, damping, traumatic failure strength, fatigue strength, creep strength, anisotropy (variation of properties with direction of loading), non-homogeneity (variation of properties with position), and viscoelasticity.

The following provides a useful and focused biomechanical subdivision for throwing injuries.

Congenital and biological factors

Congenital factors are innate musculoskeletal deformities, including alignment abnormalities, such as pes planus (flat feet).

Age (e.g. the high incidence of little leaguer's elbow in young baseball pitchers) or sex (male–female differences) may also be factors.

Fitness or training status

Insufficient training or low general fitness can increase the risk of injury, for example due to lack of flexibility or joint laxity, or a lack of, or imbalance in, muscular strength. However, the risk is also increased by excessive training for the subject's current fitness status, for instance where there is overtraining, fatigue or other training errors.

Equipment and surfaces

The footwear–surface interface is a factor in many throwing injuries to the lower extremity, because it is ever-present and because of the frequency of contact between the shoe and the surface. Changes in shoe or surface characteristics can alter not only the ground reaction force but also the activation patterns of the major leg extensor muscles. There appears to be an optimal compliance for a surface, both for performance and for reduction of injury (Greene & McMahon 1984). Although non-compliant (stiff) surfaces, which increase the impact loading,

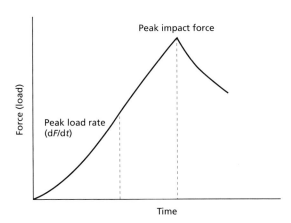

Fig. 18.10 Important impact variables. (Adapted from Bartlett 1999.)

are mostly implicated in injury, excessively compliant surfaces can lead to fatigue, which may also predispose to injury. Synthetic surfaces are also implicated in joint and tendon injuries owing to the stiffness of the surface. The important impact variables would appear to be peak vertical impact force, and the time to its occurrence; and peak vertical loading rate, and the time to its occurrence (Fig. 18.10). It is, however, not clear which of these ground reaction force measures are most important. The peak vertical impact force and peak loading rate are likely to relate to the shock wave travelling through the body. All of these variables are worsened by non-compliant (stiff) surfaces.

Technique

Throwers subject their bodies to loads that are well beyond the stresses and strains of sedentary life. The throwing techniques used, even when considered 'correct', may therefore cause injury. The use of many repetitions of these techniques in training should not therefore be undertaken lightly; the risk of injury may well override beneficial motor learning considerations. The use of an incorrect technique is usually considered to exacerbate the injury potential of sports. This has rarely been verified scientifically, although indirect evidence can often be deduced. The sport biomechanist should seek to

identify incorrect techniques to prevent injury (see e.g. Chapters 24–28). Training to improve throwing technique and to acquire appropriate strength and flexibility is likely to help to reduce injury as well as to improve performance. However, many throwing techniques are determined by the activity, reducing possible changes to technique, particularly at high standards of performance.

THE TRUNK

Low-back pain affects, at some time, most of the world's population (Rasch 1989) and has several causes. These are the weakness of the region and the loads to which it is subjected in everyday tasks and, particularly, in sport. Injury risk factors include the following three activities (Rasch 1989).
- Weight-loading, involving spinal compression. This may be exacerbated by any imbalance in the strength of the abdominal and back musculature.
- Rotation-causing activities involving forceful twisting of the trunk, such as discus throwing.
- Back-arching activities, as in many overarm throws.

Obviously, activities involving all three of these are more hazardous. An example is the 'mixed technique' used by many fast bowlers in cricket. Here the bowler counter-rotates the shoulders with respect to the hips from a more front-on position, at back foot strike in the delivery stride, to a more side-on position at front foot strike. At front foot strike, the impact forces on the foot typically reach over six times body weight. This counter-rotation, or twisting, is also associated with hyperextension of the lumbar spine. The result is commonly spondylolysis (a stress fracture of the neural arch, usually of L5) in fast bowlers with such a technique (Elliott *et al.* 1995). The incidence of spondylolysis and other lumbar abnormalities in fast bowlers is a good example of the association between technique and injury.

Relatively few incidences of spondylolysis have been reported amongst genuine side-on or front-on bowlers. A study of the 20 members of the western Australian fast bowling development squad (mean age 17.9 years) grouped the bowlers into those showing:

1 no abnormal radiological features;

2 disc degeneration or bulging on magnetic resonance imaging (MRI) scan; and

3 bony abnormalities.

This last group included spondylolysis, spondylolisthesis (forward subluxation of one vertebral body on another, usually after bilateral spondylolysis) or pedicle sclerosis (an increase in bone density of the pedicle or neural arch). The only significant difference was that between group 1 and both groups 2 and 3 for the change in shoulder alignment from back foot impact to the minimum angle, a clear indication of a mixed bowling technique (Elliott *et al.* 1992). This supported earlier research at the University of Western Australia (e.g. Foster *et al.* 1989). It might be hypothesized that incorrect coaching at a young age was responsible. British coaches and teachers have long been taught that the side-on technique is the correct one. However, as the less-coached West Indians might be held to demonstrate, the front-on technique may be more natural. Other factors (see also Elliott *et al.* 1995; Bartlett *et al.* 1996) that may contribute to lower back injury in fast bowlers include:

• overbowling, particularly by young bowlers whose epiphyses are not yet closed;

• poor footwear and hard surfaces, particularly in indoor nets;

• lack of physical conditioning;

• relatively high ball release positions;

• poor hamstring and lower back flexibility; and

• a straight front knee from front foot impact to ball release.

Soft tissue injury and avulsion fractures have been reported in the shot put from incorrect timing of the contractions of back muscles (e.g. Reilly 1992). Damage to the transverse abdominal muscle can result from errors in timing the hip 'lead' over the shoulders in the hammer throw (Reilly 1992).

THE UPPER EXTREMITY

In overarm throwing movements, such as javelin throwing and baseball pitching, the joints of the shoulder region often experience large ranges of motion at high angular velocities, often with many repetitions (Mallon & Hawkins 1994). Overuse injuries are common and frequently involve the tendons of the rotator cuff muscles that pass between the head of the humerus and the acromion process. These injuries appear to be dependent on the configuration of the acromion process and to occur more in individuals with a hook-shape configuration along the anterior portion of the acromion (e.g. Marone 1992). Examples are tendinitis of the supraspinatus, infraspinatus and subscapularis, and impingement syndrome. The latter term is used to describe the entrapment and inflammation of the rotator cuff muscles, the long head of biceps brachii and the subacromial bursa (e.g. Pecina & Bojanic 1993). Other soft-tissue injuries include supraspinatus calcification, rupture of the supraspinatus tendon, triceps brachii tendinitis, and rupture or inflammation of the long head tendon of biceps brachii. When repetitive stress exceeds the rate of tissue repair, the shoulder's stabilizing structures can de damaged leading, for example, to glenohumeral subluxation (Kvitne & Jobe 1993).

Most injuries to the upper extremity in throwing are overuse injuries, caused by repeated loading of the tissues affected (Atwater 1979). The stretch placed on the anterior soft tissues of the shoulder, at the limit of lateral rotation of the upper arm, may lead to injury. Spiral fractures, caused by torsional loading usually in combination with other loads, can occur in overarm throwing movements, owing to the inertia of the throwing object (e.g. a javelin) or large accelerations (Ogawa & Yoshida 1998). Posterior shoulder injuries are most likely during the recovery phase of throwing. Elbow injury is possible, particularly towards the end of the preparation phase, where the maximum valgus stress on the elbow occurs (e.g. Safran 1995). In overarm throwing, it appears that to achieve the goal of the movement (maximum ball or implement speed) the desire to avoid injury is relegated to second place.

Atwater (1979) proposed that sidearm as opposed to overarm throwing incurs an increased injury risk. This is well established for the javelin throw (Kuland 1982), where a round-arm throw, rather than throwing with the classic elbow lead position, can lead to sprains of the medial collateral elbow ligament, paralysis of the ulnar nerve or fractures of the olecranon. A poor technique has been implicated, starting with an incorrect position of the wrist after withdrawal and a wrong line of pull, followed by pronation during the final elbow extension in an attempt to reduce javelin flutter. Hyperextension of the elbow can damage the olecranon process; incorrect alignment of the javelin before the start of the throw can rupture the pronator teres. A faulty grip on the binding can injure the extensor pollicis longus (Reilly 1992).

Incorrect timing of the shot put can lead to injury to any of the rotator cuff muscles. Various tears of the long head tendon of biceps brachii and the wrist and finger flexors and extensors originating from the humeral epicondyles are associated with several shot-put technique faults. These include: poor co-ordination of arm and trunk muscles; the putting elbow being too low or ahead of the shot; and

'dropping' the shoulder on the non-throwing side. Incorrect positioning of the thumb can injure the extensor policis longus (Reilly 1992). Timing errors in the discus and hammer throws can also result in similar injuries to those in the shot put.

LOWER EXTREMITY

Injuries to the lower extremity caused by the trunk twisting or turning while excessive traction fixes the foot have a technique component, in addition to the properties of the shoe–surface interface. Where possible, twists and turns should be executed while the body is accelerating downwards; this technique, known as unweighting, reduces the normal component of ground contact force, for example in hammer and discus throwing.

References

Adrian, M.J. & Cooper, J.M. (1989) *Biomechanics of Human Movement*, 2nd edn. Brown & Benchmark, Madison.

Alexander, R. McN. (1991) Optimum timing of muscle activation for simple models of throwing. *Journal of Theoretical Biology* 150, 349–372.

Alexander, R. McN. (1992) *The Human Machine*. Natural History Museum Publications, London.

Andriacchi, T.P. (1989) Biomechanics and orthopaedic practice: a quantitative approach. In: *Future Directions in Exercise and Sport Science Research* (eds J.S. Skinner, C.B. Corbin, D.M. Landers, P.E. Martin & C.L. Wells), pp. 45–56. Human Kinetics Publishers, Champaign, IL.

Atwater, A.E. (1979) Biomechanics of overarm throwing movements and of throwing injuries. In: *Exercise and Sport Sciences Reviews*, Vol. 7 (eds R.S. Hutton & D.I. Miller), pp. 43–85. Franklin Institute Press, New York.

Bartlett, R.M. (1992) The biomechanics of discus throwing: a review. *Journal of Sports Sciences* 10, 467–510.

Bartlett, R.M. (1997a) *Introduction to Sports Biomechanics*. E. & F.N. Spon, London.

Bartlett, R.M. (1997b) Current issue in the mechanics of athletic activities: a position paper. *Journal of Biomechanics* 30, 477–486.

Bartlett, R.M. (1999) *Sports Biomechanics: Reducing Injury and Improving Performance*. E. & F.N. Spon, London.

Bartlett, R.M. & Best, R.J. (1988) The biomechanics of javelin throwing: a review. *Journal of Sports Sciences* 6, 1–38.

Bartlett, R.M., Stockill, N.P., Elliott, B.C. & Burnett, A.F. (1996) The biomechanics of fast bowling in cricket: a review. *Journal of Sports Sciences* 14, 403–424.

Best, R.J., Bartlett, R.M. & Morriss, C.J. (1993) A three-dimensional analysis of javelin throwing technique. *Journal of Sports Sciences* 11, 315–328.

Bober, T. (1981) Biomechanical aspects of sports techniques. In: *Biomechanics VII* (eds A. Morecki, K. Fidelus, K. Kedzior & A. Wit), pp. 501–509. University Park Press, Baltimore.

Brancazio, P.J. (1992) Physics of basketball. In: *The Physics of Sports*, Vol. I (ed. A. Armenti), pp. 86–95. American Institute of Physics, New York.

Brown, L. (ed.) (1993) *The New Shorter Oxford English Dictionary*. Clarendon Press, Oxford.

Deporte, E. & van Gheluwe, B. (1988) Ground reaction forces and moments in javelin throwing. In: *Biomechanics XI-B* (eds G. De Groot, A.P. Hollander, P.A. Huijing & G.J. van Ingen Schenau), pp. 575–581. Free University Press, Amsterdam.

Dillman, C.J., Fleisig, G.S. & Andrews, J.R. (1993) Biomechanics of pitching with emphasis upon shoulder kinematics. *Journal of Orthopaedic and Sports Physical Therapy* 18, 402–408.

Dyson, G. (1978) *The Mechanics of Athletics*,

7th edn. University of London Press, London.

Elliott, B.C., Hardcastle, P.H., Burnett, A.F. & Foster, D.H. (1992) The influence of fast bowling and physical factors on radiological features in high performance young fast bowlers. *Sports Medicine, Training and Rehabilitation* 3, 113–130.

Elliott, B.C., Burnett, A.F., Stockill, N.P. & Bartlett, R.M. (1995) The fast bowler in cricket: a sports medicine perspective. *Sports Exercise and Injury* 1, 201–206.

Foster, D.H., Elliott, B.C., Ackland, T. & Fitch, K. (1989) Back injuries to fast bowlers in cricket: a prospective study. *British Journal of Sports Medicine* 23, 150–154.

Gowitzke, B.A. & Milner, M. (1980) *Understanding the Scientific Bases of Human Movement*. Williams & Wilkins, Baltimore.

Gozna, E.R. (1982) Biomechanics of long bone injuries. In: *Biomechanics of Musculoskeletal Injury* (eds E.R. Gozna & I.J. Harrington), pp. 1–29. Williams & Wilkins, Baltimore.

Greene, P.R. & McMahon, T.A. (1984) Reflex stiffness of man's anti-gravity muscles during kneebends while carrying extra weights. In: *Sports Shoes and Playing Surfaces* (ed. E.C. Frederick), pp. 119–137. Human Kinetics Publishers, Champaign, IL.

Hatze, H. (1983) Computerised optimisation of sports motions: an overview of possibilities, methods and recent developments. *Journal of Sports Sciences* **1**, 3–12.

Herring, R.M. & Chapman, A.E. (1992) Effects of changes in segmental values and timing of both torque and torque reversal in simulated throws. *Journal of Biomechanics* **25**, 1173–1184.

Higgins (1977) *Human Movement: an Integrated Approach*. Mosby, St Louis.

Hore, I., Watts, S. & Tweed, D. (1994) Arm position constraints when throwing in 3 dimensions. *Journal of Neurophysiology* **72**, 1171–1180.

Hore, I., Watts, S. & Tweed, D. (1996) Errors in the control of joint rotations associated with inaccuracies in overarm throws. *Journal of Neurophysiology* **75**, 1013–1025.

Kanatani-Fujimoto, K., Lazareva, B.V. & Zatsiorsky, V.M. (1997) Local proportional scaling of time-series data: method and applications. *Motor Control* **1**, 20–24.

Kreighbaum, E. & Barthels, K.M. (1990) *Biomechanics: A Qualitative Approach for Studying Human Movement*, 3rd edn. MacMillan, New York.

Kuland, D.N. (1982) *The Injured Athlete*. Lippincott, Philadelphia.

Kvitne, R.S. & Jobe, F.W. (1993) The diagnosis and treatment of anterior instability in the throwing athlete. *Clinical Orthopaedics and Related Research* **291**, 107–123.

Luttgens, K., Deutsch, H. & Hamilton, N. (1992) *Kinesiology: Scientific Basis of Human Motion*, 8th edn. Brown & Benchmark, Madison.

Mallon, W.J. & Hawkins, R.J. (1994) Shoulder injuries. In: *Clinical Practice of Sports Injury: Prevention and Care* (ed. P.A.F.H. Renström), pp. 144–163. Blackwell Scientific Publications, Oxford.

Marone, P.J. (1992) *Shoulder Injuries in Sport*. Martin Dunitz, London.

Morriss, C.J. & Bartlett, R.M. (1996) Biomechanical factors critical for performance in the men's javelin throw. *Sports Medicine* **21**, 438–446.

Ogawa, K. & Yoshida, A. (1998) Throwing fracture of the humeral shaft—an analysis of 90 patients. *American Journal of Sports Medicine* **26**, 242–246.

Pecina, M.M. & Bojanic, I. (1993) *Overuse Injuries of the Musculoskeletal System*. CRC Press, Boca Raton.

Putnam, C.A. (1983) Interaction between segments during a kicking motion. In: *Biomechanics VIII-B* (eds H. Matsui & K. Kobayashi), pp. 688–694. Human Kinetics Publishers, Champaign, IL.

Putnam, C.A. (1993) Sequential motions of body segments in striking and throwing. *Journal of Biomechanics* **26** (S1), 125–135.

Rasch, P.J. (1989) *Kinesiology and Applied Anatomy*. Lea & Febiger, Philadelphia.

Rasch, P.J. & Burke, R.K. (1978) *Kinesiology and Applied Anatomy*. Lea & Febiger, Philadelphia.

Red, W.E. & Zogaib, A.J. (1977) Javelin dynamics including body interaction. *Journal of Applied Mechanics* **44**, 496–497.

Reilly, T. (1992) Track and field—2. The throws. In: *Sports Fitness and Sports Injuries* (ed. T. Reilly), pp. 145–151. Wolfe, London.

Safran, M.R. (1995) Elbow injuries in athletes—a review. *Clinical Orthopaedics and Related Research* no. 310, 257–277.

Sørensen, H., Zacho, M., Simonsen, E.B., Dhyre-Poulsen, P. & Klausen, K. (1996) Dynamics of the martial arts high front kick. *Journal of Sports Sciences* **14**, 483–495.

Tsirakos, D.T., Bartlett, R.M. & Kollias, I.A. (1995) A comparative study of the release and temporal characteristics of shot-put. *Journal of Human Movement Studies* **28**, 227–242.

Viitasalo, J.T. & Korjus, T. (1988) On-line measurement of kinematic characteristics in javelin throwing. In: *Biomechanics XI-B* (eds G. De Groot, A.P. Hollander, P.A. Huijing & G.J. van Ingen Schenau), pp. 583–587. Free University Press, Amsterdam.

Zajac, F.E. & Gordon, M.E. (1989) Determining muscle's force and action in multi-articular movement. *Exercise and Sport Sciences Reviews* **17**, 187–230.

Chapter 19

The Flight of Sports Projectiles

M. HUBBARD

Theory without experiment is vain; experiment without theory is blind.

Introduction

Many sports involve the flight of objects, typically balls or other implements but sometimes even the athletes themselves. This chapter defines and describes the important principles and features of such flight from a general point of view, frequently illustrating these general principles with specific examples. Often also in sports, the competitive nature of the activity implies that some feature of the trajectory, for example range or time aloft, should be maximized. Thus we approach much of the chapter from this point of view, asking and answering such questions as how maximum range or other optimal conditions can be achieved.

In the treatment here we are interested mainly in the flight itself and the determinants of this flight, and almost not at all with how the object is launched into flight by throwing, hitting, kicking or jumping muscular actions of the athlete. Thus we will be concerned with sensitivity of the flight to release conditions that the athlete can affect, but not specifically with how these can be achieved. Furthermore, we will consider only peripherally other second-order effects over which the athlete has little or no control, including atmospheric parameters such as wind, humidity, temperature and pressure. The rationale is that a comprehensive understanding of projectile flight is best achieved by paring the subject down to its essentials and that, even if second-order effects are considered, they may have little practical effect

since the athlete can do little or nothing to secure their existence.

Occasionally the flight must operate within or subject to constraints. Examples of this are the basketball passing through the hoop, a high-jumper or pole vaulter passing over a bar without contact, or a golf ball rolling around the rim of the hole. Only briefly will we consider constraints of these types and phenomena that link successive periods of flight such as bounces or other impacts.

Finally, we will restrict our discussion to autonomous flight of bodies, in which a knowledge of the initial (or 'release') conditions and a model for the flight characteristics enable a prediction of the ensuing motion. This precludes discussion of events that are controlled during flight by the athlete such as ski jumping, long-jumping and high-jumping, and gymnastic flight, except for models of these events which themselves neglect this real-time control.

The chapter first considers the interplay of the two main physical forces that determine flight, namely gravitational and aerodynamic ones. We discuss the special cases when one or the other of these is dominant and we try to develop an appreciation for the importance of the relative magnitudes of the two main contributors. Treated specifically is the special case when aerodynamic forces are absent entirely since this case admits closed form solutions that can supply substantial insight into the range optimization process. Next we consider how aerodynamic lift and drag forces are characterized and generated, and attempt to elaborate their general effects on flight trajectories. Finally we provide numerous examples from a variety of sports that illustrate the complexity and subtlety of the subject.

Before beginning we mention several previous general treatments of our subject in the literature. The first seven chapters of the delightful book by deMestre (1990) build the mathematical theory of ballistics towards an understanding of sports projectile flight. Although it concentrates heavily on the mathematics (having been used as a maths text) and shies away from any substantial treatment of numerical methods, in the last chapter it gives a brief review of the progress that had been made then in mathematical understanding of a wide range of sports projectiles. We highly recommend it as an introduction to the use of perturbation methods in flight mechanics.

The similar but more elementary book on projectile flight by Hart and Croft (1988) follows perhaps a more balanced approach. Although its first portion is analytical (since analytical methods when applicable can give more insight into the sensitivities and solutions than can purely numerical solutions), it ends with a tutorial on the numerical solution of differential equations and contains an entire appendix of example computer programs.

Several other relevant books on baseball (Watts & Bahill 1990; Adair 1990), golf (Jorgensen 1994) and pool (Marlow 1994) include more specialized treatments of specific sports but still devote considerable space to their flight aspects. The collection of 57 original articles on the physics of sports edited by Armenti (1992) contains many papers on projectile flight (in baseball, tennis, football, archery and long-jumping) and an even more extensive bibliography. Finally, the review of the four track and field throwing events by Hubbard (1989) takes a similar approach to the present chapter, although it is less general and less tutorial in nature.

Equations of motion

All motions in sports, and especially the flight of projectiles, are subject to Newton's Laws of Mechanics. Most simply these can be stated as: forces are required to change the velocity or state of motion of an object, with the rate of change being proportional to the magnitude of the force. Thus the equations of motion that describe flight are fundamentally *differential equations*, as opposed to algebraic relations that must be satisfied among a set of variables. The solutions of the equations of motion are the velocities and positions of the object *as functions of time*. So an inherent feature of flight is that things are changing, and understanding flight means understanding how all the relevant variables change simultaneously in time.

Without much loss in generality, we assume that the projectile is a single rigid body. The motion of such a body can be decomposed into translation of its centre of mass (COM) and rotation of the body about the COM. Translation is described by three Cartesian positions, x, y and z, and three corresponding velocities, v_x, v_y and v_z, and rotation by three orientation angles and three corresponding angular velocities that quantify the rotational speed of the object. If we lump all 12 of these variables that quantify the positions, orientations, velocities and angular velocities of the body into a single vector, x (called the state vector), the differential equations can be written compactly in schematic (or vector) form as

$$\mathrm{d}x/\mathrm{d}t = f(x,\mathbf{p}) \quad x(t=0) = x_o \qquad (19.1)$$

We distinguish in the above equation the variables (the elements of the vector x that change over time) from constant *parameters* $\mathbf{p}$, which quantify unchanging qualities of the body or the environment (such as air density, acceleration due to gravity, body mass, moment of inertia, length, etc.).

Equation 19.1 is valid at every instant during the motion. What the equation means is that how all the variables (the elements of x) are changing at every instant is dependent only on what values those variables have at that instant and on the values of the parameters describing the body. From the form of Eqn. 19.1 apparently, if the initial values x_o of the state variables are known, it should be possible to compute (either analytically or numerically) what happens, i.e. how the variables change throughout time. Equation 19.1 decomposes naturally into two subsets: a *kinetic* subset, which are simply mathematical statements of Newton's Laws, and a *kinematic* subset, which describe how the velocities cause changes in positions.

If the laws of motion are known and able to be solved, it is thus possible to think of the motion along the trajectory as a function only of the values of the state variables at the initial instant. Specifically, everything that happens (e.g. the maximum height achieved, the range when ground contact occurs, or the times when these events occur) is predetermined by the set of initial conditions x_o (and of course by Eqn. 19.1, which describes how these initial conditions evolve into the flight). Furthermore, it is also possible to calculate which set of initial conditions optimize the particular feature of interest.

One of the elements of the state vector is usually taken to be the velocity vector of the centre of mass (COM) of the body, v. The kinetic equations (the mathematical statement of Newton's Laws) for the translation of a single rigid body can be written in somewhat more detail as:

$$m \, dv/dt = F_g + F_a = -mg + F_a u_a$$

or, dividing by m,

$$dv/dt = -g(u_g - \beta u_a) \qquad (19.2)$$

where m is the mass of the body, and F_g and F_a denote the gravitational and aerodynamic force vectors acting on the body, respectively. In the simplified Eqn. 19.2 the two unit vectors, u_g and u_a,

point in the direction of the upward vertical and the aerodynamic force, respectively, and the dimensionless (variable) parameter β is the ratio of the aerodynamic to gravitational forces. This form of the equations of motion makes it clearest that the parameter β is a measure of the dominance of the varying aerodynamic forces compared to the constant gravity forces and that it is a fundamental determinant of the motion.

Forces

In general, the ratio β and the resulting aerodynamic force $\beta g u_a$ in Eqn. 19.2 vary in time as the orientation and velocity of the body change throughout flight. Nevertheless, it is useful to consider either the maximum possible value β_{max} (or alternately its average value), since this single number can give an idea of the overall importance of aerodynamic forces relative to gravitational ones and therefore which, if either, dominates the motion. Hubbard (1989) has coined the term 'aerodynamicity' for the ratio β_{max}, and it is called drag to weight ratio by deMestre (1990). It is tabulated in Table 19.1 for numerous sports balls and other objects.

Table 19.1 is modelled after, and some of its data are comparable to, similar tables for spherical and

Table 19.1 Various parameters and values of aerodynamicity for sports balls.

Sports ball	Estimated max. speed (m · s⁻¹)	Diameter (cm)	$Re \times 10^{5*}$	Mass (g)	β_{max} (aerodynamicity)
Table tennis	25	3.80	0.63	2.5	8.89
Squash	40	4.10	1.09	24	2.76
Shot put	15	11.0	1.10	7260	0.0086
Lacrosse	35	6.40	1.49	142	0.87
Cricket	35	7.20	1.68	156	1.00
Golf	65	4.30	1.86	46	4.18
Water polo	15	22.0	2.20	420	0.64
Jai lai	67	5.10	2.28	139	2.07
Baseball	50	7.30	2.43	145	2.26
Tennis	63	6.50	2.73	58	7.12
Softball	44	9.70	2.85	188	2.39
Basketball	18	24.30	2.92	600	0.79
Volleyball	30	21.0	4.20	270	3.62
Soccer	30	22.10	4.42	454	2.38

* Reynolds number.

other sports balls which appear in Frohlich (1984) and deMestre (1990). Table 19.1 includes the ball diameter and mass, a rough estimate of its maximum velocity in the particular game, the corresponding Reynolds number, and (based on a constant drag coefficient of 0.5) calculations of the aerodynamicity or maximum ratio of aerodynamic forces to weight. Since (as will be discussed below) the drag coefficient can decrease below 0.5 above the critical Reynolds number, this estimate for β_{max} is necessarily a rough and conservatively high one.

As Table 19.1 shows, however, the aerodynamicity, β_{max}, can vary over several orders of magnitude when we consider all sports projectiles. For example, for the extremely dense and relatively aerodynamically efficient shot put, $\beta = 0.0086$ and the trajectory is influenced less than 1% by aerodynamic drag. On the other hand, the very light and feathery badminton shuttlecock hit at a peak serving velocity of 68 m · s^{-1} (Tsai et al. 1997)—10 times its terminal velocity in air of about 6.8 m · s^{-1} (Peastrel et al. 1980) —experiences aerodynamic forces of roughly 100 times its weight. Thus $\beta_{max} = 100$ and the weight is negligible compared to the aerodynamic forces (but for only a short time!).

In summary, the interplay between F_g and F_a is mainly determined by β_{max}, the value of the aerodynamicity. Perturbation techniques (deMestre 1990) are applicable and can yield approximate analytical solutions to the equations of motion when β is very small or very large compared to unity but not, in general, when β is near 1. Nevertheless, even when analytical solutions to the motion equations are not available, numerical integration of the equations of motion is always possible and, more often than not, this is the approach chosen. We now turn to the characterization of the two kinds of forces.

Gravity

Perhaps the simplest fact about the flight of all autonomous bodies (regardless of their aerodynamicity, β_{max}) is that, because of the effects of gravity, everything which goes up must come down. Sports motions always take place over a small extent relative to the earth's radius so that the value of the apparent gravitational constant, g, to be used in Eqn. 19.2 is constant. Nevertheless, the value of g can vary substantially with changes in latitude and altitude on the earth's surface. The dependence of g_g, the gravitational attraction portion of g, on latitude λ is due to the oblateness of the earth and is given by Halliday and Resnick (1960) as:

$$g_g = 9.78039 + 0.05178 \sin^2 \lambda \qquad (19.3)$$

In addition it is conventional to include in the expression for g the vertical component g_c of the centripetal force due to the earth's rotation, so that Eqn. 19.3 for the apparent gravitational constant is thereby transformed to:

$$g = g_g + g_c$$
$$= 9.78039 + 0.05178 \sin^2 \lambda - 0.03373 \cos^2 \lambda \qquad (19.4)$$

Note that the centripetal correction (the coefficient $0.03373, = r\omega_e^2$, where r and ω_e are the earth's radius and spin angular velocity, respectively) is of the same order of magnitude as the oblateness gravity correction. The sum of these two terms yields a correction of almost 1% of the mean value of gravity, large enough to require careful application of Eqn. 19.4.

Changes in g also arise from altitude variations h from sea level. Since the gravitational force is proportional to the inverse square of distance, the percentage change in g due to a percentage change in radius r is given roughly by

$$dg/g = -2 \, dr/r \qquad (19.5)$$

and, since h is usually much smaller than r, the final expression for g becomes

$$g = (9.78039 + 0.05178 \sin^2 \lambda - 0.03373 \cos^2 \lambda)(1 - 2h/r) \qquad (19.6)$$

Altitude corrections ($-2h/r$) typically amount to considerably less than 0.1% and are sometimes neglected, depending on the accuracy required. Finally, as has been noted by Kirkpatrick (1944), even the eastward or westward motion of the object itself can induce centrifugal forces which, although smaller than the effects noted above, can cause differences in range exceeding the precision of the measurements by officials in track and field.

Aerodynamic forces

In general (i.e. for a complicated body shape) the dependence of the aerodynamic forces on velocities and orientation of the body must be determined experimentally, either through the use of wind tunnel tests in which the forces are measured directly, or through flight tests in which the aerodynamic forces may be deduced indirectly from their effects on the trajectory. For simple shapes (e.g. spherical balls, cylinders, flat plates, etc.) a large number of aerodynamic force results have already been obtained in the fluid mechanics literature. We will speak more about these cases in the discussion of lift and drag below.

The net aerodynamic force is the integrated effect of pressure and shear stresses acting over the surface of the body and is due partly to relative motion of the fluid (usually air) in which the body is immersed. We define the *relative wind velocity* to be the difference between the true wind velocity v_w and the velocity v of the centre of mass of the body. Thus when the body is motionless the relative wind velocity is the same as the wind velocity, while in the case of zero wind speed the relative wind velocity is merely the negative of the velocity of the body.

Because we have foresworn treatment of second-order effects, we assume henceforth that there is no wind so that the relative wind velocity is opposite to that of the object.

The total aerodynamic force is the integral of the normal pressure and shear stresses over the entire external surface of the body. This aerodynamic force is typically broken down into two components called lift and drag.

$$F_a = F_D + F_L \tag{19.7}$$

The *drag* is that component of the aerodynamic force in the direction of the relative wind, while *lift* (the remainder) is the component of the total force perpendicular to the relative wind. This decomposition is useful since the roles of drag and lift are fundamentally different. The drag force acts to decrease the speed of the object since it opposes the motion, while the role of lift is to change the direction of the velocity vector but not its magnitude.

DRAG

The drag force, F_D, is a sum of two parts: friction drag (drag due to shear stresses induced from motion of the projectile through a viscous medium) and pressure drag (drag due to the pressure in front of the object being greater than that in the rear). For the flight of most sports objects, pressure drag generally dominates and friction drag is often neglected.

At the velocities experienced by typical sports projectiles, the magnitude of the drag force F_D can be most conveniently expressed as a product of three factors: the dynamic pressure, $\rho v^2/2$ (where ρ is fluid density); a characteristic cross-sectional area, A (usually perpendicular to the mean flow or relative wind direction), and a dimensionless drag coefficient, C_D, as:

$$F_D = (\rho v^2/2)AC_D \tag{19.8}$$

Thus at a given speed and for a given characteristic cross-sectional area, only the drag coefficient is needed to completely specify the drag force.

Copious experimental fluid mechanics research has investigated the dependence of the drag coefficients of (usually non-rotating) bodies with simple shapes (spheres, cylinders, flat plates, etc.). In the first of these cases (in which there is spherical symmetry and thus no dependence on the body's orientation) it is found that the drag coefficient for a given body depends most strongly on a dimensionless number, Re, called the Reynolds number and defined as:

$$Re = \rho v d/\mu \tag{19.9}$$

where v is the relative (or free stream) wind speed, d is a characteristic distance of the object (e.g. in the case of a sphere we use the diameter $d = 2(A/\pi)^{1/2}$), and ρ and μ are the density and dynamic viscosity of the fluid (usually air), respectively. The Reynolds number (Re) can be interpreted to be the ratio of inertial to viscous forces in the flow. Even in cases when symmetry is partially or totally absent or when the attitude of the body is held constant, the drag coefficient depends strongly on the Reynolds number. Finally, we note that, for a given body and fluid, the Reynolds number is directly proportional

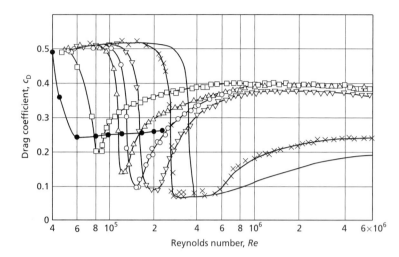

Fig. 19.1 Drag coefficient for a golf ball (black circles) (Bearman & Harvey 1976) and for spheres of varying roughness vs. Reynolds number. Although constant over a wide range of velocities, each undergoes an abrupt decrease (drag crisis) at a critical Reynolds number (and corresponding speed) which decreases with increasing roughness. (Adapted from Achenbach 1972, 1974; courtesy of Cambridge University Press.)

to speed (v), and that therefore most changes in Re are due to changes in v.

Figure 19.1 shows a typical set of such experimentally determined relations between c_D and Re for non-spinning spheres of varying roughness (a measure of the percentage deviation of the surface from that of a perfect sphere) as well as drag data for a golf ball. For purposes of preliminary discussion, consider the curve without symbols in Fig. 19.1, which is the drag curve for a nearly perfectly smooth sphere.

At very small velocities and Reynolds numbers ($Re \ll 1$) the flow field throughout the region around the sphere is laminar with flow *streamlines* (fluid particle trajectories) smoothly enveloping the body. This type of flow is called Stokes flow. The boundary layer (a thin layer near the body through which the flow velocity transitions between that of the body and that of the fluid) remains entirely attached to the surface. Over a wide range of Reynolds numbers less than about $Re = 1$, the drag force is found experimentally to be proportional to velocity and thus the drag coefficient defined by Eqn. 19.8 decreases more or less linearly with inverse velocity and hence Reynolds number. In this range of Reynolds numbers friction drag dominates, but the velocities at these Reynolds numbers are too small to be relevant to most sports. For

example, for a shot put in air $Re = 1$ at the very low speed $v = 0.00014$ m · s^{-1}.

As the Reynolds number is increased to a value somewhat larger than unity a relatively smooth transition in the drag coefficient curve occurs, until a range of Reynolds numbers is reached throughout which the drag coefficient for the sphere is nearly constant (at about $c_D = 0.5$ for a sphere), indicating the dominance of pressure drag. This gradual transition in drag coefficient is due to the initiation and gradual change in the point of separation of the laminar boundary layer from the surface of the sphere, beginning first at the rear stagnation point directly behind the sphere, and proceeding towards the front as Reynolds number and velocity increase. Beyond the Reynolds number at which the forwardmost point of separation is reached, and over a fairly wide range of Reynolds numbers ($Re = 100–250\,000$), flow conditions remain fairly stable and the drag coefficient remains nearly constant near the value of 0.5.

However, at a Reynolds number of roughly $250\,000$ (for the smooth sphere under discussion), when the Reynolds number is again increased only slightly (say by a factor of about 30%) the drag coefficient suddenly drops by a factor of more than five. The decrease in drag is due to a change of the flow conditions within the boundary layer from laminar to turbulent and a consequent shift backwards again of the separation point. This causes a consequent reduction of the size of the turbulent wake and hence decreases the pressure drag. This abrupt decrease in the drag coefficient is termed the *drag crisis* and plays an important role in many ball games, as will be discussed more fully below. Indeed the drop in drag coefficient over this relatively small range of velocities is large enough to cause even the size of the drag *force* (and not merely the drag coefficient) to decrease with speed and Reynolds number.

As the Reynolds number is increased further beyond the critical point, gradual increases in C_D are observed but the drag coefficient never returns to the value it has at precritical values of *Re*. The critical Reynolds number at which the drag crisis occurs depends strongly on surface roughness. As the relative roughness of the surface increases the drag crisis occurs at lower values of Reynolds number, as may be seen in the remainder of the family of curves presented in Fig. 19.1. Furthermore, the minimum value of drag coefficient reached increases gradually with increasing roughness, so that both the abruptness and the overall drop are less severe as roughness increases.

Return now to Table 19.1, which has been organized according to the maximum Reynolds number reached by the balls at the estimated maximum velocities thereof. We note that the Reynolds numbers of the several balls tabulated lie, to various degrees, within the critical Reynolds number range. Thus we would expect that the drag crisis affects, to a greater or lesser extent, the flight and performance of many sports balls. Frohlich (1984) has carefully investigated such effects in the case of the baseball, and Depra *et al.* (1997) have detected the drag crisis in served volleyballs. Apparently such investigations would be fruitful in many other sports.

Because air is a compressible fluid the drag coefficient technically depends on the Mach number (the ratio of the speed of the object to the speed of sound) but projectiles moving at speeds less than about $100 \text{ m} \cdot \text{s}^{-1}$ will be minimally affected by compressibility effects (Batchelor 1967). Few if any exceed this range.

There is considerable experimental evidence, however, that spin of the body directly and substantially affects the drag. For spherical objects the dimensionless *spin parameter*, S ($= \omega r/v$), is used to quantify spin, with ω being the magnitude of the angular velocity of the body. For a sphere or cylinder *r* is the radius and *S* can be interpreted as the ratio of velocity at the surface due to spin to that due to translation. Maccoll (1928), followed by Davies (1949), Bearman and Harvey (1976), Stepanek (1988), Aoyama (1990) and Smits and Smith (1994), documented the dependence of drag on the spin parameter, but for specific balls. Some general trends emerge but there is little comprehensive understanding as yet. Nevertheless, for a given object, the dependence of drag on spin and Reynolds number must be known in order to calculate accurately the motion.

Figure 19.2 shows the dependence of golf ball drag coefficient as a function of the spin parameter for various Reynolds numbers. As noted by Smits and Smith (1994), for Reynolds numbers greater than about 50 000 (corresponding to ball velocities greater than about $17 \text{ m} \cdot \text{s}^{-1}$) C_D increases monotonically as spin parameter increases, but for Reynolds numbers lower than 50 000, C_D first decreases to a minimum value as spin parameter increases, before beginning to increase with further increases in spin parameter. The complexities of these data (the most detailed yet available) show the intricate functional relationships which can be present between drag coefficient (and also lift and pitching moment coefficients as discussed below) and the two main independent variables, spin parameter and Reynolds number, even for a spherical ball.

TERMINAL VELOCITY

The drag coefficient is always positive and the drag force is quadratic in velocity. Thus for spherical objects such as those in Fig. 19.1 (and even for more general projectile shapes as long as a specific orientation with respect to the wind direction is chosen) there is always a velocity (v_t, called the *terminal velocity*) at which the drag force F_D equals the weight of the object. If the object is falling downwards, the

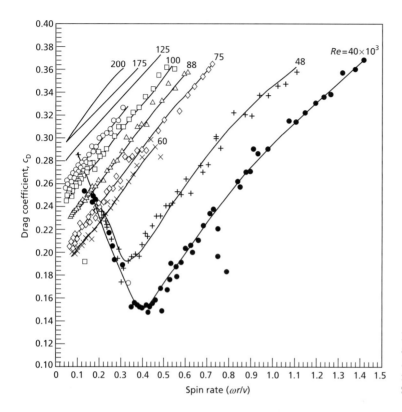

Fig. 19.2 Golf ball drag coefficient as a function of spin parameter $S = \omega r / v$, for various Reynolds numbers (Re). (Data from Smits & Smith 1994.)

drag force acts upwards, balancing the weight and bringing the body into equilibrium. Thus the terminal velocity is a measure of the maximum speed at which an object can steadily fall accelerated by gravity but retarded by drag in a given medium.

Substituting Eqn. 19.8 into the force balance $mg = F_{D}$, which expresses this equilibrium, and solving for the terminal velocity yields the expression

$$v_{t} = (2mg/\rho C_{D} A)^{1/2} \qquad (19.10)$$

The terminal velocity of an object is a property of the object and the medium, and it may even be used to characterize motions other than vertical falls. For example, if the motion is (mostly) in the horizontal direction the equation of motion for the velocity does not involve gravity and becomes

$$dv/dt = -F_{D}/m = -(\rho v^2/2)AC_{D}/m \qquad (19.11)$$

$$= -g(v^2/v_{t}^2)$$

$$= -v^2/L \qquad (19.12)$$

where $L \ (= 2m/\rho AC_{D} = v_{t}^2/g)$ is a characteristic distance of the velocity deceleration process, which is a function only of the physical and geometric parameters of the object and the fluid. The solution $v(t)$ to Eqn. 19.12 with an initial velocity v_{o} can be shown to be

$$v = v_{o}/(v_{o}t/L + 1) \qquad (19.13)$$

Thus in one characteristic time $T = L/v_{o}$ (here T depends not only on the object and medium but the initial velocity v_{o} as well) the object decreases its speed by a factor of two; in two characteristic times by a factor of three, and so on. This formulation and interpretation is most relevant in the approximate description of the motion of objects from initial velocities much larger than their terminal velocity, for example the badminton shuttlecock, and is only a good approximation if the deceleration is rapid enough to make the assumption of only horizontal motion a good one for a long enough time.

LIFT

The other major component of the aerodynamic force, lift, is characterized by a relation similar to the drag (Eqn. 19.8), namely

$$F_L = (\rho v^2/2)AC_L \qquad (19.14)$$

where the dimensionless lift coefficient C_L is a measure of the effectiveness of the body in producing aerodynamic force perpendicular to the velocity vector.

The lift coefficient (Batchelor 1967) is a function of the circulation, κ, defined to be the line integral of fluid velocity around a closed curve encircling the object. The magnitude of the lift force can be simply expressed as a product of three factors:

$$F_L = \rho v \kappa \qquad (19.15)$$

and can therefore be seen to be a direct effect of the combined translational speed of the body (v) and the circulation of the fluid around it (κ).

Circulation (κ) can arise in several ways, two of which are most important in sports applications. The most familiar of these is flow around an asymmetric body inclined to the flow direction through a non-zero *angle of attack.* This can best be illustrated by the two-dimensional case of a cambered aerofoil which, when its mean chord (the line connecting the front and rear tips) is inclined to the relative wind at an angle of attack α, generates a circulation because the air must travel further and faster around the top than the bottom. Many sports objects, although not designed to be aerofoil-like, nevertheless generate this kind of lift. Examples include bobsleds (Hubbard *et al.* 1989), javelins (Hubbard & Rust 1984) and discuses (Frohlich 1981).

Another way of creating circulation, especially for a symmetrical body such as a spherical ball, is to spin the body thereby creating a motion and velocity distribution of the fluid in the body's reference frame. This causes the circulation required for lift even though the fluid may possibly be motionless in an inertial reference frame. Although the first scientific investigation of this spin-induced lift force was accomplished by Robins (1742) it is often termed the *Magnus effect* (Magnus 1853). The Robins–

Magnus lift is a major determinant of the curvature of trajectories in golf, baseball, tennis and table tennis, volleyball and soccer, as well as many other ball games. For a discussion of this topic see the technical review by Swanson (1961), the paper by Barkla and Auchterlonie (1971) and a historical discussion of priority by Johnson (1986).

In the case of spherical balls, the spin-induced lift force can be written (Alaways 1998) using a dimensionless lift coefficient similar to Eqn. 19.8. Because the circulation is spin-induced, the direction of the force is obtainable from the cross product of the ball angular velocity vector $\boldsymbol{\omega}$ and speed vector $\mathbf{v}$ as

$$F_L = (\rho v^2/2)AC_L\,\boldsymbol{\omega} \times v/|\boldsymbol{\omega} \times v| \qquad (19.16)$$

which can be written in simpler form as

$$= (\rho v^2/2)AC_L\,u_L \qquad (19.17)$$

where u_L is the unit vector in the $\boldsymbol{\omega} \times \mathbf{v}$ direction.

Note that when the spin angular vector $\boldsymbol{\omega}$ is in the same direction as the velocity vector v there is no Robins–Magnus force or spin-induced lift.

The Robins–Magnus lift coefficient is a strong function of both the Reynolds number and the spin parameter. Maccoll (1928) apparently made some of the first direct measurements of the force on a sphere, although both Rayleigh (1877) and later Tait, in a series of papers (Tait 1890, 1891, 1893, 1896), had investigated its effect on tennis and golf trajectories, respectively. Davies (1949) and Bearman and Harvey (1976) made similar measurements specifically on golf balls. A review by Mehta (1985) covers the aerodynamics of baseballs and golf and cricket balls. Recent work by Kao *et al.* (1994) measured the Robins–Magnus force on volleyballs.

These studies have recently been extended by Aoyama (1990) and Smits and Smith (1994). Figure 19.3 shows a golf ball lift coefficient as a function of spin parameter S ($= r\omega/v$) for various Reynolds numbers. This work has shown definitively that, at least in the golf ball, substantial variations in C_L occur as a function of both S and Re. For example, at constant $Re = 40\,000$, the golf-ball lift coefficient can increase by as much as a factor of 2.5 over the range $S = 0.4–1.4$. The full fluid mechanical explanation for these changes is not yet fully understood and experiments must still play the dominant role.

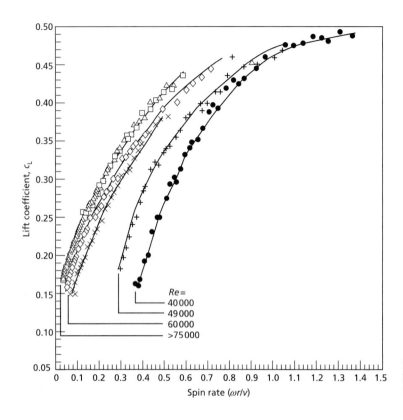

Fig. 19.3 Lift coefficients for golf balls as a function of spin parameter. (Data from Smits & Smith 1994.)

In summary, for spherically symmetrical balls the lift and drag coefficients depend substantially on Reynolds number and spin parameter, with these dependencies further complicated by surface roughness. In addition, non-symmetrical objects show dependence on body attitude relative to the mean flow.

MOMENTS OF AERODYNAMIC FORCES

Although by definition the gravity force acts at the COM, this is not the case for aerodynamic forces. Thus aerodynamic forces create moments about the COM, which cause angular acceleration of the body. These moments act as an excitation to the rotational equations of motion. For example, in motion of the javelin in a two-dimensional plane, the moment perpendicular to this plane causes rotation of the javelin within the plane. In general, both drag and lift can exert moments of this kind and their effects are frequently lumped together in expressions

which are reminiscent of the lift and drag equations (Eqns 19.14 & 19.8). The expression for the magnitude of the moment is usually given as

$$M = (\rho v^2/2)AdC_M \qquad (19.18)$$

where the moment arm distance, d, is a characteristic geometric distance of the body which is required to convert forces to moments.

The simple case of spindown of a spinning golf ball has also been investigated experimentally by Smits and Smith (1994) by measuring the torque about the axis of spin. They found no dependence on Reynolds number and a linear dependence between dimensionless spin rate decay and spin parameter, according to $(r^2/v^2)d\omega/dt = -0.00002r\omega/v$. This implies a linear differential equation for spin:

$$50\,000\ r/v\ d\omega/dt + \omega = \tau d\omega/dt + \omega = 0 \qquad (19.19)$$

For a typical speed $v = 60$ m·s^{-1} and radius $r = 0.0213$ m, the spin, ω, which is the solution to Eqn.

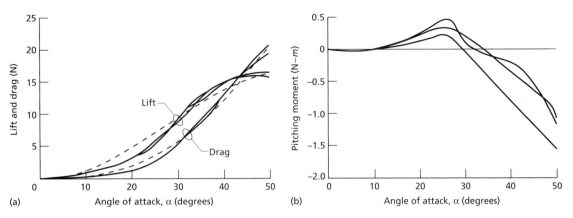

Fig. 19.4 Aerodynamic forces: (a) lift and drag; and (b) pitching moment vs. angle of attack for the old-rules javelin. (From Hubbard & Rust 1984, pp. 769–776, with permission from Elsevier Science.)

19.19 is given by $\omega = \omega_0 \exp(-t/\tau)$. The characteristic time, τ, for spin decay is in this case about 18 s and a ball loses only about 30% of its initial spin during a 6 s flight. Applying similar ideas to short flights of projectiles such as baseballs or cricket balls leads to the often used approximation that spin is roughly constant during a flight of one second or less.

Although for a spinning sphere the torque depends only on spin rate, when there is not spherical symmetry (e.g. the discus or javelin) the dimensionless moment coefficient, C_M, is a function of both the attitude of the body relative to the fluid stream and the Reynolds number, Re, and may even be a function of other parameters such as angular velocity. When the asymmetry is large the most important of these is the angle of attack.

As a real example of lift, drag and pitching moment coefficients and their dependence on attitude for an asymmetrical body, Fig. 19.4 shows these functions for three javelins (Terauds 1972). Because the asymmetry is so large for the javelin, each is plotted as a function of angle of attack, α, the primary variable of importance. They are found to be only weak functions of Reynolds number and Mach number.

VARIATIONS OF LIFT, DRAG AND MOMENTS
DURING FLIGHT

When discussing drag, lift and aerodynamic mo-

ments separately in terms of Eqns 19.8, 19.14 and 19.18, one focuses on them as algebraic relations which are functions of the variables involved. But this tends to obscure the important fact that several factors (certainly v and sometimes even C_L and C_D) in these expressions are variables during the flight. As a consequence the lift and drag forces themselves vary continuously during flight. Indeed, it is the forces that cause changes in velocities that cause changes in the forces, so that everything is coupled and changing together.

Solutions to the equations of motion

If the equations of motion are simple enough it may be possible to derive or calculate analytical, closed-form solutions (e.g. Eqn. 19.13 above) which take this simultaneous variation into account. Some examples of such cases are given in the book by deMestre (1990). It must be recognized however, that the simplifying assumptions required to make an analytical solution possible severely limit the applicability of these methods to but a few realistic problems. Even when the equations are so complex that analytical solutions are not at hand, however, it is reassuring that numerical integration techniques can always be used to obtain quantitative solutions to the equations of motion. Furthermore, one should not view numerical integration as an inferior or inadequate method of solution since this is the

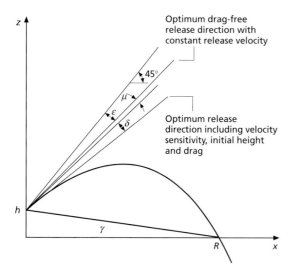

Fig. 19.5 Release variables and resulting shot put trajectory showing deviations of optimal release angle from 45° due to initial height (ε), drag (μ) and velocity sensitivity (δ).

way almost all solutions of realistic projectile flight problems are obtained.

Drag-free trajectories

We now discuss the simplest special case, namely when there is no aerodynamic force and the trajectory is completely determined by gravity. Consider the object shown in Fig. 19.5, which is released with speed v in a vertical plane from a height h above the horizontal ground plane, and with an initial velocity vector which has angle θ with respect to the horizontal. In this case the trajectory is soluble analytically. Numerous authors have presented what is perhaps the most informative single equation for motion of a drag-free projectile. It expresses the range (horizontal distance between launch point and impact point on the horizontal plane) in terms of the three release variables (v, h and θ) at the initial instant, and thus shows clearly the dependence of the range on each of these variables.

$$R(v,h,\theta) = v^2 \cos \theta \, [\sin \theta + (\sin^2 \theta + 2gh/v^2)^{1/2}]/g \tag{19.20}$$

Small drag approximations

When the aerodynamicity, β, is non-zero but small, then drag is not entirely negligible but can be treated as a small perturbation to the drag-free motion. In this case perturbation methods can supply analytical approximations to the trajectory. The good news is that these approximations are in closed form so that interpretation of the solutions is possible. The bad news is not very bad. Even though the solutions are only approximations, they are reasonably good ones when the aerodynamicity is small.

The object with perhaps the smallest aerodynamicity is the shot put (see Table 19.1). After rederiving Eqn. 19.20, Lichtenberg and Wills (1978) then added drag to the equations of motion. Using a variant of perturbation theory they derived an expression for the decrease in maximum range due to drag which, in the absence of wind, becomes

$$dR_m = -av^3/3g^2 \sin^2 \theta_m \cos \theta_m \tag{19.21}$$

where the small parameter $a = C_D A\rho v/2m$ and, since the velocity changes little over the entire flight, is roughly proportional to the aerodynamicity

$$a \approx g\beta_{max}/v \tag{19.22}$$

Dividing Eqn. 19.21 by Eqn. 19.20 and using Eqn. 19.22 we can then express the percentage reduction in the range due to drag as

$$dR_m/R_m = -av/(3g \sin \theta_m \cos^2 \theta_m)$$
$$\approx -\beta_{max} \text{ when } \theta_m \approx 45° \tag{19.23}$$

Notice that Eqn. 19.23 implies that β_{max} is a good approximation to the percentage reduction in drag, no matter what the initial velocity.

Two-dimensional motion with non-negligible aerodynamic forces

A somewhat simplified version of the most general case is that of two-dimensional (2D) motion. Here a reasonably accurate approximation may be obtained by restricting the motion to a single vertical plane, reducing the number of degrees of freedom to just

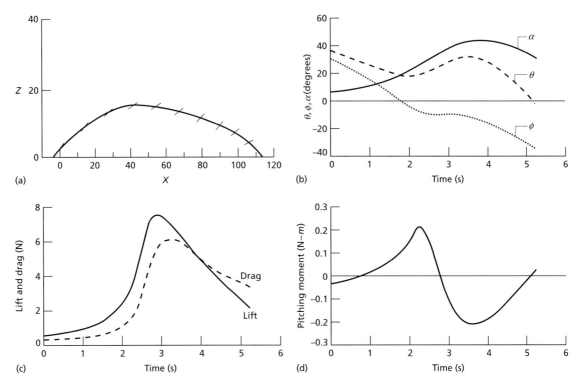

Fig. 19.6 Simulation results for flight of the javelin with aerodynamic forces and moments as in Fig. 19.4. (a) X,Z positions of the centre of mass (COM). (b) Pitch attitude (θ), angle of attack (α) and flight path angle ($\phi = \tan^{-1}(v_y/v_x)$) vs. time. (c) Aerodynamic lift and drag forces vs. time. (d) Pitching moment vs. time. (From Hubbard & Rust 1984, pp. 769–776, with permission from Elsevier Science.)

three: cartesian x,y positions of the COM in the plane and the pitch rotation, ϕ, about an axis perpendicular to the vertical plane. The translational velocity and the lift and drag forces obviously act in the vertical plane as well. But in this case the complicated dependence of lift, drag and pitching moment on angle of attack and velocity usually precludes any closed-form solution and numerical methods must be used to integrate the differential equations.

Shown in Fig. 19.6 are the results of a 2D simulation using the lift and drag forces for the javelin with aerodynamic force characteristics previously given in Fig. 19.4. Figure 19.6a depicts the x,y positions of the COM through the flight while Fig. 19.6b shows the evolution of the pitch attitude (θ), the angle of attack (α) and the flight path angle ($\phi = \tan^{-1}$

(v_y/v_x)). Finally, Figs 19.6c & 19.6d show lift and drag forces, and pitching moment, respectively, plotted as functions of time. For the particular set of initial conditions chosen, note that the lift and drag forces reach values of 7.5 and 6.1 N, respectively, at a time around $t = 3.0$ s. Since the javelin mass is only 0.8 kg, the total aerodynamic force is more than 1.5 times the javelin's weight of 7.84 N, corroborating that the aerodynamicity of the javelin is of the order of unity.

Three-dimensional motion—the general case

In the most general case, the lift and drag forces are of the same order of magnitude as the weight and they vary continuously throughout flight, but not necessarily in a single plane as the orientation and speed of the body change. An example of projectile flight which embodies this full complexity is the badminton shuttlecock. Although it is geometrically axially symmetrical, it nevertheless experiences rotations about all three axes during flight, and its trajectory is fully three-dimensional. Thus a complete description of the motion requires all six degrees of freedom and 12 state variables as well as a knowledge of how all aerodynamic forces and moments depend on all state variables. McShane *et al.* (1953) describe this approach for rotating axially symmetrical shells.

Another example of a sports projectile which, while axially symmetrical, nevertheless embodies important three-dimensional effects, is the discus. A provocative paper by Frohlich (1981) has considered this problem, which is interesting for several reasons. The discus is not only extremely aerodynamic, but also it has a large amount of spin angular momentum which must be accounted for in the analysis. The lift force does not act through the COM and it thus creates a torque which precesses the spin axis. Frolich calculates that the discus can be thrown further into the wind than with a following wind. A search for optimal release conditions which maximize range would probably show that the prominence of the lift force will allow a range exceeding that in a vacuum, even without a headwind.

Optimization of release conditions

One of the most common goals in sport is to maximize the range of a projectile. All four throwing events in track and field (shot put, hammer, discus and javelin) involve this task. Additional examples include the badminton high clear, golf driving for distance, and the baseball home run, but others have more complicated objectives (e.g. the football punt may attempt to maximize a combination of the time aloft and distance). To illustrate the general idea of range maximization we choose the drag-free range equation (Eqn. 19.19), realizing that it is actually only a very good approximation when the aerodynamicity is small, namely for the shot put.

In order to achieve maximum range in the drag-free case it is necessary to differentiate Eqn. 19.19 with respect to the three input variables and set

these derivatives to zero, since the definition of optimal implies that the sensitivity of the range with respect to each of the optimizable variables vanishes. If this is done it is easy to see that there are no optimal values for either v or h since the derivatives of range with respect to each of these variables are always positive. This is a mathematical way of saying that it is always better to have v and h as large as possible. But given some values for v and h, there is indeed an optimal value (θ_m) for the release angle which will maximize the range.

Optimal release conditions when release variables are independent

We now assume that the other two release variables, v and h, are independent of θ since this assumption simplifies the analysis considerably (the validity of this assumption and its effect on the optimal release angle results will be discussed in more detail below). Then, differentiating $R(v,h,\theta)$ with respect to θ, setting this expression equal to zero at θ_m, and solving for the function involving θ_m yields the relation

$$\sin^2 \theta_m = 1/(2 + 2gh/v^2)^{1/2} \qquad (19.24)$$

which can be substituted into Eqn. 19.20 to eliminate v (Lichtenberg & Wills 1978) and write the maximum range in particularly simple form as a function of only two variables:

$$R_m = h \tan 2\theta_m \qquad (19.25)$$

If Eqn. 19.25 is solved for the optimal release angle, θ_m, which maximizes the range,

$$\theta_m = \tan^{-1} (R_m/h)/2 \qquad (19.26)$$

it can be shown (Hubbard 1989) that θ_m deviates only slightly from 45° according to

$$\theta_m = 45° - \varepsilon \qquad (19.27)$$

where $\varepsilon = \gamma/2$ and γ is the angle between the horizontal and the line drawn from the shot put at release to the eventual landing point (see Fig. 19.5).

When $h = 0$ and the object is released from ground level, Eqn. 19.20 reduces to the well-known equation from elementary physics:

$$R = (v^2 \sin 2\theta)/2g \qquad (19.28)$$

which according to Eqn. 19.26 is maximized when $\theta_m = 45°$.

At this point it is useful to highlight a prominent feature of Eqns 19.20 and 19.28. Note that each of these expressions for range contains a factor which is quadratic in velocity and inversely proportional to the strength of gravity. The simplicity of the drag-free case and the resulting ability to derive analytical closed-form expressions make the fundamental tradeoff in projectile flight particularly apparent; flight is a struggle to prolong the time when the initial vertical velocity and resulting height are annulled by the inexorable downward pull of gravity. Even in situations where the aerodynamic forces are larger (but not dominant) and related in a complicated way to the other variables in the problem (here the equations of motion must necessarily be solved numerically), this fundamental fact remains roughly true. To first order in virtually all projectile flight, *range is quadratic in release velocity*: doubling the velocity will roughly quadruple the range.

Lichtenberg and Wills (1978) extended the analysis of drag-free optimal release discussed above by deriving an expression for the optimal release angle in the case of (small) drag. They showed that the additional deviation μ of the optimal release angle from 45° due to drag is given by

$$\mu = av(\cos \theta_m - (\sec \theta_m)/3)/g \qquad (19.29)$$

$$\approx \beta (\cos \theta_m - (\sec \theta_m)/3)/g$$

$$\approx 0.1° \text{ when } \theta_m \approx 45°$$

Thus the optimal release angle deviates from 45° according to

$$\theta_m = 45° - \varepsilon - \mu \qquad (19.30)$$

(but only when the release velocity is constant and independent of the other release conditions θ and h). The main conclusions of Lichtenberg and Wills (1978) may be summarized in Eqns 19.22 and 19.29, and in words as: drag in the shot put causes less than a 1% decrease in range and an insignificant change in the optimal release angle from the drag-free case (when the release velocity is independent of the other release conditions).

Optimal release conditions when release velocity (v) depends on release angle

The assumption that the release variables are independent of each other—which was so naturally made by Lichtenberg and Wills (1978) and in the optimization discussion of the previous section—turns out in fact not to be a good one. Its motivation, of course, was to make the mathematics simpler, since if it were true the optimal release angle is easily calculated by the above procedure given by Eqn. 19.30. But it should not be surprising that the human thrower is not necessarily able to achieve the same maximal velocity at all release angles. Therefore this fact must be taken into account in the optimal release angle calculations if the resulting optimal release angles are to be realistic.

It is interesting that this general concept was apparently first understood in the javelin throw, an event in which the drag-free equations and development above are not relevant at all. Soong (1975) presented the first simulations of the flight of the javelin. He made the same assumption as did Lichtenberg and Wills (1978), namely that release velocity was independent of release angle (actually this assumption was implicit since the converse was not explicitly stated). Soong used the simulations to determine the javelin optimal release angle, which he found to be about 43°.

Later, however, in reaction to the work of Soong (1975), Red and Zogaib (1977) presented results of experiments which measured release angle and velocity in throws of 1.14 kg balls (chosen to be nearly equal to the mass of the javelin, 0.8 kg). These results showed clearly that release velocity decreases substantially as release angle increases, at an average rate of about 0.127 m · s⁻¹ per degree. Using an actual javelin, Viitasalo and Korjus (1988) measured the same sensitivity of release velocity to release angle of 0.127 m · s⁻¹ per degree. Writing the release velocity as a function of release angle we have

$$v = v_0 + 0.127 \ (\theta° - 35°) \qquad (19.31)$$

where v_0 is the 'nominal' velocity achievable at a nominal release angle of 35°, and $\theta°$ is the release angle in degrees, the angle between the initial velocity vector and the horizontal.

Red and Zogaib (1977) then used the dependence of Eqn. 19.31 in simulations of javelin flight from which they were able to determine the optimal release angle. For a nominal release velocity of $30 \, \mathrm{m \cdot s^{-1}}$ their calculated optimal release angle of $37°$ differed by more than $6°$ from that of Soong (1975). Similar simulations including the same release velocity sensitivity were later done by Hubbard (1984) (but using aerodynamic forces and moments for the pre-1986 javelin, which had been measured by Terauds (1972), rather than classical theoretical expressions which had been assumed by Soong). Hubbard calculated an optimal release angle of $31°$, the $6°$ difference from the results of Red and Zogaib being due mostly to the differences in the aerodynamic forces assumed. Later Best et al. (1995) repeated the same calculations for five post-1986 (new rules) javelins, which have aerodynamics more like the theoretical assumptions of Soong (1975), and found optimal release angles for these javelins to be between $29°$ and $34°$ at a release velocity of $30 \, \mathrm{m \cdot s^{-1}}$.

It cannot be overemphasized that the inclusion of even a small dependence of release velocity on release angle is crucial in optimal release angle and range calculations, and that its incorporation can have a large effect on the results, as seen in the previous discussion. This applies to all the track-and-field throwing events and the flight of other sports projectiles in which maximization of range is a desirable objective. Although the masses of objects differ considerably, the general rule that achievable velocity decreases with increasing release angle might be expected to hold for all thrown projectiles.

Recently, similar experiments to those of Red and Zogaib (1975) were conducted by Hubbard et al. (2000) to measure the sensitivity of release velocity to release angle in the shot put. Preliminary results for three throwers show that the shot put release velocity decreases with release angle at a rate of about $0.031 \, \mathrm{m \cdot s^{-1}}$ per degree, a considerably smaller sensitivity than that in the javelin. Further, optimization results (deMestre et al. 2000) show that the incorporation of this sensitivity changes the optimal release angle for the shot put (assuming release velocity $v = 15 \, \mathrm{m \cdot s^{-1}}$ and release height $h = 2.0 \, \mathrm{m}$) from $42°$ to roughly $38°$, in considerably better agreement than Eqn. 19.30 with experimental measurements of release angle in the shot put by Dessureault (1978) and McCoy et al. (1984).

If we generalize the form of Eqn. 19.30 to include all three deviations of the optimal release angle from $45°$, due to release height, aerodynamic drag and release velocity sensitivity, respectively, we have

$$\theta_{\mathrm{m}} = 45° - \varepsilon - \mu - \delta \qquad (19.32)$$

and (in the shot put at least) the deviation δ due to the velocity sensitivity is in general an order of magnitude larger than μ, that part due to non-zero drag.

Major advances in the understanding of optimal release conditions which maximize the range of other sports projectiles have yet to occur. These will happen when similar velocity sensitivity measurements are made in the discus and hammer throws, and other batted and kicked projectiles where the same ideas may be expected to apply.

Lack of continuity in optimal release conditions as a function of velocity

The optimal release calculations discussed previously have all assumed either that release velocity was constant (independent of the other release conditions, such as release angle) or that the sensitivity, when it exists, is small enough that the variations in velocity are small compared to the nominal velocity achievable at the optimal release angle. For example, world-class velocities in the javelin throw are approximately $30 \, \mathrm{m \cdot s^{-1}}$, and Eqn. 19.31 predicts that deviations of $5°$ from the optimal release condition will cause changes in v of only about $0.65 \, \mathrm{m \cdot s^{-1}}$. But the capacities of elite and subelite throwers differ by considerably more than this, and the same is true of the other throwing events. Thus it is of interest to do the optimal release calculations over a range of values for nominal velocity (v_0) so that the optimal release conditions may be known to all throwers over a wide range of strength and nominal velocity capacities.

Hubbard and Alaways (1987) presented such optimal release conditions in the javelin throw as a function of nominal velocity, v_0. It was found that

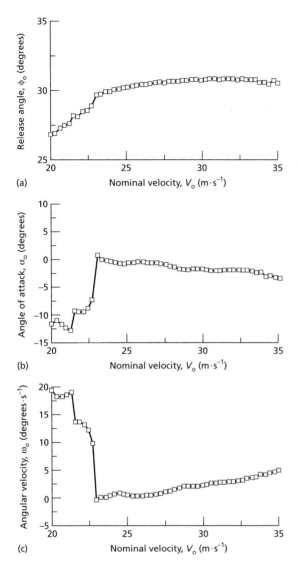

Fig. 19.7 Optimal release conditions ((a) release angle, (b) initial angle of attack and (c) pitching angular velocity) in the javelin throw vs. nominal release velocity. The discontinuities are caused by the strong aerodynamic effects and the fact that non-neighbouring trajectories become optimal as v_o is changed gradually. (From Hubbard & Alaways 1987.)

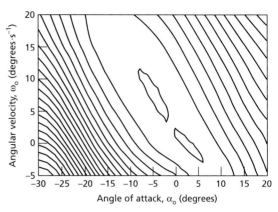

Fig. 19.8 Range contours for the new-rules javelin in the angle of attack (α_o) and pitching angular velocity (ω_o) space, at $v = 22.85$ m · s^{-1}. Two sets of initial conditions (the tops of the two hills) result in the same maximum range at this velocity. (From Hubbard & Alaways 1987.)

these optimal release conditions were not a continuous function of nominal velocity, a fact that was later verified by Best *et al.* (1995). The results of Hubbard and Alaways are shown in Fig. 19.7. Optimal release conditions may be thought of

heuristically as the 'location' of the top of the 'hill' in parameter space which maximizes the height of the hill (the range). In this case there are several hilltops, but only one which is highest. As the nominal velocity v_o is gradually changed, the second highest hill displaces the highest hill and the location of the optimum suddenly shifts to that point. Figure 19.8 depicts the two local maxima which exist in the α_o–ω_o plane for a nominal release speed v_o near 23 m · s^{-1} for the javelin range problem previously discussed in Fig. 19.7. It is thought that these discontinuities arise as a result of the substantial effects of aerodynamics (relatively large β_{max}) and that they will not be present in other events in which aerodynamics are not as important, such as the shot put.

Experimental measurement of flight trajectories

Thus far this chapter has focused on theoretical and computational aspects of sports projectile flight. Although probably more understanding has been gained from theoretical and numerical studies than from experimental ones, experiments have been a valuable source of verification of theoretical ideas and models, and much effort has been applied to studying such phenomena experimentally.

Typically the flight of the projectile is tracked using one or more film or video cameras. As video resolution and speed have increased and computers have risen to the enormous data-processing tasks that one second of video data presents (e.g. 200 frames per second $\times$ 1 000 000 pixels in each frame with 256 bits of grey scale in each pixel = about 50 000 000 bits/second), video has gradually become more popular. Furthermore, its output is inherently digital and thus can be readily dealt with by computers.

If the flight is near enough to lying in a single vertical plane and if it is possible to control carefully the experimental conditions, then a single camera orientated with the camera axis perpendicular to the flight plane can suffice. In this case, either the centre of the body (for spheres) or numerous points on the body are located in each frame and transformed by a distance scale factor (with units of metres per pixel and determined by calibration filming of an object of known size) into x,y coordinates in the plane. Almost always the resolution of the camera is low such that the entire flight cannot be filmed because the resulting uncertainty in the location of the object in each frame is an unacceptably large percentage of the total field of view. Thus usually only the first few metres of flight are tracked and the 'release' conditions are determined from these data. The concomitant increase in accuracy usually more than outweighs the loss of data for the entire trajectory.

When flight is fully three-dimensional or when the single plane of flight is not known or able to be controlled *a priori*, two or more cameras are needed orientated with their optical axes non-collinear. In this case the images from the two cameras are combined with calibration data, again determined by filming an object with several points of known positions using the DLT algorithm (Abdel-Aziz & Karara 1971) to yield fully three-dimensional x,y,z coordinates of the flight.

When the body is extended and asymmetrical (e.g. the discus and javelin) several points on the body must be tracked in order to determine not only its position but also its attitude. Indeed, the javelin is an even more complicated case since it is a body which does not remain rigid. Thus the theoretical model for flight must include not only the 12 state variables for rigid body motion (see discussion above) but also some model for the free-free vibrations which are induced by the acceleration of the javelin by the thrower. These vibrations affect the aerodynamic forces in flight (Hubbard & Bergman 1989) and also act as high-frequency noise, corrupting the quantitative determination of the trajectory from the film data. Without the incorporation of a model for the vibrations the vibratory noise completely swamps the rigid body motions, making their accurate determination impossible (Hubbard & Always 1989).

Another desirable feature of experimental determination of flight trajectories using video instead of film cameras is that it can be done quickly enough to allow the quantitative data to be used in athlete training (Hubbard & Always 1989).

Summary and conclusions

In this chapter we have attempted to give an introductory but comprehensive account of the causes and techniques for understanding the motion of sports projectiles. Aerodynamic forces cause the trajectories to deviate from the parabolic ones which would be produced by gravity alone. The size of aerodynamic forces can range roughly from 0.01 to 100 times the sports projectile's weight. The lift and drag forces are functions of body attitude relative to the wind stream, the spin of the body, the relative wind speed, and the shape and size of the projectile. Analytical solutions to the equations of motion can be determined only in the case when aerodynamic drag and lift are very small. Otherwise numerical methods must be used to generate solutions to the equations of motion and the specific solutions are functions of the particular release conditions chosen. Optimal release conditions are strongly dependent on the interdependence of release velocity with the other release variables, most importantly release angle. It is important to use experimental results to validate and verify theoretical and simulation results.

References

Abdel-Aziz, Y.I. & Karara, H.M. (1971) Direct linear transformation from comparator coordinates into object space coordinates in close-range photogrammetry. In: *ASP Symposium on Close Range Photogrammetry*, pp. 1–18. American Society of Photogrammetry, Falls Church, VA.

Achenbach, E. (1972) Experiments on the flow past spheres at very high Reynolds numbers. *Journal of Fluid Mechanics* **54**, 565–575.

Achenbach, E. (1974) The effects of surface roughness and tunnel blockage on the flow past spheres. *Journal of Fluid Mechanics* **65** (1), 113–125.

Adair, R.K. (1990) *The Physics of Baseball*. Harper & Row, New York.

Alaways, L.W. (1998) Aerodynamics of the curve-ball: an investigation of the effects of angular velocity on baseball trajectories. PhD thesis, University of California, Davis.

Aoyama, S. (1990) A modern method for the measurement of aerodynamic lift and drag on golf balls. In: *Science and Golf* (ed. A.J. Cochran), pp. 199–204. E.F. Spon, London.

Armenti, A. Jr. (ed.) (1992) *The Physics of Sports*. American Institute of Physics, New York.

Barkla, H.M. & Auchterlonie, L.J. (1971) The Magnus or Robins effect on rotating spheres. *Journal of Fluid Mechanics* **47** (3), 437–447.

Batchelor, G. (1967) *An Introduction to Fluid Dynamics*. Cambridge University Press, Cambridge.

Bearman, P.W. & Harvey, J.K. (1976) Golf ball aerodynamics. *Aeronautics Quarterly* **27**, 112–122.

Best, R.J., Bartlett, R.M. & Sawyer, R.A. (1995) Optimal javelin release. *Journal of Applied Biomechanics* **11** (4), 371–394.

Davies, J.M. (1949) The aerodynamics of golf balls. *Journal of Applied Physics* **20**, 821–828.

Depra, P., Brenzikofer, R., Barros, R. & Lima, E.C. (1997) Methodology for the 'drag crisis' detection in services executed by high level volleyball athletes. In: *Proceedings of XVIth Congress, International Society of Biomechanics, Tokyo* (eds S. Fukashiro, T. Fukunaga, Y. Hirano *et al.*), p. 157.

Dessureault, J. (1978) Selected kinetic and kinematic factors involved in shot putting. In: *Biomechanics VI-B* (eds E. Asmussen & J. Jorgensen), p. 51.

Human Kinetics Publishers, Champaign, IL.

Frohlich, C. (1984) Aerodynamic drag crisis and its possible effect on the flight of baseballs. *American Journal of Physics* **52** (4), 325–334.

Frohlich, C. (1981) Aerodynamic effects on discus flight. *American Journal of Physics* **49**, 1125–1132.

Groh, H., Kuboth, A. & Baumann, W. (1966) De la cinétique et de la dynamique des movements corporels rapides, études concernant les phases finales du lance et du javelot. *Sportartz*, 10.

Halliday, D. & Resnick, R. (1960) *Physics for Students of Science and Engineering*. John Wiley & Sons, New York.

Hart, D. & Croft, T. (1988) *Modelling with Projectiles*. Ellis Horwood, Chichester, West Sussex.

Hubbard, M. (1984) Optimal javelin trajectories. *Journal of Biomechanics* **17** (10), 777–787.

Hubbard, M. (1989) The throwing events in track and field. In: *Biomechanics of Sport* (ed. C.L. Vaughn), pp. 213–238. CRC Press, Boca Raton, FL.

Hubbard, M. & Alaways, L.W. (1987) Optimal release conditions for the new rules javelin. *International Journal of Sport Biomechanics* **3**, 207–221.

Hubbard, M. & Alaways, L.W. (1989) Rapid and accurate estimation of release conditions in the javelin throw. *Journal of Biomechanics* **22** (6/7), 583–595.

Hubbard, M. & Bergman, C.L. (1989) Effect of vibrations on javelin lift and drag. *International Journal of Sport Biomechanics* **5**, 40–59.

Hubbard, M. & Rust, H.J. (1984) Simulation of javelin flight using experimental aerodynamic data. *Journal of Biomechanics* **17** (10), 769–776.

Hubbard, M., Kallay, M. & Rowhani, P. (1989) Three-dimensional bobsled turning dynamics. *International Journal of Sport Biomechanics* **5**, 222–237.

Hubbard, M., deMestre, N. & Scott, J. (2000) Sensitivity of release variables in the shot put. *Journal of Biomechanics* (submitted).

Johnson, W. (1986) The Magnus effect – early investigations and a question of priority. *International Journal of Mechanical Sciences* **28**, 859–872.

Jorgensen, T.P. (1994) *The Physics of Golf*. American Institute of Physics, New York.

Kao, S.S., Sellens, R.W. & Stevenson, J.M. (1994) A mathematical model for the trajectory of a spiked volleyball and its coaching application. *Journal of Applied Biomechanics* **10**, 95–109.

Kirkpatrick, P. (1944) Bad physics in athletic measurement. *American Journal of Physics* **12**, 7–12.

Lichtenberg, D.B. & Wills, J.G. (1978) Maximizing the range of the shot put. *American Journal of Physics* **46** (5), 546–549.

Lieberman, B.B. (1990) Estimating lift and drag coefficients from golf ball trajectories. In: *Science and Golf* (ed. A.J. Cochran), pp. 187–192. E. & F.N. Spon, London.

Maccoll, J.W. (1928) Aerodynamics of a spinning sphere. *Journal of the Royal Aeronautical Society* **28**, 777–798.

Magnus, G. (1853) Uber die Abweichung der Geschosse und eine auffallende Erscheinung bei rotirenden Körpern. *Poggendorf Annalen der Physik und Chemie* **88**, 1.

Marlow, W.C. (1994) *The Physics of Pocket Billiards*. Marlow Advanced Systems Technologies, Palm Beach Gardens, FL.

McCoy, R.W., Gregor, R.J., Whiting, W.C., Rich, R.G. & Ward, P.E. (1984) Kinematic analysis of elite shot putters. *Track Technique* **90**, 2868–2871.

McShane, E.J., Kelley, J.L. & Reno, F.V. (1953) *Exterior Ballistics*. University of Denver Press, Denver, CO.

Mehta, R.D. (1985) Aerodynamics of sports balls. *Annual Review of Fluid Mechanics* **17**, 151–189.

deMestre, N. (1990) *The Mathematics of Projectiles in Sport*. Cambridge University Press, Cambridge.

deMestre, N., Hubbard, M. & Scott, J. (2000) Optimizing the shot put (submitted).

Peastrel, M., Lynch, R. & Armenti, A. (1980) Terminal velocity of a shuttlecock in vertical fall. *American Journal of Physics* **48**, 511–513.

Rayleigh, L. (1877) On the irregular flight of a tennis ball. *Messenger of Mathematics* **7**, 14–16.

Red, W.E. & Zogaib, A.J. (1977) Javelin dynamics including body interaction. *Journal of Applied Mechanics* **44**, 496–497.

Robins, B. (1742) *New Principles of Gunnery*. [Republished in 1972 by Richmond Publishing Company, Richmond, UK.]

Smits, A.J. & Smith, D.R. (1994) A new aerodynamic model of a golf ball in flight. In: *The 1994 World Scientific*

Congress of Golf (eds A.J. Cochran & M.R. Farrally), pp. 340–347. E. & F.N. Spon, St. Andrews, UK.

Soong, T.C. (1975) The dynamics of javelin throw. *Journal of Applied Mechanics* **42**, 257.

Stepanek, A. (1988) The aerodynamics of tennis balls – the topspin lob. *American Journal of Physics* **56**, 138–142.

Swanson, W.W. (1961) The Magnus effect; a summary of investigations to date. *Journal of Basic Engineering* **83**, Series D, 461.

Tait, P.G. (1890) Some points in the physics of golf. *Nature* **42**, 420–423.

Tait, P.G. (1891) Some points in the physics of golf. Part II. *Nature* **44**, 487–498.

Tait, P.G. (1893) Some points in the physics of golf. Part III. *Nature* **48**, 202–205.

Tait, P.G. (1896) On the path of a rotating spherical projectile. *Transactions of the Royal Society of Edinburgh* **39** (Part II), 490–506.

Terauds, J. (1972) A comparative analysis of the aerodynamics and ballistic characteristics of competition javelins. PhD thesis, University of Maryland.

Tsai, C.L., Huang, C. & Jyh, S.C. (1997) Biomechanical analysis of different badminton overhead forehand strokes of Taiwan elite players. In: *Proceedings of XVIth Congress, International Society of Biomechanics, Tokyo* (eds S. Fukashiro, T. Fukunaga, Y. Hirano *et al.*), p. 356.

Viitasalo, J.T. & Korjus, T. (1988) On-line measurement of kinematic characteristics for javelin. In: *Biomechanics XI-B* (eds G. deGroot, A.P. Hollander, P.A. Huijing *et al.*), pp. 582–587. Free University Press, Amsterdam.

Watts, R.G. & Bahill, A.T. (1990) *Keep Your Eye on the Ball*. W.H. Freeman, New York.

Chapter 20

Javelin Throwing: an Approach to Performance Development

K. BARTONIETZ

To rush on the spear point and break the enemy's ranks is great courage; to be able to open heaven and earth shows wonderful talent. [Chinese proverb (in Scarborough & Allan 1964, p. 342)]

The past, present and future of Olympic javelin throwing

Modern javelin history

To rush on the javelin point and break the competition's ranks can open heaven and earth for an athlete and coach. This feeling has undoubtedly been felt by the event's top athletes since the beginning of modern javelin history. If one compares early javelin competitions (Sweden 1792, Greece 1856, Hungary 1870, Finland 1879 and Germany 1906) with modern-day events the distance thrown has almost tripled. The javelin throw was introduced to the Olympic Games for men in 1906 and for women in 1932. Scandinavian athletes were predominant during the first three decades of Olympic javelin throwing, winning all six gold medals, four silver and four bronze medals during the period 1908–32, as well as being world-record holders until 1953. Eric Lemming of Sweden was the only athlete to win three Olympic titles—in 1906 (in Athens), 1908 (in London) and 1912 (in Stockholm). Finnish athletes developed the throwing technique during the 1920s and 1930s. Their movement pattern together with an ideal combination of speed and technique was demonstrated by Matti Järvinen and his pupil Yrjo Nikkanen, the leading athletes during this period. Light implements for young athletes were also

introduced at this time. The preoccupation of the Finns with javelin throwing was probably based, to some extent, on an ancient wartime tradition of the Ugro-Finnic people (Quercetani 1964).

A remarkable aberration in javelin-throwing technique occurred during the mid-1950s with the rotational throwing style. This technique was first used by the Spanish and Basques and was based on a popular throwing event of the Basques during folk games. The idea is to enhance the acceleration of a wooden beam (of mass 3.5 kg and length 1.5 m) by several turns. The record at that time for throwing the bar was 50.56 m, which compares with a distance for the 4 kg shot of 40 m, thrown by Czech discus thrower Imre Bugar. The javelin was thrown after two turns (F. Eraszquin, a previously unknown Basque athlete, attaining 83.40 m) or with one turn after 8–10 strides. Along with the obvious safety considerations when using this technique and the potential of throwing distances greater than 100 m, biomechanical considerations led to this technique being banned since this javelin sling was an abandonment of the classic throwing technique. Since this time, in accordance with rule 186-5-a of the International Amateur Athletics Federation (IAAF) (1996, p. 181), 'the javelin shall be held at the grip. It shall be thrown over the shoulder or upper part of the throwing arm and shall not be slung or hurled. Non-orthodox styles are not permitted.'

Coaches and athletes from the Soviet Union were the event's leaders during the 1960s and 70s, culminating in the Latvian Janis Lusis' complete set of Olympic medals (bronze in 1964, gold in 1968, silver in 1972), his four European titles and two world records. At the end of the 1970s and beginning of the 1980s, Hungarian athletes served as technical role models for other athletes to follow. Based on more than 50 years of experience, top Hungarian javelin throwers such as Miklos Nemeth (94.30 m in 1976, Olympic title in 1976) and Ferenc Paragi (96.72 m in 1980) wrote a further chapter of javelin history. After the first 100 m throw in 1984 by Uwe Hohn of Germany, the men's javelin was reconstructed to ensure a safe landing with the point. However, 10 years later the world record with the modified javelin is again close to the 100 m mark—currently standing at 98.48 m and thrown by Jan Zelezny in 1996.

Women started to throw the javelin at the beginning of the 1920s. In 1926 the 600 g implement was introduced, replacing the 800 g implement. Athletes from the former Soviet Union were the first to throw 50 m (in 1947), 60 m (in 1964), and 70 m (in 1980). Double Olympic Champion, Ruth Fuchs (1972 and 1976) of Germany and her coach took the event to a new level, setting six world records, culminating in 69.96 m. Her successor, Petra Felke, was the leading athlete of the late 1980s, setting the 80.00 m world record in 1988, prior to winning the Olympic Games. Changes to the women's javelin were made in 1999, just 13 years after similar changes to the men's implement, to eliminate illegal flat landings and with it the possibility of dubious decisions being made by judges. Such specifications have been discussed by Paish (1986) for more than 10 years. Since 1 April 1999 the 80.00 m world record is no longer recognized.

Javelins have been made from different materials, ranging from wood (using a glued laminated hollow construction) to special metallic alloys (the first metal javelins were introduced in 1954) to high-tech implements incorporating carbon fibres as a reinforcing material which, together with resins, forms a composite material with a higher strength/weight ratio than metal. The very stiff carbon javelins, when thrown by top throwers possessing a good technique (optimum angle of release, minimum angle of attack and yaw), can achieve an extra distance of 2–3 m, based on our own observations. The general increase in performance is attributable, in part, to the development of high-preformance imple-

ments for training and competition. Among 100 wooden javelins only one would have been a high-performance implement. Today, almost identical high-performance implements are produced and available for everyone. Although the choice of material does play a certain role in achieving good performance, Elvira Ozolina of the Soviet Union won the gold medal in 1960 (i.e. after the introduction of metal javelins) with an implement made of Finnish birch. So it is ultimately the thrower who has to select and be able to handle the different types of implements. The construction of synthetic runways, officially introduced at the Olympic Games of 1968 in Mexico City, has led to a faster run-up and allowed higher release velocities, based on a harder block of the thrower's left side.

Event-specific and individual performance development

The top 10 male and female athletes in 1997 came from eight countries spread over three continents, underlining the recent popularity of the event. Since Järvinen's day, different approaches have been taken to analyse the development of top performances (e.g. world records, national records, world top 10) in an attempt to forecast the evolution of the event. Regardless of international and national records, which most athletes never achieve, each athlete needs his or her respective medium- or long-term prognosis of performance improvement. It is the main aim of the present study to develop a training structure, based on biomechanical knowledge, to attain this targeted performance.

Athlete and coach must work through the following consecutive steps to achieve this goal:
• get a clear picture of the evolution of the event;
• determine the athlete's required development in the main performance parameters;
• identify individual strengths and weaknesses in throwing technique and stamina;
• construct an individual goal technique and develop the internal movement picture of the athlete (Fig. 20.1);
• ascertain the effects of the main training exercises from both a biomechanical and a physiological point of view;

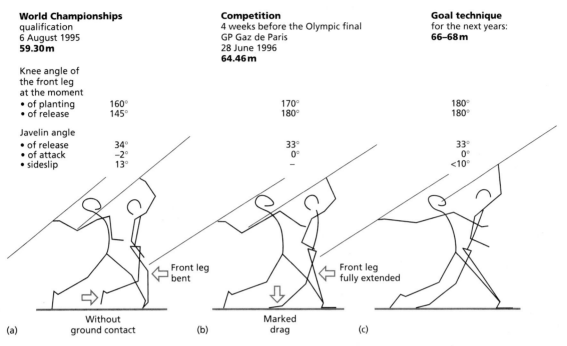

World Championships	Competition	Goal technique
qualification	4 weeks before the Olympic final	for the next years:
6 August 1995	GP Gaz de Paris	**66–68 m**
59.30 m	28 June 1996	
	64.46 m	

Knee angle of
the front leg
at the moment

• of planting	160°	170°	180°
• of release	145°	180°	180°

Javelin angle

• of release	34°	33°	33°
• of attack	−2°	0°	0°
• sideslip	13°	–	<10°

Fig. 20.1 Body positions at the moment of planting the front leg and at the moment of release for a female javelin thrower. (a) In the qualifying round at the World Championships in 1995 (the athlete did not qualify).(b) Close to the technical demands at the competition during the peaking period. The athlete reached the Olympic final and won the silver medal. (c) Target body positions for attaining a higher performance level. (From Bartonietz & Larsen 1997.)

• ascertain the achieved loads in all training areas, by recording and analysing training work, as a basis for planning the training load for the targeted performances;
• adhere to the golden rule of 'training–performance–training', based on the comparison of 'debit and credit' during training and competition; and
• performance diagnosis.

From here, the coach and the athlete can progress step by step, starting from the targeted distance via the necessary power demands of the athlete's actions to the selection of training exercises and planning the loads accordingly.

The internal ballistics of world-class performances

The main goal of javelin throwing is simply to enable an implement of specified mass (800 g for men; 600 g for women; less for younger athletes) to land in a throwing sector with the point as far as possible from the foul or scratch line. The athlete's active influence on the implement finishes at the moment of release and the javelin starts to fly according to the initial release parameters. Study of the interaction between the thrower and the implement leading up to the moment of release is called 'internal ballistics' (cf. the study of the flight of projectiles, which is called 'external ballistics'). The following section reviews the basic factors that determine the distance thrown. An analysis of the energy and power production necessary for the implement's movement and for the thrower's key actions follows. Based on this analysis, the basic demands are discussed for the coordination of movement, i.e. the movement pattern, when throwing the javelin at different performance levels. The findings of this part are supported by the basic laws of mechanics, by accumulated experimental research data, and by the practical experiences of coaches and athletes alike. The implications for training are given throughout this section. The information given is intended to enable both coach and athlete to determine, in a more detailed fashion, their own current performance level and to take the right decisions in planning the next steps to reach performance targets both in training and competition.

When interpreting the experimental research data presented below, it has to be remembered that such data are always accompanied by certain inaccuracies in measurement. The crucial moment of release, in particular, and with it the release velocity, are difficult to determine, due to the high movement velocity and the spatial movements of the thrower's limbs and the implement. Information concerning calculated average data and the statistical significance of research results can be misleading. They have to be considered with all due scepticism since they can only give information about an average level of technique and performance. This study defines the parameters for attaining a targeted high performance with an almost ideal technique. Individual variations have to be accounted for.

Parameters of release

Using a simplified approach the distance thrown is determined by the velocity of release, the height of release and the angle of release, i.e. the direction of the velocity of release. These parameters are also responsible, to a large degree, for the distance thrown in the javelin event. For a detailed analysis, for example in comparing different throws of a single athlete or comparing athletes, the more comprehensive initial conditions for the aerodynamics of the flight phase and the flight phase itself have to be taken into consideration. This issue is discussed in more detail by M. Hubbard in Chapter 19—see also the studies of Terauds (1985), Hubbard (1988) and Best et al. (1995). In contrast to throwing or putting the shot, the angle of attack, the angle of yaw, the initial pitching momentum and the air conditions (air resistance, influenced mainly by wind direction and velocity with respect to the javelin's position in the air) all influence the distance thrown. The revolutions of the javelin around its long axis and the

amplitude of its vibrations also have an influence (Fig. 20.2). All these parameters are the result of the athlete's action during delivery until the end of contact with the implement, and will be discussed in this context.

VELOCITY OF RELEASE

The most important factor influencing the distance thrown is the velocity of release, a measure of the kinetic energy given to the implement; it is the only factor that can be maximized by the athlete's action. Nevertheless, any search for a 'maximum' velocity of release produces instead an 'optimal' value because of the need for an optimal movement direction. Therefore, it is the maximum velocity within the restrictions of the optimal values of the other parameters (see below) whilst paying attention to the rules for the movement execution. Despite the squared effect of the release velocity (see Eqn. 19.20 in Chapter 19 by M. Hubbard), the linking with other parameters causes a quasi-linear relationship between release velocity and flight distance of the implement in the window targeted zone, for example from 45 to 65 m for female athletes or from 70 to 90 m for males (Bartonietz 1987; Bartonietz et al. 1996) (Fig. 20.3; see also the data of Hubbard 1989). The practical implication for coaching a targeted increase in distance thrown, say by 10%, is that it requires an equal increase of release velocity, also by 10%. But it does not mean that an improvement of the strength level to the same extent (e.g. developed by weights) leads automatically to a corresponding improvement in release velocity. As shown later (see 'Energy and power demands' below), the desired training effect involves changes in strength and power capacities, and in throwing technique as well. It is often difficult to compare release velocities and distances of throws from different competitions when considering external conditions, the implements used, release parameters and the accuracy of the measuring methods. This difficulty has to be taken into account when interpreting the data in Fig. 20.3.

The close relationship between thrown distance and velocity of release is reflected in a correlation coefficient $r = 0.90-0.97$ (data of several authors

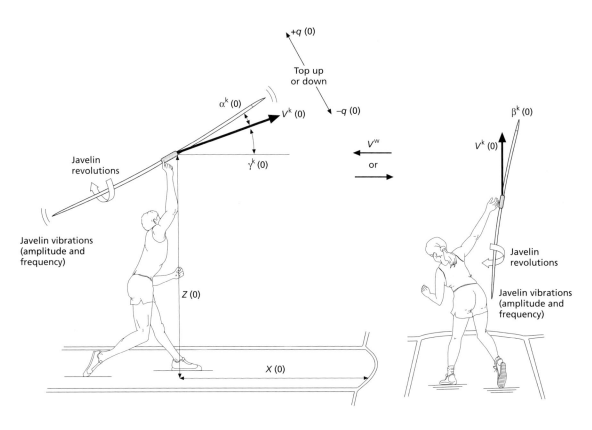

Fig. 20.2 The release parameters, side and rear view.

Parameter	Unit of measure	Name	Definition
$Z(0)$	m	Height of release	Height between ground and the javelin's mass centre at the instant of release
$X(0)$	m	Distance to foul line	Distance between the projection of the javelin's mass centre to the ground and the foul line at the instant of release
$V^k(0)$	degrees	Release velocity	Velocity of the javelin's mass centre to the ground
$\gamma^k(0)$	degrees	Release angle	Angle between direction of vector of the release velocity and the ground
$\alpha^k(0)$	degrees	Angle of attack	Angle between the javelin's longitudinal axis and the direction of the vector of the release velocity
$\beta^k(0)$	degrees	Angle of yaw	Also: angle of side attack, or angle of sideslip, angle between the vector direction of the velocity of release and the javelin's longitudinal axis (looking from behind)
$q(0)$	degrees·s^{-1}	Release pitch rate	Angular velocity of the javelin's tip at the instant of release
V^w	m·s^{-1}	Wind speed	

summarized by Borgström 1988) for the old javelin (valid before April 1986), which decreased to a correlation coefficient of between 0.80 and 0.87 for the implement with the current specifications (valid since April 1986) (Borgström & Almström 1986; quoted by Borgström 1988). The lower correlation coefficient underlines the greater role of technique with the new-style javelin, due to the fact that this implement reacts more sensitively to deviations from the optimal release parameters; a view supported

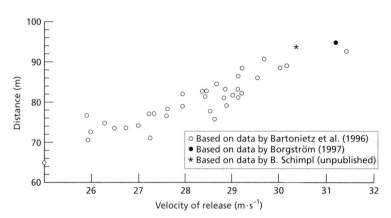

Fig. 20.3 Relationship between distance thrown and velocity of release. Based on release velocity data of Bartonietz *et al.* (1996), Borgström 1997 and Schimpl (1997). *Note:* The measured distance in competitions, from the foul line to the point of landing, is not identical with the real thrown distance, from the point of landing to the vertical projection to the ground of the point of release (see Fig. 20.2). The distances used here are 'real thrown distances', including the distances between the foul line and release position.

by the observations of Julin (1988). Because of this, the introduction of the new javelin meant increased demands on technique and a greater need for biomechanical research, contradicting some coaches' and athletes' expectations, that the demands of technique would be less with the new implement (Paish 1986; Borgström 1988). The same requirements are expected for the new women's implement from 1999 onwards.

Up to four different kinds of grip have been suggested in the relevant textbooks (Suliev 1961; Schmolinsky 1983; Sing 1984; Terauds 1985; Jarver 1987; Johnson 1987). Bankhead and Thorsen (1964) found no statistically significant differences in strength development on the grip. The unusual fork grip (also called 'first and second finger grip', 'V' or claw grip) was used by the former world-record holder, Tom Petranoff, and is used by the second-best female performer in the world in 1997 and 1998, Joanna Stone (68.64 m).

JAVELIN POSITION AT THE MOMENT
OF RELEASE WITH RESPECT TO FLIGHT
DIRECTION AND PITCH RATE

The distance thrown depends partly on the direction of the release velocity because the velocity is a vector characterized by its degree and direction: the latter is described in terms of the angle of release (as in a side view) (Fig. 20.2). Furthermore, the position of the implement in the air in relation to its flight

direction plays an important role as well as the angle of attack and the yaw angle. The optimal velocity direction, characterized by the angle of release, angle of attack and yaw angle, is the result of the correct timing of the arm/hand action, upper body action and leg action. For example, the athlete has to strive for a flatter release against a head wind, whereas a tail wind requires a steeper release. These changes can be achieved by modifying the javelin inclination, changing the position of the implement in the hand, and/or by changes in the arm position at the moment of release.

Angle of release $\gamma^k(0)$

According to data given by Mero *et al.* (1994) and Bartonietz *et al.* (1996), top male javelin throwers achieve average angles of release of between 32 and 34°, and top female javelin throwers of between 33 and 34°, as demonstrated by finalists of the Olympic Games in 1992 and of the World Championships in 1995 (see also data of Salo & Viitasalo 1995). Steeper release angles are found in less-skilled throwers. Böttcher and Kühl (1998) calculated a targeted value of 36° for throws of female athletes of about 70 m. The analysis of throws by elite female athletes by Böttcher and Kühl (1998) has shown angles of release of between 31 and 44° (in the ISTAF competition of 26 August 1997). The data of Mero *et al.* (1994) show that the standard deviation, as a measure of the parameter variability, reaches 4° (more than 10%) for throws of both men and women. (For more data see Table 20.2.)

Angle of attack $\alpha^k(0)$

The athlete has to aim for a zero angle of attack, regardless of the calculated and often, in training or competition, validated increase of the distance thrown by a positive or negative angle of attack (e.g. Hubbard 1988; Rich *et al.* 1992; Bartonietz *et al.* 1996; Böttcher & Kühl 1998). The results of Best *et al.* (1988), Bartlett *et al.* (1996), Bartonietz *et al.* (1996), Morriss *et al.* (1997) and Böttcher and Kühl (1998) underline the necessity of producing attack angles close to zero. (For more data see Table 20.2.)

Angle of yaw or sideslip $\beta^k(0)$

The yaw angle is the angle of attack, seen from behind. It is the result of a divergence between the lateral movement of the upper body and the arm and the position of the implement's long axis; it has to be at a minimum. Normally athletes achieve their best results with smaller yaw angles: for example, Joanna Stone's 63.74 m, a personal best performance in 1995, was attained with $\beta^k(0) = 1°$; similarly, Tom Pukstys threw a distance of 87.12 m, gaining a US record 1997, with $\beta^k(0) = 6°$, while Jan Zelezny's world record in 1996 had $\beta^k(0) = 10°$ (see also the data of Bartonietz *et al.* 1994, 1996; Morris *et al.* 1997; Böttcher & Kühl 1998). Regressions calculated by Böttcher and Kühl (1998) for individual female elite athletes produced an angle of yaw of <3° for throws of about 70 m. Bartlett *et al.* (1996) have established that the yaw angle was the only angular parameter at release for which a significant difference was found between club athletes ($\beta^k(0) = 2.33 \pm 2.53°$) and novices ($\beta^k(0) = 9.64 \pm 4.90°$). Table 20.1 shows the angles of release of several athletes during the years 1993–1998 and for two athletes during the six throws of a competition. The yaw angle data in Table 20.1 underline the subtle differences in throwing technique, which are related to the spatial control of the javelin's point. Following Best *et al.* (1993), the yaw angle achieved by most athletes produces an upwards-directed Magnus force component in

interaction with the javelin's spin. So the negative effect of an increased drag component by the yaw angle can be partly compensated by an increased lift component. This may be the reason why, in training and competition, yaw angles of 5–10° can be tolerated. (For more data see Table 20.2.)

Pitch rate

A pitch rate can be given to the javelin during the final stage of delivery. It allows the implement to rotate around its transverse axis in a clockwise or anticlockwise direction, nosing the javelin up or down (Terauds 1983, 1985; Hubbard 1984, 1988; Best *et al.* 1993; Bartonietz *et al.* 1996) (see Fig. 20.2). This parameter was discovered only about 20 years ago, and is very difficult to measure accurately. Athletes can use it to compensate for the undesirable effects of an oversized angle of attack (Bartonietz *et al.* 1997). The pitch rate can reach about 25–40° s^{-1} in the throws of top athletes (Bartonietz *et al.* 1996), and even up to 100° s^{-1} in the throws of young athletes (Bartonietz *et al.* 1997). Following the results of flight simulation by Hubbard (1988), the ideal pitch rate is top upward at 3° s^{-1}. Terauds (1985) noted that grip influenced the pitch rate, with a fork grip associated with the highest pitch rates, but this finding has not been confirmed by other observations of top throwers. The initial pitching momentum of the javelin, produced by the thrower as discussed above, should not be confused with the pitching-momentum profile for a javelin during flight, which is caused by initial conditions of the flight phase and by aerodynamics.

REVOLUTIONS AROUND THE JAVELIN'S
LONGITUDINAL AXIS AND VIBRATIONS

The processes of throwing the implement are very complex and include overlapping rotational movements in several planes and around different axes of the trunk, the upper arm, the lower arm and the wrist, based on a more or less horizontal movement of the centre of gravity. As a result of the final hand and forearm rotational movement and of the fingers' take off from the grip, the javelin can gain up to 30 revolutions per second (r.p.s.) around its long

Table 20.1 Release angles of throws by top athletes during the competition periods 1993–1998.

Athlete	Distances (m)	Date	Release angles (°)*			Data source
			$\gamma^k(0)$	$\alpha^k(0)$	$\beta^k(0)$	
B. Henry	86.08	13 Aug 95	35	−5	15	Bartonietz *et al.* (1996)
	86.70	17 May 97	32	−2	4	
	89.32	25 May 97	32	−2	16	
	87.40	13 Jun 97	32	−2	17	Adamczewski (1997)
	85.42	22 Jun 97	32	0	18	
	88.06	28 Jun 97	34	−2	18	
	90.44	9 Jul 97	36	−6	4	B. Schimpl (personal communication)
	86.26	16 May 98	32	−2	17	
	87.11	20 May 98	35	0	18	
	88.32	25 May 98	34	−2	12	
	88.62	4 Jul 98	33	0	22	Adamczewski (1998)
	86.66	4 Jul 98	35	−3	22	
	86.97	11 Jul 98	34	0	18	
S. Backley	81.80	16 Aug 93	33	2	13	Bartonietz & Felder (1994)
	86.30	13 Aug 95	34	1	7	Bartonietz *et al.* (1996)
	83.20	11 Aug 95	31	4	3	Bartonietz *et al.* (1996)
	86.86	22 Jun 95	38	0	0	Adamczewski (1997)
T. Hattestad	69.18	13 Aug 93	30	10	12	
	62.80	13 Aug 93	29	9	21	
	64.78	13 Aug 93	30	13	10	
	64.80	13 Aug 93	32	7	19	Present author
	61.04	13 Aug 93	30	5	21	
	66.18	13 Aug 93	31	6	13	
	64.20	26 Aug 97	31	5	9	Böttcher & Kühl (1998)
P. Boden	77.61	16 May 98	29	−3	29	
	79.63	16 May 98	34	−1	23	
	83.95	16 May 98	36	−4	29	A. Borgström (personal communication)
	81.56	16 May 98	34	0	32	
	83.54	16 May 98	36	−1	28	
	83.80	16 May 98	32	−1	34	

*Release angles: $\gamma^k(0)$, angle of release; $\alpha^k(0)$, angle of attack; $\beta^k(0)$, angle of yaw.

axis, ranging between 3 and 30 r.p.s. (Tutevich 1969; Terauds 1985). According to Terauds (1985), there are notable differences in the number of revolutions depending on the grip used—the fork grip leads to a lower number of revolutions. Indeed, complete absence of rotations can sometimes be observed in training using the fork grip (J. Gorsky, personal communication). The present author's research has shown up to about 18–20 r.p.s. using the less common 'V' or claw grip, as employed by Joanna Stone and Andreas Linden. However, the selection of grip should depend on what feels best to the individual athlete.

The positive effect of the javelin's revolutions on the distance thrown is very small. For a computed throw with revolutions of 25 r.p.s., an angle of release of 30° and velocity of release of 24 m · s⁻¹, the gain was approximately 0.5 m, when compared to a release without revolutions (Terauds 1985). To date there is no evidence that trying to rotate the javelin gives any benefit. Consequently the use of gripping agents, synthetic resins or home-made substances based on turpentine, used by some athletes in an attempt to improve the grip on the binding (Johnson 1987) or to impart a greater spin to slow down the effect of the pitching moment due to the gyroscopic effect (Paish 1986), should be viewed accordingly. The use of gripping substances also results in unequal conditions for athletes during competition: javelins with residues of such resins are practically of no use for athletes who prefer to throw without gripping agents or who use simply magnesia without any disadvantages for other athletes.

Vibrations of the javelin during flight are initiated during the final forearm sling as a result of a transverse-acting force component. They are the result of the overlapping combination of the curvilinear paths of the upper arm, forearm and hand movements around the shoulder, elbow and wrist, the trunk flexion and the more or less pronounced body raise over the front leg. Their amplitude is minimized with perfect coordination of time, space and force—'throwing though the point'—but they are never completely avoidable. Voronkin et al. (1974) measured a transverse force component of about one-third of the accelerating force component 0.05 s before release. Throws, both in training and competition, can show high-amplitude vibrations even with optimal release angles. The amplitudes also depend on the stiffness of the javelin: minimum amplitudes are achieved by using carbon fibre-reinforced implements.

HEIGHT OF RELEASE AND DISTANCE TO FOUL LINE

Theoretically, the distance thrown increases with an increase in release height (Tutevich 1969). In reality, there is an optimum height of release for each athlete, depending on his or her body dimensions and technique. In practice, a high release height is typical of athletes at a low performance level (see below for a comparison of decathletes vs. javelin specialists) or it can be linked to technical faults, for example a relatively high body position at the beginning of the delivery, caused by a steep planted front leg resulting in the implement being released over an almost vertical left leg.

The male finalists in the 1992 Olympic Games reached a release height of about 1.81 m, women of about 1.75 m with a very small standard deviation (respectively ± 0.04 m and ± 0.06 m) (Mero et al. 1994). On average, the height of release reached for top female athletes is about 105% of body height (Böttcher & Kühl 1998). The male finalists at the World Championships in 1995 released the javelins at an average height of 1.97 m (range 1.81–2.13 m; data of Morriss et al. 1997). According to the data of Salo and Viitasalo (1995), decathletes had a statistically significant higher release height (eight throws between 52.34 m and 65.70 m, athletes on average 1.85 m tall, in comparison with javelin throwers, 10 throws between 68.04 m and 75.96 m, athletes on average also 1.85 m tall). Table 20.2 shows release height data of top athletes. The calculated release height data can serve as an orientation, the real moment of release (zero javelin acceleration) can only be determined with adequate accuracy by combining kinematic methods (high-speed film or video) with dynamometric research methods. This can explain the differences between the release height data of the Olympic Games in 1992 and the World Championships in 1995, analysing almost the same athletes (see above).

The practical relevance of this parameter is limited to performance diagnosis and to technique training. However, the height of release has to be taken into account as a parameter of the movement path during special investigations, for example in determining the path of acceleration by throws with implements of different masses, due to the fact that the path of acceleration decreases with an increase of the weight thrown (Bartonietz 1987). For a detailed analysis, it is necessary to distinguish between the release height of the javelin, the centre of gravity under the front part of the grip cord, and the hand height at the moment of release behind the grip (Borgström 1997) (Table 20.2). The recovery distance from the vertical projection of the release position to the foul line (Fig. 20.2) depends on the remaining body velocity and the recovery technique. It has to be at a minimum but without any negative influence on the throwing technique (see 'Recovery'). This distance has to be taken into account for a detailed performance diagnosis.

Table 20.2 Height of release by throws of selected athletes.

Athlete	Body height (m)	Distance thrown (m)	Release height (m)	Data source
Zelezny	1.84	79.58	2.12	Morriss *et al.* (1997)
		89.06	1.81	Morriss *et al.* (1997)
		98.48	1.65	Author's calculation based on video recording of the IAT, Leipzig
		92.5 (foul)	1.65 (hand) 1.78 (implement)	Borgström (1997)
Backley	1.86	86.30	2.02	Morriss *et al.* (1997)
Hecht	1.90	83.30	2.13	Morriss *et al.* (1997)

Note: Jan Zelezny, the world's best athlete in 1995/96, reached the lowest height of release as a result of a marked upper body thrust and sideward release. As with stride length data for individual comparisons, the height of release has to be related to body height.

Energy and power demands

No sporting technique is possible without power, and conversely no power production is possible without technique. This has to be the overriding principle in both training and performance diagnosis. Technique training, including stamina, is a year-round task.

THE POWER TRANSFERRED TO THE IMPLEMENT

The velocity of release, including its direction, obtained by the implement is in essence the result of energy transfer from the body to the implement, comparable with the physical work done. In other words the velocity of release is dependent on the available power as the energy flow during a given time:

$$\Delta E_{ges}/\Delta t = P_{res}(W) \tag{20.1}$$

$$\Delta E_{kin} + \Delta E_{pot}/\Delta t = P_a + P_s \tag{20.2}$$

$$\tfrac{1}{2}m\Delta v^2 + mg\Delta h/\Delta t = P_a + P_s \tag{20.3}$$

where E_{ges} = total energy; P_{res} = total power; E_{kin} = kinetic energy; P_a = power component to accelerate; E_{pot} = potential energy; P_s = power component for shift; h = vertical path; m = mass; and t = time. The following examples will demonstrate the coaching relevance of the energetic approach to competition and training exercise analysis.

For the 800 g implement thrown with a velocity of $30 \text{ m} \cdot \text{s}^{-1}$ the ratio between the kinetic and potential energy is 30 : 1, or 360 : 12 J. Based on this ratio the potential energy component and the power portion for the vertical shift of the implement can be ignored. The athlete has only to accelerate the implement. However, when a top javelin thrower throws a 7.26 kg shot approximately 19 m with both arms a relationship of 3.7 : 1 is found between the accelerating and the shifting energy components (i.e. 522 vs. 140 J). Both energy components increase in comparison to the javelin throw, but the potential energy component increases by a factor of more than 10, and the kinetic portion by just a factor of 1.5, reaching more than 20% of the total energy and power. Table 20.3 gives an overview of these data. There are some basic differences in the movement pattern and power production of a one-arm throw after an approach speed of up to $7 \text{ m} \cdot \text{s}^{-1}$ and an overhead throw with both arms from a standing position. In the latter the power, which is necessary for the final acceleration, is produced in a simpler way from both legs, the trunk and both arms, without rotational movements around the longitudinal axis of the body. The overhead throw requires less power, but more work can be done. The differences also underline how to evaluate

Table 20.3 Energetic relationships for two different throwing-movement patterns.

Parameter	Javelin throw (competition)	Overhead throw two-handed (training)
Mass of the implement (kg)	0.8	7.26
Initial velocity (m · s^{-1})	7	0
Duration of the delivery (s)	0.12	0.35
Velocity of release (m · s^{-1})	30	12
Energy (J)		
Kinetic energy	360	522
Potential energy	12	140
Total energy	372	662
Average power (kW)		
To accelerate	3.0	1.50
To shift	0.10	0.40
Total power	3.10	1.90

the specific benefits of training using different exercises and implements of different weights. When heavy-weight work, for example explosive snatches with 130 kg or more from a hang position, is included in the analysis, further divergences are shown between the energy and power components and, correspondingly, between the training effects (Bartonietz 1987, 1995, 1996).

The above estimated power components are average values. During a real throw, as the energy transformation changes vs. the available path commensurate with the given time, the developed power changes as well, reaching a momentary maximum close to the instant of release. According to a hypothesis by Hochmuth (1984), the maximum available power to accelerate the implement, and the body, determines the sporting performance. A simple model was developed by Schwuchow (1986) to analyse the javelin's acceleration during delivery. The model is based on the mechanical dependence of the course of the velocity with respect to the acceleration path. The following assumptions were made: initial velocity 5 m · s^{-1}; duration 0.10 s; available path 1.5 m (this path has to be used during the simulations to prevent shortening the acceleration path); release velocities of 29, 31 and 33 m · s^{-1}, characteristic of the force vs. time course (impulse) close to reality. The results, presented on the left of Fig. 20.4, underline the importance of peak power. Based on the findings of Schwuchow (1986), the

following changes are achieved with increase in performance.

1 The maximum power is reached 0.003 s (or 0.115 m) earlier, by increasing the velocity of release from 29 m · s^{-1} to 31 m · s^{-1} and 0.009 s (or 0.28 m) earlier, by increasing the velocity of release from 31 m · s^{-1} to 33 m · s^{-1}.

2 Greater arm strike delay. As a result of a faster velocity increase during the start of the delivery, the available path is passed through faster, so that the maximum velocity is reached even before the available path is used to the full extent. So a delay in arm strike is essential.

Experimental data (middle and right of Fig. 20.4) and practical experience support these findings. From a practical point of view, the athlete has a number of possibilities to lengthen his or her acceleration path, or at least to conserve its length and to counteract the path shortening:

• being active with the right leg before the left leg plants;
• preventing early movement of the throwing arm;
• using a marked upper body thrust during the delivery (see Fig. 20.1, compare left with right part); and
• using special stretching exercises after maximum strength training as well as before and after throwing.

As shown by Bartonietz (1987), implements of different masses are used in training to improve

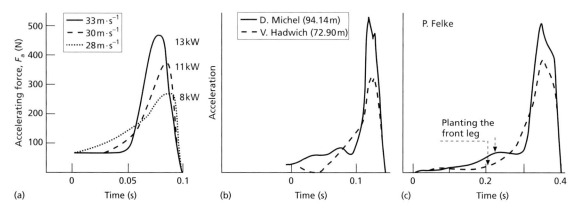

Fig. 20.4 Accelerating force and acceleration vs. time during the delivery of the javelin. (a) Accelerating force–time histories. (From Schwuchow 1986.) (b) Acceleration–time histories of two athletes of different performance levels. (From Schwuchow 1986.) (c) Acceleration–time histories of throws of a top female athlete, during throwing training (4 April 1984, continuous line) and during the maximum-strength training period (12 December 1984, broken line). (From Bartonietz 1987.)

the power level of the thrower. By using an optimal weight the athlete's maximum power can be achieved. This weight normally exceeds the weight of the competition implement. In javelin throwing, javelins of mass up to 1.3 kg are used. Also, shots with masses up to 3–4 kg are thrown with one arm, while special machines can imitate one-arm throws of 35 kg mass for women (Bartonietz *et al.* 1985; Felke 1993) or 50 kg for men, to attain maximum strength training. The data in Table 20.4 and the accompanying acceleration–time histories emphasize that higher power can be produced by the athlete, in comparison to the competition implement, by using heavy javelins. This is the result of the energy transfer to the implement in the same or even shorter time. Corresponding special investigations are necessary to find out the optimal weight for an athlete and to avoid undesirable changes in technique.

THE KINETIC ENERGY OF THE THROWER AND
THE POWER DEMANDS ON THE FRONT LEG
DURING DELIVERY

Velocity of the run-up

Apart from the weight of the thrower's body and of the implement, the body velocity is a import-

ant working condition at the beginning of the delivery, determining the thrower's kinetic energy (see below). The velocity of the body is measured by light diodes as the average velocity during measuring intervals of different length, for instance 4.0 m for men and 3.5 m women (Bartonietz *et al.* 1986), 5 m (Adamczewski 1995), corresponding to the intervals used in the horizontal jumps and pole vault, or 3 m (Schimpl 1997). The first set of two pairs of diodes measures the average body speed during the so-called 'cyclic part' of the approach, the second during the so-called 'acyclic part' to obtain information about the run-up acceleration. According to the technical model of Bartonietz and Dörr (1986), the second interval has to be passed faster than the first as the result of an accelerated run-up. Table 20.5 shows corresponding velocity data. Tidow (1994) states that beginners and decathletes often choose an approach which is too long, reaching their maximum approach run velocity too early.

Another type of information is given by analysis of the velocity of the mass centre or of a reference point in the hip area at the end of approach/beginning of delivery. According to the data of Morriss *et al.* (1997), the velocity of the centre of mass reached an average value of 6.0 m · s^{-1} (range 5.2–6.7 m · s^{-1}) for the 12 male finalists at the 1995 World Championships.

Table 20.4 Biomechanical data and the acceleration–time course of throws with javelins of different masses. (Based on data of Schwuchow 1986.)

Athlete	Javelin mass (kg)	v_{release} (m · s^{-1})	$F_{\text{a(max)}}$ (N)	E_{kin} (J)	$P_{\text{a(max)}}$ (kW)	$P_{\text{a(av)}}$ (kW)
Weissbach	0.77	18.6	157	133.2	2.4	0.33
	0.97	19.1	236	177.1	3.5	0.55
	1.17	19.5	235	222.8	3.4	0.64
Herbst	0.77	19.1	159	140.6	2.9	0.29
	0.97	19.0	195	175.2	3.1	0.42
	1.17	20.8	230	254.2	3.9	0.55
Thomä	0.77	16.8	170	108.1	2.3	0.28
	0.97	19.4	193	182.8	3.0	0.37
	1.07	20.6	218	227.9	3.7	0.51

Note: The velocity of release was calculated by integrating the *a–t* curves; the acceleration of the javelin was measured by a strain-gauge accelerometer.
v_{release}, Release velocity; $F_{\text{a(max)}}$, acceleration component of the force, acting on the javelin; E_{kin}, kinetic energy of the javelin; $P_{\text{a(max)}}$, maximum power of the javelin (acceleration component); $P_{\text{a(av)}}$, average power of the javelin (acceleration component).

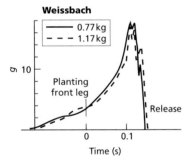 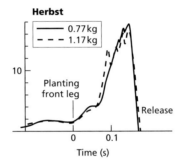 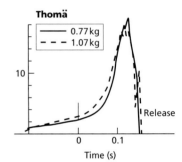

Analysis of data of average velocities and of the velocities of the mass centre by throws after full approach show the following.

1 Comparing different individuals, top athletes have a higher body velocity at the beginning of the delivery (Salo & Viitasalo 1995).

2 Comparing throws for a given athlete, the world's best athletes (e.g. Zelezny, Henry, Hattestad) achieve their longest throws with their highest run-up speeds.

According to Böttcher and Kühl (1996), longer throws are achieved with a higher speed level and with longer impulse strides.

Kinetic energy

Together with the body mass, the body speed at the end of the approach has a strong influence on the kinetic energy obtained by the thrower. The kinetic energy is an energy of motion and is defined as the work that will be done by the body possessing the energy when it is brought to rest or the velocity is changed (see Eqns 20.1–20.3). High kinetic energy is a prerequisite for a powerful javelin delivery. It is comparable with the kinetic energy of a pole vaulter, which can be stored to a large extent as elastic energy of deformation of the pole, or is comparable with the kinetic energy put into the stretching of a bow to launch an arrow. The values in Table 20.6 illustrate the squared relationship between run-up speed and kinetic energy: doubling the run-up speed results in a fourfold increase in kinetic energy, which is normal in training. Because of the relatively stable duration of the energy transfer

Table 20.5 Average body velocity over two measured intervals of the run-up, recorded during the 1993 World Championships. (From Bartonietz & Felder 1994.)

| | | Average body velocity (m · s⁻¹) over measured intervals | | | |
| | | Men | | Women | |
Athlete	Distance of throw (m)	6–12 m	12–16 m	6–11.5 m	11.5–15 m
Zelezny	81.86	7.12	6.85		
	83.82	6.56	6.49		
	85.98	6.78	6.90		
	84.62	6.90	7.02		
Kinnunen	77.46	7.10	6.50		
	77.68	7.03	6.25		
	84.78	7.12	6.81		
Hill	82.80	6.11	6.96		
	80.18	6.15	7.02		
	82.96	6.25	6.45		
Hattestad	69.18			7.00	6.14
	62.80			6.79	6.03
	64.78			6.86	6.03
	64.80			7.00	6.04
	61.04			6.73	6.04
	66.18			7.14	6.03
Forkel	65.80			6.73	5.70
N. Shikolenko	65.64			7.14	6.03

Note: The measuring system used double light diodes to prevent measuring impulses by vertical arm or javelin movements. For more data see Bartonietz and Felder (1994).

Table 20.6 Kinetic energy of the javelin-thrower at the end of the approach.

| | Kinetic energy of the body (J) | | |
Run-up velocity (m · s⁻¹)	Body mass (kg) 100	70	40
3	450	315	180
4	800	560	320
5	1250	875	500
6	1800	1260	720
7	2450	1715	980

at different initial velocities, the use of higher run-up speeds sometimes puts the athlete in great trouble (see below).

Demands on the front leg

One of the key points of javelin throwing is the work of the front leg during delivery. A male athlete of 100 kg body mass, throwing distances of between 85 and 90 m, has to brake, during a delivery duration of 0.12 s, from a body speed of about 7 m · s⁻¹ down to 3.5 m · s⁻¹ ($\Delta E_{kin} = 613$ J). It results in an average power of 5.1 kW. The peak value will be much higher and can exceed 10 kW. The high power level required of the front leg limits the number of throws which can made in workouts, although the upper body and throwing arm could continue with the throwing work. By far the greatest velocity decrease occurs during the first half or even third of the delivery in throws of top athletes, as can be shown by the

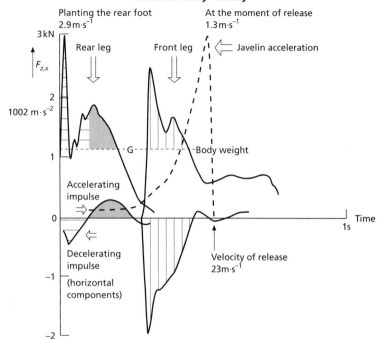

Fig. 20.5 Ground reaction force–time histories, javelin acceleration–time history and biomechanical data during the delivery phase. Athlete B.H., training session, 17 December 1993, short approach run, Institut für Angewandte Trainingswissenschaft e.V. Leipzig. (Data from Adamczweski *et al.* 1993.)

ground reaction forces (Fig. 20.5) and by kinematic data, such as velocity–time history of the mass centre (see Fig. 20.8).

Consider an intensive training throw, made after a run-up of 3–5 strides and achieving a thrown distance of some 75 m (about 83% of the targeted competition result). The body speed of around 4 m · s⁻¹ decelerates to around 2 m · s⁻¹ in a slightly longer (compared to competition) time of 0.14 s. This represents a change of the body's kinetic energy of 200 J, resulting in only 1.4 kW braking power capacity, i.e. 27% of the 5.1 kW attained in competition. This relationship can explain why athletes may experience problems in training and competition by striving for a high release velocity with the proper technique. In competitive throwing the kinetic energy increases by up to 4–5 times, from throwing after 3–5 steps in training at run-up speeds of 3–4 m · s⁻¹ to throwing with run-up speeds of 6–7 m · s⁻¹. The time to transfer this amount of kinetic energy remains almost constant, so the power needed is quadrupled because of the square influence of the body velocity on the kinetic energy and with it on the power. This is

the reason why, from the biomechanical point of view, athletes can achieve a movement pattern close to the demands of the target technique (e.g. stable front leg) at lower training speeds using a short approach, but not with increasing speeds and a full approach, whether in training or competition; they simply do not have the necessary power . The same physical relationship is valid for sprint events. According to calculations by Bartonietz and Güllich (1992), much greater physical power is required for the peak-up acceleration than for the acceleration phase after the start. The thrower has to be trained to take advantage of the increase in kinetic energy so that the necessary power capacity is at her or his disposal, otherwise the athlete becomes restricted by the following undesirable deviations in throwing technique, or a combination of them:

• reduced run-up speed or slow-down during the final strides, e.g. passive penultimate stride, which is normally an accelerating 'impulse stride' before planting the front leg;

• inactivity of the right leg, i.e. failure to push the right side forwards;

• planting the front leg with flexed knee (this makes it very hard to stabilize the knee);
• swerving the upper body to the side;
• steep planting angle of the front leg;
• short-timed delivery; and
• premature movement of the throwing arm because of a deficit in muscular pretension.

Fault correction requires power development of the front leg for the braking work, together with the development of the internal movement picture, for example how to block the left side. Power is developed by maximum strength exercises, drills, jumps and sprints and, last but not least, by throwing at approach velocities close to the competition situation. Throws with weight jackets can also be an effective additional measure for advanced athletes. The amount of body velocity lost during the delivery phase, mainly by the work of the front leg, serves as a criterion of throwing efficiency, taking into account the initial velocity. It is much easier to lose a relatively large amount of velocity at low speed (because less power is required) than losing the same amount of velocity at a much higher initial speed level; compare the data of Räty and Zelezny in Table 20.7.

Table 20.7 Velocity of the thrower's body at the beginning of the delivery (planting of the front foot) and at the moment of release. v_{FF}, velocity at the moment of planting the front foot; v_R, velocity at the moment of release.

Athlete	Distance (m)	Velocity ($m \cdot s^{-1}$)			Reduction in v_{FF} (%)	Measured or calculated point	Author
		v_{FF}	v_R	$(v_{FF} - v_R)$			
Women							
Lillak	69.00	5.5	2.3	3.2	58	Mass centre	Komi & Mero (1985)
Felke	74.94	5.7	2.1	3.6	63	Right hip	Bartonietz (1987)
IL	62.32	5.4	3.0	2.4	44	Mass centre ⎫	
T. Shikolenko	59.34	4.0	1.8	2.2	55	⎬	Best *et al.* 1993
PB	58.28	4.2	2.0	2.2	52	⎪	
ML	57.22	4.6	2.4	2.2	48	⎭	
Men							
Hohn	99.52	7.2	3.6	3.6	50	Mass centre ⎫	
Hohn	104.80	6.4	1.9	4.5	70	Right hip ⎬	Bartonietz (1987)
Michel	96.72	6.3	2.0	4.3	68	Right hip ⎭	
Backley	87.42	6.0	4.6	1.4	23	Mass centre	Best *et al.* (1993)
Backley	83.22	6.8	4.5	2.3	34	Mass centre	Best *et al.* (1993)
Backley	85.20	6.3	3.7	2.6	41	Mass centre	Morriss (1996)
Backley	86.30	6.0	3.3	2.7	45	Mass centre	Morriss *et al.* (1997)
OC	80.60	5.8	2.8	3.0	52	Mass centre	Best *et al.* (1993)
NB	69.40	6.2	4.6	1.6	26	Mass centre	Best *et al.* (1993)
Räty	82.90	4.7	1.6	2.9	66	Mass centre	Best *et al.* (1994)
Zelezny	82.58	6.3	3.6	2.7	43	Mass centre	Best *et al.* (1994)
Zelezny	92.5 (foul)	6.6	3.2	3.4	52	Mass centre	Borgström (1997)
Zelezny	89.06	6.6	3.4	3.2	48	Mass centre	Morriss *et al.* (1997)
Henry	86.08	6.2	3.9	2.3	37	Mass centre	Morriss *et al.* (1997)
SS	74.64	5.60	4.40	1.20	21	Mass centre ⎫	
ST	72.58	6.23	3.11	3.12	50	Mass centre ⎪	
HM	59.88	4.80	2.61	2.19	46	Mass centre ⎬	Ikegami *et al.* (1981)
II	51.27	4.62	4.06	0.56	12	Mass centre ⎭	

According to data from Morriss *et al.* (1997), the 12 finalists of the World Championships in 1995 decreased their body velocity on average by 46%, ranging from 31% to 59%. This variation implicates corresponding differences in the throwing technique (see next section). The data show that the highest velocities of release are reached at the lowest velocities of the centre of gravity, underlining the importance of an effective braking process. Nevertheless, it does not exclude the possibility of producing an individual maximum release velocity at a relatively high level of body velocity at the moment of release, a case in point being the performances of Boris Henry (throw of 86.08 m in 1995) (Morriss *et al.* 1997).

Basic demands of movement coordination (movement pattern): biomechanical aspects

Athletes both past and present sum up the impact of movement coordination as follows:

> I passed a multitude of bigger, better throwers on the way up . . . What they didn't realize . . . was the importance of being a technician, of getting into position. If you're just 1 degree off, you've blown it. But when you hit it right, it's like steak and potatoes. It's like going to heaven in a wheelbarrow. To make it, you improve a little here and a little there. You have to go up a hundred blind alleys to pick up a few feet.
> [Albert Cantello, world-record holder (86.04 m) in 1959 (Kirshenbaum 1969, p. 41)]

> Javelin throwing is a fine sport. But you have to train very seriously and must have complete control. If you develop an improper technique, it takes a long time to get back to doing things the right way.
> [Terje Pedersen, world-record holder (91.72 m) in 1964 (Kirshenbaum 1969, p. 41)]

> I think that the technique is my strongest weapon.
> [Jan Zelezny, current world-record holder (Vrabel 1997, p. 14)]

The athlete's body can be regarded as a kinematic chain system, in which a series of segments with different masses and mass distribution are connected by joint structures and driven by the neuromuscular system. From the biomechanical point of view, the motor output is the complex result of the interaction between muscular torque pulling around the joints—energy transfer, supported by the reinforcing potential of stored elastic energy during the stretch–shortening cycle—and external forces, namely the inertia of the implement and the body limbs and gravity. For simplicity, the movements of both legs, the trunk plus the left arm, and the throwing arm will be analysed as the main body segments in action. Knowledge about movement coordination comes from observing throws, measuring javelin performances with different kinds of equipment, and simulating throws using models of different complexity. Each approach has its benefits, but also its limitations, so the synthesis of different approaches will give a clearer picture about the movement pattern the athlete has to strive for.

The delivery phase is defined here as the movement following the moment of planting the rear leg, after the impulse stride, until the release of the implement.

LEG WORK

In javelin throwing, as in other throwing activities, the muscular actions that drive the body and the implement start with those furthest from the hand. 'To build up a throw from the legs' is a well-known principle of coaching for both strength and technique. Tom Pukstys, after throwing a US record of 87.12 m in 1997, said: 'by my sixth throw, I figured out what I did wrong on my other throws. I was trying to throw too hard with just my arm, instead of letting my legs set up the throw. So on my last throw, I let my legs set up everything' (Hendershott 1997, p. 11).

Rear leg

The approach run, including the impulse stride, has to create the conditions for delivery: i.e. the optimal amount of velocity of the centre of gravity in an optimal direction; an effective body and javelin position; suitable length of path to accelerate the implement; and control of the implement to ensure optimal release conditions. The need for high body speed before delivery implies minimal braking forces after the rear foot has been planted together with an optimal backward lean of the body. Regardless of the individual peculiarities in each athlete's technique, coaches and athletes develop technique to improve efficiency (see the inter- and intra-individual comparisons in Fig. 20.6), reducing the velocity loss after planting the rear foot and reducing back lean. The body position achieved at the moment of planting the rear foot is the result of the preceding movements, in particular of the impulse stride. Newton's Law of action and reaction dictates that a high swinging action of the right leg during the impulse stride leads to a tilted torso. In contrast, the 'target' technique is characterized by an active, 'grabbing' grounding of the left foot interacting with a short-duration, 'scissors-like' impulse from the right lower leg. Instabilities in legwork, which can occur especially during competition, underline the importance of learning the proper movements from the outset. With the use of the rear leg, the thrower has a last chance to increase body velocity, and contribute to a more pronounced body pre-tension.

It wasn't a good throw. The rear end of the javelin wasn't in the correct position. But I got my hip into the throw so well that the javelin flew to a record. But if my coach had been here to see my technique, he would have given me a scolding. [Tiina Lillak about her world record throw of 74.76 m (*Track and Field News* 1983, p. 29)]

Biomechanical research by Adamczewski (1995) into top male javelin throwers and heptathletes led to the hypothesis that the body position and the legwork have to minimize the loss of body velocity. This decrease in speed averaged $-0.31 \text{ m} \cdot \text{s}^{-1}$ and $-0.67 \text{ m} \cdot \text{s}^{-1}$, respectively. It was presumed that keeping the body speed almost constant or even increasing it was impossible to achieve. Applied research by Adamczewski et al. (1998) during an in-season training session with top javelin throwers demonstrated the possibility of increasing the body velocity by use of the action of the rear leg. Based on an active impulse stride—keeping the upper body stable in an almost vertical position—the planting of the rear leg on the ball of the foot allows the body to accelerate. Figure 20.7 shows the ground reaction forces and biomechanical data for such a throw.

The concept of a beneficial backlean is still misleading athletes and coaches. The greater the amount of backlean, the greater the loss of velocity. As shown above, Hay (1978) and Tidow (1994), labouring under a misapprehension, stated that a backward inclination allows the athlete more time and lengthens the path to exert force. The foot position of the rear leg at the instant of planting can differ from an almost straight to a squared touchdown. The first variant limits the influence of the right leg drive. The latter variant is useful, if the athlete can take full advantage of the hip drive (Sing 1984; L. Penfold, personal communication), as did such athletes as Siitonen in 1973, T. Lillak in 1982/83, and Joanna Stone in 1997. With such a landing, passivity can lead to serious knee injuries, caused by an inward bending of the knee (see 'Injury prevention' below). Most athletes therefore prefer a landing with an intermediate foot direction of about 45° to the throwing direction.

Front leg

The main demand on the front leg is maximum stability in order to achieve high efficiency of braking. For this reason, the knee joint has to be as stable as possible (Fig. 20.7 and Table 20.8). The front leg as a whole limb does not pivot like a lever around the ground support (see the leg angle data in Table 20.8). This will prevent a 'running over' of this leg. From a biomechanical and physiological point of view, a bent front leg and a leg raise do not effectively produce muscular pre-tension in the upper chest and shoulder girdle, i.e. the 'arch position'. Knee bending and leg pivoting can be combined in different proportions (see data in Table 20.8). The minimum knee angle of the front leg is related to the performance level, higher performances being associated with a more stable front leg (Menzel 1986; Salo & Viitasalo 1995; Bartonietz & Emrich 1997). The front leg has to be planted as fast as possible, within the constraints determined by the body velocity and the front leg position at the moment the rear leg is planted (Fig. 20.7), as well as the activity of the rear leg. According to data from Morriss et al. (1997), Jan Zelezny had the fastest front leg plant of all throwers, 0.14 s after planting the rear leg.

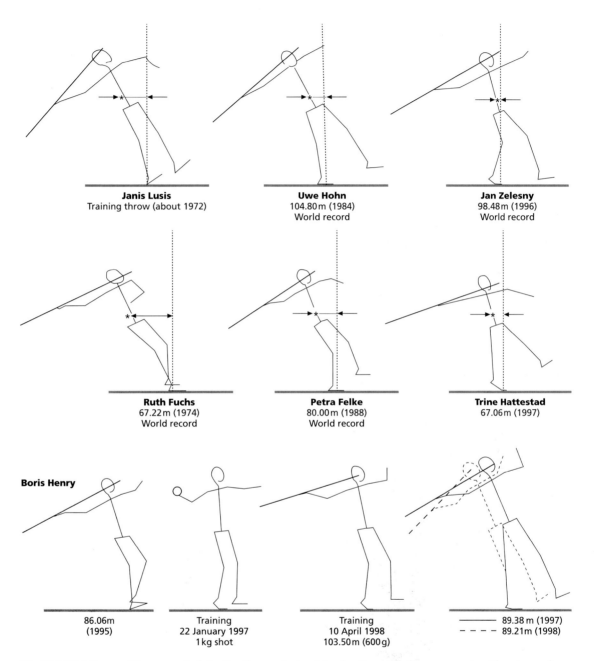

Fig. 20.6 Stick figures at the moment of planting the rear foot and decelerating path of the mass centre. *Above*: top male athletes: 1972, 1986, 1996. *Middle*: top female athletes: 1974, 1988, 1997. *Below*: top male athlete, 1995–98, in training and competition.

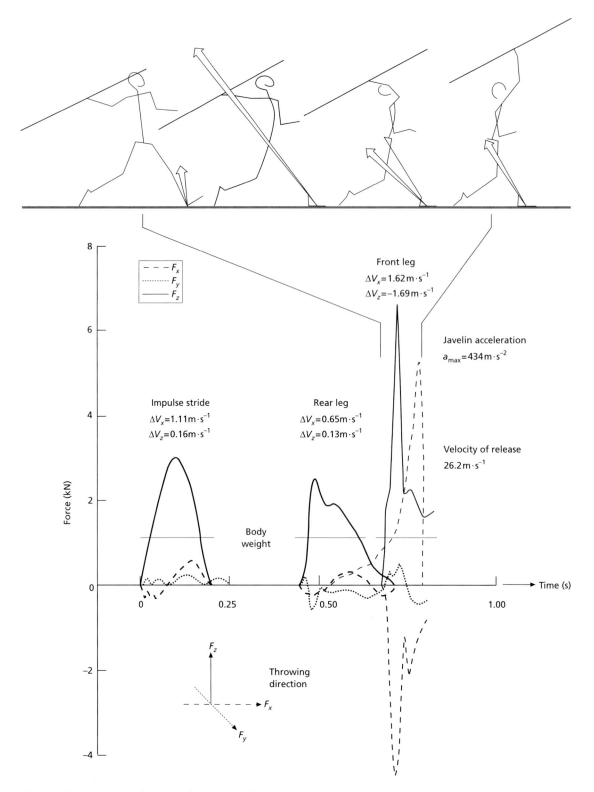

Fig. 20.7 Ground reaction force–time histories, javelin acceleration–time history and biomechanical data for training session 26 May 1998, Institut für Angewandte Trainingswissenschaft e.V, Leipzig, athlete B.H., short approach run. Position 1: 0.01 s after front foot planting; position 2: 0.04 s; position 3: 0.08 s; position 4: 0.10 s (release). The arrows show magnitude and direction of the resulting ground reaction force. (Data from Adamczewski *et al.* 1998.)

Table 20.8 Knee angle and leg angle data in determining the efficiency of front leg work. 1, Planting the front leg; 2, maximum body pretension ('bow position'); 3, release.

	Distance (m)	Year	Knee angle (°)			Leg angle (°)		Source
			1	2	3	1	3	
Men								
Hohn	104.80	1984	180	168	180	46	60 ⎫	
Zelezny	98.48	1996	175	175	180	40	53 ⎬	Present author
	89.58	1995	177	169	180*	47	55 ⎪	
	90.12	1995	175	170	180*	43	53 ⎭	
Henry	77.42	1993	180	160	152			Bartonietz & Felder 1994
	84.12	1993	180	175	180	47	60 ⎫	
	89.38	1997	180	170	180	48	60 ⎪	
	88.58	1997	180	175	180*	48	56 ⎪	
	86.26	1998	180	180	180	46	50 ⎬	Present author
	89.21	1998	180	177	180	49	58 ⎪	
Pukstys	87.12	1997	180	160	155	42	60 ⎪	
Lovegrove	88.20	1996	180	175	180	48	62 ⎭	
Backley	81.80	1993	163	145	140			Bartonietz & Felder 1994
	86.30	1995	173	152	152			Bartonietz *et al.* 1996
	86.86	1997	175	148	160	48	67 ⎫	
Women								⎬ Present author
Felke	88.00	1988	180	170	180	47	64 ⎭	
Hattestad	69.18	1993	170	170	180	52	62	Bartonietz & Felder 1994
	67.06	1997	165	180	180*	52	56 ⎫	
Stone	67.72	1997	180	178	180*	55	59 ⎬	Present author
Manjani	62.40	1995	175	156	180*		⎪	
	55.56	1995	156	149	180		⎭	

Note: The knee angle is the angle between hip, knee and ankle joints; the leg angle is the angle between the leg axis and the horizontal.
* Denotes hyperextension of the front knee joint.

Effective bracing front legwork (hard block) leads to a short travel of the centre of body mass during the delivery, as shown by data of the 1992 Olympic finalists analysed by Mero *et al.* (1994). The data in Table 20.8 illustrate that the distance thrown should not be overrated as the criterion for performance diagnosis. Even though throwing a US record, the athlete Tom Pukstys still shows potential for improvement, because he bends his front leg until the moment of release. On the other hand, the 86.26 m throw by Boris Henry at the beginning of the competition period, on 16 May 1998, was char-acterized by almost ideal front legwork. His training condition at this time, together with unfavourable wind conditions, restricted an even longer throw. The data of throws by Steve Backley are an example of development of front legwork over the years, underlining the fact that older athletes too can continue to develop their skills. The desired flat planting of the front leg demands a long bracing stride. Less-qualified throwers have a shorter bracing stride with steeper ground reaction forces than more qualified throwers (Menzel 1986; Salo & Viitasalo 1995). Figure 20.7 is a model of the ground reaction forces interacting with the thrower's movement. As the front leg is planted, an angular momentum of the upper body is created from the force direction, passing the mass centre. Immediately after a relatively steep planting of the front leg, i.e. after touchdown, the first measured impact force is applied at an angle of 85°, and an anticlockwise-directed angular momentum can be detected during the first 0.035 s, which provides a highly stable leg base, including the pelvis, and allows a build-up of body pre-tension into the 'arch' or 'bow' position (see position 2 in Fig. 20.7) with a delay of the shoulder/arm movement. During this time, the upper body and throwing arm are kept almost rigid as a result of the overlapping effects of the inertia of the upper body movement and the angular momentum, produced by the ground reaction forces. The resultant of the ground reaction forces changes its amount and direction in relation to the mass centre (see the arrows in Fig. 20.7, which illustrate the force vector). After an interval of 0.045 s after the planting, the maximum ground reaction force of 7.73 kN is applied at an angle of 60°, and acts along the biomechanical axis of the front leg. The clockwise-turning angular momentum reinforces the powerful thrust of the chest and the arm movement until release. The beginning of the upper body and arm movement coincides with the change to a clockwise direction of the momentum. LeBlank and Dapena (1998) describe this process as transfer of angular momentum from the body to the throwing arm.

Data about the angular momentum and its direction have to be related to the performance level in general and to the legwork in particular. A bent front knee reduces the magnitude of the ground reaction force and changes its direction. If we can establish essential differences in kinematic data (e.g. joint angles, joint and mass centre velocities) between different performance levels we can assume with certainty essential differences between the dynamic and kinetic parameters, which are the causes for the kinematics. Figures 20.5 and 20.7 show the ground reaction force–time histories and the javelin acceleration–time histories of throws by the same male athlete 4.5 years apart: best performance in 1993, 84.12 m; best performance in 1998, 89.29 m. In 1993, a release velocity of 23.0 m · s⁻¹ was achieved for the

throw in question, made off-season, while during the season of 1998 the release velocity was 26.2 m · s⁻¹. The performance of 1998 is characterized by:
1 lower amplitude of the ground reaction forces after the impulse stride/rear foot planting;
2 a more active landing with less back lean;
3 an increase of body velocity as a result of the work of the rear leg; and
4 very hard braking of the front leg (amplitude of the resulting force 7.45 times body weight), leading to a velocity decrease of 2.5 m · s⁻¹.

MOVEMENTS OF THE TRUNK AND THE THROWING ARM

Kinematic data by film or video show consecutive velocity maxima of hip, shoulder, elbow and implement or of the mass centres of the body limbs (Fig. 20.8). The velocity–time history of hip, shoulder, elbow and hand can be used as an external indicator of the impulse transmission to the implement. In interpreting such data, the hypothesis of momentum transfer in throwing movements is used for javelin and ball throwing (Matveev 1967; Kreighbaum & Barthels 1981; Menzel 1986). The basic physical relationship is the conservation of momentum:

$$m_1 v_1 = m_2 v_2 \qquad (20.4)$$

where m_1 and m_2 are the masses of two bodies, and v_1 and v_2 are their velocities. The idea in using this principle is to first accelerate the total body—in javelin throwing during the run-up—to obtain a certain amount of momentum (body mass multiplied by its velocity) and then to decelerate the large, proximal masses of the legs and the lower parts of the trunk to increase the velocity of the distal links, i.e. the upper part of the trunk, then to decelerate the trunk while accelerating the upper arm, forearm/hand, and the implement, by a whip-like movement. A key action in javelin throwing is the stabilization of the left leg and parts of the upper body during delivery so that the momentum can be transferred effectively from the lower parts of the body to the trunk and the throwing arm.

In training, long throws are sometimes made by athletes 'very easily', without stress on the arm and

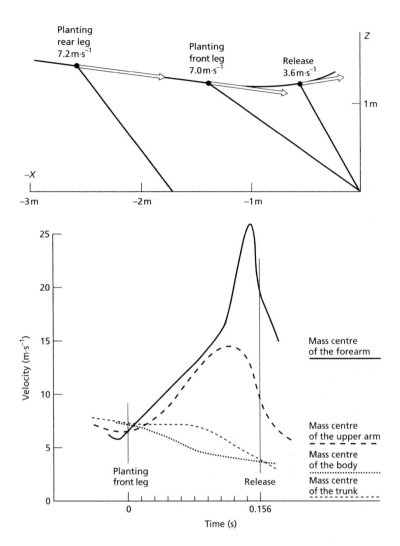

Fig. 20.8 Throw of Uwe Hohn, 99.52 m. *Above*: movement path of the mass centre of the body and its velocity at key positions. *Below*: velocity–time histories of the mass centres of the trunk, upper arm, forearm and the entire body. (From Bartonietz & Dörr 1986, Bartonietz 1987.)

trunk movements caused by conscious reinforcing actions. Sometimes the final throwing arm movement happens so quickly that the athlete misses the final opportunity to add power to the throw. This often occurs during training sessions, particularly at the beginning of throwing preparation. In these cases it is assumed that there has been effective use of momentum transfer.

The underlying hypothesis is that when throwing with effort for maximum distance, the momentum transfer is working in combination with reinforcing driving mechanisms of the thrower's muscles. The following findings support this hypothesis. Simul-

ating a simple throwing movement, Alexander (1991) illustrated the necessity of a chained delay in muscular actions, from proximal to distal. According to his findings, only an optimal delay between the activation of the more proximal muscles and the more distal muscles maximizes the velocity change to the implement. With increasing mass of the implement, there are sufficient changes in the coordination pattern. His findings can be related to the results of Hochmuth (1984) concerning an optimal delay by coordinating impulses in a link system, based on the mechanical interaction between the accelerated masses.

In the case of most of the top throwers over the last decades, the upper body works actively throughout the throw, up to the moment of release, reaching a marked forward inclination (examples include J. Kinnunen in 1969, Petranoff and Hohn and, among recent throwers, Backley, Henry, Zelezny, Stone and Damaske). This forward movement can lead to a head-first 'plunge' (see 'Recovery' below). The upper body thrust, the shoulder 'punch' or 'strike', and corresponding arm movement do not simply happen 'automatically' by virtue of a transfer of momentum. They require active muscular work, which is the result of special training. The biomechanical explanation for this upper body thrust is the production of angular momentum by the legwork during the delivery (see above). Changes in technique and performance development can be achieved during a period of several weeks between the off-season and the competition period. These changes are not brought about solely by more effective transfer of momentum, but by developing event-specific abilities and skills, including a longer delay of the final arm movement and the acquisition of 'feeling' for the implement. Any marked delay of the throwing arm movement has great relevance for increased performance, creating a pronounced body pre-tension, with an 'arched' or 'bow' position. Navarro *et al.* (1994) use as a criterion for determining the 'arched' position the instant of the change from external to internal rotation of the upper arm. This instant in time can be considered as the beginning of the final acceleration. With it, the potential of the stretch–shortening cycle is used. There is, of course an optimal initial body speed with which this mechanism works most effectively. Practice shows that an athlete is incapable of producing release velocities close to his or her maximum if the approach speed is low, even if the accumulated amount of linear momentum would be more than enough to do so. For example, consider a javelin of mass 0.8 kg and release velocity $30 \text{ m} \cdot \text{s}^{-1}$; it would have a momentum of $30 \times 0.8 = 24 \text{ kgm} \cdot \text{s}^{-1}$. The thrower, of body mass 100 kg, but with a very low approach speed of, say, $3 \text{ m} \cdot \text{s}^{-1}$, would still have a relatively large momentum of $300 \text{ kgm} \cdot \text{s}^{-1}$. Personal observations show that an athlete who should be able to throw 86–88 m, based on an approach speed of 6.5–$7 \text{ m} \cdot \text{s}^{-1}$, can throw only between 78 and 80 m if the approach speed is only $3–4 \text{ m} \cdot \text{s}^{-1}$, whether throwing after only 3–5 strides or after a slow approach. The difference in release velocity of about 10% is hypothetically caused mainly by the lower efficiency in storing and recuperating elastic energy in the muscles and tendons at low initial speeds.

When interpreting kinematic data such as velocity–time histories, it must be remembered that the movement pattern shown by kinematic data is only the end result and external picture of energy transfer in the chain system. No conclusions about energy flow mechanisms can be made without incorporating information about joint moments and joint power. Results of movement simulation of a three-link system for throwing implements of different masses by Bartonietz (1987) show that the deceleration of a proximal limb or joint (e.g. lower arm or elbow; see Figs 20.8 (lower part) & 20.9) can be interpreted as the result of the action of the distal limb, as described by Newton's Third Law (action and reaction): 'If one body exerts a force on another, there is an equal and opposite force, called a reaction, exerted on the first body by the second' (Isaacs 1996, p. 278). The connected limbs of the thrower's chain system can be regarded as being such interacting bodies. At least for the outer limbs—upper arm, forearm and hand—it can be assumed that the distal limb (e.g. forearm) is accelerated not because the corresponding proximal limb is decelerating—to ensure momentum transfer, as stated by Kreighbaum and Barthels (1981) and colleagues—but that the proximal limb is decelerated as a reaction to acceleration of the distal limb. As a result, the velocity of the elbow decreases, in spite of neuromuscular work against the decrease (Fig. 20.9). The results of ball-throwing movements on a link system, simulating the arm activity in javelin throwing and obtained by Kulig (1984) and Kulig *et al.* (1983), support this finding: distal links affect the proximal links more than vice versa. Applying this observation to trunk movement, it can be assumed that the almost constant velocity of trunk movement after planting the front leg, as shown in the lower part of Fig. 20.8, is influenced by the reaction of the arm acceleration.

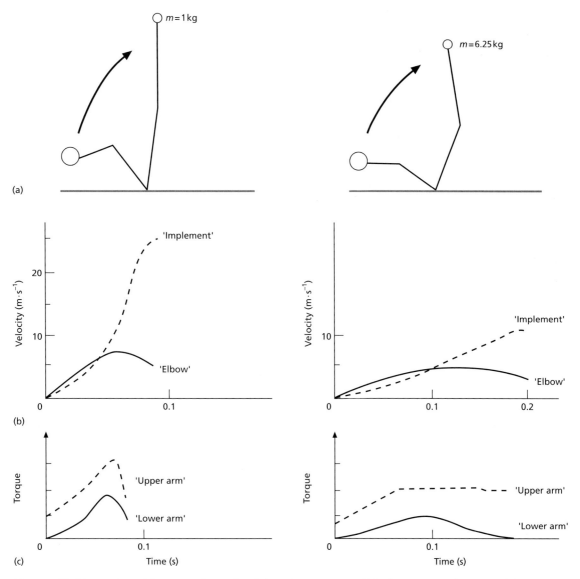

Fig. 20.9 The kinematics and dynamics of a simulated throwing movement. (a) Link positions at the start and the end. (b) Velocities of the implement and the elbow. (c) Torque vs. time. Note the positive values of the torque for the upper arm and lower arm until the instant of release, but a deceleration of the elbow joint. (From Bartonietz 1987.)

During this time interval, the athlete is 'working through' with the upper body. 'Working through', a common term in coaches' language, means not stopping the upper body or upper arm movements, but to continue working in a mechanical sense. Thus, a better support will be created for the acceleration of the subsequent limb. Without the active thrusting forward movement, the upper body remains almost in a vertical position in reaction to the arm movement. Stopping the upper body movement, as some athletes do, does not produce the maximum release velocity nor its optimal direction. Such throws are

Table 20.9 The influence of different improvement rates of the shoulder, elbow and hand drives of a simulated throwing movement. (Adapted from Bartonietz 1991.)

Simulation	Percent maximum of the joint momentum			Velocity of release (m · s^{-1})	Angle of release (°)	Calculated distance (m)	%
	'Upper arm'	'Forearm'	'Hand'				
1	100	100	100	7.96	25	4.95	100
2	110	110	110	8.58	24	5.58	113
3	115	110	105	8.82	30	6.87	139

released at too high an angle or are characterized by an ineffective arm movement at shoulder level, with a lack of 'rolling in' of the elbow.

According to data from Bartlett *et al.* (1996) and Morriss *et al.* (1997), the differences in linear joint peak velocities (absolute values and values related to the velocity of the centre of gravity) and angular velocities of the main limbs can serve as a basis for evaluating the individual throwing pattern. Interpreting similar kinematic data, the restrictions mentioned earlier have to be taken into consideration: kinematic parameters by themselves are not a sufficient basis for evaluating the contribution of each segment to the throwing movement. For a better understanding of the changes in the capacities of the prime movers necessary for improved performance, throwing movements were simulated on a three-link system. This model was developed to investigate the training effect of heavy throwing implements. Table 20.9 shows the results, with simulation 1 serving as a reference. The data show that an increase of 10% for each of the drives increased the final result by about the same extent, i.e. 13%. Using a stepwise increase in momentum of 15, 10 and 5%, the direction of the velocity becomes much more important in achieving a greater distance. The practical implication is the need to strengthen the muscle groups around the shoulder complex by special strength exercises, like pull-overs and using throws with heavy implements. Kulig (1984) and Kulig *et al.* (1983) reached similar conclusions, stating as one of the results of their throwing movement simulation that the ability to develop sufficient muscular moments primarily of the proximal link, is one

of the preconditions for achieving greater final velocities.

RECOVERY

After release of the javelin the body has to be brought to rest. When throwing heavy implements with a short approach run (Bartonietz 1987) there is enough movement amplitude to bring the arm to rest. Throwing light implements allows a longer path for acceleration. This has to be taken into consideration when decelerating the elbow extension after release, because the decelerating muscle work of the biceps, a primary elbow flexor, can be insufficient in producing the required high end-range forces. In this case, the joint stop will be achieved mechanically, which is a potential source of elbow injury (see 'Injury prevention' below). The use of light implements must be introduced so that proper care is taken to set up the appropriate movement pattern, especially for the throwing arm after release.

The residual body speed and its direction at the instant of release has an influence on the length of the stopping distance and on the movement pattern to prevent fouling. An average distance of 2.50 m for men and 2.20 m for women between the foul line and the release position (author's own data from the 1995 World Championship finalists) can be considered normal. On the one hand, the thrower does not want to sacrifice any of the distance thrown by stopping too far from the foul line. On the other hand, from a coaching point of view, there is an undesired effect of too short a stopping distance on the throwing technique both in training and competition: a short distance can unconsciously lead to starting the recovery movement before delivery is finished—right foot take-off from the ground and hip flexion. This has to be taken into account when following the suggestions of Rich *et al.* (1992), to minimize the front foot to foul line distance at the instant of release while still being able to decelerate the forward movement of the body. Some top male throwers use a head-first plunge or a movement close to this, touching the ground with the throwing hand after release. Examples include the following athletes on the occasion of their record throws: E. Danielsen (world record of 85.70 m in the 1956 Olympic Games), A. Cantello (world record of 86.04 in 1959), J. Zelezny (world record of 98.48 m in 1996), P.-A. Fagerson (Norwegian record of 85.06 in 1996), A. Currey (Australian record of 84.92 m in 1996), G. Lovegrove (New Zealand record of 88.20 m in 1996) and J. Kloek (Belgian record of 81.18 m in 1998).

Injury prevention

Health is the highest rated value in human life. A long-term training plan can only be considered effective when it also conserves the athlete's health. Good training methods prevent injuries and this should be a major goal for both athlete and coach.

The throwing motion puts the anatomical structures under a great deal of torsional, shearing and impact forces, which can reach and exceed the tolerance limits. Following Radin *et al.* (1979), damage of the joint structures and the musculoskeletal tissues can occur by repeated loadings even when each load is below the tolerance threshold of the structures. Besides the injuries that are common to other events and sports, there are some specific injuries that a thrower may sustain. The javelin thrower can consider them as 'occupational hazards' (Sing 1984). Additional sources of injuries are an incorrect throwing technique, using too heavy training loads or performing when fatigued. The nature of these stresses is better understood in the light of knowledge about the mechanics of javelin throwing. Knowledge about the sources of injury always precedes methods to prevent them.

General and special warming-up exercises must be used before throwing. General and special stretching exercises are also imperative before and after training. Many athletes in the throwing events suffer from various problems around the main joints (Fig. 20.10). The javelin thrower's injuries are mainly to the ankle of the front leg, the knees, the lower back, the shoulder and the elbow of the throwing arm. According to Goertzen and Zinser (1998), about three-quarters of all injuries to top javelin throwers occur in training. The following

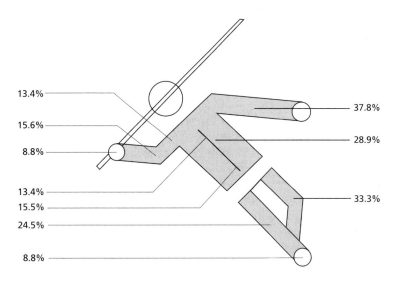

Fig. 20.10 Percentage localization of injuries in the throwing events. (From Pförringer *et al.* 1985.)

overview will show the possible relationship between javelin throwing mechanics and throwing injury, underlining the role of correct throwing technique and of proper training planning. Of course, a physician should always be consulted in case of any injury.

Ankle of the front leg

INJURIES

Injuries to the ankle joint of the front leg include ligament strain or rupture, inflammation, and loose bodies within the joint.

SOURCE

The injuries are caused by shearing forces produced when planting the foot out of line, whether inclined laterally or medially, or by impact forces on joint structures when foot planting.

PREVENTION

Various measures can be taken to prevent this type of injury. These include:
• plant the front foot straight;
• strengthen the ankles and the feet;
• exercise barefoot in sand;
• perform uniplanar and multidirectional proprioceptive exercises on one and two wobble boards to develop the neuromuscular response;
• learn to implement preinnervation prior to foot planting to control the stiffness of the whole front leg;
• use the correct footwear; different parts of the throwing shoe can exert additional stress on the foot, on Achilles tendon, arch tendons and ligaments. Most throwing shoes, based on a design for sprinters, do not take into account the forces generated by athletes whose body weight may be 100 kg or more. Additional work by orthopaedic shoemakers is generally necessary, for example reinforcement of the front-foot shoe sole, and a broad lateral belt over the instep; and
• tape the ankle before throwing in training and competition.

Knee of the rear drive leg

INJURY

The main injury to the rear drive leg is ligament damage.

SOURCE

This type of injury results from rotational stress and shearing forces produced by striking the ground at an angle of between 90 and 60° to the throwing direction, compared with the passivity of the right leg.

PREVENTION

Measures that can help to prevent this type of injury include:
• active drive of the rear leg before the foot of the front leg plants; and
• plant the foot of the rear leg at an angle of about 45° to the throwing direction.

Knee of the bracing front leg

INJURIES

The main injuries to the front-leg knee are cartilage damage and ligament damage.

SOURCE

These injuries result from high impact stresses (10 times body weight and more), torsional stresses and shearing forces if the foot is not planted straight in front of the thrower.

PREVENTION

Preventive measures for these types of injury include:
• muscular stabilization of the leg—learn the technique of preinnervation prior to planting the foot in order to control the stiffness of the whole front leg, which is increased several-fold during active muscle work; and

• avoid planting to the left, which is caused by passivity of the rear leg and a premature movement of the left arm, known as 'premature opening of the left side'.

Lower back (Alexander 1985)

INJURIES

The most common injuries to the lower back are lumbo-sacral strains and sprains, stress fractures, and slipped disc.

SOURCE

Injuries to the lower back are caused by various factors:
• hard, passive landing on the rear foot after the impulse stride in a lean-back position;
• twisted column during throwing movement, especially using the 'rotational style' of javelin throwing (Giles 1980);
• overload during weight training; and
• 'bow position', like an inverted 'C', with the maximum prestretch in the abdominal area instead of the thoraco-acromial area.

PREVENTION

Various steps can be taken to reduce the risk of injury to the lower back, including:
• an active impulse stride, keeping the upper body stable with proper control of the body position at rear-foot landing and minimizing landing impact;
• use of a belt during throwing and weightlifting—see Faigenbaum and Liatsos (1994) about the use and abuse of weightlifting belts, also Zatsiorsky (1995); and
• strengthen the back and abdominal muscle groups as a year-round task, to create a 'muscular corset', using general and special exercises.

Shoulder joint

The shoulder joint is a very complex structure of three connected joints. It is essential to strengthen

the rotator cuff and the muscles of the back part of the upper trunk by different pulling exercises, such as shrugs and chin-ups. Functional resistive exercisers (rubber bands of different elasticity, e.g. Thera bands, Deuser bands or Clini bands) and dumbbells are effective tools for strengthening the muscles and ligaments around the shoulders.

INJURIES

The main shoulder injuries encountered by the javelin thrower are shoulder sprain and rotator cuff strain.

SOURCE

These shoulder injuries are caused by traction stresses, arising from excessive momentum on the shoulder due to a long arm lever (throwing with a straight arm and minimum forearm sling).

PREVENTION

The risk of shoulder injury can be minimized by strengthening exercises aimed at better holding the shoulder joints together, such as different kinds of shrugs, internal and external rotations, and stretching exercises.

Elbow

INJURIES

The common elbow injuries for javelin throwers include:
• 'javelin thrower's elbow', which is damage/inflammation of the medial elbow structures;
• 'tennis elbow', i.e. epicondylitis or tendinitis; and
• loose bodies within the joint.

SOURCE

Elbow injuries arise due to too many throws and/or use of implements that are too heavy. Chronic stress by overuse, as described for 'tennis elbow' by Priest *et al.* (1980) and Szewczyk (1992), can also be a major cause of elbow trauma in javelin throwing. High-torque end-range forces when throwing light implements can also lead to elbow injury.

PREVENTION

It is essential to learn the correct throwing technique as a beginner since a chronic injury is often sustained during the first years of training. This observation, made by Waris (1946), has lost none of its importance. Avoid sidearm throwing, control the use of heavy implements, and perform strengthening exercises.

Rehabilitation

The specific throwing loadings, which are different for each side of the body, develop a functional asymmetry from the arms to the feet. Effective prevention of injuries and rehabilitation after injuries requires an understanding of the characteristics of the joint complexes involved. Knowledge of the strength ratio between opposing muscle groups (e.g. the hamstrings/quadriceps ratio for the legs, or the flexor/extensor ratio for the trunk) can help to counteract the development of excessive muscular imbalances. Experimental data underline the high stresses on joint structures when throwing with a reduced range of movement. According to data from Morriss *et al.* (1997), the athlete with the most bent elbow at the World Championships in 1995 was A. Linden (who threw a distance of 79.12 m), with a permanently reduced range of movement due to an elbow injury. This athlete displayed the highest angular velocity of elbow extension of all throwers analysed, and a maximum velocity of wrist flexion comparable with the throws of other athletes. The reason for the great contribution of the forearm to the final velocity is the relatively long angular path of the forearm compared with the other limbs (Kulig *et al.* 1983; Kulig 1984).

With this in mind, any training programme must:
• ensure the right order of training work and provide for recovery in general;
• ensure the right order of training exercises during the workout—for example avoid jumping and sprinting work after throwing workouts where the focus is on the braking work of the front leg;

• prevent intensive throwing training when the athlete is fatigued;
• develop the correct movement execution by throwing different implements, when sprinting and jumping and during strength training (e.g. barbell exercises, special strength exercises);
• include exercises to improve the strength of ligaments around the main joints: ankles, knees, shoulder and elbow; and
• develop muscles with stabilizing functions—legs, trunk, shoulder/arm—and the strength of opposing muscle groups, strengthening the 'muscular corset' of trunk muscles as a year-round task.

It must be remembered that ligaments and cartilage need a long adaptation period, up to 2–3 months.

Biomechanical knowledge: a must for coaching

Biomechanical knowledge about a particular sporting discipline helps to develop the internal movement picture of the athletes concerned. Athletes with knowledge about the basic biomechanical relationships of their event can develop a better sensory feedback. Although the distance thrown is the final criterion, relevant biomechanical data offer the opportunity to provide a detailed performance diagnosis. Even experienced athletes, older in years and training, have shown a capability to improve their technical skills with target-directed specific strength development. Heptathletes and decathletes that use the goal technique employed by specialists can also develop a respectable javelin technique. The world's best athletes in the multievents underline that this goal is achievable, as evidenced by the performances of the Estonian Erki Nool, European Champion for the decathlon in 1998. He threw the javelin 70.65 m with an excellent technique; this was 20% further than the distances thrown by the athletes placed second and third.

Release parameters

Optimal values of the release parameters have to be used as principal targets for the training of javelin-throwing skills and abilities. In the targeted performance window, distance improvement and the necessary increase in release velocity can be assumed as being proportional. The velocity of release has to be maximized, while for the other parameters optimal values are required. The optimal value of the angle of release—the direction of the javelin's velocity—is dependent upon the performance level. Male and female athletes must strive for 30–34° with a zero angle of attack and minimum angle of yaw. With the introduction of a modified implement for female athletes in 1999, the recommendations for the angle of release will be redefined.

Energy transfer, power demands and movement coordination

The main principle in both training and competition performance diagnosis should be that no sporting movement can exist without energy transfer and power production. This has to be considered when determining the criteria and parameters for performance diagnosis in training and competition, by selecting training exercises and by planning the training load. Understanding of the interaction between the links in the limb chain, based only on kinematic data, is limited. A kinetic-based approach to throwing movements in general and javelin throwing in particular provides deeper insights into the movement structure. Examples in this chapter have demonstrated the coaching relevance of the energetic approach.

Although researchers have comprehensively studied the kinematics and, partly, the kinetics of javelin throwing at different performance levels, the way in which complex performance is coordinated and improved, in both training and competition, requires further research. A higher velocity of release requires a higher level of power in terms of physics. With increasing performance, the limited path for accelerating the body and the javelin requires changes in the velocity–time history, leading to a more pronounced delay of the final arm movement. Because of the high power demands of the competition movement at high approach speeds, the training value of throws at lower initial approach speeds is limited. The hypothesis of mastering with performance improvement the many degrees of freedom of the neuromuscular system, developed by Bernstein

(1967), can be also applied to a complex movement such as the javelin throw. The changes associated with performance development in such movement elements as impulse stride, key body positions, spatial control of the throwing arm and javelin, and the rear and front legwork, can also be interpreted from this viewpoint. This underlines that the correct throwing movement pattern must be learnt and developed thoroughly and continuously. The evidence about gender-specific differences in ball-throwing, discovered by Geese (1997), should lead to special attention being given to skill acquisition and development with girls and advanced female athletes alike. Observations in training and competition support this conclusion.

Movement coordination

The world's leading male and female javelin throwers demonstrate a technique which, in its most important elements, corresponds very closely to the 'ideal throw'. Individual variations, due to different training philosophies, the model technique aspired to, as well as individual physical abilities and skills, lead to deviations in the movement pattern from the ideal 'target' technique.

A stable front leg is one of the main criteria in javelin performance diagnosis. The bracing work of the front leg shows a close relationship to the performance level. Athletes have to learn, from the beginning, how to decelerate about 50% of their initial body velocity effectively. A planting angle of the front leg of between 40 and 50° whilst raising the leg no more than 15°, creates the best conditions to apply braking forces and to produce an angular momentum for the upper body and arm work. The front leg should not bend more than 10°, being fully extended at the moment of release. The model for the braking legwork and experimental data suggest a clear relationship between performance and the degree of decelerated body velocity. The athlete has, within his or her individual capacity, to strive for the effective use of the potentials of the stretch–shortening cycle. Momentum transfer has to be understood as an active process occurring from proximal to distal segments. The deceleration of proximal limbs can be understood as a reaction to the acceleration of distal limbs. 'Working through' is a demand from the coaches' point of view. Effective use of the stretch–shortening cycle is crucial in high-performance javelin throwing.

Performance improvement requires changes in movement coordination. The movement complex 'delay of the arm strike/creation of a marked body pretension' has a key function in javelin throwing. The 'arched' or 'bow' position of the thrower is one of the characteristics of this important movement part.

Biomechanical aspects of injury

The assumed relationship between javelin-throwing mechanics and throwing injury underlines the role of a correct throwing technique and of proper training planning. The javelin thrower's injuries mainly affect the ankle of the front leg, the knees, the lower back, the shoulder and the elbow of the throwing arm, and occur mostly during training. Any training programme must incorporate measures to minimize the risk of injury.

Postscript

One mustn't think of the javelin as a minor sport, like curling or anything. The javelin represents the glory of Greece and it symbolizes man's search for his primitive ancestral identity. I can blink my eyes and look out at a javelin thrower and see tens of thousands of warriors marching across the field and I can hear the voices of antiquity. No, the javelin isn't some minor sport. It is classic. It is beauty. It is excellence. It is immortality.

[Steve Seymour, 1948 Olympic Games silver medal winner (Kirshenbaum 1969, p. 40)]

References

Adamczewski, H. (1995) Untersuchung-sergebnisse vom Meßplatz Speerwurf. *Die Lehre der Leichtathletik* 17, 97–100, 18, 101–104, 19, 105–108.

Adamczewski, H. (1997) Javelin throwing—competition analysis: biomechanical data. Institut für Angewandte Trainingswissenschaft e.V., Leipzig (unpublished research).

Adamczewski, H. (1998) Javelin throwing—competition analysis: biomechanical data. Institut für Angewandte Trainingswissenschaft e.V., Leipzig (unpublished research).

Adamczewski, H. & Perlt, B. (1993) Training on the 3D force plate system (MIS) for javelin throwers, December 17th 1993—biomechanical results. Institut für Angewandte Trainings-wissenschaft e.V., Leipzig (unpublished research).

Adamczewski, H., Perlt, B. & Bartonietz, K. (1998) Ground reaction force data—training support of Boris Henry and Tom Pukstys, May 27, 1998. Institut für Angewandte Trainingswissenschaft e.V., Leipzig (unpublished research).

Alexander, M.J.L. (1985) Biomechanical aspects of lumbar spine injuries in athletes: a review. *Canadian Journal of Applied Sport Science* 10 (1), 1–20.

Alexander, R. McN. (1991) Optimum timing of muscle activation for simple models in throwing. *Journal of Theoretical Biology* 150, 349–379.

Bankhead, W.H. & Thorsen, M.A. (1964) A comparison of four grips used in throwing the javelin. *Research Quarterly* 35 (Suppl.) 438–442.

Bartlett, R., Müller, E., Lindinger, S., Brunner, F. & Morriss, C. (1996) Three-dimensional evaluation of the release parameters for javelin throwers of different skill levels. *Journal of Applied Biomechanics* 12 (1), 58–71.

Bartonietz, K. (1987) Zur sportlichen Technik der Wettkampfübungen und zur Wirkungsrichtung ausgewählter Trainingsübungen in den Wurf- und Stoßdisziplinen der Leichtathletik. [The technique of competition exercises and the effect of selected training exercises in the throwing events and shot put.] PhD thesis, Deutsche Hochschule für Körperkultur, Leipzig.

Bartonietz, K. (1991) Zum Beitrag der Bio-mechanik für höhere Wirksamkeit des Trainings. In: *Trainingswissen-schaftliche Studien zur Leichtathletik* (eds M. Letzelter & W. Steinmann), pp. 197–227. Schors-Verlag, Niedernhausen.

Bartonietz, K. (1992) Spezielle Analyse der WM 1991 in Tokyo: Wurf/Stoß. *Die Lehre der Leichtathletik* 1, 2, 15–18.

Bartonietz, K. (1994) Training of technique and specific power in throwing events.

Modern Athlete and Coach, Adelaide 32 (1), 10–16.

Bartonietz, K. (1995) Moderne Auffassungen zur Entwicklung von Maximalkraftfähigkeiten. Theoretische Ansätze und praktische Umsetzung in den Wurfdisziplinen—ein Überblick. [Modern points of view on the development of maximum strength capacities. Theory and use in training practice of throwers—an overview.] *Lehre der Leichtathletik* 34 (14), 73–79, (15), 81–88, (16), 81–89.

Bartonietz, K. (1996) Strength training of throwers. *Modern Athlete and Coach, Adelaide* 34 (4), 3–8.

Bartonietz, K. & Dörr, J. (1986) *Trainer-handmaterial Technikleitbild Speerwerfen*. [*Manual for coaches: Goal technique in javelin throwing*.] FKS, Leipzig.

Bartonietz, K. & Emrich, E. (1997) Die neuralgischen Punkte der Speerwurf-fleistung. [The sore spots of javelin performance.] *Leichtathletik training* 8, 26–31.

Bartonietz, K. & Felder, H. (1994) WM 1993—Technikanalyse der weltbesten Athleten im Speerwerfen. *Lehre der Leichtathletik* 26, 15–18, 27, 18.

Bartonietz, K. & Güllich, A. (1992) Zur Bedeutung der Pick-up-Beschleunigung bei Höchstleistungen im 100-m-Sprint. Ein Beitrag zur Leistungs- und Trainingsstruktur des Kurzsprints. *Lehre der Leichtathletik* **31** (10), 17–18, (11), 15–18.

Bartonietz, K. & Hellmann, K. (1985) Empfehlungen für das Training am KTG Speerwurf mit Sollvorgaben an leistungsbestimmende biomechanische Parameter für spezielle Krafttrainings-übungen am KTG in Ableitung von den Anforderungen der Speerwurf-Wettkampfübung. Forschungsinstitut für Körperkultur und Sport, Leipzig (unpublished research).

Bartonietz, K. & Larsen, B. (1997) General and event-specific considerations in peaking for the main competition. *New Studies in Athletics* 2/3, 75–86.

Bartonietz, K., Best, R.J. & Borgström, A. (1996) The throwing events at the World Championship in Athletics 1995, Göteborg – technique of the world's best athletes, part 2: Discus and javelin throw, *New Studies in Athletics* **11** (1), 19–44.

Bernstein, N. (1967) *The Co-ordination and Regulation of Movements*. Pergamon Press, Oxford.

Best, R.J. & Bartlett, R.M. (1988) Computer flight simulation of the men's new rules javelin. In: *Biomechanics XI-B* (eds G. de Groot, A.P. Hollander, P.A. Huijing & G.J. van Ingen Schenau), pp. 588–594. Free University Press, Amsterdam.

Best, R.J., Bartlett, R.M. & Morriss, C.J. (1993) A three-dimensional analysis of javelin throwing technique. *Journal of Sports Science* **11**, 315–328.

Best, R.J., Bartlett, R.M. & Sawyer, R.A. (1995) Optimal javelin release. *Journal of Applied Biomechanics* **11**, 371–394.

Borgström, A. (1988) Two years with the new javelin. *New Studies in Athletics* **1**, 85–88.

Borgström, A. (1997) Biomekanik Spjut/Javelin January Zelezny c. 92,5 (övertram/foul) 1996–06–22 Kuortane, FIN, *Spjutkastaren* 2/3, 34–39.

Böttcher, J. & Kühl, L. (1996) Untersuchungen zum Speerwurf. *Lehre der Leichtathletik* **35** (31), 812, (32), 84–85, (33), 86–87.

Böttcher, J. & Kühl, L. (1998) The technique of the best female javelin throwers in 1997. *New Studies in Athletics* **1**, 47–61.

Faigenbaum, A.D. & Liatsos, N.S. (1994) The use and abuse of weightlifting belts. *Strength and Conditioning*, August, pp. 60–62.

Felke, P. (1993) Zur Erneuerung des Krafttrainings im Speerwerfen (Hochleist-ungsbereich). Diploma, Faculty of Sports Science, University of Leipzig.

Geese, R. (1997) Geschlechtsspezifische Unterschiede in der Wurfmotorik. *Spectrum der Sportwissenschaften* 9 (2), 31–41.

Giles, K. (1980) Rotation in javelin throwing. *Track and Field Quarterly Review* 80 (1), 21.

Goertzen, M. & Zinser, W. (1998) Langzeit-analyse der Prävalenz und 'Life-time'-Inzidenz von Wirbelsäulenbeschwerden nach Beendigung des Hochleistungs-sports. [Prevalence and lifetime incidence of back pain in athletes.] *Sportmedizin* **48**, 9–17.

Hay, J.G. (1978) *The Biomechanics of Sports Techniques*, 2nd edn. Prentice Hall, Englewood Cliffs, N.J.

Hendershott, J. (1997) Pukstys puts balance in life. *Track & Field News*, August, p. 11.

Hochmuth, G. (1984) *Biomechanics of Athletic Movements*. Sportverlag, Berlin.

Hubbard, M. (1984) Optimal javelin trajectories. *Journal of Biomechanics* **17**, 777–787.

Hubbard, M. (1988) The flight of the javelin. *Scientific American*, September, pp. 120–121.

Hubbard, M. (1989) The throwing events in track and field. In: *Biomechanics of Sport* (ed. C.L. Vaughan), pp. 213–238. CRC Press, Boca Raton, FL.

IAAF (1996) *Handbook 1996–97*. International Amateur Athletics Federation, Monaco.

Ikegami, Y., Miura, M., Matsui, H. & Hashimoto, I. (1981) Biomechanical analysis of the javelin throw. In: *Biomechanics VII B. International series on Biomechanics, Vol 3B, Proceedings of the 7th International Congress of Biomechanics* (eds A. Morecki, K. Fidelus, K. Kedzior et al.), pp. 271–276. Polish Scientific Publishers, Warsaw and University Park Press, Baltimore.

Isaacs, A. (1996) *A Dictionary of Physics*, 3rd edn. Oxford University Press, Oxford.

Jarver, J. (1987) *Track and Field Coaching Manual*. Rothmans Foundation/ National Sport Division.

Johnson, C. (1987) *Javelin Throwing*. British Amateur Athletic Board, London.

Julin, A.L. (1988) The new javelin: effects on level of performance. *New Studies in Athletics* **1**, 75–84.

Kirshenbaum, J. (1969) 'They're all out to launch'. *Sports Illustrated*, July 21, 38–41.

Komi, P.V. & Mero, A. (1985) Biomechanical analysis of Olympic javelin throwers. *Journal of Sport Biomechanics* **1**, 139–150.

Kreighbaum, E. & Barthels, K.M. (1981) *Biomechanics*. Burgess Publishing Company, Minneapolis.

Kulig, K. (1984) Koordinacija szlonów kónczyny górnej w ruchach wymag-ajacuch rozwijanija maksymalnej predkósci. [Coordination of a difficult arm movement with maximum velocity.] *Rozprawy naukowe AWF we Wroclawiu*. Wroclaw **XVIII**, 61–89.

Kulig, K., Nowacki, Z. & Bober, T. (1983) Synchronization of partial impulses as a biomechanical principle. In: *Biomechanics VIII-B. Proceedings of the Eighth International Congress of Biomechanics*, pp. 1144–1151. Human Kinetics Publishers, Champaign, IL.

LeBlank, M.K. & Dapena, J. (1998) Angular momentum flow during the javelin throw. *Medicine and Science in Sports and Exercise* **30**, 194.

Matveev, E.N. (1967) Eksperimentalnoe obosnovanie primenenija spezialnych uprzhnenij dlja razvitija skorostno-silivych kachestv u metatelej. PhD dissertation, Gozudarstvenniy Zentralniy Ordena Lenina Institut Fizicheckoj Kultury, Moscow.

Menzel, H.-J. (1986) Biomechanics of javelin throwing. *New Studies in Athletics* **3**, 85–98.

Mero, A., Komi, P.V., Korjus, T., Navarro, E. & Gregor, R.J. (1994) Body segment contribution to javelin throwing during final thrust phases. *Journal of Applied Biomechanics* **10**, 166–177.

Morriss, C. (1996) Differences in throwing style between competitors at the 1994 European Championships men's javelin final. *The Thrower*, April, pp. 19–24.

Morriss, C., Bartlett, R. & Fowler, N. (1997) Biomechanical analysis of the men's javelin throw at the 1995 World Championships in Athletics. *New Studies in Athletics* 2/3, 31–41.

Navarro, E., Campos, J., Vera, P. & Chillaron, E. (1994) A procedure for determining the acceleration phase in javelin throwing. In: *Biomechanics in Sports XII, Proceedings of the 12th International Symposium on Biomechanics in Sports, July 2–6 1994, Budapest* (eds A. Barabas & G. Fabian), pp. 357–359. International Society of Biomechanics in Sport and Hungarian University of Physical Education, Budapest.

Paish, W. (1986) Some initial observations on the new men's javelin. *New Studies in Athletics* **1**, 81–84.

Pförringer, W., Rosemeyer, B. & Bär, H.-W. (eds) (1985) *Sport—Trauma und Belastung*. Perimed Fachbuch-Verlagsgesellschaft, Erlangen.

Priest, J.D., Branden, V. & Goodwin, S.G. (1980) A study of players with pain. *Physician and Sports Medicine* **8** (5), 77–85.

Quercetani, R.L. (1964) *A World History of Track and Field Athletics 1868–1964.* Oxford University Press, London.

Radin, E.L., Simon, S.R., Rose, R.M. & Paul, I.L. (1979) *Practical Biomechanics for the Orthopedic Surgeon.* John Wiley & Sons, New York.

Rich, R.G., Whiting, W.C., McCoy, R.W. & Gregor, R.J. (1992) Analysis of release parameters in elite javelin throwers. *Track Technique*, Spring, pp. 2932–2934.

Salo, A. & Viitasalo, J.T. (1995) Vergleich kinematischer Merkmale des Speer-wurfs bei Werfern internationalen und nationalen Niveaus und bei Zehnkämp-fern. [Comparison of the kinematic characteristics of the javelin throw in throwers of international and national level and of decathletes.] *Leistungssport* **5**, 40–44.

Scarborough, W. & Allan, C.W. (1964) *A Collection of Chinese Proverbs.*

Paragon Book Reprint Corp., New York.

Schmolinsky, G. (1983) *Track and Field Textbook for Coaches and Sports Teachers.* Sportverlag, Berlin.

Schwuchow, H. (1986) Anforderungen an die Charakteristik des finalen Krafteinsatzes zum Erreichen der Prognoseleistungen im Speerwerfen. [Power demands of the javelin throw delivery for predicted record per-formances.] Diploma, Deutsche Hochschule für Körperkultur, Leipzig.

Sing, R.F. (1984) *The Dynamics of the Javelin Throw.* Reynolds Publishers, Cherry Hill, N.J.

Suliev, L. (1961) *Metanie kopja.* [Javelin throwing.] Fizkultura i sport, Moscow.

Szewczyk, J.T. (1992) Eine Übersicht zur Entstehung des sogenannten Tennisel-lebogen beim Tennisspielen. *Sport-medizin* **43** (3), 104–117.

Terauds, J. (1985) *Biomechanics of the Javelin Throw.* Academic Publishers, Del Mar, CA.

Tidow, G. (1994) Modelle für das leichtathletische Techniktraining —Speerwurf. *Lehre der Leichtathletik* **21**, 15–17, **22**, 15–18, **23**, 15–18.

Tutevich, V.N. (1969) *Teorija sportivnych matanij.* [Theory of the throwing events.] Fizkultura i Sport, Moscow.

Voronkin, V.I. & Maksimov, R.I. (1974) Metod objektivnogo kontrolja sportivno-technicheskogo masterstva metatelej kopja. *Teorija I Praktika Fizicheskogo Vospitanija* **6**, 20–22.

Vrabel, J. (1997) Zelezny, the javelin thrower. *The Thrower* **73** (April), 12–18.

Waris, W. (1946) Elbow injuries of javelin throwers. *Acta Chirurgica Scandinavica* **93**, 563–575 (cited by Sing 1984).

Zatsiorsky, V.M. (1995) *Science and Practice of Strength Training.* Human Kinetics Publishers, Champaign, IL.

Chapter 21

Shot Putting

J. LANKA

The purpose of this chapter is to summarize the results of investigations on the biomechanics of shot putting. The main emphasis is on the conventional glide technique (back-facing style) and the rotational technique (Barishnikov's style) of a right-handed shot-putter. Precise and thoroughly documented data are available on only certain aspects of shot-putting performance. Many variations in technique are based on personal opinions of athletes, coaches and researchers. In some cases they are included here in order to provide a systematic treatment of technique variations. However, their scientific merit remains to be tested.

History

Shot putting as a sport has more than a hundred years of history. Opinions about shot-putting techniques have changed throughout its history. Generally, the evolution of shot-putting technique from the beginning of this century up to the present day can be related to the four variants of movement performance that have been applied by different generations of shot-putters. These are:
• shot putting from a standing position;
• shot putting with a glide from the take-off position with one's side or back against the push direction; and
• shot putting with a rotational technique.

The history of shot-putting technique can be evaluated according to what extent the technique allows use of an athlete's speed and power (Tutevich 1969). During the first stage of technique improvement the push was mainly executed by the hand; during the

second, by means of the upper body as well as the hand; during the third stage, by including the legs and thereby all the potential sources of the body's strength and power.

The first relevant innovation after the shot put from a standing position was moving along a circle (glide) followed by a subsequent pushoff. An athlete started the glide by staying sideways with respect to the movement direction ('from the side to the push direction' technique). Athletes had used different variations of this approach for many years. The next alteration that turned out to be essential took place in the 1950s. The technique of the US athlete P. O'Brian was the basis for this change. He pushed the shot from an initial position with his back against the circle, increasing his body's bending and emphasizing the rotational movements during the pushing-off phase.

P. O'Brian's technique was further developed and perfected by other athletes (Zatsiorsky *et al.*, 1978). For example, the technique with a 'short-long rhythm' was proposed by German coaches. The preliminary movements were simplified and the path of applying force to the shot was increased. In the 1970s shot putting with a rotational technique became popular. The main idea of this technique was borrowed from discus throwing. More than four decades have passed since the first put using the rotational technique took place. This was performed by O. Chandler (USA), who threw 17.08 m (at that time the world record was 17.95 m). The following years brought some well-known performances by A. Barysnikov (USSR), B. Oldfield (USA), D. Laut (USA), R. Barnes (USA) and others.

Flight of shot

The horizontal distance travelled by a projectile released at a certain angle to the horizontal depends on its initial velocity (V_0), release angle (α_0), and release height (h_0). This can be represented by the following equation:

$$L = \frac{V_0^2}{g} \cos \alpha_0 \left(\sin \alpha_0 + \sqrt{\sin^2 \alpha_0 + \frac{2gh_0}{V_0^2}} \right) \qquad (21.1)$$

where g is the acceleration due to gravity. Air resistance is not considered in this formula, as its influence is minimal (Tutevich 1969). Optimal values of these variables in shot putting are related to individual qualities such as strength and speed as well as technique of the athlete.

The release height of the shot depends on the length of the athlete's body and arms, and the level of his/her physical and technical preparedness. An increase in release height will cause an approximately equal increase in the distance the shot flies (Tutevich 1969).

The optimal angle of shot release (37–41°) is less than 45° because the release height (usually 2.2–2.3 m) is higher than the level of landing. An increase in release height will decrease the optimal angle of release and vice versa. The value of the angle of release also depends on the release velocity. Increasing the velocity will increase the optimal angle of release (Dyson 1968). A deviation of ±3–4° from the optimal value of the angle does not greatly influence the flight distance of the device, although a deviation of 10° might diminish it by approximately 1 m (Tutevich 1969). It has been reported that great deviations were not observed in practice, even among beginners (Grigalka 1970). However, the measurements taken at the 1995 World Championship provided contrary evidence (Bartonietz 1995). Nine of the finalists had significant deviations from the optimal release angle: J. Godina, USA (21.47 m) = 31°; M. Halvari, Finland (20.93 m) = 35°; R. Barnes, USA (20.41 m) = 30°; A. Klimenko, Ukraine (18.36 m) = 31°. The same was observed during the women's match: S. Storp, Germany (18.81 m) = 29°; L. Zhang, China (19.07 m) = 33°; V. Fedyushina, Ukraine (18.03 m) = 45°.

Height and angle of release are relatively constant for an individual athlete and, from a practical standpoint, cannot be changed to improve the performance (Dyson 1968; Grigalka 1974).

The most important factor in shot putting is the release velocity, as the horizontal distance (L) covered during the flight is proportional to the release velocity squared. Increasing the initial velocity by 150% will cause the shot to fly 2.25 times further. Increasing the velocity by a factor of two will improve the performance result by a factor of four.

Release velocity depends on the magnitude and direction of the force applied to the shot, the distance over which the force is applied, and the duration of the action. This can be represented by the following equation:

$$V = \frac{Ft}{m} = \sqrt{\frac{2Fs}{m}} \qquad (21.2)$$

where V = velocity of release, F = force applied to the implement, t = duration of the force application, s = distance, and m = mass of the implement. Equation 21.2 is valid only when F is constant, which corresponds to a highly simplified ideal situation. The magnitude of the force applied to the shot is determined by the level of physical preparedness of the athlete and body position during the period of force application; the effect of force production is determined by the duration of force application and/or distance. These mechanical characteristics of the movement depend on the body dimensions and the technique of the movement. The possibilities of increasing the length of the shot path are limited by the size of circle, thus increasing the force is of great importance. All the changes in shot-putting technique have had the aim of either increasing the magnitude of force applied to the implement, or increasing the time (length of the path) of force application.

Movement of the shot prior to release

The term 'speed dynamics' is used here to mean the pattern of speed changes of the shot during shot-put performance.

Speed dynamics

Some authors (Doherty 1950; Simonyi 1973) have emphasized the importance of achieving maximum speed of the shot early in the performance. Others (Schpenke 1973; Grigalka 1980) have claimed that speed should increase gradually. In reality, the changes have an undulating character. According to the experimental data (Susanka 1974; Susanka & Stepanek 1988; Bartonietz 1994a), the shot reaches a speed of approximately 1.8–2.6 m · s⁻¹ during the initial acceleration in the onset phase (Fig. 21.1).

During the deceleration and right-foot support following the glide, the speed drops and then increases considerably after the left foot contacts the ground. The speed variation of the shot depends on the strength and speed of the shot putter (Marhold 1974), movement of the body's centre of gravity, and the speed and direction of the shot motion (Fidelus & Zienkowicz 1965; Susanka & Stepanek 1988). Measurements of the shot's speed, by means of the stereophotogrammetric method (Lanka & Shalmanov 1982), showed that during the transmission phase, the speed actually does not decrease (in elite shot-putters), and during successful attempts can even increase. The speed decrease during the transmission stage that has been reported by Susanka (1974) and other researchers seems to be connected with the fact that only the shot motion in the vertical plane has been registered. The stereophotogrammetric method enables the determination of all three vector components of the shot's velocity, including the speed acquired by the shot due to upper body turning. As stated earlier, introducing rotational movements in the middle phase of shot putting was one of P. O'Brian's most significant innovations in the shot-put technique during the 1950s. The greatest speed gains coincide with the initiation of movement of the right shoulder and arm during the final putting effort. A shot gains 70–85% of its speed from the shoulder girdle turning and the extension of the right hand (Grigalka 1980). The pattern of shot speed variations found in the glide technique is similar to the pattern when executing a rotational technique (Fig. 21.2).

In highly skilled athletes, speed increases more gradually than in less-skilled competitors (Susanka & Stepanek 1988) and their technique is distinguished by a high speed at the beginning of the final acceleration. In performances exceeding 21 m, this speed must reach 25–27% of the release velocity (Marhold 1974).

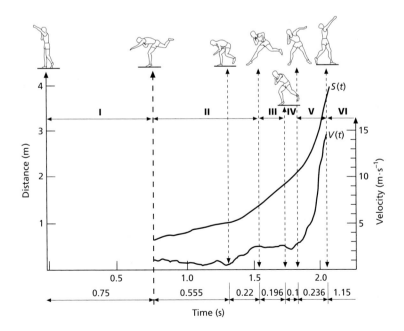

Fig. 21.1 Path length and speed of the shot of elite skilled shot-putters. I, preparatory phase; II, starting phase; III, glide phase; IV, intermediate (transition) phase; V, delivery phase; VI, final phase. J. Brabec (Czechoslovakia), 20.11 m. (Adapted from Susanka 1974.)

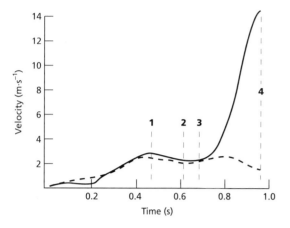

Fig. 21.2 Time-related changes in shot speed. Glide technique, W. Ginter (Switzerland), 22.23 m. 1, Takeoff, right foot; 2, planting right foot; 3, planting left foot; 4, release. (From Susanka & Stepanek 1988.)

Velocity vectors

During the glide and during the final phase, the velocity vectors point in different directions. This lack of collinearity limits the shot's release velocity. The shot's release velocity is equal to the sum of speeds that are gained by the implement during different phases of movement. Because of the different direction of the velocity vectors they need to be summed geometrically according to the parallelogram principle (Fig. 21.3).

Top shot putters can push a shot from a standing position to a distance of 19–20 m, which corresponds to a release velocity of about 13 m · s⁻¹. The shot's speed at the end of the glide is 2.0–2.5 m · s⁻¹. If athletes were able to perform the put in such a way that these speeds could be summed arithmetically (so the speeds' directions coincide), the release velocity of the shot might be 15–15.5 m · s⁻¹. This corresponds to a throw of 25–26 m (Tutevich 1969; Koltai 1973). However, the lack of collinearity of the shot velocities during the glide and delivery phases results in a considerable loss in the initial and final velocities. Losses of up to 60–70% in initial velocity were reported by Koltai (1973) and Kerssenbrock (1974).

What are the possibilities for decreasing these losses of speed? One method is to push the shot

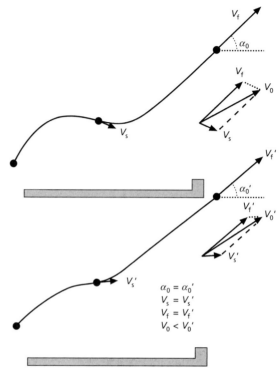

Fig. 21.3 Summarizing start and final speed in shot trajectories of different shapes, a schematic. V_s, shot speed at the end of glide; V_f, speed acquired by shot at the final part of push; V_0, resultant velocity at the moment of release; α_0, angle of release. (From Lanka & Shalmanov 1982.)

at an angle smaller than optimal. However, this is not always sensible because a decreased angle diminishes the flight distance. If the speed increase obtained by straightening the shot's trajectory exceeds the losses due to the decrease of the release angle and release height, this method would be admissible. However, the rationality of this technique has not been proven experimentally.

A second method is to straighten the legs and body more actively at the beginning of the final effort. Such a technique cannot be considered if the athlete already takes a position that is too straight at the beginning of the final acceleration. In this case, the athlete will not be fully able to make use of his/her strength.

A third method is to decrease the height of shot at

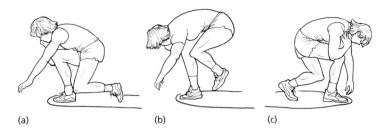

Fig. 21.4 Shot-putter's position during start: (a) I. Slupjanek, (b) S. Kratshevskaja and (c) A. Feuerbach. (From Lanka & Shalmanov 1982.)   (a)   (b)   (c)

the start position. Due to this, the shot trajectory will be straightened in the projection on the vertical plane and thus the loss of speed will be diminished. A majority of top shot putters have used this technique (Delevan 1973; Schpenke 1974; Dessureault 1978). The shot's height from the ground does not exceed 80 cm on average. This can be illustrated by the start position of two former world-record holders, I. Slupjanek (Germany) and A. Feuerbach (USA), and another athlete S. Kratshevskaja (USSR, best performance 21 m) (Fig. 21.4), as well as by the average joint angles of top athletes (Fig. 21.5).

The recommendation to decrease the shot height during the start position is also observed by the majority of the leading shot-putters who apply the

rotational technique. They use a low starting position with bent knees (about 90–120°) and lean their upper body forwards. According to Bartonietz (1994b), this variant offers some advantages: a smooth and controlled starting movement with a wide amplitude; a continuously increasing rise of the centre of gravity (shot and athlete); and a flat movement path during the non-support phase without dropping the upper body onto the right foot.

Top contemporary shot-putters more or less make use of the above-mentioned techniques, resulting in a comparatively straight, low and long trajectory of the shot (Fig. 21.6).

As mentioned before, the trunk rotation during the final part of the push phase may increase the shot's velocity. However, this rotation causes curving of the shot's trajectory in the horizontal plane projection. There is an opinion that a shot-putter should perform the movement so that the projection of the shot trajectory onto the horizontal plane is as straight as possible (Pearson 1966). However, since a shot is not on the central vertical axis of the athlete-plus-shot system, the path of the shot is close to a straight line only in poor shot putting when the shoulders are inclined too far to the left during delivery (Grigalka 1967) (path S in Fig. 21.7).

If deviation of the shot trajectory from a straight line is necessary (which inevitably involves a reduction in release velocity of the shot due to differences in the directions of the initial and final acceleration in a horizontal plane), a question arises: to attain maximum release velocity, is it necessary while turning to attempt to move the shot at the end of a large radius (as in throwing) or a small one? It is clear that employing a larger radius at the same angular velocity will result in a higher linear velocity of the shot than employing a smaller radius.

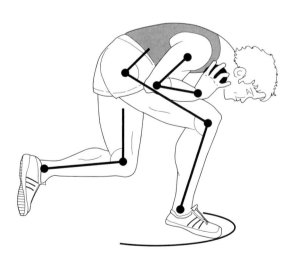

Fig. 21.5 Average values of joint angles during start: knee joint of the right leg 108° ± 11.9°; right hip joint 109° ± 24.8°; knee joint of the left leg 80° ± 10.9°; elbow joint of the right arm 65° ± 7.1°. (From Lanka & Shalmanov 1982.)

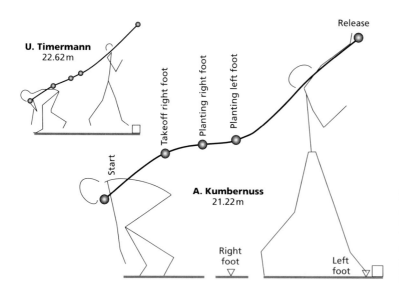

U. Timermann
22.62 m

Release

Start

Takeoff right foot

Planting right foot

Planting left foot

A. Kumbernuss
21.22 m

Right
foot

Left
foot

Fig. 21.6 Trajectory of the shot. A. Kumbernuss (21.22 m) in comparison with an ideal throw by U. Timermann (22.62 m). Inverted triangles indicate the positions of right foot and left foot. (From Bartonietz 1995.)

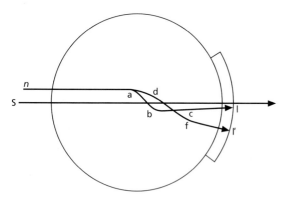

Fig. 21.7 Shot trajectories in the horizontal plane whilst in the athlete's hand, using the glide technique. S indicates a straight-line path found in poor shot-putters when their shoulders are inclined too far to the left during delivery. An *n*-a-b-c-l path is characteristic of successful performances of top athletes, and an *n*-a-d-f-l′ path of unsuccessful attempts or of less-skilled athletes. *n* indicates the position of the shot at the start. (From Grigalka 1974.)

Increasing the shot's movement radius will increase the load on muscles and a higher level of strength training is necessary (Tutevich 1969). However, if the radius of rotation is too large, it may hinder the speed at which the putting arm can be extended.

It seems that some of the problems associated with acceleration of the shot occurring during the delivery might be solved by the rotational tech-nique. Such a technique solves the problem of non-collinearity of the initial and final speed directions and theoretically makes it possible to considerably increase the path of force application during the final part of the movement (Ihring 1982; Bosen 1985) (Fig. 21.8).

During the beginning of the turn and the body-weight shift from the right to the left leg (pre-acceleration of body and shot) the velocity of the shot can reach nearly 4 m · s^{-1} (Kerssenbrock 1974, 1981). It is larger than in the glide technique. However, Kerssenbrock (1974) reported that 65% of the initial speed was lost during the 20.54 m put of A. Barishnikov. According to the data provided by Bartonietz (1983), Palm (1990) and Stepanek (1987, 1990) the shot speed before the delivery phase is between 0.6 and 1.2 m · s^{-1}. That is considerably less than the shot speed during the takeoff phase (at the beginning of body rotation). The losses of the take-off speed are explained firstly by the fact that during the transition stage (between the landing of right and left legs) the shot moves opposite to the push direction. Secondly, the problems are caused by the centripetal forces: the linear velocity has a squared influence on the centripetal force according to the following equation:

$$F = \frac{mv^2}{r}$$

(21.3)

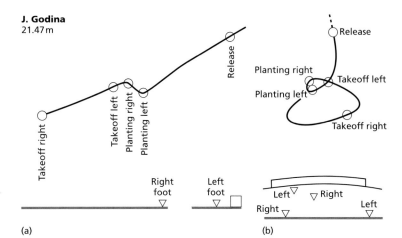

Fig. 21.8 Path of the shot, using the rotation technique, J. Godina (21.47 m). (a) Side view; (b) top view. Inverted triangles indicate the positions of the right and left feet. (From Bartonietz 1995.)

where F = centripetal force component (N); m = shot mass (kg); v = velocity of the shot (m · s^{-1}); and r = radius of the shot movement (m).

Average values of the centripetal force component of the shot can reach 300 N or higher (Bartonietz 1994b). The values of the centripetal force depend on the rotation speed and radius. The implement can move in a wide loop (radius 20 cm or higher) or cramped loop (7–10 cm), or the athlete can turn around the shot ($r = 0$). As a result of great centripetal forces in throws with a wide loop, high initial velocity often causes problems with preserving a proper throwing direction (the shot tends to land outside the right boundary).

Coordination of body segments

The shot's movement (and speed) is the outcome of the movements (and speeds) of several body segments—legs, trunk and arms. Each body segment takes part in two movements: turning around the proximal joint axis and movement together with a joint. The hand and shot velocity equals the vector sum of the velocity of the shoulder joint and the arm. Thus, there arises the following question: how should the individual movements be coordinated to make the speed of the hand and the shot maximal.

Hypothetically, there exist several ways of obtaining maximal velocity of the hand and shot. The first possibility, maximum velocity may be achieved when the speed of all body segments is maximum (Marhold 1964). According to this explanation the speed of the shot consists of two components. The first is the result of extension of the lower extremities and trunk, while the second is produced by the extension of the throwing arm. The question concerns the timing of these two velocities. According to the biomechanical principle of 'particular impulse coordination' (Hochmuth 1974), temporal coincidence of the maximum trunk and maximum arm speeds should lead to an increase in the release velocity. This leads to the following conclusions:
• the release velocity of the shot will be reduced if the maximum speed of the extending arm is added to the submaximal speed of the extending lower extremities, and vice versa; and
• the greater the difference in time between the maximum trunk and lower extremity velocities, the smaller the total velocity of the shot (this speed timing pattern, however, has yet to be confirmed experimentally).

A second possibility is that shot speed is maximal when the body segments are activated in sequence from proximal to distal.

Broer (1960) identified three types of segment interaction depending on the purpose of the movement:
1 if the speed of movement is paramount, the actions of segments are consecutive with each segment starting its action at the moment the proximal segment reaches its maximum speed;
2 if the task requires the development of maximum

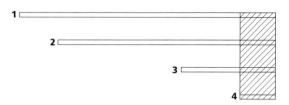

Fig. 21.9 Action of a shot-putter's body segments. Muscle activity associated with (1) lower extremities, (2) hip rotation, (3) trunk, and (4) arms and shoulders up to release is indicated. The hatched area shows the duration of simultaneous activity of all the participating segments. (From Grigalka 1970.)

force, all body segments act simultaneously, and it is not efficient to engage weaker segments; and
3 if one or more segments are engaged in the activity, the lower segments should be fixed, providing a stable base for a more effective performance by the upper segments.

The determination of the best combination of individual segment forces and their pattern of activation becomes even more complicated, as the shot-putter must combine all three types of interaction. First, the putter should provide maximum release speed to the shot. Second, maximum force is necessary to effectively accelerate the shot. And third, the put is completed with one arm. Thus, all three types

of interaction should be combined to best utilize the 'explosive power capacity' of the athlete during the 0.2–0.4 s available for the final application of force.

Grigalka (1970) presented a diagram which, from his point of view, reflects an optimal combination of the segments in a shot put (Fig. 21.9). Each segment is brought into action at a different time, but the cessation of their movements should be simultaneous and occur as close as possible to the moment the shot is released.

Our investigation (Lanka 1978) using goniometers to measure changes in joint angles of 50 putters of various skill levels has suggested two different patterns of segmental interaction during final acceleration of the shot:
1 after the initiation of the right knee extension, the angle of the right hip starts to change followed by the extension of the left knee and the elbow of the throwing arm; and
2 extension of the left knee precedes that of the right hip while the sequence of the other segments remains unchanged (Fig. 21.10).

Contrary to Grigalka's diagram, we have not found any cases in which the body segments ceased their motion simultaneously.

The theoretically ideal variations of body segment interactions that are offered by Marhold, Dyson and Grigalka probably are rational from a mechanical

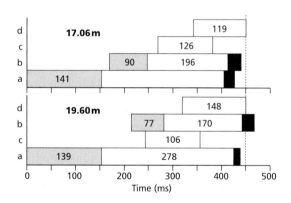

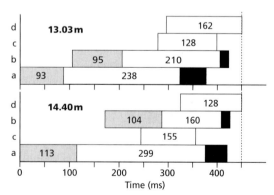

Fig. 21.10 Duration of action (milliseconds) of the main segments, and the sequence in which they are engaged during delivery of the shot. Data of putters of different skill levels are shown. The broken vertical line indicates the instant of release; the grey shading, the time from landing to the beginning of extension of the lower extremity; the clear portion, the period during which the segment is active; and the black shading, the period from the moment of maximum extension of the lower extremity until the foot leaves the ground. (a) Right foot; (b) left foot; (c) right hip; (d) right hand. (From Lanka & Shalmanov 1982.)

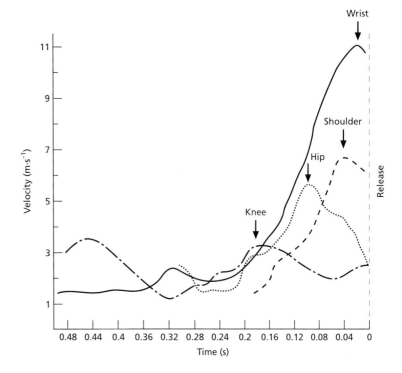

Fig. 21.11 Resultant speed of main joints (right side of the body) in shot-putting obtained by the stereophotogrammetric technique. Arrows indicate the maximum joint speeds and show that deceleration begins at the knee and proceeds progressively upwards to the hip, shoulder and wrist. (From Lanka & Shalmanov 1982.)

point of view; however, they might not be the best from a biomechanical point of view. There are many properties of the system and the muscles that must be taken into consideration. First of all the segments have different masses, and the muscles that move these segments generate different maximal forces. The time to reach maximal force also varies, and the fact that muscular force depends on movement velocity is also very important. Due to the complexity of the task, the most efficient pattern of body segment interaction cannot be determined on the basis of simple mechanical rules.

In conformity with the experimental data of many researchers, athletes executing the movements of striking, throwing a ball, discus or javelin, and putting the shot attain a maximal speed when the body segments are activated sequentially, from proximal to distal (Zatsiorsky 1997).

According to Tutevich (1969), the process of accelerating the shot is as follows. During the first period (initial and glide phases in conventional technique and turn on–take off phases in rotation technique), the whole athlete-plus-shot system gains speed.

During the second period (first half of final force application), acceleration of the shot is achieved both by contraction of the trunk muscles and through a transfer of momentum to the upper body by deceleration of the translation and rotation movement of the lower body. In the third period (which begins with the contraction of muscles of the throwing arm) the forces are directed towards accelerating the shot. The release velocity of the shot is maximal if, after the preliminary acceleration of the athlete-plus-shot system, there is a gradual upward deceleration of all body segments. At the moment the shot is released, the speed of the lower extremities, hips and trunk should be close to zero.

As a rule, investigators who experimentally study the timing of body segments in throwing movements irrespective of the type of throwing, note consecutive acceleration and deceleration of the main body segments. Our investigation (Lanka 1978, 1996) of shot putting (glide technique) using stereophotography confirmed the rationality of the consecutive upward acceleration and deceleration of the body segments (Fig. 21.11). By improving the skill of shot-putters,

Table 21.1 Speed (m · s⁻¹) of the body segments of variously skilled shot-putters.

Registered indices	Performance results in shot put (m)			
	19.60	18.30	13.30	12.26
Maximum speed of hip joint	5.74	5.13	4.28	4.81
Speed of hip joint in release	2.75	1.05	0.83	1.96
Maximum speed of shoulder joint	6.77	7.66	4.91	5.32
Speed of shoulder joint in release	6.34	5.46	3.10	4.82
Maximum speed of wrist joint	11.00	10.64	8.02	7.95
Speed of wrist joint in release	10.90	9.25	7.51	7.85
Release velocity of the shot	13.12	12.51	10.49	10.12

Table 21.2 Centre of gravity displacement of the athlete-plus-shot system during delivery in shot-putting attempts by Randy Matson. (From Ariel 1973b.)

Distance of put (m)	Duration of delivery phase (s)	Horizontal displacement (m)	Vertical displacement (m)
19.83	0.22	0.39	0.14
21.35	0.22	0.52	0.27

the maximum speed values of body segments increase, beginning with the right hip joint and finishing with the right hand (Table 21.1).

When speaking about the effectiveness of body segment deceleration, it is necessary to point out that the process of deceleration takes place most intensively in the hip joint. However, a swift hip joint deceleration has to be coordinated with the body continuously moving along a circle in the shot flight direction. This means a hip joint speed may not decrease to zero. A comparative analysis of 21.35 m and 19.83 m throws by the former world-record holder, R. Matson (USA), showed that horizontal and vertical displacement of the centre of gravity continued through release in the better throw (Ariel 1973b), whereas in the other attempt, horizontal displacement was smaller and maximal elevation of the centre of gravity was achieved after release of the shot (Table 21.2).

The effectiveness of consecutive deceleration of the body segments depends greatly on proper timing. If one of the segments reaches the maximum speed in relation to another too early or too late, the performance diminishes (Fig. 21.12). There exists an

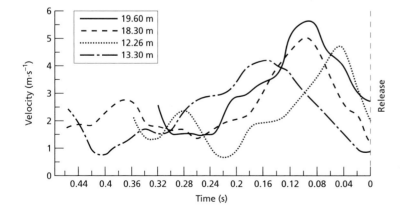

Fig. 21.12 The hip joint speed of differently skilled shot-putters. (From Lanka & Shalmanov 1982.)

Table 21.3 Time characteristics of the body segments in the final part of a put (values in milliseconds).

Time from the instant of maximal speed of a segment to the instant of release	High-skilled athletes		Low-skilled athletes	
	$\bar{X}$	σ	$\bar{X}$	σ
Right knee joint	179.2	14.3	141.6	87.3
Right hip joint	93.7	17.2	98.9	81.6
Right shoulder joint	59.3	11.6	67.1	26.2
Right wrist joint	24.4	20.2	29.3	8.9

$\bar{X}$, mean value; σ, standard deviation.

optimal timing of segment actions that maximizes shot release velocity (Table 21.3).

The main conclusion from the data presented is that the technique of skilled shot-putters is characterized by a greater and more precise segment interaction than that of less-skilled athletes. This conclusion is proved by comparing the standard deviation values for high-skilled athletes (14.3 ms and 17.2 ms, right knee and hip joint) and for low-skilled athletes (87.3 ms and 81.6 ms).

Kinetics of shot putting

The body's change in velocity is caused by the forces acting on it. The measures of a force's action are work of a force (product of the force and distance through which it is applied) and impulse of force (integral of the force over time).

Work and energy

The total mechanical energy of a shot equals the sum of its kinetic and potential energies. It is also equivalent to the mechanical work performed by a shot putter to accelerate and elevate the shot. Thus:

$$W = mgh_0 + \frac{mv_0^2}{2} + \frac{I\omega_0^2}{2} \qquad (21.4)$$

where: W is work; m is the projectile mass; h_0 is its height; and v_0 and ω_0 are linear and angular velocity, respectively. The last term in Eqn. 21.4 (kinetic rotational energy of the shot) is small and usually is neglected. Hence, the release velocity of the shot

and its height at the instant of release represent the energy the implement receives from the thrower.

Samotsvetov (1961) found that in an 18.19 m put the work was 732 Nm, 80% of which was spent in accelerating the shot and 20% in elevating it. Short duration of the delivery phase (around 0.2 s) coupled with the large amount of work performed within this short time results in high power production. The athlete performing the put described would have developed power of 5.08 kW (6.9 hp). According to Bartonietz (1996), in throws that are further than 21 m the measures are much greater: 6.2 kW (21.31 m) and 6.7 kW (21.56 m).

Force applied to the shot

Direct measurement of the force applied to the shot is rather difficult. Investigators have assessed this force by multiplying the mass of the shot by its calculated acceleration for those parts of the path that are assumed to be linear. Only the tangential component of the acceleration was measured, as the radial component was considered to be equal to zero.

Lebedev (1969) analysed the characteristics of a shot acceleration–time history during the final application of force. The slope of the first part of this curve was small, but it increased dramatically in the second part of the final force application. The author indicated two periods during which acceleration decreased. The first began in the middle of the final force application phase as arm extension was initiated. The second occurred just before the shot was released. The acceleration curve from a beginner

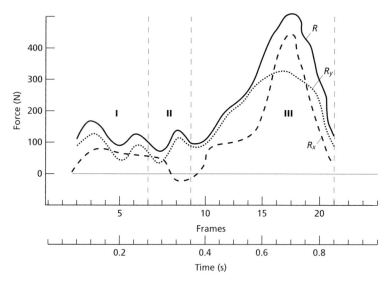

Fig. 21.13 Force applied to the shot. The solid line is the resultant force, and the dashed (R_x) and dotted (R_y) lines are its horizontal and vertical components, respectively. I, II and III indicate preparatory, glide and delivery phases, respectively. (From Fidelus & Zienkowicz 1965.)

was wavy, its slope was less steep, and its duration was longer than that of a skilled putter. The force was applied in a jerky manner such that the movement seemed to be divided into parts separated in time from one another.

In the put analysed in Fig. 21.13 (Fidelus & Zienkowicz 1965), the force had dropped almost to zero at the end of the glide and increased abruptly after left foot contact (frames 10–17). Maximum delivery force was 465 N, while the maximum vertical and horizontal force components were 298 N and 381 N, respectively.

Investigators have pointed out that the vertical and horizontal curves were also of an undulating nature. Horizontal acceleration dropped at the beginning of the glide and increased at the end due to some trunk extension, with a sharp increase observed at left-foot contact. Maximal acceleration was developed before the completion of throwing-arm extension. Vertical acceleration became negative at the end of the glide. The second decrease was observed at the moment of left-foot contact and during the deceleration phase.

Similar data were reported by Machabeli (1969), who used an instrumented shot to register horizontal (radial and tangential) and vertical acceleration. He reported considerable fluctuations in acceleration in all directions. The radial and the tangential components of acceleration were close to zero just

after right-foot takeoff was completed. They gradually increased with right-foot contact, and at the end of push reached 5.8 g for the radial and 7.8 g for the tangential component ($1 \text{ g} = 9.82 \text{ m} \cdot \text{s}^{-2}$). Vertical acceleration fluctuated from 0 to 1 g and increased sharply during delivery phase, reaching values of 5.4 g.

In the theoretical force–time curve of shot putting proposed by Kristev *et al.* (1973) (Fig. 21.14), the first

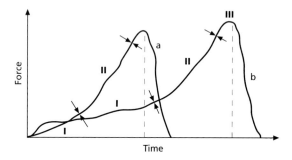

Fig. 21.14 Theoretical patterns of force application against a shot in a performance without a glide (curve a) and with a glide (curve b). The broken vertical line denotes maximum force. During stage I, the 'glide' (arrows show the margins of stage), the force is moderate. Force increases during stage II, which includes double support and the beginning of support on the left foot. During stage III, in which support is on the left foot alone, the force increases to maximum and than rapidly drops to zero corresponding with release. (From Kristev *et al.* 1973.)

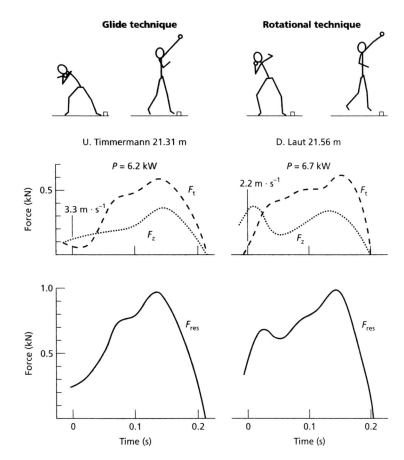

Fig. 21.15 Time-related changes of the force acting on the shot (left leg planting to release) and biomechanical parameters of the two techniques: t_0 = planting the left foot; F_t = tangential component; F_z = centripetal component; F_{res} = resultant force; P = maximum power. (From Bartonietz 1990.)

phase was the longest and was characterized by moderate forces. In the second phase, encompassing double support and single support on the left foot, the most powerful muscle groups were employed. In the third and final phase, which was the shortest of the movement, the putter was supported by only one foot. The world's top shot-putters have a similar pattern of force–time history (Fig. 21.15).

When the rotational technique is used to attain a comparable release velocity a higher acceleration must be produced because of a lower implement speed at the instant of right leg placement, and a shorter acceleration path.

The release velocity (or energy) of the shot does not depend merely on the magnitude of force, but also on the way in which the force acts. A technique is better when an athlete can apply the force along a longer path (Dyson 1968). But increasing the length of the force application path is sensible only when the shot passes this way in a minimal period of time. Thus, it is more correct to speak about an optimal path of shot acceleration rather than a maximally long path (Nett 1969). It is especially important to increase the path of force application in the final part of the shot put (Tutevich 1969). Here we might observe the advantages of tall, long-armed athletes, whose path of final acceleration can be as long as 2 m (Grigalka 1970). According to the data of Schpenke (1973), the best shot-putters typically have an acceleration path of 1.8 m. The minimum that every shot-putter has to try to attain is around 1.6 m.

The release velocity of the shot is higher when the acceleration path is long but the time taken by the shot to travel along this path is short. This is illustrated in Table 21.4. The table shows that the

Table 21.4 Several biomechanical variables and performance results of top shot-putters.

Shot-putter	Distance (m)	Time of delivery (s)	Final acceleration path (m)	Release height (m)	Release angle	Author
Briesenik, H.	21.54	0.20	1.70	2.27	40°	Schpenke (1973)
Timmermann, U.	21.31	0.22	1.65			Bartonietz (1996)
Gies, H. P.	21.07	0.25	1.78			Schpenke (1973)
Briesenik, H.	20.09	0.18	1.55	2.25	39°	Schpenke (1973)
Matson, R.	20.27	0.26	1.70	2.25	42°	Kutiev (1966)
MacGrath, D.	19.08	0.26	1.50	2.20	42°	Kutiev (1966)
Lipsnis, V.	19.00	0.28	1.55	2.25	42°	Kutiev (1966)
Karasev, N.	18.98	0.27	1.48	2.06	39°	Kutiev (1966)

distance achieved is greater in those puts where the athlete has managed to move the shot in a long path, but also in a short time. Kristev (1971) studied the change of path travelled by the shot during separate phases of the final part of a throw. The most relevant changes associated with improving skill take place in the double-support phase (which starts with planting of the left foot) and the non-support phase (losing contact with the ground just before implement release). The shot's path in the double-support phase increased from 36 cm for weaker shot-putters to 92 cm for stronger ones.

Enhancement of release velocity

Several mechanisms ensure maximal release speed of the shot.

'Whip technique'

Rotation of a distal segment is determined by: (i) the moment of force acting at the proximal joint; and (ii) accelerated movement of the joint itself. When the joint's axis accelerates the segment will turn around this axis. Both mechanisms are widely applied in throwing and striking movements. Coordinated translatory movement of the proximal joint that involves consecutive acceleration and deceleration of the joint is sometimes called 'whip technique'. At the beginning of the movement the proximal joint(s) moves quickly in the direction of the throw, but afterwards it is actively decelerated. This movement pattern evokes a quick rotation of the distal segment.

When a linear motion of a rigid object is constrained at one end, the result is a forward rotation. The other end of the object continues to move ahead and rotation begins, and consequently the velocity of the end can increase. When a shot-putter plants the left foot prior to releasing the shot, the upper body and arm (and, of course, the shot) increase their speed, aiding in increasing the shot's release speed. The axis of rotation passes through the point where the foot meets the ground. For instance, it has been proven that in high jump and long jump (Shalmanov 1986) this inverted pendulum mechanism contributes considerably to the speed of the body's centre of mass. Though this mechanism has not been addressed in scientific research in shot putting, one might suppose that at a high speed of the body and with energetic braking activity of the left leg during the final phase, its contribution could be vital.

In the event that external forces do not act on the system, the velocity of the system's centre of mass has to be constant; internal forces cannot change its movement. However, in the system itself it is possible to redistribute momentum (momentum is the product of the velocity of the body's mass centre and the body's mass). Hence, by means of internal forces is it possible to decrease the velocity of some body parts by decelerating other parts of the system. In shot putting, of course, this principle does not act alone because the shot-putter is affected by external forces (ground reaction), and the momentum of the athlete-plus-shot system is not constant. Still, the described mechanism may contribute to the increase of the hand and shot speed. Immediately before and at the beginning of the right arm extension, the consecutive deceleration of the body segments in an upward direction takes place (Ariel 1973a). It results in increased speed of the upper body as well as the hand and the shot. In other words, there is redistribution of momentum between body segments.

Reversible muscle action

The second mechanism ensuring the increase of the shot speed is a consecutive stretching and shortening of the muscles and tendons involved in the performance (Tschiene 1974). Similar to the momentum redistribution in the system, the contribution of this mechanism depends on a properly coordinated acceleration and deceleration of the body segments.

It is well known that if a muscle shortens immediately after a stretch, force and power outputs increase. Active muscles are typically prestretched to enhance force (power, velocity) output of movements. This type of activity is called the *stretch–shortening cycle* or *reversible muscle action* (Zatsiorsky 1995). Muscle and tendon elasticity, spinal reflexes and other mechanisms play a substantial role in enhancing the motor output (see Chapter 5). In

throwing, the prestretching of muscles is achieved through a windup movement and other mechanisms.

In shot putting, in addition to the stretching and shortening of the leg muscles, two other mechanisms are important: stretching of the muscles, tendons and ligaments of the shoulder girdle, and reversible muscle action of the wrist. The forceful movement of the left shoulder backwards immediately before the right arm extension, as well as an accelerated movement of the chest forwards and upwards before and at the early beginning of the delivery phase, induce stretching of the shoulder girdle. As a result, during the delivery phase the shot velocity increases. Since the movement is highly complex and executed in a very brief time, even some elite athletes fail to perform reversed muscle action correctly (Fig. 21.16).

The contribution of the wrist muscles and tendons to the shot-put performance is substantial. The difference between the maximum speed of the wrist joint and the shot release speed for the top shot-putters is about 2 m · s⁻¹. Such an increase of speed extends the flight distance by almost 5 m. The wrist and finger flexors by themselves are not strong and powerful enough to achieve such performance gains. However, if the wrist and fingers are first forcefully extended and then are permitted to flex

Distance: 21.41 m

Distance: 19.32 m

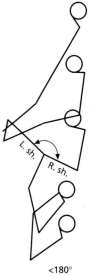

Fig. 21.16 Stick figure showing two attempts in shot putting with different results. L. sh. and R. Sh. are the left and right shoulders. In the successful attempt, the athlete managed to stretch the muscles of the shoulder girdle prior to delivery, while in the less successful attempt, this element of technique was not properly executed. (From Bartonietz 1990.)

The anterior angle between the left and right shoulder

>180°

<180°

the speed and power increases (the reader is invited to perform this simple experiment on him/herself). When the reversible muscle action is used, the elastic forces (and quite possibly other mechanisms as well) contribute to the force and power enhancement. When executing the shot delivery correctly, the contribution of the elastic forces is considerably greater than the force that can be created by the wrist muscles alone without a prestretch (Gonsales 1985).

Legwork

This section addresses two questions: (i) coordination of the instant of the shot release with the legwork; and (ii) optimal foot placement during delivery phase. Other aspects of legwork will be discussed in the subsequent section devoted to the ground reaction forces.

Shot release when an athlete is in the air

The question of whether the athlete should be in contact with the ground at the moment of shot release has been debated in the literature for decades. Some authors (Marhold, 1964; Tutevich, 1969; Shalmanov, 1977) strictly oppose an early takeoff because the largest force can be imparted onto the shot when the athlete is in contact with the support. Others (Nett, 1962) permit taking off from the support before the release. Certainly, untimely taking off from the support can decrease the shot's release velocity. However, compensation of the loss might be possible by lengthening the force application path and increasing the release height. It has been reported (Marhold 1964) that an untimely loss of contact with a support decreased the release velocity by 0.3 m · s^{-1}. That reduced the distance thrown by approximately 40 cm, while the gain from other factors was only 10–15 cm (the performance result was 16.42 m). Thus, release of the shot after contact with the support is lost is detrimental: the losses are greater than the possible gains.

Why does the shot-putter finish the put on a non-support position? One view centres on the discrepancy between the arm force and the force of the legs and body. As a result of powerful leg extension and body straightening, the shot-putter loses contact with the ground at the beginning of the arm extension. It is often observed that after release there is a jump of about 10–20 cm. In the rotational technique the jump is higher than in the glide technique (Bartonietz 1994a). However, the height of the jump does not affect the shot flight distance (Tutevich 1969).

In recent years, many top shot-putters have paid special attention to increasing the strength of the right arm. The underlying idea was to decrease the time between the moment of extending the left foot and right arm, with the intention of decreasing the duration of the non-support phase.

The duration of the non-support phase decreases with increased skill. For some low-skilled athletes it reaches 100 ms, whereas for highly skilled athletes it is close to zero (Lanka 1978; Shalmanov 1977). In the world's best athletes, the shot is released just before the left foot has left the ground (Questions to Vanegers, 1987).

Feet placement

In practice, one more variation of technique to lengthen the acceleration path of the shot is used, namely a wide stance during the final part of the put. Most authors (e.g. Tutevich 1955; Bresnahan *et al.* 1960; Kristev 1971) have recommended that the right foot be placed in the centre of the circle and the left foot near the stopboard. According to this recommendation, the distance between the feet should not exceed 1 m. These authors assumed that such a foot position would provide greater opportunity to apply lower-extremity force because of a longer knee extension period. A too narrow foot position would have the disadvantage of loss of balance during the delivery and would shorten the path of the shot.

Many top shot-putters, however, have begun to use a wider stance, including: Timmermann, Germany (22.62 m), 1.30 m; Briesenick, Germany (22.45 m), 1.45 m; Lissovskaja, Russia (22.63 m), 1.30 m; and Kumbernuss, Germany (21.22 m), 1.17 m. According to Bartonietz (1994a), the average percentage ratio for the length of the glide/stance width is 44 : 56 (glide technique). Hence, the tech-

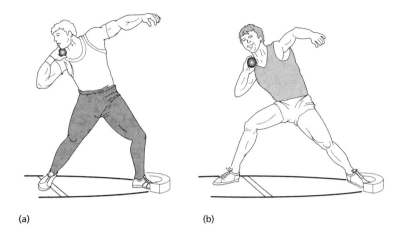

Fig. 21.17 Variations of feet placement (a, short stance; b, wide stance) in the final part of push, illustrated by the former world-record holders U. Bayer and I. Slupjanek. (From Lanka & Shalmanov 1982.)

(a)   (b)

nique is characterized by a so-called 'short–long rhythm', which has both advantages and disadvantages (Fig. 21.17).

While the 'short–long rhythm' technique reduces the amount of force that can be applied with the right leg (Tschiene 1973), it lengthens the path over which the force is applied to the shot (Schpenke 1973), improves conditions for the braking function of the left leg, and stabilizes the body (Bartonietz 1983, 1995). Analysis has shown that the advantages of increasing the path of force application outweigh the loss from incomplete use of the strength of the right leg (Schpenke 1973).

During delivery from a wide foot position, the direction of acceleration of the right lower extremity coincides to a greater degree with the direction of the shot release than in a shot put from a short stance. This convergence considerably increases the efficiency of right limb usage and helps in accelerating the shot along a straight path. In support of this view, Schpenke (1973, 1974) claimed that shot acceleration in an optimal direction and through the longest and straightest path is possible only if all the joints of the lower extremity, trunk and throwing arm extend gradually from initial position to the instant of release of the shot (knee and hip joint angles increase by 15–20° from phase to phase). Thus, most shot-putters and investigators have revised the idea, popular in the 1940s and 1950s, that the final force applied by the lower extremity should be directed upwards while that of throwing

segments should be directed forwards (i.e. 'legs put upwards, arm forwards').

Users of the rotational technique demonstrate a shorter stance width: for example, Oldfield (21.00 m), 0.90 m; Laut (21.56 m), 0.90 m; Barnes (22.00 m), 0.70 m; and Halvari (20.93), 0.73 m. It is important to note that on the one hand a narrow position of the feet helps to decrease the body's moment of inertia during body rotation. On the other hand, a wide feet position lengthens the final acceleration path and allows for better braking with the left leg. Unlike in the glide technique, the wide feet placement in the rotational technique makes it harder for the leg to work during the delivery.

The left foot contacts the ground 0.15–0.20 m (Ward 1970) or 0.20–0.35 m (Lanka 1996) to the left of the right foot. The distance depends on the delivery technique. If emphasis is placed on rotation during the delivery, the foot is shifted more to the left.

One of the shot-putter's major tasks at the beginning of final force application is to give additional acceleration to the athlete-plus-shot system in the direction of the put without losing horizontal velocity. The problem arises of when should the left foot contact the ground (time of the intermediate or transition phase), and what action the left foot should take after the right foot contacts the ground. Authorities are divided over what should be the duration of this phase. Some (Tutevich 1969; Kristev 1971; Turk 1997) assume that it should be as short as possible. In other words, they believe that it is most effective to land on both feet almost simultaneously, thereby reducing, as much as possible, this phase, which does not contribute to acceleration of the shot. Others (Simonyi 1973; Zatsiorsky *et al.* 1978; Grigalka 1980; Lanka & Shalmanov 1982) claim that a certain time interval between contact of the two feet is necessary to maintain continuity in the acceleration of the shot and thus to avoid a considerable decrease in the horizontal velocity of the athlete-plus-shot system, which might develop as a result of the braking action of the left foot.

The solution to the problem of the duration of the initial phase of the delivery is related to the roles of the left and right legs in the final acceleration of the athlete-plus-shot system. In contrast to the previously popular shot-putting technique theories, in which the right foot played the major role in accelerating the putter and the shot, many authorities now believe that the acceleration of the shot, especially its horizontal component, depends more on the action of the left leg than on the action of the right leg (e.g. Fidelus & Zienkowicz 1965; Marhold 1970; Ariel 1973a; Simonyi 1973; Vanegas 1987; Ionesku 1992).

Ground reaction forces

Force platforms are used to measure the magnitude and direction of the ground reaction forces, which are equal in magnitude and opposite in direction to those applied to the ground by the athlete.

Initial phase

The athletes action on the support during the initial phase is of interest, because the system's centre of gravity movement depends on the magnitude, direction and duration of the ground reaction forces.

The vertical and horizontal components of the ground reaction force applied against the right foot during the initial phase are characterized by a gradual increase to a maximum value followed by a sharp decrease to zero (Fig. 21.18). A more gradual increase with a sharp drop in force is typical for the top shot-putters. For the less skilled, the force curve undulates, reflecting the lack of synchronization between the actions of the left and right lower extremities.

We found (Lanka 1978) a low correlation between the duration of the right-foot force application during the initial phase before the glide, and the distance of the put. In other words, a somewhat slower initial acceleration was typical of the highly skilled putters, whereas a rapid increase in the vertical and horizontal components negatively affected the subsequent actions of the shot-putter. The magnitude of the vertical force component was twice the athlete's weight.

According to our data, the peak horizontal force reached 647 ± 240 N and correlated positively with performance. Similar conclusions were made by Marhold (1970), who found that improved perform-

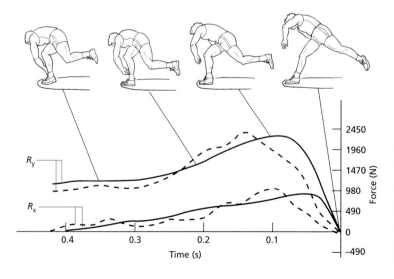

Fig. 21.18 Horizontal (R_x) and vertical (R_y) ground reaction force components exerted against the right foot during the initial phase of the shot put. The solid line is the performance of a top athlete (19.60 m) and the broken line that of a poorly skilled putter (13.50 m). (From Lanka & Shalmanov 1982.)

ance was associated with a decrease in the angle between the resultant force vector and the horizontal. The greater the angle, the greater the force during the initial upward acceleration and the higher the glide. This type of initial phase is not effective and is characteristic of beginners.

Final acceleration

Records of the vertical and horizontal ground reaction components exerted against the right foot show rather complex, undulating curves with different duration and magnitude in athletes of varying skill levels (Fig. 21.19) (Zatsiorsky *et al.* 1981). The vertical component of force has two major peaks, followed by a gradual decrease in magnitude until the foot leaves the ground. Near the beginning of foot contact with the ground, the vertical force is very high; in some athletes it was three to four times body weight.

The size of the first peak is directly related to the technique of the glide and subsequent movement of the right foot. Highly skilled shot-putters are characterized by a rapid and forceful contact of the right foot with the ground, which influences the way in which the vertical force changes. The initial slope of the force–time curve is steeper in skilled athletes than in non-skilled athletes. This leads to the conclusion that the rate of increase in the vertical force reflects the athlete's skill level to a greater degree than does the maximum force exerted.

Poorly skilled shot-putters can be divided in two groups according to the way in which the right foot contacts the ground. One group contact the ground after a high glide, and as a result their maximum vertical force is very high. Another group is characterized by a soft right-foot contact followed by a rapid weight shift to the left foot.

After the first peak the vertical force decreases to a relative minimum and then begins to increase again. With improvement in skill, the magnitude of the relative minimum increases and the magnitude of the second peak increases, exceeding the athlete's body weight by 65–75%. The second peak coincides approximately with the beginning of the right knee extension, in agreement with Payne *et al.* (1968). The horizontal ground reaction component (in the line of the put) against the right foot changes direction

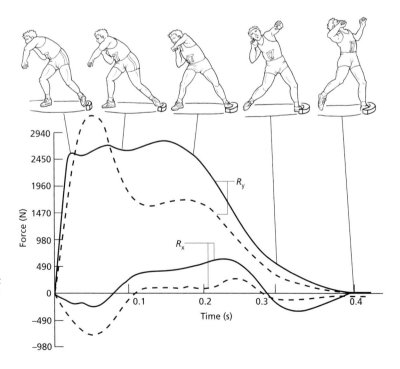

Fig. 21.19 Horizontal (R_x) and vertical (R_y) ground reaction force components exerted against the right foot during delivery. The solid line is from a 19.60 m put by a top athlete, while the broken line is a 13.50 m put of a less-skilled performer. (From Lanka & Shalmanov 1982.)

three times. As the right foot contacts the ground following the glide, the reaction force is towards the rear of the circle (shown as a negative deflection). Then its direction changes (i.e. towards the front of the circle), facilitating movement in the direction of the put. Finally, just before the right foot leaves the ground, this component again reverses direction.

The maximum value and the duration of the initial (backward-directed) portion of the horizontal ground reaction force history, corresponding with right foot contact, decreases with improvement in skill. In some athletes this force reaches 700–800 N (mean values 436 ± 146 N), resulting in a considerable decrease in horizontal velocity. Since backward horizontal ground reaction force hinders movement of the athlete across the circle, it is not efficient.

Positive horizontal ground reaction force exerted against the right foot acts in the direction of the put and accelerates the shot-putter across the circle. The maximal value of the force increases with an improvement in skill and reaches 500–600 N in top shot-putters ($r = 0.60$; $n = 50$). This force correlates negatively ($r = 0.50$; $n = 50$) with the maximum backward-directed force previously mentioned. In

some athletes, this so-called 'blocking' force reaches 700–800 N, resulting in a considerable decrease of horizontal velocity. Thus, athletes whose velocity is less hindered after the glide develop higher forces, favouring acceleration of the whole system.

At the completion of extension of the lower extremity, approximately 70–80 ms before the right foot leaves the ground and when the vertical force is still 400–600 N, the horizontal force becomes negative and reaches 200–300 N in top shot-putters. A positive correlation is found between this force and the distance of the put. The force develops as a result of sliding the right foot across the ground from the centre of the circle towards the stopboard. It is caused by the athlete's attempt to maintain contact with the ground while moving forwards and to decelerate the movement of the lower extremities across the circle.

The vertical and horizontal components of force produced by the left foot pushing against the ground also form rather complex curves (Fig. 21.20). In all athletes, the horizontal component acts sideways in relation to the direction of the put and also decelerates the forward movement of the athlete. In other

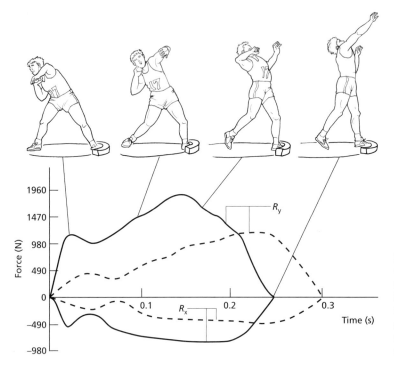

Fig. 21.20 Horizontal (R_x) and vertical (R_y) ground reaction components exerted against the left foot during delivery. The solid line is from a 19.60 m put by a top athlete and the broken line is a 13.50 m put of a less-skilled performer. (From Lanka & Shalmanov 1982.)

words, throughout the final application of force, the left foot hinders forward movement and assists in elevating the centre of mass of the system. Top athletes are characterized by high forces and steep slopes in vertical and horizontal force curves, as well as by small decreases in force during the amortisation phase (bending of the left knee after landing). A positive correlation is found between horizontal force and distance of the put. The negative force impulse ('blocking' impulse) created by the left leg is greater than for the right leg; to brake and heave up is a harder job for left leg (Simonyi 1973; Payne, 1974; Lanka & Shalmanov 1982; Ionesku 1992).

With improvement in skill, the right leg produces maximum force, while the negative force exerted by the left leg decreases. This means that the effectiveness of the right leg is determined by the activity of the left leg. Otherwise, it could turn out that when the right leg accelerates the system in a direction of shot put, the left leg decelerates it and the maximum horizontal positive force produced by the right leg could coincide in time with the maximum horizontal negative force produced by the left leg. The movement towards the direction of shot release is being retarded and a shot put by means of a glide (run-up) would actually turn into a shot put from a standing position. Thus, it is important to determine when the left leg has to be positioned on the ground, in what way it has to be positioned (actively, passively, with a forward-downward or downward 'pawing' movement, with soft or hard contact) and what its activity should be after planting. It might be sup-

posed that there exists a unique duration of the transmission phase for each athlete and an optimal coordination pattern for the activity of the right and left leg.

Experiments on the ground reaction forces during the delivery phase in the rotational and glide technique (Bartonietz 1994b; Palm 1990) revealed similar patterns. These data showed that the rotational technique is characterized by a higher vertical component of the ground reaction forces and a steeper rise in the forces.

Experimental results show that top athletes have a common pattern of interaction between the feet and the ground. The task of the right leg at the beginning of the delivery is to accelerate the athlete-plus-shot system in the direction of the put. Later, the acceleration provided by the right foot decreases and the horizontal ground reaction force component is directed towards the rear of the circle, retarding the movement of the athlete across the circle. The retarding action of the right foot coincides in time with the beginning of force application against the ground by the left foot. As the action of the left foot is of a decelerative nature, the lower body segments are decelerated even more.

Thus, during the final acceleration phase, the right foot has a two-fold task. First, it accelerates the athlete-plus-shot system and then, together with the left foot, it decelerates the movement of the lower extremities of the athlete, thereby increasing the speed of the upper body and increasing the velocity of the shot.

References

Ariel, G. (1973a) Computerized biomechanical analysis of the world's best shot-putters. *Track and Field Quarterly Review* **73**, 199–206.

Ariel, G. (1973b) Biomechanical analysis of the shotput technique utilizing the center of gravity displacement. *Track and Field Quarterly Review* **73**, 207–210.

Bartonietz, K. (1983) Zur Bewegungsstruktur der Drehtechnik im Kugelstoßen. *Theorie Praxis Leistungssport Berlin* **21** (10), 77–92.

Bartonietz, K. (1990) Drehtechnik kontra Angleittechnik? Erfahrungen, Erkenntnisse und Hypothesen zur Kugelstoß-Drehtechnik, veranschaulicht an einem

22-m-stoß von Randy Barnes. *Lehre der Leichtathletik, Berlin* **29** (19), 15–18, (20), 22.

Bartonietz, K. (1994a) Rotational shot put technique: Biomechanical findings and recommendations for training. *Track and Field Quarterly Review* **93** (3), 18–19.

Bartonietz, K. (1994b) The energy relationship in rotational and glide shot put techniques. *Modern Athlete and Coach* **32** (2), 7–10.

Bartonietz, K. (1995) The throwing events at the World Championships in Athletics 1995, Göteborg—Technique of the world's best athletes. Part 1: shot put

and hammer throw. *New Studies in Athletics* **10** (4), 43–63.

Bartonietz, K. (1996) Biomechanical aspects of the performance structure in throwing events. *Modern Athlete and Coach, Adelaide* **34** (2), 7–11.

Bosen, K. (1985) A comparative study between the conventional and rotational techniques of shot put. *Track and Field Quarterly Review, Kalamazoo* **85** (1), 7–11.

Bresnahan, G.T., Tuttle, W.W. & Cretzmeyer, F.X. (1960) *Track and Field Athletics*, 5th edn. C.V. Mosby, St. Louis.

Broer, M.R. (1960) *Efficiency of Human Movement*. W.B. Saunders, Philadelphia.

Delevan, P. (1973) Techniques of putting the shot. *Track and Field Quarterly Review* **73**, 211–213.

Dessureault, J. (1978) Étude des facteurs cinétiques et cinématiques au lancer du poids. In: *Biomechanics of Sports and Kinanthropometry* (eds F. Landry & W.A.R. Orban) pp. 91–101. Symposia Specialists, Miami.

Dyson, G.H.G. (1968) *The Mechanics of Athletics*, 4th edn. University of London Press, London.

Fidelus, K. & Zienkowicz, W. (1965) Sila I predkosc rozwijane podczas pchniecia kula. *Kultura Fizyczna (Warszawa)* **18** (2), 83–95.

Gonsaless, K.X.K. (1985) Biodynamics of palm functioning at maximum speed-strength performance. PhD dissertation, Central Institute of Physical Culture, Moscow.

Grigalka, O. (1967) The basis of modern shot putting technique (Russian). *Track and Field Events* **6**, 6–7.

Grigalka, O. (1970) Shot putting (Russian). Fizkultura i Sport, Moscow.

Grigalka, O. (1974) Shot putting and discus throwing (Russian). In: *Textbook for Track and Field Coaches*, pp. 423–447. Fizkultura i Sport, Moscow.

Grigalka, O. (1980) Thoughts on shot put technique (Russian). *Track and Field Events* **6**, 10–14.

Hochmuth, G. (1974) *Biomechanik sportlicher Bewegungen*. Sportverlag, Berlin.

Ihring, A. (1982) Rotacna technika vrhu gul'on. *Trener, Bratislava* **26** (5), 202–204.

Ionesku, R. (1992) Rotational shot put technique. *Modern Athlete and Coach, Adelaide* **30**, 41.

Kerssenbrock, K. (1974) Analysis of rotation technique. In: *The Throws* (ed. F. Wilt), pp. 39–41. Tafnews Press, Los Altos, CA.

Kerssenbrock, K. (1981) Znova vrh kouli rotacni technikou. *Atletika* **12**, 16–17.

Koltai, J. (1973) Examination of previous research in shot put technique. VI International Congress JTFCA, Madrid.

Kristev, I.N. (1971) *Shot putting* (Bulgarian). Medicine and Physical Culture (Sofia).

Kristev, I.N., Boichev, K., Nakov, K., Barzakov, P., Popov, I. & Boukov, N. (1973) Means and methods of improving shot put technique (Bulgarian). *Problems of Physical Culture* **8** (5), 268–275.

Kutiev, N. (1966) The shot put by top athletes (Russian). *Track and Field Events* **11**, 8–10.

Lanka, J.J. (1978) Biomechanical investigation of shot putting technique in athletes of different skill level (Russian). PhD dissertation, Institute of Physical Culture, Kiev.

Lanka, J. (1996) *Biomechanics of shot put* (Latvian). Latvian Academy of Sport Education, Riga.

Lanka, J. & Shalmanov, A. (1982) *Biomechanics of shot put* (Russian). F.I.S., Moscow.

Lebedev, N.A. (1969) Experimental study of explosive exercise role in preparation of athletes specializing in throwing events (shot putting) (Russian). PhD dissertation, Institute of Physical Culture, Leningrad.

Lindsay, M.R. (1994) A comparison of the rotational and O'Brian shot put techniques. *The Thrower* **63**, 12–17.

Machabeli, G.S. (1969) Dynamometric apparatus for shot putting technique (Russian). In: *The Materials of an Annual Scientific Conference of the Georgian Institute of Physical Culture of 1968*, Tbilisi, p. 160.

Marhold, G.S. (1964) Über den Absprung beim Kugelstoßen. *Theorie und Praxis der Körperkultur* **13** (8), 695.

Marhold, G. (1970) Badania nad biomechaniczna charakterystika techniki pchniecia kula. In: *Sympozjum Teorii Techniki Sportovej*, Warszawa, pp. 99–109.

Marhold G. (1974) Biomechanical analysis of the shot put. In: *Biomechanics IV* (eds R.C. Nelson & C.A. Morehouse), pp. 175–179. University Park Press, Baltimore.

Nett, T. (1962) Foot contact at the instant of release in throwing. *Track Technique* **9**, 71–74.

Oesterreich, R., Bartonietz, K. & Goldmann, W. (1997) Drehstoßtechnik: ein modell für die Langjährige Vorbereitung von Jungen Sportlern. *Die Lehre der Leichtathletik* **38**, 81–86.

Palm, V. (1990) Some biomechanical observations of the rotational shot put. *Modern Athlete and Coach, Adelaide* **28** (3), 15–18.

Payne, A.H. (1974) A force platform system for biomechanics research in sport. In: *Biomechanics IV* (eds R.C. Nelson & C.A. Morehouse), pp. 502–509. University Park Press, Baltimore.

Payne, A.H., Slater, W.J. & Telford, T. (1968) The use of a force platform in the study of athletic activities. a preliminary investigation. *Ergonomics* **11** (2), 123–143.

Pearson, G.F.D. (1966) Shot put questions and answers. *Track Technique* **24**, 760–763.

Questions to Vanegas (1987) XIV Congress of the European Athletics Coaches Association (ed. A.E.F.A.), Aix-Les-Bains, 19–23.

Samotsvetov, A.A. (1961) The shot will fly farther (Russian). *Track and Field Events* **4**, 18–20.

Schpenke, J. (1973) Zur technik des Kugelstoßens. *Der Leichtathletik* **10** (17), 8–9.

Schpenke, J. (1974) Problems of technique and training in the shot put. In: *The Throws, Contemporary Theory, Technique and Training* (ed. F. Wilt), pp. 28–33. Tafnews Press, Los Altos, CA.

Shalmanov, A.A. (1977) The study of sport technique variation (shot putting) (Russian). PhD dissertation, Central Institute of Physical Culture, Moscow.

Shalmanov, Al.A. (1986) Interaction with ground in jumps as subject of teaching. PhD dissertation, Central Institute of Physical Culture, Moscow.

Simonyi, G. (1973) Form breakdown of Wladyslaw Komar, Poland, Olympic Champion 69–6. *Scholastic Coach* **42** (7) 7–9, 94–102.

Stepanek, J. (1990) Kinematic analysis of glide and turn shot put technique. In: *Abstracts: Techniques in Athletics*. 1st International Conference, 7–9 June 1990, Cologne, Germany, pp. 65–66.

Susanka, P. (1974) Computer techniques in biomechanics of sport. In: *Biomechanics IV* (eds R.C. Nelson & C.A. Morehouse), pp. 531–534. University Park Press, Baltimore.

Susanka, P. & Stepanek, J. (1987) Biomechanical analysis of the shot put. Scientific Material presented by IAAF Research Team, II WC Rome. Part 1, Prague, Cologne, Athens.

Tschiene, P. (1973) Der Kugelstoß. *Leichtathletik* **10** (11), 378.

Tschiene, P. (1974) Perfection of shot put technique. In: *The Throws* (ed. F. Wilt), pp. 25–27. Tafnews Press, Los Altos, CA.

Turk, M. (1997) Building a technical model for the shot put. *IAAF Regional Development Centre Bulletin* **2**, 35–41.

Tutevich, V.N. (1955) *Shot put* (Russian). Fizkultura i Sport, Moscow.

Tutevich, V.N. (1969) *The theory of throwing events* (Russian). F.I.S., Moscow.

Vanegas, A. (1987) Rotational shot technique. *The Throws* XIV Congress of the European Athletics Coaches Association, Aix-Les-Bains, 13–18.

Ward, B. (1970) Analysis of Dallas Long's shot putting. *Track Technique* **39**, 1232–1234.

Zatsiorsky, V.M. (1995) *Science and Practice of Strength Training*. Human Kinetics Publishers, Champaign, IL.

Zatsiorsky, V.M. (1997) *Kinematics of Human Motion*. Human Kinetics Publishers, Champaign, IL.

Zatsiorsky, V.M., Lanka, J.J. & Shalmanov, A.A. (1978) Biomechanical problems of shot putting (Russian).

Theory and Practice of Physical Culture (Moscow) **54** (12), 6–17.

Zatsiorsky, V.M., Lanka, J.J. & Shalmanov, A.A. (1981) Biomechanical analysis of shot putting technique. *Exercise and Sport Sciences Reviews* **9**, 353–389.

Chapter 22

Hammer Throwing: Problems and Prospects

K. BARTONIETZ

By hammer and hand
All arts do stand.
[Motto on arms over Smith's Hall, Newcastle, 1771]

The first section of this chapter gives a brief outline of the history of the hammer-throwing event, focusing on the development of technique and biomechanical aspects. More about hammer-throwing history can be found by referring to Bartonietz (1985), Voronkin and Limar (1989), Dunn and McGill (1994) and Black (1999). There follows a review of the relationships between the factors that determine the distance thrown, and a description of energy transfer and movement coordination (movement pattern) in hammer throwing at different performance levels in male and female athletes. After this there is an analysis of the throwing technique of world-class male and female hammer-throwers. Findings concerning the training effects of using hammers of different weight and length are then presented. The material presented is based on mechanical and biomechanical principles, data from experimental research, and on the practical experience of coaches and athletes. Recommendations for training are given throughout, and these are summarized at the end.

The evolution of Olympic hammer throwing

The introductory motto reflects the high regard for hammer throwing over the centuries. The sources of modern hammer throwing are hidden in the dim and distant past, and draw on a combination of work, leisure and warfare. Outstanding rulers and politicans of the Middle Ages were given an epithet, partly derived from their hammer-throwing abilities, for example Charles Martel (688–741) was dubbed 'hammer Charles', Edward I (ruled 1272–1307) was 'Hammer of the Scots', and Thomas Cromwell (1485–1540) had the epithet 'hammer of the monks'. During the 18th and 19th centuries in Ireland and Scotland, hammer throwing was the sport of farmers and workmen, not in keeping with the status of the English gentry. From there, modern hammer throwing had its origin. The sequence photographs of Eadweard Muybridge are probably the first movement study of early athletic hammer throwing (see e.g. Muybridge 1955). These ancient traditions live on in the Scottish Highland Games.

The hammer throw is an event clearly based on national traditions. Athletes with an Irish background advanced the world record 33 times from 1877 until 1937 and won gold medals at five Olympic games (see Table 22.2). The rules concerning length and mass for modern competitive hammer throwing were laid down in 1887 in the USA: length 4 feet (1.22 m) and mass 15 pounds (6.8 kg), including the stick, and since about 1891 with the wire and grip, 16 pounds (7.26 kg). Nevertheless, as shown in Table 22.1, different hammers were in use during those years.

The effectiveness of the hammer-throw technique judged by the number of turns used, has been discussed since the 1920s (see the overview by Bartonietz 1985; Bondarchuk 1985). The first noted world record of 57.77 m in 1913 (Table 22.2) was established with two turns. The 'American rule' was

Table 22.1 Results from the beginning of modern hammer throwing, according to Bartonietz (1985).

Hammer mass		Distance thrown (m)	Remarks
(pounds)	(kg)		
8	3.64	67.13	With one hand in 1892
10	4.54	42.72	From standing position, with one hand
12	5.44	40.92	Two-handed
12	5.44	44.65	1889
14	6.35	35.15	From standing position
16	7.26	45.92	1897
21	9.53	27.51	1888
22	9.98	16.30	1879, one turn, one hand

recommended during the early stages: two turns for big athletes 'rolling' through the circle, and three turns for smaller athletes with better developed explosive leg power. In recent years, in the men's hammer throw, the overwhelming number of top athletes use four turns; for example the world's six best male athletes in 1995 all used four turns. The three medallists from the European Championships in 1998, the international debut of female hammer throw, used four turns, but three turns are also used by a number of female 60 m throwers. The inclusion of an additional fifth turn was discussed and tested some decades ago, but was largely discarded due to difficulties in movement coordination. However, at the World Athletics Championships in 1999, Vladislav Piskunov of the Ukraine successfully managed five turns and won the bronze medal with a result of 79.03 m.

In the beginning of competitive hammer throwing, the implement was thrown from a dirt circle, and the athletes wore shoes with spikes. The high torsional loadings led to knee injuries, so leather soles without spikes were introduced. Today the soles of shoes for hammer-throwers are made from rubber and special synthetic materials.

D. Quinn of the USA was already using a heel/toe footwork technique in 1927, demonstrating four turns for the first time. With this technique, one foot could be kept on the ground at all times during the throw, leading to faster turns. This element of technique is often attributed to the German coach S. Christmann, who developed it in conjunction

with a golf swing-like body and arm action. Soviet athletes and their coaches greatly improved performances with this technique, starting with the 63.34 m world-record throw of Krivonosov in 1954, and ultimately achieving world-record throws in 1984 by Litvinov and Sedych (see Table 22.2).

Applied biomechanical research started in the 1950s in the former Soviet Union, undertaken mainly by former top throwers—see the scientific work of M.P. Krivonosov, A.A. Baltovskij, A.A. Schechtel, A.P. Bondarchuk and Yu. Bakarinov, all of whom were world-class throwers. This is one of the reasons for the outstanding performances of athletes from the former Soviet Union. Soviet coaches and their athletes developed the 'wound up' method of hammer acceleration, characterized by a torque between shoulder and hip axis during the turns, to the leg lead, 'catch-up' technique. The latter is the basic element of modern hammer-throwing technique.

Recently (in 1999) 80 m hammer-throwers are coming out of Hungary (Géscek, European champion in 1998; Németh, Annus and Kiss), Germany (Weis, World champion in 1997; Kobs, World champion in 1999), the USA (Deal), the former Soviet republics (Skwaruk and Piskunov, Ukraine; Konovalov, Russia), Czech Republic (Maska) and Italy (Paoluzzi). They are the event's leaders. After the culmination of Jurij Sedych's and Sergeij Litvinov's excellence in the mid-1980s there has been no increase in the world record. The men's top performances during the last two Olympic Games,

Table 22.2 Performance development in men's and women's hammer throw.

Year	World record (m)	Olympic Games medal distances (m)		
		1st	2nd	3rd
Men				
1900		49.73	49.13	42.46
1904		51.23	50.26	45.73
1908		54.74	51.18	48.50
1912		54.74	48.39	48.17
1913	57.77			
1920		52.87	48.43	48.25
1924		53.29	50.84	48.87
1928		51.39	51.29	49.03
1932		53.92	52.27	50.33
1936		56.49	55.04	54.83
1938	59.00			
1948	59.02	56.07	54.27	53.73
1949	59.57			
1950	59.88			
1952	60.34, 61.25	60.34	58.86	57.74
1953	62.36			
1954	63.34, 64.05			
1955	63.33, 64.52			
1956	65.85, 66.38, 67.32, 68.54	63.19	63.03	62.56
1958	68.68			
1960	70.33	67.10	65.79	65.64
1962	70.67			
1964		69.74	69.09	68.09
1965	71.06, 71.26, 73.74			
1968	73.76	73.36	73.28	69.78
1969	74.52, 74.68, 75.48			
1971	76.40			
1972		75.50	74.96	74.04
1974	76.60, 76.66			
1975	76.70, 77.56, 78.50, 79.30			
1976		77.52	76.08	75.48
1978	80.14, 80.32			
1980	80.38, 80.46, 80.64, 81.66, 81.80	81.80	80.64	78.96
1982	83.98			
1983	84.14			
1984	86.34	78.08	77.98	76.68
1986	86.66, 86.74			
1988		84.80	83.76	81.16
1992		82.54	81.96	81.38
Women				
1993	65.40			
1994	67.34			
1995	68.16			
1996	69.46	81.24	81.12	80.02
1997	73.10			
1998	73.80			
1999	76.07			

World and European Championships have stabilized at the 80–83 m level. The rapid improvement in the women's hammer throw has to do mainly with its acceptance as an Olympic event (Table 22.2). The same effect was noted at the beginning of the 20th century, when in 1900 men's hammer throwing became an Olympic event. Experts are convinced that by the year 2000 the women's record in hammer throwing may equal 75–80 m or even more (Bartonietz *et al.* 1997; Agachi *et al.* 1997). Mihaela Melinte, the world-record holder (76.07 m, see Table 22.2) and first World champion of the event (75.20 m), reached this benchmark in 1999. In 1999, four women athletes threw the hammer over the 70 m mark (Melinte of Romania, Kusenkova and Konstantinova of Russia, and Ellerby of the USA). They are the current leaders in women's hammer throwing.

Biomechanical basics of hammer throwing

To find the balance in the field of tension of counteracting forces.

[World Champion in hammer throwing 1997, Heinz Weis (personal best 83.04 m) about the art of hammer throwing. (Frommeyer, 1999.)]

The main goal of hammer throwing is simply to propel the implement—of mass 7.26 kg and 4 kg, respectively, for men and women (less for younger athletes), with a length of 1.215 m and 1.195 m, respectively—so that it lands as far away from the thrower as possible within the landing area sector. The acceleration of the hammer occurs in a circle constructed of concrete with an inside diameter of 2.135 m ± 5 mm. The competitors have to commence the throw from a stationary position and stabilize their body after release inside the confines of the circle. No other restrictions are made concerning the movement execution itself. A cage serves for security reasons, but often limits visual movement analysis. A degree or time chart is used to describe the position of thrower and implement. This reference chart is shown in Fig. 22.1, along with the orbit of the hammer and the path of the mass centre of the thrower-hammer system. Coaches prefer the chart that resembles a clock face. When using reference charts, the movement of the thrower through the circle has to be taken into consideration. This movement does not occur in a straight line, but along a more or less curvilinear path, depending on the starting position and the feet placement during the turns (see Figs 22.1, 22.11 & 22.12; *also* Bartonietz & Borgström 1995).

Parameters of release

In the hammer throw, the distance thrown is determined by the velocity of release, the angle of release, the height of release, and air resistance, and is represented by the relationship as shown in Chapter 19, Eqn. 19.20. The most important factor for a long throw is the velocity of release, as this is a measure of the hammer's kinetic energy. It is the one factor that can be maximized by the athlete's actions, the others being the angle and height of relase, which can have optimal values. Despite the squared effect of release velocity (see Eqn. 19.20 in Chapter 19), the linking with other parameters causes a quasi-linear relationship between release velocity and flight distance of the implement in the targeted zone, i.e. from 40 to 85 m (see Fig. 22.2). Table 22.3 shows angles of release for throws by male athletes in a range between 34 and 44°.

Analysis has shown that female athletes obtain angles of release of between 29 and 42° (Bartonietz 1994b; Hildebrand & Bartonietz 1995; author's own unpublished data). However, an angle of approximately 44° is optimal (Tutevich 1969) for both male and female athletes. Female athletes tend to have a flat release, which could possibly be caused by the unfavourable relationship between the hammer length and body height compared to males, and/or ineffective legwork during the delivery phase that keeps the plane of movement too flat. A change of 5° in the angle of release corresponds with a reduction in the distance thrown of approximately 1 m.

The results of Bartonietz *et al.* (1997), presented below, show, for the women's event, a significant tendency (0.001 level of significance) towards steeper release angles with increased performance. They analysed 1–20 throws by 13 female athletes in the distance range 40.50–49.64 m. The average angle of release ($a_{o(av)}$) was found to be 36°, the

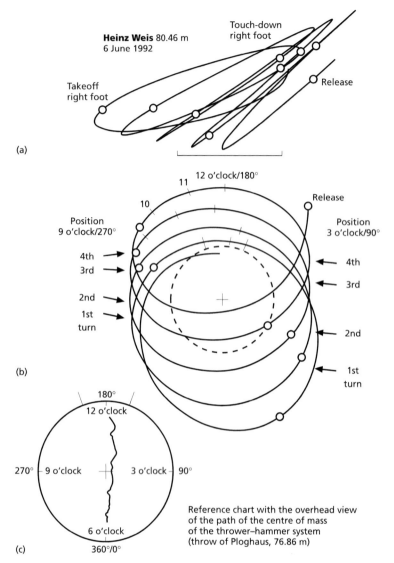

(a)

(b)

(c)

Reference chart with the overhead view
of the path of the centre of mass
of the thrower–hammer system
(throw of Ploghaus, 76.86 m)

Fig. 22.1 Reference degree and time
chart for movement analysis in the
hammer throw, incorporating the
orbit of the hammer. (a) Side view.
(b) Overhead view (throw of
Heinz Weis, 80.46 m, 6 June 1982).
(c) Reference degree and time chart.

standard deviation (SD) $\pm 3.7°$, the minimum
value $(a_{o(min)})$ was 29°, and the maximum value
$(a_{o(max)})$ was 42°. Analysis of 2 to 15 throws by
five female athletes in the distance range 50.04–
67.58 m revealed $a_{o(av)} = 40°$, $s = \pm 3°$, $a_{o(min)} = 36°$
and $a_{o(max)} = 45°$.

The hammer should leave the hands at shoulder
level. Therefore, the height of release is determined
by the athlete's constitution and technique; that
being so, the distance thrown increases by the same

amount as the height of release increases (Tutevich
1969). The height of release in male athletes was
recorded as between 1.60 and 1.70 m (Otto 1990a,b;
Morriss & Bartlett 1992). Release heights above or
below shoulder level can be related to a defective
release movement. Release heights recorded as
being much above shoulder level can be caused
by measurement inaccuracy, because the instant of
release (corresponding with maximum release
velocity) and the visible loss of grip contact are not

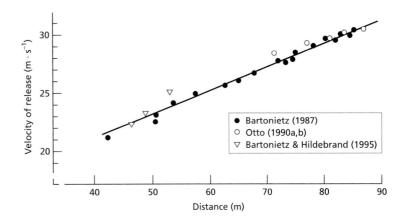

Fig. 22.2 Relationship between velocity of release and the distance thrown in hammer throwing.

Table 22.3 Men's hammer throw: angles of release.

Athlete	Distance (m)	Year	Angle of release (°)	Source
Sedych	86.74	1986	39.9	Otto (1990a)
Litvinov	83.06	1987	38.4	
Tamm	80.84	1987	43.2	
Haber	80.76	1987	40.5	Otto (1990b)
Sahner	80.58	1987	40.0	
Gescek	77.34	1987	40.1	
Nikulin	80.18	1987	44.0	
Nikulin	80.62	1992	36.9	Gutiérrez & Soto Hermoso (1995)
Weis	80.18	1987	40.2	Otto (1990b)
Weis	79.20	1991	39	Present author*
Weis	80.46	1992	40	
Astapkovich	100.67 (6.26 kg)	1992	39.8	Gutiérrez & Soto Hermoso (1995)
Sidorenko	78.82	1991	38.3	Morriss & Bartlett (1992)
Alay	77.50	1991	41.8	
Caspers	70.74	1995	45 (5.00 kg)	
Caspers	64.22	1995	39 (6.26 kg)	
Caspers	66.48	1996	34 (6.26 kg, April 27)	Present author*
Caspers	67.44	1996	42 (6.26 kg, May 29)	
Caspers	11.60	1996	34 (25 kg/0.40 m)	

* Denotes unpublished data of K. Bartonietz.
Values in brackets denote mass of the implement/length of the implement.

identical. There seems to be a correlation between performance level and release height, with less-proficient athletes attaining lower release heights. This conclusion can be drawn from the data of Morriss and Bartlett (1992), who compared throws of Soviet and British athletes with about 10 m differences in distances thrown.

Movement of the implement and the thrower

It is postulated that the general target technique for women is the same as it is for men (Bartonietz *et al.* 1997; Romanov & Vrublevsky 1998). The differences in biomechanical parameters, which have to do with the physical differences between male and female athletes, mainly body height, are taken into account in this section.

From the physical relationship between linear velocity (v_H), angular velocity (ω_H), and the radius of the hammer path (r_H), it is obvious that the thrower must strive for an optimum relationship between these parameters, which is represented by the following equation and Fig. 22.3:

$$v_H = r_H\omega_H \qquad (22.1)$$

If we assume that there is a limit set for the extension of the radius, an increase in release velocity, for example from 24 to 25 m · s⁻¹ by a radius of 1.6 m, is linked to the increase of the average angular velocity by 6 rad · s⁻¹ (Fig. 22.3). This will lead to faster turns, with the overall time for the turns being reduced. The data in Table 22.4 (part I) highlight this. Interpretation of the data is based on the

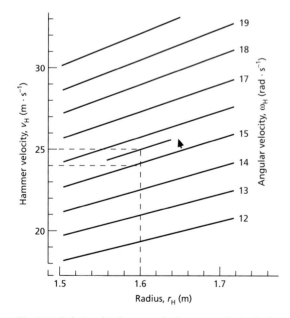

Fig. 22.3 Relationship between the hammer velocity (v_H), radius (r_H) and angular velocity (ω_H). (From Bartonietz 1990.)

assumption that differences between the angles of release can be excluded as the reason for the differences in distance thrown. Our analysis of throws in training and competition shows this assumption to be valid. Throws with a flat release caused by a faulty movement during delivery are often declared as invalid by the athlete herself or himself.

It can be noted that with improving performance some of the athletes increase or stabilize the total time used in the turns. If the athlete reaches a higher velocity of release, but the total turning time (and with it the average angular velocity) remains the same or even increases, then the movement radius must be increased. This is acceptable as it indicates that these athletes are utilizing all the potential of their technique (Table 22.4, part II). The data of Olga Kuzenkova's throws (see Table 22.12) show in more detail the changes over several years of training in the relationship between the single- and double-support phases (one foot or both feet in contact with the ground).

The following formula represents how the centripetal force component (F_{cp}) is related to the radius and the square of the angular velocity (ω_H):

$$F_{cp} = m_H r_H \omega_H{}^2 \qquad (22.2)$$

where m_H is the mass of the hammer.

From the thrower's perspective, increasing the radius would seem to be more effective than increasing the angular velocity—the latter, e.g. by assembling and declining a marked twist between the hip and shoulder axis as it was common for the technical model of the 1970s—because the centripetal force changes with the angular velocity squared. Dapena and Felter (1989) and Dapena and McDonald (1989) assumed that lower angular velocities can create better working conditions for the leg muscles, facilitating the increase of angular momentum of the thrower–hammer system.

The relationship between linear velocity of the hammer, angular velocity and radius of the hammer path is illustrated in Fig. 22.4. The representation starts with the transition into the first turn at the end of the last arm swing and ends at the instant of release. The double-support phases are marked by the bold bars. The figure shows that the increase in peripheral velocity is achieved during a single turn

Table 22.4 Duration of turns and distance thrown at varying performance levels.

Athlete	Distance (m)	Duration of turns (s)	Distance (m)	Duration of turns (s)	Date (other info.)	Source
PART I						
Females						
Kuzenkova	64.40	2.57	67.58	2.40	25 Feb 96	D. Gathercole (unpublished work)
	63.90	2.46			11 Feb 96	
	64.38	2.46			11 Feb 96	
Melinte	66.96	2.08	68.84	2.04	23 May 97	Present author*
Sosimenko	60.20	1.77	62.70	1.64	25/11 Feb 96	
	59.50	1.70	62.86	1.62	11 Feb 96	
Mathes	48.90	1.64	53.28	1.56	10 Jul 93 (3 turns)	
	54.60	2.30	57.38	2.28	14 May 94 (4 turns)	
	61.24	2.24	63.94	2.16	23 May 97	
Beyer	57.50	1.72	60.54	1.66	29 May/27 Apr 96	
Males						
Sedych	75.40	1.60	82.34	1.47		Present author*
	82.34	1.47	84.92	1.43		Otto (1990a)
			86.74	1.34		
Weis	74.88	2.23	79.20	2.13	14 May 94/28 Jul 91	
	75.06	2.18			14 May 94	
Sidorenko	78.22	2.12	80.64	2.06	6 Jun 92	Present author*
Kiss	79.02	2.12			World Championship 1995	
			81.26	2.04	European Championship 1998	
Strohschänk	66.34	2.20	69.20	2.12	15 May 94/27 Apr 96	
PART II						
Females						
McNaugthon	52.66	2.25	55.28	2.28	26 Jan 96	Gathercole (1996)
			56.00	2.38	11 Feb 96	
Suzuki	57.52	1.70	58.86	1.72	1996	
Mathes	56.12	2.16	63.94	2.16	23 May 97	
Kuzenkova	66.00	2.26	71.22	2.26	1995–1997	
Melinte	68.84	2.04			23 May 97	Present author*
			68.65	2.06	21 Aug 98	
Males						
Weis	77.72	2.22	80.46	2.22	6 Jun 92	
	76.89	2.18	80.04	2.22	19 Aug 98	

* Denotes unpublished data of K. Bartonietz.

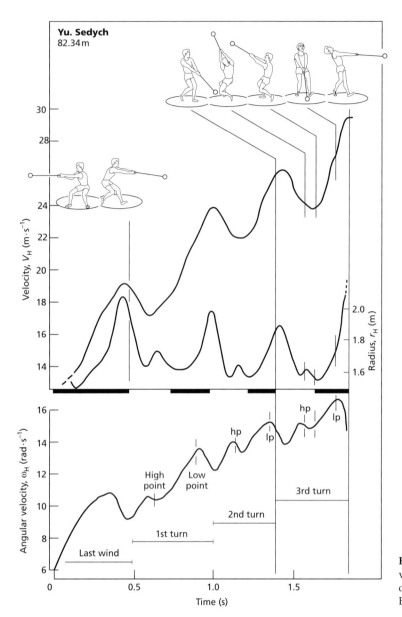

Fig. 22.4 Time-related changes of velocity, radius and angular velocity of the hammer movement. (From Bartonietz 1990.)

by an increase of the angular velocity, supported by radius extension during the double-support phases.

The angular velocity increases from turn to turn, for example from 8 rad · s⁻¹ at the beginning of the first turn to 14 rad · s⁻¹ at the beginning of the third turn, or by 175%. At the same time, the radius is slightly decreased, due to the upright-backward position of the thrower, compensating for the growing centripetal forces. This points to the effect of decreasing the moment of inertia of the thrower by an increase of the angular velocity, based on the law of conservation of momentum in a closed system. In the hammer throw, the thrower has the opportunity of adding energy to the thrower-hammer system during the double-support phases.

For the sake of completeness it should be noted that the Earth's gravitational field has an accelerating and decelerating effect on the hammer (Dapena 1984). However, it can be assumed that both acceleration and deceleration caused by gravity are in balance during the turns. During the single-support phases, the rotational energy can only be redistributed between the thrower and the implement. An acceleration of the hammer at the beginning of the single-support phases, as is noted in some throws, is caused by an ineffective deceleration of the thrower's body, leading to an 'outrun' of the hammer—radius extension, caused by an expressed transition of the thrower through the circle—and extended duration of the single-support phases with the consequence of shortening the following acceleration phase (Hildebrand & Bartonietz 1995). In such cases, an ineffective redistribution of rotational energy must then occur from the hammer to the thrower.

The legwork must be the effective drive to increase the angular velocity by keeping the radius as long as possible. It must be noted, that the increase in angular velocity does not automatically lead to an increase of linear velocity of the hammer because of the interaction with the radius.

As a result of changes in body balance, the applied ground reaction forces and the transition of the thrower through the circle, the axis of the thrower-implement system changes its support and inclination. This axis intersects the mass centre of the entire system, and the turning movement of the axis forms a curve, called an axoid (Krevald 1975). There is no need for a vertical position of the system's axis during all parts of the throw (Tutevic 1969; Pataki & Slamka 1979; Bondarchuk 1985). The athlete has to strive for an almost circular movement of the system's axis, known as 'round turning'. According to the hypothesis of Krevald (1975), the position of the system's axis greatly affects the load on the legs, or putting cause and effect in the right order, the achieved leg power and throwing technique affect the position and movement of the system's axis. Problems with 'round turning' can originate from insufficient loading on the support leg, going into the turns. The ground reaction forces (Fig. 22.5) can give deeper insights into the move-

ments of the thrower with the implement, as the results of Pozzo (1990) indicate. The data show a change in the direction of the applied forces: the forward trunk lean is characterized by flatter directed legwork. For these analysed throws, no significant differences were found in the radius of the hammer movement and in its velocity at the high and low points. Thus, leaning the trunk forwards does not automatically imply an increase in radius and hammer velocity. For this, the thrower must generate the necessary driving power (see below). Ground reaction force data recorded separately for the right and left leg would provide more detailed information about the body and hammer drive.

As in other throwing events, the work of the left leg is a key to success. The rapid grounding of the left heel reflects left leg activity, since the left heel has to be grounded faster from turn to turn. Tables 22.11–22.13 include relevant data.

FORCES ACTING ON THE HAMMER HEAD

In analysing the forces acting on the hammer head, it has to be taken into account that the athlete transfers forces through the grip via the wire to the hammer head. The forces measured on the hammer head are not identical with the forces on the grip. According to calculations of Pataki and Slamka (1979), the acceleration force component on the grip reaches about 2.9 times the value on the hammer head. There are three basic situations of energy transfer (Fig. 22.6): the athlete 'pulls' the hammer (left); the hammer is in a neutral position (middle); or the athlete is 'pulled' by the hammer (right).

Because the initial angular velocity at the beginning of each turn influences the tangential force component, the latter must increase from turn to turn (Hildebrand 1982), as the force–time history in Fig. 22.7 illustrates. The momentary maxima of the acceleration and centripetal components, of which the resulting force is composed, are achieved in the range of the low points of the hammer path (see also Susanka et al. 1987, analysing a 79.22 m throw of Yurij Sedych). The muscle groups of the legs provide the impetus, while the trunk and the arms transmit the forces to the hammer ball. The resulting force, measured tensodynamometrically with

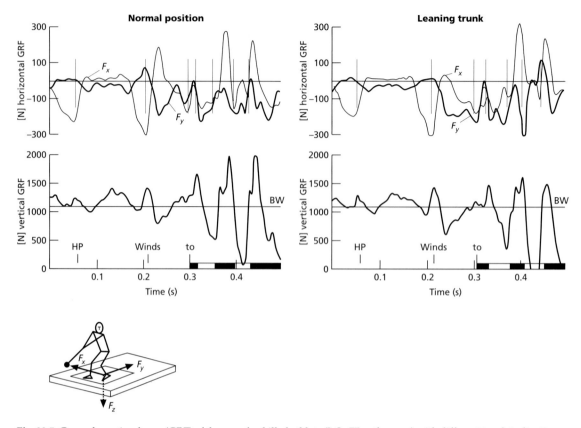

Fig. 22.5 Ground reaction forces (GRF) of throws of a skilled athlete (L.S., 77 m thrower) with different trunk inclinations during the preliminary wind-ups and the first and second turns. BW, Body weight; to, time at moment zero. (From Pozzo 1990.)

the help of special hammer handles or wires (e.g. Hwang & Adrian 1984), and its differential coefficient (called 'jerk'), can be used in training and for diagnosis as feedback information (Kollodij 1972; Stache 1980; Pozzo 1987).

The acceleration of the hammer starts during the turns at the end of the single-support phase, after the high point of the hammer trajectory is reached, and continues until the low point of the hammer trajectory is passed. Data often suggest the presence of a braking phase, close to the low point, and a second acceleration phase until the double-support phase is finished. During this braking phase energy is transferred ineffectively from the hammer to the thrower by a shortcoming in the legwork (Hildebrand & Bartonietz 1995). During such a situation, in coaching

language, the 'hammer has overtaken the thrower'. To avoid this, the angular difference between the shoulder axis and the hip axis must be relatively stable in the turns to ensure effective transfer of the legwork energy to the hammer (Fig. 22.6 (below), Fig. 22.8, Table 22.5).

A divergence between the shoulder and the hip axis at the beginning of each turn was a main element of the hammer throw technique until the mid-1970s, and was called the 'wound-up' or 'torqued' method (see above). The attempt to gain a big lead on the hammer with the lower body during each turn allows, on the one hand, a long pull with a corresponding velocity increase. On the other hand, this throwing pattern is characterized by an ineffective decrease in hammer velocity during the

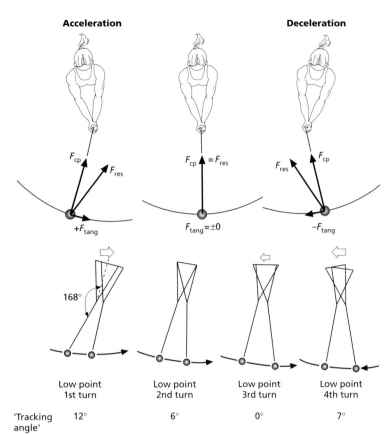

Acceleration

F_{cp} F_{res} $+F_{tang}$

$F_{cp} = F_{res}$ $F_{tang} = \pm 0$

Deceleration

F_{res} F_{cp} $-F_{tang}$

168°

| Low point 1st turn | Low point 2nd turn | Low point 3rd turn | Low point 4th turn |

'Tracking angle'   12°   6°   0°   7°

Fig. 22.6 *Top*: The main forces acting on the hammer (the accelerating and decelerating effect of gravity is not taken into account). *Bottom*: Positions of the hammer, arms and shoulder axis at the low points of the hammer trajectory (throw of O. Kuzenkova, 66.00 m, 30 June 1995). *Note:* An angle between the hammer head, grip and middle of the shoulder axis <180° (e.g. 165°) indicates an acceleration in the 1st turn: The 'tracking angle' is determined by 180−168 = 12°. The arrows above the shoulder axis show the direction of movement of the shoulder girdle. (From Bartonietz *et al.* 1997.)

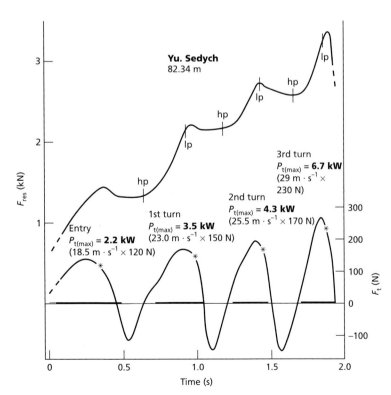

Fig. 22.7 Time-related changes of the resulting force (F_{res}) and the tangential component (F_t), peak power values during the entry and the turns. Note the differences in the force scales. The instant of achieving peak power is marked by asterisks. (Adapted from Bartonietz *et al.* 1986.)

Yu. Sedych
82.34 m

Entry
$P_{t(max)} = 2.2$ kW
(18.5 m · s^{-1} × 120 N)

1st turn
$P_{t(max)} = 3.5$ kW
(23.0 m · s^{-1} × 150 N)

2nd turn
$P_{t(max)} = 4.3$ kW
(25.5 m · s^{-1} × 170 N)

3rd turn
$P_{t(max)} = 6.7$ kW
(29 m · s^{-1} × 230 N)

F_{res} (kN)

F_t (N)

Time (s)

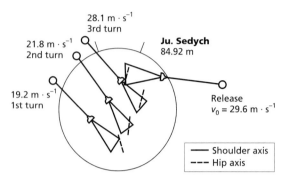

Fig. 22.8 Position of hammer, arms, and shoulder and hip axes (projection in the horizontal plane) and velocity values of the hammer, at the beginning of the double-support phases and at the instant of release. (From Bartonietz 1990.)

Table 22.5 Differences between the shoulder and hip axis (γ) in the high and low points of the hammer path (also called 'torque angle'), in the throw of Sergej Litvinov (distance = 86.04 m).

Turn no.	Shoulder/hip axis difference (γ) (°)	
	High points	Low points
1	−8	27
2	−5	25
3	−12	14
4	−25	7

Note: A negative difference is based on the shoulder axis being in front of the hip axis; a positive difference is a result of the hip axis being in front of the shoulder axis.

process of 'winding up'. The 'catch-up' technique, as demonstrated by Sedych and Litvinov, with the focus on a stable shoulder girdle and wide movement radius, has proved superior. A twist between the hip and shoulder axes is essential only in the final hammer acceleration during the release phase of the last turn. According to data of Otto (1992), in Yurij Sedych's world-record throw there was no 'torque angle' during the first turn and only 30° of difference during each of the final turns. The magnitude of his torque was reduced in favour of a stable trunk position and a controllable body posture.

In comparing two throws of Heinz Weis (World champion in 1998) at different performance levels (76.30 m in 1987 vs. 82.16 m in 1989), the better throw has much less 'torque angle' during the turns and release (Otto 1990b).

SINGLE- AND DOUBLE-SUPPORT PHASES

Applied research in the former Soviet Union led to the hypothesis that the duration of the movement phases with both legs on the ground—double-support—should be longer than the duration of the turn on one leg—single-support. It was supposed that the athlete can effectively drive his own body and the implement only in the double-support phases, increasing the angular momentum. During single-support phases it was assumed that only a redistribution of rotational kinetic energy is possible between the thrower and implement. The total amount of angular momentum of the entire system is kept almost constant during this period, except for the loss caused by ground friction and the accelerating/decelerating effect of gravity. During the double-support phases the angular momentum of the system can be increased, mainly by legwork.

Analysis of experimental data of throws of the world's best athletes seem to support this hypothesis, i.e. that the duration of double-support phases is greater than the duration of single-support phases. According to the data of Otto (1990a, 1992), Jurij Sedych had longer double-support phases than single-support phases during his world-record throw (average 55.8% of the duration of the turns). The path of the hammer during the double-support phases was longer than the path during the single-support phases. The 'early catch of the hammer' was one of Sedych's strong technical points (see Bartonietz 1987, 1994c; Otto 1990a). Other elite hammer-throwers show a similar movement pattern, including Kiss, Gécsek and Kuzenkova in 1996, and Sosimenko. Also the 1964 Olympic champion and former world-record holder, R. Klim, exhibited this legwork pattern (Shukevich & Krivonossov 1971).

However, a number of top athletes show, to varying degrees, the opposite, i.e. shorter double-

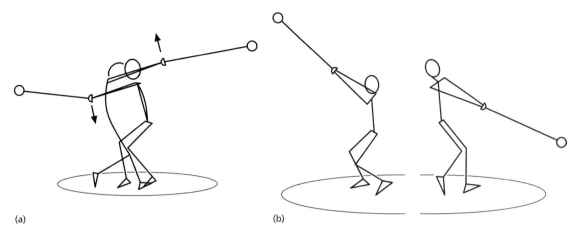

Fig. 22.9 Position of the hammer-thrower at the beginning and end of the single-support phase. (a) Female athlete, performance level 50 m. (b) O. Kuzenkova, 71.22 m in 1997.

support phases than single-support phases, especially during the penultimate and/or final turn (e.g. Abduvaliev, Weis, Melinte, Mathes, Münchow and Kuzenkova in 1997). Athletes at a low performance level or with little training overwhelmingly show a pattern of movement with shorter double-support phases (Bartonietz 1994c). Bujak (1983) recommends the duration of the double-support phases as one criterion for performance diagnosis, based on statistical analysis of elite hammer-throwers over several years of performance development. Dapena (1990) has focused on the possibilities to accelerate the hammer during the single-support phases by gravity and by the thrower's transition through the circle. Analysing the transfer of momentum between thrower and implement, Hildebrand and Bartonietz (1995) describe the hammer acceleration at the beginning of the single-support phase as ineffective, because of the necessary redistribution of angular momentum from the hammer back to the thrower. The same applies to the acceleration of the hammer before the single-support phases are finished, by falling on the double-support and pulling the hammer by radius shortening.

Video analysis can verify the external movement pattern, and provide evidence about the mechanics of hammer drive. Figure 22.9 shows the corresponding positions of the hammer and the thrower. The arrows mark the movement direction of the grip in relationship to the hammer head. They indicate an acceleration of the hammer by the thrower before the double-support phases start—pulling down— and after the double-support phases are finished— lifting up.

Although these results cannot serve as conclusive evidence that extended double-support phases are the only effective way to throw, it can be assumed that a long duration of the double-support phases can give evidence of an effective hammer drive. The data concerning the time intervals of single- and double-support phases should not be relied on too heavily. They have to be interpreted in the context of information about spatial parameters, such as radius, body and hammer positions, and path covered by the hammer during these phases. The basic assertion, that the duration of the single-support phases should be less than that of the double-support phases, must be examined from this point of view.

ROTATIONAL KINETIC ENERGY AND POWER

The velocity of the implement during the turns and at the moment of release is the result of the energy transfer by acceleration and deceleration of different parts of the thrower's body. The athlete must transfer a great amount of kinetic energy in short time intervals and must strive to shorten the braking phases, which occur mainly during the single-support phases and can be found also in the middle part or at the end of the double-support phases. In other words, the athlete must achieve a high power level:

$$\text{power} = \Delta\text{energy}/\Delta\text{time} \qquad (22.3)$$

In the case of a rotational movement, the rotational kinetic energy (W) can be calculated as:

$$W = I\omega^2/2 \qquad (22.4)$$

where I = moment of inertia and ω = angular velocity. The average power exerted on the hammer (P_H), or causally produced by the thrower (P_T), is determined by the momentum ($L_{H,T}$) and the angular velocity ($\omega_{H,T}$):

$$P_{H,T} = L_{H,T}\omega_{H,T} \qquad (22.5)$$

Based on these physical relationships, it can be assumed that M. Melinte (who achieved a distance of 73.14 m in 1998, the world's best female performance) produces the power by focusing on the angular acceleration in comparison with throws of other athletes, such as O. Kuzenkova. The long duration of the single-support phases of Melinte's throws in relationship to the double-support phases (compare the data in Tables 22.12 and 22.13) leads to the conclusion that the athlete uses a relatively short path to accelerate the hammer during the double-support phases. To accelerate the body and implement using a short path requires a much higher power level. Equation 22.5 underlines that a wider movement

path, with increased momentum of inertia, and/or faster turns, with increased angular velocity, basically require a correspondingly higher level of driving power in physical terms. An increase in angular velocity does not automatically lead to a faster hammer speed (Eqn. 22.1) if at the same time the movement radius is decreased, for example by a more upright body position or by raised arms/shoulder girdle. Only the necessary power level, developed by special training, can ensure the effective driving interaction between movement path (radius) and angular velocity.

Table 22.6 presents data about the average power for accelerating the hammer during the turns. The data show a doubling of power demands between the first and the penultimate and final turns. The final turn contains the delivery and is characterized by a relatively long duration. It can be assumed for the last turn that the average power, until the low point is passed will reach a value, clearly surpassing the value of the penultimate turn. To add an effective fourth turn, the athlete must be provided with the necessary driving power. In real-life 82 m throws of top male athletes, the peak power calculated for the hammer head during the turns can reach between 3.5 and 7 kW (see Fig. 22.7).

Table 22.7 illustrates the time duration of the turns for one of the world's best hammer-throwers over several years, using four turns. These data serve as a basis for the following calculations regarding performance development during the competition period and for long-term performance development as well. In the following, the kinetic energy for

Table 22.6 Kinetic energy of the 4 kg hammer and average power to accelerate the implement.

Parameter	1st turn		2nd turn		3rd turn		4th turn	
	Start	Finish	Start	Finish	Start	Finish	Start	Finish
Velocity of the hammer (m · s⁻¹)	15	18	18	21	21	24	24	27
Duration (s)	0.30		0.26		0.22		0.24	
Kinetic energy (J)	198		234		270		306	
Average power (W)	660		900		1227		1275	

Note: For the sake of simplicity, the velocity increase during each turn and during the delivery is assumed to be 3 m · s⁻¹.

Table 22.7 Experimental data of total duration for the turns by throws at different performance levels (*top*) and calculated power demands of hammer throws at different performance levels (*bottom*).

Athlete	Age (years)	Date	Hammer mass (kg)	Distance (m)	Total time of the turns (s)
H.W.	27	28 Jul 91	7.26	79.20	2.13
H.W.	29	14 May 94	7.26	74.88	2.23*
H.W.	34	8 Aug 98	7.26	80.04	2.22
F.C.	16	14 May 94	5.0	64.68	1.62
F.C.	17	18 Jun 95	5.0	71.08	1.58
F.C.	18	29 May 96	6.26	67.44	1.58

* (Best performance of the year 81.20 m).

Mass (kg)	Distance (m)	Initial velocity (m · s⁻¹)	Velocity of release (m · s⁻¹)	ΔKinetic energy (J)	Duration (s)	Average power (kW)
5.00	70	16.2	27	1.166	1.50	0.777
7.26	85	18.6	31	2.192	1.40	1.566 (3 turns)
7.26	82	18.0	30	2.091	2.15	0.972 (3 turns)
7.26	75	16.8	28	1.821	2.22	0.820 (4 turns)

the turns is calculated on the assumption that the throwers enter the first turn with a hammer velocity of about 60% (using three turns) or 50% (using four turns) of its release velocity. This assumption is based on experimental data of Bartonietz (1987). The data in Table 22.7 show that the change from a young athlete, throwing 70 m with the 5 kg hammer, to a world-class athlete requires a more than two-fold increase in power. The latter has to transfer much higher kinetic energy to a heavier implement in a shorter time interval. These calculations are related only to the accelerating work of the thrower. In the hammer throw, a great amount of work must be done to stabilize the body and to counteract the centripetal forces. Although this work has to be taken into account, it can be estimated only with great difficulty. For a top thrower, developing performance from the off-season level to a fully competitive level involves a 9% increase in distance, say from 75 m to 82 m, which requires roughly a 20% increase in average power.

A developing young athlete will probably add a fourth turn. With it he or she increases the path for transferring kinetic energy to the implement. In this case, the required power for a final fourth turn is less than the power required for a final third turn. This is the biomechanical basis for the preferred use of a fourth turn, in both male and female athletes. Using four turns, the slower entry allows for better movement control at the beginning. One of the problems is to maintain the correct body and hammer position after three turns for the final, fourth turn. Faults in movement coordination from the beginning have more scope for a negative influence, especially during the last two turns. The 'late catch' of the implement at the beginning of the last double-support phase is a very common fault, especially for young female athletes, reducing the effectiveness of the final turn. Table 22.8 underlines this finding; note the long duration of the single-support phases and the short duration of the double-support phases of the final and penultimate turns.

Reactive strength capabilities of the legs are a crucial part of the movement structure. The results of leg performance diagnosis for hammer-throwers underline this finding. The force–time histories and the biomechanical data show how young athletes have to improve the explosive power of their legs (Fig. 22.10, left). The parameter K characterizes the power output of the legs: the energy of the falling

Table 22.8 Duration (s) of the single- and double-support phases for two female athletes with improving performance.

Athlete	Distance	Year	Support phase*	Turns			
				1st	2nd	3rd	4th
K. Münchow	54.64	1994	Σ (I + II)	0.66	0.62	0.62	
			I	0.32	0.28	0.28	
			II	0.34	0.24	0.24	
	66.61	1998	Σ (I + II)	0.70	0.58	0.44	0.48
			I	0.34	0.22	0.24	0.26
			II	0.36	0.26	0.20	0.22
M. Priemer	50.82	1994	Σ (I + II)	0.64	0.54	0.56	
			I	0.34	0.32	0.30	
			II	0.30	0.22	0.26	
	59.15	1998	Σ (I + II)	0.56	0.50	0.48	0.56
			I	0.28	0.28	0.28	0.30
			II	0.28	0.22	0.20	0.26

Note: An almost stable duration of 0.28–0.30 s for the single-support phases during the turns in throws of M. Priemer (including the delivery) indicates a consistently later planting of the right foot, as video analysis confirms. It is recommended that the duration of the single-support phase from turn to turn is decreased.
* I, duration of the single-support phases; II, duration of the double-support phases.

body (i.e. fall height) plus the energy of the takeoff process (i.e. jumping height) divided by the necessary time interval for both the deceleration and acceleration (i.e. contact time). The differences in K between the athletes are of the same order of magnitude as the above-mentioned differences between the power demands for hammer acceleration. Figure 22.10 (right) shows the ground reaction force–time histories of drop jumps for two top female athletes. The athlete with the better performance in hammer throw achieved the poorer drop-jump performance. This indicates that athlete I.B. has not 'transferred' her physical potential, shown in the jumps, into a corresponding competition result. More specifically strength-orientated work seems to be necessary. Athlete D.S., on the other hand, demonstrates reserves in performance by developing the explosive power of her legwork.

Experimental data (Dapena & McDonald 1989; Dapena 1990; Gutiérrez & Soto Hermoso 1995; Hildebrand & Bartonietz 1995) show that the angular momentum of the implement and of the thrower—the product of the moment of inertia and the angular velocity—increases from turn to turn. This is caused by the addition of rotational energy during the double-support phases by the legwork, and its effective redistribution. The relationship between the initial and final angular momentum is one of the characteristic features of the throwing movement pattern. A throwing technique is effective when the athlete can accelerate the implement by reducing his or her moment of inertia. A perfect throwing pattern gives an additional increase of the angular momentum which reinforces the velocity outcome of the hammer. Taking into account the available time for the energy transfer, further conclusions can made about the applied power and the effectiveness of the hammer drive. The data in Table 22.9 show that the increase in hammer speed during the turns is attributed by a decrease of the moment of inertia. The increase of the moment of inertia at release is probably caused by a lack of leg power during the delivery phase. Further research may reveal if high angular velocities are limiting the increase of angular momentum by legwork.

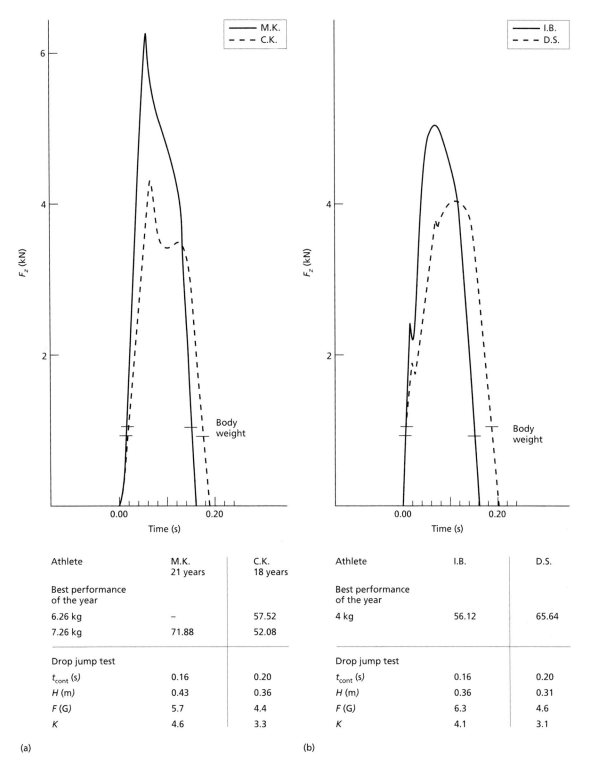

Athlete	M.K. 21 years	C.K. 18 years
Best performance of the year		
6.26 kg	–	57.52
7.26 kg	71.88	52.08
Drop jump test		
t_{cont} (s)	0.16	0.20
H (m)	0.43	0.36
F (G)	5.7	4.4
K	4.6	3.3

(a)

Athlete	I.B.	D.S.
Best performance of the year		
4 kg	56.12	65.64
Drop jump test		
t_{cont} (s)	0.16	0.20
H (m)	0.36	0.31
F (G)	6.3	4.6
K	4.1	3.1

(b)

Fig. 22.10 Ground reaction forces and biomechanical data for drop jumps of two hammer-throwers. Drop height = 0.30 m; K = (drop height + jumping height)/contact time. (a) Male athletes, test data, 19 June 1993 (immediately after the State Championships). (b) Female athletes; test data for athlete I.B., 3 March 1994 (off-season); test data for athlete D.S., 21 July 1995 (in-season).

Table 22.9 Moment of inertia (kg · m²) at the high points (HP) and low points (LP) of the hammer trajectory of throws by two female athletes (data of Hildebrand & Bartonietz 1995) and illustration of the body position at the low points.

Turn no.	Point of trajectory	Athlete (distance of throw)		
		M. (52.26 m)	R.: 3 turns (48.10 m)	R.: 4 turns (45.78 m)
1	HP	5.0	6.0	5.9
	LP	5.1	5.5	5.3
2	HP	5.2	6.5	6.2
	LP	5.1	5.5	5.3
3	HP	5.8	7.0	6.1
	LP	5.0	5.4	5.6
4	HP	–	6.4	6.4
	LP	–	–	6.0
Release		7.5	7.4	9.5

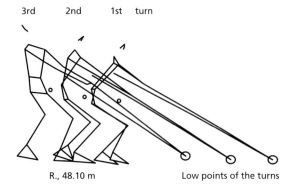

3rd   2nd   1st   turn

R., 48.10 m   Low points of the turns

Biomechanical characteristics of world-class performances

In this section we present biomechanical data of certain world-class performances (e.g. Otto 1990a,b; Morriss & Bartlett 1992; Bartonietz & Borgström 1995), and also examine the movement and biomechanical support of recent top athletes, in order to give a fuller picture of the target technique in hammer throwing. Some examples are given for performance diagnosis.

Table 22.10 Performance data of Balász Kiss in 1991 (junior age), based on data of Szabó. (From Agachi *et al.* 1997.)

Event/exercise	Result
7.26 kg hammer	68.40 m*
8 kg hammer/1.22 m	64.00 m
10 kg implement/1.0 m	49.50 m
30 m sprint, high start	3.6 s
Five hops from standing, both feet	16.98 m
Overhead throw backwards	
Two-handed 6 kg	19.66 m
7.26 kg	18.02 m
Maximum strength training	
Snatch	115 kg
Power clean	165 kg
Deep back squat	215 kg
Deep front squat	190 kg

* Junior World Championship in 1991.

Balász Kiss

STATISTICS

- Height: 1.92 m
- Weight: 115 kg
- Career highlights: 82.90 m in 1997, 83.00 m in 1998, Olympic Champion in 1996, 2nd in the World Championships in 1995, 2nd in the European Championships in 1998.
- Training performance, see Table 22.10.

TECHNIQUE

Balász Kiss has, to a large extent, a model technique, characterized by the following
- Deeply squatted body position, going into the turns and during the turns.
- Angle of the right knee at the moment of planting of the first turn 90°, keeping the forward tilting momentum low. (On other throwers, using a more upright body position, a longer lever by 20% can act.)
- 'Knee fall' of the left leg during the single-support phases: at the moment of takeoff (2nd to 4th turns) the left shank has an almost vertical position; at the

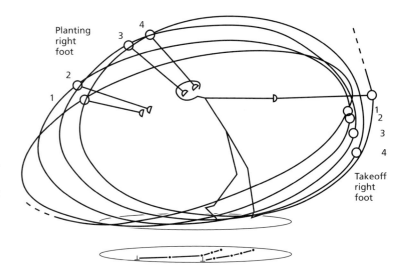

Fig. 22.11 Trajectory of the hammer movements, hammer positions at the moment of takeoff, and planting of the right foot and placement of the feet during the turns (view from behind: Balász Kiss, 79.02 m, 6 August 1995). (From Bartonietz & Borgström 1995.)

high points of the hammer path the shank is inclined by about 60° (angle between shank axis and horizontal is 30°, i.e. the left knee is dropped).

- Base shortening during the turns (Fig. 22.11).
- Perfect relationship between single- and double-support phases during the years 1995–1998.
- With each consecutive turn there is faster left heel planting before the low point of the hammer path is achieved, an element of a good rhythm (Table 22.11).
- Improving the body position: an ineffective leading head movement was noticed during the last turns in 1995, but in 1998 the head was back and looking at the hammer head.
- 'Early catch' of the hammer from the first and second turns to the third and fourth turns (Fig. 22.11).
- Powerful final leg extension, with knee angles of 90–75° for the left and right leg at the beginning of the last double-support phase, and full leg extension at the moment of release in 1998 (but the crossed legs hinder a stable body position immediately after release).

Olga Kuzenkova

STATISTICS

- Height: 1.76 m
- Weight: 70 kg
- Arm span: 1.77 m

Table 22.11 Throws of Balász Kiss: duration of legwork phases. (1995 data based on Bartonietz & Borgström 1995.)

Throw (m)	Year	Turns				Total time (s)
		1st	2nd	3rd	4th	
79.02	1995					2.12
Phase I (s)		0.30	0.24	0.18	0.18	
Phase II (s)		0.40	0.28	0.26	0.28	
81.24	1996*					2.16
Phase I (s)		0.30	0.24	0.18	0.18	
Phase II (s)		0.38	0.26	0.28	0.24	
LH touchdown (s)		0.18	0.14	0.14	0.14	
79.32	1997†					2.14
Phase I (s)		0.32	0.26	0.22	0.20	
Phase II (s)		0.40	0.26	0.24	0.24	
80.71	1998					2.14
Phase I (s)		0.34	0.24	0.20	0.20	
Phase II (s)		0.38	0.28	0.24	0.26	
LH touchdown (s)		0.18	0.16	0.14	0.12	
81.26	1998					2.12
Phase I (s)		0.30	0.24	0.22	0.20	
Phase II (s)		0.40	0.28	0.24	0.24	
LH touchdown (s)		0.20	0.16	0.14	0.12	

Note: Phase I, single-support phase; phase II, double-support phase; LH touchdown, left heel touchdown.
* Olympic Games.
† World Championships.

• Career highlights: 73.10 m in 1997 (world record), 74.40 m in 1999, 2nd in the World Championships in 1999.

TECHNIQUE

Based on data of Barclay (1996), Olga Kuzenkova has achieved training performances of 150 kg in the squat, 100 kg in the clean and 70 kg in the snatch. Olga's technique has the following characteristics.

• Two preliminary swings—used by the majority of female and male hammer-throwers—and at the high point of the second swing an active turn of the upper body towards the hammer for sweeping the implement to the front. The low point is reached in a 7 o'clock position.

• She uses a wide initial stance, 47% wider than her shoulder width, going into the first turn. The distance between the feet decreases from the base (0.55 m) up to the delivery (0.37 m), by a factor of about 35%.

• With consecutive turns there is shortening of the duration of the single-support phase, with the double-support phases being longer than the single-support phases (see Table 22.12; data of 1995 and 1996) (the best competitive throws are characterized by shortening of the single-support phases to benefit the double-support phases; Bartonietz et al. 1997). However, the performance data of 1997 and 1998 show the opposite: longer single-support phases and shorter double-support phases during the important final turns. To realize such a pattern, the athlete must have at her disposal a much higher power level for transferring a greater amount of rotational kinetic energy in shorter time intervals to her body and to the implement. In other words, Kuzenkova became stronger, but her throwing technique did not keep pace with her improved abilities.

• The head leads the movement, going into the first turn at a perfect 4.30 o'clock position (73.10 m). Looking to the ball of the hammer would be more effective for a wide hammer movement and a fast turn under the hammer (out run).

• During the four turns, at the moment of planting the right foot, the twist between the hip and shoulder axes reaches almost 40°. This occurs due to the wide path of the hammer head and the fast turn of

Table 22.12 Throws of Olga Kuzenkova: duration of legwork phases. (Data of present author and from Bartonietz et al. 1997.)

Throw (m)	Year	Turns				Total time (s)
		1st	2nd	3rd	4th	
66.00	1995					2.26
Phase I (s)		0.30	0.26	0.24	0.22	
Phase II (s)		0.50	0.30	0.26	0.30	
LH touchdown (s)		0.24	0.18	0.18	0.12	
67.58	1996					2.40
Phase I (s)		0.30	0.23	0.24	0.25	
Phase II (s)		0.50	0.35	0.23	0.30	
71.22	1997					2.26
Phase I (s)		0.34	0.28	0.26	0.24	
Phase II (s)		0.44	0.24	0.22	0.24	
69.28	1998					2.20
Phase I (s)		0.32	0.26	0.28	0.28	
Phase II (s)		0.34	0.26	0.20	0.26	
LH touchdown (s)		0.16	0.14	0.10	0.14	

Note: Phase I, single support phase; phase II, double-support phase; LH touchdown, left heel touchdown.

the right leg around the left. (In comparision, in Sedych's world-record throw of 86.74 m, accomplished with three turns, at the moment of planting the right foot there was a difference between the shoulder and hip rotation of 50°—Otto 1990a.) At the low points no more twist occurred and a 'tracking angle' was noticed (see Fig. 22.6, below), with the hip and shoulder axis being almost parallel. This shows that the legs were the effective 'engine' for driving the implement through the low points of its trajectory.

Figure 22.12 illustrates the trajectory of the hammer movement. The left heel plants before the low point of the hammer's trajectory is reached (Table 22.12), with effective work of the right against the stable left side, driving the upper body plus the triangle formed by the shoulder axis and grip. The athlete achieves an almost optimal angle of release of 41°, throwing a distance of 67.58 m.

The crossed legs during the delivery (throws of 66.00 m and 67.58 m), caused by an early hip and knee extension of the free leg towards the ground,

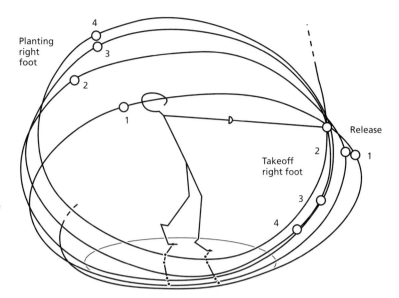

Fig. 22.12 Trajectory of the hammer movements, hammer positions at the moment of takeoff, and planting of the right foot and placement of the feet during the turns (view from behind: Olga Kuzenkova, 66.00 m, 30 June 1995). (From Bartonietz *et al.* 1997.)

possibly hinders the maximum effort of the final pull. Kuzenkova's jumping movement, with a shift in body weight to the left side after release, is an indication of residual impetus, which could be better used for a more powerful final pull.

Mihaela Melinte

STATISTICS

- Height: 1.70 m
- Weight: 89 kg
- Career highlights: 73.14 m in 1998; European Champion in 1998, World Champion in 1999.

TECHNIQUE

Melinte's throw at the European Championships in 1998 (distance 71.17 m) is characterized by the following.
- Low squatted body position going into the first turn, with a left knee joint angle of 90° at takeoff.
- Early takeoff, at the 4 o'clock position, but late planting of the right leg (9 o'clock position) due to the inward rotation of the right foot.
- Almost continuous narrowing of the stance during the turns (initial stance slightly greater than

shoulder width), with the leg base of the third turn being wider than the base of the second turn.
- Short double-support phases in relationship to the single-support phases (Table 22.13).
- Her low body position, with relatively great initial moment of inertia, and the short double-support phases for hammer acceleration indicate a high level of driving power.
- With each consecutive turn there is faster planting of the left heel, which points to a good legwork rhythm.

Table 22.13 Throws of Mihaela Melinte: duration of legwork phases.

Throw (m)	Year	Turns				Total time (s)
		1st	2nd	3rd	4th	
68.84	1997					2.04
Phase I (s)		0.32	0.30	0.28	0.26	
Phase II (s)		0.24	0.22	0.18	0.24	
71.17	1998					2.06
Phase I (s)		0.32	0.28	0.26	0.28	
Phase II (s)		0.28	0.22	0.22	0.20	
LH touchdown (s)		0.12	0.08	0.06	–	

Note: Phase I, single-support phase; phase II, double-support phase; LH touchdown, left heel touchdown.

• The short leg base and minimum backlean at release allows a wide movement radius and a high angular velocity.
• A very stable and balanced body position after release.

Biomechanical characteristics of training exercises

The need for greater power in competition is the starting point for planning and putting into practice both training of technique and improving general and specific strength capacities (maximum and specific strength, throwing training). As discussed above, to increase the distance thrown with the competition implement basically requires an increase in power of the main muscle groups. Training must be aimed at developing a perfect technique with the necessary specific strength abilities. Sporting technique and physical abilities are the two main aspects of that complex phenomenon, the athlete's movement. Technique should therefore develop as physical abilities grow, and conversely, growing abilities demand a development in technique.

Up to half of all training throws are made using hammers of various weights and lengths (Schotte & Stache 1982; Bakarinov 1987; Bartonietz 1990). It is beneficial to know what effects these different training hammers have on the competition movement. Heavy implements with reduced length are used in an effort to conserve the time pattern of the legwork, which is typical for the competition exercise. With growing physical abilities, the athletes can effectively use a longer hammer radius: the 10 kg hammer was thrown in the mid-1960s with 0.80 m length, and the 12 kg implement with a length of 0.60 m (Samosvetov 1967). Fifteen years later the 10 kg hammer was thrown with 1.0 m length and the 12.5 kg implement with a length of 0.70 m (Schotte & Stache 1982; see also the overview by Bartonietz 1987). The world record was extended during these two decades by more than 10 m (see Table 22.2). The basic idea is, from the biomechanical point of view, to transfer to the heavy implement more kinetic energy in the same or less time. Figure 22.13 shows the relationship between transferred kinetic energy and implements of different masses and lengths. The data of Losch (1990), included in Fig. 22.13, belong to an unknown number of throws of top athletes during the period 1986–88. There are counteracting effects to note of the shortening of the hammer and of the mass increase: the shorter wire reduces the path for transferring energy to the implement. But, all in all, due to the mass increase, the reduction of kinetic energy is kept within reasonable limits. For example, if moving from the

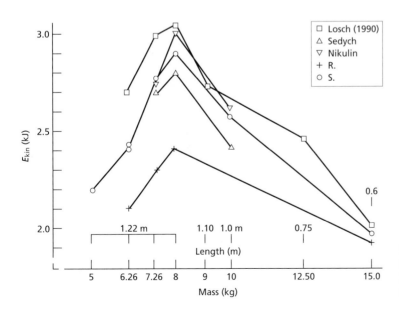

Fig. 22.13 Kinetic energy of hammers with different masses and lengths. (From Bartonietz 1987; incorporating data from Losch 1990.)

8 kg implement to the 15 kg implement, the length is decreased by 0.62 m (51%), but the kinetic energy drops by only about 21%. Thus, the athlete can achieve a great amount of physical work. Table 22.14 illustrates the energy and power relationship for such throws. The times for the double-support phases are based on experimental data obtained from one of the world's best athletes in 1998. The data underline the efficiency of the 8 kg hammer: the power needed to reach a distance of 70 m is, under the given assumptions, higher than with the 7.26 kg implement. Experimental data presented from training throws of an elite female athlete (Debbie Sosimenko; Australian record holder, distance thrown in 1999, 66.78 m) and the anticipated velocity of release, kinetic energy and average power data underline the fact that lighter implements require, at a certain stage of training, less power than the competition implement (see also Bartonietz 1987). This does not, however, mean that light implements have no place in a training system. Gutiérrez and Soto Hermoso (1995) recorded and analysed a 100.67 m throw with the 6 kg implement made by A. Astapkovich in preparation for the Olympic Games in 1992. It can be calculated that work of about 3.4 kJ must be done on this implement. This physical work could result in a velocity of release of 30.4 m · s^{-1} for the 7.26 kg hammer—enough for a throw of about 85.5 m. In 1992 A. Astapkovich reached a distance of 84.26 m, almost at this target 85 m level. To assess this result in relation to the 100 m outcome with the 6 kg implement, the training regime must be known, especially the number, intensity and time course of throws with light, normal and heavy implements. Theoretically there is a possibility that greater accelerating work could be done on the 7.26 kg implement, resulting in distances *over* 85 m. The attempt to interpret such data substantiates once more the necessity of interdisciplinary work between biomechanics and training science.

For top young athletes or adult athletes at a lower performance level, the maximum power output is achieved by throwing the 6.26 kg implement. For these athletes, the 7.26 kg implement functions as a heavy implement. For each athlete, a power–mass history can be determined as a basis for the effective use of implements of different mass and length.

For a desired training effect, the angular velocities have to be equal to or only slightly less than throws with the competition implement. This allows the development of specific strength more efficiently than by using the competition implement alone. Investigations of throws with hammers of various masses and length (Schotte & Stache 1982; Stache 1983; Bartonietz 1987; Losch 1990) indicated that coaches and athletes must consider the fact that with increased masses and shortening of the wire the working conditions for the driving muscle groups are changed, especially the relationship between the muscular work to accelerate the implement and the thrower and the quasi-static muscular work to counteract the centripetal forces and to stabilize the body. Using heavy implements with normal length, the centripetal force component increases dramatically: for example, by throwing the 10 kg implement with a length of 0.85 m, a centripetal force component of 3 kN was recorded, whereas throwing with the standard length of 1.22 m resulted in 4.3 kN (Stache 1983). Using heavier implements causes the tangential acceleration of the hammer to decrease. The change in hammer velocity—as a measure of acceleration, through virtually constant time intervals—during the third turn in throws of a top athlete were as follows: 4 m · s^{-1} with the 15 kg implement, 5 m · s^{-1} with the 10 kg implement and 6 m · s^{-1} with the 8 kg, 7.26 kg and 6.0 kg implements (Stache 1983). But the tangential force component, as a product of mass and acceleration, increases due to the dominating influence of mass.

The high level of the centripetal force component, for which the thrower has to compensate by leg and trunk work, has led to a hypothesis about a maximum strength component of the throwing training of hammer-throwers (Arbeit *et al.* 1988; Losch 1990) concerning the 8 kg/1.22 m implement. It permits the development of specific strength capacities of the legs and the trunk for maintaining the stability of the thrower-hammer system. Special investigations have to verify this hypothesis.

The data in Fig. 22.13 and Tables 22.14 and 22.15 indicate that hammers with lower mass than the competition implement are useful for developing

Table 22.14 Kinetic energy and power of the hammer movement by throws of implements of different masses and lengths.

Hammer mass (kg)	Hammer length (m)	Distance (m)	Velocity of release (m · s⁻¹)	Duration of double-support phases (s)	ΔKinetic energy (kJ)	Average power (kW)	Comments	Source
6.26	1.21	80	29	1.10	1.974	1.795	4 turns	Present author
7.26	1.21	75	28	1.10	2.134	1.940		
8	1.21	70	27	1.10	2.187	1.988		
10	1.00	55	24	1.20	2.160	1.800		
		50	23	1.20	1.984	1.653		
3	1.21	65	26.3	0.76	0.165	0.217	Experimental data, athlete D. Sosimenko, training 21 July 1995 with 3 turns (personal best in 1994 65.24 m) and estimation of the energetic data	Barclay, Gathercole, Bartonietz (unpublished work)
4	1.21	59	25	0.78	0.200	0.256		
6	1.00	39.09	21.3	1.04	0.145	0.139	Training 4 October 1995	
4	1.21	56.40	24.3	0.98	0.188	0.192		
3.5	1.21	59.35	25.1	0.92	0.175	0.190		

Table 22.15 Maximum resulting force acting on the hammer head in throws of implements of different masses and lengths (average values of 32 throws by top athletes). (From Bartonietz 1987.)

Mass (kg)	Length (m)	Maximum resulting force on the hammer head	
		(kN)	%
5	1.22	2.3	84
6.26	1.22	2.4	88
7.26	1.22	2.7	100
8	1.22	2.8	104
10	1.00	2.9	107
15	0.60	2.95	109

the movement pattern for higher speed. With such throws the athlete achieves a higher angular velocity and a longer path of acceleration. However, as a result of the low external resistance, kinetic energy, power and consequently forces are lower, and so the training effect is limited.

Implications of biomechanics for training

Based on the knowledge presented here, coach and athlete should be able to determine in more detail the current performance level of the athlete, and plan future training more effectively to reach targeted performances in both training and competition. The interpretation of data from applied biomechanical research substantiates the necessity of interdisciplinary work of biomechanics and training science. Accumulation of knowledge about the basic elements of hammer-throwing technique—the correct internal image of the technique—is fundamental for the development of coaches and athletes alike. This section will attempt to give guidance to athletes, coaches and other team members responsible for training top athletes.

The world's best female and male hammer-throwers demonstrate a high level of sporting technique. This, in association with results from other throwing events, has allowed the formulation of a 'target technique'. Even so, biomechanical analysis shows that top athletes usually have some room for performance improvement. The main requirements for male hammer-throwers are valid also for the training of female athletes:

• a high level of consciousness and execution of the training exercises corresponding with the demands of the target technique;

• optimization of the yearly training cycle, by varying the components of the training load with regard to volume, intensity and quality; and

• balancing the training loads with restorative and prophylactic measures.

Relation between skills and abilities

In the hammer throw there exists an inseparable relationship between the athlete's sporting technique and his or her mechanical performance capacity. As a result, the perfection of technique has to be a year-round process: strength must be increased within the bounds of technique, which requires special training throughout the year. The unity of skills and physical capacities underlies all strength and technique training. Biomechanical research, accompanying the training process, can improve training efficiency by covering strength training exercises into the analysis.

Angular velocity and radius of the hammer movement

The interaction between angular velocity and radius of the hammer movement produces the linear velocity of the hammer. The athlete has to find the right compromise between a long radius and a high angular velocity, based on the level of his or her event-specific skills and abilities.

Single- and double-support phases

A long duration of the double-support phases suggests an effective hammer drive. The relationship between the duration of the single-and double-leg ground-contact phases can serve as a criterion for performance diagnosis. However, such data concerning time intervals should not be over-emphasized. They have to be interpreted in close association with information about spatial parameters, such as radius, body and hammer positions, and distance covered by the hammer during these phases. Although hammer movement data can provide a yardstick to verify the biomechanical hypothesis, further research is necessary.

Energy transfer and power

Energy transfer between thrower and implement is relevant for performance diagnosis and training, but needs more research. Effective throwing involves acceleration of the implement by reducing the moment of inertia of the thrower. With a perfect throwing pattern, the additional increase of the angular momentum reinforces the velocity outcome. Knowledge about the available time for the energy transfer allows further conclusion to be made about the applied power and the effectiveness of the hammer drive. Using kinematic data—changes of hammer velocity and legwork duration—some insight into energy transfer and power production can be obtained.

Leg power is one of the crucial elements in hammer throwing. A rough estimation shows that for a 10% increase in distance thrown, the available average power must increase by 20%. During each consecutive turn, the thrower has to transfer an increasing amount of kinetic energy to the implement in a shorter time interval, hence the greater and greater power demand per turn. It can be assumed that the available power is limiting the thrower's effectiveness, especially in the final two turns. As performance improves during the training years, athletes must apply a greater amount of kinetic energy to the implement (higher release velocities and greater mass) in shorter time intervals (i.e. faster turns). The use of a fourth turn is an option for keeping the power required relatively low but places high demands on movement coordination.

Implements of different lengths and weights

For advanced athletes, throws with heavy implements are an effective means of increasing leg and trunk power, alongside special and maximum-

strength exercises. The increase in hammer mass, wire shortening and realized movement pattern influence the biomechanical component of the training effect.

Throws with lighter implements are useful in developing the speed pattern of the throw. However, they demand a lower power level in comparison with the competition implement. Hence their effectiveness is limited. For advanced male hammer-throwers, throws with the 8 kg/normal-length hammer are an effective means of improving the power capacity under event-specific conditions. Throws with heavier and shorter implements are characterized by a high amount of physical work but decreased power to accelerate the implement. With increasing mass, the centripetal and tangential force components increase. The determination of individual power–mass histories can serve as a basis for an effective use of implements with different masses and lengths. In general, throws with hammers of various lengths and masses have the same general effects on male and female athletes. But the specific movement patterns of throws using implements of different masses and lengths does not automatically cause the changes required for improvement of competition throws. These changes happen only after considering the movement pattern of throws of different implements.

Recommendations for coaches and athletes

From biomechanical analysis of the hammer throws, the following recommendations can be made.
• Strive for a wide movement path of the implement going into the first turn, based on a flexible shoulder girdle.
• Keep the body low going into the first turn, and also the subsequent turns, to minimize the tilting momentum, to create a wide movement path of the implement, and enable a powerful leg extension during the delivery.
• Strive for effective use of existing capacities in the necessary body positions, or use special strength exercises, before increasing the maximum strength level; use drills such as multiple swings and turns with weights, different in their forms and masses; imitations to feel comfortable in the position. This

is necessary to avoid a gap between non-specific capacities and skills.

• Coaches must watch for the key body positions, and should be confident about the way the thrower and hammer interact. Familiarization with the energy transfer between athlete and implement— redistribution of rotational energy—is essential. The effective training implements for each athlete have to be selected taking into account at least the duration of the turns and the velocity of release, respectively, distance thrown. Further applied research should be guided and supported by coaches.

References

Agachi, T., Bakarinov, Y., Barclay, L. *et al.* (1997) NSA Round Table 34—hammer throw. *New Studies in Athletics* **2/3**, 13–27.

Arbeit, E., Bartonietz, K., Börner, P. *et al.* (1988) *Erhöhung der Wirksamkeit des Einsatzes spezieller Kraftübungen zur Entwicklung wurfspezifischer Kraftfähigkeiten.* Research Institut for Sports (FKS), Leipzig.

Barclay, L. (1996) Olga Kuzenkova's Australian visit. *The Thrower* **71**, 22–23.

Bakarinov, Y. (1987) Metanie molota: Evoluzija i perspectivy. [Hammer throw: evolution and perspectives.] *Legkaya Atletika* **1**, 12–14.

Bartonietz, K. (1985) Diente der Schmiedehammer als Vorbild? *Der Leichtathlet* **8**, 7–9.

Bartonietz, K. (1987) Zur sportlichen Technik der Wettkampfübungen und zur Wirkungsrichtung ausgewählter Trainingsübungen in den Wurf- und Stoßdisziplinen der Leichtathletik. [The technique of competition exercises and the effect of selected training exercises in the throwing events and shot put.] Postdoctoral thesis (habilitation), Deutsche Hochschule für Körperkultur, Leipzig.

Bartonietz, K. (1990) Biomechanical analysis of throws with hammers of various weight and length as basis for an effective training technique in athletics. In: *Technique in Athletics*, The First International Conference, Cologne, 7–9 June 1990, (eds G.-P. Brüggemann & J.K. Rühl), pp. 542–551. Sport und Buch Strauss, Cologne.

Bartonietz, K. (1994a) A biomechanical analysis of throws with different weight and length hammers. *Modern Athlete and Coach* **4**, 33–36.

Bartonietz, K. (1994b) Hammerwurf der Frauen—quo vadis? *Lehre der Leichtathletik* **33** (3) 15–16, 33–34, (4), 18.

Bartonietz, K. (1994c) Werfertag Halle 14.5. 1994: Übersicht über Stützzeiten. Olympic Training Centre of Rhineland–Palatinate, Mainz (unpublished research result).

Bartonietz, K. & Borgström, A. (1995) The throwing events at the World Championships in Athletics 1995, Göteborg—Technique of the world's best athletes. Part 1: shot put and hammer throw. *New Studies in Athletics* **4**, 43–63.

Bartonietz, K., Schotte, K.H. & Stache, H.J. (1986) *Technikleitbild Hammerwurf.* Forschungsinstitut für Körperkultur und Sport, Leipzig.

Bartonietz, K., Barclay, L. & Gathercole, D. (1997) Characteristics of top performances in the women's hammer throw: basics and technique of the world's best athletes. *New Studies in Athletics* **2/3**, 101–109.

Black, C.B. (1999) *History of Hammer Throw.* http://www.saa-net.org/free/hist.html (13.02.2000).

Bondarchuk, A.P. (1985) *Metanie Molota.* Fizkultura i sport, Moscow.

Bujak, G.A. (1983) Formirovanie ritmovoj struktury dvizhenij metatelej molota v processe mnogoletnej podgotovki. [Development of movement rhythm in hammer throw during several years of preparation.] Thesis for dissertation, GZOLIFK, Moscow.

Dunn, G.D. & McGill, K. (1994) *The Throws Manual,* 2nd edn. Tafnews Press, Mountain View, CA.

Dapena, J. (1984) The pattern of hammer speed during a hammer throw and influence of gravity on its fluctuations. *Journal of Biomechanics* **17** (8), 553–559.

Dapena, J. (1990) Some biomechanical aspects of hammer throwing. *Track Technique* **111**, 3535–3539; **113**, 3620.

Dapena, J. & Felter, M.E. (1989) Influence of the direction of the cable force and of the radius of the hammer path on speed fluctuations during hammer throwing. *Journal of Biomechanics* **6/7**, 565–575.

Dapena, J. & McDonald, G. (1989) A three-dimensional analysis of angular momentum in the hammer throw. *Medicine and Science in Sports and Exercise* **21** (2), 206–220.

Gathercole, D. (1996) Biomechanical analysis of the hammer throw, Optus Grand Prix, Hobart, 25 February 96. Australian Institute of Sport, Belconnen/ACT (unpublished research result).

Gutiérrez, D.M. & Soto Hermoso, V.M. (1995) Análisis biomechánico del lanzamiento de martillo. In: *Análisis biomecánico de los lanzamientos en atletismo, Investigaciones en ciencias del deporte, number 1,* (ed. Ministerio de Education y Ciencia), pp. 3–45.

Hildebrand, F. (1982) *Eine Analyse der Technik des Hammerwerfens.* Forschungsinstitut für Körperkultur und Sport, Leipzig.

Hildebrand, F. & Bartonietz, K. (1995) Eine biomechanische Analyse des Hammerwerfens am Beispiel der Technik zweier Werferinnen. In: *Schriftenreihe zur angewandten Trainingswissenschaft* **3** pp. 45–56. Meyer & Meyer, Aachen.

Hwang, I. & Adrian, M. (1984) Biomechanical analysis of hammer throwing. In: *Proceedings of the 1984 Olympic Scientific Congress—Biomechanics* (eds M. Adrian & H. Deutsch), pp. 79–86. University of Oregon, Eugene, OR.

Kollodij, O. (1972) Specialnye uprasznenija metatelej molota. *Legkaja Atletika* **18**, 18–19.

Krevald, A.A. (1975) Biomechanicheskij analiz prostranstvennogo sportivnogo dvizhenija (na primere metanija molota). [Biomechanical analysis of spatial movements in sports.] Dissertation, Polytechnic College, Tallin.

Losch, M. (1990) Trainingsableitungen aus biomechanischen Untersuchungen im Hammerwurf. In: *Technique in Athletics. The First International Conference, Cologne, 7–9 June* (eds G.-P. Brüggemann & J.K. Rühl) Vol. 2, pp. 532–541. Sport und Buch Strauss, Cologne.

Morriss, C. & Bartlett, R. (1992) Biomechanical analysis of the hammer throw. *Athletics Coach* **26** (3), 11–17.

Muybridge, E. (1955) *The Human Figure in Motion* (introduction by Robert Taft). Dover, New York.

Otto, R. (1990a) Kinematic analysis of the World record in the hammer throw—Juri Sedych throws 86.74m. In: *Technique in Athletics. The First International Conference, Cologne, 7–9 June 1990* (eds G.-P. Brüggemann & J.K. Rühl) Vol. 2, pp. 523–531. Sport und Buch Strauss, Cologne.

Otto, R. (1990b) Biomechanical analysis of the hammer throw—Athens 1986 and Rome 1987. In: *Technique in Athletics. The First International Conference, Cologne, 7–9 June 1990* (eds G.-P. Brüggemann & J.K. Rühl) Vol. 2, pp. 561–570. Sport und Buch Strauss, Cologne.

Otto, R. (1992) NSA photosequences 22—Hammer throw, commentary. *New Studies in Athletics* 3, 51–65.

Pataki, L. & Slamka, M. (1979) Struktura vykonu v hode kladivom z hladiska pohybovych schopnosti. Teor. Praxe tel. Vych. 27 (4), 208–214.

Pozzo, R. (1987) Biomechanische Mittel für Techniktraining und -diagnostik im Hammerwerfen. *Leistungssport* 3, 35–41.

Pozzo, R. (1990) Ground reaction forces and hammer kinematics in the pre- liminary winds and in the 1st and 2nd turns during hammer throwing. In: *Technique in Athletics. The First International Conference, Cologne, 7–9 June, 1990* (eds G.-P. Brüggemann & J.K. Rühl) Vol. 2, pp. 552–560. Sport und Buch Strauss, Cologne.

Romanov, I. & Vrublevsky, J. (1998) Women and the hammer—some tech- nical and kinematic characteristics. *Modern Athlete and Coach* 4, 35–37.

Samosvetov, A. (1967) *Zamenit normalnogo molota.* [Change the normal hammer.] *Legkaja Atletika* 5, 16–17

Schotte, K.-H. & Stache, H.-J. (1982) Untersuchungen im Hammerwurf zur Bewegungsstruktur von Würfen mit Geräten unterschiedlicher Masse und Länge und ihre methodische Auswert- ung im Rahmen eines Trainings- experimentes. Forschungsinstitut für Körperkultur und Sport, Leipzig.

Shukevich, E. & Krivonossov, M. (1971) *Metanie Molota.* [Hammer throw.] Fizkultura i Sport, Moscow.

Stache, H.-J. (1980) Biomechanische Untersuchungen zur Modifizierung des Technikmodells im Hammerwurf und zur Unterstützung und Fundierung des zielgerichteten Einsatzes schwerer Wurfgeräte. Forschungsinstitut für Körperkultur und Sport, Leipzig.

Stache, H.-J. (1983) Zwischenbericht zur biomechanischen Charakteristik von Hammerwürfen mit Geräten unter- schiedlicher Masse und Länge, nachgewiesen an ausgewählten Parametern. Forschungsinstitut für Körperkultur und Sport, Leipzig.

Susanka, P., Stepanek, J., Miskos, G. & Terauds, J. (1987) Hammer-athlete relationship during the hammer throw. In: *Biomechanics in Sports III & IV. Pro- ceedings of the International Symposium of Biomechanics in Sports, Halifax/Canada 1987* (eds J. Terauds, B.A. Gowitzke & L. Holt), pp. 194–200.

Tutevich, V.N. (1969) *Teorija sportivnych matanij.* [Theory of the throwing events.] Fizkultura i Sport, Moscow.

Voronkin, V.I & Limar, P.L. (1989) Metanie molota. [Hammer throw.] *Legkaja Atletika*, Moscow 1989, 590–607.

Chapter 23

Hitting and Kicking

B.C. ELLIOTT

Introduction

Many Olympic sports involve hitting or kicking actions. In these striking skills, a distal segment such as the foot in a kick, the hand in a hit, or a racket/stick interact with a ball or object.

Coaches of high-performance athletes are constantly attempting to have their players hit or kick a ball faster, while maintaining an acceptable level of control. This chapter reviews biomechanics research which endeavours to identify factors that are integral to success in hitting and kicking. The techniques used can then be optimized, the risk of injury reduced and rehabilitation programmes better structured.

The Olympic sports of tennis, field hockey, baseball (batting), badminton, boxing and volleyball will be used to provide hitting examples; while soccer will be used to provide an understanding of kicking. To avoid repetition, the chapter integrates the preparation, backswing, forward swing, impact and follow-through phases of movement as they apply to hitting and kicking.

Preparation for movement

Generally these movement skills are poorly understood and, for this reason, are rarely practised. Effective footwork and quick movement to the ball should never be considered something that comes naturally. What then, are the key factors that assist an athlete to react to the appropriate visual cue(s) and move quickly into position and prepare to impact an object with an implement, foot, hand or head?

Unweighting

Perhaps one of the most important aspects of movement is the way that it is initiated. Groppel (1984, p. 36) stated that 'regardless of the position a skilled tennis player assumes while awaiting the opponent's shot, upon or just prior to impact by the opponent, the player will unweight'. What is this unweighting and how does it relate to rapid movement about a court or field? Before an athlete prepares to move, the force applied to the ground, and therefore the equal and opposite force applied by the ground to the feet (ground reaction force: GRF), is equal to body weight (area 1 in Fig. 23.1). Once the decision to move is made, the knees flex and the body (hip in figure) is accelerated towards the ground. Mean peak velocities of the hip for high-performance tennis players during this preparation were $0.5 \, \text{m} \cdot \text{s}^{-1}$ and $0.4 \, \text{m} \cdot \text{s}^{-1}$ for the forehand (Elliott et al. 1989a) and backhand (Elliott et al. 1989b) drives, respectively. The force of the athlete's body on the court is therefore lowered (unweighted—area 2 in Fig. 23.1). This unweighting is an integral part of the initial preparatory movement, whether it is before a return of serve in tennis/volleyball or moving to defend against an opponent in soccer/hockey.

The rapid flexion of the knees must obviously cease, otherwise the body would move into a full squat position. This deceleration of the downward movement (area 3 in Fig. 23.1) is caused by eccentric contraction of the quadriceps group. Hence tension is developed in this muscle group and elastic energy is stored (Komi & Bosco 1978). The preloading of the quadriceps, in combination with the stored energy,

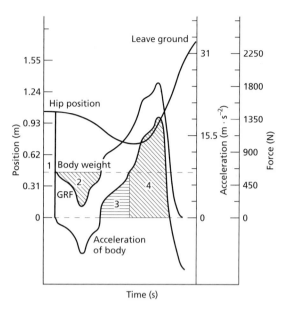

Fig. 23.1 Vertical position, acceleration and ground reaction force (GRF) in a standing jump.

is used to assist the concentric quadriceps contraction during the lower limb drive, if the movement of knee flexion is followed quickly by knee extension. Knee extension and the acceleration upwards of the body (area 4 in Fig. 23.1), increases the GRF and therefore allows the player to drive from the court/field in the direction of the next hit or kick. The key to these movements is the timing of the knee flexion-extension action to coordinate with the opponent's stroke or movement. Athlete effectiveness in this action relies on the ability to cue to key elements of the opponent's movements.

Cuing

While awaiting the ball, the batter in baseball or receiver in tennis and volleyball has two problems, namely a sensory-perceptual issue followed by a motor response. The sensory-perceptual problems consist of visually tracking a ball such that a decision must be made as to where and when to swing, and whether or not the ball should be played at all. On the motor side, the bat or limb(s) must be moved with the correct timing and sequencing so as to

ensure the swing coincides precisely with the time of arrival of the ball in the contact zone. When an object, such as a ball, is moving towards an athlete, or conversely, the athlete approaches the object, the image on the retina of the eye becomes progressively larger. The rate of dilation of the image on the retina may be the trigger for a specific motor response. It has been shown that the assessment of movement velocity of the ball (the tau: the time it takes for an object to reach a given position) is at least in part used to control the timing of movement. Hypothetical strategies used to control velocity are beyond the scope of this chapter; however, an introduction to 'tau-hypotheses' can be found in Zatsiorsky (1998) and Abernethy and Burgess-Limerick (1992). Research studies in this area clearly show that continuous time-to-contact information is critical to successful performance (Lee *et al.* 1983; Peper *et al.* 1994). Athletes do not predict where a ball can be impacted and then move the hand/implement to that position. Actions are continuously geared to source information.

A major perceptual problem facing athletes is therefore one of tracking the ball and predicting its course. Harrison (1978) wrote that visual dynamics would be greatly improved if baseball hitters adopted a sequence of visual focuses while watching the pitcher. This sequence could easily be modified for returning serve in tennis or volleyball.
1 Soft focus—watch the whole body/general area of mound.
2 Fine focus—focus on the letter on the cap or something in the plane of the ball at release.
3 Specific fine focus—focus on the area of release, i.e. the hand and ball.

Selective attention to specific areas is necessary because the attention process in fast ball sports is limited by three factors at least (Norman 1969; Jones 1972).
1 The amount of information in the display.
2 The time available to take in the required information.
3 The ability of the player.

A review of visual processes in baseball is presented by Grove (1989). Expert-novice differences in the use of perceptual strategies such as anticipation, scanning and focusing to reduce the quantity and enhance the quality of the to-be-processed input information are outlined in Abernethy (1987, 1991).

A brief review of the relevant literature on cuing in hitting sports follows. Higher performance players are able to process critical information earlier in the opponent's action, thus permitting more time to move to the ball (Goulet *et al.* 1989) and giving the impression that they 'have all the time in the world'. It also has been shown that attention to early cues provided by the actions of a baseball pitcher is critical to batting performance. High-performance players were faster than novices at responding and accurately predicting the path of the ball (Paul & Glencross 1997).

While experts and lesser skilled players may pick up different information from cues, there is no general agreement in the literature as to whether there are differences in the eye movement patterns of players of varying skill levels. Some expert-novice differences in eye movement patterns have been reported (e.g. Goulet *et al.* 1989). However, these cannot account fully for variations in anticipatory skill, as differences in the ability to anticipate exist even when visual search patterns are essentially identical (e.g. Abernethy & Russell 1987). Skilled players must be able to 'look' at the right cues and 'see' the information these cues provide.

Hubbard and Seng (1954) showed that high-performance baseball batters used pursuit movement of the eyes with the head essentially fixed when tracking a pitched ball. Tracking movement of the eyes stopped when the ball was 2.5–4.5 m from the plate. This was because the eyes are not capable of tracking at very close distances and high velocities (Bahill & La Ritz 1984). As these authors emphasized, this does not mean that coaches should minimize the importance of theoretically tracking the ball 'as long as possible'. De Lucia and Cochran (1985) showed that, while baseball batters extracted tracking information over the entire ball trajectory, the middle third of the flight seemed critical to success. Accurate processing of information from the hitting/throwing action of the opponent, together with tracking information, is obviously critical in sports when the ball approaches at high velocity. Then, one can make the precise predictions of the temporal and spatial coordinates of the approach-ing ball which are necessary for a successful impact (Abernethy 1987).

A further logical expectation with respect to hitting/kicking sports is that the expert performer will have a more precise knowledge of event probabilities than a novice. This experience will guide their selective attention, with respect to realistic outcomes, and ultimately their skilled performance. It is therefore evident that a 'knowledge structure' is established in tennis and baseball, which can make use of particular cues to guide perception and action.

Regular training has shown that a player may develop a more acute sensibility to the perceived signals and thus improve decision-making (Davids *et al.* 1989). In baseball, when varsity-level performers were tested with respect to visual cues (marked vs. unmarked baseballs), players hit a greater percentage of marked than unmarked balls (Osborne *et al.* 1990). This result, plus earlier research by Burroughs (1984), suggests that the addition of visual cues could be a significant and beneficial technique to enhance hitting performance. Research has also shown that players in all hitting and kicking games must purposefully practise cuing (Abernethy 1996). Then, prediction of ball direction, or opponent's actions, and subsequent movement to the appropriate position on the court/field can be enhanced.

Balance

Rapid movement to the impact area combined with a balanced stance, which enables a ball to be hit or kicked effectively, is a prerequisite for skilled performance. Quick movements and balance are determined by a number of factors. The first is where the line of gravity (a line from the centre of gravity perpendicular to the ground) falls with respect to the base of support. An athlete is most stable if this line is central to the base of support. If quick movement is required, the centre of gravity should be positioned near to the edge of the base towards which the action is most likely to occur. Where movement direction is uncertain the athlete generally moves this line closer to the forward edge of the base of support (body weight on the toes). This creates an unstable position and prepares one for quick movement in any direction. Players also tend to lower their centres of gravity to create more stable positions from which to kick in soccer or dig in volleyball.

Backswing

The backswing phase involves positioning the body such that selected muscles and tissues are 'stretched' and a segment or implement is displaced for the forward swing phase of the movement.

Approach

The general trend in skill development is that a backswing is initiated from a stationary position prior to including a run-up to increase the speed of the foot/hand or implement (Bloomfield *et al.* 1979; Opavsky 1988). In kicking, this run-up changes from a straight to a more curved approach as skill level improves. Isokawa and Lees (1988) reported that an angled approach of 30–40° enabled the leg to be tilted in the frontal plane so that the foot could be placed further under the ball, thereby making a better contact.

In the volleyball spike, the approach phase is characterized by 2–3 steps during which time the centre of gravity is lowered. This lowering is also linked to the storage of energy, which has been discussed previously. The approach also enables the spiker to gain horizontal momentum, which is then converted primarily to vertical momentum by actions that follow. International players bring the trailing foot forwards to join the leading foot using a 'step-close' plant style prior to the '2-foot' jump to position the body for the spike (Coleman *et al.* 1993).

Segment/implement displacement

Research into hitting/kicking skills typically has shown that the trunk and upper limb rotate in hand-based movements, while the trunk and lower limb rotate in foot-based activities to appropriately position the body for the forward swing. In tennis, almost all strokes are characterized by trunk and upper limb rotations. For example, in groundstrokes, the upper trunk rotates approximately 120° from the preparatory position to the completion of the backswing (Elliott *et al.* 1989a,b; Elliott &

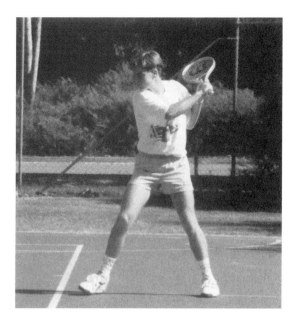

Fig. 23.2 Backswing position for a backspin backhand in tennis.

Christmass 1995) (Fig. 23.2). Takahashi *et al.* (1996) reported a trunk twist angle of approximately 30° in the tennis forehand, which showed that the upper trunk (shoulder alignment) was rotated more than the lower trunk (hips) at the completion of the backswing. This has the effect of stretching muscles and associated tissues. The racket in tennis is rotated approximately 100° in the forehand (Elliott *et al.* 1989a) and 130–180° in the backhand (Elliott *et al.* 1989b; Elliott & Christmass 1995) from a position where it was initially pointing at the opponent. A greater racket displacement was also recorded for volleys hit at the service line when compared to those played at the net (Elliott *et al.* 1988).

In baseball, Welch *et al.* (1995) showed from force plate data that the centre of pressure was moved 20 cm posterior to its original position in preparation for the transference of weight in the forward swing. A major league professional player rotated the bat by approximately 120° (Galinas & Hoshizaki 1988) in preparation for the forward swing.

Large segment and stick rotations are also apparent in the field-hockey penalty corner hit (Fig. 23.3).

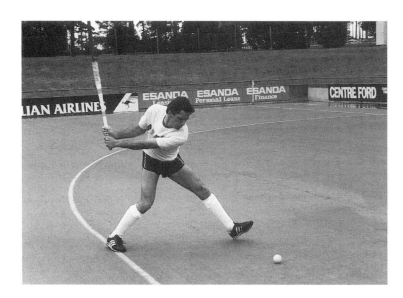

Fig. 23.3 Backswing position in the penalty corner hit in field hockey.

At the completion of the backswing, the trunk is rotated such that the hips are generally in line with the intended direction of the hit, while a line through the shoulders is further rotated. Elite performers revealed mean elbow angles of approximately 90° and 155° for the right and left elbows, respectively (Elliott & Chivers 1987). This enabled the stick to be positioned almost vertically to the ground at the completion of the backswing.

In badminton, Gowitzke and Wadell (1979) were the first to emphasize the need for upper limb, long axis rotations (forearm pronation/supination, upper arm internal/external rotation), together with hand and trunk rotations, as essential preparatory movements for effective speed generation in the forward swing. Tang *et al.* (1995) provided data to support these assertions in reporting angular displacements of 50°, 36° and 40° for pronation, ulnar flexion and palmar flexion, respectively, in the badminton smash.

In boxing, Smith and Hamill (1985a) recorded higher fist velocities than previously reported. Their subjects were permitted to use more degrees of freedom in the backswing phase of the action. That is, a forward stepping action and greater trunk rotation were used in the striking action to assist the development of fist speed.

Forward swing to impact

In the forward swing phase of hitting/kicking skills, movement is augmented if muscles have been preloaded and elastic energy stored during the backswing. Where controlled high speed is a required characteristic of the forward swing, a greater number of body segments must be coordinated than would occur if only control was required. Segment/implement speed (forward, side-to-side and up-or-down) and trajectory at impact dictate the type of collision (off-centre or through the centre of the ball), and the subsequent direction, spin and speed of the projectile (ball or shuttle). The mechanics associated with all types of impacts, whether between the hand and a ball (volleyball), a boot and a ball (soccer) or an implement and a ball (tennis) will be discussed in the impact subsection of this chapter.

Augmentation to performance

Hitting and kicking movements are generally characterized by a stretch–shortening cycle (SSC) of muscular activity. An eccentric contraction (during late backswing) is followed by concentric muscle activity in the forward swing. High levels of muscular activity during the eccentric phase of muscle action and the magnitude of prior stretch have been suggested as factors that enhance the storage of elastic energy (Wilson *et al.* 1991) and preload the muscles used in the concentric phase of the movement (van Ingen Schenau *et al.* 1997). In fact, 30% of the variance in augmentation to internal rotation of the upper arm from prior stretch was accounted for by maximum angle of external rotation (Elliott *et al.* 1999). The maximum angle recorded, either at the completion of the backswing or early in the forward swing, may represent the magnitude of prior stretch. Hence a greater prestretch might result in a better prepared muscle for consequent concentric contraction (van Ingen Schenau *et al.* 1997).

The pause period between the stretch and shorten phases of movement also has been shown to influence the level of augmentation. Mean augmentations to performance of 22% and 19%, respectively, were recorded during internal rotation of the upper arm for a no-pause compared with a 1.5 s pause condition (Elliott *et al.* 1999), and when a no-pause bench press was compared to one performed using a purely concentric movement (Wilson *et al.* 1991). These values are similar to the 21.9% augmentation to jump height when a rebound knee bend was compared to a no-rebound condition (1.5 s pause: Thys *et al.* 1972); and the 21% increase in speed for a simulated kicking action when using an SSC rather than a purely concentric muscular contraction to extend the knee (Bober *et al.* 1987). Significant relationships between pause time and augmentation from prior stretch have been shown by Aura and Komi (1987) and Wilson *et al.* (1991). Aura and Komi (1987) reported a correlation of −0.60 between pause duration and mechanical efficiency of SSC leg flexion and extension movements performed on a sledge ergometer. Wilson *et al.* (1991) found a significant relationship of −0.72 between pause duration and relative concentric impulse for the bench-press movement. In general terms, approximately 50% of the benefit from prior stretch is lost after a pause period of 1 s (Wilson *et al.* 1991).

The augmentation to performance occurs early in the forward swing phase. Chapman and Caldwell (1985) reported that augmentation to a forearm rotation movement occurred within the first 0.25 s of the action. This was similar to the 0.2 s period reported by Wilson *et al.* (1991) for a bench-press movement. It should be noted that this assistance often comes when the body segments are in positions of poor mechanical efficiency, which further enhances the significance of the augmentation.

Therefore, hitting and kicking athletes use the SSC to benefit performance. While the absolute augmentation following a prior stretch may vary, research has clearly shown that the influence is significant.

The coordination of multiple segments

Almost all hitting and kicking skills require that maximum speed is produced at the end of a distal segment in a kinematic chain. The effectiveness in this summation is determined by the manner with which each body segment moves with respect to the more proximal segment. The multitude of coordination sequences (e.g. 'kinematic chain', 'kinetic chain') can most easily be imagined as being variations on Bunn's (1972) 'summation of speed principle'. In essence, the principle states that, to produce the largest possible speed at the end of a chain of segments, the motion should start with the more proximal segments and proceed to the more distal segments. The more distal segment begins its motion at the time of the maximum speed of the proximal one and each succeeding segment generates a larger endpoint velocity than the proximal segment. Many investigators have demonstrated proximal-to-distal sequencing in terms of either linear velocities of a joint which represents a segment endpoint (e.g. malleolus of tibia: the ankle), segmental angular velocities (e.g. the leg) or joint angular velocities (e.g. the knee).

HITTING IN TENNIS

Selected strokes will be used in this section to characterize hitting in tennis. A full review of tennis stroke production can be found in Elliott (2000).

The serve

Lower limb GRFs of sufficient magnitude to drive the body 'off the ground' (Elliott & Wood 1983; van

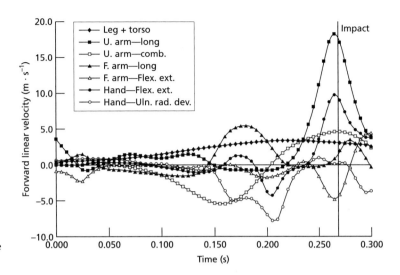

Fig. 23.4 Average linear tennis serve velocities (direction of opponent, velocity measured perpendicular to the baseline) for 11 high-performance players.

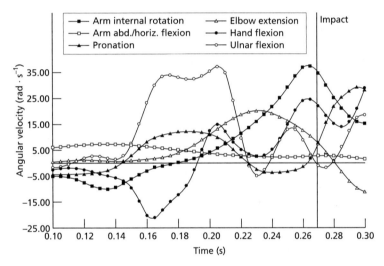

Fig. 23.5 Average upper limb segment angular velocities in the tennis serve for 11 high-performance players.

Gheluwe & Hebbelinck 1986), together with trunk rotation, produce a forward and upward shoulder speed of approximately 10–20% of the racket speed at impact (Elliott *et al*. 1986; van Gheluwe & Hebbelinck 1986; Elliott *et al*. 1995). These lower limb and trunk actions also drive the racket 'down behind the back' and away from the body such that muscles and tissues that cross the shoulder and elbow joints are 'put on stretch'. While this may enhance performance, it also creates a high level of shoulder and valgus (outward) stress at the elbow, which increases the potential for injury (Bahamonde 1997; Noffal *et al*. 1998).

The forward linear velocities of the racket-head and upper arm segment endpoints in the service action, together with their angular velocities, are shown in Figs 23.4 and 23.5, respectively. The sequence of rotations shows that upper arm flexion and abduction peaks first. This is followed by elbow extension, hand/ulnar flexion, upper arm internal rotation and hand flexion, and finally minor racket adjustments from forearm pronation (Elliott *et al*. 1995). Thus, while proximal-to-distal sequencing is demonstrated by the segment endpoints (Fig. 23.4), it is not entirely supported when all degrees of freedom for upper limb segments are considered

(Fig. 23.5). The major contributors to the mean linear forward velocity of the centre of the racket-head ($\approx$31.0 m · s^{-1}) at impact were upper arm internal rotation (30–50%) and hand flexion ($\approx$30%) (van Gheluwe *et al.* 1987; Elliott *et al.* 1995).

Groundstrokes

The roles of individual segments in the multi-segment stroke were compared to the single unit forehand by Elliott *et al.* (1989a). However, the biomechanical basis for the multi-segment stroke, with particular reference to the topspin forehand, is best provided by Takahashi *et al.* (1996) and Elliott *et al.* (1997).

Trunk rotation and extension of the lower limbs initiate the forward movement of the racket, and are responsible at impact for much of the speed of the 'hitting-shoulder'. Fujisawa *et al.* (1997) showed the importance of a vigorous trunk rotation in creating a lag in the hitting arm movement, which stretched shoulder musculature in the early forward swing. The trunk continued to rotate forwards such that by impact the shoulders were almost parallel with the baseline and the level of trunk twist was approximately 10° (shoulders forward of hips: see Fig. 23.6d). Similar forward shoulder speeds of approximately 2 m · s^{-1} at impact were observed for flat, topspin and topspin lob strokes, although upward velocity varies across strokes. Shoulder speed has been shown to contribute approximately 15% (Elliott *et al.* 1997) of the forward and upward impact speed of the racket. van Gheluwe and Hebbelinck (1986) reported low GRFs in driving the body forwards, and therefore trunk rotation and any forward movement of the body were responsible for the majority of this shoulder speed.

Forward movement of the upper arm is a key feature of forehand mechanics (Fig. 23.6a–d). It produces 20–30% of forward velocity and approximately 20% of upward velocity, depending on the grip being used. The elbow angle remains relatively constant ($\approx$100°) throughout the forward swing and therefore movement at this joint is not used in the development of racket speed for impact. The upper arm rotates internally from an externally (outward) rotated position at the completion of the backswing, in the period immediately before and after impact

(Fig. 23.6c,d). This movement, which was identified in the forehand of an elite player (Deporte *et al.* 1990), was shown by Elliott *et al.* (1997) to be an integral feature in the generation of impact racket speed (30–40%). van Gheluwe and Hebbelinck (1986) had previously shown that muscles responsible for internal rotation of the upper arm were strongly active prior to and at impact, and Bahamonde and Knudson (1998) reported that internal rotation torque at the shoulder was also high at impact.

Depending on the method of holding the racket, the hand flexes forwards and upwards and plays an important role in the generation of racket speed (Fig. 23.6b–d). Players using a western grip are able to derive a greater proportion of upward racket velocity ($\approx$20%) from hand movements when compared with those who use an eastern grip ($\approx$5%). The ability to produce upward racket velocity is an integral part of topspin stroke production and provides a distinct advantage for players using 'western-type' grips.

The mechanical basis of the topspin (Elliott *et al.* 1989b; Wang *et al.* 1998) and backspin backhand strokes is provided by Elliott and Christmass (1995). Because the general mechanics of these strokes are similar to the kinematic flow in the forehand stroke, they will not be discussed in this chapter.

The one-handed vs. two-handed backhand

This brief review summarizes research to provide a coach with the background to the strengths and weaknesses of these strokes. The speed of the racket at impact is derived from the product of the radius of rotation (distance from impact location to shoulder) and the rotational speed of the upper limb(s) and racket, plus any forward speed of the body. All else being equal, an increase in this radius (more extended hitting limb) will produce a higher forward impact speed which, theoretically, favours the one-handed technique. The reduced moment of inertia (swing weight) of the upper limb system (racket closer to hitting-shoulder) and possible increase in strength (both upper limbs) with the two-handed stroke may assist the player in attaining a higher rotational speed of the racket-limb system, thus counteracting the effect of a reduced hitting radius. However, does

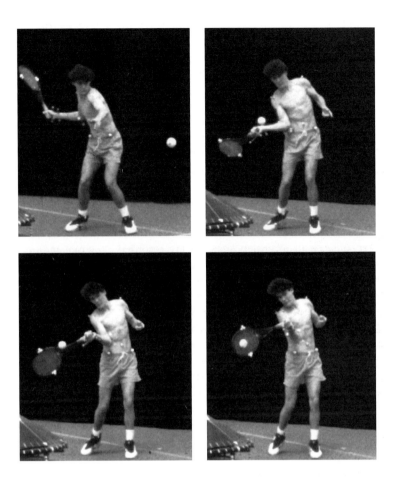

Fig. 23.6 A–D: Forward swing during the tennis forehand drive.

the increased reach of the one-handed stroke influence the reach of a player during a normal stroke? It has been shown that there is no difference in the distance between the impact location and the body (hitting radius) for the two strokes (Groppel 1978). This is providing the player was not required to run or stretch for the ball.

Giangarra *et al.* (1993) demonstrated that increased upper limb muscle activity was generally higher in the double-handed technique when compared with that recorded in the single-handed stroke. Therefore any changes in the incidence of 'tennis elbow' for players using this technique may not be related to a reduced activity in the extensor muscles. Rather, they are caused by factors associated with flawed stroke mechanics or impact conditions, particularly in the single-handed stroke.

The volley

Because this stroke involves an impact that requires more control than power, it differs from the strokes discussed previously. The small trunk rotation of 10° for the forehand volley, and the minimal change for the backhand volley, highlight the importance of general forward movement in these strokes. A shoulder speed of 2 m · s⁻¹ was reported for the forehand volley of an elite player (Deporte *et al.* 1990). When this is compared with the racket speeds of approximately 11 m · s⁻¹ for high-performance players at impact reported by Elliott *et al.* (1988), it shows that approximately 20% of the racket speed is derived from forward movement.

Upper limb movements which reach their peak levels at similar times, a characteristic of accuracy-based activities, are responsible for the development of the majority of racket speed at impact. There are only small changes in abduction/adduction shoulder joint angle, from the position in the backswing to impact. This suggests that this joint is involved in racket orientation, although horizontal flexion does increase upper arm speed. The elbow joint angle increases ($\approx 10°$) from the backswing position to impact for both forehand and backhand volleys, irrespective of court location (Elliott et al. 1988). The role of elbow extension in the generation of impact racket speed was also reported for the forehand volley of a national-level performer (Deporte et al. 1990). However, only small extension speeds were recorded at impact by Elliott et al. (1988), which stresses the need for impact stability at the elbow joint. Wrist joint flexion in the forehand volley and extension in the backhand volley showed that the hand also plays a role in speed generation of the racket. A key finding was that a line drawn from the wrist to the tip of the racket must be aligned perpendicular to the direction of the hit, both at and after impact (Elliott et al. 1988).

HITTING IN VOLLEYBALL

Coordinated actions of body segments have been shown to be an integral part of the takeoff and flight phases of the skilled volleyball spike, whereas this was not the case with lesser skilled players (Maxwell 1982). Wedaman et al. (1988) reported that while poor spikers were not uncoordinated, there were large overlaps between the segment sequencing in their actions, which led to an inefficient action.

A coordinated spiking action commenced with ankle joint plantarflexion, and extension at the knee and hip joints, such that the body is driven upwards. Relatively high hip and knee extensor angular velocities (≈ 9 rad $\cdot$ s^{-1} and 19 rad $\cdot$ s^{-1}, respectively: Sampson & Roy 1976; Coleman et al. 1993), and plantarflexion angular velocity (≈ 19 rad $\cdot$ s^{-1}: Coleman et al. 1993) were responsible for the 3.6 m $\cdot$ s^{-1} centre of mass vertical velocity at takeoff (Sampson & Roy 1976; Coleman et al. 1993).

The sequence of movements in the spike was typically reported as: trunk rotation, followed by upper arm, forearm and hand movements (Maxwell 1982). The study by Coleman et al. (1993) showed that, while the above sequence was generally true, preimpact upper arm internal rotation had the strongest correlation to ball velocity. However, elbow angular velocity did not show a significant correlation. This phenomenon has previously been discussed with reference to the tennis service action (Elliott et al. 1995). Therefore elbow extension (not to 180°) occurs earlier in the sequence to produce an extended upper limb, prior to the internal rotation which produces much of the power in the hit. The use of the non-hitting arm also is important in this sequenced action (Coleman et al. 1993). That is, the equal and opposite reaction of the non-hitting limb being rotated downwards assists the hitting action when the body is off the ground.

Maxwell (1982) indicated that the impact in the volleyball spike should occur at or near the top of the jump. The mean -0.2 m $\cdot$ s^{-1} vertical velocity of the centre of mass for 10 international players at impact supports this.

A brief review of other volleyball hitting skills is included to direct interested coaches to other research literature. Tant et al. (1993) showed that the jump spike and serve have more commonalities than differences, particularly with reference to segment angles and temporal parameters. At the point of contact, the armswing seems to be identical between the skills within each sex. However, differences were noted between the sexes. Therefore young players may expect a skill carryover from one action to the other.

Marryatt and Holt (1982) reported that the following three factors were associated with a successful contact between the forearms and the ball when initiating a return of serve.

1 The greater the angle of the left elbow ($\approx 180°$) at contact with the ball, the more successful the contact.

2 The smaller the angle formed by the left elbow, mid-grip and right elbow (effective hitting platform) the more successful the contact.

3 The smaller the difference between the path of the mid-point of the elbows through contact and the path of the rebounded ball, the more successful the contact.

Because of the time of contact between the ball and the forearms the return of serve in volleyball is a hitting action where all upper limb segments must be positioned for impact.

Ridgway and Wilkerson (1987) reported that the similarities in action when setters execute a front and back set, far exceeded any technique differences. As would be expected, the head, trunk and shoulders exhibited the greatest positional variance between sets. This study also showed that elbow extension occurred prior to ball contact, which makes setting more of a striking skill rather than a catching-throwing skill.

HITTING IN BADMINTON

It has been shown that proximal-to-distal speed generation is a key feature of badminton stroke production. While research into different strokes shows varying displacement and speed profiles (smash: Tang *et al.* 1995; drop/cut: Sakurai *et al.* 1989; smash/clear/drop spike: Ye 1991; overhead power: Gowitzke & Waddell 1979; underhand clear/serve: Gowitzke & Waddell 1986), a coordinated sequencing of motion is evident across strokes. Sakurai *et al.* (1989) reported angular velocities of 9.9, 18.1 and 14.6 rad · s^{-1} for internal rotation, pronation and ulnar flexion, respectively, for a relatively low-velocity badminton shot. Tang *et al.* (1995) reported pronation and palmar flexion angular velocity levels of 43.6 and 19.2 rad · s^{-1}, respectively, in the high-velocity jump smash. The importance of long axis rotation about the upper arm and forearm, and hand movements in velocity generation, are clearly evident. It should also be noted that internal rotation and hand flexion occur late in badminton stroke production. Therefore, summation does not completely follow a proximal-to-distal pattern.

HITTING IN BASEBALL/HOCKEY

The motion of the baseball bat is similar to the hockey stick in that it occurs in two phases. The first is the change from a vertical to a horizontal orientation of the long axis of the bat/stick, and the second is characterized by rapid rotation in the horizontal plane. The position and speed of the bat at impact is produced by a coordinated sequence of movements proceeding from the ground to the hips, shoulders, arms and, finally, the hands. Hirano (1987) reported that skilled batters (Japanese college level) recorded higher impact speeds of the centre of gravity of the bat (22.6 m · s^{-1}) when compared with lesser skilled players (19.9 m · s^{-1}). Professional players who were analysed by Welch *et al.* (1995), recorded a mean end-of-bat speed of 29 m · s^{-1} at impact when hitting a ball from a tee.

As the stride of the front limb shifts body weight forwards (0.85 m stride length) the hips rotate forwards and the shoulders continue to rotate away from the ball. This increases the 'coiling of the trunk' (Welch *et al.* 1995). Skilled players did not rotate their hips as early as lesser skilled players but were able to produce a greater lower trunk rotational speed prior to impact than the lesser skilled (Hirano 1987). Then, as the shoulders rotated forwards, the arms continued to rotate away from the ball around the axis of the trunk. Peak rotational velocities for the hips (0.075 s), followed by the shoulders and arms (0.065 s), were recorded prior to impact. Nearing the point of impact, the hitter then rotated the last link in the 'kinematic chain', i.e. the hands, such that the bat reached its maximum angular rotation 0.02 s prior to impact.

Another feature of skilled hitting performance is the delayed 'uncocking' of the wrists, which has been shown to occur in golf (Milburn 1982). This delay allows acceleration of the arms to reach a higher level and the acceleration of the stick to be summed with the existing maximum angular acceleration of the proximal segment. The skilled players analysed by Hirano (1987) and Welch *et al.* (1995) also used this technique to produce a high impact velocity. The less-skilled batters 'uncocked' the wrists earlier in the forward swing, which increased the moment of inertia of the upper limb-bat system and recorded a lesser peak angular velocity.

A study by Galinas and Hoshizaki (1988) reported changes in joint angles and the resultant bat alignment (when considered in combination with the direction of the pitch) required to hit the ball to different parts of the field. Players significantly modified the angular displacement of the bat, and reduced the level of shoulder and hip segment rotation to hit the ball to the right when compared with left sections of the field. They also noted that the high variability about the left elbow and shoulder joints, over repeated trials, was a reflection of neural adaptations needed to adapt the swing in order to make optimal contact with the ball.

In field hockey, much of the power of the hit is derived from lower limb, trunk and upper limb rotations, as is the case in baseball (Elliott & Chivers 1987). In the penalty corner hit, the two upper limbs operate in a coordinated but independent manner. The left upper limb (right-handed hitter) works primarily as a double pendulum, as described for golf, but the right upper limb works as three separate units (upper arm, forearm and hand) (Elliott & Chivers 1987). Figure 23.7 shows the delayed 'uncocking' of the left hand up to 0.04 s prior to impact. Mean speeds of 38.6 m · s⁻¹ for male strikers, and 31.5 m · s⁻¹ for female hitters, demonstrated the high quality of players studied by Elliott and Chivers (1987).

KICKING IN SOCCER

Browder *et al.* (1991) carried out a three-dimensional (3D) description of fast and slow instep kicking (ball speeds of 17.0 and 13.5 m · s⁻¹, respectively) for female players and reported greater pelvic rotational movement for the faster kick (18° vs. 13°), while hip abduction remained relatively constant (19°).

During the early forward swing, the thigh increases its angular velocity and the leg is held flexed in a relatively constant position. This decreases the moment of inertia of the lower limb and reduces the energy needed for rotation. The thigh and leg then increase their angular velocities until just prior to impact. Then, there is a marked increase in leg angular velocity and a decrease in thigh angular velocity. Wickstrom's (1975) description of the kicking skill suggests that the thigh becomes almost stationary at impact, although research data suggest that this is not entirely true. For adult players, thigh angular velocities at impact of –2.8 to 5.4 rad · s⁻¹ have been reported (Aitcheson & Lees 1983; Putnam 1993); while values for children of up to 5.9 rad · s⁻¹ also have been reported (Day 1987). However, com-

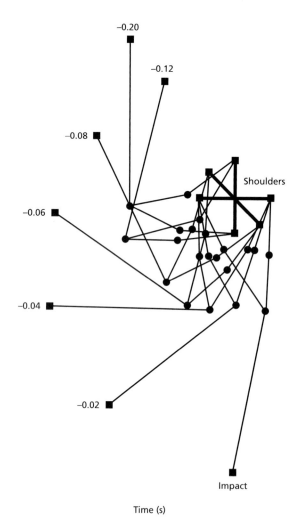

Fig. 23.7 Upper limb angular displacement during the downswing for an elite penalty corner hitter in field hockey.

pared to the 35 rad · s⁻¹ reported by these studies for the angular velocity of the leg, or 19.5 rad · s⁻¹ for knee joint angular velocity (Rodano & Tavana 1993), the thigh has a minor effect on foot speed at impact. Asami and Nolte (1983) reported a significant correlation of 0.74 for professional soccer players between ball and foot speed, which suggests that foot speed is a significant factor in the mechanics of the foot–ball impact. The section on impact (below) contains a more comprehensive review of how interactions with different parts of the foot affect ball speed. For experienced adult players, mean maximum ball speed has been reported to be in the range of 20–30 m · s⁻¹ (Asami & Nolte 1983; Robertson & Mosher 1985; Luhtanen 1988; Narici *et al.* 1988; Opavsky 1988).

Kinetic studies on kicking have provided some insight into causal mechanisms with reference to the above rotations. Zernicke and Roberts (1978) reported that the greatest muscle moments were generated about the hip (280 N m), then about the knee (140 N m) and finally about the ankle joints (30 N m), and that these reduced with decreasing speed of rotation. Robertson and Mosher (1985) reported hip and knee moments of 220 and 90 N m, respectively, for national-level players. At impact, values at all joints are relatively small, possibly indicating the level of muscle co-contraction (stability) at each joint.

Luhtanen (1988) reported that the peak knee moment occurs after the peak hip moment, whereas Putnam (1983) suggested that these occur in the reverse order. Therefore there are two lines of thought on lower limb segment interaction in the forward swing phase of a kick. One theory is that an extensor hip moment is recorded just prior to impact, which increases the rotational velocity of the leg (Luhtanen 1988). Roberts (1991), in a simulation of a toe-kick, reported that the leg could be accelerated or decelerated through its joint connection to the thigh without any muscular moment. A second line of thought is that the high level of leg rotation actually slows thigh rotation. Dunn and Putnam (1987) found that four male college-level soccer players recorded a flexor resultant joint moment at the hip over the phase where the thigh was decelerating. Thus, thigh deceleration was primarily influenced by the motion of the leg and not by the resultant joint moment at the hip, regardless of the speed of the motion. Sorensen *et al.* (1996) was also of this opinion when presenting data on martial arts kicking.

Regardless of which of the two theories is correct for soccer or kicking in general, it is apparent that players should be taught to try and continue flexing the thigh and extending the leg at as high a rate as possible at impact for an optimal result.

Impact

For the equations discussed in this section to be valid the requirement is that during the collision the colliding bodies do not interact. For this reason impacts that are considered to be of short duration and elastic (linear momentum conserved) will be discussed under the 'short-period impacts' subheading. Those where interaction between the end effector (hand, foot, implement) and the ball logically would occur are treated in the 'longer-period impact' subsection.

Short-period impacts

During the initial part of an impact both bodies deform (to some extent) and the energy stored in the deformation will be partly returned in subsequent movements (imperfectly elastic collision). Linear momentum is conserved in such direct impacts, when the velocity vectors are parallel, and the forces of impact act through the centres of mass. Such an impact may be expressed algebraically as (Newton's law of impacts):

$$V_{ball} - V_{bat} = -e\,(U_{ball} - U_{bat}) \qquad (23.1)$$

where V_{ball} and V_{bat} are velocities of the bodies after impact, U_{ball} and U_{bat} are their respective velocities before impact, and e is the coefficient of restitution (determined by the materials and construction of colliding objects).

Equation 23.1 may be used to answer the question as to whether the speed of a pitched baseball influences the postimpact speed, if all other things are equal. A 95 m.p.h. (≈ 42 m · s⁻¹) fastball pitch is hit by a batter with a preimpact bat velocity (speed in the horizontal direction) of 36 m · s⁻¹, which slows to 30 m · s⁻¹ immediately after impact. If the bat has a 0.5 coefficient of restitution and the direction of the bat and hence postimpact ball velocity is considered positive then this velocity can be calculated as follows:

$$V_{ball} - V_{bat} = -e\,(U_{ball} - U_{bat})$$
$$V_{ball} - 30 = -0.5\,(-42 - 36)$$
$$V_{ball} = 39 + 30$$
$$= 69 \text{ m · s}^{-1}$$

Similarly, a ball pitched at 38 m · s⁻¹ (≈85 m.p.h.) can be shown to produce a postimpact ball velocity of 67 m · s⁻¹. All other things being equal, and remembering that one may not be able to hit the faster pitch, and that the coefficient of restitution will be marginally lower for a higher velocity impact, you can hit the fastball with a slightly higher speed than a slower speed pitch.

Lees and Nolan (1998) described other mechanical factors that may be evaluated during the direct impact of a soccer kick:

$$V_{ball} = V_{foot} \times \frac{(M) \times (1+e)}{(M+m)} \qquad (23.2)$$

where V_{ball} is the velocity of the ball (postimpact); V_{foot} is the impact velocity of the foot; M is the effective mass of the system (the mass equivalent of the foot/leg complex); m is the mass of the ball; and e is the coefficient of restitution.

The ratio of $M/(M + m)$ in Eqn. 23.2 gives an indication of the rigidity of the foot and leg at impact, and relates to the activity and strength of the muscles involved in the kick. The force of impact serves to deform the foot at the metatarsophalangeal joints (if the foot is plantarflexed) and this deformation will have an effect on the firmness of impact.

Asami and Nolte (1983) reported that the ≈20° change in ankle joint angle did not correlate with ball speed; however, the change in angle at the metatarsophalangeal joints (≈ 30°) correlated significantly with ball speed ($r = -0.81$). To decrease this deformation, impact should be made as close as possible to the ankle joint and not on the toes of the foot. Lees and Nolan (1998) predicted that:

$$V_{ball} = 1.2 \times V_{foot} \qquad (23.3)$$

Zernicke and Roberts (1978) reported a regression equation between foot and ball speed over a ball velocity range of 16–27 m · s⁻¹ as: $V_{ball} = 1.23 \times V_{foot} + 2.72$. The relationship advocated by Lees and Nolan (1998) in Eqn. 23.3 would therefore seem a good 'rule of thumb'.

Longer-period impacts

Research by Tsaousidis and Zatsiorsky (1996) found that certain aspects of impact theory in soccer kicking need to be rethought as the contact time (≈16 ms) is longer than for tennis (≈5 ms, Brody 1987) and much longer than the ≈0.5 ms in golf (Gobush 1990). They reported that the collision phase in kicking could only barely be described as an elastic impact during which the total momentum of the system is conserved. There are three factors in favour of the idea that the energy which is supplied by the muscles during the collision cannot be disregarded.

1 During contact the ball-foot displacement is ≈ 26 cm.

2 At the instant of peak deformation, the ball possesses considerable speed (≈13 m · s⁻¹), which is more than 50% of the resulting ball speed.

3 During the ball-recoil, the foot does not decelerate in spite of the force that is acting on it from the decompressing ball (possibly due to counterbalancing muscle force).

These results supported data collected using high-speed videography (4500 f.p.s.) by Asai et al. (1995). They reported a mean contact time of the instep with the ball of approximately 9 ms and a horizontal contact distance of approximately 15 cm.

The results of these studies support the recommendation given by coaches that the 'follow-through' (continued emphasis on impact zone) increases the amount of mechanical work on the ball by the muscles during impact.

In short-period impacts, movements (speed, trajectory of racket and racket-face angle) needed to produce velocity, direction and spin must occur prior to impact. In longer-period impacts, while the above is also important, mechanical work may be applied to the ball during contact (to increase ball velocity and change direction). Therefore inappropriate movements during impact may in fact affect accuracy.

Boxing

Boxing will be considered as a special impact situation and will be discussed separately. While research has been conducted on many facets of boxing, the scope of this chapter necessitates a focus on impact between the glove and the body. As a force of 784 N for about 8 ms has been shown to produce a head acceleration sufficient to cause concussion

(Wayne State Tolerance Curve: Hodgson & Thomas 1981), the research reviewed focuses on the delivery of force during impact.

Smith and Hamill (1985a) showed that skill level did not affect fist speed (approximately 11.5 m · s⁻¹) 0.01 s prior to impact. However, with similar fist speeds, highly skilled subjects were able to impart more momentum to a boxing bag than intermediate or low-skilled subjects. The fact that a boxing glove transmitted more momentum to the bag than a bare fist is a warning for coaches. The cushioning effect of the gloves may encourage subjects to hit harder since the impact would be less painful to the person delivering the punch (Smith & Hamill 1985a). The gloves studied by these researchers could not be considered safe for boxing as the impact forces which were created were above the human tolerance to concussion (Hodgson & Thomas 1981). In a further study by Smith and Hamill (1985b) it was shown that, by the 50th trial, peak impact force had almost doubled (1484 to 2913 N). The impact forces from the gloves used in this study would attenuate forces below the concussion level (588 N for 26 ms) only on the first few impacts. The speed data presented in a 3D study by Whiting et al. (1988) compared well with previously reported data using 2D techniques. However, marginally lower values were recorded than those reported by Smith and Hamill (1985a). Data showed varying fist speeds for different punches (6 m · s⁻¹ for jab; 8 m · s⁻¹ for hook), supporting previously reported values (7 m · s⁻¹ for jab; 8 m · s⁻¹ for hook: Johnson et al. 1975).

The fist speeds and duration of impact produced in boxing give rise to concern with respect to injury. Thus, great care must be taken in all full-contact sessions. Correct headwear and gloves are a necessity, and boxers must be trained to minimize injury.

Equipment design

Although equipment such as the bat in baseball, stick in hockey, racket in tennis and badminton, and boot in soccer, are integral to performance, a full discussion of equipment design is beyond the scope of this chapter. A review of the boot in soccer can be found in Lees and Nolan (1998). In brief, the boot must be comfortable to wear, provide protection, and enable the foot to perform its impact functions. Brody (1987) reviewed all aspects of tennis racket design, including many functional considerations. Elliott (1981) reported from a practical perspective that the swing moment of inertia (primarily length) of a racket must be related to young players' physical maturity if tennis skills are to be mastered.

Noble and Walker (1994) researched the inertial and vibrational characteristics of baseball bats, and showed that the areas near the centre of pressure and distal node of the fundamental frequency of the bat are the most comfortable areas at which to impact the ball. Bat loading strategies (Noble & Eck 1985) for softball bats showed that knob end loading had the greatest effect on the displacement of the effective hitting area towards the barrel end of the bat and on enlarging the effective hitting area. Of specific interest to coaches and players are the findings by De Renne et al. (1995) on the effects of weighted bat training on swing speed. They showed that the best results were achieved by training with variable weighted implements (0.879–964 kg overweight; 0.766–822 kg underweight; 0.850 kg correct weight) in conjunction with batting practice. This practice significantly increased bat swing speed and would therefore suggest that the use of a combination of weighted bats can serve as an adjunct training method in baseball and possibly other hitting sports.

Follow-through

The follow-through phase of a hitting/kicking skill plays a number of very important roles in performance. A follow-through phase is required to slow body segments gradually to protect the body from injury. In optimizing performance it also enables the racket/foot/hand to achieve near-maximal speed at impact, while also preparing the body for the next facet of play.

Acknowledgements

The author thanks Professor Brian Blanksby from The University of Western Australia for his assistance in the general structure of this chapter, and Professor Bruce Abernethy from the University of Queensland for his guidance in the section on cuing.

References

Abernethy, B. (1987) Review: Selective attention in fast ball sports II: expert-novice differences. *Australian Journal of Science and Medicine in Sport* 19, 7–16.

Abernethy, B. (1991) Visual search strategies and decision-making in sport. *International Journal of Sport Psychology* 22, 189–210.

Abernethy, B. (1996) Training the visual-perceptual skills of athletes: Insights from the study of motor expertise. *American Journal of Sports Medicine* 24, S89–S92.

Abernethy, B. & Burgess-Limerick, R. (1992) Visual information for the timing of skilled movements: A review. In: *Approaches to the Study of Motor Control and Learning* (ed. J. Summers), pp. 343–384. Elsevier Science Publishers, London.

Abernethy, B. & Russell, D. (1987) The relationship between expertise and visual search strategy in a racquet sport. *Human Movement Science* 6, 283–319.

Aitcheson, I. & Lees, A. (1983) A biomechanical analysis of place kicking in Rugby Union Football. *Journal of Sports Sciences* 1, 136–137.

Asai, T., Akatsuka, T. & Kaga, M. (1995) Impact process in kicking in football. In: *Book of Abstracts. XVth Congress of the International Society of Biomechanics* (eds K. Häkkinen, K. Keskinen, P. Komi & A. Mero), pp. 74–75. University of Jyväskylä, Finland.

Asami, T. & Nolte, V. (1983) Analysis of powerful ball kicking. In: *Biomechanics VIII-B* (eds H. Matsui & K. Kobayashi), pp. 695–700. Human Kinetics, Champaign, IL.

Aura, O. & Komi, P. (1987) Coupling time in stretch shortening cycle: influence on mechanical efficiency and elastic characteristics of leg extensor muscles. In: *Biomechanics X-A* (ed. B. Jonsson), pp. 507–512. Human Kinetics, Champaign, IL.

Bahamonde, R. (1997) Joint power production during flat and slice tennis serves. In: *Proceedings of the XV Symposium on Biomechanics in Sports* (eds J. Wilkerson, W. Zimmermann & K. Ludwig), p. 92. Texas Woman's University, Texas.

Bahamonde, R. & Knudson, D. (1998) Upper extremity kinetics of the open and square stance tennis forehand. In: *The 4th International Conference on Sports Medicine and Science in Tennis, March.* United States Tennis Association, Miami.

Bahill, A. & La Ritz, T. (1984) Why can't batters keep their eyes on the ball? *American Scientist* 72, 249–253.

Bloomfield, J., Elliott, B. & Davies, C. (1979) Development of the soccer kick: a cinematographical analysis. *Journal of Human Movement Studies* 5, 152–159.

Bober, T., Putnam, C. & Woodworth, G.C. (1987) Factors influencing the angular velocity of a human limb segment. *Journal of Biomechanics* 20, 511–521.

Brody, H. (1987) *Tennis Science for Tennis Players.* University of Pennsylvania Press, Philadelphia.

Browder, K., Tant, C. & Wilkerson, J. (1991) A three dimensional kinematic analysis of three kicking techniques in female players. In: *Biomechanics in Sport IX* (eds C.L. Tant, P.E. Patterson & S.L. York), pp. 95–100. Iowa State University Press, Ames.

Bunn, J. (1972) *Scientific Principles of Coaching.* Prentice-Hall, Englewood Cliffs, NJ.

Burroughs, W. (1984) Visual simulation training of baseball batters. *International Journal of Sport Psychology* 15, 117–126.

Chapman, A. & Caldwell, G. (1985) The use of muscle stretch in inertial loading. In: *Biomechanics IX-A* (eds D. Winter, R. Norman, R. Wells, K. Hayes & A. Patla), pp. 44–49. Human Kinetics, Champaign, IL.

Coleman, S., Benham, A. & Northcott, S. (1993) A three-dimensional cinematographic analysis of the volleyball spike. *Journal of Sports Sciences* 11, 295–302.

Davids, W., de Palmer, D. & Savelsbergh, G. (1989) Skill level, peripheral vision and tennis volleying performance. *Journal of Human Movement Studies* 16, 191–202.

Day, P. (1987) A biomechanical analysis of the development of the mature kicking pattern in soccer. BSc thesis, Liverpool Polytechnic, Liverpool.

De Lucia, P. & Cochran, E. (1985) Perceptual information for batting can be extracted throughout a ball's trajectory. *Perceptual and Motor Skills* 61, 143–150.

Deporte, E., Van Gheluwe, B. & Hebbelinck, M. (1990) A three-dimensional cinematographical analysis of arm and racket at impact in tennis. In: *Biomechanics of Human Movement: Applications in Rehabilitation, Sport and Ergonomics* (eds N. Berme & A. Cappozzo), pp. 460–467. Bertec Corporation, Worthington, OH.

De Renne, C., Buxton, B., Hetzler, R. & Ho, K. (1995) Effects of weighted bat implement training on bat swing velocity. *Journal of Strength and Conditioning Research* 9, 247–250.

Dunn, E. & Putnam, C. (1987) The influence of the lower leg motion on thigh deceleration in kicking. In: *Biomechanics XI-B* (eds G. de Groot, A. Hollander, P. Huijing & G. van Ingen Schenau), pp. 787–790. Free University Press, Amsterdam.

Elliott, B. (1981) Tennis racquet selection: a factor in early skill development. *Australian Journal of Sport Sciences* 1, 23–35.

Elliott, B. (2000) The biomechanics of tennis. In: *The IOC Handbook on Tennis Medicine* (ed. P. Renstrom). Blackwell Science, Oxford (in publication).

Elliott, B. & Chivers, L. (1987) A three-dimensional cinematographic analysis of the penalty corner hit in field hockey. In: *Biomechanics XI-B* (eds G. de Groot, A. Hollander, P. Huijing & G. van Ingen Schenau), pp. 791–797. Free University Press, Amsterdam.

Elliott, B. & Christmass, M. (1995) A comparison of the high and low backspin backhand drives in tennis using different grips. *Journal of Sports Sciences* 13, 141–151.

Elliott, B. & Wood, G. (1983) The biomechanics of the foot-up and foot-back tennis service techniques. *Australian Journal of Sports Science* 3, 3–6.

Elliott, B., Marsh, T. & Blanksby, B. (1986) A three-dimensional cinematographic analysis of the tennis serve. *International Journal of Sports Biomechanics* 2, 260–271.

Elliott, B., Overheu, P. & Marsh, P. (1988) The service line and net volleys in tennis: a cinematographic analysis. *Australian Journal of Science and Medicine in Sport* 20, 10–18.

Elliott, B., Marsh, T. & Overheu, P. (1989a) A biomechanical comparison of the multisegment and single unit topspin forehand drives in tennis. *International Journal of Sport Biomechanics* 5, 350–364.

Elliott, B., Marsh, T. & Overheu, P. (1989b) The topspin backhand drive in tennis. *Journal of Human Movement Studies* 16, 1–16.

Elliott, B., Marshall, R. & Noffal, G. (1995) Contributions of upper limb segment rotations during the power serve in tennis. *Journal of Applied Biomechanics* 11, 433–442.

Elliott, B., Takahashi, K. & Noffal, G. (1997) The influence of grip position on upper limb contributions to racket-head speed in the tennis forehand. *Journal of Applied Biomechanics* **13**, 182–196.

Elliott, B., Baxter, K. & Besier, T. (1999) Internal rotation of the upper arm segment during a stretch-shorten cycle movement. *Journal of Applied Biomechanics* **15**, 381–395.

Fujisawa, T., Fuchimoto, T. & Kaneko, M. (1997) Joint moments during tennis forehand drive: an analysis of rotational movements on a horizontal plane. In: *Book of Abstracts, XVI Congress of the International Society of Biomechanics, Tokyo*, p. 354. International Society of Biomechanics, Tokyo.

Galinas, M. & Hoshizaki, T. (1988) Kinematic characteristics of opposite-field hitting. In: *Biomechanics in Sports VI* (eds K. Kreighbaum & A. McNeill), pp. 519–530. International Society of Biomechanics in Sports, Bozeman, MT.

van Gheluwe, B. & Hebbelinck, M. (1986) Muscle action and ground reaction forces in tennis. *International Journal of Sports Biomechanics* **2**, 88–99.

van Gheluwe, B., De Ruysscher, I. & Craenhals, J. (1987) Pronation and endorotation of the racket arm in a tennis serve. In: *Biomechanics X-B* (ed. B. Jonsson), pp. 666–672. Human Kinetics, Champaign, IL.

Giangarra, C., Conroy, G., Jobe, F., Pink, M. & Perry, J. (1993) Electromyographic and cinematographic analysis of elbow function in tennis players using single- and double-handed backhand strokes. *American Journal of Sports Medicine* **21**, 394–399.

Gobush, W. (1990) Impact force measurements on golf balls. In: *First World Scientific Congress on Golf* (ed. A. Cochran), pp. 219–224. E. & F.N. Spon, London.

Goulet, C., Bard, C. & Fleury, M. (1989) Expertise differences in preparing to return a tennis serve: a visual information processing approach. *Journal of Sport and Exercise Psychology* **11**, 382–398.

Gowitzke, B. & Wadell, D. (1979) Technique of badminton stroke production. In: *Science in Racquet Sports* (ed. J. Terauds), pp. 17–41. American Publishers, Del Mar.

Gowitzke, B. & Waddell, D. (1986) The biomechanics of underarm power strokes in badminton. In: *Proceedings of the International Conference on Sport, Physical Education, Dance and Health* (eds J. Watkins, T. Reilly & L. Burwitz), pp. 137–142. E. & F.N. Spon, Glasgow.

Groppel, J. (1978) A kinematic analysis of the tennis one-handed and two-handed backhand drives of highly skilled female competitors. PhD thesis, Florida State University, Tallahassee.

Groppel, J. (1984) *Tennis for Advanced Players and Those Who Would Like to Be.* Human Kinetics, Champaign, IL.

Grove, J. (1989) Visual processes in baseball: a glance at the literature and a comment on research possibilities. *Journal of Applied Research in Coaching and Athletics* **4**, 176–194.

Harrison, W. (1978) Visual dynamics. *Scholastic Coach* **47**, 38–40.

Hirano, Y. (1987) Biomechanical analysis of baseball hitting. In: *Biomechanics in Sports III and IV* (eds J. Terauds, B. Gowitzke & L. Holt), pp. 21–28. Academic Publishers, Del Mar, CA.

Hodgson, V. & Thomas, L. (1981) *Boxing Gloves Compared Using Dummy Head Acceleration Response.* Report to New York State Athletic Commission.

Hubbard, A. & Seng, C. (1954) Visual movements of batters. *Research Quarterly* **25**, 42–57.

van Ingen Schenau, G., Bobbert, M. & de Haan, A. (1997) Does elastic energy enhance work and efficiency in the stretch-shortening cycle? *Journal of Applied Biomechanics* **13**, 389–415.

Isokawa, M. & Lees. A. (1988) A biomechanical analysis of the instep kick motion in soccer. In: *Science and Football* (eds T. Reilly, A. Lees, K. Davids & W.J. Murphy), pp. 449–455. E. & F.N. Spon, London.

Johnson, J., Skorecki, J. & Wells, R.P. (1975) Peak accelerations of the head experienced in boxing. *Medical and Biological Engineering* **13**, 396–404.

Jones, M. (1972) Perceptual characteristics and athletic performance. In: *Readings in Sports Psychology* (ed. H.T.A. Whiting), pp. 96–115. Henry Kimpton, London.

Komi, P. & Bosco, C. (1978) Utilisation of stored elastic energy in leg extensor muscles by men and women. *Medicine and Science in Sports and Exercise* **10**, 261–269.

Lee, D., Young, D., Reddish, P. & Clayton, T. (1983) Visual timing in hitting an accelerating ball. *Quarterly Journal of Experimental Psychology* **35A**, 333–346.

Lees, A. & Nolan, L. (1998) The biomechanics of soccer: a review. *Journal of Sports Sciences* **16**, 211–234.

Luhtanen, P. (1988) Kinematics and kinetics of maximal instep kicking in junior soccer players. In: *Science and Football* (eds T. Reilly, A. Lees, K. Davids & W.J. Murphy), pp. 441–448. E. & F.N. Spon, London.

Marryatt, W. & Holt, L. (1982) Prediction of performance in volleyball forearm contact: at high incoming ball velocities. In: *Biomechanics in Sport I* (ed. J. Terauds), pp. 425–431. Research Center for Sports, Del Mar, CA.

Maxwell, T. (1982) A cinematographic analysis of the volleyball spike of selected top-class female athletes. *Volleyball Technical Journal* **7**, 43–54.

Milburn, P. (1982) Summation of segmental velocities in the golf swing. *Medicine and Science in Sports and Exercise* **14**, 60–64.

Narici, M., Sirtori, M. & Morgan, P. (1988) Maximum ball velocity and peak torques of hip flexor and knee extensor muscles. In: *Science and Football* (eds T. Reilly, A. Lees, K. Davids & W. Murphy), pp. 429–433. E. & F.N. Spon, London.

Noble, L. & Eck, J. (1985) Bat loading strategies. In: *Biomechanics in Sports II* (eds J. Terauds & J. Barham), pp. 58–71. Academic Publishers, Del Mar, CA.

Noble, L. & Walker, H. (1994) Baseball bat inertial and vibrational characteristics and discomfort following bat-ball impacts. *Journal of Applied Biomechanics* **10**, 132–144.

Noffal, G., Elliott, B. & Marshall, R. (1998) Shoulder and elbow resultant joint moments in the tennis serve. In: *4th International Conference on Sports Medicine and Science in Tennis.* United States Tennis Association, Miami.

Norman, D. (1969) *Memory and Attention.* John Wiley & Sons, New York.

Opavsky, P. (1988) An investigation of linear and angular kinematics of the leg during two types of soccer kick. In: *Science and Football* (eds T. Reilly, A. Lees, K. Davids & W. Murphy), pp. 460–467. E. & F.N. Spon, London.

Osborne, K., Rudrud, E. & Zezoney, F. (1990) Improved curveball hitting through the enhancement of visual cues. *Journal of Applied Behavior Analysis* **23**, 371–377.

Paul, G. & Glencross, D. (1997) Expert perception and decision making in baseball. *International Journal of Sport Psychology* **28** (1), 35–56.

Peper, L., Bootsma, R., Mestre, D. & Bakker, F. (1994) Catching balls: how to get the hand to the right place at the right time. *Journal of Experimental Psychology: Human Perception and Performance* **20**, 591–612.

Putnam, C. (1983) Interaction between segments during a kicking motion. In: *Biomechanics VIII-B* (eds H. Matsui

& K. Kobayashi), pp. 688–694. Human Kinetics, Champaign, IL.

Putnam, C. (1993) Sequential motions of the body segments in striking and throwing skills: descriptions and explanations. *Journal of Biomechanics* **26** (Suppl.), 125–135.

Ridgway, M. & Wilkerson, J. (1987) A kinematic analysis of the front set and back set in volleyball. In: *Biomechanics in Sport III and IV* (eds J. Terauds, B. Gowitzke & L. Holt), pp. 240–248. Academic Publishers, Del Mar, CA.

Roberts, E.M. (1991) Tracking velocity in motion. In: *Biomechanics in Sports IX* (eds C.L. Tant, P.E. Patterson & S.L. York), pp. 3–25. Iowa State Printing Service, Ames.

Robertson, D. & Mosher, R. (1985) Work and power of the leg muscles in soccer kicking. In: *Biomechanics IX-B* (ed. D. Winter), pp. 533–538. Human Kinetics, Champaign, IL.

Rodano, R. & Tavana, R. (1993) Three-dimensional analysis of the instep kick in professional soccer players. In: *Science and Football II* (eds T. Reilly, J. Clarys & A. Stibbe), pp. 357–361. E. & F.N. Spon, London.

Sakurai, S., Ikegami, Y. & Yabe, K. (1989) A three-dimensional cinematographic analysis of badminton strokes. In: *Biomechanics in Sports V* (eds L. Tsarouchas, J. Terauds, B. Gowitzke & L. Holt), pp. 357–363. Helenic Sports Research Institute, Athens.

Sampson, J. & Roy, B. (1976) Biomechanical analysis of the volleyball spike. In: *Biomechanics V-B* (ed. P. Komi), pp. 332–336. University Park Press, London, England.

Smith, P. & Hamill, J. (1985a) Karate and boxing glove impact. In: *Biomechanics in Sports II* (eds J. Terauds & J. Barham),

pp. 114–122. Academic Publishers, Del Mar, CA.

Smith, P. & Hamill, J. (1985b) Karate and boxing glove impact characteristics as functions of velocity and repeated impact. In: *Biomechanics in Sports II* (eds J. Terauds & J. Barham), pp. 123–133. Academic Publishers, Del Mar, CA.

Sorensen, H., Zacho, M., Simonsen, E., Dyhre-Poulsen, P. & Klausen, K. (1996) Dynamics of the martial arts high front kick. *Journal of Sports Sciences* **14**, 483–495.

Takahashi, K., Elliott, B. & Noffal, G. (1996) The role of upper limb segment rotations in the development of spin in the tennis forehand. *Australian Journal of Science and Medicine in Sport* **28**, 106–113.

Tang, H., Abe, K., Katoh, K. & Ae, M. (1995) Three-dimensional cinematographical analysis of the badminton forehand smash: movements of the forearm and hand. In: *Science and Racket Sports* (eds T. Reilly, M. Hughes & A. Lees), pp. 113–118. E. & F.N. Spon, London.

Tant, C., Greene, B. & Bernhardt, M. (1993) A comparison of the volleyball jump serve and the volleyball spike. In: *Biomechanics in Sports XI* (eds J. Hamill, T. Derrick & E. Elliott), pp. 344–348. University of Massachusetts Campus Center Printing, Amherst, MA.

Thys, H., Faraggiana, T. & Margaria, R. (1972) Utilization of muscle elasticity in exercise. *Journal of Applied Physiology* **32**, 491–494.

Tsaousidis, N. & Zatsiorsky, V. (1996) Two types of ball–effector interaction and their relative contribution to soccer kicking. *Human Movement Science* **15**, 861–876.

Wang, L., Su, H. & Lo, K. (1998) Kinematics of upper limb and trunk in tennis players using single handed backhand

stroke. In: *International Symposium on Biomechanics in Sports* (eds H. Riehle & M. Vieten), pp. 273–276. University of Konstanz, Germany.

Wedaman, R., Tant, C. & Wilkerson, J. (1988) Segmental coordination and temporal structure of the volleyball spike. In: *Biomechanics in Sports VI* (eds E. Kreighbaum & A. McNeill), pp. 577–586. International Society of Biomechanics in Sports, Bozeman, MT.

Welch, C., Banks, S., Cook, F. & Draovitch, P. (1995) Hitting a baseball: a biomechanical description. *Journal of Orthopaedic and Sports Physical Therapy* **22**, 193–201.

Wickstrom, R. (1975) Developmental kinesiology. *Exercise and Sports Science Reviews* **3**, 163–192.

Whiting, W., Gregor, R. & Finerman, G. (1988) Kinematic analysis of human upper extremity movements in boxing. *American Journal of Sports Medicine* **16**, 130–136.

Wilson, G., Elliott, B. & Wood, G. (1991) The effect on performance of imposing a delay during a stretch-shorten cycle movement. *Medicine and Science in Sports and Exercise* **23**, 364–370.

Ye, W. (1991) Analysis of the movement velocities of upper limb in smash, driven clear and drop spike actions in badminton. In: *XIIIth International Congress on Biomechanics, Book of Abstracts* (eds R. Marshall, G. Wood, B. Elliott, T. Ackland & P. McNair), pp. 152–154. University of Western Australia, Perth.

Zatsiorsky, V.M. (1998) *Kinematics of Human Motion.* Human Kinetics, Champaign, IL.

Zernicke, R. & Roberts, E. (1978) Lower extremity forces and torques during systematic variation of non-weight bearing motion. *Medicine and Science in Sports* **10**, 21–26.

PART 5

INJURY PREVENTION AND REHABILITATION

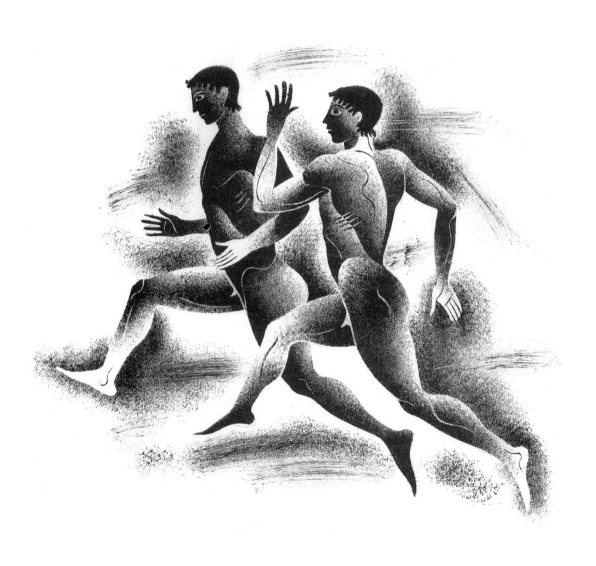

Chapter 24

Mechanisms of Musculoskeletal Injury

R.F. ZERNICKE AND W.C. WHITING

Introduction

Leonardo da Vinci noted that 'all injury leaves pain in the memory' and for Olympic-calibre athletes, the memory often is not limited to the injury itself, but frequently includes the lifelong pain of lost opportunity. Injury can affect peak performance—through the loss of a millimetre or fraction of a second—and be the deciding factor in being chosen for an Olympic team or winning an Olympic medal. As tragic as injury can be in denying an athlete the joy of Olympic competition, so too is Olympic history replete with stories of courageous athletes who have overcome injury to achieve the enduring glory of Olympic success. Al Oerter, for example, in Tokyo in 1964 won the third of his four gold medals by ignoring the pain of a dislocated cervical vertebra and torn rib cartilage and hurling the discus an Olympic record distance of 60.54 m. In receiving his unprecedented third gold medal, Oerter said, 'These are the Olympics. You die for them.' (International Amateur Athletic Federation 1997).

Injury is an undeniable facet of athletic life. Individuals across the spectrum of competitive levels, from recreational athletes to Olympic competitors, are subject to the limitations and disappointments imposed by musculoskeletal injury. Elite athletes, however, are particularly susceptible to the physical, emotional and economic costs that injury exacts. Though these costs are inconsequential for minor injuries, they can be overwhelming in cases of devastating injury that make it impossible, either temporarily or permanently, for an athlete to train and compete.

Lessening the chance of injury and facilitating the treatment and recovery of injured athletes requires an interdisciplinary approach that includes consideration of the anatomical, physiological, medical, kinesiological, psychological and mechanical aspects of athletes and their competitive environments. The injury-related problems of elite athletes are not addressed optimally by each discipline acting in isolation. The interdisciplinary team may include medical professionals, physical therapists, athletic trainers, sport scientists, psychologists, coaches and athletes.

Each of these professionals brings a specific perspective to the challenges of dealing with injuries to athletes. In addition to these individual perspectives, musculoskeletal injury can be viewed from many different general perspectives, including historical, epidemiological, economic, psychological and biomechanical.

Historical perspective

Archaeological evidence suggests that musculoskeletal injury is as old as life itself. As well, injury is endemic to athletic lore, as illustrated in the legendary tale of Phidippides, who fell dead on the plain of Marathon (490 BC) after running 40 km and proclaiming the news of the Athenian victory over the Persian forces of Darius the Great.

Injuries always have been and will continue to be a part of the athletic experience for participants at all levels of sport. Despite the inevitability of injury, athletes have benefited greatly from medical progress in the 20th century. Advances such as clinical arthroscopy, pioneered by Bircher in the early 1900s, presaged an age in which rapidly developing technologies would render tractable many problems that were previously impossible to solve. Not long ago, laser surgery, advanced imaging techniques, microsurgery and computer- or robot-assisted surgery were dismissed as futuristic dreams. Such medical advances, combined with remarkably improved rehabilitative programmes, now provide new hope where previously there was only despair. Many athletes, who in earlier times would have been unable to compete due to injury, are now able to fulfil their dreams of Olympic participation.

Epidemiological perspective

Epidemiology—the study of the incidence, distribution and control of disease and injury—documents the frequency and distribution of a particular injury in a given population. With the large number of participating nations, the huge array of sporting events and numbers of participating athletes, and the scatter in data-collection procedures, comprehensive injury data for Olympic athletes do not exist. While isolated reports of injuries to specific groups of Olympic competitors are available (e.g. Jegathesan 1973; Estwanik *et al.* 1978; Zemper & Pieter 1989; Ekeland *et al.* 1996), comprehensive documentation of injuries to Olympic athletes is unavailable and may remain so in light of the logistical constraints to gathering such data. In the general population, many injuries are never officially recorded. Thus published injury statistics are underestimates of the true injury toll. This is undoubtedly true for Olympic athletes as well; it is highly likely that many more injuries happen than are officially recorded and reported.

Psychological perspective

The most noticeable consequence of injury is the direct, physical damage to the body's tissues. Less obvious, and arguably no less important, are the psychological consequences that accompany musculoskeletal injury. Injury-related psychological factors can be involved before, during and after the actual injury, and can influence the likelihood and severity of injury, and the course of treatment and rehabilitation.

The psychological profiles of highly competitive, Olympic-calibre athletes differ in many ways from those of the general population. Psychological attributes such as high motivation, pain tolerance, goal orientation and exemplar physical training habits can benefit one's performance. On the negative side, elite athletes may be predisposed to a higher sense of loss, greater threat to their self-image, and harbour unrealistic expectations and a desire for a quick recovery from injury (Heil 1993). While some psychological factors are common to athletes across a wide range of athletic events, the risk of injury also is clearly event-dependent. An Olympic alpine skier or boxer, for example, is much more likely to suffer an injury than a participant in events such as curling or archery. Psychological factors affecting athletic performance and injury should be neither underestimated nor ignored.

Economic perspective

While injury exacts physical and emotional costs, the economic consequences of injury are often overlooked. Such costs can include direct costs (medical and non-medical), morbidity costs (lost value of goods and services as a result of injury), and mortality costs (value of remaining lifetime earnings adjusted for a person's life expectancy at the time of death). Since death due to athletic injuries is rare, the last of these costs is of minor consequence. The combination of direct and morbidity costs resulting from athletic injuries, however, is considerable. For an event such as the Olympic Games, these costs can account for a significant portion of the event's budget. At an individual level, the costs can be even more catastrophic, especially in cases where one's economic livelihood is predicated on his or her athletic success.

Biomechanical perspective

Of all scientific disciplines, physics and its subdiscipline, mechanics, are arguably most central to the study of injury, since most injuries have mechanically related causes. Forces and force-related factors (e.g. energy) are the prime agents that determine the likelihood and severity of injury. The nature of an injury and its treatment rests on the effective integration of biological and mechanical knowledge. Interdisciplinary biomechanics (i.e. the application of mechanical principles to biological problems) is ideally positioned to provide this integrated perspective. In the case of musculoskeletal injury to athletes, the problems include those related to the prevention, diagnosis and treatment of injuries so as to minimize their incidence and severity. The goal is to mitigate the negative effects of injury and allow athletes at all levels to maximize their performance potential.

Biomechanical concepts

Basic terms and principles

Movement is inherent to life and the quintessential element of our being. Without movement there would be no life. Some forms of movement developed to ensure survival, and others evolved as a means of expression. Athletic movements, in particular, are among the most demanding of all those imposed on the human body's framework.

Assessment of movement from a descriptive perspective falls within the area of mechanics known as *kinematics*. Kinematic analysis of movement involves five primary descriptive variables:
1 time (temporal characteristics of movement);
2 position or location;
3 displacement (describing what movement has occurred);
4 velocity (measuring how fast something has moved); and
5 acceleration (indicating how quickly the velocity has changed).

Movement description provides a useful tool for coaches and athletes in assessing the movement demands of their respective sports. Description alone, however, has limitations, and a comprehensive analysis of a movement pattern or skill also requires knowledge of the forces that produce the movement. Analysis of the force-related characteristics of movement falls within the area of mechanics known as *kinetics*.

FORCE AND PRESSURE

Body movements are produced and controlled by forces acting both within the body (e.g. muscle forces) and upon the body from external sources (e.g. gravity, impact). These forces, in addition to modulating movement patterns, also act on tissues in the body. Under most conditions, these forces are well tolerated by the body's tissues. Indeed, force is central to optimal growth and development of tissues, especially those such as bone that provide structural support. But when forces exceed a tissue's ability to withstand the load, injury occurs. Force therefore is the most fundamental element in injuries.

Force is defined as the mechanical action or effect applied to a body that tends to produce acceleration. The standard (SI) unit of force is the newton (N), which is defined as the amount of force necessary to accelerate a 1 kg mass at $1 \text{ m} \cdot \text{s}^{-2}$. Forces pertinent to injury analysis include those that act in or upon the human body, and include gravity, impact (e.g. a runner's foot contact with the ground), musculotendinous forces, ligamentous forces that stabilize joints, and forces applied to bones. For all injury-related forces, seven factors combine to determine the nature and severity of the injury (Whiting & Zernicke 1998). These factors are:
• magnitude (how much force is applied?);
• location (where on the body or structure is the force applied?);
• direction (where is the force directed?);
• duration (over what time interval is the force applied?);
• frequency (how often is the force applied?);
• variability (is the magnitude of the force constant or variable over the application interval?); and
• rate (how quickly is the force applied?).

Injury often occurs when one object impacts with another, such as when an ice-hockey player collides with an opponent or with the boards. Impact also occurs when an object such as a ball contacts an athlete. A sharp object (e.g. javelin) contacting the skin with a given force level will cause a different injury than a blunt object (e.g. shot put) that impacts the skin with a similar force. In general, as the area of force application increases, the likelihood of injury decreases. This relation between force and application area is measured by *pressure*, which is defined as the applied force divided by the area over which the force is applied. The standard unit of pressure is the pascal (Pa), defined as a 1 N force applied to an area of 1 m^2 (1 Pa = 1 N $\cdot$ m^{-2}). In cases where forces are applied to structures over a relatively small area, a more convenient unit of pressure is the megapascal (MPa), equal to a 1 N force applied to 1 mm^2 (1 MPa = 1 N $\cdot$ mm^{-2}).

STRESS, STRAIN AND STIFFNESS

When examining human movement, envisioning the body's segments as rigid links is sometimes useful. Such rigid-body formulations make assumptions of non-deformability, fixed centre of mass, and material homogeneity. Although biological materials are deformable, the limitations imposed by the simplifying assumptions of a rigid-body model are generally acceptable for quantifying movement mechanics. In exploring the biomechanics of musculoskeletal injury, however, tissues must be considered as deformable solids since most injuries involve some amount of material deformation. In viewing bodily tissues as deformable solids, it is essential to understand the concepts of mechanical *stress* and *strain*.

A tissue loaded by an external force develops an internal resistance. The amount of resistance depends on the material properties of the tissue. In the case of skin, the resistance may be quite low. Bone, in contrast, will develop considerable resistance. This internal resistance is mechanical *stress* (σ) and is calculated by $\sigma = F/A$, where F is the magnitude of the load, and A is the tissue cross-sectional area over which the load is distributed. Stresses are classified as one of three types: tension, compression or shear (Fig. 24.1). *Tension (tensile) stress* develops in response to tensile loads that seek to elongate, or stretch the tissue. *Compression (compressive) stress* results when the load pushes the ends of the tissue together. *Shear stress* occurs when parallel forces act to produce an angulation or slippage between two surfaces.

Tissues typically change their shape in response to loading. This change is called a deformation and is measured as a mechanical *strain* (ε). Just as there are three principal stresses, the deformational response

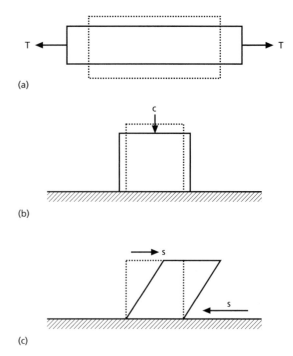

Fig. 24.1 Mechanical stress and strain. The three principal stresses and strains are: (a) tension; (b) compression; and (c) shear. Tissues deform (strain) in response to external loads for each condition as shown by the loaded condition (solid lines) compared with the unloaded condition (dashed lines). (Adapted from Whiting & Zernicke 1998.)

for each stress produces a corresponding principal strain. *Tensile strain* is a stretching or elongation of the tissue (e.g. tendon or ligament). *Compressive strain* produces a decrease in the longitudinal dimensions of a tissue, such as when a vertebra is subjected to a compressive load. *Shear strain* is an angular deformation as depicted in Fig. 24.1c.

Biological tissues have complex relations between stress and strain. Skin, for example, deforms readily under relatively low forces, whereas bone develops considerable internal resistance and deforms little. The responses of connective tissues such as tendon, ligament and cartilage fall between these two extremes. The relation between stress and strain (σ/ε) can be visualized by plotting stress as a function of strain (Fig. 24.2). The σ/ε ratio provides a single numerical value describing the relation between stress and strain. This ratio is termed the *stiffness*

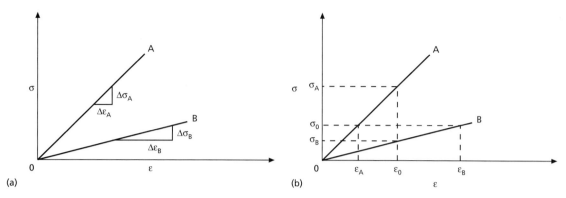

Fig. 24.2 Stress–strain (σ/ε) relation. (a) Linear σ/ε curves for two materials. The slope of each line measures the material's stiffness (e.g. A is stiffer than B). (b) The relative stiffness determines each tissue's response to loading. For a given stress level (σ_0), material B exhibits more strain than material A ($\varepsilon_B > \varepsilon_A$). For a given strain ($\varepsilon_0$), material A develops a greater stress than material B ($\sigma_A > \sigma_B$). (Adapted from Whiting & Zernicke 1998.)

of the material. Bone is relatively stiff and deforms little as loads are applied; by comparison, tendon is less stiff (more compliant) than bone. The σ/ε curves in Fig. 24.2 depict a linear relation between stress and strain. Typically, the mechanical responses of biological tissues are not linear throughout their physiological ranges, as explained in the next section.

VISCOELASTICITY

A material is said to be *elastic* if it has the ability to return to its original shape (configuration) when a mechanical load is removed. Bone, for example, is elastic since the slight bending induced by a compressive load disappears when the load is removed and the bone returns to its original shape. Body tissues are elastic within their physiological ranges of normal movement, but tissues that are deformed beyond the elastic limit are injured.

The mechanical response of any material (tissue) depends on its constituent matter. Biological tissues generally have a fluid component and therefore are influenced by the principles of fluid mechanics. One of the most important of these principles posits that the response of a tissue depends, in part, on the *rate* at which the tissue is deformed (strained). The tissue is described as being *strain-rate dependent*. A tendon, for example, that is stretched quickly will respond differently than the same tendon stretched more slowly. Specifically, the quickly stretched tendon will

be stiffer (stretches less for a given load), stronger (accepts greater forces before failing), and will absorb more energy if taken to its point of rupture.

Tissues possessing these conjoint properties of elasticity and viscous strain-rate dependency are called *viscoelastic* tissues. The nature of a tissue's viscoelastic response plays an important role in the pathomechanics of injury.

Modes of loading

During athletic activities, body tissues are continuously subjected to forces that vary in magnitude, location, direction, duration, frequency, variability and rate. In most cases, the body tolerates these forces well, but when loads exceed the normal physiological range—a not uncommon occurrence in elite athletes—tissues can experience overload and sustain injury. Injuries resulting from a single or a few overload episodes are called *acute* injuries. These injuries often happen with a violent impact, such as when a downhill skier loses control and crashes into a restraining barrier.

Where repeated loading leads to tissue damage, the injury is called an *overuse* or *chronic* injury. Calcaneal (Achilles) tendonitis in a long-distance runner provides one example of a chronic, overuse injury. Distinguishing acute from chronic injuries usually poses little difficulty. However, a relation between the two types sometimes exists. Chronic loading (overuse) may weaken a tissue and increase its susceptibility to injury. A runner with chronic inflammation of the calcaneal tendon, for example, may be predisposed to acute rupture of that tendon.

Biological tissues often are subjected to complex loading involving one or more of the three fundamental forms of loading (tension, compression, shear). Several of these complex modes of loading are described below.

AXIAL LOADING

The simplest form of force application is uniaxial loading. In this mode, forces act along a single line, most often along the primary axis of the structure, such as when a long bone (e.g. femur) is loaded in compression or a tendon is pulled in tension by the action of its skeletal muscle. The tissue's response varies with the direction of the load. As noted earlier, biological tissues can demonstrate linear σ/ε behaviour through certain loading ranges, but typically are non-linear in other ranges. A generalized stress–strain curve is presented in Fig. 24.3. As the stress (σ) increases, the tissue's behaviour changes from its initial linear response (up to σ_B) to a non-linear region beyond σ_B.

In the real world of the athlete, forces are not always (or even usually) uniaxial in nature. Forces are typically multidimensional. The concepts of stress and strain are still applicable, but they interact across more than one dimension and thus present a more complex response. The case of biaxial loading is presented in Fig. 24.4. In this case, the tissue is

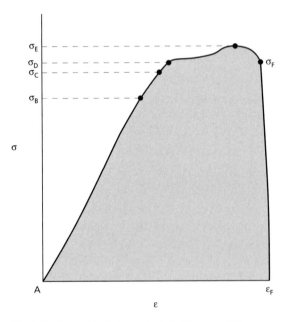

Fig. 24.3 Generalized stress–strain (σ/ε) curve. At low stress levels, the σ/ε response is linear. At stresses above the proportional limit (σ_B) the response becomes non-linear. At stresses below the elastic limit (σ_C), the tissue is elastic (i.e. returns to its original shape when the load is removed). Above σ_C the tissue experiences a permanent (plastic) deformation. Stresses above the yield point (σ_D) produce a brief region of relatively large strain for small increases in stress. This compliant yielding phenomenon is characteristic of many biological tissues. Continued increases in stress eventually reach the ultimate stress (σ_E) where tissue failure begins. Actual tissue rupture occurs at the rupture point (σ_F). The area under the curve (shaded) measures the energy to failure. (Adapted from Whiting & Zernicke 1998.)

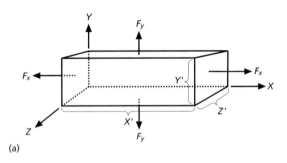

(a)

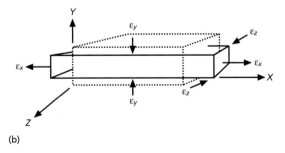

(b)

Fig. 24.4 Biaxial loading. (a) Forces applied in the x and y directions (F_x and F_y, respectively). (b) Elongation caused by F_x results in perpendicular contraction in the y and z directions (ε_y and ε_z, respectively). Solid lines indicate the loaded condition. Broken lines indicate the unloaded condition. (Adapted from Whiting & Zernicke 1998.)

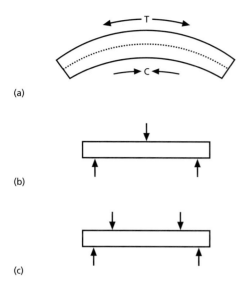

(a)

(b)

(c)

Fig. 24.5 Bending mechanisms. (a) Bending creates compressive stresses along the inner (concave) side of the beam and tensile stresses along the outer (convex) side. These stresses are maximal at the surfaces. (b) Three-point bending caused by the action of three parallel forces. The middle force is directed opposite to the two outer forces. (c) Four-point bending caused by the action of four parallel forces. The two inner forces act in the same direction and opposite to the direction of the two outer forces.

subject to simultaneous horizontal (F_x) and vertical (F_y) forces.

BENDING

A long, slender structure (e.g. long bone) can be viewed mechanically as a beam. Forces acting perpendicular to the long axis of the beam create bending. In bending, the concave (inner) surface of the bone experiences compressive stress; the convex (outer) surface of the bone is subjected to tensile stress (Fig. 24.5a). The maximal stresses occur at the surface of bone, with lower stresses developed away from the surface towards the midline (neutral axis) of the bone. The bone resists the bending moment created by external forces. Greater increases in bending loads can cause the bone to fail. Two common bending modes (three- and four-point bending) are depicted in Fig. 24.5b & c.

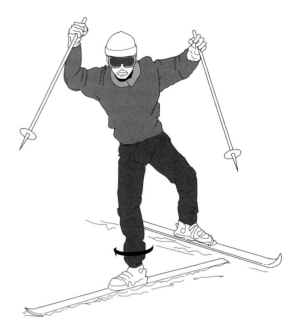

Fig. 24.6 Torsional loading. The skier's lower leg is torsionally loaded by the twisting action produced by a backward fall with the ski secured to the ground.

TORSION

A twisted structure experiences torsional loading (torque), for example when the lower leg twists during a rapid change of direction while the foot is planted on the ground. Anatomical structures in the lower leg (e.g. tibia) resist the applied torsional load. The ability of a bone to resist these applied torques depends on the bone's structural integrity. Several important principles govern a bone's torsional resistance:

1 the larger a bone's radius, the more resistance it develops and the more difficult it is to deform;

2 the stiffer the material being loaded, the harder it is to deform;

3 shear stresses develop across the bone's cross-section; and

4 torsion produces tensile and compressive stresses in the form of helical (spiral) stress trajectories, which are maximal at the bone's surface. Excessive torsional loading can result in spiral failure (fracture) along these lines (Fig. 24.6).

Mechanisms of upper-extremity injuries in athletes

Most Olympic events require athletes to perform upper-extremity movements, especially overhead movements involving lifting, throwing and striking. Among these are athletic field events such as the javelin, discus, shot put, hammer throw and pole vault, as well as weightlifting, baseball, softball, volleyball and water polo. Other events such as nordic skiing, rowing, ice hockey and swimming involve repetitive upper-extremity movements that also may predispose athletes to injury. Instability of upper-extremity joints, in particular the shoulder, and the repetitive nature of the throwing and lifting events, often lead to overuse injuries. Several such conditions and their mechanisms of injury are detailed in the following sections.

Injury mechanisms

Before examining the mechanics of specific musculoskeletal injuries, two terms require definition. The first is *injury*, defined as the damage (caused by physical trauma) sustained by tissues of the body. The second is *mechanism*, which is the fundamental physical process responsible for a given action, reaction or result (Whiting & Zernicke 1998).

Injury mechanisms are categorized according to mechanical concepts, tissue responses, or a combination of the two. The variety of injury types suggests a wide array of injury mechanisms. No single list or categorization system of mechanisms can adequately cover all types of injuries. Two exemplar classification systems, however, provide representative lists of injury mechanisms. Leadbetter (1994) listed contact or impact, dynamic overload, overuse, structural vulnerability, inflexibility, muscle imbalance and rapid growth as mechanisms of injury. The Committee on Trauma Research (1985) included crushing deformation, impulsive impact, skeletal acceleration, energy absorption, and the extent and rate of tissue deformation as causal mechanisms of injury. A sound understanding of injury mechanisms is essential for the effective assessment, treatment and prevention of musculoskeletal injuries.

Shoulder injuries

The shoulder (glenohumeral) joint is the upper extremity's most proximal articulation and influences most movements distal to it. Efficient upper-extremity throwing and lifting skills depend on adequate glenohumeral joint range of motion and neuromuscular coordination. Shoulder injury usually precludes normal movement not only of the glenohumeral joint, but also of the elbow and wrist joints, especially in multijoint movements. Anatomically, the glenohumeral joint is formed by the articulation of the head of the humerus with the shallow glenoid fossa of the scapula. The loose fit of the humeral head within the glenoid fossa permits considerable triplanar movement, but also contributes to the least stable joint in the body.

GLENOHUMERAL INSTABILITY

A joint's ability to resist luxation (dislocation) is directly related to its inherent structural stability. The glenohumeral joint is strengthened by ligaments (e.g. glenohumeral, coracohumeral) and surrounding musculature including the superficial deltoid and the deeper muscles of the rotator cuff. The glenoid labrum also contributes to joint stability, to a limited degree, by increasing the surface area and deepening the fossa, and thus improving the joint's bony fit. In spite of these supporting structural elements, the glenohumeral joint remains the least stable joint in the body, a distinction substantiated by its frequent dislocation. Simply stated, what the glenohumeral joint gains in mobility, it sacrifices in stability.

At the extremes of glenohumeral joint movement, such as at the end of the cocking phase in throwing, tension in the capsuloligamentous structures provides resistance to dislocation. During normal ranges of motion, however, laxity in these structures precludes their involvement in stabilizing the joint to a large extent. Other mechanisms are therefore needed to ensure joint stability. These mechanisms include limited joint volume, negative intra-articular pressure, concavity compression, and scapulohumeral balance.

In a normal shoulder with an uninjured joint capsule, a small negative intracapsular pressure contributes to joint stability (Speer 1995). While not particularly large, this negative pressure nonetheless helps stabilize the glenohumeral articulation. Concavity compression—the stability created when a convex object is pressed into a concave surface—also contributes to joint stability. The surfaces of the humeral head and the glenoid fossa are pressed together by multiple muscle forces. This pressure provides greater resistance to translational movement between the surfaces. Translational resistance in the glenohumeral joint is greater in the superior-inferior direction than in the anterior-posterior direction and increases with greater compressive loading (Lippitt & Matsen 1993). Despite the resistance provided by concavity compression, translation of the humeral head on the glenoid fossa will happen with the combined movements of glenohumeral horizontal abduction and external rotation associated with the cocking phase of throwing. These translational movements are relevant to skill mechanics since they indicate that the glenohumeral joint does not function purely as a ball-and-socket mechanism but allows for anterior humeral head movement during glenohumeral flexion and cross-body movements, and posterior translation with extension and external rotation (Harryman et al. 1990).

Scapulohumeral balance describes the coordinated action of muscles controlling movement of the glenohumeral joint. The muscles most immediately responsible for maintaining scapulohumeral balance are those of the rotator cuff group (subscapularis, supraspinatus, infraspinatus and teres minor). The rotator cuff muscles are assisted by action of the deltoid, latissimus dorsi, trapezius, serratus anterior, rhomboids and levator scapulae. To maintain joint stability, the net joint reaction force created by the combined action of these muscles must remain within the glenoid fossa. When muscle forces are uncoordinated, the joint reaction force may not be balanced within the glenoid fossa and thus contributes to joint instability. Fatigue in any of the muscles (e.g. from repeated throwing or lifting) compromises the ability of the musculoskeletal system to effect proper movement mechanics.

Glenohumeral instability predictably contributes to increased potential for other pathological shoulder conditions. Kvitne and Jobe (1993) described the progressive pathology of the overhand throwing athlete along a continuum from overuse inflammatory conditions to mild joint laxity with anterior subluxation (partial dislocation), to internal impingement syndrome, and finally to rotator cuff tearing.

Throwing athletes require sufficient joint flexibility to achieve the joint ranges of motion required to generate high velocities. An athlete with inadequate flexibility may be advised to focus on increasing range of motion through appropriate stretching and strengthening exercises. On the other hand, repeated throwing can lead to increased joint laxity and range of motion. Brown et al. (1988), for example, found that professional baseball pitchers exhibited 9° more external rotation in abduction in their dominant arm compared with the non-dominant side. Such increases in range of motion, conceivably, could facilitate throwing performance, but more is not necessarily better. Too much flexibility is detrimental since excessive stretching may enhance capsular laxity and lead to eventual shoulder instability (Fleisig et al. 1996).

Soft tissue adaptations (e.g. capsular laxity) may not be solely responsible for joint laxity. Recent evidence suggests that bony adaptations also may play a role in anterior glenohumeral instability. Pieper (1998) examined the degree of humeral retrotorsion in a group of male professional handball players, and found that the retrotorsional angle of the humerus in a player's throwing arm was an average of 9.4° larger in the dominant side than in the non-dominant. Even more interesting from an injury perspective was the fact that in players without chronic shoulder pain, the side-to-side difference was 14.4° greater in the throwing arm. Players with chronic shoulder pain actually showed a decrease of 5.2° of humeral retrotorsion in their throwing arm compared to the non-throwing arm. Pieper (1998) explained these results as evidence of an osseous adaptation during growth to the repetitive external rotation demands of throwing practice. He concluded that 'Athletes who do not adapt this way seem to have more strain on their anterior capsules

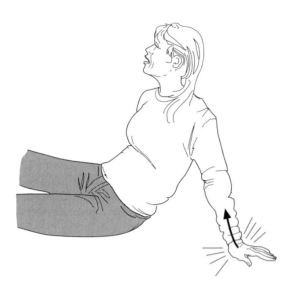

Fig. 24.7 Anterior glenohumeral luxation. The humeral head is violently dislocated from the glenoid fossa by the indirect force applied to the extended, abducted and externally rotated arm.

at less external rotation and develop chronic shoulder pain because of anterior instability' (Pieper 1998, p. 247).

As noted previously, the glenohumeral joint is susceptible to luxation or subluxation. In rare cases, individuals with congenitally lax shoulders may experience atraumatic glenohumeral luxations. Most cases of shoulder dislocation, however, result from traumatic forces applied directly or indirectly to the glenohumeral complex. Ninety percent or more of glenohumeral luxations happen anteriorly, usually as a result of indirect axial forces (e.g. ground reaction forces acting through the hand and arm during a fall) applied to an extended, abducted and externally rotated arm (Fig. 24.7). These forces effectively drive the humeral head out of its normal position in the glenoid fossa. Much less frequently, anterior glenohumeral luxation is caused by direct forces applied to the posterior aspect of the shoulder.

Mechanisms responsible for the much less common posterior luxation basically are the reverse of those causing anterior dislocation. Indirect forces transmitted through a flexed, adducted and internally rotated arm, as would be seen in landing during a

forward fall, effectively drive the humerus posteriorly. Posterior luxation also can result from direct trauma applied to the anterior aspect of the humerus.

IMPINGEMENT SYNDROME

Much of the interest in glenohumeral impingement was stimulated by the pioneering work of Neer (1972), who proposed an anatomical rationale and surgical treatment for chronic subacromial impingement syndrome. Glenohumeral (subacromial) impingement generally refers to arm abduction that results in the forcible pressing of suprahumeral structures (e.g. supraspinatus tendon, subacromial bursa) against the anterior surface of the acromion and the coracoacromial ligament that forms the coracoacromial arch (Fig. 24.8). Repeated abduction imposes large stresses on the capsuloligamentous and musculotendinous structures of the glenohumeral joint. These stresses typically lead to tissue microtrauma, which with continued mechanical insult can lead to tissue failure. Tissue failure then exacerbates joint instability and greater humeral movement. This, in turn, further aggravates the impingement condition. The athlete therefore is trapped in a negative feedback loop of compromised tissue integrity and joint function.

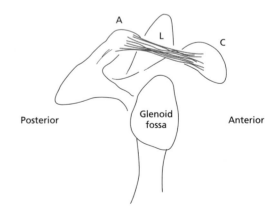

Fig. 24.8 Coracoacromial arch. The coracoacromial ligament (L) spans the acromion (A) and coracoid (C) processes of the scapula and forms an arch. In an impingement syndrome, suprahumeral structures are pressed against the arch by abduction and superior translation of the humeral head.

Impingement pathologies have been divided broadly into two age-related categories. Older individuals are most disposed to degenerative processes that promote bone spur formation, capsular thinning, decreased tissue perfusion, and muscle atrophy. More relevant to athletes is the second category, which includes individuals under 35 years who engage in sports involving extensive and repetitive overhead movements. Jobe and Pink (1993) proposed a classification system based on age-related differences.

• Group I injuries include those of isolated impingement with no instability. This group typically includes older recreational athletes and only rarely includes younger athletes.

• Group II patients exhibit instability with impingement secondary to overuse-related tissue microtrauma. This group comprises mostly young 'overhead' athletes.

• Group III injuries are closely associated with Group II pathologies common in younger athletes and are characterized by generalized ligamentous laxity and resultant shoulder instability.

• Group IV includes injuries resulting from a traumatic event such as direct impact or a fall. Injuries in this group show shoulder instability without impingement.

The mechanisms of glenohumeral impingement remain controversial. The precise role of extrinsic (e.g. forces acting outside the rotator cuff) and intrinsic (e.g. inflammatory changes within the cuff) factors remains the subject of debate (Fu *et al.* 1991; Ticker *et al.* 1995). Among the contributing factors are: the structural characteristics of the subacromial space (most notably the shape and size of the acromion; see Fig. 24.9); the presence of bone spurs that focus forces on the subacromial structures and produce a functionally smaller supraspinatus outlet (Wuelker *et al.* 1994); degenerative processes affecting the supraspinatus; eccentric overload of the supraspinatus; muscular fatigue; compromised blood flow in regions of impingement pressure and relative tissue avascularity; and thickening of the coracoacromial ligament (Soslowsky *et al.* 1994).

The risk factors for impingement closely parallel the movement characteristics of sports with extensive upper-extremity involvement (e.g. baseball, vol-

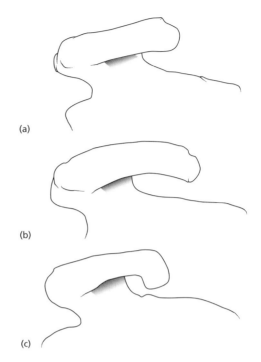

(a)

(b)

(c)

Fig. 24.9 Variation in acromion shapes. (a) Type I, flat. (b) Type II, curved. (c) Type III, hooked. A hook-shaped acromion (Type III) has been associated with a higher incidence of rotator cuff lesions. (Adapted from Whiting & Zernicke 1998.)

leyball, tennis, swimming, water polo, weightlifting). These include heavy work, direct load bearing, repetitive arm movements, working with hands above shoulder height, fatigue resulting from lack of rest, and high-velocity movements.

Impingement syndrome is not restricted to the general athletic population but afflicts special population athletes as well. Wheelchair athletes, for example, suffer a high incidence of rotator cuff impingement pathologies. Burnham *et al.* (1993) reported that paraplegic athletes demonstrated an imbalance of abduction/adduction strength with relative weakness of shoulder adduction. In addition, paraplegics' shoulders affected by impingement syndrome exhibited significant weakness of adduction, external rotation and internal rotation when compared to the uninvolved shoulders. They suggested that strengthening of shoulder adduction and internal and external rotation may be an important preventive strategy for these athletes (Burnham *et al*. 1993).

ROTATOR CUFF PATHOLOGIES

Rupture of musculotendinous structures in the rotator cuff is the final step in a chain of events that has been described as an *instability continuum* (Kvitne & Jobe 1993). The progressive pathologies of instability, subluxation and impingement lead ultimately to rotator cuff tearing in some athletes. While not common in younger athletes, rotator cuff tears can significantly affect an athlete's ability to train and perform. The loading characteristics of the rotator cuff depend on the functional demands of an athlete's sport or event. Each sport has its own specific demands. Electromyographic (EMG) data show that rapid and precise movement patterns elicit selective muscle action and periods of high muscle intensity (Perry & Glousman 1990). In spite of the unique phasic patterns particular to each throwing or striking sport motion, there is a general pattern common to most. Perry (1983) described this common pattern as starting with a gentle approach to an appropriate starting position, followed by a 'cocking' phase in which shoulder structures are tensed to provide a forceful accleration. Once the necessary acceleration has been accomplished, the system's muscles typically act eccentrically to decelerate the arm to avoid injurious forces. Repetitive attempts to decelerate the horizontal adduction, internal rotation, and glenohumeral distraction forces during the deceleration phase of throwing can lead to an eccentric tensile overload failure of the rotator cuff muscles, especially the supraspinatus (Andrews & Wilk 1994; Fleisig *et al*. 1996). Repeated movements also can lead to muscle fatigue and compromised tissue integrity (e.g. advanced inflammation and microtearing) that contribute, in turn, to altered movement mechanics. Modifications in movement control and technique can further stress the tissues and hasten additional damage and eventual failure.

As noted, the supraspinatus is the most frequently injured muscle of the rotator cuff group and is most often associated with repeated, and often violent, overhead movement patterns (e.g. throwing, striking). The other rotator cuff muscles, while less susceptible to injury, are not immune to injury.

The muscles involved depend in part on the movement pattern and the task demands placed on the shoulder. Burkhart (1993) described four patterns of rotator cuff kinematics associated with specific cuff lesions. Type I lesions exhibited tears of the supraspinatus and portions of the infraspinatus, but not to an extent that disrupted essential mechanical force couples. Patients in this group had normal motion and near-normal strength.

Patients with Type II lesions had massive tears of the superior and posterior portions of the rotator cuff. These resulted in an uncoupling of the essential force couples and led to an unstable fulcrum (axis) for glenohumeral motion. Type II patients were extremely limited and could do little more than shrug their shoulders.

Type III pathologies had partial tears of the subscapularis accompanying supraspinatus and major posterior cuff lesions. These injuries prevented the muscles from centring the humeral head in the glenoid fossa and led to superior humeral subluxation. Type IV lesions involved tears of the subscapularis and supraspinatus with no involvement of the posterior cuff muscles (infraspinatus, teres minor).

The complex shoulder movements required in many sports place considerable stress on the muscles of the rotator cuff group. The throwing motion, in particular, places extraordinary loads on the shoulder. Throwing involves considerable abduction and external rotation of the arm, a position that places the rotator cuff at risk of injury, since high supraspinatus forces have been reported with the arm in this position (Hughes & An 1996). Those loads place the rotator cuff muscles at particular risk of injury. The role of the rotator cuff in synergistically resisting distraction of the humeral head is compromised by injury or fatigue to any of these muscles. The resulting alterations in throwing mechanics increases the likelihood of further tissue damage.

Elbow injuries

The elbow joint provides the critical middle link in the kinetic chain of the upper extremity. It is a synovial hinge joint formed by the dual articulations of the capitulum of the humerus with the head of the radius and the trochlea of the humerus with the trochlear notch of the ulna. Normal elbow motion is limited to uniplanar flexion-extension, with forearm pronation-supination produced by concurrent rotation of the proximal and distal radio-ulnar joints. The elbow is reinforced by collateral ligament complexes on the medial and lateral aspects of the joint. Elbow flexion is controlled by concentric action of the biceps brachii, brachialis and brachioradialis, with joint extension controlled by the triceps brachii.

Before considering mechanisms of elbow injury, we note several catch-all terms used to describe elbow injuries. The most common of these is *tennis elbow*, a term with various meanings ranging from a general descriptor of elbow pain to a specific reference to lateral epicondylitis. As with this and other nebulous terms (e.g. little leaguer's elbow, golfer's elbow, climber's elbow), we discourage their use and prefer instead to use specific clinical descriptors (e.g. epicondylitis, tendonitis, ligamentous sprain).

EPICONDYLITIS

Most elbow injuries result from overuse and are characterized by progressive tissue degeneration that begins with asymptomatic microtrauma and evidence of intracytoplasmic calcification, collagen fibre splitting and kinking, and abnormal fibre cross-links (Kannus & Jozsa 1991). Continued loading exacerbates the tissue damage and leads to symptomatic inflammation, inflexibility, and tissue weakness.

The specific dynamics of an athletic task determine whether epicondylitis affects the medial or lateral aspect of the elbow. In tennis, for example, the lateral epicondyle experiences injury five times as often as the medial side (Leach & Miller 1987). Lateral epicondylitis is most commonly attributed to inflammation of the proximal attachment of the extensor carpi radialis brevis during execution of the backhand stroke (Morris *et al*. 1989; Giangarra *et al*. 1993; Roetert *et al*. 1995; Safran 1995). When a player strikes the ball, forces are generated in the wrist extensor muscles. These loads are transferred through the stiffened forearm musculature to the proximal attachment on the lateral humerus. Medial epicondylitis happens much less frequently in tennis players and is due largely to extreme forces developed during the forehand and service strokes when the eccentric action of wrist flexors is required to control wrist extension. In cases of both medial

and lateral epicondylitis, the suspected injury mechanisms include poor stroke mechanics, off-centre ball contact with the racket, grip tightness, wrist position at contact, and racquet vibration (e.g. Elliott 1982; Grabiner *et al*. 1983; Henning *et al*. 1992).

Lateral epicondylitis is not exclusive to tennis. Athletes in other sports that involve backhand striking movements (e.g. racquetball, golf) also are susceptible to chronic pathologies of the lateral elbow. Though less common, medial epicondylitis afflicts athletes across a wide range of sports, including archery, baseball, weightlifting, javelin, handball, swimming and racquetball. These sports involve repetitive upper-extremity movements that predispose the athlete to overuse. The forearm muscles often fatigue and the resulting muscle weakness leads to eccentric failure of the flexor-pronator mass (e.g. flexor carpi radialis and pronator teres). The confluence of this group's muscle attachments on the medial epicondyle is subjected to repetitive microtrauma and subsequent inflammation (Plancher *et al*. 1996). Athletes affected by medial epicondylitis often are aggressive players participating at elite levels who subject their elbows to extraordinary stresses (Vangsness & Jobe 1991).

VALGUS-EXTENSION MECHANISM

Medial epicondylitis and other injuries affecting the elbow (e.g. ulnar nerve injury, medial elbow instability) often result from movement patterns involving throwing. Numerous studies have explored the kinematics and kinetics of the elbow during the throwing motion, which typically is divided into five phases: windup, cocking, acceleration, deceleration and follow-through. Several of these studies (e.g. Fleisig *et al*. 1995) quantified elbow kinetics and found large and potentially injurious forces and moments (torques). Near the end of the cocking phase, the elbow experiences valgus loading as the elbow approaches terminal extension. This valgus loading is resisted by a varus torque produced by musculotendinous and periarticular tissues. Varus torques at this time have been estimated at between 64 and 120 N m, with an associated joint force of about 500 N between the humerus and radius (Werner *et al*. 1993; Fleisig *et al*. 1995).

The coupled effect of valgus torque and elbow

extension produces a *valgus-extension mechanism* that can overload the joint and lead to medial elbow injuries such as epicondylitis, ulnar (medial) collateral ligament rupture, avulsion fracture and nerve damage. The valgus stress also causes compression of the lateral radiocapitular joint and impingement of the medial aspect of the olecranon on the olecranon fossa (Caldwell & Safran 1995). Repeated impingement leads to inflammation and eventual osteophyte formation on the posteriomedial aspect of the olecranon process (Wilson *et al.* 1983).

In throwing, as in other dynamic movements, the highest loads occur during phases when eccentric muscle actions are required to control (decelerate) high-velocity motion. Repeated development of such large loads can lead to progressive tissue degeneration that culminates in failure. This process is common but not inevitable. Some athletes are able to accommodate large, repeated loads with little, if any, symptomatic response. The answer remains elusive as to why some athletes are susceptible to overload injuries while others apparently are unaffected.

ELBOW FRACTURE/DISLOCATION

In contrast to the chronic, overuse injuries just described are acute injuries caused by the rapid application of large forces. At the elbow, such acute injuries usually manifest as fractures or dislocations. Given the elbow's relative stability, it is no surprise that the elbow is more than three times less likely than the shoulder to suffer dislocation (Praemer *et al.* 1992). Elbow dislocations, however, are not uncommon. Elbow joint luxation usually is accompanied by extensive soft-tissue damage that includes complete rupture or avulsion of both the ulnar and radial collateral ligaments. The elbow's bony configuration provides considerable resistance to anterior dislocation. As a result, most elbow dislocations occur posteriorly. The most common mechanism involves axial compressive forces applied to an extended or hyperextended elbow, such as would happen when someone falls onto an extended arm. The forces in this position lever the ulna out of the trochlea and rupture the capsule and ligaments, and thus allow joint dislocation (Hotchkiss 1996).

Elbow fractures can happen to any of the three bones (humerus, radius, ulna) comprising the joint and are determined by the nature, magnitude, location and direction of the applied forces. Fracture of the distal humerus can occur in any area of the bone, including the supracondylar, intercondylar, condylar, epicondylar and articular regions. Ulnar fractures commonly involve the olecranon process, and may be caused by either direct and violent insult to the posterior elbow, or indirectly from falls that load the elbow joint through the forearm. Radial head fractures typically result from axial loading of the radius during a fall (Fig. 24.10).

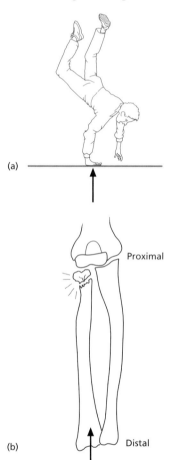

Fig. 24.10 Radial head fracture. (a) Compressive forces at impact during a fall are transmitted through the radius to the radial head. (b) Forces exceeding the bone's strength tolerance cause radial head fracture. (Adapted from Whiting & Zernicke 1998.)

Summary

Musculoskeletal injuries, while an unfortunate fact of life for everyone, have special urgency for athletes, especially those committed to competing at the highest levels. Regrettably, many athletic careers have been hampered or even ended by injury. Olympic-level athletes often depend on precise upper-extremity movements for success in their sport or event. Compromised upper-extremity function caused by injury, however slight, can have profound repercussions on the athlete's performance. A clear understanding of the mechanisms of musculoskeletal injury can aid in the effective diagnosis and treatment of the athlete, and a knowledge of injury mechanisms also may lead to better injury prevention strategies—the best injury is the one that never happens.

References

Andrews, J.R. & Wilk, K.E. (1994) Shoulder injuries in baseball. In: *The Athlete's Shoulder* (eds J.R. Andrews & K.E. Wilk), pp. 369–389. Churchill Livingstone, New York.

Brown, L.P., Niehues, S.L., Harrah, A., Yavorsky, P. & Hirshman, H.P. (1988) Upper extremity range of motion and isokinetic strength of internal and external shoulder rotators in major league baseball players. *American Journal of Sports Medicine* **16** (6), 577–585.

Burkhart, S.S. (1993) Arthroscopic debridement and decompression for selected rotator cuff tears. Clinical results, pathomechanics, and patient selection based on biomechanical parameters. *Orthopedic Clinics of North America* **24** (1), 111–123.

Burnham, R.S., May, L., Nelson, E., Steadward, R. & Reid, D.C. (1993) Shoulder pain in wheelchair athletes: The role of muscle imbalance. *American Journal of Sports Medicine* **21** (2), 238–242.

Caldwell, G.L. & Safran, M.R. (1995) Elbow problems in the athlete. *Orthopedic Clinics of North America* **26** (3), 465–485.

Committee on Trauma Research (1985) *Injury in America: a Continuing Public Health Problem*. National Academy Press, Washington, D.C.

Ekeland, A., Dimmen, S., Lystad, H. & Aune, A. (1996) Completion rates and injuries in alpine races during the 1994 Olympic Winter Games. *Scandinavian Journal of Medicine and Science in Sports* **6** (5), 287–290.

Elliott, B.C. (1982) Tennis: The influence of grip tightness on reaction impulse and rebound velocity. *Medicine and Science in Sports and Exercise* **14**, 348–352.

Estwanik, J., Bergfeld, J. & Canty, T. (1978) Report of injuries sustained during the United States Olympic wrestling trials. *American Journal of Sports Medicine* **6** (6), 335–340.

Fleisig, G.S., Andrews, J.R., Dillman, C.J. & Escamilla, R.F. (1995) Kinetics of baseball pitching with implications about injury mechanisms. *American Journal of Sports Medicine* **23** (2), 233–239.

Fleisig, G.S., Barrentine, S.W., Escamilla, R.F. & Andrews, J.R. (1996) Biomechanics of overhand throwing with implications for injuries. *Sports Medicine* **21** (6), 421–437.

Fu, F.H., Harner, C.D. & Klein, A.H. (1991) Shoulder impingement syndrome: a critical review. *Clinical Orthopaedics and Related Research* **269**, 162–173.

Giangarra, C.E., Conroy, B., Jobe, F.W., Pink, M. & Perry, J. (1993) Electromyographic and cinematographic analysis of elbow function in tennis players using single- and double-handed backhand strokes. *American Journal of Sports Medicine* **21** (3), 394–399.

Grabiner, M.D., Groppel, J.L. & Campbell, K.R. (1983) Resultant tennis ball velocity as a function of off-center impact and grip firmness. *Medicine and Science in Sports and Exercise* **15**, 542–544.

Harryman, D.T.I.I., Sidles, J.A., Clark, J.M., McQuade, K.J., Gibb, T.D. & Matsen, F.A. III (1990) Translation of the humeral head on the glenoid with passive glenohumeral motion. *Journal of Bone and Joint Surgery* **72A** (9), 1334–1343.

Heil, J. (1993) *Psychology of Sport Injury*. Human Kinetics, Champaign, IL.

Henning, E.M., Rosenbaum, D. & Milani, T.L. (1992) Transfer of tennis racket vibrations onto the human forearm. *Medicine and Science in Sports and Exercise* **24**, 1134–1140.

Hotchkiss, R.N. (1996) Fractures and dislocations of the elbow. In: *Rockwood and Green's Fractures in Adults* (eds C.A. Rockwood, D.P. Green, R.W. Bucholz & J.D. Heckman), pp. 929–1024. Lippincott-Raven, Philadelphia.

Hughes, R.E. & An, K.-N. (1996) Force analysis of rotator cuff muscles. *Clinical Orthopaedics and Related Research* **330**, 75–83.

International Amateur Athletic Federation (1997) http://www.iaaf.org/Athletes/Legends/AlOerter.html.

Jegathesan, M. (1973) Pattern of injuries and illnesses in the Malaysian Olympic Team. *Medical Journal of Malaya* **27** (4), 248–252.

Jobe, F.W. & Pink, M. (1993) Classification and treatment of shoulder dysfunction in the overhead athlete. *Journal of Orthopaedic and Sports Physical Therapy* **18** (2), 427–432.

Kannus, P. & Jozsa, L. (1991) Histopathologic changes preceding spontaneous rupture of a tendon. *Journal of Bone and Joint Surgery* **73A**, 1517–1525.

Kvitne, R.S. & Jobe, F.W. (1993) The diagnosis and treatment of anterior instability in the throwing athlete. *Clinical Orthopaedics and Related Research* **291**, 107–123.

Leach, R.E. & Miller, J.K. (1987) Lateral and medial epicondylitis of the elbow. *Clinics in Sports Medicine* **6** (2), 259–272.

Leadbetter, W. (1994) Soft tissue athletic injury. In: *Sports Injuries: Mechanisms, Prevention, Treatment* (eds F.H. Fu & D.A. Stone), pp. 733–780. Williams & Wilkins, Baltimore.

Lippitt, S. & Matsen, F. (1993) Mechanisms of glenohumeral joint stability. *Clinical Orthopaedics and Related Research* **291**, 20–28.

Morris, J., Jobe, F.W., Perry, J., Pink, M. & Healy, B.S. (1989) Electromyographic analysis of elbow function in tennis players. *American Journal of Sports Medicine* **17**, 241–247.

Neer, C.S. II (1972) Anterior acromioplasty for the chronic impingement syndrome in the shoulder: a preliminary report.

Journal of Bone and Joint Surgery **54A**, 41–50.

Perry, J. (1983) Anatomy and biomechanics of the shoulder in throwing, swimming, gymnastics and tennis: symposium on injuries to the shoulder in the athlete. *Clinics in Sports Medicine* **2** (2), 247–270.

Perry, J. & Glousman, R. (1990) Biomechanics of throwing. In: *The Upper Extremity in Sports Medicine* (eds J.A. Nicholas, E.B. Hershman & M.A. Posner), pp. 725–750. Mosby, St. Louis.

Pieper, H.-G. (1998) Humeral torsion in the throwing arm of handball players. *American Journal of Sports Medicine* **26** (2), 247–253.

Plancher, K.D., Halbrecht, J. & Lourie, G.M. (1996) Medial and lateral epicondylitis in the athlete. *Clinics in Sports Medicine* **15** (2), 283–305.

Praemer, A., Furner, S. & Rice, D.P. (1992) *Musculoskeletal Conditions in the United States.* American Academy of Orthopaedic Surgeons, Park Ridge, IL.

Roetert, E.P., Brody, H., Dillman, C.J., Groppel, J.L. & Schultheis, J.M. (1995) The biomechanics of tennis elbow. *Clinics in Sports Medicine* **14** (1), 47–57.

Safran, M.R. (1995) Elbow injuries in athletes: a review. *Clinical Orthopaedics and Related Research* **310**, 257–277.

Soslowsky, L.J., An, C.H., Johnston, S.P. & Carpenter, J.E. (1994) Geometric and mechanical properties of the coracoacromial ligament and their relationship to rotator cuff disease. *Clinical Ortho-paedics and Related Research* **304**, 10–17.

Speer, K.P. (1995) Anatomy and pathomechanics of shoulder instability. *Clinics in Sports Medicine* **14** (4), 751–760.

Ticker, J.B., Fealy, S. & Fu, F.H. (1995) Instability and impingement in the athlete's shoulder. *Sports Medicine* **19** (6), 418–426.

Vangsness, C.T. Jr & Jobe, F.W. (1991) Surgical treatment of medial epicondylitis. Results in 35 elbows. *Journal of Bone and Joint Surgery* **73B**, 409–411.

Werner, S.L., Fleisig, G.S., Dillman, C.J. & Andrews, J.R. (1993) Biomechanics of the elbow during baseball pitching. *Journal of Orthopaedic and Sports Physical Therapy* **17** (6), 274–278.

Whiting, W.C. & Zernicke, R.F. (1998) *Biomechanics of Musculoskeletal Injury.* Human Kinetics, Champaign, IL.

Wilson, F.D., Andrews, J.R., Blackburn, T.A. & McCluskey, G. (1983) Valgus extension overload in the pitching elbow. *American Journal of Sports Medicine* **11** (2), 83–88.

Wuelker, N., Plitz, W. & Roetman, B. (1994) Biomechanical data concerning the shoulder impingement syndrome. *Clinical Orthopaedics and Related Research* **303**, 242–249.

Zemper, E. & Pieter, W. (1989) Injury rates during the 1988 US Olympic team trials for taekwondo. *British Journal of Sports Medicine* **23** (3), 161–164.

Chapter 25

Musculoskeletal Loading During Landing

J.L. MCNITT-GRAY

This chapter is comprised of four sections. The first introduces the need to assess musculoskeletal loading in relation to the response of musculoskeletal structures to stress. The second section provides an overview of how the mechanical objective of the task, the individual's self-selected landing strategy, and the properties of the landing surface influence musculoskeletal loading. The following section deals with reaction forces, kinematics, joint kinetics and electromyography (EMG), quantified during landing activities performed under a variety of task, subject, and surface conditions, to provide a window on musculoskeletal loading at the total body and joint levels. In addition, exemplar data are provided to illustrate how individual subjects prepare for contact and control the moments created by the reaction force during a range of foot-first landings. The final section summarizes factors that athletes, coaches and trainers need to consider when attempting to balance loading during landing with the response to stress of musculoskeletal structures.

Introduction

During landing activities, forces and moments generated by muscle-tendon units and reaction forces are applied to the musculoskeletal structures of the lower extremity. To avoid injury, load experienced by the body needs to be kept in balance with the ability of musculoskeletal structures to respond to stress induced by loading. Absence of stress results in degeneration or muscle atrophy, whereas a single excessive load may result in acute injury (e.g. fracture, sprain) or may lead to chronic injury (e.g. cartilage

damage). Repetitive loading may produce positive effects such as increased critical limits of musculoskeletal components, even in compromised nutritional and hormonal environments, or negative effects such as fatigue fracture, muscle soreness, or chronic pain.

The need for multijoint control of moments created by these large reaction forces experienced during landing presents a significant challenge to the neuromuscular system prior to and during the landing. Although accomplished athletic populations regularly encounter repetitive high forces during training, effective and safe interaction with landing surfaces during low-velocity activity (e.g. curb descent) may present a challenge for partially disabled, normal geriatric or arthritic, as well as visually, vestibular- and proprioceptive-impaired populations.

No causal relationship has been proven between load and injury. The high incidence of injury to the lower extremities of athletes participating in landing activities (NCAA 1986, 1990), however, suggests the process of preparing athletes for the rigours of competition is out of balance with the ability of the body to positively adapt to the loads experienced (Fig. 25.1). Epidemiology data from the National Collegiate Athletic Association (NCAA) in the USA indicate that lower-extremity injuries account for 55–65% of all injuries experienced by both male and female collegiate athletes involved in repetitive landing activities. These injuries result in a significant loss of training and competition time and may lead to chronic problems over time. Despite improvements in footwear, injuries to the musculoskeletal

523

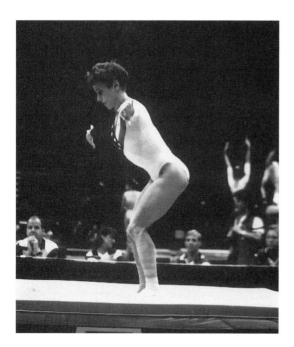

Fig. 25.1 Female gymnast landing a vault during a warm-up session preceding the 1996 Olympic Gymnastics Competition in Atlanta, Georgia. (Photograph by J. L. McNitt-Gray).

system closest to the point of contact persist (e.g. foot, shank, ankle and knee; NCAA 1986, 1990).

Methodological limitations associated with direct measurement of forces experienced by individual anatomical structures during realistic movement, as well as the assessment of the material properties of intact biological structures, currently limits development of a clear cause-effect relationship between load and musculoskeletal response (Nigg & Bobbert 1990). Load experienced by internal structures during landing, however, may be estimated at the total body and joint level by quantifying reaction forces, net joint forces (NJFs) and net joint moments (NJMs) (Elftman 1939). Comparison of total body and joint kinetics between landing tasks will also provide insight regarding differences in musculoskeletal loading (Nigg & Bobbert 1990). Distribution of these forces and moments to individual structures in the region of the joint, however, is limited by experimental and modelling approaches (Smith 1975; Crowninshield & Brand 1981; Hatze 1981; Gregor &

Abelew 1994; Herzog 1996). Assessing load experienced by an individual is further complicated by the use of self-selected multijoint neuromuscular control strategies that modulate the mechanical characteristics of the extremities in relation to the task, velocity at touchdown, and properties of the landing surface (Figs 25.2 & 25.3). In this chapter, *landing strategy* will refer to the multijoint coordination plan that an individual executes to satisfy the objectives of a landing task.

Task, human and surface interactions: an overview

Task

The mechanical goal of a landing task is to effectively convert the total body momentum at touchdown to achieve a subsequent task. For example, during the takeoff of the running long jump, the mechanical goal of the single leg landing performed during the takeoff phase is to convert a portion of the total body horizontal momentum generated during the run-up into vertical momentum at departure (Hay 1986). Like the long jump, the mechanical goal of the two-foot takeoff preceding an aerial gymnastics skill is to convert a portion of the total body horizontal and angular momentum generated during the preceding tumbling skills into vertical momentum at departure (Munkasy *et al.* 1994; Munkasy *et al.* 1997). Landings of this type are categorized in this chapter as 'Land and Go' tasks. In contrast, the mechanical goal of a two-foot gymnastics landing is to reduce the total body vertical, horizontal and angular momentum at touchdown to zero without moving the feet (Fédération Internationale de Gymnastique 1984). This type of landing task is categorized in this chapter as a 'Land and Stop' task.

The mechanical goal of Land and Go and Land and Stop tasks is achieved by the net impulse applied by body weight and the reaction force during foot contact with the surface. The magnitude, direction and duration of the impulse experienced during the landing phase of a specific task will influence musculoskeletal loading experienced during the task. The direction of impulse created by the reaction force immediately following touchdown is influenced by the body position and momentum at touchdown. The magnitude of the reaction force impulse is influenced by the muscle activation, segment motion and magnitude of the total body centre of mass (TBCM) momentum prior to contact (Lees 1981; Mizrahi & Suzak 1982; Ozguven & Berme 1988; McKinley & Pedotti 1992; Irvine & McNitt-Gray 1993; McNitt-Gray 1993; Munkasy et al. 1996). The duration of the reaction force impulse is influenced by the mechanical properties of the surface in relation to the multijoint control strategy selected by the individual to accomplish the task (Farley et al. 1998; McNitt-Gray et al. 1994c; Ferris & Farley 1997).

Human

Successful performance of a landing task requires the individual to effectively interact with the landing surface to achieve the goal of the task. Musculoskeletal loading during landing, however, depends on how the individual has chosen to interact with the surface (Fig. 25.2). The redundancy of the musculoskeletal system allows the central nervous system to choose from a set of multijoint control strategies that balance the need for effective load distribution with the need to accomplish the mechanical goal of the task. Experimental evidence indicates that human subjects can voluntarily modulate the external loading experienced during impact by as much as eight times the magnitude of their body weight (McNitt-Gray et al. 1990) by modifying their multijoint control strategy.

Performance criteria also influence the landing strategy selected, and may take precedence over reducing the musculoskeletal loading experienced. For example, during the landing of a volleyball block, decreasing the time to block a ball may take precedence over loading the lead leg by 5 BW more than the lag leg (McNitt-Gray et al. 1994b). Landing strategies that are self-selected by athletes also demonstrate individual preferences for internal distribution of load between joints, bone (Zatsiorsky & Prilutsky 1987) and recruitment of uni- and biarticular muscle-tendon units (Irvine & McNitt-Gray 1993; McNitt-Gray et al. 1993a). These clinically and experimentally observed differences in multijoint control strategies between athletes appear to be

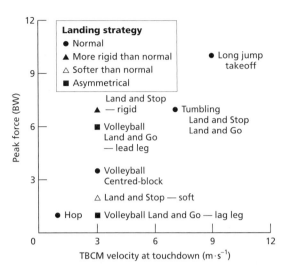

Fig. 25.2 The relationship between peak reaction forces experienced by one leg and total body centre of mass (TBCM) velocity at touchdown. The peak reaction forces and TBCM velocity at touchdown quantified during landings performed using the individual subject's normal landing strategy are represented by filled circles. These data demonstrate the tendency for peak reaction force magnitudes to increase with increases in TBCM velocity at touchdown. Landings performed using strategies more or less rigid than normal are represented by filled and open triangles, respectively. These data demonstrate the ability of an individual athlete to modify the peak reaction force by modifying their landing strategy. Differences in peak reaction forces experienced by the lead and lag legs of volleyball players performing a Land and Go block are represented by filled squares. These data reflect the potential for asymmetrical loading between legs during a landing. The observations presented are based on data acquired by McNitt-Gray et al. In the case of the long jump, a national-level decathlete performed the long jump takeoff on a force plate located at the end of the runway and landed in a sand-filled landing pit. In the case of gymnastics tumbling, the force plate was located at the end of a spring floor tumbling strip preceding a foam-filled landing pit. Gymnastics takeoffs and landings were performed by junior national team members on an isolated spring floor section fully supported by one force plate.

dependent on athlete-specific morphological, physiological and motor control capabilities that are scaled to the task, velocity and landing surface conditions (McKinley & Pedotti 1992; McNitt-Gray et al. 1993a).

Surfaces

During landing, humans rely primarily on lengthening of active muscle during joint flexion and bone deformation to attenuate and transmit forces experienced during contact (Radin & Paul 1970). As the velocity of the body at contact increases, the need for protective surfaces also increases. When the velocity of the body at touchdown is achieved with the aid of a mechanical apparatus (e.g. pole vaulting, gymnastics, etc.) or when impact with the surface is unanticipated, the need for protective landing surfaces is amplified. To promote effective interaction between the human body and landing surface, the landing surface needs to be designed to complement the ability of the human body to control body momentum during contact. During Land and Stop tasks, the surface needs to assist the body in attenuating the forces experienced during the landing phase. During Land and Go tasks, the surface needs to complement the mechanical properties of the lower extremity to facilitate achievement of the subsequent task (McMahon & Greene 1979; Farley et al. 1998).

Previous research on footwear and landing surfaces shows that humans use greater degrees of joint flexion as the rigidity of the surface increases (Denoth & Nigg 1981; Clarke et al. 1983; Gollhofer 1987; Nigg & Yeadon 1987; Nigg et al. 1988; McKinley & Pedotti 1992; McNitt-Gray et al. 1994c; Ferris & Farley 1997; Farley et al. 1998). These modifications in movement patterns associated with differences in surface properties may be related to the higher incidence of knee injury associated with harder surfaces as compared to those reported on softer surfaces. For example, the incidence of 'jumper's knee' has been reported to be greater for players playing on harder floors than softer floors (Ferretti et al. 1985). In addition, senior players who have trained over time on softer courts have reported fewer knee problems than senior players playing on hard courts (Kulund et al. 1979). Injury incidence and reports of pain have also been found to vary with friction characteristics of landing surfaces (Nigg & Yeadon 1987).

Landing surface standards established by international governing bodies are often based on the need to establish uniformity of equipment used during sanctioned competitions to ensure justice in competition (e.g. Fédération Internationale de Gymnastique 1984) and are not based on musculoskeletal loading issues. In gymnastics, as in other sports, the mechanical properties of landing surfaces currently used in competition have been characterized through standardized rigid body impact tests (Schweitzer 1985). Laboratory engineers typically perform these tests by dropping instrumented rigid bodies (10 kg, 20 kg) from predetermined heights (e.g. 0.4 m, 0.8 m). The acceleration experienced by the rigid mass, the energy absorbed by the surface, and the degree and rate of deformation of the surface are then measured during impact. Although rigid body tests provide repeatable results in characterizing the impact between inanimate objects, they fail to assess the internal loading implications of strategies used by athletes to interact with different surfaces (Nigg & Bobbert 1990; Nigg 1990).

The interaction between the athlete and equipment is critical for maximizing performance. During competition, however, athletes often have limited opportunities to demonstrate mastery of their interaction with the landing surface. In sports where athletes are unable to individualize their equipment and/or have limited exposure to their equipment prior to the competition (e.g. gymnasts), mastery of their interaction with the landing surfaces becomes more difficult. Although landing surfaces and equipment used in international competition must fall within guidelines established by the international governing body for the sport, these standards tend to be broad and allow for great variations in equipment between and within venues. For example, in baseball, the 'landing' conditions for the plant foot during pitching may be dramatically influenced by the shape, texture and height of the mound relative to the placement of the plant foot. Although the bull pen within the venue enables the pitcher to 'practise' pitching prior to entering the game, the height, shape and texture of the pitching mound in the bull pen is often different from the pitching mound on the playing field. In gymnastics, routines during competition are performed on apparatus and mats placed on a podium, whereas apparatus and mats in the warm-up area are placed directly on the existing floor. Often, years of preparation comes down to the ability of the gymnast to land without moving the feet. The success rate of gymnastics landings performed during the 1992 Olympic Games in Barcelona ($n = 644$) and during the 1996 Olympic Games in Atlanta ($n = 323$) averaged less than 50% (McNitt-Gray 1992; McNitt-Gray *et al.* 1997). Athletes can prepare themselves for variations in landing surface properties by practising landings under a variety of conditions.

Modifications in musculoskeletal loading associated with changes in landing strategies made in response to changes in landing surfaces need to be considered during skill development and when preparing for competition. For example, when gymnasts learn new skills they often land the aerial skill in a deep foam pit. As an intermediate step, gymnasts will then perform the landing onto 0.2 m crash pads placed on top of the spring floor. Although the mat thickness provides the gymnast with additional time to reduce body momentum, the deformation pattern of the surface around the foot may increase the potential for foot, subtalar and ankle instability, and create greater demand on the neuromuscular system. As the gymnast prepares for competition, landings are performed directly onto the spring floor. Since less energy is being absorbed by the surface, more energy must be absorbed by the athlete. Therefore, the intensity of training regimes needs to accommodate potential changes in musculoskeletal loading when athletes make transitions between landing surfaces.

When designing a landing surface for a particular venue, the size, maturity and skill level of the individuals interacting with the surface, as well as the mechanical goal of all tasks to be performed, need to be considered. When surfaces are used for more than one type of task (e.g. Land and Stop and Land and Go) the design of the surface becomes more complex. For example, successful performance of advanced aerial tumbling skills is dependent on the ability of the gymnast to utilize the mechanical properties of the spring floor during both the takeoff (Land and Go) and landing (Land and Stop) phases of the skill. The same spring floor system is used by growing young female gymnasts and mature male gymnasts of various skill levels and sizes. The difficulty of performing both Land and Go and Land and Stop tumbling tasks on the same spring floor is reflected in the high incidence of performance errors (McNitt-Gray 1992) and injuries associated with the floor exercise event (Garrick & Requa 1980; Riccardelli & Pettrone 1984; NCAA 1986, 1990).

Mechanical load

Musculoskeletal loading is influenced by how the individual prepares for the impending collision and distributes the load during the landing, as well as by strategies used by the individual to generate advantageous reaction forces for successful performance of the subsequent Stop or Go task. In the first part of this section, variables used to characterize musculoskeletal loading are defined. In the second part, preparation prior to touchdown is discussed. In the third part, load distribution after touchdown is addressed at the total body and the joint level using exemplar kinematic, reaction force, joint kinetic and EMG data acquired during a range of landing tasks.

Definition of variables used to characterize musculoskeletal loading

Load is defined as the forces and moments experienced by the body (Nigg 1985). Load exposure can be characterized by the amplitude, direction, duration, loading rate and frequency of forces and moments applied to the musculoskeletal system. A *force* is a push or pull and is represented by a vector that has magnitude, direction and a point of force application. During landing, reaction forces typically push and muscles pull. The magnitude of a force, illustrated by the length of the force vector, represents *how much* force is present. The direction of a force, illustrated by the angle of the force vector, is expressed as an angle relative to a frame of reference (e.g. 1 rad counterclockwise relative to the vertical). In foot-first landings, the point of force application, or *centre of pressure* (CP), is *where* the force is considered to be applied at the foot/surface interface. The CP describes the centroid of the pressure distribution at the foot/mat interface and represents the point of force application where a resultant reaction force would be applied to the foot to reflect the effect of all forces applied to the foot (Rodgers & Cavanagh 1984). If the line of action of the force vector acts a distance from the axis of rotation (e.g. segment COM), the force creates a *moment* about the axis of rotation. A *moment* is the rotation created by a force acting a distance from the axis of rotation (Rodgers & Cavanagh 1984). A moment is determined by the vector cross product of the position vector from the axis of rotation to the point of force application (*r*) and the force vector (**F**).

A free body diagram of a lower-extremity segment is a helpful tool for visualizing and accounting for all of the forces and moments acting on the segment at an instant (Rodgers & Cavanagh 1984). For example, the free body diagram of the foot reflects the reaction force applied at the centre of pressure, the segment weight vector applied at the segment centre of mass (COM), the net joint force at the ankle, and the net joint moment at the ankle. The weight vector is applied at the segment COM and reflects the acceleration of the segment mass due to gravity. The net joint force (NJF) is the net force acting at the joint. Together, the NJF and all other forces acting on the segment cause the linear acceleration of the segment COM. The NJF reflects only the net force at a joint, and in most cases is significantly less than the bone-on-bone forces that exist between the articular surfaces of the joint (Winter 1979). The net joint moment (NJM) reflects the net moment of all structures crossing the joint. The proximal (PM) and distal moments (DM) about the foot COM are created by the reaction force applied at the CP foot/plate interface (DM) and the NJF applied at the ankle (PM). The PM and DM about the shank and thigh COM are the moments about the segment COM created by the NJFs applied at the ankle and knee, and knee and hip, respectively. Together, the NJMs, PM and DM cause the angular acceleration of the segment about a mediolateral axis passing through the segment COM.

Differences in impulse, loading rate and time to peak reaction force characteristics between subjects and tasks provides insight regarding differences in musculoskeletal loading experienced by subjects when landing different tasks. The impulse created by a force is the integration of the force–time curve over an interval of time. For example, the landing phase, as defined in this chapter, is the interval of time from first contact with the plate by the foot (touchdown) until the time of last contact with the plate (departure) prior to the flight phase of the secondary movement (e.g. Land and Go tasks) or until the TBCM vertical velocity at touchdown is reduced to zero (e.g. Land and Stop tasks). Although the impulse created by a force characterizes how much force is applied over an interval of time, the distribution of the impulse during the landing phase is best characterized by the force–time curve. Loading rate is calculated by determining the time required for the force to rise by a specified magnitude (e.g. body weight ± 50 N, Munroe *et al.* 1987), whereas the time to peak force is the time elapsed after initial touchdown when the force reaches a local maximum. Observed differences in force–time characteristics between tasks have implications regarding how the musculoskeletal structures may respond to the load.

Preparation for touchdown

Because the musculoskeletal system experiences large loads immediately following contact, strategies used to attenuate and control the reaction force must be initiated prior to contact (Melvill-Jones & Watt 1971; Lees 1981). The ability of an individual to prepare for contact may be compromised by the preparation time, segment kinematics and visual conditions prior to contact (Nigg 1985; McNitt-Gray & Nelson 1988; McNitt-Gray 1991b; Sidaway *et al.* 1989). How the individual prepares for contact influences how the reaction force impulse is distributed during the landing phase (Fig. 25.3). For example, a collegiate female basketball player rebounding a ball from the same height under four different landing conditions experienced different reaction force–time characteristics after touchdown (Fig. 25.3). Muscle activation and segment kinematics prior to contact indicate preparation for impact involves multiple lower-extremity muscles and segments. Muscle activity observed prior to contact (Melvill-Jones & Watt 1971; Greenwood & Hopkins 1976; Sidaway *et al.* 1989; Dyhre-Poulsen *et al.* 1991) is thought to regulate changes in muscle length after

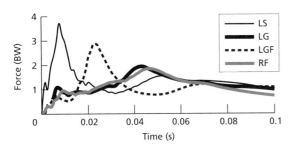

Fig. 25.3 Differences in reaction force–time characteristics for one leg during basketball rebound landings performed by the same female collegiate basketball player under four different conditions: Land and Stop using their normal strategy (LS), Land and Go using their normal strategy (LG), Land and Go under fatigued conditions induced by a series of repetitive maximum vertical jumps (LGF), Land and Stop using their reduced force landing strategy (RF) (McNitt-Gray et al. 1996). During localized muscular fatigue, the Land and Go Fatigued force–time characteristics become more like those observed for the Land and Stop landings than the Land and Go landings.

contact and the peak reaction force magnitude (Dyhre-Poulsen & Laursen 1994; Mizrahi & Susak 1982; Stacoff et al. 1987).

LANDING PREPARATION TIME

The landing preparation time during the flight phase preceding touchdown influences the ability of the athlete to prepare for contact. Preparation for contact may include placing segments in an advantageous position at touchdown, adjustment of lower-extremity segment velocity prior to contact, and/or activation of the muscles responsible for controlling the reaction force. Therefore, skills performed preceding the landing task must be performed in a way that ensures adequate preparation time is available prior to touchdown. During the flight phase of simple drop landings, joints of the lower extremity approach full extension and then flex just prior to touchdown (McKinley & Pedotti 1992; Munkasy & McNitt-Gray 1992; McNitt-Gray 1993). Landings of more complex tasks, however, may limit the time to prepare for contact. For example, examination of vaulting landings performed by men and women gymnasts during the 1984 Olympic competition (McNitt-Gray & Nelson 1988) indicated that women

achieved a smaller hip angle at touchdown than the men. This difference in hip angles at touchdown between men and women was associated with the longer flight times observed for the men as compared to the women. Longer flight times were attributed to both a higher horse height and a larger vertical velocity of the TBCM at horse departure for the men as compared to the women.

Compensatory kinematics associated with reductions in landing preparation time were also observed in a within-subject comparison of dismount landings performed by gymnasts during the 1996 Olympic Games (Fig. 25.4a,b). In general, dismounts with longer flight times provided the gymnast with more time to complete the required rotations and to extend the joints in preparation for contact, whereas dismounts with shorter flight times provided the gymnast with less time to complete both the rotation and preparation for foot first contact. For example, greater hip angles at touchdown and flight times were observed for landings of backward-rotating dismounts performed from the high bar than from the parallel bars (n = 10; McNitt-Gray et al. 1998a). The longer flight times observed for the high-bar dismounts were associated with the greater height of the apparatus and the greater TBCM vertical velocity at the time of release from the high bar as compared with the height and velocity observed at time of release from the parallel bars. Differences in the hip angle at touchdown between tasks influence the musculoskeletal loading characteristics by requiring hip muscles to generate moments at different muscle lengths.

Landing preparation time may also be compromised by decreases in time to view the landing surface. Vision is thought to play a major role when preparing for contact (Lees 1981; Sidaway et al. 1989). For example, during activities involving forward rotation, the anatomical orientation of the head and eyes contributes to a decrease in landing surface viewing time (McNitt-Gray 1992). This reduction in viewing time appears to increase the difficulty of the Land and Stop task. For example, the success rate of forward-rotating handspring vaults performed by male gymnasts during the 1992 Olympic Compulsory Competition was less than 15% (McNitt-Gray 1992). In addition, male and female

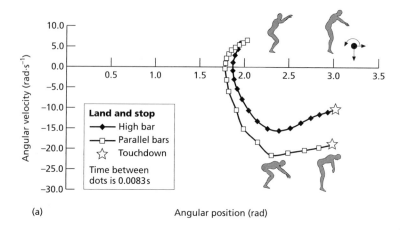

(a)   Angular position (rad)

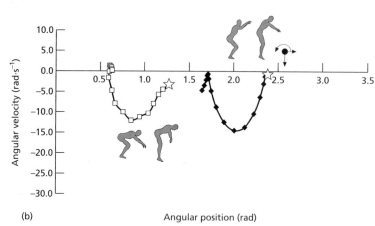

(b)   Angular position (rad)

Fig. 25.4 Knee (a) and hip (b) phase plane relationships observed during back salto landings performed from the high bar and parallel bars by the same male gymnast during the 1996 Olympic Gymnastics Competition. Similar knee angular positions were observed at touchdown (star); however, greater knee angular velocity was observed during the landing from the high bar than during the landing from the parallel bars. In contrast, greater hip extension was observed at touchdown during the landing from the high bar than from the parallel bars. (From McNitt-Gray *et al.* 1998.)

gymnasts apparently chose to avoid landings of forward-rotating skills when choreographing their optional routines for the 1992 Olympic Gymnastics Competition (McNitt-Gray 1992). Avoidance of landings of forward-rotating tasks may also reflect the difficulty in preparing for and controlling large forces and moments after touchdown.

RELATIVE SEGMENT VELOCITY PRIOR TO
TOUCHDOWN

Segment kinematics prior to touchdown in Land and Stop tasks performed by collegiate gymnasts, volleyball players and basketball players indicate that subjects prepare for contact by reducing the downward segment velocity of the lower-extremity segments relative to the TBCM vertical velocity.

Examination of the relative velocity of segments prior to touchdown indicates thigh, shank and foot COMs fell at a slower rate than hip, knee and ankle, respectively (Munkasy & McNitt-Gray 1992). Relative segment velocities of the thigh, shank and foot, and joint angular velocities of the hip, knee and ankle observed in the last 10 ms prior to contact during front and back salto landings were computed using the following relationships:

$$v_{T/H} = v_T - v_H$$

$$v_{S/K} = v_S - v_H - v_{K/H}$$

$$v_{F/A} = v_F - v_H - v_{K/H} - v_{A/K}$$

where v represents vertical velocity; the solidus (/) means with respect to; the modifiers T, S and F represent thigh, shank and foot centres of mass; and the modifiers H, K and A represent the hip, knee and ankle joints. The difference in leg and TBCM velocity averaged 0.3 m · s^{-1} for Land and Stop drop landings performed by collegiate male gymnasts from a height of 0.72 m onto a mat (0.12 m thick) (Munkasy & McNitt-Gray 1992). Qualitative examination of lower-extremity kinematics during a drop landing at 1000 frames per second performed in our laboratory also shows the toes moving up relative to the forefoot prior to touchdown.

In contrast to drop landings, the lower-extremity COM fell at a faster rate than the TBCM during the landings preceded by forward and backward rotation (Munkasy *et al.* 1996). During landings preceded by backward rotation, the ankle, knee and hip angular velocities indicated that all joints were flexing (−5 to −6 rad · s^{-1}) prior to contact. However, during landings preceded by forward rotation, the knee and hip joints were extending (+1–2 rad · s^{-1}) prior to touchdown. Examination of relative segment COM vertical velocities indicated that the foot was falling slower than the ankle, and the shank was following slower than the knee for both front and back salto landings. The thigh COM prior to touchdown, however, was falling faster (0.75 m · s^{-1}) than the hip during the front salto landings and was falling slower than the hip during the back salto landings. These differences in thigh segment kinematics when preparing for front and back salto landing suggest thigh motion ensures feet first contact and then adjusts segment COM velocity relative to the TBCM velocity. These differences between landings of front and back saltos may also reflect differences in visual conditions prior to touchdown, anatomical constraints relative to the direction of rotation, and/or joint kinetics during contact.

When athletes are asked to land 'softer' than normal an accentuated 'pull-up' of the landing gear is observed in association with the reduction in peak vertical force. For example, comparison of segment kinematics (200 Hz) prior to contact between normal and reduced force landings performed by volleyball players and basketball players resulted in differences in the degree of 'pull-up' prior to touchdown. When individuals attempted to reduce peak reaction forces after touchdown, the shank fell at an even slower rate with respect to the thigh than

during a normal landing (Munkasy & McNitt-Gray 1992). Relative leg, thigh and foot velocities, however, were not significantly different between normal and softer-than-normal landings.

Lower-extremity kinematics

JOINT ANGLES AT TOUCHDOWN

In general, all subjects performing Land and Stop tasks initiate contact with the landing surface using a forefoot-heel landing pattern. During Land and Go tasks, however, subjects may use a forefoot-heel, flat foot, or heel-toe landing pattern. The range of knee angular positions at touchdown observed during both Land and Go and Land and Stop tasks tends to be much smaller than the range of hip angles observed at touchdown (Figs 25.4–25.6). The observed differences in hip angles at touchdown reflect differences in mechanics between tasks (Fig. 25.6a–c) as well as differences in the landing pre-paration time (Fig. 25.4b). For example, the hip angle at touchdown is more flexed during the back salto landing than during the drop landing performed by the same gymnast (Fig. 25.6a,b). The more flexed hip angle allows the gymnast to position their TBCM more anterior relative to the feet than during the drop landing, and thus enables the gymnast to apply the linear and angular impulse needed to Land and Stop without steps. Similarly, the more extended hip angle during front salto landing as compared to the drop landing enables the gymnast to position their TBCM more posterior relative to the feet, enabling the gymnast to apply the linear and angular impulse needed to Land and Stop.

In contrast, the differences in hip angle at touchdown observed between the back salto landings performed from the high bar and those performed from the parallel bars may be attributed to less landing preparation time prior to touchdown when dismounting from the parallel bars as compared to the high bar (Figs 25.4a,b & 25.5a). Differences in hip angle at touchdown during vaulting landings performed during the 1984 Olympic competition, however, appeared to be independent of the body positions achieved during the flight phase of the aerial skill preceding touchdown (e.g. tucked, piked, layout) (McNitt-Gray & Nelson 1988).

JOINT KINEMATICS AFTER TOUCHDOWN

In general, joints closest to the point of force application demonstrated larger peak flexion angular velocities than those positioned farther from the application of force (McNitt-Gray 1991; McKinley & Pedotti 1992; McNitt-Gray et al. 1993b; McNitt-Gray et al. 1997) (Fig. 25.4a,b). As the TBCM velocity at touchdown increase, joint flexion velocities after touchdown also increase. The general shape of the phase plane relationships of the lower-extremity joints for a particular athlete, however, appears to exhibit some invariant qualities independent of task (McNitt-Gray et al. 1998a) (Fig. 25.4a,b). The similarities in phase plane shapes observed across tasks suggest that an individual subject may prefer a particular muscle lengthening rate when controlling joint flexion after touchdown.

All subjects tended to utilize the majority of their available ankle dorsiflexion during the landing phase. The observed differences in minimum hip and knee angles between tasks appear to be related to TBCM velocity at touchdown, surface properties, landing strategies selected by the individual, or level of fatigue (Figs 25.4a,b & 25.5a,b). Increases in knee and hip flexion observed when landing from progressively greater heights suggests that athletes regulate total body rigidity using a multijoint solution (McNitt-Gray 1993b). Comparison of minimum knee and hip angles observed during landings performed from progressively greater heights with and without landing mats indicates that landing on a mat may reduce the need for knee and hip flexion (McNitt-Gray et al. 1993). Accomplishing the landing task with less lower-extremity joint flexion may allow the athlete to generate the net joint moments needed to control the large reaction force at more advantageous muscle lengths. If less joint flexion is required to perform a landing, then more knee and hip range of motion would become available to compensate for unexpected events. Less lower-extremity joint flexion was also observed when landing on less-rigid surfaces (Ozguven & Berme 1988; McKinley & Pedotti 1992; McNitt-Gray et al. 1993b; McNitt-Gray et al. 1994c; Ferris & Farley 1997;

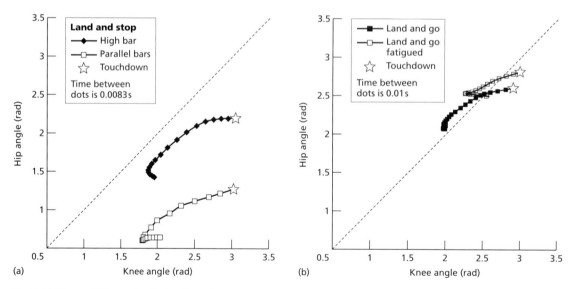

Fig. 25.5 Knee and hip angle relationships observed during (a) back salto landings performed from the high bar and parallel bars by the same male gymnast during the 1996 Olympic Gymnastics Competition and (b) female collegiate volleyball players performing block landings using their normal landing strategy under non-fatigued and fatigued conditions. In both conditions, both athletes exhibit similar relationships despite differences in initial (b) or final (a) joint angular positions between tasks.

Farley *et al.* 1998) or when wearing more energy-absorbing shoes (Clarke *et al.* 1983) at comparable TBCM vertical velocities at touchdown.

Landing strategies favouring a reduction in peak vertical reaction force exhibited greater degrees of joint flexion during the landing phase than those observed during normal landings (Lees 1981; Dufek & Bates 1990; Irvine *et al.* 1992). During these reduced peak vertical force landings, a greater percentage of the vertical impulse was applied later in the landing phase at times of greater knee flexion (Irvine *et al.* 1992). The temporal shift in impulse distribution associated with the reduced force landing strategy would most likely influence the musculoskeletal loading characteristics throughout the landing phase.

Observed modifications in landing strategy in response to changes in landing surfaces or footwear, may also contribute to a reduction in peak reaction force. For example, collegiate gymnasts experienced greater peak vertical reaction forces when landing on a mat than when landing on a rigid force plate (McNitt-Gray *et al.* 1994c). Examination of the lower-extremity kinematics during these trials revealed that the gymnasts modified their landing strategy by increasing their lower-extremity flexion when landing on the more rigid force plate than when landing on the mat (McNitt-Gray *et al.* 1994c). This observed relationship between lower-extremity flexion, surface properties and reaction force magnitude suggests that humans may choose to fix the combined rigidity of the body/surface system during landings from a given height and scale the degree of joint flexion to the properties of the landing surface (McNitt-Gray *et al.* 1994c). In addition, the mulitjoint solution used to compensate for modifications in surface appears to be somewhat invariant within subject. For example, gymnasts tending to flex the knees more than the hips when landing on a mat, tended to adjust their landing strategy when landing on a force plate by increasing knee flexion more than hip flexion (McNitt-Gray *et al.* 1994c).

Adjacent joint coordination patterns used by subjects across tasks also appear to be invariant within subject (Fig. 25.5a,b). For example, male gymnasts performing dismounts from the high bar and parallel bars appeared to use the same adjacent joint coordination patterns for both tasks, despite differences

in hip angle at touchdown (Fig. 25.5a). Female volleyball players also appear to use the same hip and knee coordination during Land and Go and Land and Go block landings performed under fatigued conditions (Fig. 25.5b) despite differences in minimum knee flexion observed between the Land and Go fatigued and the Land and Go landings (Fig. 25.5b). The invariant qualities of these knee and hip angle-angle relationships across tasks suggests that subjects may be choosing to keep changes in biarticular muscle length to a minimum.

Load distribution

LANDING PHASE DURATION

During Land and Stop tasks, the majority of the TBCM velocity at touchdown was reduced during the first 75 ms after touchdown (Fig. 25.6a–j). The duration of the impulse during Land and Go tasks appears to vary with the immediacy of the Go movement. For example, a long-jumper may need to depart from the ground in less than 0.125 s whereas a basketball player may opt to delay the initiation of the Go movement following touchdown (0.175 s). During a Land and Go movement performed on a spring floor, contact duration will correspond to the surface deformation time characteristics (e.g. diving board, trampoline vs. force plate) and the goal of the task (e.g. maintain frequency of hopping (Ferris & Farley 1997; Farley *et al.* 1998).

REACTION FORCE–TIME CHARACTERISTICS

All landings are characterized by a rapid increase in the reaction force magnitude within the first 50 ms after touchdown. However, time to peak force and loading rate between tasks, surfaces and landing strategies vary. For example, the time to peak force was observed to be similar during the landing of the front salto (Fig. 25.6c) and the takeoff of the long jump (Fig. 25.6d); however, the loading rate was significantly greater during the long-jump takeoff than during the front salto landing. Within-subject comparison of force–time characteristics observed during a Land and Stop task performed with and

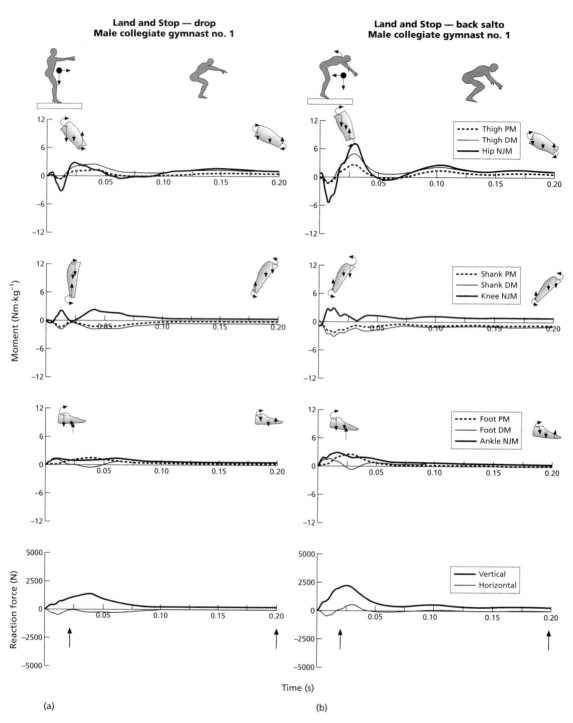

Fig. 25.6 Representative net joint moments (NJM) during landings performed by national-level collegiate gymnasts, volleyball players, basketball players and long-jumpers are displayed using data acquired by McNitt-Gray *et al.* All experiments were designed with the assistance of coaches and/or athletes to replicate the environmental context under which the landing movements are typically performed. In all cases presented here, subjects performed the landing task using their self-selected landing strategy. The human figure represents the body position at touchdown (time 0) and at the time near minimum total body centre of mass (TBCM) position during the landing phase. The TBCM vertical and horizontal velocities at touchdown for the trial are represented as vectors. Reaction forces experienced by one foot were quantified using a force plate and are expressed in newtons (N). The vertical (+) and horizontal (anterior (+)/posterior (–)) components of the reaction force applied at the foot and the NJMs at the ankle, knee and hip are presented from touchdown to 0.2 s after contact. Extensor NJMs are represented as positive quantities. The proximal (PM) and distal (DM) moments created about the segment COM by the reaction force and net joint forces (NJFs) acting on the foot, shank

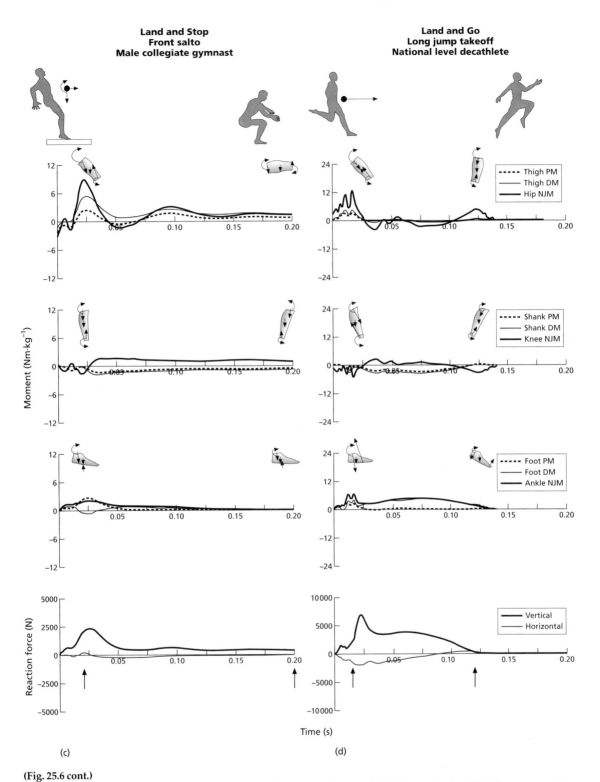

(Fig. 25.6 cont.)

and thigh are also presented from touchdown to 0.2 s after contact. Counterclockwise proximal and distal moments acting on the segment are represented as positive, whereas extensor NJMs at the ankle, knee and hip are represented as positive. Free body diagrams of the lower-extremity segments are provided early and late (noted by arrows) within the landing phase to illustrate the interrelationship between NJFs, segment orientation and adjacent NJMs.

Joint kinetics during (a) drop, (b) back salto and (c) front salto gymnastics landings performed by the same subject from a stationary platform (0.7 m) onto regulation gymnastics mats (0.12 m thick, peak vertical acceleration of 5.5 head form of 52.3 g when dropped from a height of 1.82 m) fully supported by two force plates. (d) The long jump takeoff was performed by a national level male decathlete on a force plate located at the end of the runway. The decathlete landed the jump in a sand-filled landing pit.

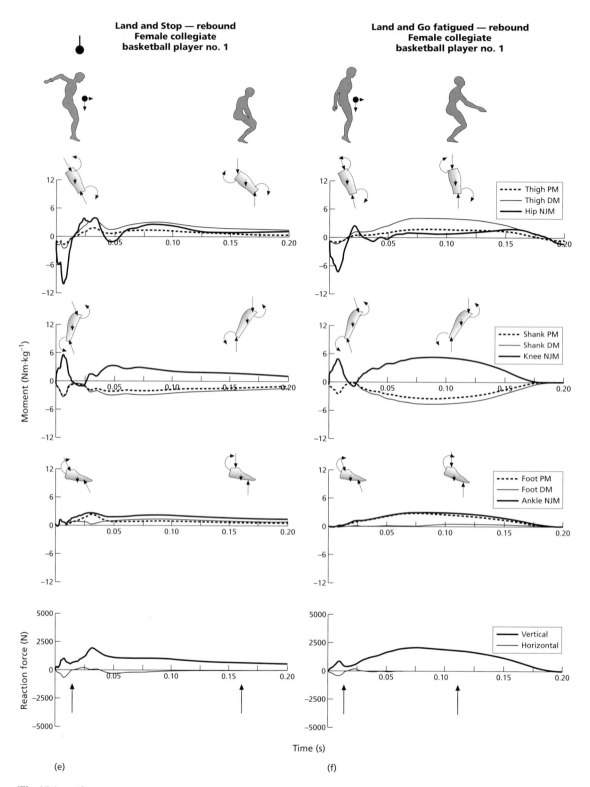

Land and Stop — rebound
Female collegiate
basketball player no. 1

Land and Go fatigued — rebound
Female collegiate
basketball player no. 1

Thigh PM
Thigh DM
Hip NJM

Shank PM
Shank DM
Knee NJM

Foot PM
Foot DM
Ankle NJM

Vertical
Horizontal

Moment (Nm·kg⁻¹)

Reaction force (N)

Time (s)

(e)

(f)

(Fig. 25.6 cont.)

(e,f) The basketball landings were performed while interacting with suspended balls overhead. Collegiate female basketball players were asked to land three different rebounding tasks using their own self-selected landing strategy. In all three tasks, the player jumped from the floor and palmed a stationary basketball suspended 0.41 m above their stand and reach height and landed on force plates. During the Land and Go tasks, each subject repeated the rebound movement and then immediately performed a second vertical jump reaching for a second ball located at 90% of the individual's maximum vertical jump and reach height. During the fatigue trial (LGF), the Land and Go task was performed after

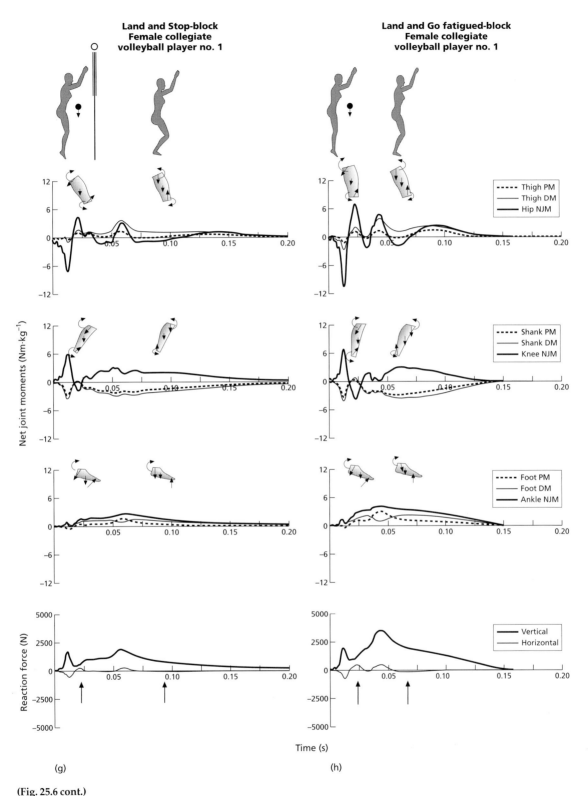

(Fig. 25.6 cont.)

moderate fatigue specific to jumping was induced immediately prior to the performance of the task. Moderate fatigue was induced by requiring the subject to perform maximum vertical jumps once every three seconds, until they were unable to obtain 80% of their maximum vertical jump and reach height. Localized muscle fatigue was induced in the volleyball players by requiring subjects to perform repetitive blocking movements along the length of the net. Localized muscle fatigue was induced in the basketball players by requiring subjects to perform maximum vertical jumps once every three seconds until they were unable to obtain 80% of the maximum jump height.

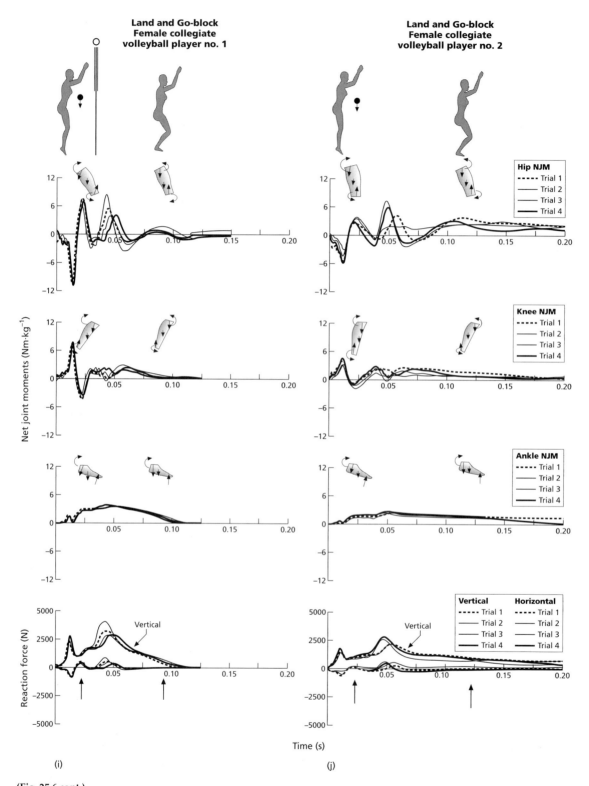

(Fig. 25.6 cont.)

(g–j) Volleyball blocking movements were performed on two force plates located alongside a regulation-height volleyball net placed in a horizontal position consistent with the individual subjects' preferred playing distance from the net. The volleyball height was standardized relative to the stand and reach height of the individual subject so that all subjects would vertically displace their TBCM approximately 19 inches during the block. During the Land and Go block, the volleyball player moved laterally to the left using her preferred footwork, jumped from the floor, blocked a suspended ball with the palms, and landed using her normal landing strategy, and then immediately moved laterally to the right and returned to her starting position.

without a landing mat, indicates that the time of peak reaction force was delayed when landing on the mat compared to when landing without the mat (McNitt-Gray et al. 1994c). Within-subject comparison of time to peak reaction force between Land and Stop and Land and Go tasks performed on sprung surfaces, indicates the time to peak force was the same between tasks (Munkasy et al. 1994). Time to peak vertical force may also be delayed when voluntarily attempting to reduce the peak reaction force magnitude by initiating contact with a more vertical foot position, as when landing softly (dancer: McNitt-Gray et al. 1992; gymnast: Irvine et al. 1992) or when initiating a Go movement following landing (McNitt-Gray et al. 1996). The more vertical foot position at touchdown appears to provide the subject with more time to reduce the velocity of the heel prior to initiating contact with the landing surface (Irvine et al. 1992). The ability to control the foot and the reaction force–time characteristics may be compromised when fatigued (McNitt-Gray et al. 1996; Fig. 25.3). During Land and Go tasks, the timing of the peak reaction force may also shift in relation to the initiation of the Go movement as selected by the subject (Fig. 25.3).

REACTION FORCE: MAGNITUDE AND DIRECTION

Reaction forces experienced by the foot during the landing phase vary with the mechanical goal of the task, the ability of the human to prepare for contact, the landing strategy and the landing surface properties (Fig. 25.6a–j). In general, the peak reaction force tends to increase in magnitude as the horizontal and/or vertical component of the TBCM velocity at touchdown increases (Hyoku et al. 1984; Nigg 1985; McNitt-Gray 1993; McNitt-Gray et al. submitted) (Fig. 25.2) and the level of control decreases (Bruggemann 1987; Panzer 1987; McNitt-Gray et al. 1993a). For example, the TBCM vertical velocity at touchdown during the tumbling takeoff (Land and Go) may be less than $-1 \text{ m} \cdot \text{s}^{-1}$ yet the reaction forces experienced by each leg may be 7 BW (Fig. 25.2). In contrast, the landing of a tumbling skill (Land and Stop) with a TBCM vertical velocity approaching $-8 \text{ m} \cdot \text{s}^{-1}$ may result in a peak vertical

reaction force of 7 BW for each leg (Fig. 25.2). A similar relationship between peak reaction forces and horizontal velocity at touchdown is observed during the takeoff phase of the long jump (Fig. 25.2). Peak reaction forces experienced by each leg during landings of vertical jumps, volleyball blocks and basketball rebounds, typically fall within these boundaries (Nigg et al. 1981; Nigg 1985; Valiant & Cavanagh 1985; Panzer 1987; Stacoff et al. 1987) and will vary with landing strategy (Fig. 25.2).

The magnitude of the peak horizontal reaction force after touchdown also increases as the magnitude of the horizontal TBCM velocity at contact increases (Fig. 25.6c,d). For example, the peak horizontal force observed during the long-jump takeoff is an order of magnitude greater than the peak horizontal force observed during the landing of the front salto.

During Land and Stop tasks, the direction of anterior/posterior reaction forces experienced during the landing phase act in opposition to the direction of the linear and angular velocity of the body at touchdown (Fig. 25.6a–j). In the case of front and back salto landings, the anterior and posterior reaction forces may change direction many times. During the back salto landing, the posterior-directed horizontal reaction forces observed after touchdown reflect the immediate reduction in angular momentum after touchdown (McNitt-Gray et al. 1991a). Whereas, during the front salto landing, the anterior-directed horizontal reaction forces observed after touchdown reflect the immediate reduction in forward rotating angular momentum after touchdown (McNitt-Gray et al. 1991a). In contrast, the direction of the net horizontal impulse applied during the entire landing phase reflects the change in horizontal momentum of the TBCM from touchdown to the end of the landing phase. For example, during the landing of the forward-travelling forward-rotating front salto the net horizontal impulse acts in the posterior direction (–), whereas during the landing of the backward-travelling backward-rotating back salto, the net horizontal impulse acts in the anterior direction (+).

During Land and Go tasks, the direction of the anterior/posterior reaction forces experienced immediately after touchdown also oppose the direction of the linear and angular velocity of the body at touchdown (Fig. 25.6d,f,h). However, later in the landing phase, the direction of the anterior/posterior reaction force applies a horizontal impulse in a direction consistent with the Go task (Fig. 25.6d,f,h).

REACTION FORCE: DIFFERENCES
BETWEEN LEGS

Musculoskeletal loading may differ between legs depending on the role of each leg in controlling and converting the TBCM momentum at touchdown. Land and Stop tasks are typically performed on two legs to provide the necessary stability for reducing the TBCM momentum at touchdown to zero. During Land and Go tasks, however, conversion of the TBCM momentum at touchdown may be achieved using one or two legs depending on the mechanical goal of the task. For example, during landings of centred Land and Stop volleyball blocks (e.g. suspended ball positioned between the hands) performed by female collegiate volleyball players, the difference in peak vertical reaction forces between legs varied between 0.5 and 1.5 BW. During Land and Stop landings performed by gymnasts, the higher degree of asymmetrical loading observed for front (0.78 (0.7) BW) and back salto (0.95 (1.1) BW) landings as compared to drop landings (0.50 (0.3) BW) suggest that the landings of more difficult skills may produce a higher degree of asymmetrical loading (McNitt-Gray et al. 1991a). In contrast, landings of late Land and Stop volleyball blocks (e.g. ball suspended beyond the lead leg) or Land and Go centred volleyball blocks, resulted in differences in peak vertical reaction forces between legs ranging from 2 to 5 BW (Fig. 25.2).

If only one leg is used to convert the TBCM momentum during the landing phase, as in the long jump, the musculoskeletal loading experienced by the takeoff leg (> 9 BW, Luhtanen & Komi 1979; McNitt-Gray et al. submitted) is substantially different than the swing leg when long jumping (0 BW). In the case of the triple jump, however, large reaction forces are experienced by both legs (Hay 1993). Differences in musculoskeletal loading between legs may still occur, however, due to differences in the way load is distributed between joints during each landing phase of the triple jump.

Over a practice session, season or career, the degree of asymmetrical loading accumulates and may produce different injury patterns between legs. Unfortunately, most epidemiological studies are retrospective and do not account for loading specific to the individual's typical movement patterns (e.g. outside hitter vs. middle blocker in volleyball).

MODIFICATION OF REACTION FORCE
MAGNITUDE

The magnitude of reaction forces can be viewed as an advantage or disadvantage depending on the goal of the landing. For example, dancers want to avoid landing 'loudly' and therefore practise landing softly and with reduced peak reaction force magnitudes. In contrast, divers initiating a dive using a 'crow hop' takeoff from the 10 m platform use the foot first impact with the tower as a way to increase their vertical reaction force, vertical impulse and jump height at departure (Miller et al. 1989; Mathiyakom et al. 1998).

Reduction of peak vertical forces, either by modifying the landing surface or by modifying the landing mechanics, has been proposed as a means of reducing the risk of injury. The magnitude of peak vertical force applied to the feet can be reduced when landing on energy-absorbing surfaces (McNitt-Gray et al. 1993b) provided the human–surface interaction does not result in maximum compression of the surface. The magnitude of the reaction force may be modified by the human, either by adopting a prescribed technique (e.g. increase knee flexion, Devita & Skelly 1992) or by asking subjects to use their own self-selected strategy (McNitt-Gray et al. 1990; Irvine et al. 1992). For example, college-age recreational athletes involved in jumping and landing activities were able to vary their peak vertical reaction force during landing by as much as 8 BW by changing their landing strategy (McNitt-Gray et al. 1990). Similar results were observed by Zatsiorsky and Prilutsky (1987). Subjects unable to reduce their peak vertical reaction force were observed to use a normal landing strategy that already favoured a relatively low peak vertical reaction force.

Although these approaches have been successful in reducing the peak vertical reaction forces, the corresponding modifications in the reaction force and the internal loads experienced throughout the duration of the contact period requires more thorough evaluation prior to implementation as a means of reducing musculoskeletal loading. Examination of joint kinetics, kinematics and simultaneously acquired muscle activation of major lower-extremity muscles provides a more complete evaluation of external and internal load implications of reduced peak vertical reaction force landings.

Landing joint kinetics

Kinematic and kinetic analyses of landings performed with self-selected strategies provide insights regarding preferred methods of force attenuation, load distribution and control of total body momentum. Quantification of kinematic and kinetic variables is also useful in evaluating specific landing techniques under a variety of circumstances (e.g. minimum knee angle less than 75°, Dufek & Bates 1990; knee angle less than 90°, Devita & Skelly 1992).

ANKLE

During all landings, the reaction force applied at the foot creates the need for an ankle extensor NJM (net joint movement) during the landing phase. Differences in ankle NJM magnitudes between tasks were directly related to foot angle at touchdown relative to the angle of the reaction force vector. Immediately following touchdown, the NJM at the ankle controls the moments created by the reaction force applied at the CP foot/plate interface (DM) and the NJF applied at the ankle (PM). When the foot touches down in a position aligned with the reaction force, the line of action of the NJF and reaction force pass near the foot COM. Consequently, the need for an ankle extensor NJM is reduced. When the alignment of the foot and the reaction force vector are less collinear, the need for an ankle extensor NJM increases.

Differences in foot position at touchdown may be observed between Land and Stop and Land and Go tasks; however, foot position at touchdown also varies between subjects. For example, six of seven female basketball players initiated a Land and Go

rebound task with a more vertical foot position than when initiating a Land and Stop rebound task. The more vertical position of the foot during the Land and Go rebound task may prove to be advantageous for initiating the subsequent 'Go' task.

More vertical foot positions at touchdown are also observed when subjects voluntarily reduce the magnitude of the peak vertical reaction force (Irvine et al. 1992) or choose to land softly (e.g. dancers) than when landing normally. The time to peak vertical force, associated with heel contact, during these 'soft' and reduced vertical force landings also tends to be longer compared to normal landings. The more vertical position of the foot at touchdown may provide additional time for the foot velocity to slow down prior to heel contact with the landing surface (McNitt-Gray et al. 1992).

After the first third of the landing phase (30–60 ms), the NJM at the ankle during Land and Stop tasks are extensor and are similar in magnitude. During this interval, the reaction force is essentially vertical. Consequently, the magnitude of the ankle NJM acts to oppose the moments created by the ankle NJF and the reaction force applied at the CP. During the Land and Go tasks, however, the reaction forces increase in magnitude in preparation for initiating the subsequent task. As a result, the ankle extensor NJM increases coincident with increases in the reaction force. Muscles responsible for creating ankle extensor NJMs also demonstrate increases in activity just prior to the increase in the reaction force (McNitt-Gray et al. 1996).

KNEE

Differences in knee NJMs between tasks are dependent on differences in both the ankle NJM magnitude and the shank angle at touchdown relative to the ankle and knee NJF vectors. This interactive relationship between adjacent joint NJMs and PM and DMs acting on a segment are illustrated in the free body diagrams for both Land and Stop and Land and Go tasks (Fig. 25.6a–j).

During both Land and Stop (e.g. front salto, Fig. 25.6c) and Land and Go (e.g. long jump, Fig. 25.6d) tasks, knee flexor NJMs were observed when the ankle NJMs were extensor and the ankle

NJFs passed anterior to the shank COM and the knee NJFs passed posterior to the shank COM. In each case, a knee flexor NJM was needed to oppose counterclockwise moments created by the ankle NJM and the shank PM and DMs. Knee flexor NJMs reach a near maximum magnitude when the ankle NJMs are large and the NJFs are nearly aligned with the shank COM.

During both Land and Stop and Land and Go tasks (e.g. volleyball, basketball; Fig. 25.6e–j), knee extensor NJMs were observed when the ankle NJMs were extensor and the ankle NJFs passed posterior to the shank COM and the knee NJFs passed anterior to the shank COM. In each case, a knee extensor NJM was needed to work with the ankle extensor NJM to oppose the clockwise shank PM and DMs (Fig. 25.6e–j). Knee extensor NJMs reach a near maximum magnitude when the ankle NJMs are small and the PM and DMs created by the ankle and knee NJFs are large and counterclockwise. This interdependency between adjacent joint moments, segment orientation, and force–time characteristics of the reaction force illustrates how musculoskeletal loading may vary between tasks.

Later in the landing phase, increases in PM and DM acting on the shank contributed to increases in extensor NJM at the knee. Subjects with more vertical shank angles at touchdown shifted more quickly from flexor NJM at the knee to extensor NJM at the knee than subjects with less vertical shank angles. The more vertical shank angle contributes to increases in moment arms for the NJF at the ankle and knee leading to increases in the PM and DM acting at the shank (McNitt-Gray *et al.*, submitted).

HIP

Differences in the hip NJM between tasks are dependent on differences in knee NJMs, as well as the thigh angle relative to the knee and hip NJFs. Immediately after touchdown, the hip NJM generally acts in opposition to the knee NJM (Fig. 25.6a–j). Later in the landing phase, the knee and hip NJM both tend to be extensor. During the basketball rebound trials (Fig. 25.6e,f), the hip NJM opposed the knee NJM, as well as the PM and DM acting on the thigh. During the Land and Stop volleyball

block, the angle of the thigh and NJF at the hip and knee were nearly the same. The collinearity of the segment and the NJFs minimized the moment arms, resulting in relatively small PM and DM. Therefore, immediately after touchdown in the Land and Stop volleyball block trial, the flexor hip NJM acted primarily to oppose the extensor knee NJM. Later in the landing phase, the extensor knee and hip NJMs tend to work together to oppose counterclockwise moments created by the knee and hip NJFs. This coordinated behaviour exhibited by adjacent joint NJMs demonstrates the ability of the lower extremity to stabilize and control the multijoint system in the presence of large external reaction forces.

TASK-DEPENDENT JOINT KINETICS

The NJM magnitude and direction is sensitive to the relative angle between the reaction force and segment orientation at touchdown and adjacent joint NJMs. For example, differences in the relative angle between the reaction force and segment position at touchdown between landings of front and back saltos contributed to differences in knee and hip net joint moments even when no significant differences in reaction force magnitude were observed between tasks. At touchdown in the front salto landing, the shank was nearly aligned with the reaction force vector and resulted in relatively small PM and DM. At touchdown in the back salto landing, however, the reaction force acted posterior to the segment COM and resulted in clockwise PM and DM. As a result, during the front salto landing, a knee flexor NJM was needed to oppose the ankle extensor NJM. In contrast, during the back salto landings, a knee extensor NJM was needed to assist the ankle in opposing the PM and DM moments created by the ankle and knee NJFs about the shank COM.

Adjacent joint NJMs also influence the NJM needed at a joint. For example, during both drop and back salto landings, a flexor NJM is needed at the hip to oppose the extensor NJM at the knee. During the drop landing, the PM and DM at the thigh were small, therefore the flexor NJM at the hip is needed to oppose the knee extensor NJM. The magnitude of the hip flexor NJM during the back salto landing is greater than during the drop landing because of the need to control greater PM, DM and knee extensor NJMs in the back salto landing as compared to the drop landing. Similarly, the magnitude of the knee flexor NJM during the long-jump takeoff is greater than the knee flexor NJM during the front salto landing because of the need to oppose greater PM, DM and ankle extensor NJM during the long jump takeoff than during the front salto landing.

Correspondence between muscle activity and joint kinetics

When accounting for a potential 50 ms electromechanical delay, associated with onset of EMG and transmission of muscle force, a good correspondence between muscle activation patterns and NJMs was observed (Fig. 25.7). For example, during the front and back salto landings, the activation patterns of muscles acting to extend (rectified +) and flex (rectified –) a joint followed the task-specific shifts in NJMs. A similar correspondence between muscle activation pattern and NJMs was also observed during landings performed by volleyball and basketball players (McNitt-Gray *et al.* 1994b, 1996).

Coactivation was observed throughout the movement and was greatest during periods when NJMs may need to quickly switch directions. The presence of muscle coactivation indicates that bone-on-bone loading at the articular surfaces will exceed the magnitude of the NJFs. In addition, the coupling of muscle activation patterns and leg kinematics at contact emphasize the need for landing preparation time to permit effective anticipation of contact.

During the propulsive phase of Go movements, the reaction force impulse and muscle activity were more pronounced than during the Land and Stop tasks (McNitt-Gray *et al.* 1996). The relationship between muscle activation patterns and NJMs was consistent within subjects over the majority of trials. Activity of the medial gastrocnemius was observed prior to contact in preparation for the ankle plantarflexor NJM following touchdown. Activity of the rectus femoris, vastus medialis and vastus lateralis were aligned with knee extensor NJMs. Later in the landing phase, when both the knee and hip NJMs

were extensor, activities of the gluteus maximus and rectus femoris were aligned with the knee and hip NJMs. Activation of biarticular muscles observed during periods where adjacent joints demonstrated opposite directions in net joint moment power create the potential for energy transfer (Prilutsky & Zatsiorsky 1994).

The net joint moment power (NJMP), represented by the product of the NJM and joint angular velocity, provides insight regarding the distribution of load between joints. In general, ankle, knee and hip flexion velocities (–) and ankle extensor NJM (+) were observed after touchdown. In contrast, the knee and hip NJMs tended to be of opposite sign immediately following touchdown. When accounting for an electromechanical delay (≈ 50 ms), medial gastrocnemius EMG was observed during periods of knee flexor and ankle plantarflexor NJMs. Biarticular muscle activity observed in correspondence with ankle (–) and knee (+) NJMPs provides the potential for energy transfer via biarticular muscle tendon units. During periods of hip (–) and knee (+) NJMPs, the activity of the semitendonosis also suggests the potential for energy transfer via a biarticular muscle tendon unit. EMG activity of biarticular muscles creating agonist moments at the knee and hip was also observed. For example, EMG activity of the rectus femoris was observed when negative NJMP was observed at the knee (extensor NJM, negative knee angular velocity) and positive NJMP was observed at the hip (flexor NJM and negative hip angular velocity). Similarly, EMG activity of the semimembranosis and the gastrocnemius were coincident with the timing of the knee flexor NJM observed later during the landing phase (McNitt-Gray *et al.* 1997). This correspondence between biarticular muscle activation and adjacent joint NJMPs provides experimental data to support distal to proximal transfer of energy via biarticular muscles as proposed by Prilutsky and Zatsiorksy (1994). Mechanical energy dissipation by more proximal muscles may prove advantageous in reducing distal lower-extremity loading during landing.

Load distribution between joints appears to be influenced by task, momentum, skill level and surface. Load distribution during landings is characterized by integrating the negative portion of the

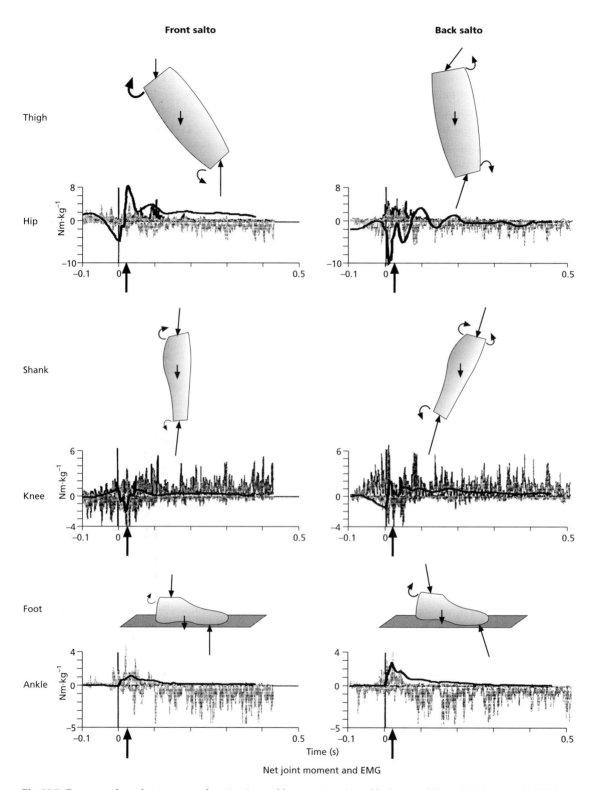

Fig. 25.7 Correspondence between muscle activation and lower-extremity ankle, knee and hip net joint moments (NJM) during forward and back salto landings performed by the same elite collegiate male. Both landings were performed from a stationary platform (0.7 m) onto a regulation gymnastics mat (0.12 m) fully supported by two force plates. Activities of muscles considered to be joint extensors are rectified, presented as positive values, and are shifted in time to account for an electromechanical delay (50 ms). Activities of muscles considered to be joint flexors are rectified, presented as negative values, and are shifted in time to account for an electromechanical delay (50 ms). In general, muscle activation patterns follow task-specific shifts in the ankle, knee and hip NJMs.

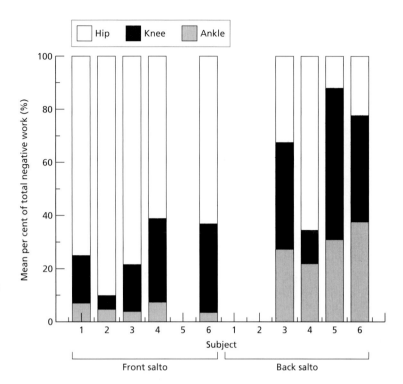

Fig. 25.8 Percentage of total lower-extremity negative work by the ankle, knee and hip NJM during the landing phase of front and back saltos. All subjects demonstrated a task-dependent difference in load distribution between tasks. In general, greater negative work was done by the hip NJM during the front salto landing compared with the back salto landing, whereas greater negative work was done by the ankle NJM during the back salto landing compared with the front salto landing.

NJMP curve for each joint from touchdown to the end of the landing phase. Examination of negative work done by net joint moments has assisted in providing an 'index of softness' (Zatsiorsky & Prilutsky 1987), evaluating the consequences of specific landing techniques (Devita & Skelly 1992), and determining differences in load distribution between tasks and subject populations (McNitt-Gray 1993). For example, task differences in load distribution were observed between front and back salto landings performed by the same gymnasts (Fig. 25.8; McNitt-Gray *et al*. 1995). The negative work by the ankle NJM comprised a greater percentage of the total negative work during the back salto landings than during the front salto landings. In contrast, work done by the hip NJM comprised a greater percentage of the total negative work during the front salto landings than during the back salto landings. In contrast, on average, 80% of the negative work done by the lower extremity NJMs was done by the ankle and knee during landings performed by basketball players (McNitt-Gray *et al*.

1996). The distribution of work done by the NJMs of joints closest to the point of force application parallels the epidemiology data reported for collegiate female basketball players.

The load distribution between joints during a task may change when an individual is required to use a specified landing technique. For example, volleyball players asked to land more softly by increasing knee flexion (Devita & Skelly 1992) redistributed the negative work within the lower extremity. During the softer landing, the negative work by the ankle and knee NJMs were nearly the same and the negative work done by the hip NJM was greater than that observed during the normal landing (Devita & Skelly 1992). During the normal landings, however, the negative work done by the ankle NJM was the greatest, followed by the knee and hip NJMs, respectively.

Examination of joint kinetics and EMG during landing activities has revealed that subjects may selectively activate biarticular muscles during periods when adjacent net joint moment powers are opposite in direction. During these intervals, power flow between adjacent joints may occur. The distal to proximal power flow may assist in distributing force to muscle tendon unit (MTU) with greater physiological cross-sectional area, thereby reducing localized stress. Examination of joint kinetics and bi- and uniarticular muscle activation patterns within-subject across task indicates these self-selected control strategies are independent of task. For example, more experienced gymnasts demonstrated reductions in biarticular muscle activity at times when adjacent net joint moments were both extensor (Irvine *et al.* 1992; McNitt-Gray *et al.* 1993a). Elite gymnasts have demonstrated different muscular recruitment patterns, despite similar joint kinetics (Fig. 25.7). For example, some gymnasts choose to activate the hamstrings rather than the gluteals when generating a hip extensor NJM in the presence of a knee extensor NJM. While this strategy may be contra-dictory from a generation of joint torque and knee compression point of view, the activation of the hamstring may serve as a strategy for joint stabilization, stress reduction of bone, or fatigue-resistant strategy. Selective recruitment of biarticular muscles during intervals when distal to proximal power transfer may also be advantageous for distribution of load within the lower extremity. Assessment of advantages and/or disadvantages of different control strategies in regard to load distribution and musculoskeletal loading, however, requires more sophisticated modelling of the musculoskeletal system. These results do however, emphasize the redundancy of the musculoskeletal system and the ability of individuals to choose from a variety of multijoint control strategies that may balance the need for effective load distribution with the need to accomplish the mechanical goal of the task.

Clinical summary

To avoid injury, the load experienced by the body needs to be kept in balance with the ability of musculoskeletal structures to respond to stress induced by loading. Visual, vestibular and proprioceptive impaired populations may have difficulty in controlling the lower-extremity moments created by large reaction forces during landing. Establishing a causal relationship between load and injury is currently compromised by methodological limitations associated with the quantification of material properties of intact biological materials and the forces experienced by anatomical structures during realistic movements. Assessment of the musculoskeletal loading experienced by an individual is further complicated by the use of multiple multijoint neuromuscular control strategies that modulate the mechanical characteristics of the extremities in relation to the task, velocity at touchdown, and properties of the landing surface. Systematic examination of the selective process by which individuals prepare for landing and dissipate load during landing, hoever, may assist in identifying advantageous subject-specific techniques for distributing musculoskeletal load.

During landing, humans rely primarily on lengthening of active muscle during joint flexion and bone deformation to attenuate and transmit forces experienced during contact. The redundancy of the musculoskeletal system allows the central nervous system to choose from a set of multijoint control strategies that balance the need for effective load distribution with the need to accomplish the mechanical goal of the task. The mechanical goal of a landing task is to effectively convert the total body momentum at touchdown to achieve a subsequent task. Musculoskeletal loading during the landing task, however, depends on how the individual has chosen to interact with the surface given performance and load-distribution goals. Landing-surface standards are often based on the need to establish uniformity of equipment during sanctioned competitions and are not based on musculoskeletal loading issues. Therefore, training regimes need to consider modifications in musculoskeletal loading when athletes make transitions between landing surfaces.

Athletes, coaches and trainers need to recognize the unique challenges imposed by each landing condition and encourage athletes to prepare for and practise landings under a variety of velocity, surface and body orientations. This can be better accomplished by following certain guidelines.

1 Clearly define the mechanical objective of the landing tasks in the context in which they are to be performed.

2 Evaluate the structure and capacity of the musculoskeletal system to control reaction forces experienced during landing.

3 Identify characteristic movement patterns used by the individual prior to, during and following touchdown as a means of identifying individual loading preferences, limitations and assets that the individual is choosing to avoid or exploit.

4 Design and follow a training programme specific to the current state of the musculoskeletal system that corresponds with the skill development time line.

5 Be aware that more than one landing strategy may be used to satisfy the mechanical and/or the load distribution goals of the landing task.

Appendix: biomechanical data acquisition and processing methods

Kinematic data are typically acquired by manually or automatically digitizing body landmarks consistent with body segment parameters used for segment masses and centre of masses (COM). These position data are then filtered using a fourth-order non-recursive filter (e.g. Butterworth) or a spline. Cut-off frequency selection criteria for each x and y coordinate typically varies between studies and may range from 4 to 20 Hz. The forces applied to the body are measured using a force plate. Kinematic and reaction force data are then synchronized using a common event observed in both sets of data (e.g. contact, a signal recorded from a light-emitting diode (LED) visible within the video image while digitally sampled along with the force data). The CP is typically determined using force plate geometry, foot position relative to the plate, and transducer output in accordance with the force plate manufacturer's specifications. The CP location relative to the foot is then projected into the kinematic reference system. The ankle, knee and hip net joint forces (NJFs) and net joint moments (NJMs) of the landing leg are then determined from segment kinematics, body segment parameters, the sagittal plane reaction force and centre of pressure (CP) using inverse dynamics (Elftman 1939). Surface or indwelling electrodes are used to monitor muscle activation patterns of lower-extremity muscles in accordance with standards established by the International Society of Electrokinesiology (1985).

Acknowledgements

The author would like to thank Philip Requejo, Witaya Mathiyakom, and Kathleen Costa for their assistance in generating the figures in this chapter and their comments regarding early versions of this manuscript.

References

Bruggemann, P. (1987) Biomechanics in gymnastics. In: *Current Research in Sports Biomechanics Medicine and Sport Science* (eds B. van Gheluwe & J. Atha), **25**, 142–176. Karger, Basel.

Clarke, T.E., Frederick, E.C. & Cooper, L.B. (1983) Effects of shoe cushioning upon ground reaction forces in running. *International Journal of Sports Medicine* **4**, 247–251.

Crowninshield, R.D. & Brand, R.A. (1981) A physiologically based criterion of muscle force prediction in locomotion. *Journal of Biomechanics* **14** (11), 793–801.

Denoth, J. & Nigg, B.M. (1981) The influence of various sport floors on the load on the lower extremities. In: *Biomechanics VII-B* (eds A. Morecki, K. Fidelus, K. Kedzior & A. Wit), pp. 100–105. University Park Press, Baltimore.

Devita, P. & Skelly, W.A. (1992) Effect of landing stiffness on joint kinetics and energetics in the lower extremity. *Medicine and Science in Sports and Exercise* **24** (1), 108–115.

Dufek, J.S. & Bates, B.T. (1990) The evaluation and prediction of impact forces during landings. *Medicine and Science in Sports and Exercise* **22**, 370–377.

Dyhre-Poulsen, P. & Laursen, A.M. (1984) Programmed electromyographic activity and negative incremental muscle stiffness in monkeys jumping downward. *Journal of Physiology* **350**, 121–136.

Elftman, H. (1939) Forces and energy changes in the leg during walking. *American Journal of Physiology* **124**, 339–356.

Farley, C.T., Houdijk, H.H., Van Strein, C. & Louie, M. (1998) Mechanism of leg stiffness adjustment for hopping on surfaces of different stiffnesses. *Journal of Applied Physiology* **85** (3), 1044–1055.

Fédération Internationale de Gymnastique (1984) *Code of Points*. International Gymnastics Federation, Bericht, West Germany.

Ferretti, A., Puddu, G., Mariani, P.P. & Neri, M. (1985) The natural history of jumper's knee. Patellar or quadriceps tendonitis. *International Orthopaedics* **8** (4), 239–242.

Ferris, D.P. & Farley, C.T. (1997) Interaction of leg stiffness and surface stiffness during human hopping. *Journal of Applied Physiology* **82**, 15–22.

Ferris, D.P., Louie, M. & Farley, C.T. (1997) Adjustments in running mechanics to accommodate different surface stiffnesses. *Physiologist* **39**, A59.

Garrick, J.G. & Requa, R.K. (1980) Epidemiology of women's gymnastics injuries. *The American Journal of Sports Medicine* 8 (4), 261–264.

Gollhofer, A. (1987) Innervation characteristics of m. gastrocnemius during landing on different surfaces. In: *Biomechanics X-B* (ed. B. Jonsson), pp. 701–706. Human Kinetics, Champaign, IL.

Greenwood, R.G. & Hopkins, A. (1976) Muscle responses during sudden falls in man. *Journal of Physiology* (Lond.) **254**, 507–518.

Gregor, R.J. & Abelew, T.A. (1994) Tendon force measurements and movement control: a review. *Medicine and Science in Sports and Exercise* **26**, 1359–1372.

Hatze, H. (1981) Estimation of myo-dynamic parameter values from observations on isometrically contracting muscle groups. *European Journal of Applied Physiology* 46 (4), 325–338.

Hay, J.G. (1986) The biomechanics of the long jump. *Exercise and Sport Sciences Reviews* **14**, 401–446.

Hay, J.G. (1993) Citius, Altius, Longius (Faster, Higher, Longer): The biomechanics of jumping for distance. *Journal of Biomechanics* **26**, 7–21.

Herzog, W. (1996) Force-sharing among synergistic muscles: theoretical considerations and experimental approaches. *Exercise and Sport Science Reviews* **24**, 173–202.

Hyoku, C., Shibukawa, K., Ae, M., Hashihara, Y., Yokoi, T. & Kawabata, A. (1984) Effect of dropping height on a buffer action in landing. Paper presented at the Japanese Society of Biomechanics, Nagoya, Japan.

International Society of Electrokinesiology (ISEK) Standards (1985). *Journal of Electromyography and Kinesiology* (1999) **9** (2), I.

Irvine, D.M.E. & McNitt-Gray, J.L. (1993) Muscle recruitment patterns in landings with reduced vertical reaction forces. In: *Proceedings of the XVIIth American Society of Biomechanics (ASB) Meeting*, pp. 111–112.

Irvine, D.M.E., McNitt-Gray, J.L., Munkasy, B.A., Barbieri, C.A. & Welch, M.D. (1992) Muscle activity and kinetics during landings with reduced vertical reaction forces. In: *Proceedings of the Second North American Congress of Biomechanics (NACOB II)*, pp. 547–548.

Kulund, D.N., McCue, F.C., Rockwell, D.A. & Gieck, J.H. (1979) Tennis injuries: prevention and treatment. *American Journal of Sports Medicine* 7, 249–253.

Lees, A. (1981) Methods of impact absorption when landing from a jump. *Engineering in Medicine* 10 (4), 207–211.

Luhtanen, P. & Komi, P.V. (1979) Mechanical power and segmental contribution to force impulses in long jump take-off. *European Journal of Applied Physiology* **41**, 267–274.

Mathiyakom, W., McNitt-Gray, J.L., Munkasy, B.A., Eagle, J. & Gabriele, J. (1998) Joint kinetics differences during take-off of forward and backward rotating dives. In: *Proceedings of the 3rd North American Congress on Biomechanics* (NACOB III), Waterloo, Canada.

McKinley, P. & Pedotti, A. (1992) Motor strategies in landing from a jump: the role of skill in task execution. *Experimental Brain Research* **90**, 427–440.

McMahon, T.A. & Greene, P.R. (1979) The influence of track compliance on running. *Journal of Biomechanics* **12**, 893–904.

McNitt-Gray, J.L. (1991) Kinematics and impulse characteristics of drop landings from three heights. *International Journal of Sport Biomechanics* **7**, 201–224.

McNitt-Gray, J.L. (1992) Biomechanical factors contributing to successful landings. *USGF Sports Science Publication* **9**, 19–25.

McNitt-Gray, J.L. (1993) Kinetics of the lower extremities during drop landings from three heights. *Journal of Biomechanics* **25**, 1037–1046.

McNitt-Gray, J.L. & Nelson, R.C. (1988) Segment and joint kinematics of Olympic vault landings. *Medicine and Science in Sport and Exercise*, (**Suppl. 20**) (2), S48.

McNitt-Gray, J.L., Anderson, D.D., Barbieri, C.A. & Cvengos, K.W. (1990) Adjustments in kinematics and kinetics during modified landings. In: *Proceedings of XIVth ASB Meeting*, pp. 75–76.

McNitt-Gray, J.L., Barbieri, C.A., Anderson, D.D. & Irvine, D.M.E. (1991a) Differences in reaction forces experienced by gymnasts during landings in front and back saltos. *Proceedings of XVth ASB Meeting*, pp. 228–229.

McNitt-Gray, J.L., Irvine, D.M.E., Barbiere, C.A. & Anderson, D.D. (1991b) The effect of landing surface on muscle activity in preparation for landing. In: *Proceedings of XVth ASB Meeting*, pp. 230–231.

McNitt-Gray, J.L., Koff, S.R. & Hall, B.L. (1992) The influence of dance training and foot position on landing mechanics. *Medical Problems of Performing Artists* **7** (3), 87–91.

McNitt-Gray, J.L., Irvine, D.M.E., Munkasy, B., Welch, M., Barbieri, C.A. & Anderson, D.D. (1993a) Lower extremity joint kinetics and muscle activation

patterns during landings of front and back saltos. In: *Proceedings of the XVIIth ASB Meeting*, pp. 11–12.

McNitt-Gray, J.L., Yokoi, T. & Millward, C. (1993b) Landing strategy adjustments made by female gymnasts in response to drop height and mat composition. *Journal of Applied Biomechanics* **9** (3), 173–190.

McNitt-Gray, J.L., Munkasy, B.A. & Welch, M. (1994a) External reaction forces experienced by gymnasts during the take-off and landing of tumbling skills. *Technique* **14** (9), 10–16.

McNitt-Gray, J.L., Munkasy, B.A., Heino, J., Eagle, J. & Smith, T. (1994b) Net joint moments and powers during stop and go movements. In: *Proceedings of the XVIIIth American Society of Biomechanics (ASB) Meeting*, pp. 131–132.

McNitt-Gray, J.L., Yokoi, T. & Millward, C. (1994c) Landing strategies used by gymnasts on different surfaces. *Journal of Applied Biomechanics* **10**, 237–252.

McNitt-Gray, J.L., Irvine, D.M.E. & Eagle, J. (1995) Relative work of net joint moments during landings of front and back saltos. In: *Proceedings of the XIXth American Society of Biomechanics (ASB) Meeting*.

McNitt-Gray, J.L., Eagle, J., Elkins, S. & Munkasy, B.A. (1996) Modifications in joint kinetics during stop and go landing movements under fatigued and non-fatigued conditions. In: *Proceedings of the XXth American Society of Biomechanics (ASB) Meeting*, pp. 47–48.

McNitt-Gray, J.L., Irvine, D.M.E., Munkasy, B.A., Smith, T. & Chin, Y.T. (1997) Biomechanics of landings. In: *FIG Scientific Symposium Proceedings, Berlin, Germany*.

McNitt-Gray, J.L., Munkasy, B.A., Costa, K.E., Mathiyakom, W., Eagle, J. & Ryan, M.M. (1998a) Invariant features of multijoint control strategies used by gymnasts during landings performed in Olympic competition. In: *Proceedings of the Third North American Congress on Biomechanics* (NACOB III), Waterloo, Canada.

McNitt-Gray, J.L., Munkasy, B.A., Mathiyakom, W. & Somera, N.H. (1998b) Asymmetrical loading of lead and lag legs during landings of blocking movements. *Volleyball USA* **26**, 14–16.

McNitt-Gray, J.L., Requejo, P., Munkasy, B.A. & Eagle, J. (2000) Multijoint control of the reaction force during the take-off phase of the long jump. *Journal of Biomechanics* (submitted).

Melvill-Jones, G. & Watt, D.G.D. (1971) Muscular control of landing from unexpected falls in man. *Journal of Physiology (London)* **219**, 729–737.

Miller, D.I., Hennig, E., Pizzimenti, M.A., Jones, I.C. & Nelson, R.C. (1989) Kinetic and kinematic characteristics of 10-m platform performances of elite divers: I. Back takeoffs. *International Journal of Sport Biomechanics* **5**, 60–88.

Mizrahi, J. & Suzak, Z. (1982) In-vivo elastic and damping response of the human leg to impact forces. *Journal of Biomechanical Engineering* **104**, 63–66.

Munkasy, B.A. & McNitt-Gray, J.L. (1992) Segment velocity prior to contact in normal and softer than normal landings. In: *Proceedings of the Second North American Congress of Biomechanics (NACOB II)*, pp. 257–258.

Munkasy, B.A., McNitt-Gray, J.L. & Welch, M. (1994) Reaction forces and impulses experienced during the take-off and landing of tumbling skills. In: *Proceedings of the XVIIIth American Society of Biomechanics (ASB) Meeting*, pp. 97–98.

Munkasy, B.A., McNitt-Gray, J.L. & Welch, M.D. (1996) Kinematics prior to contact in landings preceded by rotation. In: *Proceedings of the XXth American Society of Biomechanics (ASB) Meeting*, pp. 159–160.

Munkasy, B.A., McNitt-Gray, J.L., Eagle, J. & Ryan, M.M. (1997) Generation and control of momentum during tumbling by Olympic gymnasts. In: *Proceedings of the XXIth American Society of Biomechanics (ASB) Meeting*, pp. 89–90.

Munroe, C.F., Miller, D.I. & Fuglevand, A.J. (1987) Ground reaction forces in running: a reexamination. *Journal of Biomechanics* **20** (2), 147–155.

NCAA (National Collegiate Athletic Association) (1986) *NCAA Injury Surveillance System Report: 1982–86*. NCAA, Mission, KS.

NCAA (National Collegiate Athletic Association) (1990) *NCAA Injury Surveillance System Report: 1989–90*. NCAA, Mission, KS.

Nigg, B.M. (1985) Biomechanics, load analysis and sport injuries in the lower extremities. *Sports Medicine* **2**, 367–379.

Nigg, B.M. (1990) The validity and relevance of test used for the assessment of sports surfaces. *Medicine and Science in Sports and Exercise* **22** (1), 131–139.

Nigg, B.M. & Bobbert, M. (1990) On the potential of various approaches in load analysis to reduce the frequency of sports injuries. *Journal of Biomechanics* **23** (1), 3–12.

Nigg, B.M., Denoth, J. & Neukomm, P.A. (1981) Quantifying the load on the human body: Problems and some possible solutions. In: *Biomechanics VII-B* (ed. B. Jonsson), pp. 88–89. Human Kinetics, Champaign, IL.

Nigg, B.M. & Yeadon, M.R. (1987) Biomechanical aspects of playing surfaces. *Journal of Sports Sciences* **5**, 117–145.

Nigg, B.M., Yeadon, M.R. & Herzog, W. (1988) The influence of construction strategies of sprung surfaces on deformation during vertical jumps. *Medicine and Science in Sports and Exercise* **20** (4), 396–402.

Ozguven, H.N. & Berme, N. (1988) An experimental and analytical study of impact forces during human jumping. *Journal of Biomechanics* **21** (12), 1061–1066.

Panzer, V.P. (1987) Lower extremity loads in landing of elite gymnasts. Doctoral dissertation, University of Oregon.

Prilutsky, B.I. & Zatsiorsky, V.M. (1994) Tendon action of two-joint muscles: Transfer of mechanical energy between joints during jumping, landing, and running. *Journal of Biomechanics* **27** (1), 25–34.

Radin, E.L. & Paul, I.L. (1970) Does cartilage compliance reduce skeletal impact loads? Relative force attenuating properties of articular cartilage, synovial fluid, periarticular soft tissues and bones. *Arthritis and Rheumatism* **13**, 139–144.

Riccardelli, E. & Pettrone, F.A. (1984) Gymnastics injuries: The Virginia experience. *Technique* **2**, 16–18.

Rodgers, M.M. & Cavanagh, P.R. (1984) Glossary of biomechanical terms, concepts, and units. *The Journal of the American Physical Therapy Association* **63** (2), 1886–1902.

Schweitzer, L. (1985) *Test Procedures for Low Springs, Mats, Floor Gym Surfaces, and Springboards*. Technical Report, Freiburg University, Germany.

Sidaway, B., McNitt-Gray, J.L. & Davis, G. (1989) Visual timing of muscle preactivation in press for landing. *Ecological Psychology* **1** (3), 253–264.

Smith, A.J. (1975) Estimates of muscle and joint forces at the knee and ankle during a jumping activity. *Journal of Human Movement Studies* **1**, 78–86.

Stacoff, A., Kaelin, X. & Stuessi, E. (1987) Load at impact after a volleyball block. *Deutsche Zeitschrift Fur Sportmedizin* **11**, 458–464.

Valiant, G.A. & Cavanagh, P.R. (1985) A study of landing from a jump: Implications for the design of a basketball shoe. In: *Biomechanics IX-B, International Series on Biomechanics* (eds D. Winter, R.W. Norman, R.P. Wells, R.C. Hayes & A. Patla), pp. 117–122. Human Kinetic Publishers, Champaign, IL.

Winter, D.A. (1979) *Biomechanics of Human Movement*. John Wiley & Sons, New York.

Zatsiorsky, V.M. & Prilutsky, B.I. (1987) Soft and stiff landing. In: *Biomechanics X-B* (ed. B. Jonsson), pp. 739–743. Human Kinetics, Champaign, IL.

Chapter 26

Sport-Related Spinal Injuries and Their Prevention

G.-P. BRÜGGEMANN

Introduction

The association between physical loading and the incidence of back problems has been shown by several studies. Heavy physical exercise has been correlated with back injuries and degenerative changes of the spine (e.g. Andersson 1991). The majority of reports have focused on occupational loading, and relatively little work has been published on athletic activities which may accelerate spinal degeneration (Granhed & Morelli 1988). Long-term effects of physical loading due to exercise on back-related symptoms, disability and spine pathology in 937 former male athletes and 620 controls were analysed by Videman *et al.* (1995). Weightlifting using maximum loads was found to be associated with greater degeneration throughout the entire spine, and soccer with degeneration in the lower lumbar region. No signs of accelerated disc degeneration or injury were identified in former competitive runners. Interestingly, back pain was less common in athletes than in the control subjects. Very similar results regarding back pain in former elite athletes were reported by Tsai and Wredemark (1993) who compared the occurrence and frequency of back pain in former elite female gymnasts with that of the normal population. These studies provide evidence that participation in exercise and sports is associated with less back pain in later adulthood, despite an increase in degenerative changes in the lumbar spine of athletes participating in some sports.

During the active phase of sport the athlete's spine is often subjected to considerable mechanical load, which could be a risk factor for subsequent back injuries and back pain. Some authors reported a high incidence of back pain, of up to 65%, especially in young athletes (e.g. Horne *et al.* 1987; Swärd *et al.* 1990b). On the other hand Raspe and Kohlmann (1993) found that 31–40% of adults in the normal population suffer from back pain. The majority of pain occurred in the younger age groups (25–40 years of age). In addition, Balagué *et al.* (1988, 1993) found back pain in 44.5% of children at an age of 10–16 years. From all these findings it can be concluded that sport and physical activity do not seem to be the ultimate cause of back pain and spine injuries. But the additional and frequent load acting on the biological structures of the spine during sport may constitute the prerequisite for an injury, or at least a partial overloading. Therefore the relation between spine injuries, vertebra deformation and accelerated tissue degeneration and mechanical load related to sport is of both scientific and practical relevance. A better understanding of this relationship is a prerequisite for preventive strategies.

Over the past decades the age of training onset for many sports has become younger. At the same time the training volume, or the hours practised per week, has increased in many Olympic sports in most countries worldwide. Elite training from a young age is based on the fact that regular physical training in young, prepubescent age groups ensures a strong development of physical and motor control abilities. However, the early introduction of repetitive loading during growth may increase the risk of injury (Caine & Lindner 1985).

The strength and flexibility demands on the spine are extreme in a number of sports and intuitively seem to be combined with obvious risks of overloading and overuse injuries. The vulnerability of the spinal structures in growing individuals is known and described to be highest during the growth spurt (e.g. Schmorl & Junghanns 1971; Alexander 1977). Hellström *et al.* (1990) reported various types of radiological abnormalities which occurred in both athletes and non-athletes but were more common in athletes. In sports such as gymnastics and wrestling, in which training often starts at a young age, a higher frequency of abnormalities was found.

Therefore this chapter will not be primarily focused on catastrophic or fatal spine injuries in sport, but rather on overuse and chronic injuries with accelerated tissue damage and degeneration. In order to establish a basis for the prevention of sport-related injuries of the spine, biomechanical research should provide a better understanding of injury mechanisms.

Mechanical loading and tissue response

Mechanical load acting on the biological structures of the human locomotor system during sport is one possible stimulus to maintain and/or increase the strength of biological material. Excessive load may lead to microscopic or macroscopic damage of the anatomical structures. From this perspective mechanical overload is the cause of the damage of one or more biological structures, and an injury can generally be defined as the damage of biological tissue caused by physical loading. Injury can result from a single overload exceeding an individual tissue's maximum tolerance. Such a situation may lead to catastrophic spine injuries. The term 'catastrophic injury' is defined as any injury incurred during participation in sport in which there is a permanent severe functional neurological disability (non-fatal) or a transient but not permanent functional neurological (serious) disability (Cantu & Mueller 1990). A chronic injury is initiated by microscopic damage of the tissue's structure. Long-term repeated loading can worsen the injury, which eventually becomes macroscopic and/or results in tissue degeneration. Based on this definition a relationship between injuries and mechanical energy can be concluded.

The principal relationship between mechanical energy and injury gives us reason to examine the causes of musculoskeletal injury, especially in sports where large amounts of mechanical energy and mechanical forces are necessary for successful activity and performance. In addition, exercise and sport participation often involve twisted and bent postures combined with high external forces which increase the risk of sudden traumatic injuries and spinal pathology or mechanical overuse (Farfan *et al.* 1970; Kelsey *et al.* 1984; Andersson 1991).

Several epidemiological studies have shown that certain activities such as weightlifting (Granhed & Morelli 1988), soccer (Swärd *et al.* 1990b) and gymnastics (Goldstein *et al.* 1991) may accelerate the degeneration of spinal structures. Swärd *et al.* (1990b), for example, investigated 142 top Swedish athletes who competed in wrestling, gymnastics, soccer and tennis. All groups of athletes reported previous or present back pain at a higher frequency than found in previous studies of the general population. Radiological abnormalities of the thoracolumbar spine occurred in 36–55% of the athletes. The results may suggest a causative relationship between athletic activities and radiological abnormalities, and the radiological findings indicated both direct traumatic changes as well as disturbed vertebral growth. Swärd *et al.* (1990b) concluded that both the age at onset of athletic activity and the degree of mechanical load on the skeleton are important factors in the development of these abnormalities.

Kujala *et al.* (1992) investigated the relationship between the amount of time spent on physical activity and low back pain in 100 adolescent athletes (10.3–13.3 years) and 18 non-athletes. They found some evidence that intense physical activity in the young increases the occurrence of low back pain.

Quantification of the injury-related responses of biological structures of the human body plays a vital part in determining the mechanisms that lead to tissue damage. Knowledge of the limits of human tissue tolerances is a prerequisite in assessing the mechanical load due to physical activity. This is particularly true of individuals for whom tissue tolerance data are limited due to biological growth or other individual factors. As many sports are practised at a young age, the consideration of limited tissue strength is of major importance when studying spinal injuries and trauma in adolescents. A number of scientific papers report a remarkably high frequency of spinal abnormalities and damage, especially in young athletes. This may be an indicator of the vulnerability of the growing spinal structures. On the one hand there are the positive effects of physical activity and sport in adolescents, while on the other there are findings regarding the limited load capacity of the developing system. It is known that the musculoskeletal system needs some mechanical load to function in an optimal way. Damage occurs or is assumed to occur when a high or repeated mechanical load exceeds the strength of a biological structure. It is possible that free radical formation in connection with strenuous exercise could accelerate ageing and degeneration of the structures (Sohal & Allan 1978). Experimental and clinical studies have clearly demonstrated that inactivity causes degeneration and weakening of connective tissues and that spinal movement enhances disc metabolism (Holm & Rosenqvist 1986; Troup & Videman 1989). New bone formation (McLeod *et al.* 1990) and the increase of bone mineral density (e.g. Welten *et al.* 1994) are highly correlated with mechanical loading of the bones.

The dual role of physical activity/mechanical loading as both a positive and negative influence on the passive structures of the spine, and of how beneficial effects of training interact with potential harmful effects of mechanical loading has received relatively little attention. Moderate mechanical loading through physical activity, even when performed at a high frequency as in running, appears to have no degenerative effect even over a long period of time. Videman *et al.* (1997) found no differences in MRI examinations of the discs between co-twins discordant to lifetime endurance exercise.

Genetics may also be an important factor in the degeneration process. In a study on monozygotic twins, Battié *et al.* (1995) demonstrated the importance of genetics in relation to a lifetime of physical activity with regard to disc degeneration. Therefore the individual, genetically determined, mechanical properties of the biological material should not be underestimated.

A better understanding of the relationship between mechanical loading due to sports and the damage or injuries of spinal structures requires that the frequency and severity of an injury or a group of injuries should be evaluated. From these figures it should be determined which factors lead to a particular type of damage. The next step is to examine the relation between these factors and the specific injury to understand better the factors responsible for the injury. Consequently strategies should be considered in terms of possible changes in the injury patterns and/or injury frequency. The first step and the last step of such an approach will use prospective epidemiological studies. Concerning the factors influencing a specific injury, three steps can contribute to solving such issues:

1 identifiy structures and tissues damaged by a single or repeated mechanical load;
2 determine critical tissue strength tolerances; and
3 the mechanical load acting on the tissue in the specific exercise situation should be quantified/ estimated and compared with the critical limits.

Based on the identification of potential critical loading in specific sports, factors influencing the mechanical loading should be identified and strategies developed to ensure that the mechanical stress stays below the critical limits. However, such a research strategy has its weaknesses, as outlined below.

Damaged tissue

The determination of injured structures may be difficult in some cases. A medical diagnosis does not always allow for the precise identification of the injured anatomical structure, or may include different structural lesions in one clinical category (e.g. Scheuermann's disease). Conventional diagnostics (e.g. radiographs) may remain normal following traumatic injury, as reported by Swärd *et al.* (1990a). They reported an acute injury of the vertebral ring apophysis and intervertebral disc although the conventional radiograph was normal for the first months. Ten months after the trauma the disc height was clearly reduced, the upper anterior corner of the vertebrae was excavated and the ring apophysis separated.

A more or less accurate determination of the overloaded biological structure or the damaged tissue is a prerequisite for a cause-effect approach to spinal injury. In other words the quantification of the injury-related responses of biological structures of the human body is of major importance in identifying the mechanisms leading to tissue damage.

Critical limits

The determination of the individual critical limits of a particular tissue is an important step in attempting to identify mechanical overload. Mean critical force or strength boundaries have been determined experimentally in cadaveric tissue experiments (Yamada 1970; Hutton & Adams 1982; Genaidy et al. 1993). Callaghan and McGill (1994) showed in an in vitro study in animal models that the compressive tolerance of a porcine vertebra increased by 40% when the specimen was loaded in a pressurized wet fluid environment in comparison to the traditional testing procedure. In addition it was found that the critical limits are influenced by immobilization (Woo et al. 1984), inactivity (Brinckmann et al. 1989), age, skeletal maturity and other factors. The individual differences might exceed 100% if compared to the minimal values measured. Although the determination of critical strength limits of the involved tissue is difficult and weak, a rough estimation of the range of tolerances may be primarily helpful in identifying the most critical areas of loading in exercise and sport. The development of criteria to estimate individual strength tolerances (e.g. for spinal structures or connective tissue) should establish a basis for an individual load control, especially during growth in the future.

Internal loading

The methods used to estimate the forces acting on internal structures of the locomotor system, or more specifically of the human spine, regularly consist of two steps. In the first step the resultant moment and force in a joint is calculated using the inverse dynamic approach. Based on a multisegment model of rigid bodies, resultant moments and force can be calculated using ground reaction force measure-

ments and kinematic methods. When the resultant forces and moments at a given joint are known they have to be distributed to force-carrying structures in the vicinity of the joint. The different structures (e.g. muscles, ligaments, capsules) acting and transmitting force around a joint have an infinite number of possibilities for producing a specific movement or the resultant moments. Mathematically this results in an indeterminate system of equations. To solve the indeterminate problem Nigg and Bobbert (1990) distinguished the reduction and addition strategies. The reduction strategy solves the problem by reducing the number of force-carrying structures crossing a joint. The addition strategy adds equations based on physiological considerations or mathematical optimization techniques (Crowninshield & Brand 1981). A substantial number of different models to quantify or to estimate spinal load with various degrees of sophistication are currently used. The sensitivity and the numerical results of the models are strongly dependent on the model's strategy, the precision of the model input data (resultant moments and forces, anatomical data) and—using optimization strategies—the chosen cost function. From this it can be concluded that the determination of mechanical loads on internal structures should be used more as estimates than as absolute values. Even if the estimates do not provide absolute values of tissue load during activity and sport, a load estimation for different skills, movements, manoeuvres and training drills is important for identifying substantial and critical activities in a specific sport. The prerequisites for such a comparison are the use of the same model with the same optimization cost function and sufficient individual anatomical data.

Sport-related spine injuries and damaged biological structures

The majority of injuries associated with sports are injuries of the extremities, with most of those occurring at the knee, shank, ankle and foot. About 65% of all sport-related injuries are classified as acute or chronic injuries of the lower extremities. About 5% of acute sports injuries affect the torso and spine (Steinbrück 1987). Although spinal injuries are not the most common sport-related injuries they are very important because spinal injuries have the greatest potential for causing catastrophic injuries with dangerous effects on essential body functions, which can lead to both paralysis and death. Furthermore the structures of the spine are often related to chronic damage, long-term pain, and discomfort. Accordingly this discussion will focus not only on catastrophic injuries but also on the overuse injuries which lead to degenerative changes of the biomaterials.

In relation to other parts of the body the spine is seldom broken and accounts for only 0.5–1% of all fractures. Fractures of the vertebrae are of particular concern because of their proximity to the spinal cord. Bone fragments can be pushed into the spinal canal and impinge on the cord causing severe neural damage. Reid and Saboe (1991) presented a review of 1081 spine fractures, of which 12% had sporting or recreational causes. Sports and recreation constituted the fourth most common cause of spinal fractures and the second most frequent cause of associated paralysis. Motor vehicle accidents are reported to constitute the majority (more than 50%) of all reviewed spinal fractures. Diving is the sport with the highest frequency of catastrophic injuries (about 25% of the reported fractures) (Reid & Saboe 1991). The profile of an average diving injury is a cervical fracture usually between C4 and C6 with associated complete motor and sensory damage. Equestrian and parachute/skydiving are connected with 10–12% of all the spinal fractures. Older sources reported a high frequency of American football-related catastrophic injuries. An axial loading with the cervical spine slightly flexed aligns the spine in such a way that a burst-type injury is frequently the result of a high impact. In the past the fulcrum supplied by a single-bar face mask (Schneider's hyperflexion injury) as well as the guillotine mechanism of hyperextension with the posterior ridge of the football helmet forming a fulcrum in the upper cervical area have been gradually eliminated (Schneider 1973). The number of permanent quadriplegics in football decreased from 34 in 1976 to five in 1984 (Murphy 1985).

Fatal and catastrophic spinal injuries reported from other sports are relatively rare in relation to hours of activity. They primarily happen in high-velocity sports (e.g. snowmobile driving, luge, alpine skiing) but also in artistic sports like trampoline or gymnastics. The injury rate per athlete or per hour of activity is low, but the consequences are dramatic.

As far as sport-related acute spinal trauma without and with neurological injury is concerned the majority of cases affect the cervical spine. The most common mechanisms are the flexion–compression mechanism and extension–tension mechanism. More commonly cervical injury manifests itself as a temporary sensorimotor lesion caused by the pinching of cervical nerve roots or brachial plexus. Of all cervical disorders the whiplash injuries are the most frequent ones. Sturzenegger *et al.* (1994, p. 688) defined whiplash as 'trauma causing cervical musculoligamental sprain or strain due to acceleration/deceleration of the head relative to the trunk in any plane'. Whiplash may result from a rear-end collision of a vehicle or from a high-impact collision in contact sports.

Cervical spine injuries

Injury to the cervical spinal cord can be identified as failure of the intervertebral discs, the vertebral bodies and the processes of the vertebrae. In addition, ruptures of spinous ligaments are observed. Following injuries to these structures, further flexion or rotation of the cervical spine permits vertebral dislocation.

Flexion–compression loading of the cervical spine can cause fractures of the antero-inferior corner of the cervical vertebral body (teardrop fracture). The extension–tension mechanism creates stresses in the anterior cervical structures and may involve disruption of the anterior longitudinal ligament, intervertebral disc or even a horizontal fracture of the vertebral body. High-impact loading can result in a posterior vertebral displacement (Whiting & Zernicke 1998).

In contrast to these potentially catastrophic injuries, the most common chronic cervical injury is cervical spondylosis. Cervical spondylosis summarizes the degenerative changes of intervertebral discs and surrounding structures.

Thoracic and lumbar spine injuries

The most common types of thoraco-lumbar spinal injuries in athletes are muscle strains, ligament sprains, vertebral fractures, disc injuries and neural arch fractures. Neural arch fractures at the pars interarticularis or the isthmus between the superior and inferior articular processes are known and summarized as spondylolysis.

One of the most common types of spinal injury in sport is the compression fracture, which occurs primarily at the anterior vertebral body. Compression fracture induces a defect of the anterior column of the spine (Denis 1983). When the compression fracture is extended to the middle column of the spine the motion segment tends to become unstable. Vertebrae in the thoraco-lumbar region (T11–L3) are especially susceptible to fracture because of the spine's relatively neutral alignment in this region and because this region is a transition zone between the relatively rigid thoracic spine and the more flexible lumbar region. In general, acute and traumatic fractures directed to the thoracic and lumbar spine are not very often reported in sports. Exceptions are injuries due to extreme impacts directed to the spine. Rodrigo and Boyd (1979) reported a 50% incidence of lumbar vertebral body fractures by bad landings in military parachute-jumpers. Hirsch and Nachemson (1963) examined pilots' ejections from a jet and found a total of 35% sustained traumatic vertebral fractures with the most frequently affected vertebrae being those of the thoraco-lumbar junction.

Geffen et al. (1997) reported an extremely rare case of a rugby thoracic spinal fracture. All three vertebral columns were affected in a complex multilevel injury with no neurological complication. The injury was sustained as a result of a legal shoulder tackle.

A common fracture in young athletes is a vertebral endplate fracture, which is a compression fracture due to herniation of the nucleus pulposus into the vertebral body. The compressive strength of the disc is greater than that of the cartilaginous endplate. Therefore under excessive compressive force the endplate will fracture first. The endplate is the most vulnerable part of the vertebra and wears down first when subjected to compressive load. As the plate becomes worn and fractures the disc begins to dehydrate at an accelerated rate. Especially during the adolescent growth spurt (Alexander 1976) the cartilaginous junction between the vertebral body and the ring apophysis at the upper and lower border of the vertebra is a weak point in the disco-vertebral complex. Abnormalities in the anterior ring apophysis are generally considered to result from intravertebral disc herniation (marginal Schmorl's node) (Schmorl & Junghanns 1971). Abnormalities in the posterior part of the ring apophysis are infrequent. Hellström et al. (1990) found 26 abnormalities in the anterior and two in the posterior part of the ring apophysis in 143 young athletes.

Abnormalities of the vertebral bodies, including abnormal configuration, Schmorl's nodes and apophysial changes are common among athletes (Swärd 1992). Hellström et al. (1990) reported a higher frequency of vertebrae with abnormal configuration (e.g. flattening, wedging and increased sagittal diameter) in young athletes than in non-athletes. They argued that healing of moderate vertebral fractures in children may be disturbed by high-intensity loading and can explain the abnormal configuration.

Roy et al. (1985) have suggested that the initial disc injury in athletes is a shearing injury which leads to separation of the hyaline cartilaginous plate from the adjacent vertebral bodies. Further stress leads to fissuring and weakness of the annulus. Subsequent injury is followed by the nucleus pulposus protruding or extruding through the torn fibres of the annulus, usually at the posterolateral corner.

Disc degeneration due to mechanical load is reported controversially in the literature. Tertti et al. (1990) found no difference in disc degeneration evaluated with magnetic resonance imaging (MRI) between young gymnasts and controls. However, Goldstein et al. (1991) reported more abnormalities in subjects (gymnasts and swimmers) subjected to increased and lengthened training than for athletes subjected to lesser loads. Swärd et al. (1991) found a reduced disc MRI signal intensity more than twice as common in male (adult) gymnasts (mean age 23 years) than in non-athletes. Hellström et al. (1990) reported disc height reduction in wrestlers and gymnasts in comparison with non-athletes. The reason for the different results may be that the young individuals in Tertti's sample had not passed the growth spurt, a time when the growth plates and apophyses are most sensitive to trauma. From these findings one can conclude that participation in sports with high demands on the spine increases the risk for disc injuries. Moreover, the adolescent growth spurt may be the most vulnerable period of life (Swärd 1992). Assuming that disc degeneration is identifiable by the MRI signal and that shear forces play a role in the mechanical stress of the discs (Roy & Irmi 1983), anterior-posterior shear forces should be considered when quantifying the mechanical load of the motion segments during physical activity and sports.

Compressive load on the motion segment can lead to overload injuries in the endplates of the vertebrae. Acute traumatic or chronic injuries may produce herniation of disc material into the vertebral body forming Schmorl's nodes (Schmorl & Junghanns 1971). Schmorl's nodes are a very common finding in the spine, and their frequency has been reported equally in athletes and non-athletes. The cartilaginous junction between the vertebral body and the ring apophysis at the upper and lower border of the vertebra is a weak area in the disco-vertebral complex during growth. Hellström et al. (1990) identified apophysial abnormalities in all groups of athletes examined (wrestlers, soccer players, tennis players, gymnasts) but not one case in non-athletes. Apophysial abnormalities have been reported by different authors, mostly in young, physically active subjects. These findings have been suggested to result from trauma or chronic overload (e.g. McCall et al. 1985; Blumenthal et al. 1987) or from growth disorder (e.g. Rogge & Nieman 1976).

Swärd et al. (1990a) described an injury at the anterior part of the ring apophysis of T12 of two adolescent female gymnasts. In both cases of apophysial ring injury, normal disc heights were found at initial examination after trauma. However, marked disc height reduction with disc degeneration was identified 10–12 months after the injury. Swärd et al. (1990a) explained this history of tissue changes by an initial injury of the endplate with replacement of the cartilaginous layer between the anterior part of the ring apophysis and the vertebral body. This allowed loss of disc material through the rupture.

Abnormal vertebral configurations (flattening, wedging, increased sagittal diameter) are of higher frequency in athletes than in non-athletes (Hellström et al. 1990). Athletes with abnormal vertebral configurations appear to have more back pain than athletes without abnormalities. Swärd et al. (1990b) reported a covariance between Schmorl's nodes, disc height reduction, and abnormal configuration of vertebral bodies. These changes are recognized as parts of Scheuermann's disease, the classic form of which has its peak incidence at T7–10. Swärd's data, including wrestlers, gymnasts, soccer and tennis players, indicate a peak incidence at a lower level, at about the thoraco-lumbar junction. The thoraco-lumbar type of Scheuermann's disease is considered to be more strongly associated with trauma and back pain (Alexander 1977). Radiological abnormalities of the thoraco-lumbar spine occurred in 36–55% of the athletes—wrestlers ($n = 29$), 55.2%; male gymnasts ($n = 26$), 42.3%; soccer players ($n = 31$), 35.5%; tennis players ($n = 30$), 46.7%; female gymnasts ($n = 26$), 42.8%.

Swärd et al. (1990b) concluded that their findings were highly suggestive of a causative relationship between rigorous athletic activities, radiological abnormalities, and back pain. The radiological findings indicate both direct traumatic changes as well as disturbed vertebral growth. A recently performed clinical and radiological examination of former elite gymnasts (Fröhner 2000) supported Swärd's data in principle, and reported the majority of severe and moderate vertebral deformities to be in the region of the thoraco-lumbar junction. About one-third of the former female gymnasts examined ($n = 37$) had severe vertebral deformities, while another third showed moderate findings. Among the male gymnasts ($n = 23$) severe deformities were identified in 50% of the former athletes. The examination of 135 young female gymnasts of elite level (11–19 years of age) showed one or more osteochondrotic changes in 44.4% of the athletes. The majority of the findings were at the thoraco-lumbar junction, and osteochondroses were most frequent in the age group 12–15 years of age. These data on the examination of traumatic changes and abnormalities emphasize

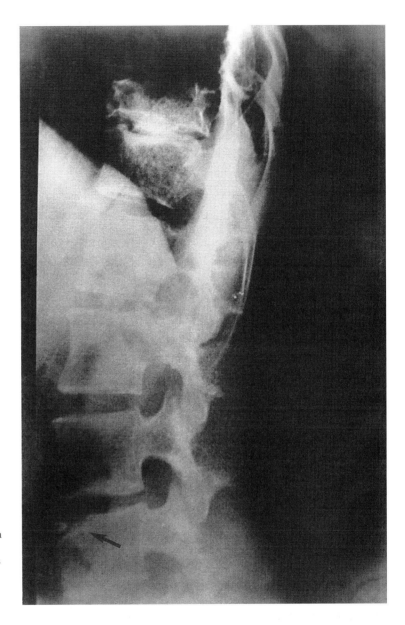

Fig. 26.1 A 14-year-old female gymnast. Reduced disc height at thoracic-lumbar junction, excavation of the upper anterior corner of L1, and separation of the ring apophysis due to frequent high compressive loading in bent trunk position by landings from dismounts.

the vulnerability of the spine, especially during the growth period. Both the age of onset of physical activity and the degree of mechanical load on the skeleton should intuitively be regarded as causal factors in the development of the described abnormalities (Fig. 26.1).

In addition to the spinal deformities already discussed, the young and athletic population is confronted with two specific conditions: spondylolysis and spondylolisthesis. These conditions affect the bony structures of the vertebrae, mostly at L4/L5 and L5/S1 levels. *Spondylolysis* is defined as a defect in the area of the lamina between the superior and inferior articular facets of the pars interarticularis. *Spondylolisthesis* is the translational movement or slippage between the adjacent vertebral bodies. Of greatest concern to young athletes is the isthmoid type of spondylolysis/spondylolisthesis in which repeated loading of the pars area causes microfractures and eventual bone failure. The high incidence of spondylolysis in sports with hyperextension and compressive loading is frequently reported. Repeated overuse may produce stress or fatigue fractures in the pars interarticularis and prevent healing, resulting in a permanent non-union and the development of spondylolysis (Cyron & Hutton 1978). This accords with the findings of a higher frequency of spondylolysis in athletes than in the general population (Swärd et al. 1992).

Sports with repeated high compressive spinal loading combined with forcible hyperextension and lumbar spine rotation pose a risk for this kind of injury. Schmitt et al. (1998) reported a frequency of spondylolysis of 61.9% and of spondylolisthesis in 47.6% of former elite javelin throwers. Elliott et al. (1992) published data showing a high incidence of pars interarticularis abnormalities in young fast-bowlers in cricket. This activity combines lateral flexion of the spine with extreme spinal extension and rotation to assist the generation of a high ball release speed. Very recent data on female gymnasts (Lohrer et al. 2000) reported slip instability in 15 of 135 (11.1%) individuals, which is in the range of the normal population. Spondylolisthesis was identified in 2.9% of the gymnasts examined. This frequency does not differ from that reported for the normal population. These data are different from those presented earlier and are a good example of how changes in the demands of a specific sport are able to influence injury characteristics. Whereas formerly in gymnastics hyperextension (e.g. frequent walkovers) figured large, modern artistic gymnastics is no longer focused on extreme reclination of the lumbar spine. Instead, the modern sport concentrates on a fixed and well-controlled spinal movement. Hyperextension does not increase the score; on the contrary, it leads to a reduced score. The low rate of spondylolysis may also be related to early examination of gymnasts and the early advice to quit gymnastics when the athlete suffers from significant disturbance of the neural arch at the pars interarticularis. Spondylolysis has been reported in up to 50% of athletes with back pain. This damage

or tissue weakness is therefore of relevance when discussing mechanical causes for overloading.

Scoliosis has been found in up to 80% of athletes with asymmetric load of the trunk and shoulders. Examples of asymmetric sports with a high incidence of scoliosis are javelin throwing (Schmitt et al. 1998) and tennis (Hainline 1995). In general, scoliosis among athletes involves only a small curvature and does not cause back pain.

The total number of vertebral deformities in the thoracic and lumbar region with diffuse onset reported in the literature is a major health problem in sports. The clinical and radiological findings associated with mechanical loading during sport activities will be the focus of the following section.

Mechanical load and injury mechanisms

Mechanical load of the spine in sports

It is remarkable that relatively few quantitative data or estimates on mechanical loading of the spine in different sports are available in the literature. While mathematical models estimating the spinal load are frequently applied to workplaces and work-related activities such as lifting and materials handling, very few applications can be identified concerning sport movements. Due to the model-dependent quantities of load estimations one must be extremely careful when comparing the absolute results calculated using different types of mathematical models. Therefore the sporting activities with the heaviest loads were analysed by reviewing the literature and adding the author's own data to allow at least some estimates of spinal mechanical loading. The focus will be on physical activities which are intuitively related to extreme spinal loading and to injuries or overuse, such as lifting heavy weights, blocking in football, jumping, landing from heights, and dynamic flexion-extension of the thoraco-lumbar spine. In addition, running at different speeds will be taken as a kind of reference for less critical loads.

LIFTING

Lander et al. (1990) carried out a detailed investigation of the parallel squat using an anatomically simplified lumbo-sacral joint model. The model utilized a single muscle equivalent in concert with an intra-abdominal pressure-relieving force, which together were used to estimate the compressive and shear forces acting at the L5/S1 joint. However, as the subjects ($n = 6$) lifted much lower weights (150–175 kg) than competitive lifters the data can only be used for the purpose of this chapter to give a very first approximation of load occurring while weight-lifting. A maximum L5/S1 moment of 669 N m resulting in 10 473 N of joint compression and 3843 N of shear force was reported.

Granhed et al. (1987) calculated an average disc compressive load of 21 457 N for six male com-petitors at the World Powerlifting Championships under the average barbell load of 284.5 kg. Using the WATBAK model, Cholewicki et al. (1991) calcu-lated the compression and shear forces acting on the motion segments of the lumbar spine under extreme weights. The WATBAK consists of a nine-segment rigid body model for symmetrical lifts and a single muscle equivalent of the spinal musculature required to support the extensor reaction moment of the low back. The muscle equivalent had an effect-ive moment arm of 0.06 m and a line of action that was inclined 5° in relation to the compressive axis of the intervertebral joint (McGill & Norman 1985, 1986, 1987). Data were taken from 13 female and 44 male powerlifters performing deadlifts at the Canadian Powerlifting Championships. Compress-ive forces of between 7442 and 18 449 N (14 times body weight, BW) at the L4/L5 level were found for male powerlifters (barbell loads: 190–320 kg). The compressive force at the motion segment L4/L5 for women (barbell loads: 120–180 kg) ranged from 5090 to 8019 N. The means of maximum shear force at the L4/L5 level were observed to be 1666 N ($\pm$ 229 N) for women and 2832 N ($\pm$ 413 N) for men. Maximum shear force load was calculated to be 3539 N. The maximum compression values obtained by Granhed et al. (1987) (21 457 N) were slightly higher than the data presented by Cholewicki et al. (1991) for similar loads (14 350–17 192 N). If Granhed et al. (1987) used a 5 cm extensor musculature moment arm, which is not specified in the paper, as suggested by Schultz and Andersson (1981) it would account for the discrepancy. Cholewicki et al.

(1991) had a 0.06 m moment arm, which results in 20% less compressive force due to the muscle activity.

FOOTBALL BLOCKING

Gatt et al. (1997) modified the models from Cappozzo (1984) and Schultz et al. (1982), and calcu-lated compressive and shear forces at the L4–5 motion segment during football blocking. The aver-age peak compression force at L4/5 was estimated at 8579 $\pm$ 1965 N (7 times BW). Maximum com-pressive force occurred about 67 ms after the impact. An anterior-posterior (ap)-shear force of 3304 $\pm$ 1116 N (2.6 BW) and a lateral shear force of 1709 $\pm$ 411 N were simultaneously applied to the motion segment. Gatt et al. (1997) discussed the flexed trunk position in a decrease of lumbar lordosis and the resultant compression in relation to anterior disc narrowing and additional stress on the pars interarticularis. The drive forwards and upwards and the extension of the lumbar spine dur-ing the collision were seen to create a shearing force at the apophysial joints. The authors concluded that repetitive tackling and loading at the apophysial joints may contribute to the development of the pars interarticularis defect.

The same model was also applied to professional golfers and rowers: the average compression forces were reported by Hosea et al. (1989) at 7500 N and 6086 N, respectively.

To estimate the mechanical load of the spine during different sports and drills, a mathematical model (Gao & Brüggemann 1995) that distributes the resultant forces and moments at the spine levels L5/S1 and T12/L1 was applied. The resultant moments and forces at L5/S1 and/or T12/L1 were calculated using inverse dynamic techniques. Indi-vidual anatomical data—lever arms and PCSA (phy-siological cross-sectional areas) for the eight muscle groups—were taken or approximated (PCSA) from MRI of all the subjects. The subjects volunteering in the studies were experienced athletes in athletics and gymnastics competing at national and inter-national level. For the distribution of the resultant forces and moments at the motion segments L5/S1 and T12/L1 to muscles, ligaments and contact forces,

Table 26.1 Compression and shear (a-p) forces at different running speeds. Force data are given as times body weight, means and standard deviations ($n = 8$).

Forces at L5/S1	Running speed (m · s^{-1})				
	2.5	3.5	4.5	5.5	6.5
Max. compression	7.40 ± 1.31	10.14 ± 1.62	12.01 ± 3.24	14.14 ± 2.91	14.42 ± 2.56
Average compression*	2.76 ± 1.95	3.58 ± 0.63	4.25 ± 0.66	4.57 ± 0.51	4.49 ± 0.14
Maximum shear (a-p)	1.75 ± 0.76	2.06 ± 0.69	2.57 ± 0.22	2.46 ± 0.23	3.31 ± 1.41
Average shear (a-p)*	0.18 ± 0.06	0.29 ± 0.14	0.32 ± 0.07	0.55 ± 0.16	0.53 ± 0.19

* Average forces in the stance phase.

an electromyograph (EMG)-based switch technique was combined with optimization methods. As cost function for the optimization the square of the total muscle stresses (the muscle force normalized to PCSA) was taken. Joint contact forces of the lumbar motion segments (compressive, anterior-posterior shear (a-p), lateral) were calculated. Although the values are probably some distance from the real *in vivo* mechanical forces acting on the spinal tissues, they will nonetheless allow an estimate of the relative magnitudes.

RUNNING

Running was studied as a reference for the jumping and landing activities because running is known or assumed to produce spinal loading within the physiological tissue tolerances (Videman *et al*. 1995). As expected the compression force on the lumbar spine increased generally with an increase in running speed. Maximum load clearly occurred during the impact phase shortly after the foot hits the ground. The heel strike indicates a linear increase of spinal load up to a running speed of 4.5 m · s^{-1}. When the subjects changed the running style to forefoot running at higher speeds the rate of load increase slowed down. The maximum compression force is about 14.5 BW at a running speed of 6.5 m · s^{-1}. In comparison with materials-handling tasks, such compression data can be identified during heavy lifting (e.g. lifting a box of >35 kg) in a forward bend trunk position (Brüggemann 1997). The average of the spinal compressive load values during the entire stance phase increased from 2.8 BW to 4.6 BW,

which is less than the average load during heavy lifting. The compressive force on the lumbar spine shown in the study represents a dynamic loading at a high amplitude acting over a short period of time in relation to lifting tasks. The maximum anterior-posterior shear force (a-p) was estimated at 3.3 BW, which is about 2 kN. An increase of the shear forces with increasing running speed was shown in the peak as well as in the average forces acting in the entire stance phase (Table 26.1).

Even if running does not produce the highest spinal load of the exercises and drills being examined the maximum value should not be underestimated when considering the high rate of load repetition at a frequency of about 1 Hz. The data may help to explain why runners with insufficient musculature or with muscular dysbalance and thus an unstable lumbar spine tend to exhibit back pain. From the data of Videman *et al*. (1995) one can conclude that the spinal load in running seems to be below the critical limits for the long-term. In general, competitive runners seem to tolerate such compressive loads even if these loads are very repetitive and reach the levels of loads induced by heavy lifting. Long-term and gradual increases of load in sport and exercise may lead to tissue adaptations and to an increase of strength tolerances.

JUMPING

Drop jumps are a commonly used training exercise for various sports. They cause an extreme increase of spinal loading. Even drop jumping after falling from 20 cm produces spinal forces which are sig-

Table 26.2 Compression and shear (a-p) forces in drop jumps from different heights. Force data are given as times body weight, means and standard deviations ($n = 8$).

Forces at L5/S1	Drop height (cm)		
	20	40	60
Max. compression	19.20 ± 8.94	23.56 ± 7.71	36.53 ± 8.69
Average compression*	5.79 ± 1.16	6.42 ± 0.78	8.40 ± 1.27
Maximum shear (a-p)	3.14 ± 0.81	3.54 ± 0.98	3.22 ± 0.69
Average shear (a-p)*	0.57 ± 0.18	0.63 ± 0.12	0.79 ± 0.16

* Average forces in the stance phase.

Table 26.3 Compression and shear (a-p) forces in gymnastic landings from different heights and with somersaults. Force data are given as times body weight, means and standard deviations ($n = 8$).

Forces at L5/S1	DJ51	DJ91	DJ171	FS91	BS91
Max. compression	22.91 ± 4.73	25.93 ± 6.02	32.22 ± 5.86	35.13 ± 6.84	40.53 ± 7.48
Average compression	8.76 ± 1.59	9.57 ± 1.79	11.59 ± 1.40	11.58 ± 1.40	14.83 ± 2.94
Maximum shear (a-p)	3.55 ± 0.96	3.28 ± 0.63	3.66 ± 0.47	3.79 ± 1.20	5.46 ± 1.5
Average shear (a-p)*	1.41 ± 0.11	1.58 ± 0.20	1.84 ± 0.31	1.42 ± 0.23	2.16 ± 0.32

* During the first 80 ms after touchdown.

nificantly higher than those in running (Table 26.2). The variability within the sample (see standard deviations in Table 26.2) was shown to be relatively high due to different leg stiffnesses of the athletes, and the identified compressive load on the spine increased with an increase in leg stiffness. The spinal load in drop jumping (from higher than 20 cm), a very popular drill used in training for many jumping-type sports, is about twice that of running. Increased height of the initial fall and increasing initial energy cause the compressive load and the load rate of the spine to increase. Maximum values of up to 40 BW were calculated, and such forces should not be underestimated when considering lumbar spine or low back pain in athletes practising all kinds of jumping events. Competitive skills like the high jump or long jump are practised only a few times with a low frequency per day or week in relation to training drills like hurdle jumps, multiple jumps and drop jumps. Therefore the major loading for the spinal tissues may be induced by training drills. These are known to produce highly dynamic spinal loads, especially compressive forces. Table 26.2 summarizes the most relevant data from drop jumping tests.

LANDING

The major and most dramatic clinical and radiological findings in gymnastics concern the thoraco-lumbar junction. There is controversy about which skill or drill in gymnastics produces the highest loading in regard to the thoraco-lumbar spine. Simmelbauer (1992) discussed the fast changes between flexion and extension of the thoraco-lumbar junction during swings on the rings and horizontal bar as a cause for the growth disturbances in the growing apophysis. Other authors considered the damage at the apophyses in gymnasts (e.g. Swärd *et al.* 1990b) as a flexion trauma and speculated that this could be caused by incorrect landing. This controversy led to the inclusion of gymnastic landings and long swings combined with dynamic flexion and extension of the thoraco-lumbar spine in this chapter.

The influence of different initial mechanical energies on landing and the resulting spinal loads are shown by the data summarized in Table 26.3. These numbers describe the peak values for compression and shear forces at L5/S1 during landings from different heights without (DJ51 = 51 cm; DJ91 = 91 cm;

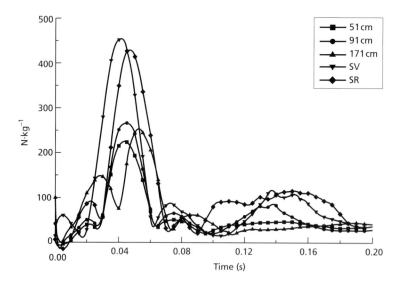

Fig. 26.2 Compressive forces at the lumbar spine (level L5/S1) in landings from different heights (51 cm, 91 cm and 171 cm) without and with somersault (forward somersault, SV; backward somersault, SR) from a height of 91 cm. The graph represents trials of a single subject. The data are normalized to the subject's body mass. Maximum compression occurs immediately after touchdown at 40–45 ms.

DJ171 = 171 cm) and with a somersault (BS = backward somersault; FS = forward somersault) during the flight prior to landing. The data are normalized to body weight and therefore allow comparison between the treatments. The estimated compression forces are relatively high in comparison to data calculated for lifting and materials handling. The compressive forces in landings without a somersault are significantly ($P \leq 0.01$) higher than in running but lower than the loads identified in the drop-jump drills (> 40 cm falling height). This should be affected by the energy absorption of the landing mat. The mechanical characteristics of gymnastics mats has recently changed due to intensive research and technical development in this area (Fig. 26.2, Tables 26.3 & 26.4).

Landings from a height of 91 cm show maximum compression forces of over 10 kN. Falling from 171 cm, which is not the ultimate height for gymnastics dismounts, induces compression forces of more than 30 BW. As expected, the compression forces increase significantly ($P < 0.05$) with increasing kinetic energy at touchdown. The shear forces were more or less constant. In addition to spinal forces, the forces of the trunk muscles were also estimated: the forces of the ventral muscle groups do not vary with the height of the fall, but the muscle force of m. erector spinae increases significantly ($P \leq 0.05$) with

higher energy during the collision between the athlete and the ground. A force of about 5 kN is necessary to decelerate and control the forward bend of the trunk. The EMG patterns indicate that highly trained athletes are able to switch off those muscles that are unnecessary for trunk stabilization at ground contact (see Fig. 26.3). With such motor patterns the subjects decrease the compression of the lumbar spine due to muscle force. Furthermore, the EMG analysis indicates that trained athletes optimize the neuromuscular drive following the used cost function in terms of minimizing the summed muscular stress (Fig. 26.3).

In the initial phase of landing the precise neuromuscular control of m. erector spinae and m. latissimus dorsi allows for a central positioning of the point of application, the force at the intervertebral disc, and a more or less homogeneous pressure distribution at the disc's endplate. Less trained subjects do not have such precise muscle coordination or muscle micro-tuning. This may result in higher muscular force, higher spinal compression, and a less homogeneous pressure distribution on disc and vertebra endplates.

When the landings are performed after a flight with a somersault, both the compression and shear forces (a-p) increase significantly ($P \leq 0.05$). During the landing from a backward somersault the max-

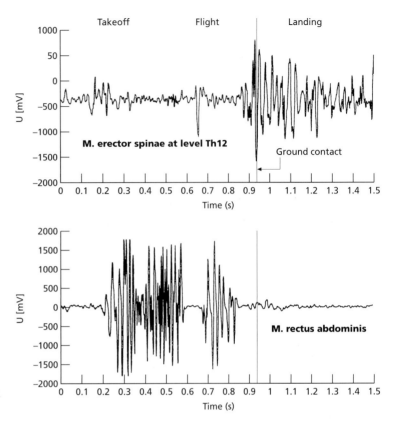

Fig. 26.3 EMG time histories of selected trunk muscles prior to and during the landing of a highly trained female gymnast on a gymnastics mat.

imum compressive force at L5/S1 was estimated to be as high as 40 BW, an amount of normalized mechanical load never before reported in the literature. Simultaneously the load for the m. erector spinae reaches nearly 14 BW. The absolute value of the compression force was at a maximum of 17 800 N. Table 26.3 demonstrates the influence of initial energy and the body position at landing. If the gymnasts use soft complementary mats on top of the landing mats the spinal load is reduced by about 20%. The cause for this decrease in mechanical spinal load is the change in stiffness of the lower extremities and the energy dissipation through the muscles. In addition the energy-absorbing capacity of the supplementary mat plays a role in the peak load reduction.

Initial energy at touchdown, body position at landing and trunk angular momentum prior to landing are all shown to determine the compression (and shear) force at the lumbar spine on landing. A proper technique (e.g. an upright trunk position), well-tuned leg muscle stiffness for muscular energy absorption, and a soft, cushioning landing mat contribute to reducing spinal loading at landing. The effect of the landing surface in terms of landing mats is shown in Table 26.4, which demonstrates the maximum compression and shear forces when landing on just a standard gymnastics mat and with a supplementary mat on top (Table 26.4).

DYNAMIC EXTENSION/FLEXION

The giant swings on the high bar and uneven bars prior to dismount and flight elements with regrasp, can be intuitively regarded as imposing high loads on the spine. Compression and shear forces were calculated over the whole skills and maximum values were summarized for the instants:
A—first maximum deflection of the bar (first maximum of bar reaction force);

Table 26.4 Compressive and shear (a-p) forces at L5/S1 while landing on a gymnastics mat without and with a supplementary soft mat. Force data are given as times body weight, means and standard deviations ($n = 8$).

Forces at L5/S1	DJ91		DJ171	
	Without	With	Without	With
Maximum compression	25.93 ± 6.02*	21.26 ± 2.54	32.22 ± 5.86*	25.25 ± 4.96
Average compression†	9.57 ± 1.79*	8.13 ± 0.96	11.59 ± 1.40	9.33 ± 1.40
Maximum shear (a-p)	3285 ± 0.63	3.57 ± 0.23	3.66 ± 0.47	3.48 ± 0.23
Average shear (a-p)†	1.58 ± 0.20	1.67 ± 0.18	1.84 ± 0.31	1.65 ± 0.08

* Indicates significant ($P \leq 0.05$) differences.
† During the first 80 ms after touchdown.

B—second peak deflection of the bar (second peak of bar reaction force); and
C—countermovement (change of the direction of angular momentum) in the Tkatchev straddle prior to release and passing the bar.

Table 26.5 summarizes the data, and demonstrates that the spinal loading is compressive during the whole drill, that muscle force is therefore higher than the inertial forces, and that compression and shear forces are counterintuitively low in comparison to the activities considered previously. Health problems due to swings and giants (e.g. on high bar and rings) should be explained by overloading mechanisms other than compression and shear loading (Table 26.5; Fig. 26.4).

OVERVIEW

Spinal compression and shear forces differ considerably in the activities analysed above. These differences are reflected in the maximum or peak values, in the force rates, and in the load duration. All the

analyses and data presented were taken from normal, anticipated activities, jumps and landings. No unexpected loads, as often occur in contact sports or happen occasionally as falls and other accidents, were studied. More or less unexpected loading induced by externally initiated forces, for example in contact sports, may lead to much higher internal loading. Mechanical stress in such activities is hard to study in a scientifically controlled way. However, the data presented will help in determining limits of load acceptance or physiological tolerances.

Comparison of spinal forces with critical strength limits

The comparison of estimates of the *in vivo* load during running, landing, drop jumps and lifting heavy weights with the critical tolerance limits of vertebrae and discs taken from the literature shows that the values are relatively close to one another. Genaidy *et al.* (1993) summarized the data of maximum compressive strength from the literature.

Table 26.5 Compression and shear (a-p) forces at L5/S1 during giants prior to the Tkatchev straddle. Data are given as times body weight, means and standard deviations.

Force at L5/S1	Sex	n	Phase A*	Phase B*	Phase C*
Maximum compression	Male	15	4.97 ± 1.08	4.32 ± 1.40	4.05 ± 1.22
	Female	20	3.02 ± 1.70	4.11 ± 1.79	2.32 ± 1.08
Maximum shear force (a-p)	Male	15	1.27 ± 0.49	2.62 ± 0.62	0.87 ± 0.49
	Female	20	1.85 ± 0.91	1.97 ± 0.71	0.98 ± 0.29

* For explanation of phases, see text.

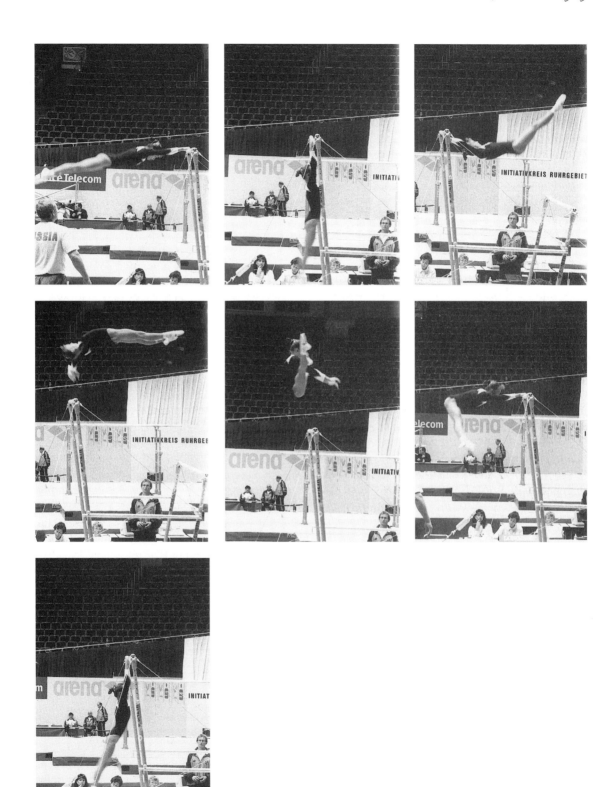

Fig. 26.4 The Tkatchev straddle.

They documented an average of 7915 N for males of 20–29 years of age. Hutton and Adams (1982) reported the highest measured values, with a mean of 9665 N for the same age group, with one specimen exceeding 12 000 N. Callaghan and McGill (1994) presented the effect of a pressurized wet (physiological) environment on porcine vertebral specimens. They demonstrated a significant increase of vertebral strength as well as capacity of energy absorption prior to failure compared to traditional test conditions in the air with no additional pressure above ambient. If human vertebrae behave in a similar fashion then estimates of compressive tolerance may be increased by 40%. Assuming the maximum reported values of Hutton and Adams are valid the tolerance limits should be at about 17 000 N for compressive loading.

It can be assumed that cadaveric studies are based on not very well-adapted specimens or often on specimens with reduced mechanical properties due to bedrest or sickness. Therefore the cadaver studies may underestimate the material strengths of healthy subjects. This hypothesis is supported by the data on bone mineral density, vertebral endplate area and material compressive strength presented by Brinckmann *et al.* (1989). Brinckmann's results indicate that subjects with no physical activities in the last two years of life were found to be clearly below the regression line of the relationship between the vertebral compressive strength and the product of vertebral mineral density and endplate area. Inactive or sick subjects demonstrated less material strength and less vertebral mineral density endplate area product. Vertebral strengths of physically inactive subjects are significantly lower than predicted by the regression equation. Therefore, the compressive strength limits of the vertebrae of healthy subjects should be about 15 000–17 000 N or more.

With this in mind the estimates of Cholewicki *et al.* (1991) of spinal compressive loading during lifting extremely heavy weights are conservative and provide underestimates of the spinal forces; the *in vivo* strength of the vertebrae of trained subjects should exceed 18 000 N. During Cholewicki's experiments no acute vertebral fractures were identified, and reviewing the literature no vertebral fractures are reported during expected and in controlled

movements. Although the mathematical estimates of loading forces are conservative the maximum compressive forces will not touch the ultimate values in the analysed sport activities in general. In summary, the calculated compression forces in jumping and landing are just within the boundaries of acceptable loads but lie very close to the upper limits. Running induces a mechanical load which is within the tolerance range, but when considering the repetitive form of the loading it may actually be relatively high.

The number of repetitions and the frequency of loading seems to play a role in the strength limit. Brinckmann *et al.* (1988) reported a significant decrease of vertebral compressive strength when the tissue is loaded over an increasing number of loading cycles. This may be one reason why even in activities with relatively low loads, such as running, injury sometimes occurs, as evidenced by a report of isolated cases of sacral stress fracture in female long-distance runners (Eller *et al.* 1997). Because no data on short-term bone healing are available, such fatigue fractures may indicate that moderate loading (10 BW) may—if applied over a long loading time at a relatively high frequency—lead to overuse of the spinal bone structures. Therefore both maximum loading and repetitive frequent loading should be considered when discussing strength limits and tolerances.

Shear force tolerances of a motion segment are given by Lamy *et al.* (1975). The authors found that one-third of the failures of the neural arch were through the pars interarticularis when a load of 3000 N shear force was applied at the facet joint. The strength was found to be same for male and female subjects as well as for those with either normal or degenerated discs. The shear forces found in the experimental studies presented above were all below the given limits of failure.

Battié *et al.* (1995) investigated the degeneration of intervertebral discs in 135 monozygotic twin pairs. The amount of the variance of disc degeneration by physical loading attributed to work (job code) and sport was relatively low. A much higher percentage of disc degeneration was found to be explained by familial aggregation. From these findings the authors concluded that genetics is an important factor in the degeneration process. Genetically determined mechanical properties of the involved biological structures are not to be underestimated or excluded from the discussion of ultimate strength limits of an individual. Even minor anatomical abnormalities of spinal structures may predispose to weakness and increase the probability of failure. Cyron and Hutton (1978) found significant differences in the cross-sectional distribution of cortical and cancellous bone in the partes interarticulares of specimens with and without fracturing when subjected to repetitive cyclic mechanical loading. The data were interpreted to suggest that a thin pars interarticularis may predispose to spondylolysis through the mechanism of fatigue failure.

From the studies of Brinckmann et al. (1989) it is known that the compressive strength of human lumbar vertebrae is strongly dependent on trabecular bone density and endplate area. Grimston and Hanley (1992) reported significantly higher bone mineral densities (BMD) of the lumbar spine in young gymnasts in comparison to less mechanically loaded swimmers. These results were supported by data from Theiss et al. (1993) studying BMDs of former elite gymnasts. Brüggemann and Krahl (2000) reported an increase in sagittal diameter of lumbar vertebrae of young female gymnasts in relation to the normal population. Kraemer (1999) compared the endplate area of lumbar and thoracic vertebrae of female gymnasts ($n = 16$) and controls ($n = 16$) of the same biological age using MRI techniques. Significantly higher values for the normalized endplate areas were identified for the gymnasts. In addition, Kraemer reported greater normalized heights of the intervertebral discs for gymnasts when compared with the controls. This was highly significant ($P \leq 0.01$) for the younger gymnasts (11–14 years of age). These studies indicate the possible adaptation of the bony structure of the spine and the intervertebral discs due to long-term mechanical loading through sport and exercise.

Nevertheless, the identified mechanical loading in association with physical activities should not be underestimated. Mechanical loading of vulnerable structures during growth should be carefully examined to avoid local overloading, which may cause morphological and functional disorders.

Overload and injury mechanisms

Mechanical loading of the spinal structures in different sports seems to be high but in the majority of cases it stays within the tolerance limits of the tissue. Contact sports are predominantly affected by unexpected and often uncontrollable external loading. Analysis of loads experienced by participants in real situations does not seem feasible, and the cause–effect relation of a collision and the resulting injury remains a matter for speculation. The mechanisms of injury in these sports are hard to differentiate and to analyse. It can be assumed that the risk of injury to the cervical and lumbar spine in sports with a high degree of contact, as well as in uncontrolled and unexpected collisions, is a priori high and difficult to estimate or quantify.

Clinical and radiological data of spine deformities and injuries focus on the thoraco-lumbar anterior areas and the posterior structures of the lumbar spine. From these findings one can differentiate between flexion and hyperextension injuries.

FLEXION INJURIES

The most frequent deformities or abnormal vertebral configurations in athletes are located in the thoraco-lumbar spine. Hellström et al. (1990) reported significant differences in the frequency of radiological abnormalities between elite athletes from different sports, such as wrestling, soccer, tennis and gymnastics, and in non-athletes. Abnormalities in the vertebral ring apophysis occurred exclusively in athletes. The different types of abnormalities were most common in male gymnasts and wrestlers. Fröhner (2000) reported similar findings of abnormalities on the anterior column of the thoraco-lumbar transition in male and female former gymnasts. During the vulnerable phase of the growth spurt the mechanism of mechanical overload seems to be trunk flexion combined with high compressive forces. When the trunk is bent forwards the centre of mass and the inertial force of the upper torso act with a long lever arm on the motion segment and the joint between the flexible lumbar spine and the compact thoracic cage. The pressure distribution will indicate peak pressures on the anterior column of the vertebrae at level T12/L1.

The finite element model of the motion segment including disc, presented by Lu *et al.* (1996), calculates the compressive and tensile stress distribution at the inferior endplate interface. The data clearly identify both peak compressive and tensile stress distribution at the inferior endplate interface. Peak compressive stress for the bend condition is located at the anterior endplate. Model simulations found the maximum tensile stress in the annulus fibres at the inner posterior annulus at the junction of the disc and the endplate. Flexion of 7° had a greater effect on posterior and posterolateral annulus fibre tensile stress than twisting of 2°. For the anterior and anterolateral regions of the disc and the junction with the endplate, 2° of twisting was shown to have a slightly greater effect than bending. The model simulation data help to explain both the mechanical compression loading of the anterior vertebral corner at the apophysis and the tensile stress on the posterior disc. A high compression force acting on the thoraco-lumbar junction with a bent and twisted trunk position may cause a mechanical load exceeding the tissue tolerances of the individual. More-over, the simulation results of Lu *et al.* (1996) illustrate that increased loading rates lead to reduction in the load at which initial fibre rupture occurred. This result indicates the importance of loading rate to tissue response.

Several authors have described the apophysial abnormalities considered to result from intravertebral disc herniations in young physically active individuals. These may result from a trauma with acute mechanical overloading, for example in a flexed landing. This is supported by data from Swärd *et al.* (1990b), who demonstrated the development of such changes after trauma in two female gymnasts. However, as the longitudinal and the intervertebral ligaments are attached to the apophysis the traction at the apophysis induced by the ligament during spinal extension may be an additional cause for apophysial injury. Knowledge of the quantity of compressive force and the inhomogeneous pressure distribution shown lead to speculation that the flexion mechanism seems to be the

most plausible cause for the most common spinal injury in young athletes.

HYPEREXTENSION INJURIES

Two specific conditions that afflict young and athletic populations are spondylolysis and spondylolisthesis. These failures or injuries effect the bony structures especially at L4/L5 and L5/S1 levels. As noted above, spondylolysis is a unilateral or bilateral fracture of the pars interarticularis, whereas spondylolisthesis involves slippage between L4 and L5 or L5 and S1 vertebrae. Classification of spondylolysis and spondylolisthesis identifies five types: dysplastic, isthmoid, degenerative, traumatic and pathological (Newman & Stone 1963). Of greatest concern for the young and athletic population is the isthmoid type, in which repeated mechanical loading of the pars area may cause microfractures and bone failure. Forcible hyperextension combined with a high compressive force produces high mechanical stress at the pars interarticularis when compressive forces are transmitted through the facet joints and eventually the processus spinosus. Increased forward tilt of the pelvis increases the lumbo-sacral angle, exaggerates the lumbar lordosis, and promotes the risk of overloading. Unilateral loading may be due to additional twisting of the motion segment. The populations which are most at risk for hyperextension injuries are those whose sport exposes them to repeated high compressive spinal loading in combination with extreme extension and rotational movements and positions. These include fast-bowlers, wrestlers, gymnasts, divers, trampolinists and javelin throwers.

Prevention of spinal injuries

The mechanical load of the spine in many sports may approach or reach the limits of tissue tolerances. When these limits are exceeded, injury or tissue damage will occur, either as a single traumatic failure or as repeated microfailures. Equipment, sporting technique and training determine the mechanical load of the spinal structures induced by any specific sport. In order to prevent spinal injuries these factors have to be addressed in order to reduce the risk of loads exceeding the physiological limits. In addition, medical examination of the athletes for early identification of possible temporary weakness (e.g. during the growth spurt) must be a part of any preventive strategy, especially for young athletes. However, preventive strategies are generally ineffective against unexpected loading caused by collisions in contact sports. For these sports the physical preparation of the athletes plays the major role in the prevention of spinal injuries.

Equipment

In dynamic loading the spine is subjected to high compression and shear forces with extreme force rates. As shown above, jumping and landing from a jump or a dismount (e.g. in gymnastics) are the manoeuvres with the greatest loads. The proper equipment contributes to shock absorption during the impact and decreases the peak forces acting on the spinal structures. For example, the use of soft landing mats can significantly reduce spinal loading. The mechanical properties of the surface influence the damping properties of the motor system, primarily of the lower extremities. Therefore the landing technique is influenced by the surface. Based on biomechanical studies on the effect of landing mats on mechanical loading of body tissue (bone, cartilage, spine) the International Gymnastic Federation changed the thickness of landing mats

from 12 cm to 20 cm. For the most stressful landings, which occur in the men's high bar, women's uneven bars, and the vaults, the Federation stipulated that 10 cm supplementary mats be used on top of the 20 cm landing mats (Fig. 26.5). Epidemiological studies have to evaluate how these strategies contribute to reducing the risk of spinal overloading as well as lower-extremity injuries, both in severity and frequency.

In repetitive footfalls and impacts the footwear quality is as important as the surface. Cushioning midsoles contribute to a decrease in impact loading of the spine. For such activities it should be mentioned that the leg stiffness plays a more important role than the footwear cushioning capacity for the peak spinal loading.

When learning difficult skills, such as high-bar dismounts, diving pits filled with soft materials (cube-shaped low-density foam) are used to ensure soft and safe landing during unexpected and uncontrolled falls. This equipment can be used in the very early stages of learning the difficult skills but it is not appropriate for learning landings controlled by the neuromuscular system.

In high-velocity sports and contact sports, helmets play an important role in the prevention of head and neck injuries. The design of the helmet has to ensure that the posterior rim does not act as a pivot during cervical hyperextension. This 'guillotine' effect of the ridge of the football helmet was

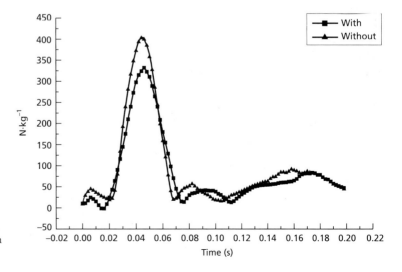

Fig. 26.5 The use of supplementary soft mats in gymnastic landing from heights of 91 and 171 cm can significantly ($P \leq 0.05$) decrease the maximum compression forces of the lumbar spine. The graph shows the landings from a height of 171 cm of a single subject with and without a thin supplementary mat.

identified as primary cause of cervical injuries in football (Schneider 1973). By changing the design of the helmets the number of severe cervical injuries in this sport clearly decreased.

In more static spinal loading, as in weight-training, weightlifting belts increase the intra-abdominal pressure. This increase of the intra-abdominal pressure leads to a reduction of compressive loading of the lumbar spine. However, the primary role of the belt is more to ensure an increase of intra-abdominal pressure than to support against spinal deformation, which was traditionally argued when using such weightlifting belts.

Technique

The proper sporting technique can contribute to the reduction and control of mechanical load of the spine. This is especially valid for the posterior column of the lumbar spine, the lumbo-sacral junction, and the anterior column of the thoraco-lumbar spine. Forwards bending or inclining the trunk when high external forces are applied to the body leads to an increase of peak pressure on the anterior area of the vertebrae at the thoraco-lumbar junction. This may be the mechanism which damages the apophysial ring when landing from a jump or a dismount in gymnastics with forward lean and bent trunk position. The technique for landing and the phases prior to landing has a major influence on the pelvis and spine posture and therefore on peak pressure and pressure distribution at the motion segment. When bending with lumbar spine flexion up to 45° to the horizontal the trunk is counterbalanced by the erector spinae muscles. If the flexion increases to about 60° the passive posterior ligaments become taut. In continuing the forward movement the pelvis rotates forwards until the pelvis rotation is passively restricted by the gluteus and hamstring muscles. In this deep forward lean position no activity of the back muscles can be registered. The inertial force and the weight of the trunk are counterbalanced by passive forces of ligaments, fasciae and muscles. Therefore, landings with an extreme forward lean contribute to the load of the passive posterior structures. Landings with a more or less upright trunk position are controlled by the

erector spinae muscles, which must clearly be activated prior to landing. Well-prepared athletes show a high preactivation of the m. erector spinae before the collision with the floor or the mat. Less-skilled athletes do not activate the back muscles prior to touchdown, which leads to an accelerated forward inclination until the ligaments and other passive structures decelerate the forward movement of the trunk. In order to minimize the total muscle force and the resulting compression force of the motion segment, well-prepared athletes do not coactivate the abdominal muscle in landing.

The peak impact force acting on the spine at landing can be influenced by the mechanical properties of the surface or footwear and the damping properties of the motor system, primarily at the foot and knee joints. These cushioning capacities strongly depend on the muscle force of the leg extensor muscles and the joint stiffness regulation. With a controlled and 'soft' landing technique, in which ankle plantarflexion and knee flexion are coordinated, the peak impact force is strongly reduced. During 'stiff' landings the body's mechanical energy is absorbed through the deformation of bone, cartilage and spine. In soft and well-coordinated landings only little energy is spent on deformation of the passive biological structures. Soft or moderately firm surfaces can contribute to use the energy absorption capacity of the musculature by prolonging the time to peak force after touchdown. Practice of landing technique in order to avoid a stiff landing is an important strategy to prevent spinal overloads and injuries. Soft and controlled landings can only be performed when the movement in the air prior to landing is well controlled. Therefore, proper technical execution of airborne manoeuvres is a major requirement for safe landings, and for prevention of spinal injuries. It has been shown that under-rotated somersaults and asymmetric landings lead to dramatic increases in the mechanical load of the tissue involved. In asymmetric landings from under-rotated twisting somersaults the Achilles tendon force increased up to about 40 kN. During correct landings the load was calculated to be about 10 kN (Panzer 1987). It can be speculated that spinal load dramatically increases in such landings from under-rotated twisting somersaults, especially when the

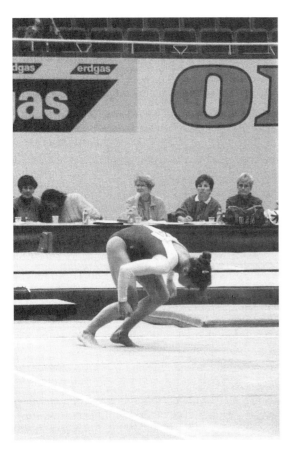

Fig. 26.6 Asymmetric landing from under-rotated twisting somersaults (e.g. double backward somersault with full twist) increases the mechanical load of the biological structures.

landing is combined with lateral flexion and torsion of the spine (Fig. 26.6).

The major cause of injuries of the posterior lumbar spine is forced hyperextension. Reclination of the lumbar spine combined with high compression and eventually lateral bending and torsion was shown to produce high mechanical stress on the neural arch at the pars interarticularis. Techniques should be carefully reviewed to minimize this kind of loading. Elliott *et al.* (1992) have shown that counter-rotation of the trunk between the back and the front foot impact in fast-bowlers in cricket predisposes the bowlers to an increased incidence of bony and disc abnormalities in the lumbar region.

A short-term programme aimed at modifying the technique was found to be unsuccessful (Elliott *et al.* 1995). Therefore a longer-term programme had to be structured to educate bowlers how to participate in a relatively injury-free environment. Any sport technique is a long-term and stable learnt pattern. It takes a long time and considerable effort in practice to relearn and change the automated movements. Learning the proper techniques at an early stage of motor learning is vital for the prevention of spinal injuries.

Gymnastics is often discussed in relation to hyperextension. The exclusion of hyperextension techniques in this sport has caused the incidence of spondylolisthesis to decrease to that of the normal population. The performance of slow walkovers has been generally reduced and the techniques used for many moves are now more focused on the extension of shoulder joints and all spinal motion segments. Hyperextension techniques combined with high compression forces can nowadays be observed in less-skilled and badly prepared athletes (e.g. in front handspring vaults in horse-vaulting).

There are a number of other sports in which—from a biomechanical point of view—critical techniques are being used. Examples are the tennis serve or the smash in volleyball. There is a need to evaluate such techniques, to develop alternatives, and to at least educate recreational athletes about techniques which produce less spinal loading.

Training

The physical preparation of the athlete is a major concern in the prevention of spine injuries. This is true for expected loading as well as for unexpected collisions, attacks and tackles. The development of a muscular 'corset' for the thoraco-lumbar spine seems to be the most effective strategy to ensure a controlled mechanical loading. The strengthened back muscles are able to control and counterbalance the trunk's weight and inertial force during impact loading. A properly developed abdominal wall also plays a large role in stabilizing the spine. The fasciae, together with the erector spinae muscle and the latissimus dorsi, build the 'corset', which helps to reduce and control shear and torsion forces acting

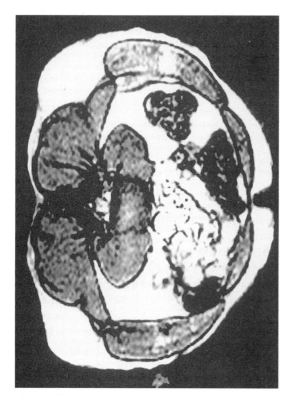

Fig. 26.7 Sectional view of the torso at level L3/L4 by a magnetic resonance image. The muscular corset including the fasciae helps to control spinal movement and to prevent uncontrolled shear and torsion.

on the motion segments. In addition, the abdominal muscles play an important role in increasing intra-abdominal pressure, which may lead to a decrease of spinal compression force (Fig. 26.7).

The issue of strengthening the trunk muscles becomes complicated because the exercises aimed at strengthening the muscular corset are associated with large compressive and sometimes shear loadings of the lumbar spine. To prevent spinal overloading during the strengthening of spine erector muscles, extreme caution is necessary. Development of the muscle corset should avoid any imbalance between the musculature of the abdominal wall and the spine extensor back muscles, the left and right lateral flexor muscles, and the left and right torsion muscle groups. When strengthening these muscles

one has to be careful not to shorten muscles which lead to posture modification. A typical example is the shortened iliopsoas muscle, which results in an increased lumbar lordosis.

Due to the high mechanical loading of the trunk-muscle strengthening exercises, the development of the trunk muscular corset has to be a long-term strategy associated with a gradual onset and well-organized training over years. The progression of loading must be slow but continuous, especially when training young athletes.

The periods of rest between the training sessions should be long enough for tissue recovery. Healing times for microlesions to bone, cartilage and connective tissue are longer than for muscles. Therefore a long-term training strategy should contain well-organized periods of rest for tissue adaptation.

The physical preparation of the athlete has to include posture corrections and the development of flexibility of the entire spine. A late and fast start to spinal strength training and the imitation of training patterns from other sports without the necessary preparation and experience can dangerously overload the spinal structures. The mobilization has to include all levels of the spine and the shoulder joints. Flexibility is especially important for the motion segments of the thoraco-lumbar junction and the thoracic spine. Posture corrections should be focused on lumbar lordosis because increased lordosis coincides with a higher risk of overload. Lordosis compensates for the tilt of the sacrum with respect to the vertical: the smaller the sacro-vertebral angle the better the mechanical loading situation. A more vertical position of the sacrum is favourable for the stability of the lumbo-sacral junction, and the tilt of the sacrum can be modified by strength development of the corresponding muscle group. The rectus abdominis muscle and the hip extensors can decrease the sacral angle by rotating the sacrum into a more vertical position. Muscle strengthening is an appropriate strategy for posture correction and thus for spinal modification and control.

Medical survey

A medical survey and clinical examination helps

with identification of early signs of dysfunction or abnormalities. Often the clinical signs can be identified earlier than radiological findings (see e.g. Swärd *et al.* 1990b). When an early dysfunction is identified and there is prompt reduction of sporting load, changes in training strategies and movement techniques, and implementation of physiotherapeutic preventive measures, the majority of microlesions and functional disturbances will heal and totally disappear. Lohrer *et al.* (2000) reported that 50% of positive clinical diagnoses of 57 young female gymnasts examined showed complete healing. Twenty-five percent of the findings were constant over the period of survey and 25% became worse. Remarkably, most of the subjects who showed a definite healing and reduction of clinical findings were directly subjected to load reduction, therapy and strengthening. From the same prospective study it was shown that the total number of positive clinical and radiological findings decreased over the five years of research, and it was speculated that this was due to early medical control and intervention.

During the growth spurt, when spinal structures are sensitive to overuse, a regular and thorough clinical control can be especially helpful in identifying any decrease in tissue tolerance. In addition the risk factors described by Fröhner (2000) indicating reduced strength during pubertal growth provide a practical basis for preventive interventions. Endogenetic factors were strongly related to the development of osteochondrosis in young female gymnasts. Some of the observed factors were 'hypermobility' and 'weak connective tissue', 'leptomorph body form', 'low body height/body mass relation', 'late maturity' and 'dysharmonic growth' (Fröhner 2000). Standing height and body weight during adolescence provide easy measures to identify dysharmonic growth and disturbance of the body height/body mass relation, which may indicate temporarily reduced tissue strength.

Summary

The use of shock-absorbing equipment (playing surfaces, mats, footwear) and protective helmets, and the development of proper sports techniques can contribute significantly to reducing the mechanical loads experienced by the spine and the consequent risk of overloading in a variety of sports. Early and long-term physical preparation plays a dominant role in the control and balance of spinal loading. It can be shown that the development of a so-called 'muscle corset' is an adequate strategy for the prevention of spinal injuries. But any such strengthening of the trunk musculature is itself necessarily coupled with high spinal loading, hence caution is important when starting trunk muscle strength programmes. The onset should be early and gradual, and the programme carried out over the long term. Physical preparation is a precondition in most sports to prevent spinal overloading in the athletes. The strength of the spine is reduced during growth spurts in adolescents, and this factor must be considered when planning the training programmes of young athletes. The principles employed in training adult athletes (e.g. continuous increase of training loads) cannot be used in training the young athlete. Regular and thorough clinical surveys of young elite athletes can help to identify periods of reduced strength and dysfunction. Such surveys are a prerequisite for reducing the sport-related loads and initiating strengthening and physiotherapy. The clinical and radiological evaluation of spinal morphology prior to the onset of training at the elite level ensures the identification of subjects who are morphologically ill-suited for the stresses associated with loading in some sports.

References

Alexander, C.J. (1976) Effect of growth rate on the strength of the growth plate-shaft junction. *Skeletal Radiology* **1**, 67–76.

Alexander, C.J. (1977) Scheuermann's disease: a traumatic spondylodystrophy? *Skeletal Radiology* **1**, 209–221.

Andersson, G. (1991) The epidemiology of spinal disorders. In: *The Adult Spine: Principles and Practice* (ed. W. Frymoyer), pp. 107–146. Raven Press, New York.

Balagué, F., Dutoit, G. & Waldburger, M. (1988) Low back pain in school children. *Scandinavian Journal of Rehabilitation and Medicine* **10**, 175–179.

Balagué, F., Damidot, P., Nordin, M., Parnianpour, M. & Waldburger, M. (1993) Cross-sectional study of isokinetic muscle trunk strength among school children. *Spine* **18**, 1199–1205.

Battié, M.C., Videman, T., Gibbons, L.E., Fisher, L.D., Manninen, H. & Gill, K.

(1995) Determinants of lumbar disc degeneration: a study relating lifetime exposures and magnetic resonance imaging findings in identical twins. *Spine* **20**, 2601–2612.

Blumenthal, S.L., Roach, J. & Herring, J.A. (1987) Lumbar Scheuermann's: a clinical series and classification. *Spine* **12**, 929–932.

Brinckmann, P., Biggemann, M. & Hilweg, D. (1988) Fatigue fracture of human lumbar vertebrae. *Clinical Biomechanics* **3** (Suppl. 1), S1–S23.

Brinckmann, P., Biggemann, M. & Hilweg, D. (1989) Prediction of the compressive strength of human lumbar vertebrae. *Clinical Biomechanics* **4** (Suppl. 2), S1–S27.

Brüggemann, G.-P. (1997) Analyse verschiedener Ansätze zur Belastungs-quantifizierung der lumbalen Wirbelsäule bei Trage- und Hebebewegungen. In: *Prävention von arbeitsbedingten Gesundheitsgefahren – 3* (eds S. Radandt, R. Griehaber & W. Schneider), pp. 233–248. Erfurter Tage Monade, Leipzig.

Brüggemann, G.-P. & Krahl, H. (2000) Belastungen und Risiken im Kunstturnen. *Schriftenreihe des Bundesinstituts für Sportwissenschaft*, **111**. Hofmann-Verlag, Schorndorf.

Caine, D.J. & Lindner, K.J. (1985) Overuse injuries of growing bones: the young female gymnast at risk? *Physician and Sports Medicine* **13**, 51–64.

Callaghan, J.P. & McGill, S. (1994) Compression tolerance of a porcine vertebral fracture model exposed to physiological pressures. In: *Proceedings of the Eighth Biennial Conference of the Canadian Society of Biomechanics, Calgary* (eds W. Herzog, B.M. Nigg & T. van den Bogert), pp. 76–77. University of Calgary, Calgary.

Cantu, R.C. & Mueller, F.O. (1990) Catastrophic spine injuries in football. *Journal of Spinal Disorders* **3**, 227–231.

Cappozzo, A. (1984) Compressive loads in the lumbar vertebral column during normal walking. *Journal of Orthopaedic Research* **1**, 234–238.

Cholewicki, J., McGill, S.M. & Norman, R.W. (1991) Lumbar spine loads during the lifting of extremely heavy weights. *Medicine and Science in Sports and Exercise* **23**, 1179–1186.

Crowninshield, R.D. & Brand, R.A. (1981) The prediction of forces in joint structures: Distribution of intersegmental resultants. *Exercise and Sport Sciences Review* **9**, 159–181.

Cyron, B.M. & Hutton, W.C. (1978) The fatigue strength of the lumbar neural arch in spondylolysis. *Journal of Bone and Joint Surgery* **60B**, 234–238.

Denis, F. (1983) The three column spine and its significance in the classification of acute thoracolumbar spinal injuries. *Spine* **8**, 817–831.

Eller, D.J., Katz, D.S., Bergman, A.G., Fredericson, M. & Beaulieu, C.F. (1997) Sacral stress fractures in long-distance runners. *Clinical Journal of Sport Medicine* **7**, 222–225.

Elliott, B., Hardcastle, P., Burnett, A. & Forster, D. (1992) The influence of fast bowling and physical factors on radiological features in high performance fast bowlers. *Journal of Sports Medicine and Training Rehabilitation* **3**, 113–130.

Elliott, B., Burnett, A., Khangure, M. & Hardcastle, P. (1995) The influence of fast bowling technique in cricket on disk degeneration: a follow-up study. In: *XVth Congress of the International Society of Biomechanics, University of Jyväskylä, Finland* (eds K. Häkkinen, K.L. Keskinen, P.V. Komi & A. Mero), pp. 244–245. University of Jyväskylä, Jyväskylä.

Farfan, H.F., Cossette, J.W., Robertson, G.H., Wells, R.V. & Kraus, H. (1970) The effects of torsion on the lumbar intervertebral joints. The role of torsion in the production of disc degeneration. *Journal of Bone and Joint Surgery* **52A**, 468–497.

Fröhner (2000) Zustand des Stütz- und Bewegungsapparates nach mehr-jährigem Hochleistungstraining. In: *Belastungen und Risiken im Kunstturnen Schriftenreihe des Bundesinstituts für Sportwissenschaft*, **111** (eds G.-P. Brüggemann & H. Krahl), pp. 67–90. Hofmann-Verlag, Schorndorf.

Frymoyer, J.W., Pope, M.H., Clements, J.H., Wilder, D.G., MacPherson, B. & Ashikaga, T. (1983) Risk factors in low-back pain. *Journal of Bone and Joint Surgery* **65A/2**, 213–218.

Gao, J. & Brüggemann, G.-P. (1995) Distribution problem at lumbar joint L5/S1 – an optimization method combined with EMG-based switch technique. In: *XVth Congress of the International Society of Biomechanics University of Jyväskylä, Finland* (eds K. Häkkinen, K.L. Keskinen, P.V. Komi & A. Mero), pp. 310–311. University of Jyväskylä, Jyväskylä.

Gatt, C.J., Hosea, T.M., Palumbo, R.C. & Zwadsky, J.P. (1997) Impact loading of the lumbar spine during football blocking. *American Journal of Sports Medicine* **25**, 317–321.

Geffen, S., Gibbs, N. & Geffen, L. (1997) Thoracic spinal fracture in a rugby league footballer. *Clinical Journal of Sports Medicine* **7**, 144–146.

Genaidy, A.M., Waly, S.M., Khalil, T.M. & Hidalgo, J. (1993) Spinal compression limits for the design of manual material handling operations in the workplace. *Ergonomics* **36**, 415–434.

Goldstein, J.D., Berger, P.E., Windler, G.F. & Jackson, D.M. (1991) Spine injuries in gymnasts and swimmers. An epidemiologic investigation. *American Journal of Sports Medicine* **19** (5), 463–468.

Granhed, H. & Morelli, B. (1988) Low back pain among retired wrestlers and heavy-weight lifters. *American Journal of Sports Medicine* **16**, 530–533.

Granhed, H., Jonson, R. & Hansson, T. (1987) The loads on the lumbar spine during extreme weight lifting. *Spine* **12**, 146–149.

Grimston, S.K. & Hanley, D.A. (1992) Bone mineral density in children is related to mechanical loading regime. *Medicine and Science in Sports and Exercise* **24** (Suppl.), 101.

Hainline, B. (1995) Low back injury. *Clinics in Sports Medicine* **14**, 241–265.

Hellström, M., Jacobbson, B., Swärd, L. & Peterson, L. (1990) Radiologic abnormalities of the thoraco-lumbar spine in athletes. *Acta Radiologica* **31**, 127–132.

Hirsch, C. & Nachemson, A. (1963) Clinical observations on the spine in ejected pilots. *Aerospace Medicine* **34**, 629–632.

Holm, S. & Rosenqvist, A.-L. (1986) Morphological and nutritional changes in the intervertebral disc after spinal motion. *Scandinavian Journal of Rheumatology* (Suppl. 60), A117.

Horne, J., Cockshott, W.P. & Shannon, H.S. (1987) Spinal column damage from water ski jumping. *Skeletal Radiology* **16**, 612–616.

Hosea, T.M., Gatt, C.J. & McCarthy, K.E. (1989) Analytic computation of rapid dynamic loading of the lumbar spine. *Transactions of the Orthopedic Research Society* **14**, 358.

Hutton, W.C. & Adams, M.A. (1982) Can the lumbar spine be crushed in heavy lifting? *Spine* **7**, 586–590.

Kelsey, J.L., Githens, P.B., White, A.A. *et al.* (1984) An epidemiologic study of lifting and twistings on the job and risk for acute prolapsed intervertebral disc. *Journal of Orthopaedic Research* **2**, 61–66.

Kraemer, U.B. (1999) Belastungsinduzierte Veränderungen an Wirbelkörpern und Bandscheiben bei Kindern und Jugendlichen: Kernspintomographischer Vergleich von Kunstturnerinnen und nicht turnenden Mädchen. Dissertation, Deutsche Sporthochschule, Köln.

Kujala, U.M., Salminen, J.J., Taimela, S., Oksanen, A. & Jaakkola, L. (1992) Subject characteristics and low back pain in young athletes and nonathletes. *Medicine and Science in Sports and Exercise* **24**, 627–632.

Lamy, C., Bazergui, A., Kraus, H. & Farfan, H.F. (1975) The strength of the neural arch and the etiology of spondylolysis. *Orthopedic Clinics of North America* **6**, 215–219.

Lander, J.E., Simonton, R.L. & Giacobbe, J.F.K. (1990) The effectiveness of weightbelts during the squat exercise. *Medicine and Science in Sports and Exercise* **22**, 117–126.

Lohrer, H., Eckhardt, R., Gruppe, V. & Theiss, P. (2000) Zustand des Stütz- und Bewegungsapparates von aktuellen Kunstturnerinnen des Hochleistungsbereiches: Eine prospektive Studie 1993–97. In: *Belastungen und Risiken im Kunstturnen Schriftenreihe des Bundesinstituts für Sportwissenschaft*, **111** (eds G.-P. Brüggemann & H. Krahl), pp. 100–122. Hofmann-Verlag, Schorndorf.

Lu, Y.M., Hutton, W.C. & Gharpuray, V.M. (1996) Do bending, twisting, and diurnal fluid changes in the disc affect propensity to prolapse? A viscoelastic finite element model. *Spine* **21**, 2570–2579.

McCall, I.W., Park, W.M. & O'Brien, J.P. (1985) Acute traumatic intraosseous disc herniation. *Spine* **10**, 134–137.

McGill, S.M. & Norman, R.W. (1985) Dynamically and statically determined low back moments during lifting. *Journal of Biomechanics* **18**, 877–885.

McGill, S.M. & Norman, R.W. (1986) Partitioning of the L4–L5 dynamic moment into disc, ligamentous and muscular components during lifting. *Spine* **11**, 666–677.

McGill, S.M. & Norman, R.W. (1987) Effects of an anatomically detailed erector spinae model on L4/L5 disc compression and shear. *Journal of Biomechanics* **20**, 591–600.

McLeod, K.J., Bain, S.D. & Rubin, C.T. (1990) Dependence of bone adaptation on the frequency of induced dynamic strains. *Transactions of the Orthopaedic Research Society* **15**, 103.

Murphy, P. (1985) Still too many neck injuries. *Physician and Sports Medicine* **13**, 29–30.

Nigg, B.M. & Bobbert, M. (1990) On the potential of various approaches in load analysis to reduce the frequency of sports injuries. *Journal of Biomechanics* **23** (Suppl. 1), 3–12.

Panzer, V.P. (1987) Dynamic assessment of lower extremity load characteristics during landing. Dissertation, University of Oregon.

Raspe, H. & Kohlmann, T. (1993) Rückenschmerzen – eine Epidemie unserer Tage? *Deutsches Ärzteblatt* **90** (44), C1963–C1967.

Reid, D.C. & Saboe, L. (1991) Spinal trauma in sports and recreation. *Journal of Clinical Sports Medicine* **1**, 75–82.

Rodrigo, J. & Boyd, R. (1979) Lumbar spine injuries in military parachute jumpers. *Physician and Sports Medicine* **7**, 9–12.

Rogge, C.W.I. & Niemann, A. (1976) Isolated and atypical manifestations of Scheuermann's disease. *Archivum Chirurgicum Neerlandicum* **28**, 140–160.

Roy, S., Caine, D. & Singer, K.M. (1985) Stress changes in the distal epiphysis in young gymnasts. *American Journal of Sports Medicine* **13**, 301–308.

Schmitt, H., Hausmann, J., Brocai, D.R.C. & Loew, M. (1998) Spätschäden am Bewegungsapparat nach Hochleistungssport am Beispiel der Speerwerfer. *Deutsche Zeitschrift für Sportmedizin* **49** (S1), 295–299.

Schmorl, G. & Junghanns, H. (1971) *The Human Spine in Health and Disease*, 2nd edn. Grune & Stratton, New York.

Schneider, R.C. (ed.) (1973) Head and neck injuries. In: *Football: Mechanisms, Treatment and Prevention*, pp. 77–125. Williams & Wilkins, Baltimore.

Schultz, A.B. & Andersson, G.B.J. (1981) Analysis of loads on the lumbar spine. *Spine* **6**, 76–82.

Schultz, A.B., Andersson, G.B.J., Prtengren, R., Haderspeck, K. & Nachemson, A. (1982) Loads on the lumbar spine. *Journal of Bone and Joint Surgery* **64**, 713–720.

Simmelbauer, B. (1992) *Knorpelverknöcherungsstörungen der Wirbelkörper bei jugendlichen Kunstturnern*. Ecomed, Landsberg.

Sohal, R.S. & Allan, R.G. (1978) Oxidative stress as a causal factor in differentiation and aging: a unifying hypothesis. *Journal of Gerontology* **25**, 499–522.

Steinbrück, K. (1987) Epidemiologie von Sportverletzungen: 15-Jahres-Analyse einer sportorthopädischen Ambulanz. *Sportverletzung – Sportschaden* **1**, 2–12.

Sturzenegger, M., DiStefano, G., Radanov, B.P. & Schnidrig, A. (1994) Presenting symptoms and signs after whiplash injury: the influence of accident mechanisms. *Neurology* **44**, 688–693.

Swärd, L. (1992) The thoracolumbar spine in young elite athletes: Current concepts on the effects of physical training. *Sports Medicine* **13** (5), 357–364.

Swärd, L., Hellström, M., Jacobsson, B., Nyman, R. & Peterson, L. (1990a) Acute injury of the vertebral ring apophysis and intervertebral disc in adolescent gymnasts. *Spine* **15**, 144–148.

Swärd, L., Hellström, M., Jacobsson, B. & Peterson, L. (1990b) Back pain and radiologic changes in the thoracolumbar spine of athletes. *Spine* **15** (2), 124–129.

Swärd, L., Hellström, M., Jacobsson, B., Nyman, R. & Peterson, L. (1991) Disc degeneration and associated abnormalities of the spine in elite gymnasts. A magnetic resonance imaging study. *Spine* **16** (4), 437–443.

Swärd, L., Hellström, M., Jacobsson, B. & Karlsson, L. (1993) Vertebral ring apophysis injury in athletes: Is the etiology different in the thoracic and lumbar spine? *American Journal of Sports Medicine* **21** (6), 841–845.

Tertti, M., Paajanen, H., Kujala, U.M. et al. (1990) Disc degeneration in young gymnasts. *American Journal of Sports Medicine* **18**, 206–208.

Theiss, P., Lohrer, H. & Keck, E. (1993) Knochendichtemessungen bei Kunstturnerinnen. In: *Biomechanics in Gymnastics* (eds G.-P. Brüggemann & H.J. Rühl), pp. 291–299. Strauss, Köln.

Troup, J.D.G. & Videman, T. (1989) Inactivity and the aetiopathogenesis of musculoskeletal disorders. *Clinical Biomechanics* **4**, 173–178.

Tsai, L. & Wredemark, T. (1993) Spinal posture, sagittal mobility, and subjective rating of back problems in former elite gymnasts. *Spine* **18**, 872–875.

Videman, T., Sarna, S., Battié, M.C. et al. (1995) The long-term effect of physical loading and exercise lifestyles on back-related symptoms, disability, and spinal pathology among men. *Spine* **20** (6), 699–709.

Videman, T., Battié, M.C., Gibbons, L.E. et al. (1997) Lifetime exercise and disk degeneration: an MRI study of monozygotic twins. *Medicine and Science in Sports and Exercise* **29**, 1350–1356.

Welten, D.C., Kemper, H.C.G., Post, G.B. et al. (1994) Weight-bearing activity during growth is a more important factor for peak bone mass than calcium intake. *Journal of Bone and Mineral Research* **9**, 1089–1096.

Whiting, W.C. & Zernicke, R.F. (1998) *Biomechanics of Musculoskeletal Injury.* Human Kinetics, Champaign, IL.

Woo, S.L.-Y., Newton, P.O., Gomez, M.A. & Akeson, W.H. (1984) Responses of medial collateral ligament to immobilization and remobilization. *Transactions of the Orthopaedic Research Society* **9**, 131.

Yamada, H. (1970) *Strength of Biological Material* (eds F. Evans & F. Gaynor). Williams & Wilkins, Baltimore.

Chapter 27

Impact Propagation and its Effects on the Human Body

A.S. VOLOSHIN

This chapter deals with a phenomenon that affects the human body during everyday physical activities, such as walking and jogging. This phenomenon, however, is one whose effect is not immediately felt by, or visible on, the body. It consists of shock waves that are generated during each contact of a part of the human body, such as the foot, with a rigid body, such as the ground. While one cannot see or directly feel them, these waves play important and seemingly contradictory roles in the process of bone growth and in the development of various joint degenerative diseases.

Introduction

Fundamental study of human motion began in prehistoric times. Drawings from the Palaeolithic period often depict various human activities and are a testimony to this fact (Andriacchi & Mikosz 1991). Attempts to describe and understand the driving force for motion were made as early as the 4th century BC by Aristotle (Steindler 1953), who observed the relationship between muscular contraction and associated joint motion. Systematic study of human locomotion based on the known physical laws, however, was not recorded until the late 17th century. Borelli (1680) was the first to approach the challenge of identifying and estimating the forces that arise during human locomotion via mathematical modelling. He generated the first models of bones and skeletal muscles integrated as one machine responsible for motion generation.

It is well known that bones provide a framework for the body by supporting the soft tissues and by providing points of attachment for the skeletal muscles. This framework, which integrates muscles, is an essential mechanism for the generation of motion—when muscles contract, they pull on bones and thus produce movement. This muscular pull, together with forces applied by other bones, constantly loads a bone, which in turn may change its properties in response to such external loading. It is the unique structural material of a bone that allows it to constantly change and self-repair. This ability to mutate is a remarkable ability, since it allows for adaptation to the environment. Wolff's law states that changes in the function of the bone are accompanied by an alteration in its structure; this process, however, occurs over a long period of time (Martin 1993). It is well documented that a bone decreases in its thickness and density as a direct response to a decrease in loading. For example, Dalen and Olsson (1974) found that runners with 25 years of experience had bones with mineral content 20% higher in appendicular sites (subject to greater amount of shock waves), but less than 10% higher in axial sites, in comparison with a control group. Additional findings that 54% of professional male and female dancers display a pronounced thickening of the cortex of the second metatarsal may also be explained by Wolff's law (Huwyler 1989). Such hypertrophy of the bone occurs in response to the stresses of dancing—specifically, dancing on half and three-quarter points, the most frequent foot positions in dance. It is also documented that in zero-gravity space flight there is significant bone demineralization (Anderson & Cohn 1985). These findings suggest that dynamic loading may be of great importance in maintaining the bone mass.

This chapter will introduce the notion of dynamic loading on the human musculoskeletal system and describe the means for its evaluation. It will elaborate on the possible destructive effects of this loading on the well-being of the human musculoskeletal system, and mention some means of protection. The possible effects of insufficient loading will be discussed as well, and some ways to deal with this problem will be proposed.

Dynamic loading on the human musculoskeletal system

Whether an athlete is running on the track, playing on grass or artificial turf, or performing a high or long jump, his foot eventually meets the surface. Each such event generates a shock, or impact, wave that propagates from the foot through the whole human musculoskeletal system, finally reaching the skull. The impact occurs for a relatively short time span of 10–40 ms, and its effect is barely evident in conventional force plate or pressure transducer recordings, where they appear as minor irregularities (Kim & Voloshin 1992). Nearly two decades ago Light (1979) suggested that the foot strike-initiated shock waves may play a direct physiological role. Since the propagation velocity of those waves through the human musculoskeletal system exceeds that of nerve conduction, they could play a role in feedback mechanisms to allow for rapid reaction to failure to make a proper foot ground contact.

While the above suggestion implies a positive role of the foot strike-generated shock waves in maintaining the well-being of the human musculoskeletal system, there have existed, for more than a quarter of a century, notions of a potentially negative role of the same waves. It was Radin *et al.* (1972) who noticed that while the incidence of osteoarthritis increases with age (Wolfe *et al.* 1968), it is also clearly activity related: pneumatic tool operators get arthritis of the elbows and shoulders, riders of heavy machinery with poor shock protection have increased incidence of arthritis of the hip, soccer players have severe arthritis of the feet, ankles and knees, etc. It was suggested that the repetitive

impulsive loading is a significant factor in the development of the osteoarthritis.

One of the important roles played by the joints of the human musculoskeletal system is that of shock absorber. The joints attenuate and dissipate the foot strike-initiated shock waves; thus, they serve a protective role for the joints located further along the path of shock-wave propagation towards the skull (Wosk & Voloshin 1981). A biomechanical study of the shock-absorbing capacity of cadaveric knees was carried out by first applying an impact load and measuring the shock wave transmitted over the intact knee joint. Next, the lateral and medial menisci were removed, which increased the transmitted peak force to 113% of the original impact. The transmitted peak force reached 121% of original after the meniscus and all the soft tissues had been removed. Finally, the articular cartilage and subchondral bone were removed and their absence resulted in the transmitted peak force increasing to 135% (Hoshino & Wallace 1987). These results show that the knee joint has a complex and substantial impact-absorbing property. They also reveal that the osteoarthritic joint is less capable of shock absorption than the normal knee with its soft tissue intact.

Much of the wear and tear on the human musculoskeletal system is not usually due to sudden, traumatic actions or serious ailments; rather, it is due to a cumulative effect of dynamic loading that is not commonly noticed. The average person takes over 6000 steps per day, making a cumulative 2.5 million steps per year. With each one of these steps sending a shock wave through the whole human musculoskeletal system, there may be sufficient damage done to the system for development of osteoarthritis or joint degeneration.

The stress fracture is a common injury seen by healthcare professionals caring for athletes (Reeder *et al.* 1996). This injury has been identified in numerous areas of the skeletal system and it has resulted from a variety of athletic activities. However, it is most commonly seen in the lower extremities, with running being the reported cause in most cases. Stress fractures result from repetitive, cyclic loading of bone, which overwhelms the reparative ability of the skeletal system. Mechanically speaking, both increases of the applied load and increases in the frequency of this load application may lead to stress fractures. It is the degree by which each of these increases, however, that truly correlates to the resulting effect; therefore an effective measurement technique is vital.

Measurement of the shock waves

As stated earlier, an impact between the foot and ground generates a shock wave that propagates through the whole human musculoskeletal system and reaches the forehead (Wosk & Voloshin 1981). Due to the significant difference in the stiffness of bones and soft tissues, it is reasonable to assume that the main carrier of these waves will be the bone. Thus, the only logical way to measure those waves is by the attachment of a wave sensor to the bone. However, such an approach has not found widespread application due to the obvious inconvenience and, more importantly, the possible danger to the well-being of the subject. An alternative approach, attaching the sensor *externally*, enables the evaluation of the effects of soft tissue on acquired data and avoids the above mentioned inconveniences and dangers (Saha & Lakes 1977; Ziegert & Lewis 1979; Voloshin *et al.* 1981).

A lightweight accelerometer can be attached at the tibial tuberosity, on the sacrum, forehead or any other location where there is a relatively thin layer of skin over the underlying bone. The uniaxial accelerometer should be aligned along the longitudinal axis of the tibia to provide axial components of tibial acceleration; the accelerometer on the sacrum should be orientated in the longitudinal direction, along the spine, etc. (Verbitsky *et al.* 1998). These accelerometers measure the frequency and intensity of shock waves propagated in the longitudinal directions of the tibia, spine and at the forehead. It was shown by Gerritsen *et al.* (1995) that during a heel strike the tibia makes an angle measuring between 91.7° and 94.6° to the horizontal, while the angle of the trunk (sacrum) to horizontal varies between 81.3 and 86.4°. Thus, the near-vertical component of acceleration is recorded (Fig. 27.1).

Each accelerometer is attached externally to the point of measurement by a metal holder tightly strapped to the skin by elastic strips (Fig. 27.1). Such

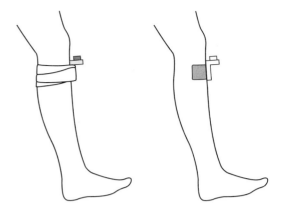

Fig. 27.1 Attachment of the accelerometer to the tibial tuberosity via holder and elastic strap.

an attachment is capable of faithfully measuring the amplitude of a shock wave (Kim *et al.* 1993). The subject then walks (Wosk & Voloshin 1981) or runs on a treadmill (Verbitsky *et al.* 1998) or over ground (Kim & Voloshin 1992) at a prescribed speed and the acceleration data are acquired. During the test, acceleration data may be recorded continuously or at specified time intervals. The accelerometers (Fig. 27.2) may be attached to the recording devices by wires (Helliwell *et al.* 1989). Alternatively, data may be stored in a memory device carried by the subject (Kim & Voloshin 1992), or the data may be transmitted via telemetry (Forner *et al.* 1995). A sample of the data recorded by an accelerometer attached at the tibial tuberosity and by the pressure transducer placed under the heel of the walking subject is shown in Fig. 27.3. The increase in the pressure (H) between the heel and ground corresponds to a peak in the acceleration curve (T), which indicates that the heel impact with the ground is the source of the shock wave.

The acceleration data are recorded and analysed usually after the completion of the experiment. Two main parameters may be extracted from each shock-wave pattern resulting from the heel strike measurement: the amplitude and the shape of the signal. The amplitude of the recorded acceleration provides information on the amount of energy transferred through the point of measurement. Increase in the amplitude means increase in the loading on

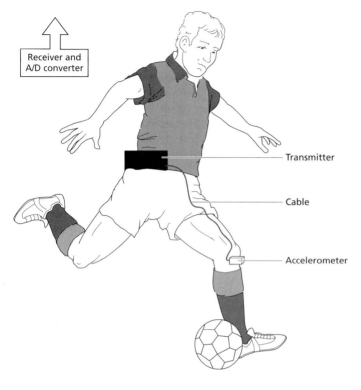

Fig. 27.2 Schematic of the acceleration data acquisition setup.

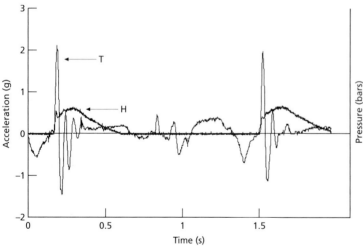

Fig. 27.3 Typical recording of the acceleration (T) and pressure (H) during walking.

the subsequent joints. Analysis of the signal's shape reveals information on the frequency content of the passing shock wave. While not much is known about the significance of various frequency components, there are some indications that higher frequencies are more damaging to the joint. Since the majority of human activities, such as running and walking, are periodic in nature, one can acquire a number of the heel strike-initiated shock waves, analyse each one of them and calculate the average acceleration amplitude. In walking, the acceleration measured at the tibial tuberosity was 1–5 g, while in

Table 27.1 Acceleration recorded at various locations in the human musculoskeletal system during walking.

Location	Acceleration (m · s⁻²)	
	Mean	Standard deviation
Tibial tuberosity	17.31	3.48
Medial femoral condyle	12.72	3.09
Forehead	5.67	1.82

running, values in the range 5–15 g were recorded, whereas jumping produced values of over 25 g (Loy & Voloshin 1991).

Analysis of the shock-wave amplitudes recorded by accelerometers attached at the tibial tuberosity, medial femoral condyle and forehead of the walking subjects reveals that the wave amplitude is decreased as it moves away from the point of foot-ground contact (Wosk & Voloshin 1981). Table 27.1 shows the data recorded from 39 healthy young subjects. These results support the idea that the repetitive loading during walking generates intermittent waves that are propagated through the human musculoskeletal system and are attenuated and dissipated by the body's natural shock absorbers (bones and soft tissues) on their way towards the skull.

Exercise and dynamic loading

The human musculoskeletal system is subjected to dynamic loading not only during running, walking and jumping, but also during other physical activities, such as swinging a racket and hitting a ball, as in tennis. Here, the hand is the extremity that absorbs most of the dynamic loading. An X-ray study of the upper extremities of 84 active professional tennis players revealed a significant increase in the diameter of the humerus in the playing hand in comparison to the non-hand (Jones *et al.* 1977). The results indicate a highly significant humeral hypertrophy as a consequence of the chronic stimulus of professional tennis playing. Thus, it is apparent that dramatic changes in bone geometry can occur in response to any exercise.

It has been shown in experiments on animals that the diameters of load-bearing bones are increased by increased activity (Woo *et al.* 1981). However, static and dynamic loading influence bone development at different rates. Some experiments demonstrate that dynamic loading has a stronger influence than static loading on bone remodelling (Hert *et al.* 1971a,b). Therefore, exercise and its associated dynamic loading may have effects undiscovered by static loading experiments. A discussion of the dual nature of these effects follows.

DESTRUCTIVE EFFECTS

Some authorities say 'Exercise is medicine'. While exercise usually promotes health and may indeed be instrumental in the treatment of some chronic diseases, under certain conditions it may lead to the development of osteoarthritis (OA), which is a disorder that confines itself to shock-wave affected joints. OA occurs when there is disruption of normal cartilage structure and homeostasis. OA results from a complex interaction of biochemical and biomechanical factors that occur concurrently and serve to perpetuate the degradative change characteristic of OA.

However, impairment, functional limitation, and disability related to OA can reach far beyond the perimeters of articular cartilage and subchondral bone. It has become increasingly obvious that the excess of dynamic loading on the human musculoskeletal system (due to exercise or everyday activities) may lead to the development of a variety of musculoskeletal disorders. Many health specialists have suggested that exercise carried out within the limits of normal joint motion and comfort does not predispose one to osteoarthritis. However, the lack of a scientific definition for 'normal joint motion and comfort' precludes the design of a safe and effective exercise programme, insofar as OA is concerned. Thus, several investigations have been initiated to study the dynamic loading effects on the human musculoskeletal system resulting from various exercises (running, walking, aerobics, etc.).

Athletes and an increasing number of middle-aged and older people who want to participate in athletics may question whether regular vigorous physical activity increases their risk of developing osteoarthritis. To answer this question the clinical syndrome of osteoarthritis must be distinguished from periarticular soft tissue pain associated with certain activity and from the development of osteophytes. Sports that subject joints to repetitive high levels of impact and torsional loading increase the risk of articular cartilage degeneration and the resulting clinical syndrome of osteoarthritis (Buckwalter & Lane 1997).

The mechanisms by which OA develops remain poorly understood; however, there is evidence that moderate use of normal joints does not increase the risk of developing OA. Contrary to popular belief, the degeneration of normal articular cartilage is not simply the result of ageing. It has been suggested that, regardless of age, high-impact and torsional loads may increase the risk of normal joint degeneration, and individuals who have an abnormal joint anatomy, joint instability, disturbances of joint or muscle innervation, or inadequate muscle strength or endurance probably will have a greater risk of degenerative joint disease (Buckwalter & Mankin 1998). Aside from the expected development of degenerative joint disease in the above-mentioned circumstances, simple overuse may lead to injuries.

Analysing ground reaction forces produced during commonly used high- and low-impact aerobic dance manoeuvres revealed that maximum vertical active peak and vertical impact peak forces were lower for the low-impact manoeuvres. The lower vertical loads produced in low-impact dancing may make this type of dance better for minimizing lower-extremity overuse injuries in aerobic dance (Michaud et al. 1993).

Another example of overuse injury is a stress fracture, which is caused by muscle forces together with bending and impact forces acting on the bone (Orava et al. 1995). A stress fracture is a series of tiny microscopic cracks in bone. They are commonly found in the lower extremities, but occur in many other bones of the body as well (i.e. hip and lower spine). The history of stress-fracture patients often reveals a considerable amount of running exercise. The symptoms are stress pain and aching at rest after training. Typical findings are local palpation pain, and sometimes tender resistance is felt. With early identification of the symptoms and diagnosis,

the acceptable treatment is simply a long training pause. The prevention of stress fractures has proved to be difficult; however, if running is substituted with some other kind of non-impact sport, the incidence of stress fractures is reduced. The exact causes of stress fractures are not yet known, but such fractures commonly result from one of the following: repetitive stress, change in the reaction force (i.e. when changing running from one surface to another), and increased bone load due to muscle fatigue or disregard of pain, etc.

Muscle and general fatigue seems to be of particular importance. Fatigued muscles are less capable of storing and dissipating energy and protecting bone against overloading by heel strike-initiated shock waves. When tired, muscles fail to carry their intended load and the skeletal system absorbs more of the shock, which may lead to stress fractures.

A recent study was aimed at analysing the effects of fatigue on the ability of the human musculoskeletal system to attenuate the heel strike-generated shock waves. Twenty-two healthy male subjects participated in this research. Each subject was instrumented with a lightweight accelerometer placed externally over the tibial tuberosity. Each subject ran on a treadmill for 30 min at a speed corresponding to the anaerobic threshold level. The acceleration data were acquired every five minutes, while the subjects were not aware of when the data were acquired to exclude possible gait modifications. The results showed that whenever general fatigue occurred, the amplitude of the acceleration signal steadily increased. Thus, one may conclude that the human musculoskeletal system becomes less capable of handling the heel strike-induced shock waves when affected by fatigue (Mizrahi et al. 1997).

Thus, it appears that participation in high-impact sports or in physical activities that involve similarly high-impact dynamic loading on and fatigue of the human musculoskeletal system, leads to the development of joint disorders such as osteoarthritis or bone stress fractures.

PROTECTION FROM OVERLOADING

The magnitude of a shock wave initiated at the heel strike is activity dependent, subject to the particu-

Table 27.2 Dynamic load on the human musculoskeletal system while running on various surfaces.

Surface type	Acceleration ($m \cdot s^{-2}$)	
	Mean	SD
Asphalt	134.1	30.6
Track	140.9	27.3
Grass	167.5	31.5

lar characteristics and mechanical properties of the footwear and the ground surface. To control the amplitude of this shock wave, without altering the activity, one must modify either the footwear or the surface. Several studies show that surfaces play a significant role in the dynamic loading experienced by a subject (Kim & Voloshin 1992; Stussi *et al.* 1997). The last study was focused on the three common running surfaces: grass, asphalt and polyurethane track. Approximately 40–60 heel strikes were recorded from nine young subjects running on those surfaces. The results (Table 27.2) show that running on grass resulted in significantly higher values of acceleration than that recorded on the asphalt or track. Since grass surface is intrinsically more uneven than the other two surfaces, one may hypothesize that this unevenness may be a reason for overall increase in dynamic loading. Running on a relatively smooth, consistent surface results in the impacts being very similar to one another. However, the grass surface changes its profile more drastically and the runner cannot see those changes since they are obscured by grass. This uncertainty may be a reason for increased impacts experienced while running on a grass surface. In the past, the development of surface materials has hardly been viewed from this aspect, but it may become increasingly important in the future.

Since prehistoric times footwear has been used to protect the feet from the ground surfaces and from bad weather. Humans have also modified the protective footwear to add decorative effects, such as high heels for women's shoes. Women have particularly favoured the addition of the heel because the anatomical effects of such a heel elevation increase femininity.

A study of 11 athletes during submaximal heel-strike running on a treadmill in identical shoes with and without a firm heel counter demonstrated the effect of a firm heel counter in the shoe. The heel counter caused a significant decrease of 2.4% in V_{O_2}, a reduction in the amplitude of the heel strike-initiated shock waves, and a decrease in the activity of the triceps surae and quadriceps muscles at heel strike. These changes reflect the kinematic adaptations the body undergoes in response to increased or decreased load and provide functional evidence for the loading factor in the pathophysiology of overuse injuries (Jorgensen 1990).

The modern running shoe has a number of features aimed to reduce the possibility of injury and increase performance. A lighter shoe generally means a lower expenditure of energy by the runner. On the other hand, the need to provide adequate shock absorption, especially at higher speeds, demands thicker and heavier soles. Interestingly enough, a light shoe that has improper cushioning will raise the energy requirement. Theoretically, one could design a shoe that would have a sole thick enough to absorb the energy and return nothing to the foot. The result would be low running efficiency. At the other end of spectrum, one could design the perfectly elastic sole that would return 100% of the impact energy. However, if the rate of return is not comparable with the motion of the foot, little of the energy will be utilized for propulsion. The materials used in modern footwear fall somewhere in the middle of the range. More research is needed to determine the winning combination of optimal rate of energy return and lightness.

Typical sports shoes incorporate various means of shock absorption: some utilize various plastics, while others structurally combine materials (i.e. the air-sole). A number of researchers have analysed and quantified the effect of various shock-absorbing techniques. Two main approaches were used: analysis of the inherent attenuational capacity of the shoe sole material and measurements of the shock waves invading the human musculoskeletal system while using the particular footwear. Tests conducted on materials show poor correlation with the *in vivo* measurements of the shock-absorbing properties of the shoe. Material testing does not account for interference between the material of the insole and the living tissue, and this was the main reason for poor correlation. Such interference is very hard, or even impossible to model in material testing.

The shoe can be thought of as a powerful tool for controlling human movement. A well-designed shoe can assist in reducing the number of lower limb injuries arising from sport and training activities. However, one has to be very cautious when looking for a shoe with 'superior shock-absorbing properties'. Recent studies by Robbins and Waked (1997) reveal a surprising and dramatic correlation between the advertising of a shoe's shock-absorbing potential and its actual performance. It turns out that exaggerated advertising claims create a false sense of security while using such athletic shoes. Fifteen healthy males confronted four surfaces: a bare force-moment platform, and three in which this platform was covered by identical shoe sole material made to appear different and advertised differently. Of the three advertising messages, one suggested superior impact absorption and protection (deceptive message), one poor impact absorption and high injury risk (warning message), and the last one indicated unknown impact absorption and suggested safety (neutral message). The measured impact varied as a function of the advertising message ($P < 0.001$). The deceptive message equalled the neutral message in eliciting a higher impact than the warning message and the bare platform. Subjects actually altered their behaviour in response to the advertised shock absorption, which led to increased impact. This sort of advertising-induced behaviour may result in injury.

More than a decade ago, the effect of various shoe insoles on injury prevention was analysed during basic military training (Smith et al. 1985). The study included three groups of randomly selected subjects during eight-week recruit training. Group A was designated as the control group, while groups B and C were issued with different types of shoe insoles. Control group A had a higher percentage (62.5%) of injuries than group B (26%) or group C (14.2%). Those results confirm the notion that properly made footwear may attenuate the heel strike-initiated shock waves and reduce the degree of injures.

Choice of footwear and surfaces, however, are not solely responsible for influencing the amount of dynamic loading experienced by the human musculoskeletal system: the choice of exercise itself alters the degree of loading. A recent study of the dynamic loading on the human musculoskeletal system during in-line skating illustrates this fact (Mahar et al. 1997). The study showed that an average acceleration experienced by the subjects while in-line skating was 2 g, whereas subjects who ran experienced 4.2 g of acceleration. Similar differences were found between high- and low-impact aerobics exercises (Michaud et al. 1993).

Effects of underloading

As illustrated above, much effort in the design of surfaces and footwear is aimed at decreasing the dynamic loading on the human musculoskeletal system. However, for people who do not actively participate in physical activities, just the opposite goal should be the aim of design, namely, increasing dynamic loading. A significant body of evidence supports the notion that a certain amount of loading is necessary to improve the strength and structure of biological materials (Stussi et al. 1997). Loading has many attributes; it is not defined only by its amplitude but also by its dynamic characteristics, such as frequency and rate of repetition. Bone, like all living tissues, is constantly growing and self-remodelling. In some tissues, such as cartilage and tendon, deformation due to external load may directly stimulate cells to produce a mechanically beneficial response. Bone, however, has a modulus that is relatively high compared with these tissues, thus the functional strains are relatively small, of the order of 0.003–0.004. Such strains seemingly cannot affect the cells responsible for remodelling, but remodelling has been shown to take place. Thus, it is not enough to measure only the overall strain acting on the bone; the strain distribution and strain rate also need to be considered (Lanyon 1987). With this consideration, Lanyon suggested a concept of a 'minimum effective strain-related stimulus'. His findings show that remodelling behaviour of bone cells may be substantially influenced by small variations from the normal pattern of dynamic strain within the bone.

Osteoporosis, characterized by bone loss leading to fractures, represents a significant health concern. Women are at particular risk of osteoporosis due to an accelerated bone loss of 2.0–6.5% per year within the first 5–8 years after menopause. The aetiology of osteoporosis includes ageing, hormones, nutrition, genetics, and mechanical loading via exercise. Of these factors, only increased mechanical loading has been shown to stimulate bone formation. Conversely, it has been shown that significant bone loss occurs because of prolonged space flight, immobilization or bed-rest. Russian cosmonauts experienced losses in bone mineral density (BMD) of 0–10% at the lumbar spine, 1.3–11.4% at the femoral neck and 0.4–9.5% at the tibia after 4.5–6.0 months aboard an orbital space station (Oganov et al. 1992). Significant decreases in pelvis, femoral neck, trochanter and calcaneus BMD after 131–312 days in space have also been reported. Recently, Nishimura et al. (1994) observed a 4.6% decrease in lumbar spine BMD and 3.6% decrease in metacarpal BMD in nine subjects after 20 days of bed-rest.

A cross-sectional study by Alfredson et al. (1997) aimed to investigate the effect of dynamic loading on bone mass in young females. The study compared 23 females, participating in aerobic workout for about 3 h per week with identically matched (age, weight and height) non-active females. Bone mineral density (BMD) was measured at several key locations in both groups. The aerobic workout group had significantly higher BMD ($P < 0.05$) in the total body (3.7%), lumbar spine (7.8%), femoral neck (11.6%), Ward's triangle (11.7%), trochanter femoris (9.6%), proximal tibia (6.8%) and tibia diaphysis (5.9%) compared to the non-active controls. It appears that aerobic exercise containing high- and low-impact movements for the lower body is associated with a higher bone mass in clinically important sites like the lumbar spine and hip. However, the muscle-strengthening exercises such as push-ups and soft-glove boxing were not associated with a higher bone mass. It appears that there is a beneficial skeletal adaptation to the loads of aerobic activity.

A similar conclusion resulted from a study to examine the role of athletic activity on BMD accretion, and the longitudinal changes in regional and whole body BMD in collegiate women gymnasts and competitive athletes whose skeletons were exposed to differential loading patterns. Runners and swimmers were monitored for a period of 8 months (Taaffe et al. 1997).

The above studies show that exercise incorporating a significant amount of impacts may increase the BMD in young women. Most interestingly, the study by Dook et al. (1997) in which BMD in a number of mature female athletes was analysed demonstrated that the group engaging in a high-impact sport (volleyball and basketball) showed a significantly higher BMD than the groups engaged in non-impact sports (swimming) and no sports at all. These results suggest that females who participate regularly in high-impact physical activity during the premenopausal years tend to have higher BMD than non-athletic controls.

It is thus apparent that the age-related bone loss from lumbar vertebrae in normal women can be successfully inhibited or reversed by bodily exercise (Krolner et al. 1983). However, any reduction of dynamic loading due to bed-rest (Krolner & Toff 1983), various immobilizations, space flight (Tilton et al. 1980) or stress shielding due to implants was shown to cause bone loss.

One of the conclusions from the Surgeon General's report on Physical Activity and Health 1996 (U.S. Department of Health and Human Services) was that it is unclear whether resistance training can reduce the rate of bone loss in postmenopausal women in the absence of oestrogen replacement therapy. Such a conclusion supports the idea that resistance training may only affect the development of the muscular mass, while it may have little, if any, effect on bone loss. Animal studies have proved that repeated impulsive loading can lead to an increase of subchondral bone density. Both animal and human exercise trials have concluded that even the very old can derive skeletal benefit from increased levels of physical activity. A number of researchers have studied the effects of rate of strain, load magnitude and load frequency on the adaptive response of bone (Lanyon 1987; Rubin et al. 1993; Gross & Rubin 1995; Riggs et al. 1998). The data suggest that all those variables interact with one another. For example, it was initially thought that increasing strain magnitudes was the optimal method of stimulating osteogenesis, until it was found that very low strains are osteogenic if applied at high rates. Strain gradients were also found to be an important factor in the bone growth process.

Conclusions

The human musculoskeletal system is in a constant process of bone remodelling. Studies show that a bone is a highly complex system that is subjected to a large number of interrelated biological, biophysical and biochemical processes. The very complex nature of the human musculoskeletal system with its multiplicity of variables means that exact measurements of the forces, accelerations and other parameters which may affect the system's behaviour are generally difficult, if not impossible, to make. Thus, because of this uncertainty, firm conclusions based on the available results are not easy to make.

While dynamic loading of the human musculoskeletal system is clearly beneficial due to its contribution to the increase in BMD, at the same time it may lead to the development of osteoarthritis. Thus, it is of great importance to develop a scientifically sound methodology to evaluate the safe and useful upper and lower boundaries of dynamic loading.

The upper loading boundary will define the limit of dynamic excitation that the human musculoskeletal system can maintain for a long time without development of osteoarthritis. The lower boundary, on the other hand, will prescribe the minimum amount of dynamic excitation needed by bone to maintain a healthy level of mineral content. These boundaries will ensure that exercise routines provide sufficient stimulus to maintain BMD at an appropriate level while avoiding the development of osteoarthritis. Knowledge of these boundaries will allow for the development of proper exercise routines. Moreover, this knowledge may help to solve the problems associated with long space flights. Current exercise routines do not provide efficient means for maintaining BMD at the proper level during prolonged exposure to zero-gravity environments, such as exist at an orbiting space station. These exercises should be augmented by adding a carefully researched and verified set of dynamic loading sequences to simulate the loading experienced by humans on Earth during everyday physiological activities. Similarly, bed-ridden patients who suffer from significant loss of BMD may be subjected to an externally applied loading sequence. One can develop an apparatus capable of providing such stimulation at a prescribed amplitude and frequency for a given time period. Such a development will be of great importance to millions of patients currently suffering from bone loss resulting from their immobilization.

Summaries, simple as this one, clearly neglect the complexity of the biomechanical and biochemical processes involved in bone remodelling, but, nonetheless, it may provide a rational starting point for future research initiatives.

References

Alfredson, H., Nordstrom, P. & Lorentzon, R. (1997) Aerobic workout and bone mass in females. *Scandinavian Journal of Medicine and Science in Sports* 7 (6), 336–341.

Anderson, S.A. & Cohn, S.H. (1985) Bone demineralization during space flight. *Physiologist* 28 (4), 212–217.

Andriacchi, T.P. & Mikosz, R.P. (1991) Musculoskeletal dynamics, locomotion and clinical applications. In: *Basic Orthopaedic Biomechanics* (eds V.C. Mow & W.C. Hayes), pp. 51–92. Raven Press, New York.

Borelli, A. (1680) *De motu animalum*. Angeli Bernabo, Rome.

Buckwalter, J.A. & Lane, N.E. (1997) Athletics and osteoarthritis. *American Journal of Sports Medicine* 25 (6), 873–881.

Buckwalter, J.A. & Mankin, H.J. (1998) Articular cartilage: degeneration and osteoarthritis, repair, regeneration, and transplantation. *Instructional Course Lectures* 47, 487–504.

Dalen, N. & Olsson, K.E. (1974) Bone mineral content and physical activity. *Acta Orthopaedica Scandinavica* 45 (2), 170–174.

Dook, J.E., James, C., Henderson, N.K. & Price, R.I. (1997) Exercise and bone mineral density in mature female athletes. *Medicine and Science in Sports and Exercise* 29 (3), 291–296.

Forner, A., Garcia, A.C., Alcantara, E., Ramiro, J., Hoyos, J.V. & Vera, P. (1995) Properties of shoe insert materials related to shock wave transmission during gait. *Foot and Ankle International* 16 (12), 778–786.

Gerritsen, K.G.M., Bogert, A.J. & Nigg, B.M. (1995) Direct dynamics simulation of the impact phase in heel–toe running. *Journal of Biomechanics* 28 (6), 661–668.

Gross, T.S. & Rubin, C.T. (1995) Uniformity of resorptive bone loss induced by disuse. *Journal of Orthopaedic Research* 13 (5), 708–714.

Helliwell, P.S., Smeathers, J.E. & Wright, V. (1989) Shock absorption by the spinal column in normals and in ankylosing spondylitis. *Proceedings of the Institute of Mechanical Engineers* 203 (4), 187–190.

Hert, J., Selenska, A. & Liskova, M. (1971a) Reaction of bone to mechanical stimuli (Part V): Effect of intermittent stress on the rabbit tibia after resection of the peripheral nerves. *Folia Morphologica* **19**, 378–387.

Hert, J., Liskova, M. & Landa, J. (1971b) Reaction of bone to mechanical stimuli (Part I): Continuous and intermittent loading of tibia in rabbit. *Folia Morphologica* **19**, 290–300.

Hoshino, A. & Wallace, W.A. (1987) Impact-absorbing properties of the human knee. *Journal of Bone and Joint Surgery* **69** (5), 807–811.

Huwyler, J. (1989) Veranderungen am Skelett des Mittelfusses durch professionelles klassisches Tanzen. [Changes in the skeleton of the middle foot caused by professional classical dancing.] *Sportverletz Sportschaden* **3** (1), 14–20.

Jones, H.H., Priest, J.D., Hayes, W.C., Tichenor, C.C. & Nagel, D.A. (1977) Humeral hypertrophy in response to exercise. *Journal of Bone and Joint Surgery* **59A**, 204–208.

Jorgensen, U. (1990) Body load in heel-strike running: the effect of a firm heel counter. *American Journal of Sports Medicine* **18** (2), 177–181.

Kim, W. & Voloshin, A.S. (1992) Dynamic loading during running on various surfaces. *Human Movement Science* **11** (6), 675–689.

Kim, W., Voloshin, A.S., Johnson, S.H. & Simkin, A. (1993) Measurement of the impulsive bone motion by skin-mounted accelerometers. *Journal of Biomechanical Engineering* **5**, 47–52.

Krolner, B. & Toff, B. (1983) Vertebral bone loss: an unheeded side effect of therapeutic bed rest. *Clinical Science* **64**, 537–540.

Krolner, B., Toff, B., Nielsen, S.P. & Tondevold, E. (1983) Physical exercise as prophylaxis against involutional vertebral bone loss: a controlled trial. *Clinical Science* **64**, 541–546.

Lanyon, L.E. (1987) Functional strain in bone tissue as an objective, and controlling stimulus for adaptive bone remodelling. *Journal of Biomechanics* **20**, 1083–1093.

Light, L.H. (1979) Potential implications of heel strike transients. *Journal of Physiology* **292**, 31–32.

Loy, D.J. & Voloshin, A.S. (1991) Biomechanics of stair walking and jumping. *Journal of Sport Sciences* **9**, 137–149.

Mahar, A.T., Derrick, T.R., Hamill, J. & Caldwell, G.E. (1997) Impact shock and attenuation during in-line skating.

Medicine and Science in Sports and Exercise **29** (8), 1069–1075.

Martin, B. (1993) Aging and strength of bone as a structural material. *Calcified Tissue International* **53** (Suppl. 1), S34–S40.

Michaud, T.J., Rodriguez-Zayas, J., Armstrong, C. & Hartnig, M. (1993) Ground reaction forces in high impact and low impact aerobic dance. *Journal of Sports Medicine and Physical Fitness* **33** (4), 359–366.

Mizrahi, J., Voloshin, A.S., Russek, D., Verbitsky, O. & Isakov, E. (1997) The influence of fatigue on EMG and impact acceleration in running. *Basic and Applied Myology* **7** (2), 119–126.

Nishimura, Y., Fukuoka, H., Kiriyama, M. *et al.* (1994) Bone turnover and calcium metabolism during 20 days bed rest in young healthy males and females. *Acta Physiologica Scandinavica* (Suppl.) **616**, 27–35.

Oganov, V.S., Grigor'ev, A.I., Voronin, L.I. *et al.* (1992) Mineral'naia plotnost' kostno-i tkani u kosmonavtov posle poletov dlitel'nost'iu 4,5–6 mesiatsev na orbital'no-i stantsii 'Mir'. [Bone mineral density in cosmonauts after flights lasting 4.5–6 months on the Mir orbital station.] *Aviakosm Ekolog Medicine* **26** (5–6), 20–24.

Orava, S., Hulkko, A., Koskinen, S. & Taimela, S. (1995) Stressfrakturen bei Sportlern und Militarrekruten. Eine Ubersicht. [Stress fractures in athletes and military recruits. An overview.] *Orthopade* **24** (5), 457–466.

Radin, E.R., Paul, I.L. & Rose, R.M. (1972) Pathogenesis of primary osteoarthritis. *Lancet* **1**, 1395–1396.

Reeder, M.T., Dick, B.H., Atkins, J.K., Pribis, A.B. & Martinez, J.M. (1996) Stress fractures. Current concepts of diagnosis and treatment. *Sports Medicine* **22** (3), 198–212.

Riggs, B.L., O'Fallon, W.M., Muhs, J., O'Connor, M.K., Kumar, R. & Melton, L.J. III (1998) Long-term effects of calcium supplementation on serum parathyroid hormone level, bone turnover, and bone loss in elderly women. *Journal of Bone Mineral Research* **13** (2), 168–174.

Robbins, S. & Waked, E. (1997) Hazard of deceptive advertising of athletic footwear. *British Journal of Sports Medicine* **31** (4), 299–303.

Rubin, C.T., Donahue, H.J., Rubin, J.E. & McLeod, K.J. (1993) Optimization of electric field parameters for the control of bone remodeling: exploitation of an indigenous mechanism for

the preven-tion of osteopenia. *Journal of Bone Mineral Research* (Suppl. 2), S573–S581.

Saha, S. & Lakes, R.S. (1977) The effect of soft tissue on wave propagation and vibration tests for determining the *in-vivo* properties of bone. *Journal of Biomechanics* **10**, 393–401.

Smith, W., Walter, J. & Bailey, M. (1985) Effects of insoles in coast guard basic training footwear. *Journal of the American Podiatric Medical Association* **75** (12), 644–647.

Steindler, A. (1953) A historical review of the studies and investigations made in relation to human gait. *Journal of Bone and Joint Surgery* **35A**, 540–542.

Stussi, E., Denoth, J., Muller, R. & Stacoff, A. (1997) Sportmedizin und Rehabilitation. Boden und Schuhe. [Sports medicine and rehabilitation. Surface and footwear.] *Orthopade* **26** (11), 993–998.

Taaffe, D.R., Robinson, T.L., Snow, C.M. & Marcus, R. (1997) High-impact exercise promotes bone gain in well-trained female athletes. *Journal of Bone Mineral Research* **12** (2), 255–260.

Tilton, F.E., Degionanni, T.T.C. & Schneider, V.S. (1980) Long-term follow-up of skylab bone demineralization. *Aviation, Space and Environmental Medicine* **51**, 1209–1213.

Verbitsky, O., Mizrahi, J., Voloshin, A., Triger, J. & Isakov, E. (1998) Shock transmission and fatigue in human running. *Journal of Applied Biomechanics* **14** (3), 300–311.

Voloshin, A.S., Wosk, J. & Brull, M. (1981) Force wave transmission through the human locomotor system. *Journal of Biomedical Engineering* **103**, 48–50.

Wolfe, A.M., Kellgren, J.H. & Masi, A.T. (1968) The epidemiology of rheumatoid arthritis: a review. II. Incidence and diagnostic criteria. *Bulletin of Rheumatic Disease* **19** (3), 524–529.

Woo, S.L.Y., Kuei, S.C., Amiel, D., Gomez, M.A., Hayes, W.C. & Akeson, W.H. (1981) The effect of prolonged physical training on the properties of long bone – a study of Wolff's law. *Journal of Bone and Joint Surgery* **63A**, 780–787.

Wosk, J. & Voloshin, A.S. (1981) Wave attenuation in skeletons of young healthy persons. *Journal of Biomechanics* **4** (4), 261–268.

Ziegert, J.C. & Lewis, J.L. (1979) The effect of soft tissue on measurements of vibrational bone motion by skin-mounted accelerometers. *Transactions of the ASME, Journal of Biomechanical Engineering* **101**, 218–220.

Chapter 28

Neuromechanics of the Initial Phase of Eccentric Contraction-Induced Muscle Injury

M.D. GRABINER

Introduction

Eccentric contraction is pervasive in the library of human motor performance. One role played by eccentric contraction is protecting articular and skeletal structures through the attenuation of forces transmitted to and through the body during even benign daily activities. For example, eccentric contraction of the knee extensors during the initial stance phase of gait is a regulated lengthening by which these muscles absorb energy and attenuate the impulse of heel contact. Similar conditions, although with much larger magnitudes, occur during running. Anyone who has unexpectedly stepped off a curb has experienced the type of non-attenuated impulse that is typically dissipated by eccentrically contracting muscle. Similarly, the following scenario also may be all too familiar. Following a period during which one has not participated in regular exercise, an initial exercise session can often be associated with muscle soreness. Symptoms of muscle soreness can appear quickly after the exercise and/or the symptoms may not emerge until days after the exercise. The intensity of the symptoms can range from mild to functionally disabling, and the time course during which the symptoms diminish can last one or more weeks. Although muscle damage and subsequent muscle soreness can be the result of both concentric and eccentric contractions (Gibala et al. 1995), eccentric contractions are generally associated with significantly larger levels of damage and soreness.

From a mechanical standpoint, eccentric contractions of *untrained* muscle are more likely to cause muscle injury than isometric or concentric contractions (Faulkner et al. 1993). The extent of the damage is a function of multiple variables, including the intensity and duration of the exercise and the training status of the muscle. There is a continuum of functional outcomes associated with the injury and a well-defined time course of the processes associated with healing that may or may not be accelerated by various interventions. Systematic investigation of eccentric contraction-related muscle injury may be traced to the beginning of the 20th century (Hough 1902), and the literature currently offers a number of excellent reviews on the topic (Fridén 1984; Stauber 1989; Armstrong et al. 1991; Faulkner et al. 1993; MacIntyre et al. 1995). The integration of biomechanics with the areas of cellular and molecular biology, and cellular and molecular mechanics has resulted in the confirmation of many previously hypothesized mechanisms and sites associated with eccentric contraction-related muscle injury and, furthermore, has led to many new hypotheses. The purpose of this brief chapter is to present a research update that focuses primarily on some of the findings that have emerged during the 1990s. In particular, the chapter addresses issues related to mechanisms underlying muscle injury caused by eccentric contractions and the structural sites of the injury.

Evidence of eccentric contraction-related muscle injury

Injury caused by eccentric contraction can be observed to occur at the molecular, cellular and tissue levels and is associated with distinct functional outcomes. Some forms of direct evidence of injury, marked by ultrastructural changes, are acquired using histological methods or using electron or light microscopy. Indirect evidence of injury is marked by the presence of various enzymes (particularly plasma creatine kinase), changes in calcium concentrations, muscle soreness/pain, swelling and force and power deficits. The time course of changes in these markers supports the contention of multiple phases associated with eccentric contraction-related muscle injury. The initial phase of injury can be related to the damage induced to the muscle by the exercise. The second stage of injury, associated with the inflammatory responses to the initial injury, is followed by the regeneration stage (see Stauber 1990; MacIntyre *et al*. 1995).

Direct evidence

A key to eccentric contraction-related injury is thought to be the cytoskeleton of the skeletal muscle fibres. The cytoskeleton of eukaryotic cells plays a number of roles. One role is to provide a scaffold for the cell and its contents. By providing this scaffold, the cytoskeleton plays a role in organizing the contents of the cell. Cellular components are not suspended in the sarcoplasm but rather are maintained in a spatial organization that may have cell specificity. A third role of the cytoskeleton in eukaryotic cells is to facilitate movement.

The cytoskeleton is a dynamic organelle that is capable of large-scale and rather rapid reorganization. The eukaryotic cytoskeleton comprises three elements: microfilaments, intermediate filaments and microtubules. The designation, in part, is a function of the size of the elements. Microtubules are hollow cylinders having an outer wall diameter of about 250 Å. Microfilaments have a diameter of about 60 Å and are composed of the protein actin. Intermediate filaments have a diameter of approximately 100 Å. There are five classes of intermediate filaments. Keratin-containing intermediate filaments are associated with epithelial cells. Glial filaments are associated with glial cells such as astrocytes, oligodendrocytes, microglia and ependyma. Neurofilaments are found in nerve cell axons. Of the five classes of intermediate filaments, the desmin-containing filaments and vimentin-containing filaments have relevance to skeletal muscle.

Two sets of filaments compose the cytoskeleton of muscle fibres. They are referred to as the exosarcomeric and the endosarcomeric cytoskeleton. The *exosarcomeric cytoskeleton* is composed of desmin, vimentin and synemin. These elements, which are peripheral to the muscle fibre, are considered responsible for maintaining the longitudinal register of sarcomeres. The *endosarcomeric cytoskeleton*, found within the sarcomere and co-localized with actin and myosin, is made up of titin and nebulin. The endosarcomeric cytoskeleton is responsible, in part, for maintaining the register of the actin and myosin filaments (see reviews by Waterman-Storer 1991; Patel & Lieber 1997). Together, the endosarcomeric and exosarcomeric cytoskeletons provide the mechanical framework through which contractile force may be transmitted in directions beyond that conventionally considered, i.e. longitudinally towards the myotendinous junction (Patel & Lieber 1997). In particular, radially directed contraction force can be transmitted to the endomysium and subsequently towards the myotendinous junction. This is a particularly exciting line of inquiry and one that has potential application to questions in areas such as ageing, exercise and space biology. Human ageing and exposure to microgravity both result in losses in muscle strength exceeding that which would be predicted by the loss of muscle mass. While altered neuromuscular control accounts for some of the difference, an additional hypothesis that may ultimately be tested is that the disproportionate losses of strength and mass reflect some type of cytoskeletal reorganization that diminishes the ability of skeletal muscle to transmit contraction force radially. Figure 28.1 illustrates the location of titin, nebulin and desmin with regard to sarcomere architecture as well as a hypothesized representation of costamere structure.

Following eccentric contraction protocols, the disruption of the cytoskeleton is characterized most frequently by the loss of the between-sarcomere Z-disc register (Fridén *et al*. 1981). This physical evidence, called Z-disc streaming, suggests that the connection between Z-discs has been disrupted (Fig. 28.2). The physical link between Z-discs is

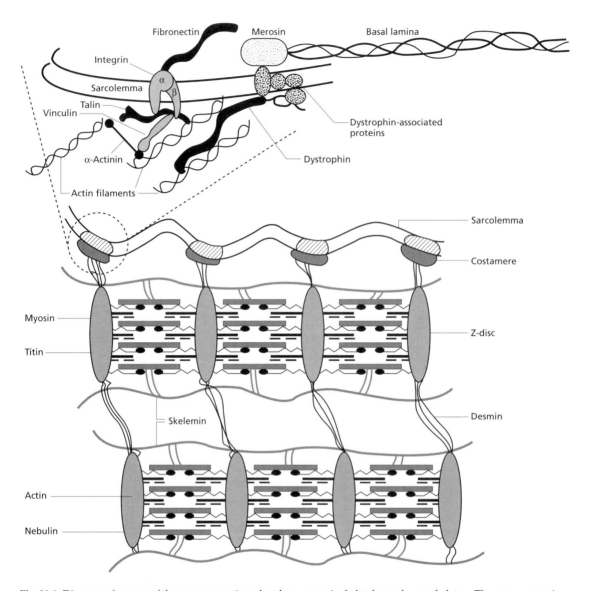

Fig. 28.1 Diagram of aspects of the exosarcomeric and endosarcomeric skeletal muscle cytoskeleton. The exosarcomeric elements underpin the ability of muscle to transmit contraction force radially from sarcomere to sarcomere and from the muscle fibre, through the costamere to extracellular tissues. (From Patel & Lieber 1997.)

provided by the intermediate filament desmin. The effect of eccentric exercise on desmin was demonstrated by Lieber *et al.* (1994). In this experiment, the tibialis anterior and extensor digitorum longus muscles of rabbits were subjected to 900 repetitions of maximum eccentric contraction over a period of 30 min. There was a substantial loss of desmin stain-

ing in both muscles although the loss of desmin staining was larger in the extensor digitorum longus than in the tibialis anterior. A significant relationship was discovered between muscle-specific loss of desmin staining and loss of tetanic tension, which suggested a causal relationship. Lieber *et al.* (1996) used a protocol in which the tibialis anterior and

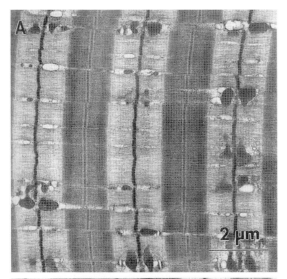

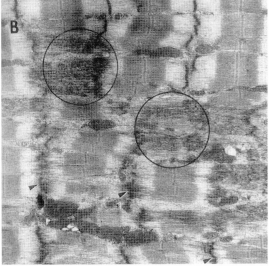

Fig. 28.2 Electron micrographs of a longitudinal section of rabbit tibialis anterior. The top panel illustrates a normal striation pattern. The bottom panel, taken from an animal that had been subjected to an eccentric exercise protocol, illustrates locations at which Z-disc streaming and smearing are evident (arrows) and areas (circles) in which the Z-discs have extended into the A-band. (From Lieber *et al.* 1991.)

extensor digitorum longus muscles of rabbits were subjected to repetitions of maximum eccentric contraction over a period of 5, 15 or 30 min. The extensor digitorum longus demonstrated a significant loss of

desmin staining after only 5 min of eccentric contractions. The tibialis anterior demonstrated significant loss of desmin staining after 15 min. Although the mechanism of the loss of desmin staining has not yet been described, these two studies underscore both the importance of the cytoskeletal protein desmin in the sequela of this type of muscle injury, and the rapidity with which this type of muscle injury can occur.

Indirect evidence

The loss of intramuscular proteins secondary to skeletal muscle damage can be detected in blood. The presence of these proteins in blood may be delayed up to 72 h after exercise and may not reach a peak until seven days after exercise (Clarkson & Newham 1995). Creatine kinase, the catalyst for the reaction in which creatine phosphate transfers its phosphoryl group to ATP, is the most commonly studied of these proteins (Clarkson *et al.* 1992).

Although creatine kinase may be the most often reported, elevated serum myoglobin (the oxygen carrier in skeletal muscle), lactate dehydrogenase (catalyses the reduction of pyruvate by the reduced form of nicotinamide adenine dinucleotide (NADH) to form lactate), aspartate aminotranferase and alanine aminotransferase (both of which are involved in amino acid degradation by transfer of amino groups from aspartate and alanine, respectively), and myosin heavy chain fragments are also evident after eccentric exercise. It is not clear as to why the presence of these substances in the blood is delayed. Nevertheless, there is interest in establishing a relationship between the increase in serum levels of these substances and the extent of muscle damage. A general but not highly specific relationship between serum creatine kinase levels and some indirect measures of muscle damage was reported by Clarkson *et al.* (1992). Notably, Sorichter *et al.* (1997) reported on the time course of plasma levels of skeletal muscle troponin I following eccentric exercises. Troponin I, a regulatory protein present only in skeletal muscle, was demonstrated to be an initial marker of muscle injury and, contrary to other plasma markers, displayed high specificity.

What is the cause of eccentric contraction-related muscle injury?

Broadly, the initiation of injury to muscle due to eccentric contraction has been related to the larger contractile forces that may be achieved during concentric contraction. McCulley and Faulkner (1985) subjected mouse extensor digitorum longus muscle to varying levels of peak eccentric contraction force and found a correlation of –0.70 between the peak force of the first eccentric contraction of the protocol and the maximum isometric force (an indirect measure of muscle injury) measured three days after the protocol. Further, a correlation of –0.79 was found between the maximum isometric force and the extent to which the muscle was injured (represented as the number of injured muscle fibres in the cross-section through the muscle belly) measured three days after the protocol. Warren *et al.* (1991) also manipulated the peak force during a protocol of five eccentric contractions using rat soleus muscle. Their criterion of muscle injury included peak isometric twitch, tetanic tension and rate of creatine kinase release. Muscles that were subjected to peak eccentric forces of less than 125% of tetanic tension demonstrated minimal indications of muscle injury. In contrast, muscles that had been subjected to peak eccentric forces of 150% of tetanic tension demonstrated reductions of peak isometric twitch and tetanic tension of 26% and 14%, respectively. These changes did not return to preprotocol values after 15 min. These muscles also demonstrated an increased rate of creatine kinase release.

Lieber *et al.* (1991) subjected rabbit tibialis anterior muscles to a protocol of cyclical isometric loading, passive stretch, or eccentric loading. Subsequent to 30 min of loading, the passive, isometric and eccentric protocols reduced maximum tetanic tension by 13, 31 and 69%, respectively. The induced muscle injury, marked by the change in contractile properties such as maximum tetanic tension, was observed to occur during the first minutes of the protocol.

Lieber and Fridén (1993) offered evidence that challenges the contention that eccentric contraction-related muscle injury is related to the contraction force. Rabbit tibialis anterior muscles were strained 25% at 125% of optimal fibre length per second.

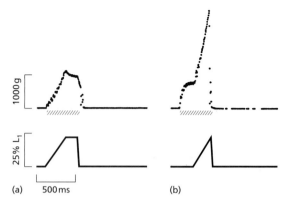

Fig. 28.3 Using a novel protocol, Lieber and Fridén manipulated the peak eccentric contraction force but maintained identical muscle strain and strain rates. The trace in the top panel represents muscle force and the shaded bar along the time axis represents the time during which the muscle was electrically stimulated. The trace in the bottom panel represents the stretch applied to the stimulated muscle. In panel (a) the stretch is applied coincident with the stimulation. In panel (b) the stretch is applied after the onset of stimulation. Although each muscle was subjected to similar strain and strain rate, the muscle in (b) was subjected to much greater stress. (From Lieber & Fridén 1993.)

However, a novel muscle stimulation pattern allowed the investigators to manipulate the peak eccentric contraction force (Fig. 28.3). The results revealed that strain accounted for approximately 50% of the variability in postprotocol peak tetanic tension, a measure of muscle injury, whereas the peak eccentric contraction force accounted for less than 10% additional variability. The authors interpreted these findings as indicative of an important role of strain in determining the extent of muscle damage. In this vein, eccentric contractions are associated with increased strain on individual cross-bridges. Lombardi and Piazzesi (1990) reported that the total number of cross-bridges formed during maximum eccentric contraction is approximately 10% higher than that during maximum isometric contraction. Structurally, the much larger increment in force compared to the increased number of cross-bridges suggests increased average strain on individual cross-bridges.

Warren *et al.* (1993a) investigated the influence of peak eccentric contraction force (100, 125 and 150%

of preinjury maximum isometric tension), muscle length change (10, 20 and 30% of resting muscle length), and lengthening velocity (50, 100 and 150% of resting length per second) on rat soleus injury. The initial muscle lengths from which the contractions were initiated were 85 or 90% of resting muscle length. The indices of muscle injury included maximal isometric tension, peak isometric twitch tension, rate of tetanic tension generation, and relaxation measured immediately following the eccentric contraction protocols. Generally, the peak eccentric contraction force explained the largest amount of variance in declines of the dependent variables observed immediately following the protocol. Lengthening velocity accounted for a modest amount of total variance and initial muscle length did not account for any variance in the dependent variables. Thus, peak eccentric force, independent of lengthening velocity, length change, and initial and final muscle length was pointed to as the factor initiating the injury. Because the injury protocol consisted of only five eccentric contractions, the results demonstrate that just a few contractions can result in significant muscle injury. In humans, Brown et al. (1997) reported that bouts of 30 or 50 eccentric maximum voluntary contractions of the knee extensor muscles were associated with significant increases in serum creatine kinase levels. This was not found for a bout of 10 maximum voluntary eccentric contractions. Most human subjects cannot maximally activate skeletal muscle during eccentric contractions. Thus, human studies will vary substantially from animal model studies in which maximum activation of the muscle preparations can be obtained. Nevertheless, the finding provides an idea of the number of eccentric maximum voluntary contractions that is necessary to result in increased values of indirect measures of muscle injury.

The relationship between the initial muscle length from which eccentric contractions are initiated and the extent to which the muscle is damaged has been contested. Warren et al. (1993a; see above) reported that initial muscle length did not account for any variance in the variables associated with muscle injury immediately following the protocol. Hunter and Faulkner (1997) subjected mouse extensor digitorum longus muscles to maximum eccentric con-

tractions initiated from 90, 100 or 120% of resting muscle fibre length. The velocity of stretch was two fibre lengths per second. Muscles were stretched to a final length of 150, 160 or 170% of resting muscle fibre length. Generally, muscle damage, as measured by a force deficit, was defined as a function of the initial muscle length, the final muscle length, and the work input to the muscle during the eccentric contraction. These findings, as well as those of Warren et al. (1993a), who reported no relationship of muscle damage to initial muscle length, are consistent with the role of sarcomere length heterogeneities resulting from muscle length extending into the descending limb of the length–tension curve.

Warren et al. (1993b) subsequently addressed the question of whether a single eccentric contraction could initiate muscle injury or whether multiple contractions were necessary. Rat soleus muscles were subjected to between zero and 10 maximum eccentric contractions. The contractions were performed at an initial starting length of 90% of resting length, through a maximum length change of 25% of resting length, at a lengthening velocity of 150% resting length per second, and having a peak eccentric contraction force of 180% of the maximum isometric tetanic tension. The results of the statistical analysis (change point regression) revealed that injury protocols having less than eight eccentric contractions generally had values for the dependent variables (indices of muscle injury) that were no different than those muscles that had not performed any eccentric contractions. These results caused the authors to conclude that the eccentric contraction-induced muscle injury is consistent with a materials fatigue model, i.e. a result of exposure to multiple contractions rather than a single contraction. There are three predictions associated with the materials fatigue model that maintains a non-linear, inverse relationship between muscle stress and the number of repetitions required for material failure of skeletal muscle (Armstrong et al. 1995). First, only a few repetitions of contractions having high stress are required to cause failure of critical muscle components. Indeed, there is evidence that a single eccentric contraction can be associated with muscle damage (Brooks et al. 1995; MacPherson et al. 1996).

Second, there is a threshold stress below which injury will not occur. Third, muscle conditioning or deconditioning will shift the relationship to the right or left, respectively.

The site of injury

The role of mechanical factors as the cause of the initial injury is clear from the experimental results. The site(s) of the initial injury, however, have not been fully determined. The model proposed by Armstrong *et al.* (1990, 1991) and later adapted by Armstrong *et al.* (1995) has served as a framework for systematic research of the early events associ-

ated with muscle injury. The model includes three phases of injury (Fig. 28.4):
1 the initial phase;
2 the calcium overload phase; and
3 the autogenic phase.
These phases of the early events of muscle injury occur prior to the arrival of inflammatory and phagocytic cells, which precedes the regenerative phase. During the initial phase a mechanical, or metabolic, insult results in damage of contractile and/or structural elements. This is the damage that results in the reduced contractile capacity commonly observed following the experimental protocols. However, the model also predicts damage to the sarcolemma,

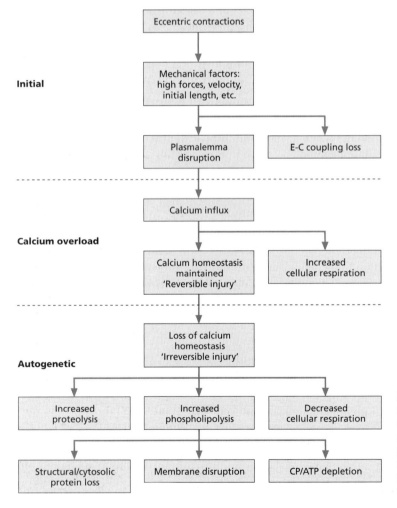

Fig. 28.4 Model of the initial and subsequent phases of eccentric contraction-induced injury. The events depicted in the model occur prior to the arrival at the damaged muscle of inflammatory and phagocytic cells. (From Armstrong *et al.* 1995.)

T-tubule system and sarcoplasmic reticulum* that gives rise to loss of Ca^{2+} homeostasis, a result of which is the increase in the concentration of total muscle Ca^{2+}. The loss of Ca^{2+} can give rise to conditions during which Ca^{2+} uptake by the sarcoplasmic reticulum and mitochondria, and Ca^{2+} binding by proteins and the calcium pump cannot extract Ca^{2+} faster than the rate of increase of free cytosolic Ca^{2+}.† The autogenic phase begins when Ca^{2+} concentration rises above a threshold value and activates Ca^{2+}-sensitive proteolytic and phospholipolytic pathways.

There are a number of confirmed sites presently associated with the initial injury. At the subcellular level, Lieber *et al.* (1994, 1996) demonstrated the loss of desmin staining following eccentric contractions. Further, as described in a previous section, the extent to which desmin staining was lost was associated with the reduction in maximum tetanic tension. This work, performed using animal models of injury, is consistent with observations made in human subjects. For example, Fridén *et al.* (1983) had subjects perform a 30 min protocol of concentric or eccentric pedalling on a bicycle ergometer at 80–100% of their maximum oxygen uptake. Biopsies were taken from the vastus lateralis muscle following the protocol and up to 6 days after the protocol. Histochemical and electron microscopic analyses revealed sarcomeric disruptions, particularly at the Z-band and myofilamentous elements in the subjects who performed the eccentric exercise. This type of damage seems consistent with disruption to the desmin scaffold described by Lieber *et al.*

The cytoskeletal disruptions provide a logical explanation for force degradation following eccen-

tric contraction-induced injury. However, the magnitude of the force degradation following injury has been suggested to be larger than can be accounted for by the number of muscle fibres that sustain damage. Warren *et al.* (1993c) conducted an experiment to determine if the maximum tetanic force deficit observed subsequent to an eccentric contraction protocol, and generally associated with damage to the contractile machinery, could be attributed to excitation failure. These authors reasoned that the increased serum levels of intracellular enzymes (e.g. creatine kinase), myoglobin and myosin heavy chain fragments reflect a loss of sarcolemmal integrity. The resulting disturbance to excitation coupling, specifically events prior to Ca^{2+} release from the sarcoplasmic reticulum, could then reduce maximum tetanic force. Isolated mouse soleus muscles were subjected to 10 or 20 eccentric contractions or 20 isometric contractions. Following the protocol, isometric tetanic force decreased by 20, 43 and 4%, respectively. For the muscles that performed 10 or 20 eccentric contractions or 20 isometric contractions, the isometric tetanic force generated following immersion in a buffer containing 50 mM caffeine, was 80, 118 and 72% of the postprotocol isometric tetanic force, respectively. Exposure to caffeine in adequate concentrations causes muscle contraction without a change in sarcolemma potential. The high caffeine-elicited force, relative to the postprotocol value, thus indicates failure of the excitation sequence up to but not including Ca^{2+} release by the sarcoplasmic reticulum. Therefore, the results demonstrate that the early force loss subsequent to eccentric contraction-induced injury may be largely attributable to an inability to activate undamaged contractile machinery. Notably, the results of a second experiment demonstrated that the force deficit following the eccentric protocol could not be attributed to impaired action potential propagation along the sarcolemma or through the T-tubule system.

Recent results of Patel *et al.* (1999), however, have refocused attention on cytoskeletal disruption as a source of force degradation following eccentric contractions. Fibre bundles from toad anterior tibialis muscle were subjected to 10 maximum eccentric contractions associated with nominal muscle fibre

---

*The review by Byrd (1992) on the influence of exercise-induced muscle damage on the sarcoplasmic reticulum (SR) links strenuous exercise to structural damage of the SR, to release and uptake of Ca^{2+} by the SR, how SR damage and dysfunction can contribute to muscle cell damage, and the events occurring during exercise associated with the initiation of structural and functional SR changes.

†Notably, Lowe *et al.* (1994) found that mouse soleus muscle injured with an eccentric contraction protocol was capable of buffering increased infusion of extracellular Ca^{2+}, thereby preventing activation of the Ca^{2+}-sensitive proteolytic and phospholipolytic pathways.

strains of 10, 25 or 35%. During the contractions, sarcomere length changes were measured using laser defraction. Subsequent to the eccentric contraction protocols, maximum isometric tetanic force decreased by 16, 40 and 60% for the 10, 25 and 35% strain conditions, respectively. Multiple regression revealed that 87% of the variation in the reduction in maximum isometric tetanic force was accounted for by sarcomere strain. The relationship between the reduction in maximum isometric tetanic force and muscle fibre stress was not significant and accounted for well below one percent of the total variation. These unique data on sarcomere strain and eccentric contraction-induced injury provide further, albeit indirect, support for the hypothesis that cytoskeletal disruption plays a dominant role in eccentric contraction-induced injury.

Ingalls et al. (1998) extended the previously described in vitro work of Warren et al. (1993c) to an in vivo model to determine if excitation-contraction coupling failure is the mechanism of eccentric contraction-induced injury. Mouse extensor digitorum longus muscles were injured using a protocol consisting of 150 eccentric contractions. The postprotocol isometric tetanic force was 53% lower than the preprotocol value. However, the postprotocol isometric tetanic force increased substantially when induced with caffeine and 4-chloro-m-cresol.‡ Thus, these data supported the previous in vitro experimental findings that excitation coupling is the cause of the immediate postprotocol reduction in isometric tetanic tension. Indeed, the authors estimated that 75% of the force impairment was due to excitation-coupling failure.

The basement membrane has been suggested as an injury site due to eccentric contractions. Tidball (1986) measured material properties of frog semitendinosus muscle fibres during sinusoidal stretch before and after enzymatic digestion of the basement membrane. Cells with basement membranes dissipated more than three times the energy of cells without basement membranes. This evidence that basement membranes provide considerable passive

resistance to muscle lengthening makes it a candidate for eccentric contraction-induced injury.

Injury to the extracellular matrix has also been reported subsequent to eccentric exercise. The extracellular matrix contributes to the passive force resisting muscle lengthening, and subsequent to muscle fibre damage serves as a scaffold during the regeneration processes. Stauber et al. (1990) reported the results of an experiment in which subjects performed a single bout of 70 maximum voluntary eccentric elbow joint flexions at $120° \cdot s^{-1}$ (Fig. 28.5). Forty-eight hours after the exercise protocol, immunohistochemical evidence that the extracellular matrix was physically torn away from the surface of muscle fibres was observed from samples of all subjects.

The ultrastructural damage described by Fridén et al. (1983) was observed primarily, but not entirely, in type II (fast twitch, glycolytic) muscle fibres. Soon after the exercise session the ratio of type II : type I damage (measured as Z-line disturbances) was nearly 3 : 1 in 666 randomly selected samples. Selective damage to type II muscle fibres as a result of eccentric contraction has been a recurrent theme in the literature (Jones et al. 1986; Lieber & Fridén 1988; Lieber et al. 1991). This is especially notable in view of evidence suggesting that eccentric contractions are associated with selective activation of high threshold (i.e. type II) motor units, which is discussed in the next section of this chapter.

Lieber (1992) has proposed an explanation for the observations of selective damage to these fibres. During contractions of sufficiently high intensity, muscle fibres of high-threshold motor units fatigue before the muscle fibres of low-threshold motor units. Lieber proposed that these fatigued fibres experience reduced capacity to regenerate ATP, which results in the failure of the actomyosin bond to be broken. This would subsequently be associated with a higher mechanical stiffness of the myofibrils in these fibres which, upon stretch, would give rise to the higher stress associated with cytoskeletal and then myofibrillar disruption. Alternatively, reduced mitochondrial calcium buffering could activate calcium-mediated neutral proteases and lysosomal proteases. The former explanation represents a mechanism associated with the period

---

‡4-Chloro-m-cresol activates the sarcoplasmic reticulum Ca^{2+} release channel and reportedly has much greater sensitivity than caffeine (Herrmann-Frank et al. 1996).

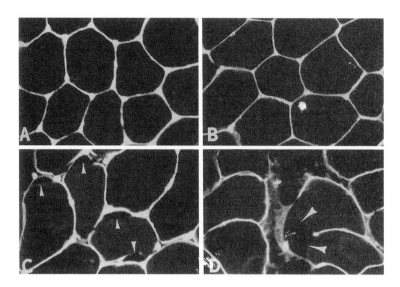

Fig. 28.5 Cross-section of human biceps brachii muscle prior to and 48 h following an eccentric contraction protocol. Panels (A) and (B) show chondroitin 6-sulphate proteoglycan localization and fluorescein-conjugated concanavalin A staining, respectively, in normal muscle. Panels (C) and (D) were similarly treated samples of exercised muscle and illustrate (arrows) locations at which the extracellular matrix has been separated from the surface of muscle fibres. (From Stauber *et al.* 1990.)

during which the contractions are performed. In contrast, the latter explanation, which occurs intracellularly and independently of the inflammatory processes, would continue to occur after the insult (see Fielding 1995). Armstrong *et al.* (1995) have suggested that the increased resistance to muscle injury evident after exposure to a single bout of eccentric exercise argues against Lieber's first explanation. The basis for this suggestion is that increased resistance to injury occurs much faster than training-related increases in oxidative capability.

Patel *et al.* (1998) specifically tested the hypothesis that injury due to eccentric contraction is a function of oxidative capacity. As part of the study, rabbit extensor digitorum longus muscle was subjected to a three-week training protocol during which the muscles were electrically stimulated to perform isometric contractions. The training protocol had the desired effect of increasing oxidative capacity as measured, in part, by citrate synthase activity (an index of whole muscle oxidative capacity). However, subsequent to the eccentric contraction injury protocol, consisting of 900 eccentric contractions over a period of 30 min, the electrical stimulation-trained muscle and the control muscle did not differ significantly relative to force deficit thereby refuting the hypothesis.

Neuromuscular factors of eccentric contraction and related injury

The literature presents evidence that eccentric contraction preferentially injures fast-twitch muscle fibres. A question that may be raised relates to whether the neuromuscular control of eccentric contractions, which can be substantially different than that of concentric or isometric contractions, is a factor that contributes to the selective damage. There are a number of curiosities associated with eccentric contraction that span the neuromechanical domain, two of which relate to central nervous system control of voluntary eccentric contractions. First, during maximum voluntary contractions (MVC) the level of muscle activation, as measured by the surface EMG, is generally observed to be lower than that of a concentric MVC. This suggests that the central nervous system is unwilling to fully activate eccentrically contracting muscle. Second, exercise protocols consisting of repeated eccentric MVCs do not result in fatigue, i.e. reductions in force generation, to the same extent or at the same rate as exercise protocols consisting of repeated concentric MCVs. These and other neurally related distinctions of eccentric contractions have been the subject of a recent review (Enoka 1996).

CNS is unwilling to fully activate skeletal muscle during eccentric MVC

A basic physiological question in the area of motor performance and rehabilitation relates to the conditions under which an individual may be capable of voluntarily maximally activating a muscle or muscle group. The ability to maximally activate muscle is considered a motor skill, one that becomes manifest in the measure of maximum voluntary muscle strength. The rapid and significant increases in muscle strength observed during the initial period of a training protocol and that occur in the absence of changes to muscle size or muscle histochemistry are testimony to the role of the nervous system. Abbott *et al.* (1952) demonstrated that eccentric contractions require less metabolic energy than concentric contractions. This work was later followed by a report describing lower activation levels during comparable concentric and eccentric workloads (Bigland & Lippold 1954).

During eccentric MVC, the larger contraction force is generally associated with lower activation levels than that of a concentric MVC. However, this appears to be a neurally mediated effect that demonstrates substantial between-subject variability. In addition, there seems to be substantial experiment-specific sensitivities. It is likely, although unsubstantiated in the literature, that this neurally mediated effect can be reduced or even abolished with training. The findings of Grabiner and Owings (1999) indirectly support this suggestion. Two groups of subjects participated in an experiment during which a concentric or eccentric fatigue protocol was performed unilaterally with the knee extensor muscles. The protocol was performed using a customized isokinetic dynamometer that allowed isokinetic knee extension to be performed either unilaterally or bilaterally and allowed independent measurement of the knee joint moments generated by each limb (Owings & Grabiner 1998a,b). Prior to and following the fatigue protocol, the concentric and eccentric MVCs of the contralateral, unexercised limb were measured. Following the concentric fatigue protocol the MVC of the contralateral, unexercised limb was unchanged. In contrast, following the eccentric fatigue protocol the MVC of the contralateral, unexercised limb increased 11% ($P = 0.028$). One interpretation of this finding is that the level of neural drive to the knee extensor musculature of the contralateral limb was altered as a result of the eccentric, but not the concentric, fatigue protocol. Altered neural drive could be manifest as increased neural drive to the agonist muscles and/or a decreased level of antagonist coactivation. Nevertheless, it appears that the fatigue protocol consisting of 75 repetitions influenced the quality of the motor command to the knee extension musculature of the contralateral limb. Thus, indirectly, these findings suggest that the neurally mediated effect that tends to limit full activation of muscle during maximum voluntary contractions can be reduced or even abolished with training.

Compelling data illustrating incomplete muscle activation during maximum eccentric contraction were reported by Westing *et al.* (1990). In this experiment, isometric MVC and concentric and eccentric MVCs performed isokinetically were compared to those obtained when supramaximal electrical stimulation was superimposed on the voluntary effort. Eccentric MVC increased significantly, over 22% on average, during conditions in which the electrical stimulation was superimposed on maximum voluntary activation. No such increases were observed for the concentric and isometric MVCs. Given the athletic nature of the subjects in the study, the results are strong evidence that under normal conditions, eccentric MVCs do not represent complete activation of the muscle. Therefore, it is reasonable that the EMG measured from the skin surface should be lower during these conditions compared to concentric MVC.

Differences in the time course of fatigue

Eccentric MVCs demonstrate resistance to fatigue to a greater extent, in human subjects, compared with concentric MVCs. Gray and Chandler (1989) and Tesch *et al.* (1990) reported that three bouts of 32 repetitions of isokinetic eccentric knee extension MVCs (performed at $180° \cdot s^{-1}$) did not decrease eccentric MVC. In contrast, the same protocol performed concentrically was associated with an approximately 40% decrease in concentric MVC. Grabiner and

Owings (1999) used a protocol consisting of 75 eccentric or concentric isokinetic knee extension MVCs performed at $30° \cdot s^{-1}$. Concentric decreases in MVC were 38%, a value similar to that reported by Gray and Chandler and Tesch *et al.* However, for the eccentric contractions, a 12% decrease in MVC was observed. This decrease in eccentric MVC was significantly smaller than the decrease in concentric MVC and it was significantly different from zero.

The observed fatigue resistance of eccentric contractions is consistent with predictions based on the submaximal level of neural drive that can be delivered to the contracting muscles. Thus, the question arises as to whether eccentric contractions would be less resistant to fatigue if the level of voluntary neural drive to the muscle could be increased. Studies using animal muscle preparations suggest that this may be true. For example, the decline of peak contraction force generated by isolated mouse extensor digitorum longus following an isometric, concentric or eccentric MVC protocol was 56.3, 53.3 and 66.7%, respectively (McCulley & Faulkner 1985). Following a submaximal isometric or eccentric contraction protocol the maximum isometric force of the isometric and eccentric contractions of rabbit tibialis anterior muscles were reduced 31 and 69%, respectively (Lieber *et al.* 1991). Further, the maximum rate of isometric tension generation of the isometric and eccentric contraction protocols were reduced 63.5 and 89.3%, respectively. Thus, in the studies of McCulley and Faulkner and Lieber *et al.* the eccentric contraction conditions did not demonstrate fatigue resistance as measured by a force deficit after the protocol. However, it must be recognized that force deficits in these types of protocols reflect an interaction of fatigue and injury.

The hypothesis linking fatigue resistance of eccentric contractions with voluntary levels of neural drive was partially supported by the data of Hortobágyi *et al.* (1996). These authors measured the influence of a six-week training protocol on fatigability of the knee extensor muscles during eccentric MVC. The greater than 40% increase in eccentric MVC and 100% increase in the fatigability of the knee extensor muscles were associated with an increase in the level of neural drive during voluntary contractions.

The extent to which muscle fatigues during eccentric protocols has been reported to be affected by the length of the muscle during the eccentric exercises. Newham *et al.* (1988) reported that fatigue is greater when eccentric exercise is performed at long muscle lengths compared to short muscle lengths. In the experiment, subjects performed 180 eccentric MVCs with the elbow flexor muscles. Each contraction required approximately one second to complete. The contractions were performed through a range of motion associated with either a long muscle length (from about 60° of flexion to full extension) or a short muscle length (from about 135° of flexion to about 90° of flexion, see their Fig. 1). The short length exercises were performed using one limb and the long length exercises were performed using the contralateral limb. Following the protocol, the MVC of the arm performing the short length exercises was unaffected but the MVC of the arm performing the long length exercises decreased 30% ($P < 0.05$). Further, muscle tenderness, the measure used to reflect muscle damage, was significantly greater for the long length exercises compared to the short length exercises 48 h after the protocol. Talbot and Morgan (1998) have demonstrated that the extent of muscle damage following eccentric contraction is related to the length of the muscle during the contraction. Isolated toad sartorius muscle was the experimental model. Muscle damage was measured as a reduction in contraction force and a shift, to longer lengths, of the optimum length for force generation. These authors confirmed for the experimental model that greater amounts of muscle injury result when eccentric contractions occur in the descending limb of the length–tension curve. This point is of particular relevance with regard to the influence of exercise training on the ability of skeletal muscle to undergo eccentric contractions without sustaining damage.

With respect to the length–tension curve, Saxton and Donnely (1996) had human subjects perform 70 eccentric maximum voluntary contractions of the elbow flexors at an isokinetic speed of $100° \cdot s^{-1}$. Following the protocol the isometric maximum voluntary contraction was affected to a greater extent at short muscle lengths compared to long muscle lengths. The authors attributed the larger force deficits observed at the short muscle lengths to an acute alteration of the length–tension characteristics of the muscles. Similarly, Child *et al.* (1998) had subjects perform a protocol of 75 maximal voluntary contractions of the knee extensor muscles at an isokinetic speed of $90° \cdot s^{-1}$. One set of exercises was performed through a range of motion in which the knee extensor muscles remained relatively short. A second set was performed through a range of motion in which the knee extensor muscles were relatively long. Immediately following the exercise protocol, the isometric maximum voluntary contraction was affected to a greater extent by the exercises performed with the longer muscle lengths. This finding was attributed to an acute increase in muscle length due to the exercise, the result of which would be a change in the length–tension characteristics.

An abundant body of literature exists that addresses observations that previous exposure to eccentric contractions decreases the extent of muscle damage following subsequent exposures. Until recently, these observations had not been associated with structural changes to the muscle that may have accounted for the increased resistance to damage (Lynn *et al.* 1998). However, Morgan (1990) proposed that a training-induced increase in the number of sarcomeres in series would have the effect of shifting the operating length of a muscle to the left, away from the descending limb of the length–tension curve, which is associated with sarcomere instabilities. Lynn and Morgan (1994) subsequently tested the proposal by exercising rats on a treadmill, either inclined or declined at an angle of 16°. The rats were exercised over a period of 5 days at a velocity of about $16 \text{ m} \cdot \text{min}^{-1}$. Over the 5-day period the duration of the exercise session increased from 15 to 35 min. The results demonstrated that the muscles of the rats exercised on the declined treadmill had about 12% more sarcomeres in series than the rats trained on the inclined treadmill.

The protocol used by Lynn and Morgan (1994) was also used by Lynn *et al.* (1998) in a study undertaken to determine if the training-induced increase in the number of sarcomeres in series was associated with a decrease in the muscle damage subsequent to a series of 20 eccentric contractions. The rats

trained on the declined treadmill had an increase of about 9% in the number of sarcomeres in series, and this was associated with decreased muscle damage following the series of 20 eccentric contractions. Thus, these results demonstrate a rapidly occurring structural change to skeletal muscle that causes the muscle to have increased resistance to eccentric contraction-induced injury.

The above mentioned rapidly occurring structural changes to skeletal muscle represent a facet of what is conventionally and broadly referred to as 'rapid adaptation' (Clarkson *et al.* 1992). Rapid adaptation refers to observations that a bout of eccentric exercise is associated with diminished muscle damage, measured with variables such as muscle soreness, serum creatine kinase and muscle strength, following previous exposure to a similar, or even a less structurally stressful bout of eccentric contractions (Clarkson & Tremblay 1988; Ebbeling & Clarkson 1990; Nosaka *et al.* 1991). Clarkson *et al.* (1992) suggested that neural factors, in addition to molecular and cellular factors, may be involved in the observed rapid adaptation. Hortobágyi *et al.* (1998) directly addressed the question of whether neural factors underlie in part the rapid adaptation, by quantifying muscle damage via muscle biopsy and transmission electron microscopy. The experiment was designed to determine whether muscle injury, as measured primarily by myofibrillar disruption, recurs after the muscle has been exposed to an initial, damaging bout of eccentric contractions, and whether the recurrence of myofibrillar disruption was associated with a voluntary muscle force deficit.

Subjects participated in two eccentric contraction protocols consisting of 100 eccentric MVCs with the knee extensor muscles, performed against a resistance of about 80% of the anisometric eccentric MVC. The protocols were separated by two weeks, which allowed recovery from the first protocol. The intention was to describe the relationship between myofibrillar disruption after the second protocol to voluntary force deficits, serum creatine kinase levels, muscle soreness, and voluntary and reflexive neural drive to the knee extensor muscles. The authors reasoned that unaffected muscle forces in the presence of myofibrillar damage may be indicative of a neurally mediated adaptation allowing increased voluntary neural drive to be delivered to the musculature. Two days after the first protocol, the expected indices of muscle damage, myofibrillar disruption, increased serum creatine kinase level and increased muscle soreness, were evident. These indices accompanied an approximately 37% decrease in the average of voluntary isometric, eccentric and concentric knee extension force. The change in force was mirrored by the change in voluntary neural drive. Two days after the second eccentric contraction protocol, which occurred after a 2-week recovery period, there was evidence of myofibrillar disruption. There was no change in serum creatine kinase levels nor was there a change in the average of voluntary isometric, eccentric and concentric knee extension force. However, there was no change in voluntary neural drive.

The data, unfortunately, could not provide an unambiguous solution to the questions that were posed. The second bout of eccentric exercise was associated with a recurrence of myofibrillar disruption but there was no change in the voluntary muscle force. However, there was also no change in the levels of neural drive to the muscles during the voluntary contractions. Thus, collectively, the data do not provide convincing support for a role of the nervous system in the rapid adaptation. However, the work does provide a framework by which further human study can be conducted and identifies specific methodological gaps that limit these types of human studies. Presently, direct measures of structural changes to human muscle represent technological challenges. Future systematic, direct and mechanistic study of rapid adaptation in humans will be reliant on being able to measure the structural changes to skeletal muscle similar to those studied in animal models. For example, increased numbers of sarcomeres in series is a structural adaptation that can be directly related to the increased resistance to damage. However, this type of measurement, i.e. *in vivo*, is presently not feasible in the human subject.

Another issue related to the role of the nervous system in eccentric contraction-related injury is whether neural factors, in part, are associated with the initial predisposition to muscle damage. That is, during the formulation and subsequent delivery of activation commands does the central nervous system give consideration to potentially injurious conditions arising from eccentric contractions? The question arises from the convergence of two independent observations. First, in experiments during which eccentric protocols have been used to induce muscle injury in the elbow flexor muscles, elbow flexors of the arm, biceps brachii and brachialis, experience substantially greater soreness than the elbow flexors of the forearm, brachioradialis (P. Clarkson, personal communication). Secondly, activation of the biceps brachii and the brachioradialis shows significant differences from one muscle to another during concentric and eccentric contractions (Grabiner & Kasprisin, submitted). Further, the differences are consistent with the observations of between-muscle differences in muscle soreness and consistent with the observations that skeletal muscle is more prone to eccentric contraction-induced injury when the eccentric contractions are performed at long muscle lengths.

In the study of Grabiner and Kasprisin, subjects performed a non-fatiguing protocol that included concentric and eccentric isokinetic MVCs of the elbow flexor muscles. The contractions were performed at $65° \cdot s^{-1}$ through an $85°$ range of motion. Elbow flexion was initiated from approximately $5°$ of flexion or $90°$ of flexion for concentric and eccentric contractions, respectively. Spatially averaged muscle activation detected using an array of surface electrodes (Kasprisin & Grabiner 1998) was collected from the biceps brachii and brachioradialis muscles. Activation of the two halves of the range of motion for each muscle was quantified separately (Fig. 28.6).

The results appear somewhat consistent with the greater predisposition of the biceps brachii to muscle soreness subsequent to eccentric contraction protocols. The observed 13% increase in activation level of the biceps brachii during the second half of the range of motion did not achieve statistical significance.§ Nevertheless, the qualitative increase

§The observed *P*-value of 0.04 was greater than the value of 0.013 required by the Bonferonni-adjustment. *A posteriori* power analysis revealed that the observed variability about the mean values limited our ability to detect significant differences between the means of less than 51%.

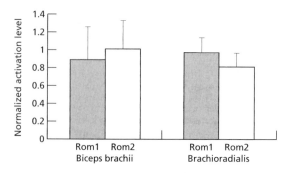

Fig. 28.6 The spatially averaged activation levels (Kasprisin & Grabiner 1998) of the brachioradialis and biceps brachii during maximum voluntary eccentric contraction are influenced differently by elbow joint angle. The activation level on the vertical axis is expressed as a percentage of the activation level observed during the first half of the elbow joint range of motion during a maximum voluntary concentric contraction. The increase in biceps brachii activation level at the joint angle, or muscle length, most associated with eccentric contraction-induced injury raises the question whether the aspect of neural control is associated with the higher predisposition to eccentric contraction-induced injury of this muscle compared with brachioradialis. Rom1 and Rom2 represent the first and second halves of the 85° range of motion.

in activation level was notable in view of the significant decrease of the activation level of the brachioradialis muscle ($P < 0.001$).

The statistical similarity of the biceps brachii activation level and the decrease of the level of brachioradialis activation during the second half of the range of motion during eccentric MVC is curious in light of the evidence that the biceps brachii is predisposed to greater muscle soreness than brachioradialis. The data broadly suggest that during the second half of the range of motion the biceps brachii stress increased to a greater extent than that of the brachioradialis. However, these observations are hypothesis generating. The hypothesis can be stated as follows: voluntary muscle activation patterns during maximum voluntary contractions are not related to the predisposition of the muscle to eccentric contraction-induced muscle injury. This is one of two broad questions that do not appear to have been widely addressed in the literature. Specifically, (i) are voluntary activation patterns associated with

the extent of injury subsequent to a muscle injury protocol? and (ii) do voluntary muscle activation patterns change subsequent to recovery from eccentric contraction injury? The second question has been partially addressed (Hortobágyi et al. 1998).

An issue raised in an earlier section will now be addressed in terms of its relevance to neuromuscular control. This concerns the evidence of preferential damage demonstrated by fast-twitch motor units as a result of exposure to eccentric contraction protocols. This preferential damage has been demonstrated in both animal models (Lieber & Fridén 1988; Lieber et al. 1991) and human models (Fridén et al. 1983; Jones et al. 1986).

The literature provides compelling evidence that the manner in which skeletal muscle is activated during voluntary contractions can be very different than that which occurs during concentric and isometric contraction. Some of these differences were addressed in a previous section and related to the lower level of voluntary activation and the greater resistance to fatigue of eccentric contractions compared to concentric contractions. However, there is emerging evidence suggesting that the disparate activation patterns associated with eccentric contraction can predispose muscle to damage. Enoka (1996) has proposed the hypothesis that 'the neural commands controlling eccentric contractions are unique'. To qualify as unique, Enoka provided criteria against which an activation pattern could be judged. The activation patterns must specify which motor units should be activated, to what extent they are activated, when they should be activated, and how the activity is distributed across muscles. The literature provides evidence supporting the contention that the uniqueness of the neural commands associated with eccentric contractions is manifest by a preferential activation, under specific conditions, of high-threshold motor units. In addition, this phenomenon has been observed in large and small muscles. For example, Nardone and Schieppati (1988) and Nardone et al. (1989) reported preferential activation of high-threshold motor units of the triceps surae in human subjects performing eccentric plantarflexion contractions. Tax et al. (1989) reported that during eccentric contraction, motor unit discharge frequency was lower than that during concentric and isometric contractions. This observation was confirmed by Sögaard *et al.* (1996). Howell *et al.* (1995) reported preferential activation of high-threshold motor units during eccentric contractions of the first dorsal interosseus, a small hand muscle. The above findings confirm, for a variety of muscles, that the central nervous system can implement a different motor unit activation strategy during isometric, concentric and eccentric contractions. However, it must be recognized that the number of published papers reporting preferential activation of high-threshold motor units is presently small, and the frequency with which these patterns have been observed is somewhat low. For example, Howell *et al.* (1995) reported preferential recruitment in three of 21 motor units, or about 14%. In contrast, there is a more sizeable, but older body of literature that presents evidence of selective activation of muscles that are composed primarily of high-threshold, or fast motor units. For example, preferential muscle activation has been reported during rapidly performed motor tasks including bicycling at high rates (Citterio & Agostini 1984) and maximum-effort hopping in humans (Moritani *et al.* 1990), paw-shaking in cats (Smith *et al.* 1980; Fowler *et al.* 1988), and rapid breathing in rabbits subjected to respiratory distress (Citterio *et al.* 1982; Citterio *et al.* 1983).

Using a novel protocol, Grabiner and Owings (in review) have reported findings that further support the contention that the neural control of eccentric contractions is unique. Subjects performed series of concentric and eccentric maximum voluntary isokinetic knee extension MVCs ($60° \cdot s^{-1}$). Both concentric and eccentric contractions were initiated from the same initial knee-joint position. Analysis of muscle activation (vastus lateralis) and knee extension force data was conducted during the isometric phase, approximately 100 ms, occurring prior to the onset of dynamometer motion. Because the quantification of the activation level and knee extension force occurred prior to motion, any influence of stretch-mediated feedback on activation during the eccentric contractions was precluded.

The results revealed that the rate of knee extension force generation measured during the isometric phase preceding the onset of dynamometer motion was similar for both concentric and eccentric contractions. These values were 0.93 ± 0.43 and $0.93 \pm 0.35 \, N \, m \cdot ms^{-1}$. However, the activation level, measured during the same period, was significantly lower (26%) during the eccentric contractions than during the concentric contractions.

Because all contractions were initiated from the same knee joint angle and because the differences between concentric and eccentric activation patterns were evident during an isometric phase prior to the onset of dynamometer motion, the quantified activation levels could not have been influenced by afferent feedback. Rather, the data suggest that the observed differences originated during the formulation of the motor command and that information in the motor command distinguishes between concentric and eccentric contractions.

Further experiments using this protocol have confirmed these findings in the vastus lateralis and, moreover, have revealed similar effects in the rectus femoris, a biarticular knee joint extensor muscle (Grabiner & Owings, in review). The question arises, however, as to how similar knee extension forces can be generated with significantly lower levels of voluntary neural drive to an agonist group. To answer these questions a mathematical model of a motor unit pool adapted from Fuglevand *et al.* (1993) has been used in simulations. These were conducted to provide feasible solutions to questions regarding the underlying motor unit behaviour necessary to give rise to the observed activation–force relationships during the initial isometric phase. The solution provided by these simulations and that best fits the experimentally derived data during eccentric MVCs is derived when more than 50% of the smallest motor units in the pool remain quiescent, i.e. high-threshold motor units are preferentially activated whereas during the concentric contraction the smaller motor units are active. This finding is notable in extending the previously referred to electrophysiological work of others that has identified disparate motor unit behaviour during eccentric contractions. Further, it has generated testable hypotheses that may elucidate potential neural aspects of training that serve to protect skeletal muscle from eccentric contraction-related injury.

Concluding remarks

Injury to skeletal muscle due to eccentric contraction has been systematically studied for nearly the entire 20th century. Driven by technological advancements, observations and simple measures of the muscle soreness, limb swelling and joint stiffness that accompanied force deficits and motor dysfunction were followed by studies of the biochemistry, cellular and molecular biology, cellular and molecular mechanics and neurophysiology of injury and healing. At the threshold of the 21st century, it would appear that many of the mechanisms and sites of the injury have been elucidated. Yet there remain substantial questions to be asked, many of which must await the development of appropriate technology. One such question for example, from the biological side, is whether the number of sarcomeres in series adapts to exercise in humans as has been observed in animals. Clearly, answers to this question must await the development of technology that will allow *in vivo* measurement of the number of sarcomeres in series in the human, and in response to training. That sequence of events is likely to extend well into the 21st century.

References

Abbott, B.C., Bigland, B. & Ritchie, J.M. (1952) The physiological cost of negative work. *Journal of Physiology (London)* **117**, 380–390.

Armstrong, R.B. (1990) Initial events in exercise-induced muscular injury. *Medicine and Science in Sports and Exercise* **22**, 429–435.

Armstrong, R.B., Warren, G.L. & Warren, J.A. (1991) Mechanisms of exercise-induced muscle fiber injury. *Sports Medicine* **12**, 184–207.

Armstrong, R.B., Warren, G.L. & Lowe, D.A. (1995) Mechanisms in the initiation of contraction-induced skeletal muscle injury. In: *Repetitive Motion Disorders of the Upper Extremity* (eds S.L. Gordon, S.J. Blair & L.J. Fine), pp. 339–349. American Academy of Orthopaedic Surgeons, Rosemont, IL.

Bigland, B. & Lippold, O.C.J. (1954) The relationship between force, velocity, and integrated electrical activity in human muscles. *Journal of Physiology (London)* **123**, 214–224.

Brooks, S.V., Zerba, E. & Faulkner, J.A. (1995) Injury to muscle fibers after single stretches of passive and maximally stimulated muscles in mice. *Journal of Physiology (London)* **488**, 459–469.

Byrd, S.K. (1992) Alterations in the sarcoplasmic reticulum: a possible link to exercise-induced muscle injury. *Medicine and Science in Sports and Exercise* **24**, 531–536.

Child, R.B., Saxton, J.M. & Donnely, A.E. (1998) Comparison of eccentric knee extensor muscle actions at two muscle lengths on indices of damage and angle-specific force production in humans. *Journal of Sports Sciences* **16**, 301–308.

Citterio, G. & Agostini, E. (1984) Selective activation of quadriceps muscle fibers according to bicycling rate. *Journal of Applied Physiology* **57**, 371–379.

Citterio, G., Agostini, E., Piccoli, S. & Sironi, S. (1982) Selective activation of parasternal muscle fibers according to breathing rate. *Respiration Physiology* **48**, 281–295.

Citterio, G., Sironi, S., Piccoli, S. & Agostini, E. (1983) Slow to fast shift in inspiratory muscle fibers during heat tachypnea. *Respiration Physiology* **51**, 259–274.

Clarkson, P.M. & Tremblay, I. (1988) Rapid adaptation to exercise induced muscle damage. *Journal of Applied Physiology* **65**, 1–6.

Clarkson, P.M., Nosaka, K. & Braun, B. (1992) Muscle function after exercise-induced muscle damage and rapid adaptation. *Medicine and Science in Sports and Exercise* **24**, 512–520.

Clarkson, P.M. & Newham, D.J. (1995) Associations between muscle soreness, damage, and fatigue. In: *Fatigue* (eds S.C. Gandevia, R.M. Enoka, A.J. McComas, D.G. Stuart & C.K. Thomas), pp. 457–469. Plenum Press, New York.

Ebbeling, C.B. & Clarkson, P.M. (1990) Muscle adaptation prior to recovery following eccentric exercise. *European Journal of Applied Physiology* **60**, 26–31.

Enoka, R.M. (1996) Eccentric contractions require unique activation strategies by the nervous system. *Journal of Applied Physiology* **81**, 2339–2346.

Faulkner, J.A., Brooks, S.V. & Opiteck, J.A. (1993) Injury to skeletal muscle fibers during contractions: conditions of occurrence and prevention. *Physical Therapy* **73**, 911–920.

Fielding, R.A. (1995) The role of inflammatory processes in exercise-induced muscle injury: implications for changes in skeletal muscle protein turnover. In: *Repetitive Motion Disorders of the Upper Extremity* (eds S.L. Gordon, S.J. Blair & L.J. Fine), pp. 323–338. American Academy of Orthopaedic Surgeons, Rosemont, IL.

Fowler, E.G., Gregor, R.J. & Roy, R.R. (1988) Differential kinetics of fast and slow ankle extensors during the paw-shake in the cat. *Experimental Neurology* **99**, 219–224.

Fridén, J. (1984) Muscle soreness after exercise: implications of morphological changes. *International Journal of Sports Medicine* **5**, 57–66.

Fridén, J., Sjostrom, M. & Ekblom, B. (1981) A morphological study of delayed muscle soreness. *Experientia* **37**, 506–507.

Fridén, J., Sjöström, M. & Ekblom, B. (1983) Myofibrillar damage following intense eccentric exercise in man. *International Journal of Sports Medicine* **4**, 170–176.

Fuglevand, A.J., Winter, D.A. & Patla, A.E. (1993) Models of recruitment and rate coding in motor unit pools. *Journal of Neurophysiology* **70**, 2470–2488.

Gibala, M.J., MacDougall, J.D., Tarnopolsky, M.A. & Stauber, W.T. (1995) Changes in human skeletal muscle ultrastructure and force production after acute resistance exercise. *Journal of Applied Physiology* **78**, 702–708.

Grabiner, M.D. & Kasprisin, J.E. (2000) Joint angle-dependencies of elbow flexor activation levels during maximum voluntary isometric and anisometric contractions. *Clinical Biomechanics* (in press).

Grabiner, M.D. & Owings, T.M. (1999) Effects of eccentrically and concentrically induced unilateral fatigue on the involved and uninvolved limbs. *Journal of Electromyography and Kinesiology* 9, 185–189.

Grabiner, M.D. & Owings, T.M. (2000) Activation differences between concentric and eccentric maximum voluntary contractions are evident prior to movement onset (in press).

Gray, J.C. & Chandler, J.M. (1989) Percent decline in peak torque production during repeated concentric and eccentric contractions of the quadriceps femoris muscle. *Journal of Orthopaedic and Sports Physical Therapy* 2, 309–314.

Hermann-Frank, A., Richter, M., Sarközi, S., Mohor, U. & Lehmann-Horn, F. (1996) 4-chloro-*m*-cresol, a potent and specific activator of skeletal muscle ryanodine receptor, *Biochimica et Biophysica Acta* 1289, 31–40.

Hortobágyi, T., Barrier, J., Beard, D. *et al.* (1996) Greater initial adaptations to submaximum muscle lengthening than maximal shortening. *Journal of Applied Physiology* 81, 1677–1682.

Hortobágyi, T., Houmard, J., Fraser, D., Dudek, R., Lambert, J. & Tracy, J. (1998) Normal forces and myofibrillar disruption after repeated eccentric exercise. *Journal of Applied Physiology* 84, 492–498.

Hough, T. (1902) Ergographic studies in muscular soreness. *American Journal of Physiology* 7, 76–92.

Howell, J.N., Fuglevand, A.J., Walsh, M.L. & Bigland-Ritchie, B. (1995) Motor unit activity during isometric and concentric-eccentric contractions of the human first dorsal interosseus muscle. *Journal of Neurophysiology* 74, 901–904.

Hunter, K.D. & Faulkner, J.A. (1997) Pliometric contraction-induced injury of mouse skeletal muscle: effect of initial length. *Journal of Applied Physiology* 82, 278–283.

Ingalls, C.P., Warren, G.L., Williams, J.H., Ward, C.W. & Armstrong, R.B. (1998) E-C coupling failure in mouse EDL muscle after in vivo eccentric contractions. *Journal of Applied Physiology* 85, 58–67.

Jones, D.A., Newham, D.J., Round, J.M. & Tolfree, S.E. (1986) Experimental human muscle damage: morphological changes in relation to other indices of damage. *Journal of Physiology (London)* 375, 435–448.

Kasprisin, J.E. & Grabiner, M.D. (1998) EMG. variability during maximum voluntary isometric and anisometric contractions is reduced using spatial averaging. *Journal of Electromyography and Kinesiology* 8, 45–50.

Lieber, R.L. (1992) *Skeletal Muscle Structure and Function*. Williams & Wilkins, Baltimore.

Lieber, R.L. & Fridén, J. (1988) Selective damage of fast glycolytic muscle fibers with eccentric contractions of the rabbit tibialis anterior. *Acta Physiologica Scandinavica* 133, 587–588.

Lieber, R.L. & Fridén, J. (1993) Muscle damage is not a function of muscle force but active muscle strain. *Journal of Applied Physiology* 74, 520–526.

Lieber, R.L., Woodburn, T.M. & Fridén, J. (1991) Muscle damage induced by eccentric contractions of 25 percent strain. *Journal of Applied Physiology* 70, 2498–2507.

Lieber, R.L., Schmitz, M.C., Mishra, D.K. & Fridén, J. (1994) Contractile and cellular remodeling in rabbit skeletal muscle after cyclic eccentric contractions. *Journal of Applied Physiology* 77, 1926–1934.

Lieber, R.L., Thornell, L.-E. & Fridén, J. (1996) Muscle cytoskeleton disruption occurs within the first 15 min of cyclic eccentric contraction. *Journal of Applied Physiology* 80, 278–284.

Lombardi, V. & Piazzesi, G. (1990) The contractile response during steady lengthening of stimulated frog muscle fibers. *Journal of Physiology (London)* 431, 141–171.

Lowe, D.A., Warren, G.L., Hayes, D.A., Farmer, M.A. & Armstrong, R.B. (1994) Eccentric contraction-induced injury of mouse soleus muscle: effect of varying $[Ca^{2+}]$. *Journal of Applied Physiology* 76, 1445–1453.

Lynn, R. & Morgan, D.L. (1994) Decline running produces more sarcomeres in rat vastus intermedius muscle fibers than does incline running. *Journal of Applied Physiology* 77, 1439–1444.

Lynn, R., Talbot, J.A. & Morgan, D.L. (1998) Differences in rat skeletal muscles after incline and decline running. *Journal of Applied Physiology* 85, 98–104.

MacIntyre, D.L., Reid, W.D. & McKenzie, D.C. (1995) Delayed muscle soreness. The inflammatory response to muscle injury and its clinical implications. *Sports Medicine* 20, 24–40.

MacPherson, C.D., Schork, A.M. & Faulkner, J.A. (1996) Contraction-induced injury to single permeabilized muscle fibers from fast and slow muscles

of the rat following single stretches. *American Journal of Physiology* 271 (*Cell Physiology* 40), C1438–C1446.

McCulley, K.K. & Faulkner, J.A. (1985) Injury to skeletal muscle fibers of mice following lengthening contractions. *Journal of Applied Physiology* 59, 119–126.

Morgan, D.L. (1990) New insights into the behavior of muscle during active lengthening. *Biophysical Journal* 57 (2), 209–221.

Moritani, T., Oddson, L. & Thorstensson, A. (1990) Electromyographic evidence of selective fatigue during the eccentric phase of stretch/shortening cycles in man. *European Journal of Applied Physiology* 60, 425–429.

Nardone, A. & Schieppati, M. (1988) Shift of activity from slow to fast muscle during voluntary lengthening contractions of the triceps surae in humans. *Journal of Physiology (London)* 395, 363–381.

Nardone, A., Romano, C. & Schieppati, M. (1989) Selective recruitment of high-threshold motor units during voluntary isotonic lengthening of active muscles. *Journal of Physiology (London)* 409, 451–471.

Newham, D.J., Jones, D.A., Ghosh, G. & Aurora, P. (1988) Muscle fatigue and pain after eccentric contractions at long and short length. *Journal of Clinical Science* 74, 553–557.

Nosaka, K., Clarkson, P.M., McGuiggin, M.E. & Byrne, J.M. (1991) Time course of muscle adaptation after high-force eccentric exercise. *European Journal of Applied Physiology* 63, 70–76.

Owings, T.M. & Grabiner, M.D. (1998a) Fatigue effects on the bilateral deficit are speed dependent. *Medicine and Science in Sports and Exercise* 30, 1257–1262.

Owings, T.M. & Grabiner, M.D. (1998b) Normally aging older adults demonstrate the bilateral deficit during ramp and hold contractions. *Journal of Gerontology: Biological Sciences* 53A, B425–B429.

Patel, T.J. & Lieber, R.L. (1997) Force transmission in skeletal muscle: from actomyosin to external tendons. In: *Exercise and Sports Sciences Reviews* (ed. J.O. Holloszy), 25, pp. 321–363. Williams & Wilkins, Baltimore.

Patel, T.J., Cuizon, D., Mthieu-Costello, O., Fridén, J. & Lieber, R.L. (1998) Increased oxidative capacity does not protect skeletal muscle fibers from eccentric contraction-induced injury. *American Journal of Physiology* 274 (*Regulatory*

Integrative Comparative Physiology) **43**, R1300–R1308.

Patel, T.J., Fridén, J. & Lieber, R.L. (1999) Sarcomere strain causes muscle injury during eccentric contractions. In: *Transactions of the 45th Meeting of the Orthopaedic Research Society, February 1–4, Anaheim, California* (ed. T.D. Brown), p. 141. Orthopaedic Research Society, Rosemont, IL.

Saxton, J.M. & Donnely, A.E. (1996) Length-specific impairment of skeletal muscle contractile function after eccentric muscle actions in man. *Clinical Science* **90**, 119–125.

Smith, J.L., Betts, B., Edgerton, V.R. & Zernicke, R.F. (1980) Rapid ankle extension during paw shakes: selective recruitment of fast ankle extensors. *Journal of Neurophysiology* **43**, 612–620.

Sögaard, K., Christensen, H., Jensen, B.R., Finsen, L. & Sjögaard, G. (1996) Motor control and kinetics during low level concentric and eccentric contractions in man. *Electroencephalography and Clinical Neurophysiology* **101**, 453–460.

Sorichter, S., Mair, J., Koller, A. *et al.* (1997) Skeletal troponin I as a marker of exercise-induced muscle damage. *Journal of Applied Physiology* **83**, 1076–1082.

Stauber, W.T. (1989) Eccentric action of muscles: physiology, injury, and adaptation. In: *Exercise and Sport Sciences Reviews* (ed. K.B. Pandolf), **17**. Williams & Wilkins, Baltimore.

Stauber, W.T. (1990) Repair models and specific tissue responses in muscle injury. In: *Sports-Induced Inflammation* (eds W.B. Leadbetter, J.A. Buckwalter & S.L. Gordon), pp. 205–213. American Academy of Orthopaedic Surgeons, Park Ridge, IL.

Stauber, W.T., Clarkson, P.M., Fritz, V.K. & Evans, W.J. (1990) Extracellular matrix disruption after eccentric muscle action. *Journal of Applied Physiology* **69**, 868–874.

Talbot, J.A. & Morgan, D.L. (1998) The effects of stretch parameters on eccentric exercise-induced damage to toad skeletal muscle. *Journal of Muscle Research and Cell Motility* **19**, 237–245.

Tax, A.A.M., Denier van der Gon, J.J., Gielen, C.C.A.M. & van den Tempel, C.M.M. (1989) Differences in the activation of M. biceps brachii in the control of slow isotonic movements and isometric contractions. *Experimental Brain Research* **76**, 55–63.

Tesch, P.A., Dudley, G.A., Duvosin, M.R., Hather, B.M. & Harris, R.T. (1990) Force and EMG signal patterns during repeated bouts of concentric or eccentric muscle actions. *Acta Physiologica Scandinavica* **138**, 263–271.

Tidball, J.G. (1986) Energy stored and dissipated in skeletal muscle basement membranes during sinusoidal oscillations. *Biophysical Journal* **50**, 1127–1138.

Warren, G., Hayes, D., Lowe, D., Guo, W. & Armstrong, R. (1991) Mechanical factors in exercise-induced muscle injury. *FASEB Journal* **5**, A1036.

Warren, G.L., Hayes, D.A., Lowe, D.A. & Armstrong, R.B. (1993a) Mechanical factors in the initiation of eccentric contraction-induced injury in rat soleus muscle. *Journal of Physiology (London)* **464**, 457–475.

Warren, G.L., Hayes, D.A., Lowe, D.A., Prior, B.M. & Armstrong, R.B. (1993b) Materials fatigue initiates eccentric contraction-induced injury in rat soleus muscle. *Journal of Physiology (London)* **464**, 477–489.

Warren, G.L., Lowe, D.A., Hayes, D.A., Karwoski, C.J., Prior, B.M. & Armstrong, R.B. (1993c) Excitation failure in eccentric contraction-induced injury of mouse soleus muscle. *Journal of Physiology (London)* **468**, 487–499.

Waterman-Storer, C.M. (1991) The cytoskeleton of skeletal muscle: is it affected by exercise? A brief review. *Medicine and Science in Sports and Exercise* **11**, 1240–1249.

Westing, S.H., Seger, J.Y. & Thorstensson, A. (1990) Effects of electrical stimulation on eccentric and concentric torque-velocity relationships during knee extension in man. *Acta Physiologica Scandinavica* **140**, 17–22.

PART 6

SPECIAL OLYMPIC SPORTS

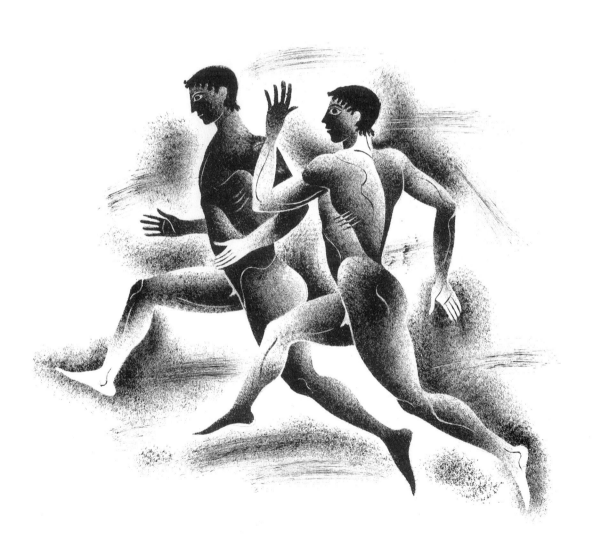

Chapter 29

Manual Wheelchair Propulsion

L.H.V. VAN DER WOUDE, H.E.J. VEEGER AND A.J. DALLMEIJER

Introduction

Among the Olympic sports for individuals with a disability, wheelchair sports historically have taken a central position. Apart from track and field events, typical wheelchair sports include tennis, basketball and quad-rugby. Wheelchair sports have developed strongly since World War II.* Simultaneously, sports performance has evolved dramatically during these decades, and consequentially competition levels have improved greatly.

Over the years, wheelchairs used in sports events have changed from, in the early 1960s, the chromium-plated wheelchairs intended for everyday use, to the current high-tech sports-specific devices. Initially, the athletes themselves largely implemented design changes and improved the fitting procedures. At a later stage wheelchair manufacturers took over this process and now custom-made wheelchairs, accurately tuned to the individual as well as to the conditions of wheelchair use, are available in all sports disciplines (Fig. 29.1). During the last decade, researchers have contributed significantly to the understanding of wheelchair arm work and sports performance. Research initially started from a mechanical point of view, and concentrated on materials, durability, safety and vehicle mechanics. At a later stage interest in manual wheelchair propulsion

was directed towards physiological responses, and more recently the focus has been on biomechanical aspects.

Three basic elements of the wheelchair–athlete combination determine the final performance in wheelchair sports (Woude 1989):

1 the athlete, who essentially produces the energy and power for propulsion;

2 the technical status and vehicle mechanics of the wheelchair itself, which determine the power requirements; and

3 the wheelchair–user interaction, which determines the efficiency of power transfer from the 'engine' to the wheelchair.

The contribution of biomechanics to the understanding of these three elements and in attaining and improving maximum performance in wheelchair sports is exemplified in this chapter.

Obviously, a wide variety of hand-propelled wheelchairs is available on the market. One cannot speak of 'the wheelchair', even if we isolate the hand rim-propelled wheelchair, which is used in 99% of the wheelchair sports events. Even small variations in wheelchair configuration will lead to differences in the man–machine interaction and in vehicle mechanics. This influences physiological and biomechanical measures of performance.

Wheelchair sports are subject to regulations. Pro-pelling mechanisms other than hand rims are not allowed in official events and competition. Only recently, the advantages of crank- and lever-propelled wheelchairs (tricycles) have become evident to the athletes. These propulsion mechanisms

*The development of wheelchair sports was accom-panied by the appearance of new magazines for wheel-chair sports, such as *Sports 'n' Spokes*.

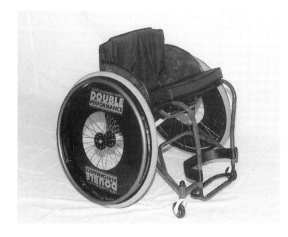

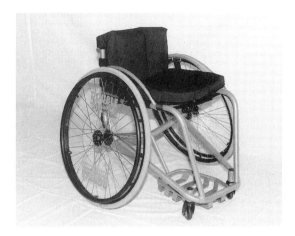

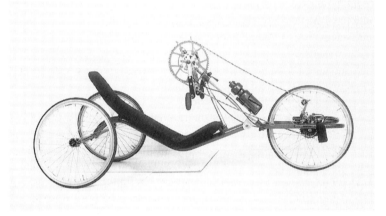

Fig. 29.1 Typical wheelchair designs: ADL wheelchair (top left), sport wheelchair (top right), crank wheelchair (bottom). (Courtesy of Double Performance in Gouda, The Netherlands.)

are used in open competitions and events only. However, given the dominance of hand rim propulsion, the biomechanics in this section will primarily focus on this type of interface.

Wheelchair propulsion and wheelchair sports have been studied from a wide variety of perspectives, i.e. sports, athlete and task specific. The biomechanics of manual wheelchair propulsion has predominantly been centred on the cyclic nature of this bimanual movement pattern. The following section will address largely the biomechanics of manual wheelchair propulsion within the concepts of cyclic movement analyses.

Research strategy

Cyclic movement

Manual wheelchair propulsion is frequently studied as a cyclic movement pattern (Woude *et al.* 1986; Ingen Schenau 1988); a given propelling motion is repeated over time at a given frequency (f), generally to maintain a certain stationary velocity (v). This implies that in each stroke or push of the wheel the athlete produces a more or less equal amount of work (A). The advantage of this approach is that physiological measures (i.e. energy cost, physical strain) can elegantly be linked with biomechanical measures (i.e. power output, work, force and torque production). The product of push frequency and work gives the average external power output (P_o, measured in watts), according to:

$$P_o = f \times A \qquad (29.1)$$

The work produced in each push constitutes the integral of the momentary torque (M) applied by the hands to the hand rim over a more or less fixed angular displacement (Q). The push is discontinuous, under steady-state conditions highly reproducible, and generally limited to an angle of 70–80°. Based on these parameters the above Eqn. 29.1 can be rewritten as:

$$P_o = f \times \int M dQ \qquad (29.2)$$

where torque is the product of the bimanual tangential force which is applied on the hand rim, and the radius of the hand rim.

Measurement of angular displacement and the torque around the wheel-axle requires specialized experimental techniques for motion analysis and force measurement, which are not widely available. Therefore a different approach to determine P_o is frequently employed. Here the forces resisting the wheelchair–athlete combination are taken as the starting point for the calculation of power output. The wheelchair–athlete combination is approached as a free body that moves at a given speed (v) and encounters the following (drag) forces: rolling friction (F_{roll}), air resistance (F_{air}), gravitational effects when going up/down a slope ($mg \sin \alpha$) and internal friction (F_{int}) (Fig. 29.2). Details of these forces are discussed below (see 'Vehicle mechanics'). The product of the sum of these drag forces (F_{drag}) and the velocity of the free body equals the power output that must be produced to maintain a constant velocity, according to:

$$P_o = F_{drag} \times v \qquad (29.3)$$

The drag force can fairly easily be determined through a drag test (Bennedik *et al.* 1978; Woude *et al.* 1986).

Armwork and mechanical efficiency

Power production during wheelchair propulsion is achieved by armwork. The relatively small muscle

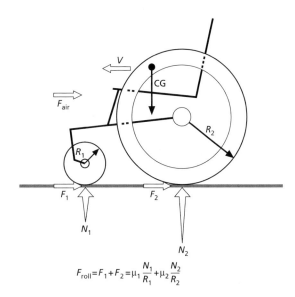

Fig. 29.2 Wheelchair–user combination as a free body diagram (see text for explanation). (From Woude 1987.)

mass of the upper extremities and increased tendency for local fatigue leads to a much lower maximal work capacity in comparison to legwork. Peak oxygen uptake is usually 20–40% lower in armwork compared to legwork. Measurement of power output in wheelchair exercise testing, in combination with physiological measurements, gives information on the physical capacity of the person, but is also required for the calculation of the efficiency of the wheelchair–user system. The gross mechanical efficiency (GME) is defined as the ratio between externally produced energy (power out) and internally liberated energy (En:, i.e. oxygen cost under submaximal, physiological steady state conditions), according to:

$$\text{GME} = (P_o/\text{En}) \times 100 \, (\%) \qquad (29.4)$$

The mechanical efficiency of wheelchair propulsion is as low as 2–10% (Woude *et al.* 1986), which is lower than in arm cranking, where values of around 15% are commonly found (Sawka 1986). The low efficiency of hand rim wheelchair propulsion may be explained by the small muscle mass in comparison with legwork, the complex movement pattern, and the complex functional anatomy of the upper

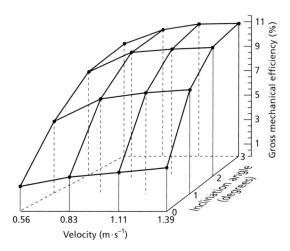

Fig. 29.3 Mechanical efficiency in relation to speed and resistance. (From Woude *et al.* 1988a.)

extremity. The mechanical efficiency is highly influenced by propulsion conditions, such as (hand rim) velocity and resistance: efficiency increases with higher velocities and higher workloads (Woude *et al.* 1988a; Veeger *et al.* 1992a) (Fig. 29.3). The configuration of the wheelchair, such as propulsion mechanism, seat height, and differences in individual

propelling technique, can also affect the mechanical efficiency (Woude *et al.* 1988a,b, 1989, 1995; Brown *et al.* 1990).

Experimental set-ups to study wheelchair propulsion

As mentioned before, in order to study performance capacity and propulsion proficiency of wheelchair athletes, a physiological and/or biomechanical analysis is required. Standardized laboratory experiments are conducted with the help of specially designed equipment, which varies in terms of reliability and validity. In Table 29.1 an overview is given of different experimental set-ups in relation to reliability and validity, with certain feasible research purposes. Obviously, the choice of experimental set-up is dependent on the research purpose, but also on the availability of measurement systems. Wheelchair tests are generally performed to investigate the physical capacity of wheelchair users, to analyse wheelchair propulsion technique, to assess different wheelchair–user systems, or to evaluate load on the upper-extremity joints. For physical capacity testing, physiological responses and, preferably, power output have to be measured. Power

Table 29.1 Reliability, validity and research purposes for different experimental set-ups to investigate wheelchair performance.

			Research purpose*				
Experimental set-up	Reliability	Validity	1: kinematics/ EMG	2: work capacity	3: efficiency	4: forces	5: modelling
Track	–	++	+/–	–	–	–	–
Treadmill	+/–	+	+	+	+	–	–
Electrical or mechanical braked wheelchair ergometer	+	–	–	+	–	–	–
3D instrumented wheel	+	+	+	+	+	+	+
Wheelchair simulator	++	+/–	+	+	+	–	–
3D wheelchair simulator	++	+/–	+	+	+	+	+

*Research purpose:
1. To evaluate kinematics and EMG.
2. To evaluate work capacity of wheelchair users (physiology and power output).
3. To evaluate efficiency of wheelchair-user system (physiology and power output).
4. To evaluate force application (biomechanics).
5. To evaluate mechanical load on the upper extremity (biomechanics and kinematics).

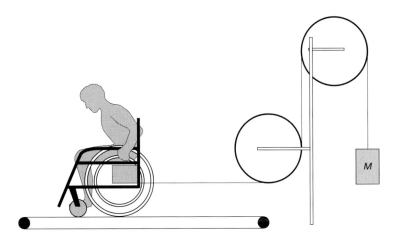

Fig. 29.4 Treadmill.

output and physiological parameters are required for the evaluation of different wheelchair–user systems. If wheelchair propulsion technique is the object of research, kinematics, electromyography (EMG), and probably force application are of interest. For evaluation of mechanical load on the upper extremity, 3D force measurements and kinematics are required as input for a biomechanical model.

Track and treadmill

The least standardized but most realistic testing condition is a simple wheelchair (racing) track. Evidently, it is complicated to control experimental conditions and procedures, such as velocity and power output, which reduces reliability for this experimental set-up. Since the wheelchair–user com-

bination is non-stationary, physiological measures and kinematics are complicated to measure. Clearly, the validity of a wheelchair track is high and it may be a useful set-up to investigate biomechanics in combination with an instrumented wheelchair wheel that allows 3D force measurements (Cooper *et al.* 1997).

Second best in terms of validity is a motor-driven treadmill (Fig. 29.4). This device is widely used for research purposes. It allows valid physiological exercise testing, and the study of kinematics and muscle activity (e.g. Gass & Camp 1979; Sanderson & Sommer 1985; Woude *et al.* 1986). Power output can be determined in the form of a simple drag test, in which the drag force of a wheelchair–user system can be determined (Bennedik *et al.* 1978; Woude *et al.* 1986) (Fig. 29.5). Workload can be varied with an

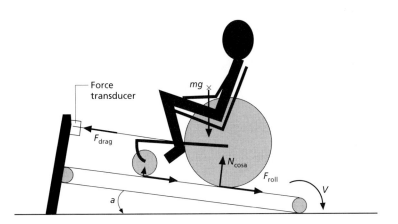

Fig. 29.5 Drag test on a treadmill; the drag force (F_{drag}) of a wheelchair–user combination is measured with a force transducer at different slopes (a) and a constant velocity (V).

inclination of the belt, or by applying a resistance force on the back of the wheelchair by means of a pulley system. Calculation of power output from drag force and velocity enables the evaluation of efficiency parameters for a given wheelchair system or configuration at submaximal, steady-state exercise conditions. Variations in calculated drag force are generally small but may, due to oscillations of the trunk, arms and head and the consequent effect on rolling friction, increase up to 10%. Treadmill wheelchair propulsion is mechanically realistic, showing a natural form of wheelchair propulsion—with additional small steering corrections—while rolling friction and inertia are realistic. Absence of air drag, however, reduces validity, and probably has an (unstudied) effect on

performance and propulsion technique. The treadmill set-up and track require the use of an actual (individual) wheelchair. This has advantages—the wheelchair–athlete combination is highly trained and is realistic within the context of wheelchair sports. A disadvantage is that it does not easily allow individual optimization of configurations of the wheelchair. If an instrumented wheel (Cooper *et al.* 1997; Wu *et al.* 1998) is available, the study of force production is also possible.

Wheelchair ergometers and simulators

Many different wheelchair ergometers have been developed, either with or without the actual use of a wheelchair, sometimes linked to an existing (cycle)

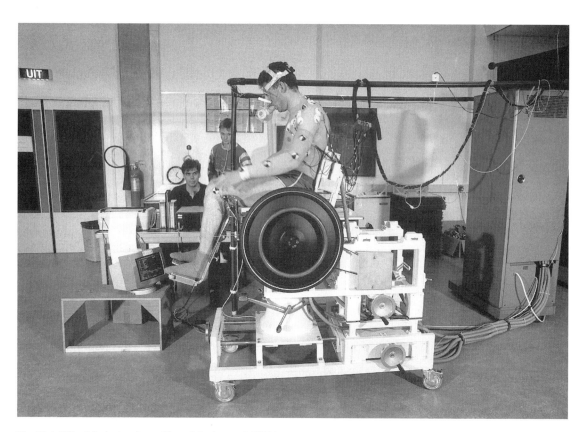

Fig. 29.6 Wheelchair simulator. (From Niesing *et al.* 1990.)

ergometer, or based on a roller system (e.g. Glaser 1985). These set-ups use mechanical or electric brakes for resistance, while inertia is not known, which limits the evaluation of realistic wheelchair propulsion characteristics. Since testing conditions are highly reproducible, these types of wheelchair ergometer are adequate for reliable exercise testing and evaluation of physical work capacity, in particular if the system can accurately measure external power.

The final category of wheelchair ergometer is the wheelchair simulator. Most of these are computer-controlled devices that accurately simulate wheelchair propulsion with an adjustable propulsion mechanism and seat configuration. Essentially it comes down to the simulation of wheelchair propulsion in terms of friction (rolling resistance, and sometimes air friction) and slope, and simulation of inertia of the wheelchair–user system. Most systems enable measurement of momentary torque and velocity, and thus power output (McLaurin & Brubaker 1991; Traut & Schmauder 1993), and sometimes the measurement of 3D forces applied by the hand on the propulsion system (Niesing *et al.* 1990) (Fig. 29.6). Power, torque and force acquisition and analysis enable rather detailed studies of propulsion technique in conjunction with different standard physiological measures, while the system does allow careful standardization of the wheelchair–user configuration. In combination with kinematic input, 3D force data can be used for biomechanical modelling (see 'Biomechanics of wheelchair propulsion'). This can provide information on forces acting on the joints of the upper extremity, which can contribute to the understanding of the high incidence of musculoskeletal disorders in wheelchair athletes.

An instrumented wheelchair wheel also allows reliable measurement of 3D force application under highly realistic conditions (Cooper *et al.* 1997; Wu *et al.* 1998). This device can be used for evaluation of propulsion forces and muscular activity on a wheelchair track. In combination with a treadmill, kinematics and physiology can be easily measured, while velocity and workload can be controlled.

Physical capacity of the wheelchair athlete

Exercise testing

The study of wheelchair propulsion is hampered not only by the large variety of research methods (see above), but also by the marked variability in ability among studied subject groups. To overcome the problem of the large heterogeneity of the disabled population, it seems quite appropriate to study non-wheelchair users first, since they will be equally well (un-) trained on all tested conditions and obviously will be quite physically homogeneous. In the evaluation of design aspects of wheelchairs, such as propulsion mechanisms, this seems a useful initial strategy. Furthermore, the effects of wheelchair armwork on the cardiovascular and/or musculoskeletal systems of non-disabled persons can be determined.

As in legwork, both maximum aerobic and anaerobic capacity tests are used in evaluating the wheelchair athlete population. Wheelchair exercise experiments have been conducted on a varied mixture of wheelchair athletes and users. The strong variability in the population requires a flexible set of exercise tests. Various aerobic and anaerobic tests have been described, but little standardization is yet apparent. In general, the findings appear more or less consistent, but may be rather susceptible to the specifics of the testing protocol. Most frequently, groups of athletes have been studied (Gass & Camp 1979; Veeger *et al.* 1991a), whereas a few studies are available on sedentary wheelchair users (Janssen *et al.* 1993), while groups of elderly subjects and children have hardly been studied (Sawka *et al.* 1981; Bednarczyk & Sanderson 1994). Also, measurements usually focused on male subjects. As a consequence data for female subjects are scarce.

Since wheelchair athletes not only differ in disability but also in age, gender, sports discipline and expertise, classification is common in wheelchair competition. Classification of subjects is a major issue in wheelchair sports and subject to strong debate. Functional classification is, however, a prerequisite for competition and important

Table 29.2 Aerobic capacity in wheelchair athletes (men) of some selected armcrank and wheelchair ergometry studies.

Authors	Mode	n	ISMGF	Disability	Vo_2 ($l \cdot min^{-1}$)	Vo_2 ($ml \cdot kg^{-1} \cdot min^{-1}$)	Heart rate (beats $\cdot min^{-1}$)	Power output (W)
Davis & Shephard (1988)	ACE	15	III–V	T6–L5	2.24	–	182	97
Veeger *et al.* (1991a)	MDT	1	Ic	C7–C8	1.64	27.3	150	–
		6	II	T1–T5	1.84	23.0	170	66
		10	III	T6–T10	1.97	26.8	175	80
		13	IV	T11–L3	2.42	36.9	182	85
		7	V	L4–S1	2.38	40.6	182	79
		3	Other	POL	2.94	39.4	160	93
Woude *et al.* (unpublished)	WCE	3	T1	C5/6–C7	0.67	–	110	22
		4	T2	C7	1.30	–	133	51
		8	T3	T5–L1	2.04	–	183	86
		23	T4	T6–S1 POL, SB	2.29	–	187	106
		6 (1F)	CP	CP	0.91	–	150	27
		6 (1F)	AMP	AMP, KA, HEM	2.38	–	186	88
Huonker *et al.* (1998)	WCE	29	II–VI	T1–S2	–	34.5	183	89

Key: ACE, armcrank ergometry; MDT, motor-driven treadmill; WCE, wheelchair ergometry.
T1–T4, ISMGF functional classification; AMP, amputees; CP, cerebral palsy; HEM, hemiplegia; KA, knee arthrodesis; POL, polio; SB, spina bifida; F, female.

in experimental research, since performance characteristics always must be placed within the framework of functional level of the subject (impairment, disability and handicap). Studies such as that performed by Higgs *et al.* (1990) led to a reduction in the number of classes in the International Stoke Mandeville Games Federation (ISMGF) classification system, and finally to the introduction of a functional classification system at world sports events.

Numerically large studies investigating performance capacity are scarce (Veeger *et al.* 1991a). One of them concerns a group of 68 athletes participating in the World Games and Championships in 1990 (Woude *et al.* 1997). Subjects conducted both aerobic and anaerobic wheelchair exercise tests on a computer-controlled wheelchair ergometer. Results stress the high variability among the wheelchair athlete population (Table 29.2).

Aerobic capacity

The aerobic capacity of wheelchair athletes has been subject to study over the years. However, not all authors present power output values next to cardiorespiratory results, like peak oxygen uptake and heart rate (Fig. 29.7). Tables 29.2 and 29.3 show the results of studies in which peak cardiorespiratory responses as well as power output were determined in male and female wheelchair athletes. Dependent on disability, values for maximal power output vary from around 20 W for persons with a cervical spinal cord injury or cerebral palsy, to around 100 W for persons with less severe disabilities (low paraplegia and amputees). For peak oxygen uptake, values ranging from less than $1 l \cdot min^{-1}$ to more than $3 l \cdot min^{-1}$ are reported (Table 29.2). Physical capacity is considerably lower in female athletes (Table 29.3). Variations in power output can also be influenced by the mode of exercise testing. Arm cranking is a widely used testing mode for persons with disabilities. However, because of the

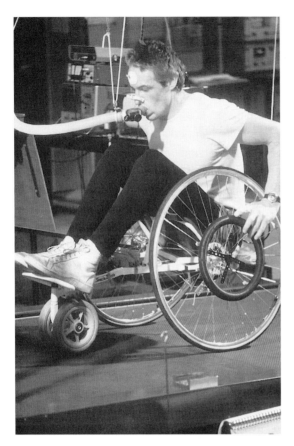

Fig. 29.7 Oxygen uptake in a maximal aerobic exercise test.

higher efficiency in comparison with wheelchair ergometry, higher peak power outputs are found in arm cranking tests, whereas peak oxygen consumption is not affected. Therefore, when the interest is focused on sport performance or daily wheelchair use, wheelchair exercise testing is greatly preferred.

Anaerobic capacity

Results of anaerobic capacity tests in wheelchair athletes are listed in Table 29.4. Values again do show considerable interstudy variation, which is not solely the consequence of population variation, but is also influenced by the experimental set-up and protocol used. In general the sprint power output is calculated over a 30 s full-out sprinting test, indicative of anaerobic power output. However, sprint performance is highly dependent on the resistance that subjects are exposed to; Veeger *et al.* (1989a) showed decreases in mean sprint power output as a consequence of a lower resistance. This decline is the consequence of a higher mean linear hand velocity (in the push phase) with a lower resistance. Again, in arm cranking, higher maximal power outputs are found in comparison with wheelchair armwork. Mean anaerobic power production in the wheelchair sprint test did not exceed 200 W. Extremely low values for power output were seen in subjects with cerebral palsy or with a cervical spinal cord injury.

Table 29.3 Aerobic capacity in wheelchair athletes (women) of some selected armcrank and wheelchair ergometry studies.

Authors	Mode	n	ISMGF	Disability	V_{O_2} ($l \cdot min^{-1}$)	V_{O_2} ($ml \cdot kg^{-1} \cdot min^{-1}$)	Heart rate (beats $\cdot$ min^{-1})	Power output (W)
Veeger *et al.* (1991a)	MDT	1	Ic	C7/8	0.80	–	–	–
		7	III–V	T6–S1	1.28	–	–	–
		8	All (Ic, III–V)	C7/8–S1	1.22	20.7	172	39
Woude *et al.* (unpublished)	WCE	4	T2	C5–C7, POL	0.74	–	143	30
		3	T3	T8, SB	1.30	–	184	64
		3	T4	T12–S1, SB, POL	1.15	–	187	61

Key: MDT, motor-driven treadmill; WCE, wheelchair ergometry.
T2–T4, ISMGF functional classification; POL, polio; SB, spina bifida.

Table 29.4 Wheelchair sprint power production in wheelchair athletes (men and women) for a number of studies.

Authors	Mode	n	ISMGF	Disability	Peak sprint P_o (W)	Peak sprint P_o (W · kg^{-1})
Coutts & Stogryn (1987)	WCE	2	Ia, Ib	C6–C7	46	0.77
		3	III–V	T9–T12, POL	143	2.02
		1 (F)	IV	T10	85	1.73
Lees & Arthur (1988)	WCE	6	II–V	T1–L5	102–149*	–
Woude et al. (1997)	WCE	3	T1	C5/6–C7	23	0.36
		4	T2	C7	68	1.03
		8	T3	T5–L1	100	1.65
		23	T4	T6–S1, POL, SB	138	2.36
		6 (1F)	CP	CP	35	0.51
		6 (1F)	AMP	AMP, KA, HEM	121	1.85
		4 (F)	T2	C5–C7, POL	38	0.83
		3 (F)	T3	T8, SB	77	1.47
		3 (F)	T4	T12–S1, SB, POL	76	1.51
Hutzler et al. (1998)	ACE	13	II	T1–T5	280	–
		15	III–VI	T6–S5	336	–
		10	AMP	AMP	443	–
		12	POL	POL	394	–
		40	All		341	–

*Values dependent on different workloads.
Key: ACE, armcrank ergometry; WCE, wheelchair ergometry.
T1–T4, ISMGF functional classification; AMP, amputees; CP, cerebral palsy; HEM, hemiplegia; KA, knee arthrodesis; POL, polio; SB, spina bifida; F, female.

Biomechanics of wheelchair propulsion

Introduction

Over the last decade, manual wheelchair propulsion and wheelchair sports have increasingly become subjects of biomechanical analyses. One of the main reasons for this increased interest is the fact that wheelchair propulsion appears to be related to high mechanical loads on the upper extremity, which often lead to overload injuries in arms and shoulders (Burnham et al. 1993; Boninger et al. 1996). To gain insight into the causes and consequences of these high loads, as well as to study propulsion technique as such, biomechanical analysis is a prerequisite.

Of course, propulsion techniques are highly dependent on the type of wheelchair used, as well as the functional capacity of the athlete. As a consequence, direct application of most of the findings is rather difficult. However, the use of general biomechanical principles, as well as the usefulness of look-ing at wheelchair propulsion from a biomechanical perspective, are the most important elements in this paragraph. It should be kept in mind, however, that almost all available information is based on studies of daily-use, tennis or basketball hand-rim wheelchairs. As a consequence, little will be said about the 'butterfly' technique, a typical wheelchair racing technique which was recently introduced. This (butterfly-like) beating technique deviates considerably from the more general 'grabbing' technique and has not been studied yet.

In hand-rim wheelchair propulsion the mechanical burden on the musculoskeletal system is high. As a consequence, shoulder pain and carpal tunnel syndrome are common problems for wheelchair athletes (Burnham & Steadward 1994; Jackson et al. 1996), although the wheelchair racing population does not appear to be at higher risk than the general wheelchair user population (Boninger et al. 1997).

The high mechanical load on the upper extremity can, at least partially, be explained by the complex

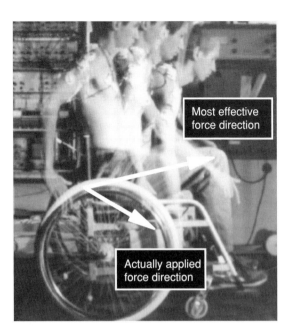

Most effective
force direction

Actually applied
force direction

Fig. 29.8 Illustration of the direction of the propulsion force during 'normal' wheelchair propulsion and the relation with the most effective force direction.

anatomy of arm and shoulder. More specifically, the complaints might be related to the need to stabilize the glenohumeral (GH) joint (usually loosely referred to as the 'shoulder joint') during wheelchair propulsion. Also, the way in which forces are applied to the hand rims appears to play an important role. Experiments in which the propulsion forces were measured have shown that the direction of the applied forces did not agree with the most optimal direction in terms of power production, i.e. the direction tangential to the hand rims. Figure 29.8 illustrates the different force components. Surprisingly, this apparently suboptimal direction of force application was found for athletes as well as untrained subjects (Veeger *et al.* 1992b; Roeleveld *et al.* 1994; Boninger *et al.* 1997; Wu 1998). It appears that this particular manner of force application is the most efficient force application technique. In other words, subjects appear to adopt the technique which demands the least energy, given the mechanical constraints of the wheelchair–user combination (Veeger & Woude 1994).

For a better insight into the causes of the high load on the upper extremity and the consequences for propulsion technique, a biomechanical analysis of the wheelchair push is required. Some of the findings, in particular the propulsion force, the torque of the hand onto the hand rim surface, and mechanical load on shoulders and wrists will be discussed. First, a brief introduction regarding the anatomy of the upper extremity will be given.

Anatomy

In contrast to the human leg, the human arm is not specialized as an extremity that is adapted for a specific category of tasks. Unlike the leg it can be used for a large diversity of tasks, varying from manipulation of small objects to handling of heavy materials. In addition, the human arm has a large range of motion. From an anatomical view, the difference in function between arms and legs is well reflected in the difference in structure between the shoulder girdle and the pelvis. Figure 29.9 illustrates the elements of arm and shoulder girdle.

As stated before, the arm has a large range of motion. This is caused by the fact that the arm is connected to the scapula, which has a loose connection to the trunk. Because the scapula is able to slide and rotate over the surface of the rib cage, it is possible to move the base of the arm; the GH joint. This leads to a dramatic increase in the reach of the arm (Fig. 29.10). Of course, the intermuscular coordination of the muscles that connect the scapula to the trunk is extremely important in this.

A second reason for the large range of motion of the arm is the fact that the GH joint is shaped as a small and shallow cup (the glenoid) and a large saucer (the humeral head). Cup and saucer are connected by strong, but loose, ligamentous tissue. The joint structure allows rotations in three directions, as well as some translation. As a result, the range of motion of the arm is already quite considerable, even if the scapula is fixed (Fig. 29.10).

Despite the fact that the glenohumeral joint is loose, spontaneous (sub)luxation seldom occurs. It is assumed that this is the result of muscular control by the rotator cuff muscles, hence good coordination between these muscles is very important. Also,

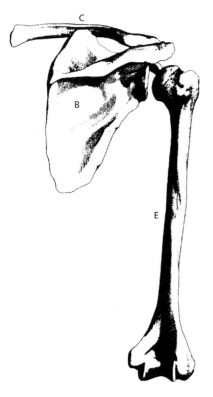

Fig. 29.9 Frontal view of the bony parts of the human shoulder. B, Shoulder blade, or scapula; E, upper arm, or humerus; C, clavicle.

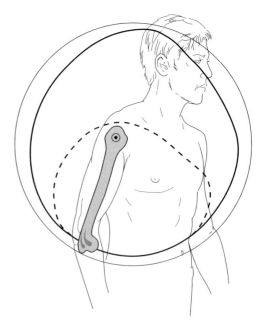

Fig. 29.10 Range of motion curves for the distal end of the humerus, projected as a sphere with the shoulder as centre. Dashed line represents scapular movement only; bold line represents glenohumeral movement; and solid line represents total movement. (From Rozendal *et al.* 1974.)

athletes who have an incomplete shoulder muscle system, and for whom muscular control is hampered, will be at risk of shoulder (sub)luxations (Campbell & Koris 1996).

Shoulder and wrist complaints are very common within the wheelchair–user combination. At least 50% of wheelchair users suffer from wrist complaints, and about 30–50% of the wheelchair users have problems with their shoulders (Sie *et al.* 1992). A later study indicated even higher prevalence rates, of up to 72% for complaints in one or both areas (Subbarao *et al.* 1995). The high prevalence of complaints is a clear indication that the mechanical load of wheelchair propulsion must be unfavourably high. One of the most likely reasons for the high mechanical load is the need for considerable muscular effort to stabilize the shoulder mechanism and especially to prevent shoulder luxations. These

additional muscular forces would then lead to overload of one or more of those muscles, but also to high compression forces in the GH joint, which in turn might damage joint cartilage.

To get an impression of the mechanical load and the underlying mechanisms, a biomechanical model is a prerequisite. In order to calculate the extra forces that would be necessary to stabilize the shoulder, a model is required that is able to calculate not only net joint torque but also individual muscle forces.

Biomechanics

Biomechanics is a powerful tool in mechanical analyses of the human musculoskeletal system. In biomechanics one often uses the inverse-dynamic modelling approach. This takes as its starting point —contrary to the direct-dynamic approach—the resulting movements and (external) forces. Starting from there, the approach then tries to estimate

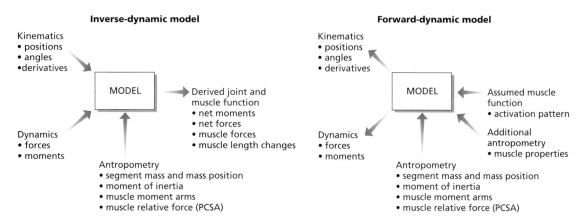

Fig. 29.11 Differences between inverse-dynamic and forward-dynamic models.

the forces and torques that have been applied by internal structures and that led to the given movement and forces. This approach can also be used to estimate the contribution of individual muscles to driving forces and torques (Fig. 29.11). The input of an inverse-dynamic model comprises the (externally) visible movements and forces. This means, of course, that these have to be measured. Movements can be measured with simple equipment such as video cameras, but also with sophisticated high-speed automatic systems. Important factors in the quality of input data are the frame frequency and image accuracy. If the movements studied are predominantly planar, such as long jumping, a two-dimensional analysis and recording of the movement usually suffices. The underlying assumption in that case is that movements in other planes are small and of lesser importance. For wheelchair propulsion this obviously is not the case. The movements do not occur in one plane and recordings from more than one view are necessary. With the help of special computer algorithms† two or more combinations of views can be used to reconstruct a three-dimensional description of the movement.

The other sources of input required are the forces.

† These algorithms are generally based on the direct linear transformation (DLT). In the DLT procedure, a reference frame with known markers is used to define the relationship between cameras and three-dimensional (3D) positions. Subsequently, the 3D positions of unknown markers can be estimated when at least two camera views are available.

In wheelchair propulsion studies, the forces can only be measured with highly specialized equipment, which is found in only a few research centres around the world. Both in the USA and in Taiwan, research groups use an instrumented wheel for their research (Cooper *et al.* 1997; Wu 1998). At the Vrije Universiteit in Amsterdam, we have a wheelchair simulator available (Niesing *et al.* 1990). An overview of the drawbacks and advantages of the different measurement systems is given above (see 'Experimental set-ups to study wheelchair propulsion').

Most inverse-dynamic models are capable of calculating the net joint torque and power. Net torques are a good indication of the muscular forces that are needed around a joint. However, these torques are net values, which implies that they are the sum of all muscle forces around that joint. Net torque values are thus likely to be underestimations of the actual muscle forces. For instance, if two antagonists produce the same force against the same torque arm, the resulting net torque will be zero, while the sum of muscles forces is not. In the shoulder, it is highly likely that, because of the need for sufficient joint stability, antagonists will be active at the same time. In analyses of muscle function in the shoulder therefore, a biomechanical model will be needed that estimates the contribution of muscles to net torques and resulting movements. Recently, a biomechanical model has been developed which includes muscles of the arm and shoulder. This model can now

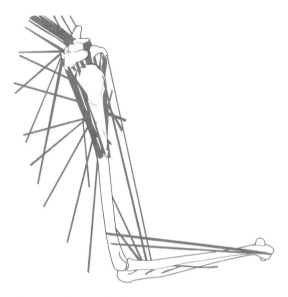

Fig. 29.12 The musculoskeletal model.

also be applied to manual wheelchair propulsion (Helm *et al.* 1997). Figure 29.12 is a graphical representation of the model.

Despite the fact that new wheelchair research tools have recently become available, most of the available data are still based on one measurement device, the wheelchair simulator. This situation is, however, likely to change in the near future. Although these data have been collected for modelling, the data in themselves have provided more insight into the characteristics of wheelchair propulsion. In the following, we will discuss the propulsion forces and the hand torque on the rims.

Propulsion forces

Wheelchair propulsion comprises a pushing phase and a recovery phase. During the pushing phase, the hands make contact with the rims and force is applied by the athlete to those rims. Since the hands hold the rims and therefore automatically follow the circular movement of those rims, the movement of the hands and arms can be characterized as a guided movement. In guided movements the forces that are applied by the hands do not directly influence the trajectory of the hands. As a consequence, it is

possible to apply force that is not tangential to the hand rims. Any force that has a tangential force component will contribute to propulsion. The propulsive force can, but does not have to be applied tangential to the hand rims.

Experimental results have shown that propulsion forces are indeed not tangentially directed. Veeger *et al.* (1991b) introduced the term 'fraction effective force' (FEF) as a measure for the effectiveness of force application. The fraction effective force is defined as:

$$FEF = \frac{F_m}{F_{tot}} \times 100\% \qquad (29.5)$$

where F_m is the tangential force component and F_{tot} is the magnitude of the propulsion force.

Table 29.5 gives an overview of FEF values as found in our own experiments. In general the FEF was below 80%. The data in Table 29.5 seem to agree with results from Wu (1998), who reported values of 47–49% for riding at a self-selected pace on level ground, and average FEF values of 63–74% for riding on a ramp of 2.9–7.1°. They also appear to agree with results of Boninger *et al.* (1997), who found values of 52–54% for the force ratio F_m^2/F^2, which is a slightly different definition for the FEF than is used here.

Both Boninger *et al.* (1997) and Wu (1998), use the term 'mechanical efficiency' when describing the force direction. Also, they view the force as being misdirected. Since mechanical efficiency has historically been used in physiology to describe the ratio between external energy production and consumed metabolic energy, the term efficiency should not be used. But more important, the suggestion that the force direction is inefficient and misdirected might well be based on a misconception of the interaction between athlete and wheelchair. In our view (Roeleveld *et al.* 1994; Helm & Veeger 1996) the force direction is in fact the most optimal force direction, given the mechanical constraints of the human musculoskeletal system and the interaction with the wheelchair propulsion system. In other words, the chosen force direction is the result of the most efficient propulsion technique possible.

To illustrate this concept, Fig. 29.13 depicts two possible conditions. One is the condition in which

Table 29.5 Torque, power and fraction effective force (FEF) for isometric, submaximal and 30-s sprint tests on a stationary wheelchair ergometer.

Test	Subject	(*n*)	Speed (m · s⁻¹)	(SD)	Power output (W)	(SD)	FEF (%)	(SD)
Submaximal	AB	8	0.56		26.6	(4.9)	81	(7)
			0.83		36.4	(5.7)	78	(7)
			1.11		46.7	(7.1)	73	(9)
			1.39		58.9	(7.7)	75	(10)
Submaximal Veeger *et al.* (1991a)	AB	9	0.83		18.2	(3.2)	72	(9)
			1.11		19.1	(4.3)	68	(13)
			1.39		18.7	(3.1)	67	(10)
			1.67		19.2	(4.6)	61	(10)
			0.83		37.1	(4.1)	70	(11)
			1.11		38.1	(6.4)	72	(9)
			1.39		38.1	(6.8)	72	(13)
			1.67		38.3	(7.1)	67	(8)
30 s tests Woude *et al.* (1998)	WA (male)	50	2.20	(0.50)	108	(45)	52	(9)
	WA (female)	17	2.0	(0.50)	66	(32)	53	(10)
Veeger *et al.* (1992b)	AB	10	1.97	(0.10)	96.0	(8.8)	57	(4)
	NWA	9	2.2	(0.40)	100	(29.4)	61	(16)
Dallmeijer *et al.* (1994)	NWA (C4–C8)	6	1.45	(0.28)	43.8	(24.6)	50	(12)
	(T1–T5)	5	1.95	(0.29)	94.4	(30.2)	59	(6)
	(T6–T10)	5	2.35	(0.37)	122	(20.4)	59	(7)
	(T11–L4)	7	2.15	(0.45)	98.3	(22.5)	59	(12)

Key: AB, able-bodied; NWA, non-wheelchair athletes; WA, wheelchair athletes.

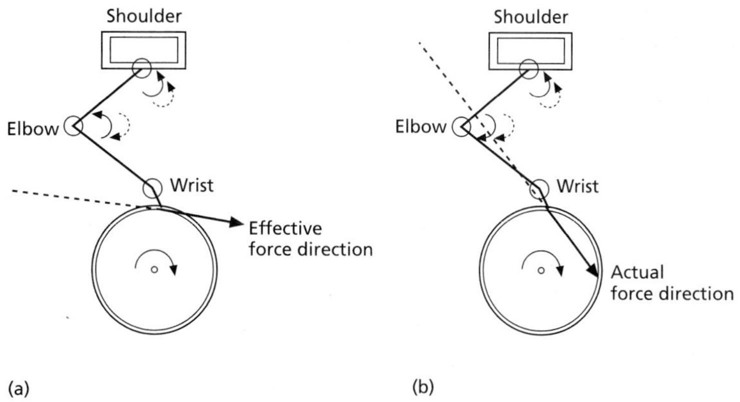

Fig. 29.13 The mechanically most effective force direction (a) and the actually applied force direction (b). The solid lines indicate the net moments around the shoulder and elbow. The dashed lines indicate the rotation direction in those joints. (From Veeger & Woude 1996.)

the mechanically most effective force is applied (a) and the other is the usually measured condition (b). If a wheelchair user were to propel her chair with a force that was directed following (a), the force would have to be generated through an anteflexion torque around the shoulder, in combination with an elbow flexion torque. These torques are shown as solid lines. On the other hand, the elbow has to be extended (dashed lines) to follow the hand rims in order to be able to apply force on those rims. As a consequence, the elbow flexors have to apply force against stretch, which is highly inefficient. It will be clear that the contribution of elbow flexors will increase the effectiveness of the propulsion force, but that the total force will be smaller. A second aspect of this force direction is that the strong elbow extensors cannot be used.

The conditions in (b) depict the force direction in which there is no conflict between torque direction and movement direction. This is the direction that is generally found. The assumption seems justified that this apparently inefficient form of propulsion is based on the most efficient solution, given the mechanical constraints of the system. The production of negative power is prevented and the strong elbow extensors can be used.

The above assumption has consequences for choosing methods to raise the low level of efficiency of wheelchair propulsion. Training of wheelchair propulsion technique may not simply focus on improving the effectiveness of force application—in cycling it has been shown that instruction to direct forces more effectively did not lead to higher efficiency levels (Lafortune & Cavanagh 1983). Instead, aspects of wheelchair configuration should be looked for in which the forces can be more effectively applied (with prevention of the conflict between movement direction and torque production around the elbow).

Torque applied by the hands onto the hand rims

Besides a propulsion force, the hands can also apply a torque on the hand rims. This torque can be imagined as a combination of a pushing force at the level of the wrist and a pulling force at the level of the index finger. The magnitude of the torque applied

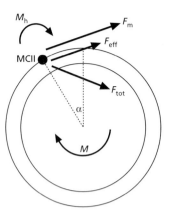

Fig. 29.14 Illustration of the principle of the hand moment. M_h, hand moment. F_{eff}, effective component of the propulsion force (F_{tot}). F_m, effective force determined from the propulsion torque (M). MCII is the (arbitrary) point of application.

by the hands to the hand rim surface can be derived from the differences between forces applied on the hand rims and the torque around the wheel axis (Fig. 29.14). If only a force is applied by the hands (F_{tot} in Fig. 29.13), the tangential component of the force that is applied on the rims (F_{eff}) should equal the torque divided by the wheel radius (F_m). The difference between F_{eff} and F_m equals the hand moment (M_h). There is some uncertainty in these estimations, however, since the exact value will depend on the point of force application in the hands (Linden et al. 1996).

From our estimations it became clear that the magnitude of this torque could be as high as 40% of the total propulsion torque. Unfortunately, the torque is generally directed against the propulsion torque for most of the push phase. Subjects appeared to work against themselves (Linden et al. 1996). One of the possible reasons for this activity might be the need to maintain sufficient contact with the rims to be able to apply force on those rims. As a consequence, the hands are being forced from radial deviation to ulnar deviation while the wrist flexors are likely to be active (Linden et al. 1996).

The application of a counterproductive hand torque is not only likely to be inefficient, but also

Table 29.6 Peak wrist angles, averaged over nine subjects and six experimental conditions. Peak wrist angles were either calculated over the full push angle, or over that part of the push angle where finger flexor activity is recorded. (From Veeger *et al*. 1998.)

Angle	Peak angle (°) (SD)	Peak angle + FA (°) (SD)	Active range of motion (average from literature)
Flexion	−14 (18)	−16 (15)	−76
Extension	34 (16)	32 (16)	66
Ulnar deviation	−24 (11)	−22 (11)	−35
Radial deviation	13 (12)	13 (10)	21

FA, flexor activity.

likely to be an important factor in the occurrence of carpal tunnel syndrome (CTS). Important predisposing factors for carpal tunnel syndrome are direct pressure on the carpal tunnel, extreme wrist positions and finger flexion activity (or tension on the tendons running through the carpal tunnel). Recent experiments (Veeger *et al*. 1998) have shown that during wheelchair propulsion, large wrist angles occur, even in combination with finger flexor activity. Peak ulnar and radial deviations were close to the range of motion seen in the general population. Table 29.6 gives the average peak values, in combination with typical values for the active range of motion in the wrist joint. The authors concluded that at least three possible contributory factors for CTS occur during wheelchair propulsion: extreme wrist excursions, occurring in combination with finger flexor activity, and a highly repetitive movement. Thus, in combination with the likelihood of considerable direct pressure of the rim on the carpal tunnel, a clear combination of three predisposing factors for CTS can be discerned in hand rim wheelchair propulsion. The suggestion, however, that a glove might reduce the risk for CTS (Veeger *et al*. 1998), could not be proven (Burnham *et al*. 1994).

Regarding the influence of the hand torque on efficiency, it should be mentioned here that in experiments in which a slightly wider rim tube was used, efficiency was significantly improved. However, no significant reductions of the magnitude of the hand torque were found (Linden *et al*. 1996).

Modelling results

Modelling results from several authors have indicated that the largest joint torques are produced around the shoulder complex. Veeger *et al*. (1991b) reported peak shoulder flexion torques of 35 N m, in combination with peak adduction torques of 20 N m. Peak elbow extension torques were 10 N m. Wu (1998) also reported largest torques around the shoulder joint, but predominantly as a shoulder flexion torque. The peak elbow extension torques were surprisingly small (43 N m and 6.1 N m, for shoulder and elbow respectively, for riding up a 2.9° ramp). Rodgers *et al*. (1998) found a large shoulder flexion torque of approx. 30 N m and elbow extension torque of approximately 10 N m.

When these values are interpreted, it should be kept in mind that the shoulder data are in fact based on a simplification of the shoulder complex as a single ball-and-socket joint. It is likely that inclusion of the scapula as a separate segment will have a lowering effect on the torques estimated in this way. However, the large torques around the shoulder complex indicate large muscle forces. This is supported by electromyographic data of Mulroy *et al*. (1996), who found the highest EMG activity in the supraspinatus muscle and sternal part of pectoralis major.

Wrist joint torques were reported by Boninger *et al*. (1997), who calculated the largest peak torques around the wrist in the direction of ulnar deviation (16.6 N m at 1.3 m · s⁻¹ travelling velocity in a standard wheelchair). The peak wrist extension torque

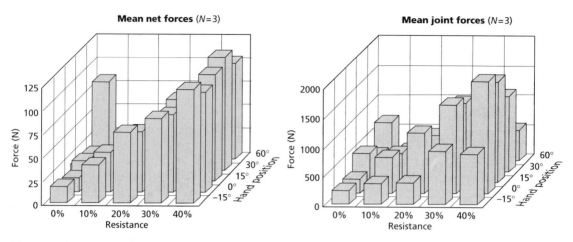

Fig. 29.15 Average results for the net forces on the GH joint (*left*) and the compression forces in the joint (*right*). (Reprinted from Helm & Veeger 1996, p. 49, with permission from Elsevier Science.)

was smaller, but still 10.4 N m (1.3 m · s⁻¹). These relationships between ulnar deviation and extension are supported in other publications (Rodgers *et al.* 1998). The large wrist torques and especially the large ulnar deviation torque can be seen as another risk factor for the occurrence of CTS.

The previously mentioned musculoskeletal model of the upper extremity has been applied to a quasi-static approximation of wheelchair propulsion (Helm & Veeger 1996). The wheelchair push was simulated by asking the subjects to push their chair with their hands on different positions of the hand rims (−15°, 0°, 15°, 30°, 45° and 60°). Also, measurements were performed against different resistances, from 0% to 40% of the maximal push force on the rims (244 ± 20 N, $n = 10$). The model was then used

to estimate the compression force in the GH joint and to compare those values with the net forces that work on the joint. Net forces are defined as the result of all external forces, generally the combination of the propulsion force and gravity. Compression forces are the net forces and the forces that work on the joint internally, i.e. by muscles and ligaments that work together to produce the propulsion force. Results of these calculations are given in Fig. 29.15. The calculations showed that the compression force in the GH joint could be as high as 2000 N or 200 kg. One of the main reasons for this high compression force was the additional muscle force that was needed to stabilize the GH joint (Fig. 29.16). Forces in the rotator cuff muscles were high, while at the same time their contribution to the external torque

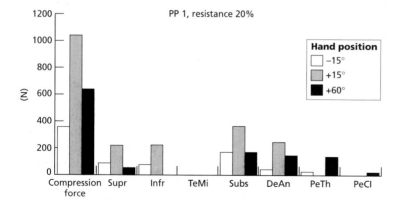

Fig. 29.16 Estimated muscle forces of a selection of shoulder muscles, plotted together with the compression force in the glenohumeral joint. Supr, supraspinatus; Infr, infraspinatus; TeMi, teres minor; Subs, subscapularis; DeAn, deltoideus pars anterior; PeTh, pectoralis major, pars thoracale; PeCl, pectoralis major, pars claviculare. (From Veeger & Woude 1996.)

around the GH joint was small. This implied that they were primarily active to compensate destabilizing effects of the 'prime movers', the deltoid and pectoral muscles.

Effect of an incomplete muscle system

Until now, the descriptions of biomechanical factors influencing wheelchair propulsion have been of a general nature and based on a user group with full control over their upper extremities and trunk. It is expected that for wheelchair users with an incomplete musculoskeletal system, the problems will be exacerbated. Adequate stabilization of the GH joint will, for instance, become more difficult and the risk of dislocation of the joint will be high. So far, there is no direct proof for this assumption, but a study by Campbell and Koris (1996) may serve as an illustration. In this study a group of 24 patients with cervical spinal cord injury were studied, eight of whom were diagnosed with a chronically unstable shoulder. Recently, Dallmeijer *et al.* (1998) found that the effectiveness of force application in submaximal wheelchair propulsion of persons with tetraplegia is even lower than in persons with unimpaired arm function; FEF values of around 50% were found. The total force vector showed a larger, inward-directed, ineffective force component.

Vehicle mechanics

Vehicle mechanics is an essential element in wheelchair sports performance. This specialty should, of course, focus on optimizing or maximizing the performance of the athlete. Hence, not only are the mechanical properties *per se* important, but also their interaction with the capacities of the musculoskeletal system of the athlete. When looking at the mechanical properties of the wheelchair, one should always consider the effect of those properties on the interaction with the user.

The mechanical performance of a wheelchair will be dominated by rolling friction, air drag and internal friction of the wheelchair–user combination. Task load can be expressed as external power, or the energy per unit time that is required to maintain the speed of the wheelchair–user combination. With the help of a so-called 'power balance', the forces and energy sources responsible can be systematically evaluated (Woude *et al.* 1986; Ingen Schenau 1988).

The power balance for wheelchair propulsion can be expressed in the following equation:

$$P_o = (F_{roll} + F_{air} + F_{int} + mg \sin \alpha + ma) \times v \qquad (29.6)$$

where P_o is external power output (expressed in watts), a is acceleration of the system and m is mass of the wheelchair and user.

If a wheelchair is kept at a constant speed, the athlete has to produce a certain amount of energy per unit time, or power. This is called external power (P_o). This external power is produced by the musculoskeletal system of the athlete and requires a certain amount of internal power. The external power output is necessary to overcome energy losses in the system. The wheelchair–user combination will lose energy in the form of rolling resistance, air resistance and internal resistance in the mechanical structures of the chair. When more external power is produced than is needed to overcome losses, the chair will accelerate. The magnitude of acceleration will be dependent on the weight of the chair (ma). Also, the surplus of external power can be used to overcome a slope ($mg \sin \alpha$). On the other hand, negotiating a slope will, at a given external power output, lead to slowing down of the system. The terms ma and $mg \sin \alpha$ should not be considered as straight losses since they will work both ways. Energy that has been invested in acceleration or climbing, will be 'harvested' when coasting or descending. In the following we will briefly discuss the sources of energy losses; rolling resistance, air resistance and internal friction.

Rolling resistance

In daily use, rolling resistance generally is the major resisting force. Below relative head wind conditions of $2 \text{ m} \cdot \text{s}^{-1}$ air drag is still negligible. Rolling resistance can be determined in different ways. A coast-down technique—as described by McLaurin (1983)—is frequently used to determine rolling friction characteristics of the wheelchair in combination with different floor surfaces, or the effect of combined

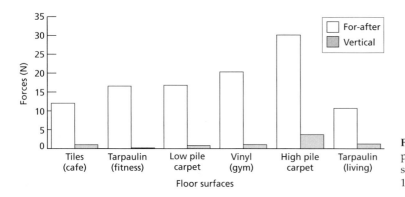

Fig. 29.17 Rolling resistance of a push wheelchair on different floor surfaces. (Adapted from Woude *et al.* 1999.)

air and rolling resistance. A second method is the drag test (see 'Track and treadmill' above). Also, rolling resistance can be measured by determining the push force exerted by a wheelchair attendant, to evaluate different floor surfaces (Fig. 29.17).

Apart from floor surface, rolling friction is essentially dependent on the characteristics of the wheels and tyres; rolling resistance is lower for wheels with a larger radius and for harder tires. Rolling resistance (measured in newtons) can be expressed by the following equation:

$$F_{\text{roll}} = \mu_1\left(\frac{N_1}{R_1}\frac{N_2}{R_2}\right) + \mu_2\left(N_2 R_2^{-1}\right) \qquad (29.7)$$

where R_1 and R_2 are the radii of the front and rear wheels, N_1 and N_2 indicate the relative weight on those wheels, and μ_1 and μ_2 are the friction coefficients.

The magnitude of the friction coefficients is related to the amount of deformation of tyre and floor surface. This deformation dissipates energy (Kauzlarich & Thacker 1985). Deformation is dependent on tyre pressure, thread and profile, or wheel diameter, but also on wheel alignment (Table 29.7). Wheel toe-in or toe-out has a considerable effect on rolling resistance (O'Reagan *et al.* 1981). For camber this is not so clear. It appears that, according to experimental results of Veeger *et al.* (1989b) and O'Reagan *et al.* (1981), camber of the rear wheels has no negative effect on rolling friction (Fig. 29.18). However, Weege (1985) advocates the opposite on the basis of theoretical considerations.

A special, frequently encountered problem is the effect of a side slope (Weege 1985; Brubaker *et al.* 1986). The wheelchair generally will tend to coast down a slope, which makes steering the wheelchair complicated and increases rolling resistance due to the effect on the alignment of the front castors. For that purpose, track and racing wheelchairs are equipped with steering mechanisms

Table 29.7 Factors influencing rolling friction.

Factor	Effect on rolling friction
Mass of athlete ↑	↑
Mass of wheelchair ↑	↑
Tyre pressure ↑	↓
Wheel size ↓	↑
Hardness of floor ↑	↓
Camber angle ↑	?
Toe-in/out ↑	↑↑
Castor shimmy ↑	↑
Centre of mass over large rear wheels	↓
Folding frame (vs. box frame)	↑

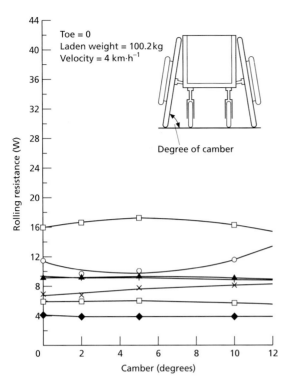

Fig. 29.18 Wheelchair rolling resistance as a function of camber. (From O'Reagan *et al*. 1981.)

that fix the direction of the front wheel in a preset direction.

Air resistance

The second important factor in the power balance equation (Eqn. 29.6) is air resistance. In wheelchair racing this factor is by far the most important source of energy losses. Air resistance (measured in newtons) is dependent on the drag coefficient (C_d), frontal plane area (A), air density (δ) and velocity of the air flow relative to the object (v):

$$F_{air} = \tfrac{1}{2}\delta A C_d v^2 \qquad (29.8)$$

As mentioned earlier, air resistance will be of minor importance at low speeds, but at high speeds and/or wind velocities air resistance will be the most important source of resistance. Following Abel and Frank (1991), at a slow speed (1 m · s⁻¹) air drag will be below 1 N, while at 5 m · s⁻¹ the drag force

due to air resistance is ± 14 N, which implies an average power output of (5 × 14 =) 70 W for wind resistance only at that wheelchair speed. It is obvious that the frontal plane area is dependent on the posture of the athlete. Although a wind tunnel experiment has been performed (Coe 1979), no recent figures on air resistance have been published with regard to contemporary wheelchair sitting posture and propulsion technique. However, many new developments have been transferred to wheelchair racing from cycling or speed skating. Besides frontal area reduction, adaptation of the seat position, orientation of the body segments, and the wearing of skin suits will all influence the drag coefficient. The introduction of strips in speed skating during the 1998 Olympics in Nagano has shown that even very small variations in design can have a significant effect on the drag coefficient and thus on the overall air resistance and performance.

Internal friction

Energy losses within the wheelchair are caused by bearing friction around the wheel axles, in the suspension of the castor wheels, and possibly, in folding wheelchairs, by deformation of the frame during force exertion in the push phase. Bearing friction generally is very small, and provided that the hubs have annular bearings and are well maintained and lubricated, this friction will not exceed 0.001 of the rolling resistance (Frank & Abel 1993). However, the losses in ill-maintained bearings can be considerable, as is indicated in Fig. 29.19, which represents the effect on external power output of a worn castor wheel-bearing of the wheelchair of subject GP. A comparison is made in this graph with the mean values for power output of seven subjects (with a higher overall mean body weight) in a similar model wheelchair. The consequence of this for the subject in Fig. 29.18 is an increase in required external power production of 20 W at a velocity of 3.3 m · s⁻¹, which implies—at a theoretical gross mechanical efficiency of 8%—an increase in oxygen consumption of 0.75 l · min⁻¹. This, despite the fact that subject GP had a lower body weight than the other seven subjects.

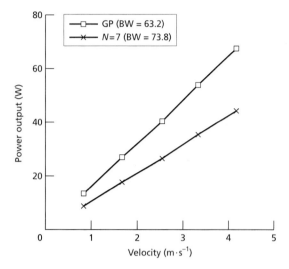

Fig. 29.19 Effect of maintenance on power output. Results of drag test on subject GP; N is the number of subjects. (From Woude 1987.)

An unknown aspect of internal energy dissipation is the loss of propulsion energy due to deformation of the frame. This will clearly be possible in folding wheelchairs, but has not been addressed empirically.

Slope and acceleration

Neither slope nor acceleration effects are straight loss components in the power balance equation. Energy invested in overcoming a hill, or increasing velocity will be returned in descents and when coasting. It should, however, be kept in mind that the invested potential energy will be returned against a greater head wind and thus incur larger power losses due to air resistance (Eqn. 29.8). As a result, maintaining the same average velocity will require more energy than compared with wheeling on a level surface.

Although body weight and wheelchair weight have a small effect on rolling resistance, they have a considerable effect on the slope component and the acceleration component. Acceleration potential is inversely related to total weight at a given power output (acceleration will be slower when the weight of the system is larger). Also, weight is linearly related to power output in climbing. Of course, this extra investment will be returned partially during descents, but will still lead to higher losses. Wheelchair weight can be influenced through use of appropriate technology and lightweight materials. It is, however, obvious that body weight is at least as important.

Given the factors that influence rolling resistance, a racing wheelchair should meet the following criteria:
- fixed, customized frame;
- fixed foot/leg support;
- custom-made and tapered front end;
- customized frame angle of 80° or more;
- camber bar;
- fixed backrest;
- fixed clothes protectors;
- weight: as low as possible;
- rear axis: customized seat angle and height; and
- rear wheel camber angle of 6–12°.

Weight distribution should be such that dynamic balance is maintained, even at high acceleration and when negotiating slopes. In other words, the centre of gravity should not be too close to the rear axis.

Wheelchair–athlete interface

The interface between wheelchair and athlete will influence performance. The interaction of the musculoskeletal system with the form and geometry of the propulsion mechanism and the seat configuration has been shown to influence the energy cost, physical strain and the gross mechanical efficiency. Experiments focusing on this interface have proved its importance with regard to propulsion technique. Crucial aspects of this interface include: rim size (Woude *et al.* 1988c), gear ratio (Veeger *et al.* 1992a), rim tube diameter (McLaurin & Brubaker 1991; Traut & Schmauder 1993) and seat height (Woude *et al.* 1989). Of course, the propulsion mechanism (levers, rims or cranks) also has an influence on performance (Woude *et al.* 1986, 1993).

Rim radius or gear ratio

The hand rim radius is in fact a gearing level. Smaller hand rims will result in a larger force and smaller hand velocity at a given travelling speed. It

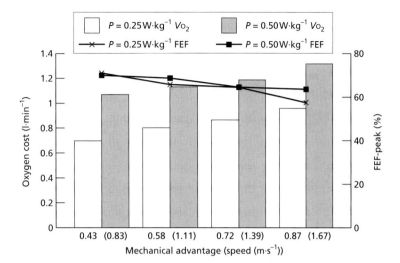

Fig. 29.20 Oxygen cost and fraction of effective force for different mechanical advantages. (Data from Veeger *et al.* 1992a.)

is logical that different task conditions will require different hand rim diameters or gearing levels: groups of well-trained subjects may want a gearing which enables them to compete at high velocities, whereas a steep incline for physically less able subjects will demand a low gear. The relevance of different gear ratios in hand rim wheelchairs is stressed by the results of different experimental studies (McLaurin & Brubaker 1991; Veeger *et al.* 1992a; Traut & Schmauder 1993).

Veeger *et al.* (1992a) showed that at equal submaximal power output, a higher mechanical advantage (0.43 compared with 0.87), i.e. a higher hand velocity—and simultaneously a lower mean resisting force—led to a higher cardiorespiratory response. Simultaneously, the increase in linear hand velocity during the push phase led to a decrease in effective force, from 71 to 58%. In addition, the amount of negative work at the beginning and end of the push increased with a higher mechanical advantage (Fig. 29.20). Application of a variable gearing in hand rim wheelchairs is worth considering. However, the choice of ratio will be power and velocity dependent.

Variable gear ratios are rarely seen in hand rim wheelchairs, but different rim diameters are more common, especially in track wheelchairs. In wheelchair sports, athletes tend to individualize their choice of hand rim size, tube diameter and profile.

To study the physiological effects of rim size, Woude *et al.* (1988b) conducted an experiment with a racing wheelchair and five different rim diameters in which track athletes participated at speeds up to 4.2 m · s[-1]. Rim diameter varied from 0.30 to 0.56 m. Results showed that the largest rim led to the highest physiological strain and lowest efficiency levels. Heart rate showed a mean difference of 20% (10–20 beats · min[-1]) between the smallest and the largest rim size. Again the linear speed of the hand rim limited performance: five out of eight athletes were unable to perform at a velocity of 4.2 m · s[-1] (power output did not exceed 50 W!).

More systematic studies should be conducted with respect to the effects of rim size, tube diameter, form and profile in a physiological and biomechanical context for different groups of wheelchair-confined subjects. The need for a choice in (exchangeable) rims is, however, clear.

Camber

The majority of sports wheelchairs are equipped with cambered rear wheels. Wheelchairs with cambered wheels are generally said to perform better in track events than wheelchairs without. The biomechanical rationale for this suggested performance advantage is as follows: with the top of the wheels as near as possible to the trunk the rims are in a plane more or less passing through the shoulder joint. This would prevent the upper arms from abducting in the frontal plane, thus reducing static effort of the shoulder muscles. The effective force vector can also be directed as closely as possible to the shoulder joint. Whether these assumptions are valid was studied by Veeger *et al.* (1989b), for a basketball wheelchair during propulsion at speeds of 0.56–1.39 m · s^{-1} on a motor-driven treadmill ($n =$ 8 non-wheelchair users). During four subsequent exercise tests the camber angle varied randomly from 0 to 3, 6 and 9°. The cardiorespiratory parameters indicated no positive or negative effect of camber angle in this wheelchair model. Similar findings were seen for the kinematics: no change in abduction angle was evident with camber angle. The electromyography signal even showed an absence of activity of the major shoulder abductor (m. deltoideus pars medialis) during the push phase. The authors explained this phenomenon by stating that the abduction which occurs during the push phase is not an active process, but a side-effect of the action of the major shoulder muscles (mm. pectoralis major and the deltoideus pars anterior). Their activity would lead both to anteflexion as well as abduction and endorotation, because of the closed kinetic chain that exists between the hand and the shoulder in the push phase. It thus appears that camber does not affect the functional load. However, the positive

effect of camber on stability is also relevant, as well as the fact that the hands are protected when the wheelchair passes alongside other objects.

Other propelling mechanisms

A relatively unknown propulsion mechanism is the hubcrank, a device that allows a continuous motion of the hand around the wheel hub of the rear wheels of a track or racing wheelchair (Fig. 29.21). Thus, hubcranks allow 'continuous' force exertion onto the wheel hubs. The hubcrank has a well-fitted handgrip that rotates freely around an axle perpendicular to the crank and adapts itself to the orientation of the hand. The crank has a free wheel. It is typically used in training of athletes, in open-competition sports events and in recreation. The efficacy of this device was studied in a group of non-wheelchair users. It was shown that the cranks led to a significantly lower strain (Fig. 29.22). Gross mechanical efficiency was up to 3% higher than for hand rims. Comparable trends were seen in a pilot study of a small group of trained wheelchair athletes (Woude *et al.* 1995). The positive effects of using the hubcrank may be explained by the following.
• The continuous circular motion allows both push and pull actions, thus reducing the periods during which no power is generated (as in hand rim propulsion during the recovery phase).

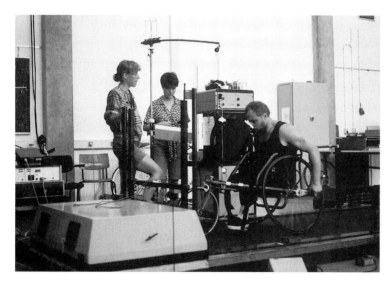

Fig. 29.21 Wheelchair with hubcrank propelling system.

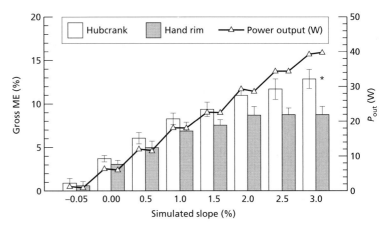

Fig. 29.22 Gross mechanical efficiency in hubcrank and hand rim propulsion. (Adapted from Woude et al. 1995.)

Racing wheelchair; $N = 10$ non-wheelchair users
$P < 0.001$; Speed $5 \, km \cdot h^{-1}$; computer-controlled roller ergometer
* Incomplete dataset

Table 29.8 Characteristics of different propulsion mechanisms.

Characteristic	Hand rim		Crank	Lever	Hub
	Basket	Racing			
Max. ME (%)	± 10	± 8	± 13	± 13	± 12
Strain CVS	High	High	Low	Low	Low?
Strain MSS	High	High	Low	Low	Low?
Risk RSI	High	High	Low?	Low?	Low?
Top speed (km · u⁻¹)	15	30	> 30	> 30	30
Mass (kg)	< 10	< 8	>>> 15	>>> 15	< 8
Coupling hand	–	– –	++	++	+
Force direction	–	–	+	++	+
Bimodal	–	+	+	+	+
Continuous	–	+	+	+	+
Manoeuvrability	++	+	–	–	–
Steering	++	+	±	±	–
Brake	±	–	+	+	–

CVS, cardiovascular system; MSS, musculoskeletal system; RSI, repetitive strain injury.

• The continuous circular motion allows for contributions of both flexor and extensor groups, and thus spreads out the load over more muscle groups.
• The hand and wrist have a more natural orientation to the lower arm (the handgrip adapts to the spatial hand orientation). As a consequence, the coupling of the hand to the propulsion mechanism is easier, with no counteracting hand moment. In addition, the grip force of the finger flexors might be lower. This may lead to a reduction of strain in the carpal tunnel.

In conclusion, the hubcrank has some clear advantages over the hand rim. Its use to date is, however, restricted to track wheelchairs, outdoor use, and to proficient wheelchair users. The hubcrank wheelchair is hard to steer, braking is more complicated, and its increased width (+ 0.15 m) complicates indoor use (Table 29.8).

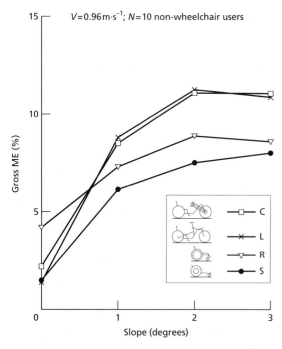

Fig. 29.23 Gross mechanical efficiency (ME) in different propelling systems. (From Woude 1987; data from Woude *et al.* 1986.)

propelled wheelchairs are inefficient, as is shown for instance in Fig. 29.23, where a comparison between a three-wheeled synchronous lever, a conventional crank-propelled wheelchair and two hand rim-propelled wheelchairs (one daily-use and one sports wheelchair) has been made with respect to oxygen uptake ($n = 10$ non-disabled subjects, $v = 0.96$ m · s^{-1}, slope of 0–3°). Despite the higher power output of the quite heavy tricycles, heart rate and oxygen cost were significantly lower. The crank and lever propulsion mechanisms seem appropriate for outside use at relatively high velocities, as well as for longer distances (Table 29.8). Optimization of gear ratio, lever length, handgrip and spatial orientation of the lever should, however, receive some attention (Woude *et al.* 1986, 1993; McLaurin & Brubaker 1991). Currently, considerable efforts are being made in the development of lever and crank-propelled wheelchairs for (open category) sports events and recreational purposes.

In conclusion, the systematic study of the wheelchair–athlete combination helps us to understand and identify determinants of performance in wheelchair athletes and may help to increase performance in sports. Interface characteristics, both those considered above and others (e.g. seat height/orientation), require detailed further analysis in relation to functionality. In this way, long-term ailments of the musculoskeletal system, related to a wheelchair-dependent lifestyle, may be prevented.

These aspects may be improved with simple design alterations.

In regular wheelchair track events propulsion mechanisms other than hand rims are not allowed. This is rather unfortunate. In general, hand rim-

References

Abel, E.W. & Frank, T.G. (1991) The design of attendant propelled wheelchairs. *Prosthetics and Orthotics International* **15** (1), 38–45.

Bednarczyk, J.H. & Sanderson, D.J. (1994) Kinematics of wheelchair propulsion in adults and children with spinal cord injury. *Archives of Physical Medicine and Rehabilitation* **75** (12), 1327–1334.

Bennedik, K., Engel, P. & Hildebrandt, G. (1978) *Der Rollstuhl. Experimentelle Grundlagen zur Technischen und Ergometrischen Beurteilung Handbetriebener Krankfahrzeuge.* Schindele-Verlag, Rheinstetten.

Boninger, M.L., Robertson, R.N. *et al.* (1996) Upper limb nerve entrapments in

elite wheelchair racers. *American Journal of Physical Medicine and Rehabilitation* **75**, 170–176.

Boninger, M.L., Cooper, R.A., Robertson, R.N. & Shimada, S.D. (1997) Three-dimensional pushrim forces during two speeds of wheelchair propulsion. *American Journal of Physical Medicine and Rehabilitation* **76** (5), 420–426.

Brown, D.D., Knowlton, R.G., Hamill, J., Schneider, T.L. & Hetzler, R.K. (1990) Physiological and biomechanical differences between wheelchair-dependent and able-bodied subjects during wheelchair ergometry. *European Journal of Applied Physiology and Occupational Physiology* **60** (3), 179–182.

Brubaker, C.E., McLaurin, C.A. & McClay, I.S. (1986) Effects of side slope on wheelchair performance. *Journal of Rehabilitation Research and Development* **23** (2), 55–58.

Burnham, R.S. & Steadward, R.D. (1994) Upper extremity peripheral nerve entrapments among wheelchair athletes: prevalence, location and risk factors. *Archives of Physical Medicine and Rehabilitation* **75**, 519–524.

Burnham, R.S., May, L., Nelson, E., Steadward, R.D. & Reid, D.C. (1993) Shoulder pain in wheelchair athletes: the role of muscle imbalance. *American Journal of Sports Medicine* **21** (2), 238–242.

Burnham, R.S., Chan, M., Hazlett, C., Laskin, J. & Steadward, R.D. (1994) Acute median nerve dysfunction from wheelchair propulsion: the development of a model and study of the effect of hand protection. *Archives of Physical Medicine and Rehabilitation* **75**, 513–518.

Campbell, C.C. & Koris, M.J. (1996) Etiologies of shoulder pain in cervical spinal cord injury. *Clinical Orthopaedics and Related Research* **322**, 140–145.

Coe, P.L. (1979) *Aerodynamic Characteristics of Wheelchairs* (80191). NASA Technical Memorandum.

Cooper, R.A., Robertson, R.N., VanSickle, D.P., Boninger, M.L. & Shimada, S.D. (1997) Methods for determining three-dimensional wheelchair pushrim forces and moments: a technical note. *Journal of Rehabilitation Research and Development* **34** (2), 162–170.

Coutts, K.D. & Stogryn, J.L. (1987) Aerobic and anaerobic power of Canadian wheelchair track athletes. *Medicine and Science in Sports and Exercise* **19** (1), 62–65.

Dallmeijer, A.J., Kappe, Y.J., Veeger, H.E.J., Janssen, T.W. & Woude, L.H.V.v.d. (1994) Anaerobic power output and propulsion technique in spinal cord injured subjects during wheelchair ergometry. *Journal of Rehabilitation Research and Development* **31** (2), 120–128.

Dallmeijer, A.J., van der Woude, L.H.V.v.d., Veeger, H.E.J. & Hollander, A.P. (1998) Effectiveness of force application in manual wheelchair propulsion in persons with spinal cord injuries. *American Journal of Physical Medicine and Rehabilitation* **77** (3), 213–221.

Davis, G.M. & Shephard, R.J. (1988) Cardiorespiratory fitness in highly active versus inactive paraplegics. *Medicine and Science in Sports and Exercise* **20** (5), 463–468.

Frank, T.G. & Abel, E.W. (1993) Drag forces in wheelchairs. In: *Ergonomics of Manual Wheelchair Propulsion: State of the Art* (eds L.H.V.v.d. Woude, P.J.M. Meijs & B.A.v.d. Grinten), pp. 255–267. IOS Press, Amsterdam.

Gass, G.C. & Camp, E.M. (1979) Physiological characteristics of trained Australian paraplegic and tetraplegic subjects. *Medicine and Science in Sports and Exercise* **11** (3), 256–259.

Glaser, R.M. (1985) Exercise and locomotion for the spinal cord injured. *Exercise and Sport Sciences Reviews* **13**, 263–303.

Helm, F.C.T.v.d. & Veeger, H.E.J. (1996) Quasi-static analysis of muscle forces in the shoulder mechanism during wheelchair propulsion. *Journal of Biomechanics* **29** (1), 39–52.

Helm, F.C.T.v.d., Veeger, H.E.J. *et al.* (1997) Analysis of the power balance during wheelchair propulsion using a 3-D musculoskeletal shoulder and elbow model. In: *XVIth Congress of the International Society of Biomechanics.* University of Tokyo, Tokyo.

Higgs, C., Babstock, P., Buck, J., Parsons, C. & Brewer, J. (1990) Wheelchair classification for track and field events: a performance approach. *Adapted Physical Activity Quarterly* **7** (1), 22–40.

Huonker, M., Schmid, A., Sorichter, S., Schmidt-Trucksab, A., Mrosek, P. & Keul, J. (1998) Cardiovascular differences between sedentary and wheelchair-trained subjects with paraplegia. *Medicine and Science in Sports and Exercise* **30** (4), 609–613.

Hutzler, Y., Ochana, S., Bolotin, R. & Kalina, E. (1998) Aerobic and anaerobic arm-cranking power outputs of males with lower limb impairments: relationship with sport participation intensity, age, impairment and functional classification. *Spinal Cord* **36** (3), 205–212.

Ingen Schenau, G.J.v. (1988) Cycle power: a predictive model. *Endeavour* **12** (1), 44–47.

Jackson, D.L., Hynninen, B.C., Caborn, D.N. & McLean, J. (1996) Electrodiagnostic study of carpal tunnel syndrome in wheelchair basketball players. *Clinical Journal of Sports Medicine* **6** (1), 27–31.

Janssen, T.W.J., van Oers, C.A.J.M., Hollander, A.P., Veeger, H.E.J. & van der Woude, L.H.V. (1993) Isometric strength, sprint power, and aerobic power in individuals with a spinal cord injury. *Medicine and Science in Sports and Exercise* **25** (7), 863–870.

Kauzlarich, J.J. & Thacker, J.G. (1985) Wheelchair tire rolling resistance and fatigue. *Journal of Rehabilitation Research and Development* **22** (3), 25–41.

Lafortune, M.A. & Cavanagh, P.R. (1983) Effectiveness and efficiency during bicycle riding. In: *Biomechanics VII-B.* Human Kinetics Publishers, Champaign, IL.

Lees, A. & Arthur, S. (1988) An investigation into anaerobic performance of wheelchair athletes. *Ergonomics* **31** (11), 1529–1537.

Linden, M.L.V., Valent, L., Veeger, H.E. & Woude, L.H. V.v.d. (1996) The effect of wheelchair handrim tube diameter on propulsion efficiency and force application. *IEEE Transactions on Rehabilitation Engineering* **4** (3), 123–132.

McLaurin, C.A. (1983) Determination of rolling resistance of manual wheelchairs. PhD Thesis, University of Virginia.

McLaurin, C.A. & Brubaker, C.E. (1991) Biomechanics and the wheelchair. *Prosthetics and Orthotics International* **15** (1), 24–37.

Mulroy, S.J., Gronley, J.K., Newsam, C.J. & Perry, J. (1996) Electromyographic activity of shoulder muscles during wheelchair propulsion by paraplegic persons. *Archives of Physical Medicine and Rehabilitation* **77**, 187–193.

Niesing, R., Eijskoot, F., Kranse, R. *et al.* (1990) Computer-controlled wheelchair ergometer. *Medical and Biological Engineering and Computing* **28** (4), 329–338.

O'Reagan, J., Thacker, J., Kauzlarich, J., Mochel, E., Carmine, D. & Bryant, M. (1981) Wheelchair dynamics. In: *Wheelchair Mobility: A Summary of Activities at the University of Virginia, Rehabilitation Engineering Centre 1976–1981* (eds C.A. McLaurin & C.K. Brubaker), pp. 33–41. REC, University of Virginia.

Rodgers, M.M., Tummarakota, S. *et al.* (1998) Three-dimensional analysis of wheelchair propulsion. *Journal of Applied Biomechanics* **14**, 80–92.

Roeleveld, K., Lute, E., Veeger, H.E.J. & Woude, L.H.V.v.d. (1994) Power output and technique of wheelchair athletes. *Adapted Physical Activity Quarterly* **11** (1), 71–85.

Rozendal, R.H. *et al.* (1974) *Inleiding in de Kinesiologie*, 3rd edn. Educa boek-Stam Technische Boeken, Culemborg.

Sanderson, D.J. & Sommer, H.J. (1985) Kinematic features of wheelchair propulsion. *Journal of Biomechanics* **18** (6), 423–429.

Sawka, M.N. (1986) Physiology of upper body-exercise. *Exercise and Sport Sciences Reviews* **14**, 175–211.

Sawka, M.N., Glaser, R.M., Laubach, L.L., Al-Samkari, O. & Suryaprasad, A.G. (1981) Wheelchair exercise performance of the young, middle-aged and elderly. *Journal of Applied Physiology: Respiratory Environmental Exercise Physiology* **50** (4), 824–828.

Sie, I.H., Waters, R.L., Adkins, R.H. & Gellmann, H. (1992) Upper extremity pain in the postrehabilitation spinal cord patient. *Archives of Physical Medicine and Rehabilitation* **73**, 44–48.

Subbarao, J.V., Klopfstein, J. & Turpin, R. (1995) Prevalence and impact of wrist and shoulder pain in patients with spinal cord injury. *Journal of Spinal Cord Medicine* **18** (1), 9–13.

Traut, L. & Schmauder, M. (1993) Ergonomic design of the hand–machine interface for wheelchairs. In: *Ergonomics of Manual Wheel-Chair Propulsion: State of the Art* (eds L.H.V.v.d. Woude, P.J.M. Meijs, B.A.v.d. Grinten *et al.*), pp. 335–348.: IOS Press, Amsterdam.

Veeger, H.E.J. (1994) Force generation in manual wheelchair propulsion. In: *XIII Southern Biomedical Engineering Conference* (ed. D. Vossoughi), pp. 779–782.

Veeger, H.E.J. & Woude, L.H.V.v.d. (1996) Fysiologische en mechanische belasting—van rolstoelrijden. *T v Fysiotherapie* **106** (3), 66–73.

Veeger, H.E.J., Woude, L.H.V.v.d. & Rozendal, R.H. (1989a) Wheelchair propulsion technique at different speeds. *Scandinavian Journal of Rehabilitation Medicine* **21** (4), 197–203.

Veeger, D., van der Woude, L.H. & Rozendal, R.H. (1989b) The effect of rear wheel camber in manual wheelchair propulsion. *Journal of Rehabilitation Research and Development* **26** (2), 37–46.

Veeger, H.E.J., Hadj Yahmed, M., Woude, L.H.V.v.d. & Charpentier, P. (1991a) Peak oxygen uptake and maximal power output of Olympic wheelchair-dependent athletes. *Medicine and Science in Sports and Exercise* **23** (10), 1201–1209.

Veeger, H.E.J., Woude, L.H.V.v.d. *et al.* (1991b) Load on the upper extremity in manual wheelchair propulsion. *Journal of Electromyography and Kinesiology* **1**, 270–280.

Veeger, H.E.J., Woude, L.H.V.v.d. & Rozendal, R.H. (1992a) Effect of hand rim velocity on mechanical efficiency in wheelchair propulsion. *Medicine and Science in Sports and Exercise* **24** (1), 100–107.

Veeger, H.E.J., Lute, E.M., Roeleveld, K. & van der Woude, L.H.V. (1992b) Differ-

ences in performance between trained and untrained subjects during a 30-s sprint test in a wheelchair ergometer. *European Journal of Applied Physiology and Occupational Physiology* **64** (2), 158–164.

Veeger, H.E.J., Meershoek, L.S., Woude, L.H.V.v.d. & Langenhoff, J. (1998) Wrist motion in handrim wheelchair propulsion. *Journal of Rehabilitation Research and Development* **35** (3), 305–313.

Weege, R.D.V. (1985) Technische Voraussetzungen fur den Aktivsport im Rollstuhl. *Orthopaedie Technik* **36** (6), 395–402.

Woude, L.H.V.v.d. (1987) Wheelchair examination. In: *Sports for the Disabled: Res-po 86, Proceedings of the International Congress on Recreation and Leisure* (ed. A. Vermeer), pp. 45–61. Vrieseborgh, Haarlem.

Woude, L.H.V.v.d. (1989) Manual wheelchair propulsion: An ergonomic perspective. PhD Thesis, Vrije Universiteit Amsterdam. Free University Press, Amsterdam.

Woude, L.H.V.v.d., Groot, G.d, Hollander, A.P., Ingen Schenau, G.J.v. & Rozendal, R.H. (1986) Wheelchair ergonomics and physiology of prototypes testing. *Ergonomics* **29** (1), 1561–1573.

Woude, L.H.V.v.d., Hendrich, K.M., Veeger, H.E. *et al.* (1988a) Manual wheelchair propulsion: effects of power output on physiology and technique. *Medicine and Science in Sports and Exercise* **20** (1), 70–78.

Woude, L.H.V.v.d., Veeger, H.E., Rozendal, R.H., Ingen Schenau, G.J.v., Rooth, F. & Nierop, P.V. (1988b) Wheelchair racing: effects of rim diameter and speed on physiology and technique. *Medicine and Science in Sports and Exercise* **20** (5), 492–500.

Woude, L.H.V.v.d., Veeger, H.E.J., Rozendal, R.H., Ingen Schenau, G.J.v., Rooth, F. & Nierop, P.V. (1988c) Wheelchair racing: effects of rim diameter and speed on physiology and technique. *Medicine and Science in Sports and Exercise* **20** (5), 492–500.

Woude, L.H.V.v.d., Veeger, D.J., Rozendal, R.H. & Sargeant, T.J. (1989) Seat height in handrim wheelchair propulsion. *Journal of Rehabilitation Research and Development* **26** (4), 31–50.

Woude, L.H.V.v.d., Veeger, H.E., Boer, Y.d. & Rozendal, R.H. (1993) Physiological evaluation of a newly designed lever mechanism for wheelchairs. *Journal of Medical Engineering and Technology* **17** (6), 232–240.

Woude, L.H.V.v.d., van Kranen, E., Ariens, G., Rozendal, R.H. & Veeger, H.E. (1995) Physical strain and mechanical efficiency in hubcrank and handrim wheelchair propulsion. *Journal of Medical Engineering and Technology* **19** (4), 123–131.

Woude, L.H.V.v.d., Bakker, W.H., Elkhuizen, J.W., Veeger, H.E. & Gwinn, T. (1997) Anaerobic work capacity in elite wheelchair athletes. *American Journal of Physical Medicine and Rehabilitation* **76** (5), 355–365.

Woude, L.H.V.v.d., Bakker, W.H., Elkhuizen, J.W., Veeger, H.E.J. & Gwinn, T. (1998) Propulsion technique and anaerobic work capacity in elite wheelchair athletes: cross-sectional analysis. *American Journal of Physical Medicine and Rehabilitation* **77** (3), 222–234.

Woude, L.H.V.v.d., Geurts, C., Winkelman, H. & Veeger, H.E.J. (1999) Measurement of wheelchair rolling resistance with a push technique. In: *Biomedical Aspects of Manual Wheelchair Propulsion: State of the Art II* (eds L.H.V.v.d. Woude, P.J.M. Meijs & B.A.v.d. Guuten), pp. 194–196. IOS Press, Amsterdam.

Wu, H.W. (1998) Biomechanics in upper extremity during wheelchair propulsion. PhD Thesis, National Cheng Kung University, Taiwan.

Wu, H.W., Berglund, L.J., Su, F.C. *et al.* (1998) An instrumented wheel for the kinetic analysis of wheelchair propulsion. *Journal of Biomechanical Engineering* **120** (4), 533–535.

Chapter 30

Sports after Amputation

A.S. ARUIN

Introduction

The history of athletic competition of individuals with physical disability started in 1948 during the Stoke Mandeville Games in England and continues to this day. Numerous sporting events around the world have contributed to the popularity of sports for the disabled. In 1996 more than 4000 athletes from 102 countries competed in the Atlanta Paralympics (Miller & Rucker 1997). Today, approximately 20 000 amputees participate actively in various sports, with more than 5000 participating in organized competitive sporting events in the USA (Michael *et al.* 1990). It is no longer merely 'inspirational' to have a disabled individual competing in sports, and there are many amputee athletes.

Approximately 500 000 individuals in the USA have had an amputation (Sherril 1997). This number includes both acquired amputation and amputation as a result of malformed body parts in individuals born with limb deficiencies on whom prostheses can be fitted at an early age (Krementz 1992). Acquired amputations usually occur in the middle-aged and elderly because of circulatory problems in the lower extremities, sometimes precipitated by diabetes. The leading causes of acquired amputation in children are trauma (vehicular, power and farm tool accidents, and gunshot explosions), as well as cancer and infection. Car accidents, armed conflicts, civil wars and landmine explosions are significant contributors to the increasing number of amputees all around the world.

Following an amputation, individuals are confronted with the necessity to be fitted with a prosthesis to restore function. This, however, requires that they literally learn anew how to perform activities such as walking using prosthetic devices. Different rehabilitation techniques are used to help amputees return to their previous levels of activity. For those individuals who were athletic prior to becoming an amputee and who want to continue sports or recreational activities, the need for individual rehabilitation and specially designed sporting equipment and prostheses becomes extremely important.

These challenges require creative prescription and design of the lower- and upper-extremity prostheses provided to such active individuals.

Lower-extremity prostheses: locomotion and balance

The oldest known artificial leg, constructed of copper and wood and thought to have been made about 300 BC, was discovered in Capua, Italy in 1958 (Wilson 1989). Many ancient prostheses displayed in museums in various parts of the world, were the work of armourers and were made of iron. There were also many 'civilian' prostheses used successfully down the centuries. A significant step towards a successful amputation technique was made by a French surgeon, Ambroise Paré, who in 1529 reintroduced the use of ligatures for amputation surgery. Paré, as a talented inventor, devised a new prosthesis for amputation through the thigh (Fig. 30.1), which is the first known to employ articulated joints. Since that pioneering work, surgical procedures and fitting with prostheses began to be

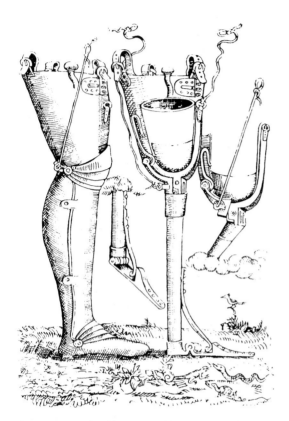

Fig. 30.1 An artificial leg invented by Ambroise Paré (mid-16th century). (From Paré 1575, courtesy of the National Library of Medicine, Bethesda, MD.)

more accessible for those who lost their limbs. Today there are many amputee-clinic teams in operation throughout the world.

Components of lower-limb prostheses

Each element of the prosthesis affects the biomechanics of locomotion, but certain of them have the most significant influence on the ability to move and participate in athletic activity.

PROSTHETIC SOCKET

This is one of the most important factors in prosthetic use because it provides the surface for contact and transfers body weight from the residual limb to the prosthesis. A good prosthetic socket must be

designed to permit efficient transference of force and motion from the residual limb and proximal joints to the prosthesis. It should do this in a way which will provide adequate comfort by ensuring that the forces are transmitted in a painless and stable manner not exceeding the residual limb's tissue tolerance. For active individuals the prosthesis can be held in place by suction provided by a close fit between stump and socket. Young, active amputees who participate in sports often use this type of suspension. A flexible socket can more readily adapt to the variation in muscular shape, which occurs with athletic activity.

Different materials are now used for socket fabrication. Newer thermoplastic materials provide a socket with lighter weight, improved fit, greater strength and less cost. In addition to the use of advanced plastic materials, new computer-aided design (CAD) and computer-aided manufacturing (CAM) techniques are used extensively to create individualized sockets, reducing design and production errors (Klasson 1985; Leonardo 1994). With the aid of a computer program, the socket is designed on the computer screen using measurements taken from the patient. Then, after necessary modification, a computer-driven milling machine shapes a solid blank into a stump model, which is used to fabricate the socket. The potential advantages of this new technique include uniform quality of prosthetic sockets, less time, and lower cost (Lilja *et al.* 1995).

KNEE MECHANISM

All knee mechanisms can be classified into five groups by their ability to restore locomotor mechanics. The oldest and the simplest model of the knee joint consists of a single axle connecting the shank and the thigh segments, which is dependent on alignment in hyperextension for stability. It is inexpensive and very durable, but provides low stability and fixed cadence (Wilson 1989). The stance control knee, or 'safety knee', is another type of knee mechanism. Artificial joints of this type use a weight-activated braking mechanism that adds additional resistance to knee motion during weight bearing to increase stability (Michael 1994). Polycentric knees are characterized by multiple centres of rotation and provide good knee stability. Manual locking knees provide more stability, but require release of the mechanism prior to seating and create an energy-consuming uncosmetic gait (Michael 1988). Fluid/air-controlled knees have a piston within a fluid- or air-filled cylinder, which allows the amputee to vary the cadence of walking. They can also provide resistance to flexion on weight bearing. Highly active individuals involved in a broad range of athletic activity can use hydraulic knees. However, the most versatile artificial joint designs combine the properties of two or more different types of knees. For example, combining the cadence responsiveness of a fluid-filled swing phase control with the reliability of a polycentric knee could provide some advantages for users (Patil & Chkraborty 1991).

PROSTHETIC FOOT

This is the element of the prosthetic that provides contact with the ground. The design of a prosthetic foot, ankle and shank should reproduce a locomotion pattern as near normal as possible, and provide the amputee with enhanced performance abilities. Mechanically a prosthetic foot should simulate the following functions of a biological human foot:

1 shock absorption;
2 the propulsion or push-off function;
3 the balance function or eversion-inversion; and
4 deceleration of dorsiflexion (Pitkin 1995).

Depending on the predominance of specialized biomechanical functions, the design of prosthetic feet is focused on one of these functions or on a combination of two or more functions. This can be broadly divided into the categories of conventional, force-absorbing, and energy storage and return.

The most exciting among these are the so-called 'energy-storing prosthetic feet', which function as a cantilevered spring (Fig. 30.2). The main component of the 'energy-storing prosthetic foot', the prosthetic keel, is deflected in the midstance phase, thereby increasing potential energy in the prosthetic keel. At toe-off the keel returns to its original position, releasing a portion of the absorbed energy. The keel stiffness of the prosthetic foot must be adequate for the activity level and body weight of a particular individual (Czerniecki & Gitter 1994). In order to meet the needs of individual patients, the companies manufacturing energy-storing prosthetic feet fabricate a spectrum of keel characteristics. To provide an amputee with a foot that could be used for both higher load sporting activities and lower load

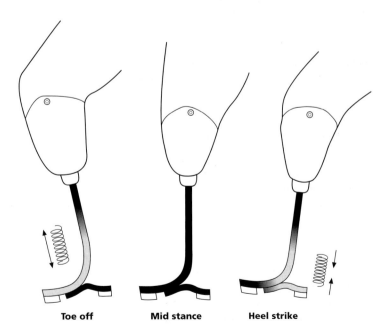

Fig. 30.2 A schematic illustration of the functional characteristics of energy-storing prosthetic feet. At heel contact, the keel bends absorbing heel strike energy. When the foot is unloaded, the keel restores its original shape, returning a portion of energy previously stored.

Toe off   **Mid stance**   **Heel strike**

activities of daily living, the foot offered by the Flex-Foot® Company (Aliso Viejo, CA) includes an air bag between two forefoot keels. By inflating or deflating the airbag, the amputee can adjust toe stiffness depending on the type of activity. To obtain sufficient deflection for sprinting and avoid drop-off past midstance, it may be necessary to have a prosthetic foot plantarflexed, making such a prosthesis only ideal for running.

ALIGNMENT

All the elements of the prosthesis should be properly aligned. Alignment refers to the positioning or state of adjustment of the prosthetic parts in relation to each other. With below-knee alignment the focus is primarily on establishing the optimal angular and linear relationship between the socket and the prosthetic foot, while with above-knee alignment the presence of a prosthetic knee joint poses some additional considerations.

Postural reorganization following lower limb amputation

Maintenance of vertical posture in the field of gravity is probably the most common component of a variety of motor tasks. Movements performed by a standing person, even low-amplitude arm movements, lead to perturbations of equilibrium because of joint coupling and also because of a change in the body configuration leading to a shift in the projection of the centre of mass. In healthy individuals equilibrium maintenance is under the control of three different sensory systems: visual, vestibular and somatosensory. After a lower-limb amputation a significant number of somatosensory sources (ankle joint, lower leg muscles, footsole) have been cut off, leading to problems with maintenance of vertical posture. One of the sources of adaptation during early rehabilitation after amputation may be an increased contribution of other sensory modalities to maintenance of posture. In particular the visual system has been shown to increase its contribution to postural sway reduction and fall prevention in cases of deficiency of information from somatosensory sources (Geurts et al. 1992).

Another potential means of improving balance in individuals with amputation is a reacquisition of balance skills. Central control of posture is expressed through two types of postural adjustments: compensatory and anticipatory adjustments. Compensatory postural adjustments deal with actual perturbation of balance that occurs because the body configuration was changed, for example, during gait initiation. Anticipatory postural adjustments are characterized by changes in the activity of postural muscles that are generated by the central nervous system in a feedforward manner, and can be seen prior to the planned movement (Aruin & Latash 1995, 1996). The apparent purpose of anticipatory postural adjustments is to counteract the predictable effects of an upcoming voluntary action on postural equilibrium.

Both compensatory and anticipatory postural adjustments may be changed in individuals with a leg amputation. After a unilateral below-knee amputation (BKA), control of the ankle joint is limited to the intact side. This can hypothetically lead to an increase in the role of the intact ankle joint, to compensatory changes in the role of other postural muscles, to a shift in the overall pattern of standing including a shift of the centre of mass, and to changes in anticipatory patterns compensating for rotational perturbations induced by the asymmetry of the motor apparatus.

Thus different anticipatory postural adjustments could be expected in individuals with below-knee amputation compared with able-bodied individuals. In particular, clear asymmetry of anticipatory postural adjustments has been found in unilateral below-knee amputees performing voluntary arm movements while standing. Activity of postural muscles was larger on the intact side of the body, but was small or absent on the side of amputation (Aruin et al. 1997) (Fig. 30.3). Such an asymmetry in postural adjustments could represent central adaptive changes secondary to the amputation.

Elements of biomechanics of prosthetic locomotion

The ideal prosthesis would effectively substitute for all of the normal functions of the human

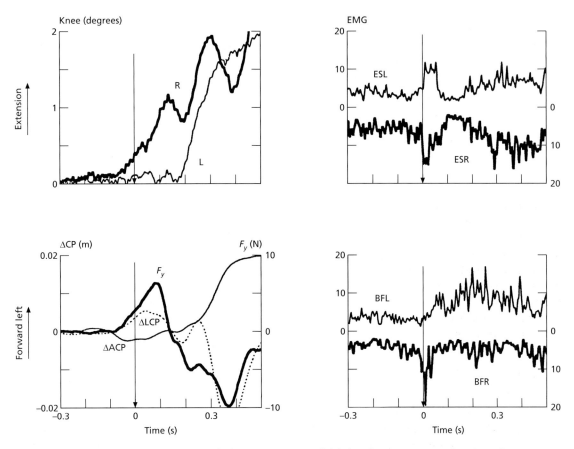

Fig. 30.3 Asymmetry of anticipatory postural adjustments seen in a left below-knee amputee performing voluntary arm movements while standing. Displacements of the knee, displacements of the centre of pressure in the anteroposterior (ΔACP) and mediolateral (ΔLCP) directions, lateral component of the ground reaction force (F_y) and EMG patterns of erector spinae (ES) and biceps femoris (BF) muscles are shown. The arrows show the start of arm movements. Note an anticipatory increase in the EMG activity in both left and right erector spinae but only in the right biceps femoris. Note also apparent anticipatory components of force in the mediolateral direction (F_y) and the displacement of the centre of pressure in the ΔACP and ΔLCP directions. There is an anticipatory movement in the right knee joint but not in the left knee joint. (Reprinted from *Clinical Biomechanics* **12**, Aruin, A.S., Nicholas, J.J. & Latash, M.L., Anticipatory postural adjustments during standing in below the knee amputees, pp. 52–59, copyright 1997, with permission from Elsevier Science.)

extremity. Unfortunately, despite progress in prosthetic design, no currently manufactured prostheses substitute even partially for the complex of normal functions of the lost arm or leg. There are many constraints, including technological and financial, which prevent the production of a prosthesis that restores most of the functions of the healthy extremity. Each prosthesis has advantages and disadvantages in the major biomechanical categories, such as force absorption and transmission. Many other elements have effects on prosthetic locomotion, such as the level of amputation and prosthesis mass.

SHOCK ABSORPTION

Most types of motions, such as walking, running, stair climbing, etc., initiate shock waves, which spread across the ankle, knee and hip joints, and along the spine. It has been shown that high-impact forces associated with the heel strike might damage articular cartilage (Radin *et al.* 1973). Another study indicated that osteoarthritis results mainly from poorly handled mechanical load, rather than from disease (Radin *et al.* 1975).

The human musculoskeletal system attenuates and dissipates these shock waves very effectively, using several mechanisms such as structures of joints, soft tissues of the lower extremities (i.e. calcaneal heel pads), or eccentric muscle contractions, for example knee flexions. These mechanisms in a healthy individual are able to attenuate up to 90% of the heel strike impact by the time the wave reaches the head (Aruin *et al.* 1989). The efficiency of the natural shock absorption mechanisms is reduced in the presence of musculoskeletal disease and fatigue (Voloshin *et al.* 1997; Verbitsky *et al.* 1998), and it is simply absent in cases of amputation when lower limbs are replaced with rigid prostheses.

Manufacturers of the lower-extremity prosthesis use several techniques to reduce impact through the residual limb. For example, the multiaxial force-absorbing prosthetic foot allows motion in three planes: sagittal, transverse and frontal, therefore allowing absorption of forces similar to that seen in the normal foot and ankle (Czerniecki & Gitter 1994). An impact-reducing pylon could attenuate maximum force levels normally transmitted to the residual limb by 30% (Anon 1996). Some shank components used in conjunction with energy-storing foot components may reduce torsional forces about the shank, and are also helpful in eliminating forces transmitted through the prosthesis (Czerniecki & Gitter 1994).

As was shown by Wirta *et al.* (1991), amputees prefer devices that have greater damping properties and transmit less shock. Thus the use of prostheses with improved force-absorption parameters provides amputees with more comfort and confidence while participating in sports and recreational activities. Shoes, especially those with compressible heels and viscoelastic insoles, also help in reducing impact on the residual limb and skeletal structures (Aruin *et al.* 1987; Lohrer 1989).

FORCE TRANSMISSION

Muscular forces transmitted through the skeleton to the ground are an integral element in producing motion. In the intact lower extremity the bony skeleton moves at joints that are stabilized by muscles and ligaments. The transverse tarsal joint in the normal foot changes its position during the push-off phase to allow force transmission. As the foot supinates during this phase, there is increasing obligatory stability of the axes of the talonavicular and calcaneocuboid joints. This reduces motion and enhances stiffness of the midtarsal region to allow more effective push-off as the gastrocnemius is generating large dynamic forces (Czerniecki & Gitter 1994). During ambulation on prostheses, multiple aspects of locomotion are affected by changes in biomechanics of the body and the effect of the prostheses. For example, in a study of amputees and able-bodied individuals during running across a force platform at a speed of $2.7 \text{ m} \cdot \text{s}^{-1}$, the prosthetic leg showed a decreased range of motions at the ankle joint. Ground reaction forces were also lower for the prosthetic limb in comparison with the intact and non-amputee limbs (Sanderson & Martin 1996) (Fig. 30.4).

Energetics of locomotion

The inability of the prosthetic foot to comply with kinematic demands and produce a powerful plantarflexion moment, and the asymmetry of locomotion due to prosthetic use increase the energy expenditure of gait and running (Fig. 30.5). It is well documented that lower-extremity amputees who walk using a prosthesis have greater energy requirements to travel a given distance than adults with no amputation during normal walking (Gonzalez *et al.* 1974). Children with below-knee amputation also have higher energy expenditures per unit distance than children without amputation (Herbert *et al.* 1994). Amputees typically adapt to this increased energy demand by slowing their gait under most circumstances to avoid oxygen debt.

Several parameters related to prosthetic design may affect energy requirements. For example, the length of the residual limb is an important parameter

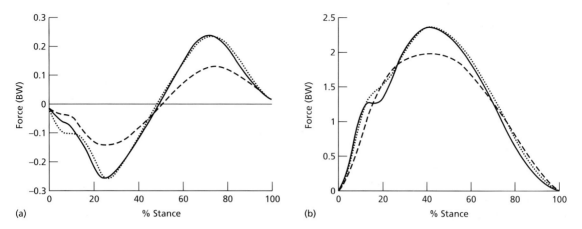

Fig. 30.4 Normalized horizontal (a) and vertical (b) components of the ground reaction force recorded in a below-knee amputee and a control subject during running at 2.7 m · s⁻¹. The solid line is the control subject, the dotted line is the intact leg of the amputee, and the broken line is the prosthetic leg. (From Sanderson & Martin 1996.)

Fig. 30.5 Energy cost (millilitres of oxygen or kilocalories per kilogram of body weight per minute) and gait efficiency (millilitres of oxygen or kilocalories per kilogram of body weight per metre walked) for normal, 'healthy' individuals (solid line) and for groups of individuals having amputation, hemiplegia, paraplegia, or using a wheelchair for mobility. The solid square represents the 'preferred' walking speed for normal subjects (BK, below-knee amputee; AK, above-knee amputee). (From Shurr & Cook 1990; with permission from Appleton & Lange.)

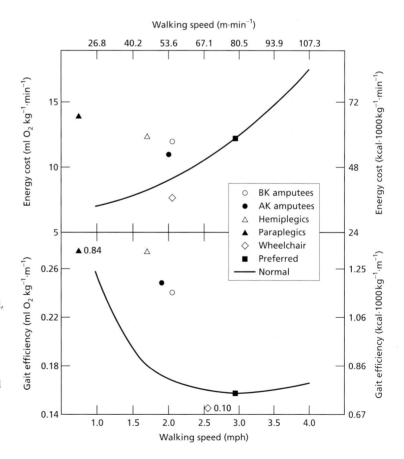

in oxygen consumption during locomotion; individuals with a higher level of unilateral and bilateral amputation expend greater energy per unit distance than those with lower-level amputations (Gonzalez *et al.* 1974; Pinzur *et al.* 1992). It has been demonstrated that a so called 'intelligent prosthesis', with microprocessor-controlled knee movements, lowers the energy cost of above-knee amputees during walking (Buckley *et al.* 1997). A study of the amount of energy being stored into and released from 14 kinds of prosthetic feet demonstrated that so-called 'energy-storing prosthetic feet' showed the highest values of both stored and released energy during level and slope walking (Ehara *et al.* 1993). Practical experience shows that many lower-limb amputees benefit from energy-storing foot systems (Alaranta *et al.* 1994).

Both logic and previous reports suggest that prosthetic mass influences energy expenditure and speed of ambulation in amputees. In order to eliminate additional energy expenditure from this source and the effect of prosthesis mass on the temporal and kinematic characteristics of locomotion, one solution is to match the mass–inertia characteristics of the stump plus prosthesis to the mass–inertia characteristics of the intact leg. This can be done by using literature data (Zatsiorsky *et al.* 1984; Winter 1991). However, this solution probably is not as simple as it seems, because lack of muscle activity in the amputated extremity might contribute to the asymmetries seen in the amputee gait. This leads to the suggestion that prostheses should be designed to minimize their distal weighting (Tashman *et al.* 1985) or to be as light as possible (Wilson 1989). On the other hand, the addition of up to 907 g of mass to prostheses of non-vascular transtibial amputees did not alter the energy cost of walking at normal speed (Gailey *et al.* 1997). The latter findings support the idea that prosthetists have a 'window of mass' in which to work when designing a prosthesis that includes additional components or accessories (Gailey *et al.* 1994).

Rehabilitation after lower limb amputation

Two major factors determine to a large extent future mobility and motor performance of an individual with amputation: the level of amputation and the number of limbs missing. Substantial strength and endurance of the proximal muscles of the residual limb and the trunk are also very important in rehabilitation after amputation. Young people are more likely to possess such capacities and are able to develop them quickly with exercise. The design of a prosthesis and the effectiveness of rehabilitation influence motor performance of an individual with amputation and have a significant impact on the number of amputees actively involved in sport and recreation activities.

Several aspects have an impact on the functional outcome of the rehabilitation process after amputation. The most critical are the election of surgical technique and level of amputation. The levels of amputation include Syme's (ankle disarticulation), below-knee amputation, knee disarticulations, and above-knee amputations. Age, gender, previous health, vocational status and recreational interests also play significant roles in returning an amputee to the highest level of function.

Several phases of rehabilitation after amputation have been defined. Each phase should be carefully designed to achieve practical goals.

In *acute phase* management, wound healing, maintenance of range of motion and prevention of deconditioning are very important. The use of an immediate postoperative rigid dressing that controls oedema and protects the limb may allow for early partial weight bearing and facilitates wound healing (Folsom *et al.* 1992). Early initiation of a physical therapy programme combined with appropriate positioning to avoid knee and hip contractures helps prevent deconditioning (Micheo & Lopez 1994).

The *preprosthetic phase* usually emphasizes strengthening of muscles of the uninvolved extremities and the trunk, residual limb preparation, and ambulation with assistance. Specific exercises focus on key muscle groups of the residual limb as well as on the muscles of the unaffected leg and arms, to train them to function as needed. For example, below-knee amputee training usually emphasizes strengthening of the hamstring muscles to provide proper deceleration of the knee at the end of the swing phase, and of the quadriceps muscles to stabilize the knee during the stance phase while walking. Strengthening of the hip abductors, hip extensors and hip flexors helps above-knee amputees to stabilize the pelvis and the knee during stance and to accelerate the prosthesis into swing phase during locomotion. A variety of assistive devices, such as parallel bars, walkers or crutches used in rehabilitation programmes of individuals with amputation are usually very effective in mobility training, decreasing the effects of deconditioning.

When the preprosthetic phase is completed, the patient should have normal strength in muscles of the uninvolved limbs and trunk, functional strength and range of motion of the residual limb, and should be independent in ambulation with assistive devices.

The *prosthetic phase* usually starts with prescription of a temporary prosthesis. The use of a temporary prosthesis provides the amputee with the ability to participate in early gait training while helping to optimally shape the residual limb and stabilize its volume. Initially the trauma of amputation produces oedema, and the disrupted venous and lymphatic systems must re-establish themselves. When the residual limb volume is stabilized, a patient is provided with a permanent prosthesis and preparation for sporting and recreational activities can start.

Numerous factors influence the ability of an individual with amputation to continue or start a new sporting activity. In addition to the level of amputation and the number of limbs missing (mentioned above), age, type of prosthesis, motivation, physical conditions, preliminary experience, etc. all play significant roles when an individual is making decisions about sporting or recreational activity after amputation. For example, age and time span since amputation influence cycling: in one study, persons who continued cycling after the amputation were 4–5.5 years younger at the time of amputation than amputees who stopped cycling (Burger *et al.* 1997).

Positive motivation plays a very important role in continuation of athletic activity after amputation, and even in choosing an appropriate new sport in which there was no previous participation. The individual's ability to handle the stress and trauma of amputation is probably the main factor which causes one amputee to became an elite athlete (i.e. in cross-country skiing or in track and field), while another with the same level of physical disability is unable to return to productive employment. Those who are highly motivated and have a strong desire to overcompensate for their disability could rehabilitate themselves with little help in achieving their goals, both in their personal lives and in sports. Other individuals with amputation require the influence of a positive attitude, to show them that their limitations are what they allow them to be. Meeting another amputee with a positive attitude helps by giving inspiration, emotional support and information. In particular, it has been demonstrated that patients with recent amputation who have been visited by volunteers with previous amputation have strong positive responses to the rehabilitation programme (Wells *et al.* 1993). The positive role of the athletic amputee has even greater impact.

Sporting and recreational activity of individuals with lower-leg amputation

For thousands of years, sports and competition have been an important component of human life. However, most of the time there has been no room for athletic competition for individuals with physical disabilities. Even 20 years ago the athletic amputee was a unique phenomenon in athletic competition. Now the number of amputees actively involved in sports and recreational activities is significant and tending to increase. (Michael *et al.* 1990). This phenomenon has attracted increased attention of physicians, psychologists, scientists and manufacturers.

There are limitations for an amputee in deciding which sport or recreational activity to choose. For those individuals who were athletic prior to becoming an amputee and who want to continue the same athletic activity, the question of whether to continue depends on a number of factors, including the level of amputation, physical ability and motivation.

When a decision to continue or start athletic activity is made, the right prosthesis should be designed for the particular athletic needs of the amputee. The usefulness of lower-limb prostheses has improved tremendously since the 1980s, when advances in composite materials flooded the prosthetics industry.

Carbon composite materials, used extensively in the aerospace industry, have brought lightness, flexibility and superior strength to the design of prosthetic feet, pylons and sockets. As a result, new developments in sporting and recreational prostheses have given many amputees the opportunity to continue sporting activity. The following paragraphs describe examples of participation of amputees in athletic competitions.

RUNNING

Running is the most difficult skill for an amputee to acquire. Poor fit, inadequate suspension or alignment of the prosthesis, incommensurate weight, suboptimal shock-absorbing properties, etc., can produce discomfort, discouraging most amputees from pursuing running-based activities. The use of advanced prostheses and proper training help to overcome most difficulties.

Tony Volpentest was born with short malformed legs and arms, but with prostheses, he worked-out and ran with an able-bodied team, though he was slower than his peers, running 100 m in only 14.3 s. Later, when provided with Flex-Foot® prostheses, he ran the 100 m in about 11.26 s and the 200 m in about 22.67 s (Sherrill 1997). This exemplifies how hard work, motivation and advanced prostheses

make it possible for a leg amputee to beat able-bodied competitors (Fig. 30.6).

WINTER SPORTS

Snow skiing is a popular sport for amputees because it offers freedom and speed, and allows many amputees to participate in a competitive sport while using adaptive equipment. While able-bodied individuals use forward lean and increased ankle dorsiflexion to maintain balance while skiing, amputees often cannot do this because of rigidity of their prosthesis. The simplest way of solving this problem for below-knee and Syme's amputees while using a conventional prosthesis is to place a wedge under the heel of the prosthetic foot. Another way to accomplish the desired position of the centre of gravity involves using a specially designed prosthesis having 15 to 25° of ankle dorsiflexion (Michael *et al.* 1990). One other way of snow skiing is to use a fibreglass kayak-like sled, monoski or three-track ski along with two ski poles or crutch outriggers. Each of the three (kayak-like sled, monoski or three-track ski) can be used with or without the prosthesis. However, in some cases special design of ski equipment has eliminated the need for using a prosthesis while skiing. It is common for the sit-skier to ski with the aid of a partner, who provides

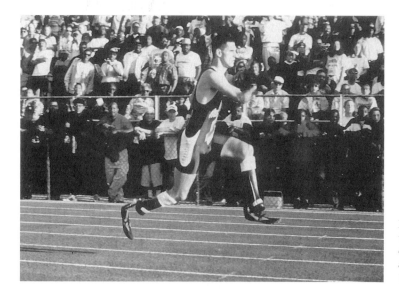

Fig. 30.6 Tony Volpentest, bilateral transtibial amputee sprinter, who currently holds the world record for amputee sprinters in the 100 m at 11.36 s. (Courtesy of Flex-Foot, Inc.)

assistance on flat areas and on mountain slopes when it is needed.

It is not an easy task for an amputee to learn how to ski. Without enough momentum due to altered biomechanics it is difficult to perform leans and weight shifts, and to use ski poles to turn or stop a sled or monoski. In many cases individuals with amputation participate in special 'Learn to Ski' programmes prior to starting actively to ski.

CYCLING

Compared to running, which is characterized by impact to the prosthetic limb during locomotion, cycling offers good aerobic conditioning with no impact while pedalling. Riding a bike requires both hip and knee flexion through a wide range of motion. Loss of either knee or hip extension or flexion in an amputee produces some problems related to the prosthetic socket and difficulties in achieving maximum power when pushing downwards on the pedal. Other problems are related to the position of the feet on the pedals and keeping their position during pedalling. Toe clips attached to the pedals (or a 'clipless pedal' if the amputee can use it) help keep the front foot in place and enable the amputee to use the power of their residual limb during both downward and upward strikes. There are differences in adaptation to biking for below- and above-knee amputees. While below-knee amputees experience minimum difficulties in biking with a prosthesis, above-knee amputees may have some balance problems due to difficulties with seating and hip range of motion. The saddle should be wide enough to permit balance and narrow enough to help avoid pinching the upper thigh between the socket and the saddle. Many cyclists with below-knee amputation have been successful in competitive racing using a prosthesis, a regular biking shoe, toe clips and a suprapatellar cuff strap. Others have utilized a modified peg leg that attaches directly to the pedal, increasing ankle mobility by incorporating a U-joint (Burgess & Rappoport 1996).

There is no doubt, though, that many amputee athletes would not be participating in sports and athletic competitions if there were no sponsors to cover the cost of advanced prostheses.

Upper-extremity prostheses for sports and recreation

The history of artificial arms and hands is not as well documented as for lower extremities. Probably the first example of use of relative motions of body parts to control movements of artificial arms and hands was introduced by Balif in 1812 (Fig. 30.7) (Wilson 1989). Since that time the design of upper-extremity prostheses has changed due to the introduction of new materials and techniques.

Sound limb design is a major component in amputee performance potential. Holding a spoon or a book, grasping a ski pole, or steering a car or bike may be necessary achievements for an individual missing one or both hands. The artificial device, which provides the ability to grasp and hold objects, can be designed as a hook or a hand. A hook-type terminal device permits more visualization of the object to be grasped; however, it is significantly less cosmetically desirable. Both hook and hand-type terminal devices can be body-powered, which requires activation through body-controlled movements, or external power. Devices which are exter-

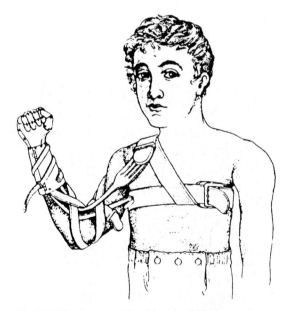

Fig. 30.7 The first example of the use of relative motion between parts of the body to obtain power for operation of an artificial arm. (From Gourdon 1924).

nally powered provide greater pinch force than the body-powered ones (Meier 1994).

There are approximately 90 000 people in the USA who have lost an upper limb. About 90% of these amputees use body-powered prostheses with a cable-operable hook, which require extensive harnessing for function and suspension (Frey et al. 1995). Myoelectric prostheses, which were introduced in the mid-1960s, provide freedom from a harness, superior punch force, and improved function for high-level amputees. Such prostheses use electrical activity of flexor and extensor muscles of the remaining limb to control the battery-powered motor, which operates the terminal device.

Recreational activities and sports are function specific, and universal prostheses cannot always provide adequate functioning, strength and control. That is why some amputees participate in sports without a prosthesis by developing great unilateral skills. However, customized designs of upper limb prostheses for specific sports and recreation activities such as canoeing or kayaking, golfing, playing hockey, sailing, skiing, etc., allow amputees to develop their skills more easily and demonstrate better results. Some sports require only minimal modification of the equipment, while others require development of a special prosthesis.

For example, archery equipment is easily adapted to a prosthesis using voluntary closing prehensors or externally powered hands with appropriate prehension configuration. In other cases prosthesis adapters, which provide a firm and controlled draw of the bowstring, are used (Adams et al. 1982). Made of wood with a single groove, in which the bowstring is held, the device has two tracks on the opposite end where the hooked finger of the prosthesis is placed to hold the device (Paciorek & Jones 1989).

Passive prostheses, which employ no cable, allow safe participation in vigorous activities. For example, a prosthesis that is anatomically proportioned to a 'cupped' hand and fabricated from unbreakable polymer (TRS Inc., Boulder, CO.), flexes and extends with external pressure enabling two-handed performance in basketball, volleyball, soccer, etc. (Fig. 30.8).

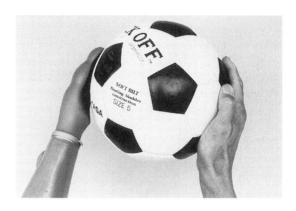

Fig. 30.8 Adult Super Sport hand prostheses with soccer ball. (Courtesy of TRS Inc., Boulder, CO.)

For baseball, the sport which is so much a part of the American heritage, prosthetic requirements vary depending on the batting or fielding role of the player. For batting, the prosthesis should be adapted for performance of a wrist/forearm action including 'wrist brake' in a normal swing. For fielding, a specialized body-powered terminal device which controls the opening of a glove or a basket-type device has been described, which allows either forehanded or backhanded catching techniques (Radocy 1992).

Another example of how minor modifications can overcome problems related to the use of conventional terminals has been described by Radocy (1987), who depicted his own experience in kayaking with a double-bladed paddle which required only coordination and practice (Fig. 30.9). Indeed, kayakers with upper-extremity amputations are faced with difficulties of holding the paddle, because most conventional terminal devices cannot hold oars or paddles. In addition, terminal devices that lock should never be used in aquatic activities (Paciorek & Jones 1989). Using modified terminal devices and simple modifications to the paddle— such as a rubber ring to prevent excess water running onto the paddle shaft, and tape to stabilize the grip—can help an upper-extremity amputee to efficiently use a kayaking paddle (Paciorek & Jones 1989).

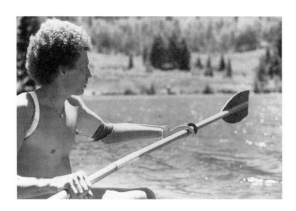

Fig. 30.9 Adaptation of a grip voluntary-closing prehensor on a kayak paddle. (From Radocy (1988) *Palaestra* **4** (2), 27.)

Summary

The goal of amputee rehabilitation is to return each individual to their highest possible level of functioning. The specific goals of treatment and rehabilitation of amputees will vary from patient to patient, depending on the particular needs of the individual. For an elderly amputee it could be independent walking; for young or middle-aged and active amputees the desire to participate in sports or recreational activity may be a major goal.

A recent trend in the rehabilitation of people after amputation has been toward supplying them with prostheses which provide for independence in living. Today there are many examples of how providing amputees with special prostheses and devices helps enable their participation in active recreational activities and sports.

Athletic competition and sports provide amputees with unique opportunities to reach goals, improve self-esteem, and to demonstrate their abilities to other amputees and the able-bodied. This positive experience can provide other amputees with the confidence to actively participate in sports, even with an amputation.

References

Adams, R.C., Daniel, A.N., McCubbin, J.A. & Rullman, L. (1982) *Games, Sports and Exercises for the Physically Handicapped*, 3rd edn. Lea & Febiger, Philadelphia.

Alaranta, H., Lempinen, V.-M., Haavisto, E., Pohjolainen, T. & Hurri, H. (1994) Subjective benefits of energy storing prostheses. *Prosthetics and Orthotics International* **18**, 92–97.

Anon (1996) Impact-reducing pylon system. *Journal of Prosthetics and Orthotics* **8**, 11A.

Aruin, A.S. & Latash, M.L. (1995) The role of motor action in anticipatory postural adjustments studied with self-induced and externally triggered perturbations. *Experimental Brain Research* **106**, 291–300.

Aruin, A.S. & Latash, M.L. (1996) Anticipatory postural adjustments during self-initiated perturbations of different magnitude triggered by standard motor action. *Electroencephalography and Clinical Neurophysiology* **101**, 497–503.

Aruin, A.S., Zatsiorsky, V.M., Koretsky, A.V. & Potjemkin, B.A. (1987) Investigation of shock absorption properties of shoes using vibration tests. *Kozevenno-Obuvnaja Promislennost (Leather Footwear Industry)* **4**, 22–23 [in Russian].

Aruin, A.S., Zatsiorsky, V.M. & Potjemkin, B.A. (1989) Damping of dynamic loads during locomotion. In: *Modern Problems of Biomechanics* (ed. K. Frolov), F 6, pp. 63–78. Zinatne, Riga [in Russian].

Aruin, A.S., Nicholas, J.J. & Latash, M.L. (1997) Anticipatory postural adjustments during standing in below the knee amputees. *Clinical Biomechanics* **12**, 52–59.

Buckley, J.G., Spence, W.D. & Solomonidis, S.E. (1997) Energy cost of walking: comparison of 'Intelligent Prosthesis' with conventional mechanism. *Archives of Physical Medicine and Rehabilitation* **78**, 330–333.

Burger, H., Marincek, C. & Isakov, E. (1997) Mobility of persons after traumatic lower limb amputation. *Disability and Rehabilitation* **19**, 272–277.

Burgess, E. & Rappoport, A. (1996) *Physical Fitness: a Guide for Individuals with Lower Limb Loss*. Department of Veterans Affairs, Baltimore.

Czerniecki, J.M. & Gitter, A. (1994) Prosthetic feet: a scientific and clinical review of current components. In: *Physical Medicine and Rehabilitation: State of the Art Reviews* (ed. A. Esquinazi), Vol. 8, pp. 109–128. Hanley & Belfus, PA.

Ehara, Y., Beppu, M., Nomura, S., Kunimi, Y. & Takahashi, S. (1993) Energy storing property of so-called energy-storing prosthetic feet. *Archives of Physical Medicine and Rehabilitation* **74**, 68–72.

Folsom, D., King, T. & Rubin, J.R. (1992) Lower extremity amputation with immediate post operative prosthetic placement. *American Journal of Surgery* **164**, 320–322.

Frey, D., Carlson, L. & Ramaswamy, V. (1995) Voluntary-opening prehensors with adjustable grip force. *Journal of Prosthetics and Orthotics* **7**, 124–131.

Gailey, R.S., Nash, M.S., Atchley, T.A. *et al.* (1997) The effect of prosthesis mass on metabolic cost of ambulation in non-vascular trans-tibial amputees. *Prosthetics and Orthotics International* **21**, 9–16.

Gailey, R.S., Wenger, M.A., Raya, M. *et al.* (1994) Energy expenditure of trans-tibial amputees during ambulation at a self selected pace. *Prosthetics and Orthotics International* **18**, 84–91.

Geurts, A.C., Mulder, T.W., Nienhuis, B. & Rijken, R.A. (1992) Postural reorganization following lower limb amputation. Possible motor and sensory determinants of recovery. *Scandinavian Journal of Rehabilitation and Medicine* **24**, 83–90.

Gonzales, E.G., Corcoran, P.J. & Peters, R.L. (1974) Energy expenditure in below-knee amputees: correlation with stump length. *Archives of Physical Medicine and Rehabilitation* **55**, 111–119.

Gourdon, J. (1924) Avant-bras de Baillif dans lequel les doigts de la main sont actionnes par un lacs relie a une ceinture throacique. *Journal de Medecine de Bordeaux et de la Region du Sud-Ouest* **3**, 85.

Herbert, L.M., Engsberg, J.R., Tedford, K.G. & Grimston, S.K. (1994) A comparison of oxygen consumption during walking between children with and without below-knee amputation. *Physical Therapy* **74**, 945–950.

Klasson, B. (1985) Computer aided design-computer aided manufacture and other computer aids in prosthetic and orthotics. *Prosthetics and Orthotics International* **9**, 3–11.

Krementz, J. (1992) *How It Feels to Live with a Physical Disability*. Simon & Schuster, New York.

Leonard, J.A. (1994) Lower limb prosthetic sockets. In: *Physical Medicine and Rehabilitation: State of the Art Reviews* (ed. A. Esquinazi), Vol. 8, pp. 129–145. Hanley & Belfus, PA.

Lilja, M., Sci, M.L. & Oberg, T. (1995) Volumetric determination with CAD/CAM in prosthetics and orthotics. Errors of measurement. *Journal of Rehabilitation Research and Development* **32**, 141–148.

Lohrer, H. (1989) Design and effect of sports shoe insoles for the runner. *Sportverletz Sportschaden* **3**, 106–111 [in German].

Meier, R.H. (1994) Upper limb amputee rehabilitation. In: *Physical Medicine and Rehabilitation: State of the Art Reviews* (ed. A. Esquinazi), Vol. 8, pp. 165–185. Hanley & Belfus, PA.

Michael, J.W. (1988) Component selection criteria: Lower limb disarticulation. *Clinical Prosthetics and Orthotics* **12**, 99–108.

Michael, J.W. (1994) Prosthetic knee mechanisms. In: *Physical Medicine and Rehabilitation: State of the Art Reviews* (ed. A. Esquinazi), Vol. 8, pp. 147–164, Hanley & Belfus, PA.

Michael, J.W., Gailey, R.S. & Bowker, J.H. (1990) New development in recreational prostheses and adaptive devices for the amputee. *Clinical Orthopedics and Related Research* **256**, 64–75.

Micheo, W.F. & Lopez, C.E. (1994) Rehabilitation of lower extremity traumatic amputees. In: *Physical Medicine and Rehabilitation: State of the Art Reviews* (ed. A. Esquinazi), Vol. 8, pp. 193–199. Hanley & Belfus, PA.

Miller, M.A. & Rucker, K.S. (1997) Disabled athletes. In: *Physical Medicine and Rehabilitation: State of the Art Reviews* (eds J.D. Fortin, F.J. Falco & H.A. Jacob), Vol. 11, pp. 465–488. Hanley & Belfus, PA.

Paciorek, M.J. & Jones, J.A. (1989) *Sport and Recreation for Disabled: a Resource Handbook*. Benchmark Press, Indianapolis.

Paré, A. (1575) *Pourtract Des Iambes Artificielles*. Gabriel Buon, Paris. [From the copy in the National Library of Medicine, Bethesda.]

Patil, K.M. & Chkraborty, J.K. (1991) Analysis of a new polycentric above-knee prosthesis with pneumatic swing phase control. *Journal of Biomechanics* **24**, 223–233.

Pinzur, M.S., Gold, J., Schwartz, D. & Gross, N. (1992) Energy demands for walking in dysvascular amputees as related to the level of amputation. *Orthopedics* **15**, 1033–1036.

Pitkin, M.R. (1995) Mechanical outcomes of a rolling-joint prosthetic foot and its performance in the dorsiflexion phase of transtibial amputee gait. *Journal of Prosthetics and Orthotics* **7**, 114–123.

Radin, E.L., Parker, H.G., Pugh, G.V., Steinberg, R.S., Paul, I.L. & Rose, R.M. (1973) Response of joints to impact loading. *Journal of Biomechnaics* **6**, 51–57.

Radin, E.L., Paul, I.L. & Rose, R.M. (1975) Mechanical factors in the aetiology of osteoarthritis. *Annals of Rheumatic Diseases* **34**, 132–133.

Radocy, B. (1987) Upper-extremity prosthesis: considerations and design for sports and recreation. *Clinical Prosthetics and Orthotics* **11**, 131–153.

Radocy, B. (1992) Upper-limb prosthetic adaptations for sports and recreation. In: *Atlas of Limb Prosthetics: Surgical, Prosthetic, and Rehabilitation Principles* (eds J. Bowker & J. Michael), pp. 325–344. Mosby Year Book, St. Louis.

Sanderson, D. & Martin, F. (1996) Joint kinematics in unilateral below-knee amputee patients during running. *Archives of Physical Medicine and Rehabilitation* **77**, 1279–1285.

Sherrill, C. (1997) *Adapted Physical Activity, Recreation and Sport: Crossdisciplinary and Lifespan*. WCB/McGraw-Hill, Boston.

Shurr, D.G. & Cook, T.M. (1990) *Prosthetics and Orthotics*. Appleton & Lange, Norwalk.

Tashman, S., Hicks, R. & Jendrzejczyk, D.J. (1985) Evaluation of prosthetic shank with variable inertial properties. *Clinical Prosthetic Orthotics* **9**, 23–28.

Verbitsky, O., Mizrahi, J., Voloshin, A., Treiger, J. & Isakov, E. (1998) Shock transmission and fatigue in human running. *Journal of Applied Biomechanics* **14**, 300–311.

Voloshin, A.S., Mizrahi, J., Verbitsky, O. & Isakov, E. (1997) Dynamic loading of the human musculoskeletal system – effect of fatigue. *Clinical Biomechanics* **13**, 515–520.

Wells, L.M., Schachter, B., Little, S., Whylie, B. & Balogh, P.A. (1993) Enhancing rehabilitation through mutual aid: outreach to people with recent amputation. *Health and Social Work* **18**, 221–229.

Wilson, B.A. (1989) *Limb Prosthetics*. Demos Publications, New York.

Winter, D. (1991) *Biomechanics and Motor Control of Human Movement*. John Wiley & Sons, New York.

Wirta, R.W., Mason, R., Calvo, K. & Golbranson, F.L. (1991) Effect of gait using various prosthetic ankle-foot devices. *Journal of Rehabilitation Research and Development* **28**, 13–24.

Zatsiorsky, V.M., Aruin, A.S. & Selujanov, V.N. (1984) *Biomechanik des Menschlichen Bewegungsapparates*. [Biomechanics of the Human Musculo-Skeletal System.] Sportverlag, Berlin.

Index

Note: page numbers in *italics* refer to figures, those in **bold** refer to tables.

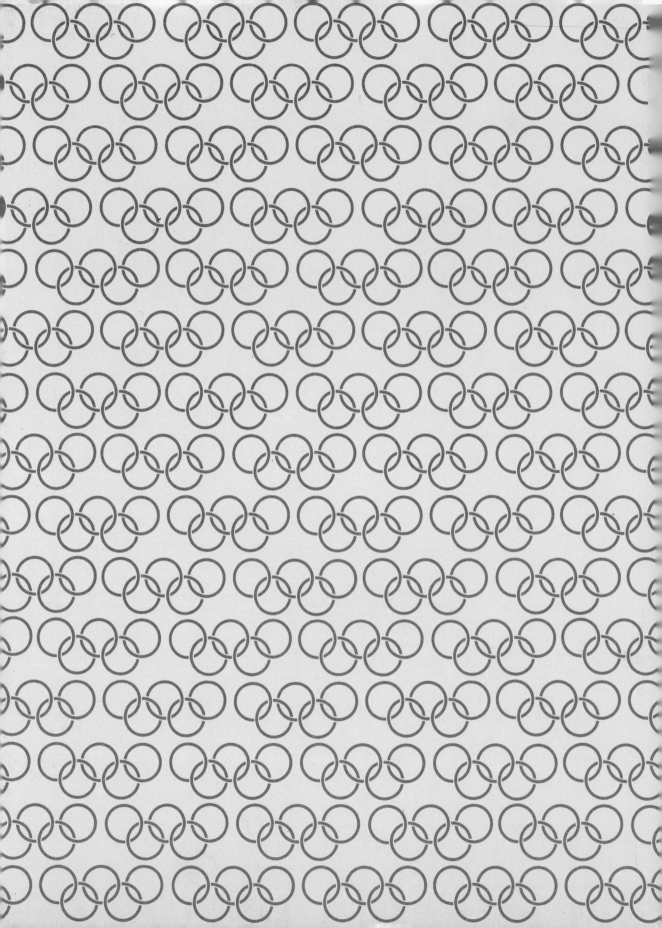